Nanomedical Device and Systems Design

Challenges, Possibilities, Visions

Nanomedical Device and Systems Design

Challenges, Possibilities, Visions

Edited by
Frank J. Boehm

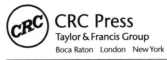

CRC Press
Taylor & Francis Group
Boca Raton London New York

CRC Press is an imprint of the
Taylor & Francis Group, an **informa** business

CRC Press
Taylor & Francis Group
6000 Broken Sound Parkway NW, Suite 300
Boca Raton, FL 33487-2742

First issued in paperback 2017

© 2014 by Taylor & Francis Group, LLC
CRC Press is an imprint of Taylor & Francis Group, an Informa business

No claim to original U.S. Government works

Version Date: 20130910

ISBN 13: 978-1-138-07260-2 (pbk)
ISBN 13: 978-0-8493-7498-2 (hbk)

Library of Congress Cataloging-in-Publication Data

Nanomedical device and systems design : challenges, possibilities, visions / edited by Frank J. Boehm.
        pages cm
    Includes bibliographical references and index.
    ISBN 978-0-8493-7498-2 (hardback)
    1. Nanomedicine. 2. Nanostructured materials--Design. 3. Nanotechnology--Health aspects. 4. Biomedical engineering. I. Boehm, Frank J.

    R857.N34N3525 2014
    610.28--dc23   2013023891

Visit the Taylor & Francis Web site at
http://www.taylorandfrancis.com

and the CRC Press Web site at
http://www.crcpress.com

I lovingly dedicate this book to the memory of my recently passed father, Josef Boehm, who ignited in me the flame of imagination by example of his unquenchable curiosity, quest for knowledge, and fascination with life and the universe; to my mother, Charlotte Boehm, whose amazing fortitude, generosity, and contagious enthusiasm for life continues to inspire all around her to never give up on their dreams and to always look up; and to my sweeties, Liz Balfour and Jazmyn Balfour-Boehm, whose unconditional love and support has allowed me to realize one of my dreams.

Contents

Section I Envisaged Nanomedical Device and System Design Strategies

Section II Merging with Reality: Nascent Nanomedical Diagnostics and Therapeutics

Section III   Beyond the Event Horizon: Nanomedical Visions

Preface

It would seem that the unfathomable wellsprings of cumulative human imagination, ingenuity, passion, and effort are not subject to any tether or constraint that cannot, over time, be unbound or circumvented. This tenet may certainly be applied to the continuously evolving field of medicine generally and particularly to the rapidly emerging discipline of nanomedicine. The incessant drive for more compact, robust, powerful, sophisticated, and effective diagnostic and therapeutic strategies within the purview of medicine has been and increasingly continues to be a critical and potent motivator for radical innovation. There is an underlying and omnipresent sense of urgency toward the investigation and development of tangible and efficacious solutions for the most vexing of humankind's medical challenges. These include heart disease, cancer, HIV/AIDS, diabetes, Alzheimer's, and a host of other serious maladies and pathogenic afflictions that relentlessly threaten to undermine the innate integrity and optimal functionality of the human body.

The rapidly emerging discipline of nanomedicine has unprecedented potential to dramatically transmute current medical paradigms, spanning diagnostics, therapeutics, and surgical procedures. Since nanomedical devices and systems will be designed and engineered to operate and impart beneficial influence at cellular, organellar, molecular, and (hypothetically) atomic domains, the realms within which diseases originate, it may be envisaged that sophisticated autonomous nanodevices and systems can be imbued with capacities for the accurate diagnoses and meticulous and thorough eradication of virtually any disease state and pathogenic or toxic threat. Further, due to facilitative nanotechnological self-assembly processes, and in light of the inevitable future advent of advanced molecular manufacturing, elegant and cost-effective nanomedical technologies might be readily accessible to those in the developing as well as developed worlds.

Concomitantly, the requirement for invasive surgeries might be relegated to obsolescence, as all corrective activities would be conducted in vivo by interactive multitudes of nanomedical cell repair devices. Myriad options for human cognitive and physiological augmentation, and the potential slowing, prevention, or possible (to a degree) reversal of the *disease* of aging may become reality. In conjunction with the option for radically increased life spans, those who are driven to venture out to the stars may undergo additional specialized nanomedical enhancements to enable efficient protective countermeasures against the degradative effects of microgravity and deep space radiation and to facilitate (barring the discovery of highly advanced spacecraft propulsion systems that approach the speed of light), if required, prolonged suspended animation.

This book is divided into three sections. Section I utilizes a conceptual exemplar nanodevice and system (Vascular Cartographic Scanning Nanodevice VCSN), which I have envisaged, to explore various prospective design considerations that might enable selected functionalities of advanced autonomous nanomedical devices. Section II is comprised of seven chapters, which have been submitted by a diverse group of expert contributing authors, describing actual laboratory-based research toward the advancement of nanomedical capabilities. Section III delves into more highly conceptual nanomedical possibilities and visions relating to the implementation of nanomedical technologies in remote regions and the developing world, as well as nanomedicine in space applications, human augmentation, and longevity.

It is hoped that this book might assist in some small measure to serve as a preliminary guide to possibly inspire specific investigative pathways that may lead to meaningful discourse and significant advances in this nascent but potentially very powerful discipline.

Acknowledgments

I am indeed deeply appreciative to all the individuals and organizations who assisted in the evolution of this book. Initially, I would like to express my gratitude to K. Eric Drexler for forging the original vision of the boundless possibilities of nanotechnology, molecular manufacturing, and nanomedicine as laid out in his highly inspirational book *Engines of Creation*. Eric subsequently translated these possibilities into technical/practical terms with his book *Nanosystems: Molecular Machinery, Manufacturing, and Computation*. Second, I would like to extend my true appreciation to Robert A. Freitas Jr. for further enlightening me as to the virtually limitless potential of nanomedicine with his excellent and groundbreaking Nanomedicine book series. Robert has been very generous and patient in responding to my many queries over the years. Both of these visionaries have contributed greatly to the illumination of my mind toward the formulation of the nanomedical concepts that inhabit these pages. It is hoped that these prospective concepts may further inspire others to one day make such nanomedical diagnostic and therapeutic devices and systems a reality for the benefit of humankind.

I would like to express my deep appreciation to the following individuals for providing information, insights, and other forms of support and assistance in facilitating the realization of this project: Kellar Autumn, Elizabeth Balfour, Jazmyn Balfour-Boehm, Scott Cheadle, Aicheng Chen, Gautam Das, Angelika Domschke, Eric Drexler, Ted Duke, Barb Eccles, Robert Freitas Jr., Billy Garrioch, Aubrey de Grey, Rose Hayeshi, Bruce Johnson, Challa Kumar, Sylvain Martel, Gina Miller (nanogirl), Bruce Philips, Chris Phoenix, Judy Sander, Ottilia Saxl, Mark Schultz, Ned Seeman, Mohsen Shahinpoor, Vesselin Shanov, Hayat Sindi, Michael Slaughter, Zach Suntres, Yuriy Svidinenko, Hulda Swai, Jessica Vakili, Dennis Wood, and Kai Yan. I apologize to any individuals whom I may have unintentionally overlooked.

My sincere thanks and gratitude go out to my publisher, Taylor & Francis Group/CRC Press, for taking a chance, having the confidence and trust in me to see this project through, and allowing me the complete freedom to explore some of the exciting possibilities of the nascent discipline of nanomedicine. In particular, I wish to convey my appreciation to Michael Slaughter and Jessica Vakili for their incredible patience and support throughout the writing process. In addition, I very much appreciate the efforts of the staff at Taylor & Francis Group/CRC Press in the production of this book.

I would also like to express my heartfelt gratitude to my dear friend Angelika Domschke, an accomplished scientist and visionary artist, for her continual encouragement, understanding, and smiles that helped to keep me going to the completion of the project. I sincerely thank Angelika for both her excellent chapter and her amazing cover art, *Angstroms in Space*.

Last, I am forever grateful to my truly inspiring and wise father, Josef Boehm; my ever sweet and generous mother, Charlotte Boehm; my loving sister, Renata Swanson, and brother, John Boehm; Jackie Balfour, Elizabeth Balfour, and our incredible daughter Jazmyn Balfour-Boehm for their unconditional love, encouragement, and unwavering support without which this book could not have been written.

Editor

Frank J. Boehm has been involved with nanotechnology and especially nanomedicine since 1996, which has inspired the development of numerous concepts and designs for advanced nanomedical diagnostic and therapeutic components, devices and systems to potentially address myriad disease states. His aim is to develop and transform these concepts into real-world applications for global benefit.

Frank serendipitously encountered the concept of nanotechnology on the Internet and immediately become fascinated with its virtually limitless potential, particularly as relates to the field of medicine. He passionately proceeded to evolve and textually articulate various advanced near-term and longer-term nanomedical concepts and designs. Concomitantly, he initiated correspondence with numerous nanotechnology and nanomedicine research scientists and thought leaders from across the globe.

In recognizing the immense potential of nanomedicine to impart positive paradigm shifts across the medical domain (e.g., precisely targeted drug delivery, vascular/neurological/cellular plaque removal, totally non-invasive surgical procedures, enhancement of physiological systems, and extended longevity), Frank was deeply motivated to write more extensively on the topic. The result has culminated in the generation of this text. In parallel, he managed to engage the interest of several researchers in the United States and Canada in his nanomedical concepts, and in 2009 he formed the startup company NanoApps Medical, Inc. The aim of this company is to investigate and develop advanced, innovative, and cost-effective nanomedical diagnostic and therapeutic devices and systems for the benefit of individuals in both the developing and developed worlds.

Contributors

Asieh Ahmadalinezhad
Department of Chemistry
Lakehead University
Thunder Bay, Ontario, Canada

Misagh Alipour
Medical Sciences Division
Northern Ontario School of Medicine
Lakehead University
Thunder Bay, Ontario, Canada

and

Programme of Biomolecular Sciences
Laurentian University
Sudbury, Ontario, Canada

Frank J. Boehm
NanoApps Medical Inc.
and
NanoApps Consulting
and
Lakehead University
Thunder Bay, Ontario, Canada

Aicheng Chen
Department of Chemistry
Lakehead University
Thunder Bay, Ontario, Canada

Wondong Cho
Nanoworld Smart Materials and Devices
Laboratory
University of Cincinnati
Cincinnati, Ohio

Gautam Das
Photonics Research Group
Department of Physics
Lakehead University
Thunder Bay, Ontario, Canada

Angelika Domschke
Angelika Domschke Consulting, LLC
Duluth, Georgia

Zhongyun Dong
Nanoworld Smart Materials and Devices
Laboratory
University of Cincinnati
Cincinnati, Ohio

Rose Hayeshi
Polymers and Composites
Council for Scientific and Industrial
Research
Pretoria, South Africa

Jianjun Hu
Department of Chemical and Materials
Engineering
University of Dayton
and
Air Force Research Laboratory
Wright-Patterson Air Force Base
Dayton, Ohio

Lonji Kalombo
Polymers and Composites
Council for Scientific and Industrial
Research
Pretoria, South Africa

Lebogang Katata
Polymers and Composites
Council for Scientific and Industrial
Research
Pretoria, South Africa

Yolandy Lemmer
Polymers and Composites
Council for Scientific and Industrial
Research
Pretoria, South Africa

Weifeng Li
Nanoworld Smart Materials and Devices
Laboratory
University of Cincinnati
Cincinnati, Ohio

Sylvain Martel
NanoRobotics Laboratory
Department of Computer and Software
    Engineering
Institute of Biomedical Engineering
Polytechnic School of Montreal
University of Montréal
Montréal, Québec, Canada

David Mast
Nanoworld Smart Materials and Devices
    Laboratory
University of Cincinnati
Cincinnati, Ohio

Chris Muratore
Department of Chemical and Materials
Engineering
University of Dayton
and
Air Force Research Laboratory
Wright-Patterson Air Force Base
Dayton, Ohio

Abdelwahab Omri
Programme of Biomolecular Sciences
Laurentian University
Sudbury, Ontario, Canada

Sarah Pixley
Nanoworld Smart Materials and Devices
    Laboratory
University of Cincinnati
Cincinnati, Ohio

Brad Ruff
Nanoworld Smart Materials and Devices
    Laboratory
University of Cincinnati
Cincinnati, Ohio

Pravahan Salunke
Nanoworld Smart Materials and Devices
    Laboratory
University of Cincinnati
Cincinnati, Ohio

Mark J. Schulz
Nanoworld Smart Materials and Devices
    Laboratory
University of Cincinnati
Cincinnati, Ohio

Boitumelo Semete
Polymers and Composites
Council for Scientific and Industrial
    Research
Pretoria, South Africa

Vesselin Shanov
Nanoworld Smart Materials and Devices
    Laboratory
University of Cincinnati
Cincinnati, Ohio

Hayat Sindi
Founder and CEO of i2 Institute of
    Imagination and Ingenuity

and

UNESCO Goodwill Ambassador for
    Sciences

and

Member of Shura Council of Saudi Arabia

and

Visiting Scholar
Department of Chemistry and Chemical
    Biology
Harvard University
Cambridge, Massachusetts

Yi Song
Nanoworld Smart Materials and Devices
    Laboratory
University of Cincinnati
Cincinnati, Ohio

Anshuman Sowani
Nanoworld Smart Materials and Devices
    Laboratory
University of Cincinnati
Cincinnati, Ohio

Bolaji Suberu
Nanoworld Smart Materials and Devices
    Laboratory
University of Cincinnati
Cincinnati, Ohio

Zacharias E. Suntres
Medical Sciences Division
Northern Ontario School of Medicine
Lakehead University
Thunder Bay, Ontario, Canada

and

Programme of Biomolecular Sciences
Laurentian University
Sudbury, Ontario, Canada

Hulda Swai
Polymers and Composites
Council for Scientific and Industrial
    Research
Pretoria, South Africa

Rajiv Venkatasubramanian
Nanoworld Smart Materials and Devices
    Laboratory
University of Cincinnati
Cincinnati, Ohio

John Yin
Nanoworld Smart Materials and Devices
    Laboratory
University of Cincinnati
Cincinnati, Ohio

Section I

Envisaged Nanomedical Device and System Design Strategies

1

Exemplar Nanomedical Vascular Cartographic Scanning Nanodevice

Frank J. Boehm

CONTENTS

1.1 Introduction

Envisioners and designers of nanomedical devices may draw their inspiration from a number of sources. These might include the myriad mechanisms and processes that operate both at macroscale and nanoscale domains in the natural world, which may be interpreted and transformed into functional synthetic analogs via biomimetics. Other inspirational sparks may emanate from purely anthropogenic dreamscapes, which reside within the realms of fantasy and science fiction. There is always the chance that completely unexpected serendipitous discovery might arrive from "nowhere" to the utter joy of long toiling recipients who might have been looking for answers for many years in one area, only to have a pivotal insight surprisingly light up, when triggered by a completely unrelated event, as if a gift from some parallel universe that has "crossed over." Incremental inspirational glimmers, and much more rarely, dramatic brilliant bursts thereof may indeed be gleaned through voluminous thoughtful, disciplined, and deliberate experimentation. From whatever quarter such inspiration may appear, it may be suggested that a certain "cognitive stance" might serve as a useful prerequisite to facilitate and breed the flames of inspiration, creativity, and innovation, which may likely percolate into reality. This attitude might encompass in varying degrees, a blend of excitement and prospective adventure, an insatiable childlike curiosity, open mindedness and playfulness, enthusiasm and positiveness, combined with responsibility, integrity; and importantly, persistence, interspersed with a modicum of naivety, and humbleness in the recognition that one can clearly never "know it all."

In actual terms, the development of innovative nanomedical concepts and designs may consist of the heterogeneous fusion of many of the above elements in combination with, from an engineering perspective, what may be perceived to be practically achieved in a manner that is not cost prohibitive. These considerations may encompass the selection of appropriate materials, as well as the development of optimized techniques that are to be employed for the synthesis of nanoscale components and devices from the "bottom–up" (e.g., utilizing advanced chemistries [1,2], or via still conceptual, albeit steadily advancing nanomanufacturing technologies [3–5]), or "top–down" strategies that include microelectromechancial systems (MEMs) [6,7] and nanoelectromechanical systems (NEMs) [8,9], lithographic patterning techniques [10,11] that may achieve features with resolutions from 10 to 100 nm, and nanoscale/molecular imprinting [12–15], stamping [16,17], and molding [18,19], which can provide 20–40 nm features.

1.2 Conceptual Exemplar Nanodevice Design

In order to facilitate the conveyance of potential strategies and thought processes that might be involved with the conceptualization and design of advanced nanomedical components, devices, and systems; two hypothetical exemplar nanomedical devices and systems, which are being evolved by the author, will be interspersed throughout this volume. The intent will be to introduce a number of potential design themes that might be considered to have utility for imparting specific functionalities when integrated into nanomedical devices. Other critical elements will include the demarcation and nurturing of a sustainable vision as to what the intended functionalities and applications for these elements will be, as well as the attempt to evolve effective and pragmatic designs that may be reasonably produced.

1.3 Vascular Cartographic Scanning Nanodevice

The first of these conceptual exemplars, the Vascular Cartographic Scanning Nanodevice (VCSN) (Figure 1.1), will be manifest as an advanced autonomous, ~1 μm in diameter nanomedical device for in vivo imaging applications. Its description throughout this text will be inclusive of its envisaged individual components and external "outbody" control infrastructures. A far less complex/rudimentary, albeit still nanocomponent-driven precursor to the VCSN device, would be manifest as a much physically larger (~3 mm in diameter) in vivo nanomedical imaging instrument, called the Gastrointestinal Micro Scanning Device (GMSD).

It is hoped that the incremental investigation of conceptual nanomedical device components laid out within these pages via these exemplars may serve as a preliminary template to perhaps illustrate how conceptualists and designers of future sophisticated nanomedical

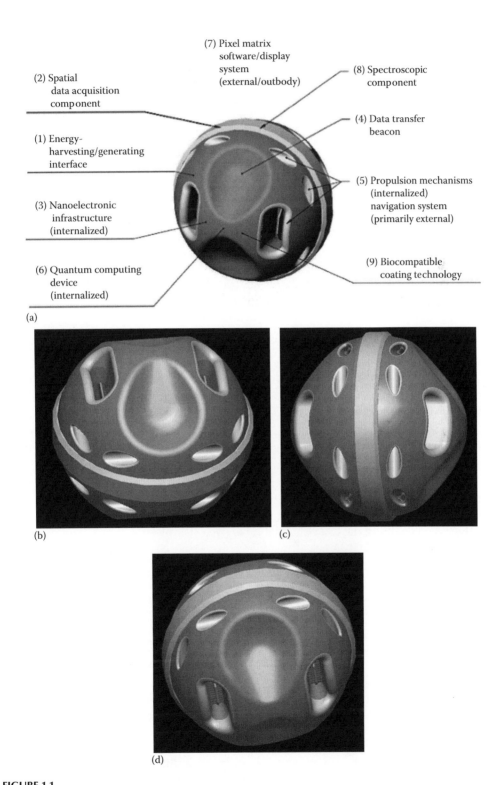

FIGURE 1.1
(a) Anatomy of conceptual Vascular Cartographic Scanning Nanodevice (VCSN). (b–d) Various VCSN orientations.

components, devices, and systems might approach the tremendous challenges that will confront them. Far more intensive and demanding tasks will be allotted to nanomedical engineers who are charged with the daunting task of devising real-world strategies as relates to the actual fabrication and functionalization of these nanoscale "medical dream machines." A few examples of the many tasks involved may include, as described earlier, the selection of appropriate nanomaterials; the design and development of robust, dependable, and scalable self-assembly (nanomanufacturing) capabilities; self-quality control verification and test strategies; the development of pragmatic component designs that will operate effectively under myriad constraints imposed by human physiology in vivo; novel approaches for modular nanocomponent/nanoelectronics integration; and the interfacing of multiple nanometric components with outbody computers and a conceptual "NanoNav" dedicated nanomedical device navigation system.

The conceptual VCSN constitutes a fully autonomous nanoscale in vivo medical imaging device and system. The ~1 µm in diameter nanodevice, or more likely, many thousands of identical such nanodevices working in parallel, would function to scan/image the entire human vasculature down to the level of the smallest capillary lumen (e.g., ~3 µm diameter) in high-resolution three-dimensional (3D) digitized format.

1.3.1 Overview of Envisaged VCSN Capabilities

1. Capacity for the generation of a very high-resolution (less than ~1 µm) 3D rendering of the complete human vasculature down to the capillary level. It may also be applied to the imaging of the lymphatic system, and in a simplified form (e.g., GMSD), the gastrointestinal tract (GIT).

2. Ability to distinguish and superimpose vascular and neurological plaque deposits and lesions with high accuracy against the topographically rendered backdrop of healthy endothelial wall surfaces.

3. Quantification of vascular wall thicknesses along with the identification and highlighting of "hot spots" at any site within the vasculature, such as imminent blockages or aneurysms that are at risk of rupturing. This capacity will be of particular value when enabling the clear elucidation of such risk sites for subsequent mitigation in situ, within the brain.

4. Capacity for physicians to "fly-through" all scanned areas via a joystick and computer display for the highly detailed inspection of any desired site within the system. The acquired spatial data may also enable holographic rendering and virtual travel through all imaged systems.

5. Ability to facilitate the targeting of tumors by revealing instances of nascent angiogenesis in close proximity to tumor growth sites.

The VCSN will comprise multiple modularly integrated nanoscale components, subsystems, and primary systems that are connected via a dynamic nanoelectronic/nanophotonic infrastructure. These entities will be organized and assembled in a prioritized and sequentially hierarchical manner. An intrinsic developmental process that may drive the conceptualization and evolution of individual functional modules, such as the propulsion system, may initially encompass several potential candidate technologies. The most promising of these candidates would be selected on the basis of their demonstration of superior performance when applied to specific tasks and when challenged with a variety of dedicated trials.

A preliminary research and discovery phase would serve to thoroughly define the perceived scope and developmental timeline of the VCSN. This might consist of a strategy that involves the preliminary identification and description, in as much detail as is possible, of every primary and secondary nanometric component, mechanism, and system. It will be a necessary and prudent step toward realistically discerning exactly which potential elements of each system might be feasible insofar as manufacturability and functionality when scaled down to the nanometer range. This exercise may manifest itself as a process of elimination, or may result in a superior hybrid design whereby several of the most desirable elements that are extracted from a number of options may ultimately prove to be the most favorable solution. The fundamental physics, chemistry, electronics, thermodynamics, and mechanics behind each of the selected component attributes will be systematically tested, theoretically, through the implementation of task-specific computer modeling, in conjunction with hands-on experimentation against predetermined parameters and a protocol checklist. This organization will assist in the determination and generation of proof-of-principal guidelines, while also serving to verifiably refute the feasibility of the use of certain components in particular applications, or negating the combination of specific elements.

1.3.2 Summary of VCSN Components

Each envisaged nanoscale element and system comprising the VCSN will embody its own specific set of investigative, conceptualization, design pathways, and associated tasks. These components, in order of perceived importance, are as follows:

1. *Energy-harvesting/generating components.* Constitute the primary and auxiliary power-harvesting/generating sources for all primary, secondary, and multiple redundant VCSN systems. These mechanisms might harvest and catalyze readily available molecular biofuels (e.g., glucose, hydrogen) from the in vivo environment, and convert them into electron flow. There are many additional potential nanoscale energy harvesting and generating technologies (e.g., thermopiles, piezoelectronics, hydrostatics, and biomimetic entities and processes) that will be worthy of exploration (Chapter 4).

2. *Spatial data acquisition component.* Functions as the spatial data acquisition signal emitter and receiver that will constitute the scanning mechanism. With this component as well, several potential technologies exist, or might be extrapolated (e.g., capacitive ultrasound, nanoscale time-of-flight LIDAR), which will warrant serious investigation (Chapter 6).

3. *Nanoelectronic/nanophotonic infrastructure.* Conveys and modulates the electrical current and photonic streams that enable myriad critical VCSN functions (e.g., propulsion, onboard navigation controls, computing, and communications) including the emission and reception of scanning pulses from the spatial data acquisition array, and to facilitate the transfer of acquired spatial information to a data transfer beacon for transmission to outbody computers for final processing, image reconstruction, and display. Various nanoelectronic/nanophotonic components and conveyance conduits such as highly conductive carbon nanotubes, organic/inorganic nanowires or conductive polymeric nanofibers, and nanoscale chalcogenide (photoconductive glass)-derived optical nanofibers might electronically and photonically interconnect and interface all nanodevice elements (Chapter 5).

4. *Data transfer beacon.* Transmits collected spatial data to an "outbody" receiver, which is interfaced with the Pixel Matrix (PM) image reconstruction system. It is also utilized as the primary communications node for receiving external commands as well as for inter-nanodevice coordination. In addition, it would serve to lock onto an external homing signal upon completion of the scanning procedure, or for emergency egress from the patient.

5. *Propulsion and navigational systems.* Endows the nanodevice with autonomy in vivo and enables travel in any orientation and direction while within this environment. Movement is initiated and guided by transmitted command signals under external computer control via a dedicated "NanoNav" navigation system, perhaps akin to a miniaturized GPS system. An onboard computer (quantum or possibly DNA based) will assist in this regard by emanating positional coordinate feedback data.

6. *Nanoscale computation.* Enables the capacity for command data storage, working protocols, and spatial data backup at a high level of redundancy for fail-safe nanodevice operation, propulsion, and navigation including internal, inter-device, and external communications. This component might be manifest as a solid-state quantum computer or an organized biomolecular device comprising restriction nuclease and ligase hardware working in conjunction with software-encoded DNA duplex arrays. Alternatively, all optical nanoscale computing may be implemented to reduce the cumulative thermal footprint that may conceivably be generated by possibly millions of in vivo nanodevices.

7. *PM display system.* Translates acquired spatial data into digitized display format with high image resolution. Each endothelial wall target "hit" that is initiated and measured by onboard ultrasonic transducer arrays (or other selected spatial data acquisition mechanisms) would be represented by a pixel, assigned to a calculated position in 3D space on a display. This software might also have the capacity for discerning vascular wall thicknesses so as to facilitate aneurysm detection via the isolation of secondary echo signatures from the spatial data set.

8. *Spectroscopic component.* Elucidates the chemical composition of scanned entities so as to accurately differentiate plaque deposits and lesions from healthy (background) vascular endothelial or lymphatic constituents by utilizing mass spectroscopic analysis. This capability may assist in the whole-body mapping and compositional analysis of pathogenic aggregates, regardless of their makeup (e.g., vascular plaques, neurological beta amyloid plaques, lipofuscin, cholesterol, and oxysterols).

9. *Biocompatible coating technology.* Endows nanodevices with reliable stealth qualities so that they may circumvent any level of immune response while they operate in vivo, through the utilization of inert and biocompatible materials (e.g., diamondoid, sapphire materials) as the main building materials of nanodevices, or via the use of bioinert diamondoid or polymeric thin film coatings.

1.3.3 Discussion

As a critical part of their development, each individual component of the VCSN will be subjected to stringent testing for safety, reliable functionality, and robustness. Further rigorous testing will take place as subsequent entities are developed and integrated with various other dedicated components to eventually comprise a complete and fully functional autonomous nanomedical scanning device.

A practical deficiency that might be addressed in global healthcare through the proposed development of the conceptual VCSN would be the potential alleviation of the very limited or non-availability of advanced medical imaging technologies in remote and impoverished regions of the world. The envisaged sophisticated nature of this innovative medical imaging technology combined with its inherent miniaturization might cost effectively facilitate access to important and medical diagnostic tools for virtually any individual on the globe.

As an autonomous nanodevice with finite energy storage capacity due to extreme physical constraints on available real estate, the VCSN will be designed with several strata of operational redundancy, particularly where the harvesting and conversion of energy is concerned, to ensure uninterrupted operation and the capacity for continuous in vivo/outbody communications. The VCSN might harvest power via the chemical catalysis of glucose, hydrogen, other appropriate biomolecules or ions within the in vivo environment of patients, thereby having the advantageous attribute of self-sustainability while in operation. Alternately, the VCSN may be induced to generate onboard power through activation by external sources. It may be possible that a hybrid, three-tiered energy capability might also evolve, whereby primary power is generated via external activation; onboard energy harvesting serves as a secondary supplementary source, and stored battery power provides a sufficient backup, should the very rare instance occur where both higher echelon systems go offline, or are otherwise disrupted or incapacitated.

The bulk of conventional power that is necessary to sustain the VCSN infrastructure would be for the operation of external computers that house the PM image reconstruction software, along with additional modular and compact hardware that is required for NanoNav guidance beacons, and communications infrastructure. These power requirements might be met via a dedicated, hybrid power-harvesting/generating "kit" that integrates solar, wind, fuel cell, mechanical crank, or other practicable/robust/efficient power-generating sources. Thus, the entire setup for VCSN scanning procedures may achieve fully functionality in remote, and if necessary, physically confined areas.

The implementation of the scanning procedure would be quite straightforward as a prescribed dose of thousands of identical VCSN units may be injected, diffused through an adhered patch or topical gel, swallowed as a pill, or administered as oral thin film wafers or drops. Once the nanodevices ingress to the bloodstream, they will self-organize, orient themselves, and report their positions using micron resolution X-, Y-, Z-coordinates relative to an established external reference point. This "confluence fiducial" may be established via the intersection of several propagating electromagnetic beams, which emanate from dedicated beacons, utilized to demarcate the patient scanning volume in 3D space. When the scanning procedure has been completed (e.g., ~5 minutes), an externally activated homing signal would direct all nanodevices to a predetermined "outbody" egress site where they would be collected and stored for subsequent molecular disassembly and recycling.

An imperative infrastructural element inherent to the VCSN developmental strategy will be the focus on an optimized and highly efficient nanomanufacturing capability, to ensure that VCSN units may be produced cost effectively via massively parallel fabrication (e.g., DNA-mediated self-assembly) techniques [2,20–26], such that they can be economically administered as "single-use" entities, and recyclable for reuse in non-medical applications. This strategy would negate a range of cumulative expenditures and time-consuming procedures involved with nanodevice sterilization and storage for eventual reuse. The latter prospect, however, will likely elicit an understandably strong psychological resistance, even if there should be a qualified assurance of safety provided. This is, no doubt, firmly grounded on innate concerns regarding undesirable and indeed, unacceptable pathogenic biotransmission. As the VCSN units will comprise biocompatible elements in accordance with established nanomedical protocols, they might be disposed of under similarly stringent procedures, as exists for standardized medical refuse, though due to their small physical size they might undergo separate processing, or ideally, recycling for benign integration into bulk products. As an option to a targeted egress strategy, once a scanning procedure has been completed, the nanodevices may be allowed to diffuse naturally from the patient via various bodily fluids, though they would be tagged for tracking to ensure that their removal from the patient is complete.

1.3.4 VCSN Advantages

The envisaged practical advantages offered by the VCSN and its associated infrastructure will include

1. Compactness and portability, as its operation will require a relatively small footprint. This would enable simple and quick setup and power-up procedures in developing countries and remote terrestrial environments. In the aerospace domain, it may be utilized as an element of an onboard medical diagnostics suite on military and medical aircraft, and for space travel if reconfigured for integration into spacesuits and spacecraft, and to provide a compact yet powerful medical imaging capability for future Moon and Mars habitats (Chapter 16).

2. Frugal energy consumption.

3. Relatively inexpensive to administer and operate.

4. Rapid scanning time (e.g., ~5 minutes).

5. Ultra-high resolution digital spatial data. Inherent flexibility for display in several different formats, and ease of file transmission to medical personnel internationally, via secure telecommunications connectivity.

6. Potential for enabling the drastic reduction or elimination of long waiting queues for critical imaging technologies.

Conventional medical imaging technologies such as magnetic resonance imaging (MRI) and computed tomography (CT) are very expensive and, hence, out of reach for developing countries. They are also physically unwieldy, power hungry, and have long waiting times for their use. Although current ultrasound imaging technology is improving, it is still relatively crude in resolution and administration, and the resulting imagery is segmental in nature, in contrast to whole-body scanning. The VCSN is envisioned as having the capability for rendering complete systems (e.g., vascular, lymphatic, or gastrointestinal) in ultrafine detail, displaying all luminal surfaces and wall thicknesses with the possibility of also distinguishing their chemical compositions.

Since there is an increasingly strong demand for smaller and more compact medical technologies that are endowed with enhanced and more complex capabilities, the VCSN would constitute an exponential step in this direction. The investigation and eventual development of initial and subsequent generations of components aimed at implementation for VCSN technology may conceivably be applied to "any" future nanomedical device and system. These components might be designed in such a way that they can be fabricated in modular form and, to some extent, adhere to a predetermined standardized format to assist in enabling future specialized nanomedical diagnostic and therapeutic capabilities and devices (e.g., ultrafine in vivo spectroscopic biopsy, cell-targeted drug delivery, vascular/neurological plaque removal devices, lysosome lipofuscin dissolution or removal, chromosome repair or replacement, bone mineral delivery and repair devices for the remediation of osteoporosis, and prospective cell repair devices).

1.4 Gastrointestinal Micro Scanning Device

The Gastrointestinal Micro Scanning Device (GMSD) (Figure 1.2) will serve as a formative and far less complex precursor to the VCSN in that it will not have the capacity for
propulsion or navigation. It will, however, utilize nascent forms of the quantum computing, nanoelectronics, spatial data acquisition, and PM technologies that are envisaged for the VCSN. Hence, the GMSD, in addition to serving as spatial data acquisition
device, may also have utility as a test bed of sorts that is employed to identify and resolve

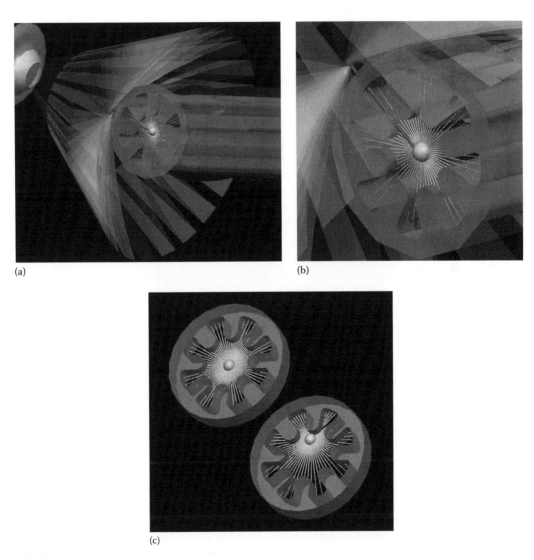

(a) (b)

(c)

FIGURE 1.2
(a) Artistic representation of conceptual Gastrointestinal Micro Scanning Device (GMSD) depicting communication link between the pulse generator/data transfer unit (PGDT) and the bright ball (BB) internal scanning
device. (b, c) Auto-adjustment of BB acquisition interrogating signals in response to a shift from central position
within lumen of GIT.

technical, integrative, and functional issues toward the further evolution of the VCSN. The GMSD system will consist of three distinct components working in unison to generate a very high-resolution 3D topography of the entire internal surface of the GIT. The GMSD would accomplish this task by employing

1. An internalized (via ingestion) scanning device
2. An external pulse generator/data transfer unit
3. A PM display element

1.4.1 Bright Ball Scanning Device

The bright ball (BB) scanning device would have a spherical morphology of ~3 mm in diameter. (A thorough assessment would be conducted using computer modeling and in vitro testing to ascertain the optimal physical parameters for the device to eliminate the possibility of the BB getting physically "snagged" en route through the GIT.) Most of the outer surface of the device, save the area required for acoustic communications beacons, will consist of a continuous tessellated array of ~1 μm in diameter emitter/receiver (ER) units, which may take the form of micron-scale capacitive ultrasonic transducers, each of which would constitute a standalone measuring instrument. Individual units might be positioned and bonded to their neighbors with a polymeric adhesive that is both biocompatible and biodegradable (e.g., 3,4-dihydroxybenzoic acid combined with chitosan). This bonding material would encapsulate all of the ER units to comprise a solid sphere, which might be finished with a translucent thin film of gold to impart a highly polished and reflective surface. The ER units would be calibrated beforehand, and distance measurements of the internal topography of the GIT would be performed using time-of-flight calculations. The resulting imagery could be reconstructed via the quantification of variances in relation to the initial reference calibration.

1.4.2 Pulse Generator/Data Transfer Unit

The pulse generator/data transfer (PGDT) unit is the component that would trigger the activity of the internalized BB device with an appropriate, specifically encrypted signal. The BB would be activated to scan subsequent to receiving this specific signal only. Once active, the BB would transmit a constant data stream to the PGDT. The PGDT would serve as the data transfer device when linked to a computer and the PM software. It would be affixed to an appropriate area of the patient's abdominal surface and would stay in place for the duration of the scan.

1.4.3 PM Display

The PM display would process the data supplied to it by the PGDT to reconstruct a high-resolution "pixel per hit" 3D rendering of the total scanned area that has been traveled by the BB. The software would enable "fly-through" and cross-sectional capabilities, allowing physicians (using a joystick, computer mouse, or touch screen display) to traverse the entire GIT to investigate any potential problem areas in great detail. One may envision that the acquired digitized information might be translated to holographic and virtual reality formats as well. The physician would thus recognize any anomalous topography consistent with tumor growth, lesions, and other abnormal features that may exist in the GIT using this procedure.

1.4.4 Description of Scanning Procedure

The setup for the GMSD operational procedure would be relatively simple to implement. Initially, the BB would be administered orally to the patient in the same manner as a pill. Next, an adhesive and waterproof PGDT thin film patch would be affixed to the skin of patient's abdomen. At this juncture, a system's calibration would be performed to assure that the communication link between the BB and the PGDT is functioning properly. A test scan would also be performed to configure the image resolution. Following these procedures, the patient would be allowed to leave the physician's office, clinic, or hospital to go about his/her normal routine. The internalized BB would now progress along with the natural peristaltic rhythms of the GIT and be naturally eliminated at the conclusion of the transit duration. The patient would subsequently return to the facility in two or three days (contingent on the assessed GIT transit time) to have the PGDT patch removed.

The PGDT will have continually accumulated all of the data acquired by the BB during the designated scanning period. This device would then be interfaced with a computer via a USB port to stream all of the acquired data to the PM software housed within the computer. The data would now be translated into high-resolution 3D imagery on a display. The interrogating signals emitted by the BB would have the capacity for passing through the contents of the small and large intestines, as if transparent, through the utilization of a selective signal filtering algorithm. The scanning signals would have no harmful effect on any cell or tissue, even with prolonged exposure. The PGDT would emit a unique pulsed signal (e.g., ultrasonic, near-infrared), which when received by sensors embedded within the surface of the BB would trigger all of the ERs embedded to fire and emit their scanning beams simultaneously in every direction. The PM software would calculate BB orientation and would correlate the hits obtained within predetermined parameters to construct a cross section of the GIT representing its internal topography. These digitized segments would be sequentially pieced together to form a seamless spatially accurate rendering of the system.

1.4.5 Additional Issues

The BB device would be stored in a sterilized environment until it is ready for use to negate any risk of infection. Additionally, due to the fairly rapid transit time (~two days) from ingestion to elimination, the chances of eliciting an immune response should be very low. Following elimination, the BB will cease to function as it will require the specialized PGDT-generated pulsed signals for activation and function. The shell of the BB, as described earlier, might include a biodegradable and environment/ecosystem-compatible polymeric binding compound that may be formulated to break down after seven days of exposure to an aqueous environment, releasing the physical support of all ER units. The ER units would subsequently separate, becoming in essence, nonfunctional micron-sized particulates that may break down further into harmless elements.

The GMSD would serve as a beneficial, minimally invasive, biocompatible diagnostic system for generating high-resolution 3D imagery of the GIT. It would be relatively simple to implement, minimize any chance of infection or discomfort, and the scanning would not be disruptive to the patient, who could carry on with his/her normal affairs. In addition, the GMSD would be biodegradable and environmentally compatible. This novel nanomedical imaging system would serve as a boon to physicians via the provision of a new and more precise method of imaging the GIT. It would aid them by offering more detailed information as to the health status of the GIT in order to prescribe the appropriate preventative or therapeutic care, and would assist by acting as an accurate diagnostic tool, thereby increasing the efficacy of their treatments.

References

1. Gu, H., Chao, J., Xiao, S.J., and Seeman, N.C., A proximity-based programmable DNA nanoscale assembly line. *Nature.* 465(7295), 202–205, 2010.
2. Boehm, F.J., An investigation of nucleic acid/DNA-based manufacturing, Thirty Essential Nanotechnology Studies: #10. Center for Responsible Nanotechnology, Menlo Park, CA, August 2004. http://wise-nano.org/w/Boehm_DNA_Study (accessed 06/17/13)
3. Freitas, R.A. Jr., Diamondoid mechanosynthesis for tip-based nanofabrication, Chapter 11, in Tseng, A., ed., *Tip-Based Nanofabrication: Fundamentals and Applications.* Springer, New York, 387–400, 2011.
4. Tarasov, D., Akberova, N., Izotova, E., Alisheva, D., Astafiev, M., and Freitas, R.A. Jr., Optimal tool tip trajectories in a hydrogen abstraction tool recharge reaction sequence for positionally controlled diamond mechanosynthesis. *J Comput Theor Nanosci.* 7, 325–353, 2010.
5. Chen, Y., Xu, Z., Gartia, M.R., Whitlock, D., Lian, Y., and Liu, G.L., Ultrahigh throughput silicon nanomanufacturing by simultaneous reactive ion synthesis and etching. *ACS Nano.* 5(10), 8002–8012, 2011.
6. Butler, E.J., Folk, C., Cohen, A., Vasilyev, N.V., Chen, R., Del Nido, P.J., and Dupont, P.E., Metal MEMS tools for beating-heart tissue approximation. *IEEE Int Conf Robot Autom.* 411–416, 2011.
7. Wheeler, J.W., Dabling, J.G., Chinn, D., Turner, T., Filatov, A., Anderson, L., and Rohrer, B., MEMS-based bubble pressure sensor for prosthetic socket interface pressure measurement. *Conf Proc IEEE Eng Med Biol Soc.* 2011, 2925–2928, 2011.
8. Basarir, O., Bramhavar, S., and Ekinci, K.L., Motion transduction in nanoelectromechanical systems (NEMS) arrays using near-field optomechanical coupling. *Nano Lett.* 12(2), 534–539, 2012.
9. Khaleque, T., Abu-Salih, S., Saunders, J.R., and Moussa, W., Experimental methods of actuation, characterization and prototyping of hydrogels for bioMEMS/NEMS applications. *J Nanosci Nanotechnol.* 11(3), 2470–2479, 2011.
10. Basnar, B. and Willner, I., Dip-pen-nanolithographic patterning of metallic, semiconductor, and metal oxide nanostructures on surfaces. *Small.* 5(1), 28–44, 2009.
11. Zhou, X., Boey, F., Huo, F., Huang, L., and Zhang, H., Chemically functionalized surface patterning. *Small.* 7(16), 2273–2289, 2011.
12. Shi, G., Lu, N., Xu, H., Wang, Y., Shi, S., Li, H., Li, Y., and Chi, L., Fabrication of hierarchical structures by unconventional two-step imprinting. *J Colloid Interface Sci.* 368(1), 655–659, 2012.
13. Villegas, J.E., Swiecicki, I., Bernard, R., Crassous, A., Briatico, J., Wolf, T., Bergeal, N. et al., Imprinting nanoporous alumina patterns into the magneto-transport of oxide superconductors. *Nanotechnology.* 22(7), 075302, 2011.
14. Hien Nguyen, T. and Ansell, R.J., *N*-Isopropylacrylamide as a functional monomer for noncovalent molecular imprinting. *J Mol Recognit.* 25(1), 1–10, 2012.
15. Xu, H., Schönhoff, M., and Zhang, X., Unconventional layer-by-layer assembly: Surface molecular imprinting and its applications. *Small.* 8(4), 517–523, 2011.
16. Taylor, C., Marega, E., Stach, E.A., Salamo, G., Hussey, L., Muñoz, M., and Malshe, A., Directed self-assembly of quantum structures by nanomechanical stamping using probe tips. *Nanotechnology.* 19(1), 015301, 2008.
17. Zeira, A., Berson, J., Feldman, I., Maoz, R., and Sagiv, J., A bipolar electrochemical approach to constructive lithography: Metal/monolayer patterns via consecutive site-defined oxidation and reduction. *Langmuir.* 27(13), 8562–8575, 2011.
18. Bass, J.D., Schaper, C.D., Rettner, C.T., Arellano, N., Alharbi, F.H., Miller, R.D., and Kim, H.C., Transfer molding of nanoscale oxides using water-soluble templates. *ACS Nano.* 5(5), 4065–4072, 2011.
19. De Marco, C., Eaton, S.M., Levi, M., Cerullo, G., Turri, S., and Osellame, R., High-fidelity solvent-resistant replica molding of hydrophobic polymer surfaces produced by femtosecond laser nanofabrication. *Langmuir.* 27(13), 8391–8395, 2011.

20. Hadorn, M. and Eggenberger Hotz, P., DNA-mediated self-assembly of artificial vesicles. *PLoS One*. 5(3), e9886, 2010.
21. Maune, H.T., Han, S.P., Barish, R.D., Bockrath, M., Iii, W.A. Rothemund, P.W., and Winfree, E., Self-assembly of carbon nanotubes into two-dimensional geometries using DNA origami templates. *Nat Nanotechnol*. 5(1), 61–66, 2010.
22. Sun, X., Hyeon Ko, S., Zhang, C., Ribbe, A.E., and Mao, C., Surface-mediated DNA self assembly. *J Am Chem Soc*. 131(37), 13248–13249, 2009.
23. Cheng, W., Campolongo, M.J., Cha, J.J., Tan, S.J., Umbach, C.C., Muller, D.A., and Luo, D., Free-standing nanoparticle superlattice sheets controlled by DNA. *Nat Mater*. 8(6), 519–525, 2009.
24. Ofir, Y., Samanta, B., and Rotello, V.M., Polymer and biopolymer mediated self-assembly of gold nanoparticles. *Chem Soc Rev*. 37(9), 1814–1825, 2008.
25. Samanta, D., Shanmugaraju, S., Joshi, S.A., Patil, Y.P., Nethaji, M., and Mukherjee, P.S., Pillar height dependent formation of unprecedented Pd(8) molecular swing and Pd(6) molecular boat via multicomponent self-assembly. *Chem Commun (Camb)*. 48, 2298–2300, 2012.
26. Breen, J.M., Clérac, R., Zhang, L., Cloonan, S.M., Kennedy, E., Feeney, M., McCabe, T., Williams, D.C., and Schmitt, W., Self-assembly of hybrid organic–inorganic polyoxovanadates: Functionalised mixed-valent clusters and molecular cages. *Dalton Trans*. 41(10), 2918–2926, 2012.

2

Design Challenges and Considerations for Nanomedical Ingress and Egress

Frank J. Boehm

CONTENTS

2.1 Introduction: Accessing Inner Sanctums

In nanomedicine, two strategies of critical importance will involve the development of methodologies to facilitate the safe entry (ingress) of nanomedical devices into a patient at the onset of any diagnostic or therapeutic procedure, and their subsequent exit (egress) from the patient at the conclusion of these activities. Envisaged sequential nanomedical operations may be considered as analogous to tactical military missions, in that nano-medical devices will be deployed in vivo, rapidly advance to the site(s) of operations to accomplish their assigned tasks, such as the destruction of cancer cells; the dissolution of vascular or neurological plaque materials; or the filling of voids in bones that have been ravaged by osteoporosis, and then quickly vacate. An alternative to instructing nanode-vices to exit the patient directly following a procedure by strategic relocation to facilitate egress via natural excretion processes may be the initiation of a hibernative protocol. This default procedure might be spontaneously engaged should a defect be detected in any nanodevice at the systems level, or if for some reason external computer or navigation systems happen to go offline. Following this protocol, the nanodevices would congregate at predetermined "homing" sites (e.g., dermal pores, tear ducts, finger/toe nail beds) to power down and initiate a "hibersleep" status. Dermal pores and tear ducts would likely provide the most immediate means of egress, whereas in the most protracted instances when nanodevices may be embedded in nail beds, they would remain nonactive to safely egress the patient through the normal course of cuticle growth.

Undoubtedly, there will also exist a wide variety of external nanomedical procedures, which may encompass dermal wound repair and maintenance (e.g., the eradication of skin cancers, removal of dermal polyps, warts, or aging spots, the treatment of psoriasis; and in the cosmetic domain, the repair of wrinkles, varicose and spider veins, acne protuberances or blackheads). Nanomedical devices may also be administered within the oral cavity in order to conduct dental repair or routine maintenance. Indeed, long residing oral-class nanodevices might regularly "patrol" the gums, teeth, tongue, salivary ducts, and glands and be charged with the restoration and maintenance of pristine oral health and hygiene. In addition, nanodevices may be programmed to imperceptibly traverse auditory chan-nels to repair ear drum or cochlear damage, address tinnitus, or perform routine mainte-nance tasks such as ear wax degradation and removal. In more sophisticated procedures, highly orchestrated collections of specialized nanomedical devices might be tasked with the remodeling of lenses of the eyes or repair of retinas of patients to improve vision, or they may be tasked with the dissolution of cataracts. Preservatory classes of nanodevices may be assigned to the removal of nonpathological proteinaceous "floaters" that are sus-pended within the vitreous humor.

This chapter will survey a number of potential nanodevice ingress strategies, and will examine possible options and venues as relates to nanomedical egress.

2.2 Prospective Advanced Nanomedical Device Ingress Strategies

Every strategy that is conceived in regard to the administration of advanced nanomedical devices into the human body will be coupled with its own particular set of challenges. As contemporary medicine advances, it is likely that increasingly convenient, noninvasive, and painless administration techniques will move to be preferential. The most probable methodologies to be employed for the "ingress," or entry, of nanomedical devices into the human in vivo milieu may include oral ingestion, intravenous injection, nasal and lung aerosol inhalation, transfer through a transdermal patch, or topically applied cutaneous colloidal gel, and aqueous ocular, nasal, or ear drops. In each instance, for example, in direct intravenous hypodermic injection, some form of barrier will have to be traversed in order to gain access to the bloodstream, thereby enabling penetration into various tissue types and internal organ systems. Hence, the composition, physical size, morphology, and surface-resident electrical charges of medical nanodevices will play a critical role in either facilitating or hindering their capacity for negotiating various types of biological structures.

The above said, in contrast to conventional drug administration routes that are exploited in order to achieve certain therapeutic advantages, such as desired localized effects, or the expedited arrival of drugs at disease-related targets, sufficiently advanced nanomedical devices will have the agility and programmable capacity to rapidly access any site within the human body with high positional accuracy (<1 μm), which may ultimately render a preferred method of ingress as inconsequential.

2.3 Oral Ingestion

One of the most straightforward, relatively noninvasive, and patient amenable nano-medical device ingress strategies may be via the ingestion of an orally prescribed dose of nanodevices that is swallowed in tablet, capsule, or liquid form. Nanodevices that are intended for oral delivery will be coated with, or encapsulated within materials that protect them from the acidic environment of the stomach. Human gastric juice comprises a highly acidic (0.1 M with a pH of 1) solution of ~0.5% hydrochloric acid (H^+Cl^-), which is secreted by parietal (oxyntic) cells that reside in the gastric lining. This acid initially breaks down consumed proteins in preparation for further degradation by the proteolytic enzyme, pepsin [1]. Hard and rigid "solid class" nanodevices constructed of diamondoid or sapphire will be highly resilient to corrosion, and hence, will not be affected by the acidic environment of the stomach. However, "flex class" nanodevices that comprising softer materials in order to accomplish specific types of procedures that require a certain degree of flexibility or deformability can likely be protected with thin film coatings of natural or synthetic polymeric biocompatible and biodegradable encapsulating materials. These coatings will enable such nanodevices to briefly reside within the stomach while their encompassing tablet or capsule degrades, leaving them unscathed by the highly caustic gastric environment before traversing the stomach wall.

When considering the oral ingestive ingress route for prescribed dosages of nanomedical devices in conveyance forms such as tablets, capsules, or ingestible films, the primary goal to be accomplished is the simple and rapid physical positioning of nanodevices within the stomach, through which they will traverse into the bloodstream. First generation nano-medical tablets may accommodate a compacted mass of nanodevices that will self-release once gastric acid dissolves the inter-device polymeric binding material. In the same manner, nanomedical capsules will likely comprise a thin outer gel wall that is designed to be rapidly dissolved in the stomach to release its payload of nanodevices, which will comprise a dense colloidal suspension. Contingent on the particular diagnostic or therapeutic assignment, the physical dimensions of the tablets or capsules will vary. At a mean individual dimension of ~1 μm³, a 1 cm³ (1 cc) spherical delivery tablet/capsule might accommodate ~100 billion nanodevices. A significant advantage that advanced nanomedical devices will have over conventional orally administered therapeutic drugs, which must endure the time-consuming prerequisite journey through the stomach and the gastrointestinal tract (GIT), and the potential for degradation prior to the release of their payloads, is that shortly after ingestion, nanodevices will expeditiously exit the stomach for ingress into the circulation.

Ultrathin film materials that are utilized to coat softer classes of nanodevices might include chitosan, alginate, cellulose acetate phthalate, carboxymethyl cellulose, hydroxy-propylmethyl cellulose, poly(methylmethacrylate-acrylic acid) (poly(MMA-AA)), eudragit, carrageenan, gelatin, or pectin [2,3]. Hydrogels, such as methacrylic acid (MAA) and poly(ethylene glycol) macromonomer (PEGMEMA), which are cross-linked, hydrophilic, three-dimensional (3D) polymeric networks, may also withstand the harsh acidic environment of the stomach [4–7]. Ulbrich et al. synthesized hydrophilic gels that comprised copolymers, N-hydroxypropyl-methacrylamide and N,O-dimethacryloylhydroxylamine, which were shown to be stable at acidic pH > 5, yet were subject to hydrolyzation at neutral and mild alkaline pH. The pace of hydrolysis was dependent on the degree of the cross-linking density of the gel, and a correlation could be made between the rate of in vivo and in vitro hydrolysis [8]. Since hydrogels may be formulated to degrade at various levels of pH, it is conceivable that dynamic hydrogel thin films might be utilized to protect nanodevices for the time that they do spend in the stomach. The hydrogel might be formulated to be stable at the low pH 1 of the stomach for a predetermined time period so as to facilitate the safe passage of the nanodevice through the stomach wall into the bloodstream. Once within the circulation, where the blood pH is 7.35–7.45, the hydrogel would be engineered such as to rapidly degrade, thereby enabling the nanodevices to conduct their assigned procedures.

It will be essential to elucidate and quantify the effects that exposure, albeit fleeting, to gastric juices, such as hydrochloric acid, mucin, and enzymes such as pepsin, rennin, and lipase, may have on nanodevices. The determination of the possible negative impacts that this type of chemical environment might impart to external nanodevice surfaces, biocompatible coatings, and exposed propulsive elements would be a worthwhile endeavor.

Upon dissolution of a nanotablet or nanocapsule in the stomach, the nanodevices will power up and transit through junctions between a layer of surface columnar epithelial mucous cells, utilizing a technique described below, and into the lamina propria, which comprises loose cellular connective tissue infused with immune cells, wherein reside the capillaries [9]. Upon arrival at this location, the nanodevices would pass between a tessellated, tightly abutting monolayer of squamous endothelial cells that comprise the capillary walls by mimicking a paracellular traversal process that is called transendothelial migration (TEM), or diapedesis, which is employed by inflammatory immune cells (leukocytes) that include neutrophils, lymphocytes, monocytes, and mast cells (Figure 2.1). Diapedesis is a multistep procedure by which leukocyte cells cross endothelial cell boundaries from within the bloodstream in ameboid fashion to access sites of inflammation within tissues. In humans, leukocyte TEM through interfacial junctions between tight, laterally apposed ($\leq$0.5 μm thick) endothelial cells involves a number of sequential steps including the organized activity of molecules upon and within the endothelial cells themselves. Additionally, the dual roles that endothelial cells must play include facilitating the traversal of (~7–10 μm in diameter) leukocytes, while sustaining tight apposing seals at the leading and trailing edges of these "passengers" as they are transferred through the junction to negate the leakage of plasma into the interstitial domain [10].

Leukocytes are also known to travel directly "through" endothelial cells when cellular junctions are too tight, as is the case with the blood–brain barrier (BBB), or should they encounter difficulty in reaching a junction. To perform transcellular migration, a temporary protrusive pseudopod is extended by the leukocyte into the endothelial cell body in order to facilitate passage [10]. Typically, cross-linked vascular cell adhesion molecule 1 (VCAM-1) [11] and intercellular adhesion molecule 1 (ICAM-1) [12], which are present on the outer surfaces of endothelial cells, initiate the generation of cytosolic-free calcium ions, which appear to be critical for diapedesis [13]. This influx of calcium ions triggers

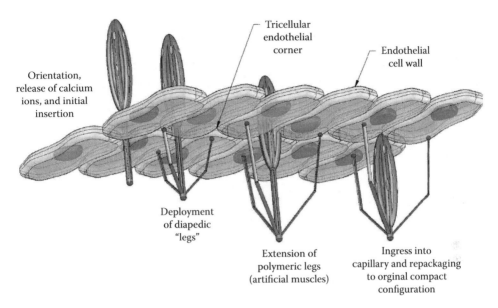

**Orientation,
release of calcium
ions, and initial
insertion**

**Tricellular
endothelial
corner**

**Endothelial
cell wall**

**Deployment
of diapedic
"legs"**

**Extension of
polymeric legs
(artificial muscles)**

**Ingress into
capillary and repackaging
to orginal compact
configuration**

FIGURE 2.1
Conceptual nanomechanical diapedesis sequence for conceptual tri-legged nanodevice.

the activity of myosin light-chain kinase (MLCK), which in turn incites the contraction of actin–myosin fibers. It is this actin–myosin fiber recoiling action that is thought to facilitate the temporary separation of endothelial cells to enable leukocyte transfer [14]. An intriguing observation by Burns et al., is that neutrophil leukocytes preferentially perform TEM through the ~2.5 μm tricellular corner apertures of three abutting endothelial cells, and that "Immunofluorescence studies confirmed that both tight junctions and adherens junctions are discontinuous at tricellular corners" [15].

In oral ingress, stomach-resident nanodevices will be programmed to emulate a reverse diapedesic maneuver, whereby they will be activated to traverse the inner stomach lining, as described earlier, in order to gain access to the capillary lumen (Figures 2.1 through 2.4). Several challenges to overcome, should the nanodevices be transiting through the tight cellular junctions of abutting endothelial cells, will include the judicious release of appropriate chemical signaling entities to mimic leukocyte activity prior to TEM, and subsequently to induce the relaxation of vascular endothelial (VE) cadherins, which are the major adhesion molecules of the adherens junction. A less problematic route, as alluded to earlier, might be traversal through the gaps that exist at endothelial tricellular corners (Figure 2.1). This may constitute an optimal "path of least resistance" for the traversal of nanomedical devices into the capillaries. Once the nanodevices reside within the lumen of the capillaries, they will travel through the mucosa, a thin muscularis mucosae layer and then into the arterioles, which reside within the submucosal bed, and into the bloodstream proper [9].

To perform the nanomechanical diapedesis maneuver, conceptual tri-legged "tripedyte"-type nanomedical devices (Figure 2.2) will approach the endothelial barrier via microfluidic propulsion and position themselves perpendicular to the surface utilizing onboard nanogyroscopic mediated orientation. A leading mandrel probe, within which the three "legs" (or extenders) of the nanodevice are stowed, will prepare for initial insertion into a nearby tricelluar corner while a colloidal cloud of calcium ions is ejected from a series of tiny ports that are located where the mandrel meets the main body of the nanodevice. The calcium ions, as described earlier, facilitate the temporary

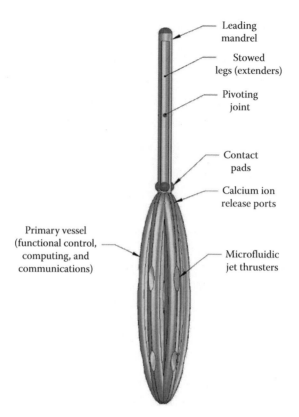

Leading
mandrel

Stowed
legs (extenders)

Pivoting
joint

Contact
pads

Calcium ion
release ports

Primary vessel
(functional control,
computing, and
communications)

Microfluidic
jet thrusters

FIGURE 2.2
Anatomy of conceptual "tripedyte" nanomedical device.

separation of adjoining endothelial cells, thereby allowing the insertion of the leading
mandrel and enabling the subsequent passage of the nanodevice. Access may be significantly less problematic at the tricellular corners as there will be fewer tight junctions
present to manage at these locations.

When the leading mandrel has attained a predetermined depth that is required for leg
clearance, they will be deployed and their contact pads will gain purchase on the surfaces
of the external membranes of the endothelial wall opposite to that where the main nanodevice body temporarily resides. The legs, which comprise a conducting polymeric artificial
muscle material, will subsequently expand in length (to slightly longer than the length of
the vessel body) in response to an applied piezoelectric voltage, and will proceed to pull
the main vessel through the barrier. This will be accomplished via the retraction of the
leading mandrel into the body of the nanodevice. Once the nanodevice body has cleared
the surface of the membrane, the legs will return to their original length and be repack-
aged into dedicated stowing cavities within the leading mandrel.

An alternate strategy for nanodevice diapedesis might be through the use of a helical configuration as is depicted for a conceptual "augeryte"-type nanodevice (Figures 2.3 and 2.4).
The augeryte would employ a helical geometry that endows its surface with the capacity for
rotating its way through the endothelial barrier. Rotation would be enabled by strategically
positioned microfluidic flow-through jets located on one side of the helical structure. They
will cumulatively provide the force necessary for the rotation of the nanodevice and will
operate on the principal similar to that of a fireworks pinwheel mechanism. An alternate

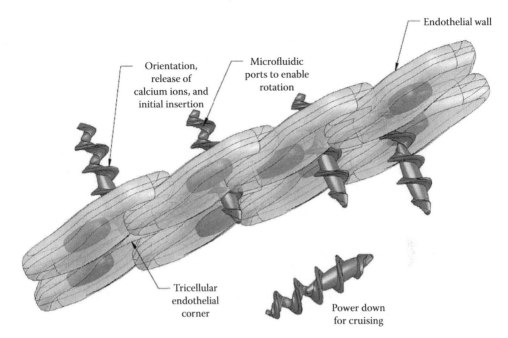

FIGURE 2.3
Nanomechanical diapedesis sequence for conceptual "augeryte" nanodevice.

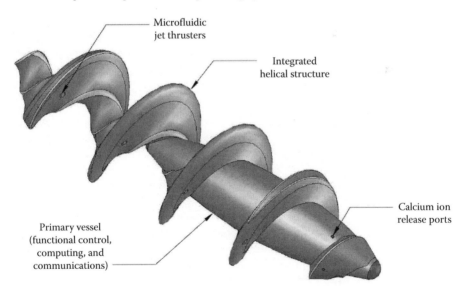

FIGURE 2.4
Anatomy of conceptual "augeryte" nanodevice.

actuation strategy might utilize superparamagnetic elements embedded within the helical tail section that may be actuated by specific external magnetic frequencies. The diapedesis sequence for the augeryte would proceed in a similar manner as that of the tripedyte, which will involve the initial positioning, orientation, and release of calcium ions. Traversal through the endothelial barrier will be quite straightforward; however, in comparison to the tripedyte, as there will be no appendages to manage.

One issue to be investigated insofar as nanodevice ingress via diapedesis is related to sustaining positional stability over an endothelial tricellular corner prior to the initiation of the traversal sequence. Although nanodevices will not be entering from the lumen of the capillaries as do leukocytes and other immune cells, and thus will not be subjected to shear forces of the capillaries blood flow, they may still encounter aqueous turbulence of some kind, contingent on the specific conditions that are present at the site of ingress (e.g., stomach, salivary glands). Therefore, a strategy will likely be required for counteracting/ preventing the possibility that they will be swept away via localized turbulence events. Some type of temporary tethering anchor could be deployed, or the engagement of laterally oriented microfluidic thrusters may be triggered in response to structural perturbations that are detected by integrated nanoscale accelerometers and gyroscopes.

2.3.1 Ingress via Structures of the Oral Cavity

The oral ingress of sufficiently advanced nanomedical devices may allow for alternate strategies that enable them to forgo having to being swallowed at all. These options might include the practically immediate transfer of nanodevices directly through the structures of the oral cavity, such as entry through the buccal walls, tongue, soft palate, or through the interfacial gingiva between the teeth and gums.

2.3.1.1 Buccal Mucosa Ingress

The human oral cavity, with a surface area of about 214.7 ± 12.9 cm² [16], is lined with a mucous membrane, and since the buccal (cheek) mucosa is highly vascularized, it may serve as an easily accessible and patient amenable site for nanodevice ingress. The buccal mucosa, with a total surface area of about 50 cm² [17], also has enhanced permeability in comparison to the epidermis, and has been estimated to be from 4- to 4000-fold or more so [18]. Beginning at the interior of the mouth and moving into the buccal wall, the salivary film that coats the mouth is between 0.07 and 0.10 mm thick [16]. The inner oral surface of buccal mucosa comprises stratified squamous epithelium, which consists of ~50 variably arranged layers of keratinocytes, surrounded by a hydrophilic intercellular matrix, that are cumulatively ~500 to 600 μm thick. This is followed by a continuous 1–2 μm thick basement membrane that separates the epithelium from the deeper connective tissue (e.g., lamina propria and submucosa) [19–24].

Advantages for drug delivery via this route include that blood from the oral mucosa flows directly into the jugular vein, thereby allowing for almost immediate access to the systemic circulation that circumvents hepatic first-pass metabolism [23,25]. Thus, the buccal mucosa may serve as an optimal site for rapid nanomedical drug delivery via a passive diffusion process, or for advanced nanodevice ingress. In vitro studies porcine oral mucosa revealed that aqueous pathway pore sizes were between 18–22 and 30–53 Å [26]. Porcine oral mucosa is typically employed for such studies as it is histologically and biochemically similar to human oral mucosa [27–29].

A spray for the administration of insulin that is delivered to the buccal mucosa has been developed by Paolo Pozzilli et al. This spray comprises a mixture of microscale micelles with thin film membranes that consist of insulin and protective absorption enhancers, which are applied within the patient's mouth as a high-velocity aerosol. The insulin-laced aerosol microdroplets rapidly traverse the superficial layers of the buccal mucosa with the assistance of the absorption enhancers. Hence, the insulin is present within the bloodstream in ~10 min. The buccal spray was shown to have a somewhat quicker absorption capacity than did a conventional subcutaneous insulin injection [30].

The drug delivery techniques utilized in the administration of certain drugs through the buccal mucosa may serve as useful guides toward the development of strategies for nanodevice ingress. Heemstra et al. investigated the delivery of risperidone (an antipsychotic for the treatment of schizophrenia) through the buccal mucosa using a mucoadhesive gel. In vitro studies demonstrated that a gel-resident risperidone dose equivalent to 2.5 mg enabled a flux of 64.65 mg/cm^2/h. It was calculated that the appropriate application area to achieve a therapeutic plasma concentration was about 2–10 cm^2 [31]. This site was also useful in the delivery of testosterone [32] and prochlorperazine [33]. Other delivery modes that may be amenable for this area are mucoadhesive tablets or patches. A potentially limiting factor and area of investigation for this method of ingress might include the dilution effects of saliva clearance as this may indeed vary from patient to patient.

A possible scheme to facilitate nanomedical ingress via the buccal mucosa may be involved in the use of agents that enhance its permeability, such as surfactants, bile salts, and fatty acids [34–44]. These compounds may act by disrupting the intercellular lipid lamellae of the non-keratinized buccal mucosa and might assist with the transfer of nanodevices to the circulation via the paracellular route [45]. Fick's first law of diffusion states that the transfer of compounds across biological membranes may be enhanced by either "increasing the diffusivity through the tissue, the partitioning into the tissue, or the concentration (or thermodynamic activity) of the permeant at the mucosal surface" [19]. It was demonstrated in an in vitro study that the permeability of 2′,3′-dideoxycytidine was facilitated with the addition of sodium glycodeoxycholate, but only when it was above its critical micelle concentration (CMC) [44]. The CMC pertains to a certain concentration of a surfactant, above which it will spontaneously form micelles. In a comparable study, the improved permeability of caffeine was observed only when the level of sodium dodecyl sulfate was above the CMC [46]. It might be surmised that proximal lipids within the buccal mucosa may be contributing to the formation of micelles that are initiated by the CMC, and in so doing, may be disrupting the interstices between cells such that they have enhanced permeability [47].

2.3.1.2 Salivary Duct Ingress

An additional option for potential nanodevice ingress within the oral cavity might be through the variously situated salivary ducts (Figure 2.5). The primary salivary ducts emanate from three pairs of primary salivary glands that include the parotid, which is located in front of and below the ears; submandibular/submaxillary (SM), which is positioned somewhat beneath the jaw bone; and sublingual (SL) glands, which reside beneath the floor of the mouth. In addition, approximately 600–1000 (1–2 mm in diameter) minor salivary glands terminate into, and are widely dispersed throughout the buccal, labial, distal palatal, and lingual regions of the oral cavity [48]. Considering the multitude of salivary ducts available across the entire oral domain, including under the tongue at the floor of the mouth, nanodevice ingress may be quite rapid as many hundreds of ducts might be utilized in parallel.

Four distinct types of cells comprise human salivary glands, which have differing morphologies and functions. These include cuboidal duct cells, spindle myoepithelial cells, flattened squamous cells, and polygonal acinar cells [49]. The typical structures of the salivary glands take the form of aggregated lobular *racemose* glands, which are geometrically akin to bunches of grapes. The *acinus* are multiple saliva-secreting units, each of which comprises a ring of glandular cells that circumscribe and dispense saliva into an inner core cavity (Figure 2.6). Adjoining *acini* are linked together via short interpolated ducts, which themselves join to shape the primary duct systems [50].

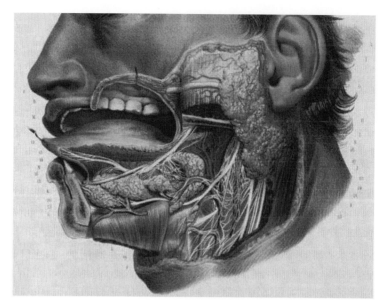

FIGURE 2.5
Location of the salivary glands. (From Bourgery, M.J., Traité complet de l'anatomie de l'homme, C. Delaunay, Paris, France, 1831–1854.)

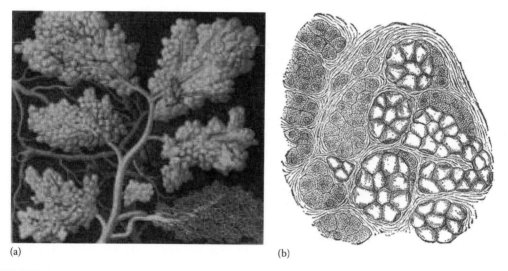

(a)   (b)

FIGURE 2.6
Depiction of racemose glands: (a) serous alveoli and (b) mucous alveoli. (From Bourgery, M.J., Traité complet de l'anatomie de l'homme, C. Delaunay, Paris, France, 1831–1854; Williams, P.L. et al., *Gray's Anatomy. International Student Edition*, 28th edn., Churchill Livingstone, London, U.K. pp. 1692–1699, 1995.)

The SM and SL, as well as the minor salivary glands, are more or less in a constant state of secretion, whereas the parotid glands are only active when stimulated [51]. According to a two-stage hypothesis put forward by Thaysen and colleagues, "… primary saliva, a NaCl-rich plasma-like isotonic fluid is secreted by salivary acinar cells and its ionic composition becomes modified in the duct system. The ducts secrete K^+ and HCO_3^- and reabsorb Na^+ and Cl^- without any water movement, thus establishing a hypotonic final saliva" [51,52].

The parotid (Stenson's) ducts are embedded in buccal mucosa apposed to each second upper molar tooth, whose ~7 cm long ductal channels emanate from the parotid gland. Although the parotid duct orifice (ostium) that enters the mouth can be rather diminutive (~0.5 mm median), the lumen that leaves the mouth toward the parotid gland is larger in diameter (~0.9 to 2 mm) with relatively thick dense walls that comprise contractile fibers lined with short columnar epithelial cells [54–56]. The SM (Wharton's) ducts terminate at small (~0.2–0.8) mm orifices located just below the bottom of the frenulum, which is a small ridge of tissue that runs from the base and underside of the tongue to its midpoint. These ducts are ~50 to 62.0 mm long with walls that are less substantial than those of the parotid duct. From 7 to 20 major SL ducts and minor SL Rivinus ducts terminate in close proximity to the SM ducts at the base of the mouth and straddle the frenulum, opening at the SL caruncle. Some of the major SL ducts also fuse with the SM ducts. The terminating surface orifices of the major SL ducts are ~2.13 mm in diameter, whereas the smaller ducts are ~1 mm in diameter with a length of ~1.3 mm [57].

Salivary secretions may be distinguished as serous, mucous, or mixed, which emanate from the parotid glands, minor glands, and SL and submandibular glands, respectively [58,59]. Saliva comprises ~99.5% water, cations including sodium, potassium, calcium, and anions such as chloride, bicarbonate, fluoride, and inorganic phosphate; metabolic by-products such as urea, and up to 1400 proteins that consist of four major groups of specific secretory proteins. These include proline-rich proteins (PRPs), statherins, cystatins and histatins, antibacterial peroxidases and mucins, digestive amylases and lipases, and epidermal and nerve growth factors [60–62] (Figure 2.7). The pH of saliva ranges from 5.75 to 7.05 [50], and as it emanates from multiple sources its exact composition can be quite variable.

For example, parotid saliva secretions have lower calcium and higher phosphate levels than do submandibular and SL secretions, and the majority of salivary amylase comes from the parotid glands. The secretions of the minor salivary glands are distinctive in that the primary anion produced is chloride. They also contain very little biocarbonate or phosphate, and have no amylase [64]. Unstimulated parotid glands supply ~25% of whole

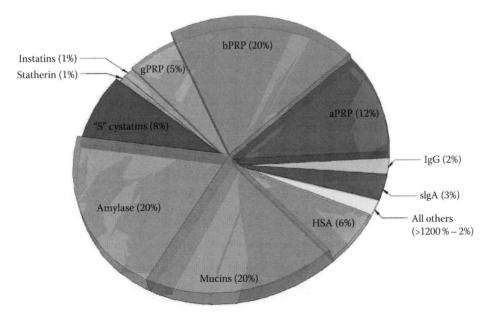

FIGURE 2.7
Primary saliva proteins. (Redrawn from Scarano, E. et al., *Acta Otorhinolaryngol. Ital.*, 30(3), 125, 2010.)

saliva, whereas in a stimulated state they can contribute up to 49%. The SM and SL glands typically contribute 67%, and the minor mucous glands about 8% [65–67].

Nanodevices that ingress via the salivary ducts will likely traverse their lumen under autonomous propulsive power, either by harvesting energy from their immediate environment or being induced to generate onboard energy via activation by external sources (Chapter 4). As described earlier, all of the terminating ducts, for example, the parotid ducts, are continually excreting saliva, with a total output per day ranging from 500 to 1500 mL [50]. Hence, salivary secretion outflows with variable velocities from these ducts may act to hydrodynamically resist entry by 1 μm in diameter nanodevices (Table 2.1). The secretion of saliva is induced by parasympathetic stimulation, with a higher release level of intracellular calcium and the activation of calcium-activated ion channels [69]. The acinar cells (Figure 2.3), from which saliva originates, shrink significantly in response to stimulation and the majority water moves via osmosis as a consequence of the presence of Na^+. Water also enters the saliva from both between and through the epithelial cells within the salivary glands via membrane-embedded aquaporin water channels, typically Aquaporin 1 and Aquaporin 5 [70].

The SM glands with their long ducts have slow output flow rates that work against gravity [71–73]. This may, therefore, allow for relatively effortless nanodevice access. An in-depth knowledge of the composition of saliva, and indeed, of all physiological biofluids within the human body will be critical for nanodevices that are scavenging for particular high-energy molecules such as glucose, or ions such as sodium to generate power for propulsion, navigation, and other critical functions, from their immediate environment. Integrated nanosensor arrays might be designed with the capacity for recalibrating on the fly in order to adapt to rapidly changing chemistries they encounter while engaged with in vivo diagnostic or therapeutic assignments, which may require them to traverse vastly different terrains within the human body.

Potential energy sources contained within human saliva, which are available for harvesting and conversion by nanodevices into useful locomotive power, include glucose, which may serve as an optimal fuel due to its relative abundance and high-energy density. An onboard 1 μm³ reservoir of glucose that is filled via arrays of onboard molecular sortation rotors [74]

TABLE 2.1

Median Saliva Flow Rates from Various Glands

Saliva Source	Resting (mL/min)		Activated (mL/min)	
	Median	**Min/Max**	**Median**	**Min/Max**
Whole saliva [93]	0.32	0.1–0.5	1.7	1.1–30
Parotid gland [93]	0.04	0.01–0.07	1.5	0.7–2.3
Submandibular/ sublingual glands [93]	0.10	0.02–0.20	0.8	0.4–1.3
Minor glands (μL/ cm²/min) [94]	Palatal (median) 0.91 ± 0.08	Buccal (median) 16.0 ± 0.7	Labial (median) 4.76 ± 0.31	
	Male (median)	Female (median)	Male (median)	Female (median)
Minor glands cumulative (μL/cm²/ min) [95]	0.82 ± 0.17	0.82 ± 0.11	2.17 ± 0.14	1.67 ± 0.11

Sources: Edgar, M., *Clinical Oral Science*, Harris, M. et al., eds., Reed Educational and Professional Publishing, Ltd., Oxford, U.K., p. 179, 1998; Eliasson, L. et al., *Arch. Oral Biol.*, 41(12), 1179, 1996; Ferguson, D.B., *Arch. Oral Biol.*, 44(Suppl. 1), S11, 1999.

(Chapter 16) might allow for the in vivo operation of a 10 pW nanodevice for ~40 min [75]. Biomimetic analogs of flagellar motors that function within bacteria, which utilize electrochemical gradients [76,77], may also power nanodevices using saliva-resident protons (H^+) and Na^+ ions. Protons drive flagellar motors in the bacterial species *Bacillus subtilis*, *Streptococcus* spp., *Escherichia coli*, and *Salmonella typhimurium*) [78–83] whereas Na^+ ions fuel the flagella of *Bacillus firmus* and *Vibrio alginolyticus* [84–90]. Molecular-scale biological motors such as ATP synthase are also powered by protons and sodium ions [91,92]. The concentration ranges of saliva-resident glucose, H^+, and Na^+ are quite variable from the resting state to activated state, and also exhibit contrasts between males and females (Table 2.2).

Being mindful of the brief transit time (several seconds) that would be required by autonomous nanodevices to traverse any of the salivary ducts, there would be a very limited draw on ambient resources. Freitas suggests that a nominal "speed limit" for in vivo nanodevices that are transiting through circulation might be ~1 to 2 cm/s [75]. Thus, it seems reasonable that a similar transit velocity might be applicable for nanodevices within the salivary ducts. Once the nanodevices enter the salivary glands themselves, they will traverse the epithelia and capillary walls via nanomechanochemical diapedesis.

TABLE 2.2

Potential Nanodevice Fuels in Saliva

Potential Nanodevice Fuels in Saliva	Resting Concentration (μM)	Activated Concentration (μM)	Resting Secretion (nmol/min)	Activated Secretion (nmol/min)
Glucose (male) [96]	78.7 ± 9.2	29.7 ± 8.1	60.9 ± 7.1	59.8 ± 16.5
Glucose (female) [96]	80.4 ± 7.9	34.4 ± 5.0	71.3 ± 9.3	55.2 ± 8.2
Hydrogen ions (H^+) [97]		20–30 (mmol/L)		
Sodium (Na^+) [50]	305 ± 99 (μg/cm³)	5–100 (mEq/L)		
Sodium (Na^+) [98]	(range 149–461)			
Cholesterol (μmol/L) [99]		Mean: 1.20 ± 0.75	Activated secretion (mL/min)	
		Men: 1.36 ± 0.85	Low quartile	1.9 ± 0.8
		Women: 1.06 ± 0.64	Intermediate quartile	1.7 ± 0.7
			High quartile	1.8 ± 1.1
			Cholesterol (μmol/L) range	
			Low quartile	0.02–0.69
			Intermediate quartile	0.70–1.48
			High quartile	1.49–5.45
Total proteins (mg/mL) [100]	0.72–2.45	1.11–5.40 (baseline)		
[101]		0.58 ± 0.186 (immediately after exercise)		
[102]		1.745 ± 0.566		

Sources: Srivastava, L.M., *Textbook of Biochemistry and Human Biology*, Talwar, G.P. and Srivastava, L.M., eds., Prentice Hall, New Delhi, India, 2006; Jurysta, C. et al., *J. Biomed. Biotechnol.*, 430426, 2009; Fejerskov, O. et al., *Dental Caries: The Disease and Its Clinical Management*, Gray Publishing, Tunbridge Wells, U.K., 2008; Jiménez-Reyes, M. and Sánchez-Aguirre, F.J., *Appl. Radiat. Isot.*, 47(3), 273, 1996; Karjalainen, S. et al., *J. Dent. Res.*, 76(10), 1637, 1997; Lin, L.Y. and Chang, C.C., *Gaoxiong Yi Xue Ke Xue Za Zhi.*, 5(7), 389, 1989; Arneberg, P., *Scand. J. Dent. Res.*, 79(1), 60, 1971; Bortolini, M.J. et al., *Res. Q. Exerc. Sport.*, 80(3), 604, 2009.

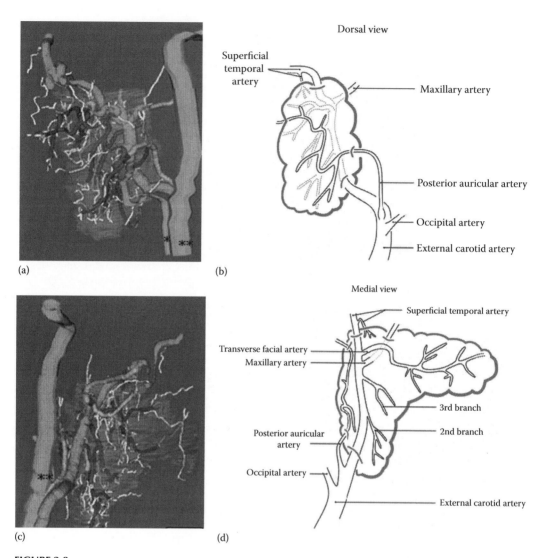

Superficial temporal artery

Maxillary artery

Posterior auricular artery

Occipital artery

External carotid artery

Dorsal view

Medial view

Superficial temporal artery

Transverse facial artery
Maxillary artery

3rd branch

2nd branch

Posterior auricular artery

Occipital artery

External carotid artery

(a)   (b)   (c)   (d)

FIGURE 2.8
(a–d) 3D reconstructions and illustrations of vasculature of the parotid salivary gland. *, denotes external carotid artery and **, denotes internal carotid artery. (Reproduced from van Holten, M.J. et al., *Head Neck*, 32(7), 837, 2010. With permission.)

The vasculature that supplies the parotid salivary gland includes arteries that extend from the external carotid primarily into the upper portion of the gland (Figure 2.8), which enters the posteromedial surface prior to bifurcating to the maxillary and superficial temporal arteries. The maxillary artery exits the parotid at the anteromedial surface, whereas the superficial temporal artery translates to the transverse facial artery. In addition, the posterior auricular artery appears to branch from the external carotid artery within the parotid and exits via its posteromedial surface. The lumen of the parotid arteries can range in size from 0.6 to 2 mm in diameter. This should provide ample space for the traversal of nanodevices once they have achieved entry through the endothelial barrier via diapedesis. The veins of the parotid proceed to the external jugular via branched pathways [103–107].

The submaxillary salivary gland is supplied with blood via branches of the facial and lingual arteries and the submental vein that drains it traces the same path. The SL salivary gland receives oxygenated blood from the SL and submental arteries and the SL and submental veins drain it [54].

2.3.1.3 Gingivial Ingress

It may be possible to administer nanomedical devices for oral ingress via the application of a mucoadhesive patch, dissolving film or hydrogels to the gingiva. The gingiva serves as a mucous membrane that lines and seals the teeth at their base and is securely tethered to the periosteum (a membrane that coats most bone surfaces), of the mandibular and maxillary bones. At the cellular level, the gingiva comprises stratified squamous epithelium and contains a high density of cylindrical connective tissue papillary bodies. The epithelium is attached to the enamel of the tooth by an extracellular matrix layer of substantial thickness that constitutes what is known as the "epithelial attachment of Gottlieb," to which the epithelial cells are anchored by hemidesmosomes [108].

Nanodevices might enter via the gingivial sulcus (crevis), where the teeth abut with the gums, and traverse the epithelial barrier via diapedesis. The gingiva is amply vascularized with a basketlike matrix of gingival arteries that branch from the dental artery, which is derived from the maxillary artery (Figure 2.9). The arrangement for venous drainage traces a similar path as the arteries. The lumen of the gingival arteries range from ~15 to 100 μm in diameter, and hence will provide ample space for resident nanodevices to maneuver [109].

It may be advantageous, in several respects for nanodevices that enter through the capillaries via any of these oral structures to utilize the arterial rather than venous capillaries.

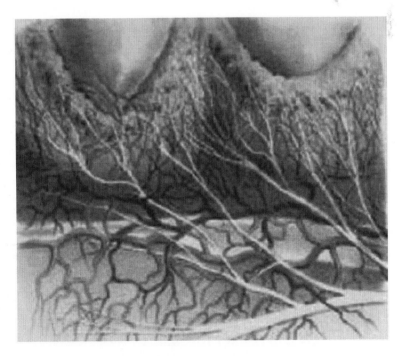

FIGURE 2.9
Artistic rendering of the vascularization of the gingival. (From Bourgery, M.J., Traité complet de l'anatomie de l'homme, C. Delaunay, Paris, France, 1831–1854.)

Variances in blood pressures and hence blood velocities are increased in arterial capillaries in contrast to venous capillaries, and this disparity is more pronounced between the arteries and veins at different sites throughout the human body. Capillary pressures range from 10 (venous) to 30 mm Hg (arterial), whereas primary venous pressures range from <1 mm Hg in the large veins leading to the heart to 7 mm Hg in the overall venous system, in contrast to a minimum for arteries of 60 mm Hg (diastole) and a maximum of 140 mm Hg (systole) [110].

To illustrate examples of blood velocity variations in different vessels, the blood flow velocity in the capillaries of the oral buccal mucosa was found to be ~0.4 mm/s [111]; the blood flow velocity of the brachial artery of the forearm with a diameter of 0.32 ± 0.01 cm has been quantified to be 8.3 ± 1.3 cm/s [112]. The main portal vein of a male, with a diameter of 1.34 ± 0.32 cm, showed a blood flow velocity of 21.58 ± 7.64 cm/s, whereas the inferior vena cava with a diameter of 2.22 ± 0.30 exhibited a blood flow velocity of 20.84 ± 0.39 cm/s. For a female subject, main portal vein with a diameter of 1.54 ± 0.4 cm had a blood flow velocity of 20.37 ± 8.73 cm/s, whereas the inferior vena cava with a diameter of 2.33 ± 0.54 exhibited a blood flow velocity of 16.26 ± 5.28 cm/s [113]. The superior caval blood flow velocity ranged between 12.4 ± 2.2 and 35.2 ± 7.3 cm/s, contingent on the states of atrial and ventricular relaxation and contraction [114]. As is demonstrated by the examples earlier, there are significant disparities that exist as per the velocities with which nanomedical devices will be transmitted through the vasculature. Therefore, one of the critical issues toward the realization of advanced autonomous nanomedical devices will be the development of robust and efficient propulsive components to counteract in vivo vascular shear forces to facilitate complete and unencumbered freedom of movement and control within the human body.

2.4 Pulmonary Ingress

The lungs represent one of the most attractive, noninvasive, unencumbered, and expeditious routes for the ingress of both nascent nanomedicine therapeutics (in the form of functional aerosolized colloids and engineered nanoparticles) and advanced medical nanodevices, as they will provide practically instantaneous access to the bloodstream via absorption at the alveoli, and the traversal of the interalveolar septum (gas/blood-exchange barrier) to reach the capillaries. Additional advantages include the circumvention of the first-pass effect (metabolism in the gut wall and liver) and a high level of bioavailability.

Physiologically, the trachea bifurcates into left and right bronchi (Figure 2.10), which further subdivide into ciliated respiratory bronchioles that terminate in multitudes alveolar clusters (Figure 2.11), which are populated by masses of polyhedral-shaped alveoli. There are approximately 274–790 million (mean ~480 million) alveoli that inhabit the lungs, which constitute a cumulative alveolocapillary surface area that ranges from ~97 to 194 m² (mean ~143 m²) [115,116]. Proceeding from the interior of the lungs, nanodevices will be tasked with the traversal of various cellular and biomaterial layers with diverse permeabilities that make up the interalveolar septum, which encapsulates and separates each alveolar pocket. Initially, the pulmonary surfactant layer will be encountered and traversed. This thin film plays a critical role for the stabilization of pulmonary alveoli and the prevention of respiratory failure as it acts to reduce interfacial air–liquid surface tension and thereby reduces the effort required to fill the alveoli upon inhalation. This thin

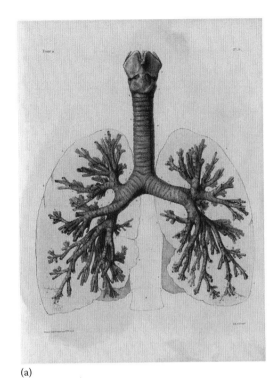
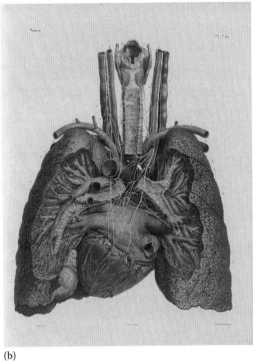

(a)   (b)

FIGURE 2.10
(a, b) Artistic rendering of the physiology of the human lungs. (From Bourgery, M.J., Traité complet de l'anatomie de l'homme, C. Delaunay, Paris, France, 1831–1854.)

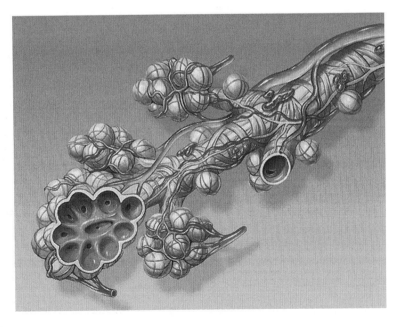

FIGURE 2.11
Simplified artistic rendering of alveoli and pulmonary circulation. (From Lynch, P.J., Wikimedia Commons, 2006.)

100 nm surfactant film is generated by cuboidal alveolar type II cells and comprises a complex of phospholipids and proteins inclusive of dipalmitoyl phosphatidylcholine (DPPC) and phosphatidylglycerol and four species of hydrophilic (HPI) and hydrophobic (HPO) surfactant proteins (SP)-SP-A (HPI), SP-B (HPO), SP-C (HPO), and SP-D (HPI), which are involved in immune functions [108,117].

In experiments, latex beads of ~8 μm in diameter and larger were deposited on the surface of a DPPC film to demonstrate that smaller particle sizes and lower surface tensions facilitated the rate of immersion into the aqueous phase. It was also observed via electron microscopy that particulates in the alveoli were found below the surface of the surfactant film. This submersion of particulates through the surfactant toward the epithelial layer is thought to facilitate clearance by macrophages [118]. Hence, it may be assumed that 1 μm in diameter nanodevices may encounter little resistance to penetration at the surfactant film surface and that the film will remain continuous once the nanodevices proceed through the epithelial layer.

The interalveolar septum is lined on either side by an epithelial layer that comprises very flat and thin (thinnest regions at ~25 nm) type I squamous alveolar cells, which are associated with gas exchange, and type II alveolar cells. Between these layers is the interstitium within which a dense network of alveolar capillaries resides to make up the main bulk of the interalveolar septum. Matrixes of elastic and reticular fibers are contained within the interstitium to support the capillaries, and this is also where macrophages and dust cells may be found. The thinner interfacial regions of the interalveolar septum, where air/blood exchange takes place between the alveoli and capillaries, contain an epithelial layer on the alveoli side and an endothelial layer on the capillary side with two fused basal laminae positioned between them. This composite layer ranges from 0.1 to 1.5 μm thick [108,119,116]. The median diameter at the mouth of the alveoli has been determined to be ~278 ± 53 μm [120], whereas the cavity of the alveoli itself is ~200 to 300 μm [121]. There are also ~10 to 15 μm in diameter pores that run between adjoining alveoli compartments.

The pulmonary vascularization begins at the pulmonary trunk that emanates from the right ventricle and then bifurcates into the right and left pulmonary arteries, which are the only arteries in the human body to carry deoxygenated blood. Within the mass of the lungs the pulmonary arteries undergo multiple bifurcations to reach the capillary level, where the blood releases its payload of CO^2 for exhalation. The opposite occurs starting with newly oxygenated blood via inhalation, which courses through the venous capillaries that continue to debifurcate to the primary, right, and left pulmonary veins, being the only veins in the human body that transport oxygenated blood and which terminate into the left atrium where the blood is pumped into the circulation [122].

In regard to the finer pulmonary vasculature, which will be the focus for ingressing nanomedical devices, lobular microvessels are evenly distributed throughout the lungs and have diameters in the 90 μm range [120], and the lumen of the pulmonary capillaries has been determined to range in diameter from 2.76 to 4.05 μm [123]. There are a staggering number of pulmonary capillaries (~280 billion), which translates to ~1000 per alveoli [124]. The epithelium layer forms the primary obstruction to permeability into the bloodstream due to the presence of plasma protein–based tight junctions that comprise three to five sets of interlocking microchannels and promontories that completely encircle the cells. In contrast, the endothelium possesses from one to three rows of particles with heterogeneously spaced proteinaceous strand-like connections. These strands are composed of claudins, which are transmembrane proteins that are engaged with cellular contractile fibers. In some areas between the endothelial cells, there is absence of connectivity. For these reasons, this barrier is to some extent more permeable [116].

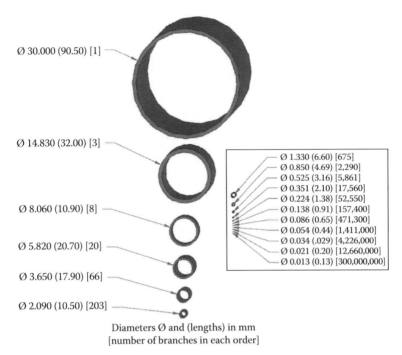

Ø 30.000 (90.50) [1]

Ø 14.830 (32.00) [3]

Ø 8.060 (10.90) [8]

Ø 5.820 (20.70) [20]

Ø 3.650 (17.90) [66]

Ø 2.090 (10.50) [203]

Ø 1.330 (6.60) [675]
Ø 0.850 (4.69) [2,290]
Ø 0.525 (3.16) [5,861]
Ø 0.351 (2.10) [17,560]
Ø 0.224 (1.38) [52,550]
Ø 0.138 (0.91) [157,400]
Ø 0.086 (0.65) [471,300]
Ø 0.054 (0.44) [1,411,000]
Ø 0.034 (.029) [4,226,000]
Ø 0.021 (0.20) [12,660,000]
Ø 0.013 (0.13) [300,000,000]

Diameters Ø and (lengths) in mm
[number of branches in each order]

FIGURE 2.12
Components of the pulmonary arterial system. (Adapted from Singhal, S. et al., *Circ. Res.*, 33(2), 190, 1973. Cited in Freitas, R.A. Jr., *Nanomedicine, Volume I: Basic Capabilities*, Landes Bioscience, Georgetown, TX, 1999.)

Although the pulmonary pathway serves as a potentially vast accessible domain that is available for the ingress of aerosolized nanodevices into the circulation (Figure 2.12), there will undoubtedly be considerable challenges to surmount toward the development and implementation of effective pulmonary nanodevice ingress strategies. A number of central premises for these nanometric medical entities will encompass safety, efficacy, controllability, and precision. Hence, in contrast to nanoengineered therapeutic particles whose rate of ingress will be contingent solely on natural pulmonary diffusion processes, first generation–advanced autonomous nanodevices will be under continuous and complete external control by physicians and computers. As operational capabilities and functionalities are increasingly expanded with subsequent generations of nanodevices, they will be programmable to a degree where they may be ingressed into the patient through the most appropriate route and perform their procedures without the requirement of external intervention. Nevertheless, they will always be tracked and their progress monitored. There will always remain the option of aborting any procedure at any juncture, or relaying a shutdown, and thereby automatically engaging an auto-egress protocol sequence.

For this venue of ingress as well, dedicated medical nanodevices will employ nanomechanical diapedesis to transfer their slim and virtually frictionless frames through the multiple barriers as described earlier. In the case of pulmonary ingress, special consideration must be taken in the design of nanodevices to ensure that they conform to certain dimensional and morphologic specifications so as to exploit and optimize the nuances of pulmonary aerodynamics. Due to pulmonary turbulence, only nanodevices within specific size limits will be enabled with the capacity for accessing the alveoli. Researchers at the Aerosol Research Laboratory of Alberta at the University of Alberta, Canada, have investigated this phenomenon utilizing the inhaled aerosolized asthma drug (Ventolin) droplets (~4 µm median diameter) to elucidate the probabilities for their deposition within particular pulmonary regions. It was observed that for alveolar deposition the optimal probability was for droplets at ~6 µm in diameter, which was reduced to 0 at diameters of ~15 µm. Conversely, droplets with diameters of ~15 µm were most likely to deposit within the extrathoracic area and those at ~9 µm in diameter were most likely to deposit in the tracheobronchial region. The most commonly recommended diameters for conventional inhaled pharmaceuticals range from ~1 to 5 µm [126].

Wiebert et al. demonstrated that ~99% of a dose of <100 nm in diameter technetium 99 m (99 mTc)-labeled carbonaceous nanoparticles were retained in the lungs after 46 h. Therefore, unless inhaled therapeutic nanoparticles are intended to specifically treat lung conditions, they should be smaller than 100 nm to evade clearance by macrophages [127]. Other considerations for nanoparticles in regard to their interactions with biological cells and tissues are attributes related to their surface areas, morphologies, and potentials for initiating degradative oxidation and proinflammatory effects [128–131]. The prospects of being phagocytized or initiating inflammation will likely not be applicable to advanced nanodevices as the lungs will be utilized as a transitory ingress gateway. Nanomechanical diapedesis will commence immediately upon nanodevice access to alveolar walls, hence their residency in the lungs will be relatively fleeting (several minutes). Ingressing nanodevices will, to a certain degree, be biomimetically modeled after leukocytes, which can complete diapedesis through the endothelial barrier in ~90 s [132]. Hence, it is likely that in view of the much more substantive pulmonary barrier that exists at the alveolar wall (e.g., the multiple tight junctions of the epithelium) nanodevices may require several minutes to complete the transfer into the circulation.

There are a number of factors that will have an influence on the distribution of pulmonary deposition sites for nanodevices. Pulmonary ingress may be facilitated by inertial impaction, gravitational sedimentation, Brownian diffusion or, if the particulate is carrying a charge, electrostatic forces. For conventional aerosolized pharmaceuticals, deposition profiles also vary between microscale aqueous droplets and dry powder particulates. Likewise, physically dense nanometric particles and nanodevices will be subjected to the vagaries of pulmonary turbulent flow, and hence the computer modeling of these entities under expected parameters may facilitate the optimization of the design process. Experimental data and pulmonary flow parameters derived from conventional aerosol delivery studies will be useful and translatable toward the development of nanomedical pulmonary deposition strategies and will likely encompass aerosol density, air temperature, pulmonary physiology, and capacity as well as inhalation velocity and dosage concentration (e.g., nanoscale droplets, nanoparticles, and nanodevices per cc).

Nanocarrier-based therapeutic formulations involving liposomes, niosomes, proniosomes, microemulsions, lipidic micelles, solid lipid nanoparticles, vault nanocapsules, polymeric micelles and nanoparticles, peptides, dendrimers, cyclodextrins, colloidal suspensions, and nanogels may be utilized for the delivery of drugs via the pulmonary route. A detailed examination of nanomedical drug delivery is beyond the scope of this book. However, there is a rapidly increasing accumulation of knowledge on this topic in the literature [133–139].

Acquired data related to deposition profiles, kinetics, and overall in vivo dispersion efficacy associated with the delivery of these nanomedical forerunners will be of great value for the establishment of ingress and egress approaches for advanced nanomedical devices. In addition, various species of nanocarriers might be employed to provide stealth and targeting capabilities for the ingress of early generations of nanodevices. They may serve as "chaperones" in guiding nanodevices to treatment sites via biochemical affinity-mediated binding (e.g., monoclonal antibodies [MAbs]) and to ensure that they will not elicit an immune response.

Various techniques for the aerosolized administration of nanodevices may include those that are similar in function to contemporary pressurized metered-dose inhalers. The original chlorofluorocarbon propellant used in these inhalers was banned, via the 1987 Montreal protocol, and was replaced with hydrofluoroalkane, which allowed for the administration of smaller drug constituents to presumably enable further reach into the peripheral airways. Other devices include propellant-free, dry powder inhalers, and nebulizers, which generate droplets that are several microns in diameter [140,141]. The electrohydrodynamic spray (electrospray) technique has the capacity for dispersing high concentrations of nanopharmaceuticals in the ~10–100 nm range for inhalation therapy, whereas a collision atomizer may generate a stable aerosol that is appropriate for nanoparticles that are larger than 100 nm [142].

For effective administration by these mechanisms, nanodevice doses will likely be monodispersed within an aqueous colloidal suspension carrier to optimize equal distribution across the fine pulmonary surface. Dynamics considerations will include the physical segmentation of the solution, coulombic force–mediated droplet dispersion, and critically, the establishment of a scaling law to encompass droplet size, liquid flow rate, and the physical attributes of the aqueous media. Although advanced nanodevices will be solidly fabricated at atomic resolution, experimental trials will determine if the aerosol ejection velocity might damage external peripheral structures, propulsive ports or jostle internal computing, navigation, or communication systems. Researchers have utilized high-speed video to elucidate the velocity of conventional metered-dose inhalers and have determined that the initial aerosol "jet" travels at 20 m/s, but rapidly slows to a 10 m/s "cloud" after 5 ms with the total distance traversed at 5–7 cm. A subsequent deceleration to 2–3 m/s occurred after 30 ms after traveling a total distance of 10–12 cm [143].

The pulmonary absorption of lipophilic molecules can take place within ~1 to 2 min, whereas water-soluble molecule absorption is on the order of ~1 h. Much longer pulmonary residency (days) might be possible via the utilization of molecules that are extremely insoluble or cationic [144]. Fluticasone propionate (a synthetic corticosteroid) [145], amphotericin B (a polyene antifungal drug) [146], and all-*trans* retinoic acid (a chemotherapeutic drug) [147] exhibit sustained pulmonary residency for many hours due to their very sluggish dissolution kinetics. Similarly, self-assembling and slow release liposomes may be "tuned" during synthesis to control the rate of absorption for the drug payloads that are encapsulated within them (Chapter 12). It is conceivable that nanodevice doses that have been prescribed to be released incrementally over a period of days or weeks (contingent on the particular condition and associated treatment regimen) might be encapsulated within liposomes and delivered by a single aerosol administration. The liposome nanocarrier dosage may be formulated such that the liposomes will have disparate pulmonary residency time lines, based on their lipid structures, with cascading dissolution rates, whereby only specific fractions of the total dose will be released on a daily basis until the entire complement has been delivered.

Natural peptides are short (<30) chains of amino acids and carboxyl groups that are smaller in size than proteins at 3000 Da. These entities are easily degraded by pulmonary-resident enzymes (peptidases); hence, their bioavailability is negligible. However, peptides of approx. <1600 Da may be chemically modified to resist attack by peptidases, enabling a high degree of bioavailability in the lungs. Cytokines (interferon α) and growth factors (human growth hormone [hGH]), which have molecular weights in the 18,000–33,000 Da range, demonstrate the best bioavailabilities for peptides and proteins, whereas larger proteins (approx. >50,000) exhibit low to nil bioavailability values [144]. The molecular weights of peptides and proteins are shown to have a strong bearing on their bioavailability (Figure 2.13) when administered

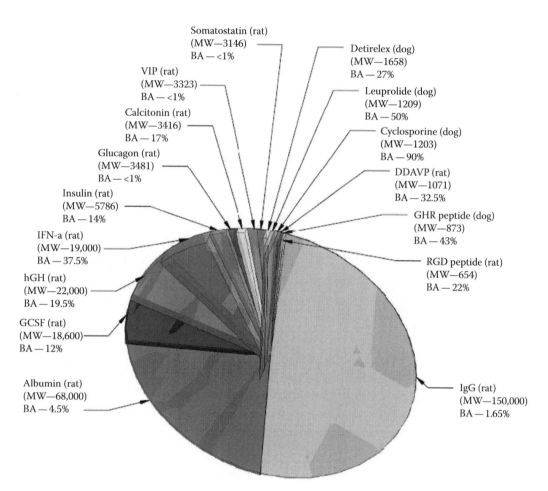

FIGURE 2.13
Bioavailability of selected peptides and proteins via the pulmonary route. MW, molecular weight; BA, bio-availability abbreviations; DDVAP (desamino-Cys1, D-arg8) vasopressin; GCSF, granulocyte colony-stimulating factor; GHR, growth hormone releasing; hGH, human growth hormone; IFN-α, interferon-α; IgG, immuno-globulin G; RGD, Arg, Gly, Asp; VIP, vasoactive intestinal peptide. (Adapted from Patton, J.S. et al., *Proc. Am. Thorac. Soc.*, 1(4), 338, 2004; Patton, J.S., *Adv. Drug Deliv. Rev.*, 19, 3, 1996; Adjei, L.A. and Gupta, P.K., Lenfant, C., executive ed., *Lung Biology in Health and Disease*, Marcel Dekker, New York, pp. 1–913, 1997.)

to the lungs, which are the most permeable route of ingress for macromolecules [148,149]. For instance, hydrophobic molecules may enter the bloodstream within seconds of inhalation [144,150–152]. These data might serve as useful preliminary guidelines for the dimensional parameters for nanodevices that are designed for the pulmonary ingress route.

Particulates must typically be within the 1–7 μm size range to effectively reach the alveoli [153]. Hence, nanodevices within this dimensional range might further facilitate pulmonary ingress by virtue of their morphology, external charge, and aerodynamic attri-butes. Access into the pulmonary vasculature may be further enhanced when they are administered in conjunction with absorption enhancing adjuvants. For example, absorp-tion enhancers such as *N*-lauryl-β-D-maltopyranoside and bacitracin are shown to increase the pulmonary bioavailablility of insulin [154].

Researchers at the Ludwig-Maximilians University in Germany have been investigat-ing "nanomagnetosols," which comprise superparamagnetic iron oxide nanoparticles

(SPIONs). The SPIONs were dispersed within ~3.5 μm droplets and computer simulations extrapolated that there were ~3000 within each aerosol droplet. The SPIONs were subjected to an external magnetic field to facilitate their transfer into the lungs of mice. It was found that the magnetic field enhanced the delivery of the SPIONs threefold, and that they successfully reached alveolar cells [155].

The benefits that are conveyed to future patients via safe and effective pulmonary ingressed nanodevice systems may indeed be tremendous and incalculable. For nanomedical drug delivery devices, a minimal volume of drug would be wasted in contrast to "flooding" the patient with conventional chemotherapeutic drugs. Much more powerful or concentrated drug compounds might also be considered for a given condition as they may be released in a highly localized fashion exclusively to diseased cells and tissues without the initiation of otherwise associated side effects.

2.4.1 Intranasal Ingress

The nasal passages may serve as unique ingress pathways to facilitate the ingress of aerosolized nanoparticulate drug formulations or special classes of dedicated nanodevices for rapid access to the systemic circulation, or to circumvent the BBB for direct access to the central nervous system (CNS) and the brain. Within the dual cavities of the nose are slit-like hollow spaces that are formed by turbinates (conchae), which are curled protuberances of tissue that emanate into the interior of the nasal passage, act to moisturize, and regulate the temperature of inhaled air. The extensively vascularized and absorptive nasal/respiratory mucosa, with a surface area of about ~150 to 180 cm², provides a readily accessible portal for the ingress of nanodevices, and capillaries are easily permeated as they lie directly beneath the skin [156–158] (Figure 2.14). The cells that make up the nasal respiratory mucosa include both ciliated and non-ciliated columnar cells, goblet cells and basal cells, which are disposed on a basal membrane. Of the columnar cells, about 20% are ciliated, and each is populated by ~300 microvilli [159–161]. The cilia are ~4 to 6 μm in length that beat ~1000

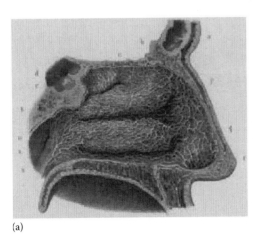
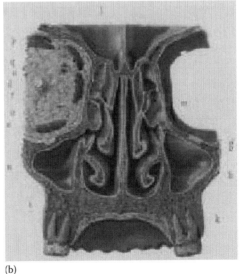

(a)   (b)

FIGURE 2.14
(a, b) Artististic depictions of nasal passage vascularization and cross section of turbinates. (From Bourgery, M.J., Traité complet de l'anatomie de l'homme, C. Delaunay, Paris, France, 1831–1854.)

times per minute to transport mucous at ~5 mm/min toward the posterior of the nasal cavity, continually replenishing the mucous layer every 15 or 20 min [162].

Insofar as drugs that are delivered via the nasal route are concerned, drug molecules enter the circulation through either passive transcellular or paracellular diffusion, active carrier/receptor-mediated transport, or endocytosis. Efficient transport across the nasal mucosa is contingent on a number of factors; some of which might be translatable to nanodevices, such as surface charge, lipophilicity, and molecular weight. Diminutive lipophilic drugs, for instance, typically undergo transcellular transference, whereas the entry of larger hydrophilic drugs paracellularly is constrained by the presence of tight junctions [162]. A number of absorption enhancers such as chitosan, cyclodextrins, and certain phospholipids may be utilized to enhance bioadhesiveness and for the delay of mucociliary clearance [163].

Hypothetically, a novel strategy may be employed by nanodevices in order to gain access to the circulation in a manner that is similar to that of drug molecules. It may facilitate nanodevice passage through tight junctions via their initial administration as molecular-scale constituents that would self-assemble into larger functional assemblies once they have traversed the barriers. Hence, this class of multicomponent "aggrecyte" nanodevice (Figure 2.15) may enable transfer through the epithelium, albeit in fragmented form, through especially recalcitrant barriers as they would comprise perhaps tens to hundreds of constituents that may be activated and directed to reassemble via external stimuli and/or computer commands.

An important step in this direction has recently (2011) been achieved through the work of researchers at Duke University, the University of California, Berkeley, and Dartmouth College, who utilized a global signal to elicit slightly altered responses from multiple (260 μm × 60 μm × 14 μm) stress-engineered electrostatic microrobots (Figure 2.16). Thus, they demonstrated that a single electronic signal could be utilized to instruct a collection of microrobots via algorithm-mediated voltage sequences, to self-assemble into larger structures [164]. "By exploiting differences in the designs and the resulting electromechanical interaction with the control signal, the behaviour of the individual robots can be differentiated" [165]. The notion of functional aggregated nanodevices

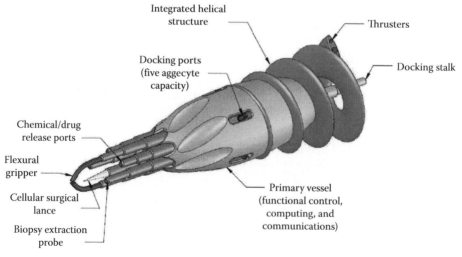

FIGURE 2.15
Anatomy of a conceptual "aggrecyte" class nanodevice.

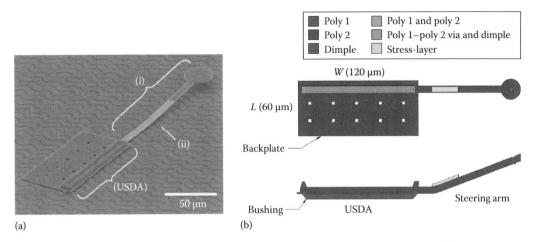

FIGURE 2.16
(a, b) Stress-engineered electrostatic microrobot that can controllably form larger structures. The untethered scratch drive actuator (USDA) enables inchworm like forward locomotion, whereas a curved steering-arm actuator enables linear travel or turning (i). The curvature of the steering arm is contingent on a lithographically applied chrome layer. ((a) Reproduced and (b) redrawn with permission from Donald, B.R. et al., *J. Microelectromech. Syst.*, 17(4), 789, 2008; Donald, B.R. et al., *The Eighth International Workshop on the Algorithmic Foundations of Robotics (WAFR)*, Guanajuato, Mexico, December 7–9, 2008.)

can also be considered as analogous to a limited application of "utility fog," which is a theoretical construct devised by John Starrs Hall. The utility fog concept envisions intelligent interlocking nanoscale robots that may shape shift on command to any desired configuration [166,167].

The conceptual aggrecyte medical nanodevice might be endowed with a number of specialized retractable telescopic "tooltips" to facilitate a myriad of medical procedures, ranging from real-time cellular level diagnostics and therapeutics to nanosurgical cell repair procedures. The envisaged complement of nanomedical tooltips might encompass

1. *Flexural articulating gripper*, comprising artificial muscle nanomaterials (e.g., carbon nanotubes, biocompatible electroactive polymers), to mechanically and orientationally secure targeted cells or organelles for diagnosis or treatment, or conceivably for the mechanical extraction of undesired biomaterials (e.g., plaque, lipofuscin).

2. *Surgical lance*, for physically penetrating the cell membranes of diseased cells or bacterial/viral pathogens in order to initiate their eradication. It may also have the capacity for imparting a highly localized electrical charge or engaging an integrated laser to enhance this utility.

3. *Biopsy extraction probe* would have the ability to retrieve (via the administration of a slight vacuum or electrostatics combined with an integrated incising tool) tiny biological samples for virtually instantaneous onboard chemical assessment and quantification. These data would be transferred to external computers for analysis by attending physicians, who would then dispatch further commands to onsite aggrecytes, in appropriate response contingent on biopsy results.

4. *Chemical/drug release ports* would discharge precise volumes of ions or pharmacologically active molecules, to facilitate the temporary relaxation of the tight junctions that line epithelial cells (for ingress purposes), or for the administration of powerful, albeit, highly localized therapeutics, respectively.

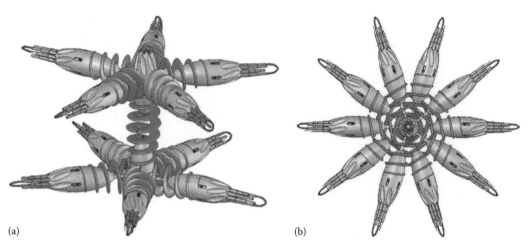

(a)   (b)

FIGURE 2.17
Depiction of aggrecyte "cluster": (a) perspective and (b) top views.

Although individual aggrecytes may function as independent units, their genuine potency, which translates to enhanced medical benefit, may be realized when they are mechanically linked to operate in conjunction with their counterparts to perform medical procedures in parallel (Figure 2.16). Each aggrecyte would be endowed with onboard docking ports with which additional aggrecytes (in this design, five in total) may link via telescoping docking stalks that are extendable from the sterns of each unit (Figure 2.17).

An example of this cooperative functionality may be illustrated through the hypothetical eradication of neurological β-amyloid plaque material, which is thought to be linked with the onset of Alzheimer's disease. Once constituent aggrecytes have successfully traversed the BBB, they would proceed to follow preprogrammed reorientation maneuvers to sequentially dock with two central "pillar" aggrecytes. These internally differentiated and enhanced aggrecytes would initially lock together at the termination of their helical structures to serve as transferral nodes through which all commands, communications, and distributed power would be supplied. Plaque material sites might be located when the nanodevices proceed to precise coordinates provided by previously acquired spatial cartographic data (e.g., via dedicated cartographic scanning nanodevices such as the vascular cartographic scanning nanodevice [VCSN]) that has been uploaded to onboard quantum computers.

Alternately, an advanced form of targeted drug delivery by which specific biomolecules or chemical groups, which are known to have a robust binding affinities for amyloid plaque (e.g., ligands such as 6-iodo-2-(4′-dimethylamino-)phenyl-imidazo[1,2]pyridine [IMPY], and 4-N-methylamino-4′-hydroxystilbene [SB-13]) may be exploited to guide and bind aggre-cyte clusters to plaque materials [168]. Once in close proximity to the plaque sites, several operations would ensue; grippers would physically anchor to the plaque, while nanoscopic lances might conduct perforative operations on the material so as to reduce its density. Concomitantly, the highly localized release of compounds that preferentially degrade β-amyloid peptides (AβPs) would ensue. For example, it has been shown that high-affinity MAbs such as MAb 6C6 and/or 10D5 have a high binding affinity for the N-terminal region of the AβP (residues 1–28) and can disassociate Aβ fibrils to reestablish the solubility of the peptides. Specifically, it was found that "site-directed antibodies toward peptide (glutamic acid, phenyl alanine, arginine, histidine) EFRH sequences 3–6 of the N-terminal region of AβP suppress in vitro formation of Aβ and dissolve already formed fibrillar amyloid" [169]. The proviso here is that any agent with the capacity for initiating the dissolution of plaque material should impart none, or very negligible collateral damage to neighboring neurons and glial cells (e.g., oligodendrocytes, microglia, astrocytes).

2.4.2 Intranasal Ingress through the BBB

The BBB presents one of the most impermeable ingress routes within the human body for the in vivo traversal of nanodevices. It encompasses the endothelium of the cerebral capillaries, the choroid plexus epithelium, and the arachnoid membranes [170]. It is estimated that there are ~100 billion capillaries within the human brain with a combined surface area of ~20 m². Nevertheless, only a small fraction of drug species may traverse this barrier [171–173].

The cerebral microvasculature that establishes this membrane comprises endothelial cells that possess tight junctions (zonula occludens), which are typically exhibited by epithelial cells. Small molecules and lipophilic drugs may traverse this barrier via free diffusion. However, other entities such as plasma proteins, peptides, viruses undergo carrier-mediated or receptor-mediated transport [174].

Though the impermeability of the BBB is typically attributed to the endothelial plasma membrane, this functionality has significant contributions from capillary pericytes that populate the same basement membrane as endothelial cells, leptomeningeal cells, parenchymal coverings; astrocyte foot processes that tesselate about 99% of the outer surfaces of the capillaries (Figure 2.18) as well as efflux transporters and enzymes [175]. An additional, less impermeable membrane that protects the spine is the blood–cerebrospinal fluid (CSF) barrier, which comprises a uninterrupted layer of tight junction–fortified epithelial cells that sheath the choroid plexus, which generates CSF and is situated within the brain ventricles [159,176,177].

There may be several approaches for the ingress of nanodevices, or constituents thereof, into the brain tissues. These may include their introduction into the systemic circulation through nasal mucosa through which they may reach the brain via minimally invasive

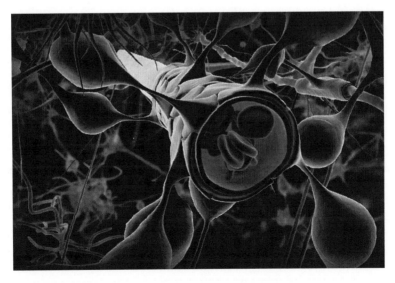

FIGURE 2.18
Artistic depiction of the arrangement of the blood–brain barrier with tessellated astrocyte foot processes. (From Mohammed BB, Wikimedia Commons, 2010-10-1.)

(nanomechanochemical diapedesis) traversal of the cerebral capillary tight junctions. Envisaged administration methods may include atomized nasal spray, vapoinhaler, drops, swab application, mucoadhesive gel, or thin film patch. A preferable ingress route might involve the circumvention of the BBB through the intranasal pathways such as traversal within the olfactory neuron cells via intracellular axons that extend through small orifices in the cribriform plate of the ethmoid bone to interface at synaptic connections within the olfactory bulb [162,178,179]. This intimate connection between the nasal structures and the brain has developed for the sensing of odors and chemical stimuli [170].

The latter route appears to be amenable to the transfer of certain metals [180], viruses, macromolecules [181], particulates, and proteins [182]. The existence of an intranasal extracellular route to the brain was first verified by Balin, who used a 40 kDa protein tracer (horseradish peroxidase) to demarcate the pathway [183]. The uptake of drugs via this path, however, is shown to be quite slow and is contingent on the composition of a compound. For example, progress may range from a relatively rapid 20–400 mm/day, to a snails pace of 0.1–4 mm/day [184]. Once drug molecules enter the olfactory bulb, they are transferred to the triangle-shaped mitral neuron cells via glomeruli-situated synapses and into the proximal structures of brain, some of which include the hippocampus, hypothalamus, and thalamus [161].

The ophthalmic and maxillary branches of the trigeminal cranial nerve provide sensory connectivity throughout the nasal mucosa and olfactory mucosa, and hence, may also be exploited as an avenue for aggrecyte component transfer [178,185–187]. Hunter and Dey demonstrated the translocation of intranasally administered rhodamine-labeled microspheres (20–200 nm in diameter) in rats [188]. Oberdörster et al. found that carbon 13 (^{13}C) nanoparticles with median diameters of 36 nm were found to increase in concentration in the olfactory bulb, cerebrum, and cerebellum of rats over 7 days, subsequent to being exposed to ^{13}C for 6 h. They determined that the nanoparticles were likely being transferred by the olfactory nerves [185]. Contingent on the complexity of fully assembled ~1 μm in diameter aggrecyte nanodevices, its constituent elements may be in the dimensional range of ~25 to 200 nm.

An additional entry option for the ingress of nanodevices to bypass the BBB may be via the olfactory epithelium, which is a 10 cm^2 region about 100 μm thick [108] located in the uppermost portion of the nasal cavity, within which reside olfactory chemoreceptors. This area interfaces directly with the brain as the normal BBB is absent [178].

The nanometric aggrecyte components, as described earlier, may traverse olfactory nerve cells to circumvent the BBB, and be activated by external commands to reassemble once inside the brain to facilitate neurological plaque removal/dissolution, the repair of imminent aneurysms, or the repair or upgrade of individual neurons (Chapter 17).

2.5 Ocular Ingress

The potential for ingress of medical nanodevices via the ocular route may have advantages such as ease of administration, through the use of eye drops, the capacity for precise dosages, and rapid access to the systemic circulation, which is comparable to that of parenteral injection [189]. There are two distinct vascular courses in the eye that include the retinal vessels and the uveal vessels. The retinal vessels typically transport drugs, metabolites, and species such as prostaglandins from the retina and the vitreous humor, a gelatinous substance comprised of 99% water, combined small concentrations of collagen and heavily hydrated hyaluronic acid molecules, which are synthesized by resident hyalocytes [108,190]. The uveal vessels facilitate the mass transport of drugs from the iris and ciliary body.

An additional transit route is provided by aqueous humor outflow via the trabecular meshwork and canal of Schlemm, which empty into the episcleral vessels. Regarding the possibility of delivering nanodevices directly to the eye itself, there exist continuous tight junctions throughout the retinal capillaries with a similar functionality as the BBB within the retinal pigment epithelium that negate the entry of hydrophilic drugs and many other substances. Glucose, however, appears to cross readily with the assistance of active transmembrane chaperones [190]. The traversal of nanodevices across this barrier, similar to the BBB, may necessitate the design of ruggedized nanomechanical diapedesis mechanisms working in conjunction with ion and molecular compound release capabilities to chemically coax the transient loosening of tight junction elements to facilitate transit.

It was found in studies with rabbits that systemic peptide drug (α-melanocyte-stimulating hormone) entry through the ocular route could be enhanced by ~10-fold through the use of surfactant permeation enhancers such as polyoxyethylene 9-lauryl ether (BL-9) and polyoxyethylene 20-stearyl ether (Brij-78). Subsequent to drug instillation, peak blood concentration for BL-9 was 5–20 min whereas for Brij-78 it was 10–60 min [191]. Xuan et al. demonstrated an increased systemic uptake of insulin by altering pH (to 8.0) through the use of absorption enhancers such as glycocholate and fusidic acid [192].

Optimal eye drop formulations should include both low-viscosity hydrophilic (lacrimal/tear fluid soluble) and hydrophobic (lipid soluble) properties, allowing for the permeation of the lipophilic corneal epithelium, the corneal stroma, and the lipophilic endothelium prior to reaching the aqueous humor [193–195]. Hence, the passage of conventional drugs and future nanomedicines and nanodevices through the cornea, which is deemed to be the primary conduit for ocular ingress, is contingent on their n-octanol–water partition coefficient, which is a surrogate model for organism drug uptake wherein using a series of compounds, higher levels of partitioning into n-octanol corresponds to enhanced accumulation within an organism. When the partition coefficient is between 10 and 100, drugs may most easily pass through the five layers of the cornea (epithelium, Bowman's membrane stroma, Descement's membrane, and endothelium) [196]. Cyclodextrins may also be used as such excipients to facilitate the delivery of drugs and perhaps nanodevices or components thereof through the ocular route as they can endow water-insoluble lipophilic entities with increased capabilities for solubility and bioavailability [197].

Akhter et al. studied the topical ocular delivery of mucoadhesive nanoformulations of ganciclovir, which is an antiviral compound for ocular infections, using mucoadhesive nanoemulsions, chitosan nanoparticles, and mucoadhesive niosomal dispersions. The nanoparticles were typically spherical in shape, in order to minimize irritation, with dimensions that ranged from 23 to 200 nm. The results indicated that the nanoformulations could be useful for the topical delivery of ganciclovir with no irritation or toxicity, which is of benefit since ganciclovir may be toxic when administered in higher doses, leading to neutropenia and bone marrow suppression [198]. Das and Suresh loaded the antifungal agent amphotericin B into slightly cationic polymeric Eudragit RS 100 nanoparticles (150–290 nm) with a zeta potential of +19–28 mV, which were topically administered to rabbit eyes as a nanosuspension. Studies showed that 60% of the drug payload was discharged in dissolution over a 24 h period, and there were no indications of irritation in the rabbits [199].

There are several issues that will work to inhibit the progress of nanodevices, as they do drugs, to ingress ocularly. The constant flow of tear fluid at a rate of 1.2–1.5 μL/min can dramatically reduce the time of residency on the surface of the eye (e.g., 15–30 s) [200,201]. This continual lacrimal rinsing has been shown to diminish the transfer of drugs across the cornea to 5% [202,203]. It has been demonstrated, however, in a comparative study between conventional eye drops that contained indomethacin, and a chitosan nanoparticle/indomethacin formulation that the nanoparticles had good interaction with the cornea (a four to five times higher permeation coefficient) and were not immediately washed away [204,205].

Hence, contingent on various factors, including chemical composition, hydrophilicity, hydrophobicity, morphology, and charge, nanodevices may simply be swept away from the surface of the eye via nasolacrimal drainage to end up in the stomach and GIT. Tear fluid emanates from the lacrimal gland (Figure 2.19) within the upper eyelid and proceeds laterally across the eye surface, via blinking, to lacrimal drainage pores called puncta, which are positioned at the inside corners of the upper and lower eyelids. The lacrimal fluid then proceeds, via capillary forces and gravity, through dual drainage ducts called canalicula

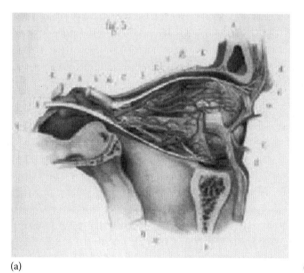

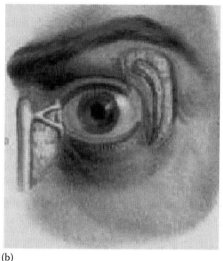

(a)   (b)

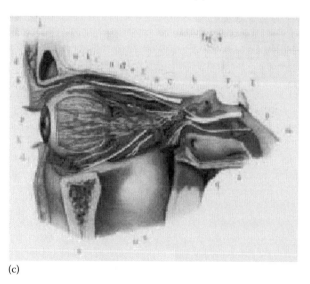

(c)

FIGURE 2.19
Artistic renderings of ocular vascularization (a) and (c), and the lacrimal gland and lacrimal fluid drainage pathway (b). (From Bourgery, M.J., Traité complet de l'anatomie de l'homme, C. Delaunay, Paris, France, 1831–1854.)

into the lacrimal drainage sac, directly into the inferior nasal passage and to the back of the throat via the nasolacrimal duct.

An alternate, though indirect, ocular ingress route to the systemic circulation for nanodevices that are administered in eye drop form would involve their transit via tear fluid and subsequent attachment to the walls of the highly vascularized inferior nasal passage "on the fly," to enter via nanomechanical diapedesis into local capillaries.

Note: The lacrimal fluid drainage pathway may serve as a viable option for nanodevice egress from the patient through natural elimination. Diapedesis-mediated egress that proceeds from the ophthalmic and lacrimal arteries into the lacrimal gland would place nanodevices in position to follow the tear fluid flow as described earlier, ultimately into the GIT.

A potential additional nanomedical ocular ingress strategy might utilize topically applied soft nanodevice-eluting contact lenses. There are currently a number of drug-eluting contact lenses under development, (Chapter 10) which include those that are hydrogel based for the delivery of antiglaucoma drugs such as acetazolamide or ethoxzolamide [206]. Molecular imprinting technology, by which drug affinities are imparted to the polymeric networks of soft contact lenses, via molecular impression templating, was used to deliver the anti-inflammatory drug flurbiprofen [207–211]. Medical nanodevices might be similarly loaded into contact lens "docking reservoirs" and stored until use, whereupon they would self-release from micron-scale cavities upon instantaneous activation on contact with ocular physiological fluids, or are triggered to do so by external stimuli.

2.6 Nanodevice Ingress through the Inner Ear

The inner ear (Figure 2.20) is scarcely accessible by conventional drugs via the systemic circulation as there are several considerable physiological barriers such as the blood–inner ear barrier that prevent passage [212]. The blood flow is also quite limited toward the inner and subsequently to the brain [213]. However, this route is quite attractive from the standpoint of its intimate proximity to the cerebral tissues and structures. The primary components of the inner ear encompass two fluid-filled multi-cavitied labyrinths that are designated bony and membranous. The membranous labyrinth is lined with continuous epithelia cells and contains two particular domains known as the utricle, which contains semicircular ducts and the saccule that houses the cochlear duct. In this region, the epithelial cells give way to sensory elements such as the maculae, cristae, and organ of Corti. The central space of the bony labyrinth is called the vestibule that encompasses the utricle and saccule, and behind which resides three semicircular canals that house the semicircular ducts, whereas the cochlea encapsulates the cochlear duct. The cochlea makes two and a half circumscribed turns around the modiolus, which is a bony core area. It is within the modiolus that is contained blood vessels, cells, and nerve processes and it is from this domain, contingent on the selected approach, that nanodevices might ingress into the systemic vasculature or travel into the brain via the vestibulocochlear cranial nerve [110].

Chinese researchers have conducted a comparative study on the delivery of anti-inflammatory drug, dexamethasone acetate–loaded solid lipid nanoparticles, to brain tissues via the intra-cochlear administration by intratympanic injection in contrast to intravenous injection. It was found that the intra-cochlear route provided a drug presence in the CSF that was four times higher than what was detected when the drug was administered intravenously [214]. Zhang et al. investigated the delivery of lipid core nanocapsules (LCNs) (50 nm) for

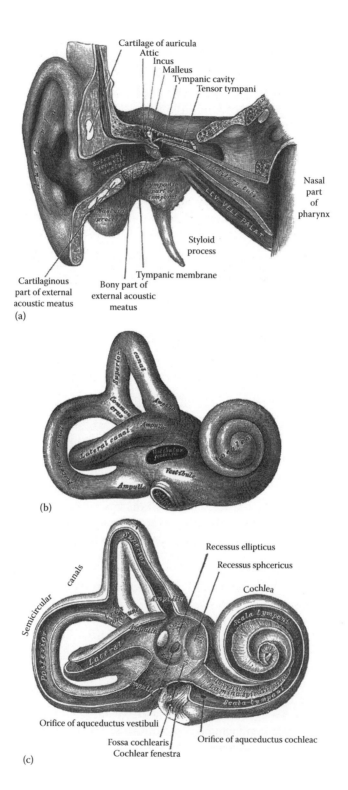

FIGURE 2.20
(a–c) Artistic renderings of the inner ear and cochlear structures. (From Gray, H., *Anatomy of the Human Body*, Lea & Febiger, Philadelphia, PA, 1918, Bartleby.com, 2000.)

the treatment of sensorineural hearing loss, and demonstrated that they had the capacity for traversing the round window membrane (*fenestra cochleae*) within the osseous labyrinth to access nerve fibers and spiral ganglion cells, among other cells, within the inner ear [215]. This may facilitate and improve hearing performance outcomes subsequent to cochlear implantation [216].

The pharmacokinetics of the LCNs may be controlled by modifying the concentrations of the core elements and it was observed that LCNs can maintain their stability as a suspension for up to 1 year [217–219]. It was shown by Zou et al. that biodegradable LCNs, which entered through the tympanic cavity resident, round window via paracellular pathways, were well distributed within the inner ear in ~30 min and established contact with the "vestibule, middle ear mucosa, and the adjacent artery." [220].

Hence, this potential noninvasive strategy raises the possibility of their use for the delivery of drug molecules to permeate spiral ganglion cells, nerve fibers, inner hair cells, pillar cells, and the spiral ligament [220]. Genes may also be delivered to the cochlea when combined with polyethyleneimine [221], and drugs (lidocaine) were shown to be sustainably discharged within the inner ear by utilizing poly lactic/glycolic acid (PLGA) nanoparticles [222]. It was indicated, however, that polyethyleneimine can impart toxicity to cells [223] and that PGLA requires further testing to verify its safety. Though much further work remains in order to ensure the safety and efficacy for permeation into the inner ear and conceivably the brain, this domain presents yet another option for the ingress on nanomedical devices or constituent nanometric elements thereof.

2.7 Hypodermic Injection

Externally controlled autonomous nanomedical devices employed for the benefit of human patients will utilize ~19,000 km of arterial, venous, and capillary vasculature to accurately locate and conduct nanomedical diagnostic or therapeutic procedures on cells, tissues, and organs at virtually any site within the human body at <1 µm spatial resolution [75]. An important second-tier access route or reconnaissance pathway would comprise the cumulative ~3500 km of the lymphatic system. Hence, an intimate knowledge of the microkinetics and functionalities inherent to these systems will be indispensable. Reliable onboard propulsive mechanisms with inbuilt multiple redundancies will enable nanodevices, perhaps administered by the thousands, to be controlled simultaneously with high precision by dedicated "outbody" navigational computer systems. For large-scale medical procedures that might require billions of nanodevices to conduct massively parallel tasks, these nanodevices would be preprogrammed with the full compliment of in vivo cartographic data that is unique to the individual patient. These spatial data sets will have been acquired previously by dedicated cartographic classes of nanodevices, such as the VCSN.

Dependent on the prescribed course of treatment, various concentrations of nanodevices will constitute a colloidal suspension that is diffused within an aqueous carrier media for injection into the patient. There are several forms of injection that may be utilized including intradermal, subcutaneous, intramuscular, intravenous, intraperitoneal, and intraosseous [224]. A modular Magnetic Plungerless Injection System has been developed for injections, which employs a magnetically actuated piston to push liquids through a sealed, single-use cartridge and into a sterile needle. An advantage for this type of injection device is that the sealed doses may be stored for extended time periods. A similar strategy might facilitate the long-term storage of doses of nanomedical devices, perhaps for decades [225].

Hypodermic injection will comprise an uncomplicated means for the administration of early generations of nanomedical devices. When viewed in retrospect from the perspective of mature nanomedicine (e.g., autonomous nanodevices), however, injection of any sort will likely be considered as unacceptably invasive. It is possible that within the next few decades, concomitant with the advent of advanced nanodevices that are enabled with the capacity for traversing the skin layers via autonomous burrowing to access the bloodstream, hypodermic injection will likely have long been consigned to the archives of medical history.

2.7.1 Parenteral Compression Jet Injection

Advanced configurations of compression jet injectors [226] such as DERMOJET [227], MED-JET [228], Prelude SkinPrep System [229] or Madajet [230], SQ-PEN [231] might be employed for the intradermal, subcutaneous, and intramuscular transfer of nanodevice-infused aqueous dosages. These devices exploit pressurized high-velocity liquid jets that may be powered by coil springs or compressed CO_2, to penetrate the epidermis and deliver drugs without the requirement of a needle. The orifices typically utilized in these devices are in the ~30 to 560 μm range, with jet velocities of 100–200 m/s. In operation, the output orifice is typically positioned slightly (~1/8′) above the epithelium. As per the resulting injected dispersal pattern, the depth of the microdroplet penetration into the intradermal tissue is in the ~4 to 4.5 mm range, whereas the medication wheel diameter is ~5 to 6 mm [230]. This depth would be sufficient to propel nanomedical devices directly into the bloodstream via the capillaries, which reside at depths of ~45 to 70 μm beneath the skin surface [232].

There are, however, a number of issues in regard to jet injectors that have prevented their widespread adoption. These include some attendant stinging pain and bruising at injection sites, which may be due to the splash back caused by high velocities combined with sizable doses (tens to hundreds of microliters), and the lack of measures to compensate for significant differences in the mechanical characteristics of human skin [233–235].

Also, although jet injectors have been available for the delivery of insulin since 1979, insurance companies are reluctant to cover patients who use them. In addition, they are not recommended for certain patients: "People taking anti-coagulant medicine, those with hemophilia, and those on dialysis are among those who should avoid using a jet injector as it could cause a bleeding problem" [236]. One study examined "eight skin specimens taken by shave biopsy after injection of local anesthetic with the Madajet. An unusual histologic feature was noted in all specimens. Irregularly shaped, variably sized holes resembling 'Swiss cheese' were noted in the papillary and midreticular dermis ..." [237].

It is possible that the jet injection of solid or semisolid ~1 μm in diameter nanomedical devices may result in physical impact damage to cells and tissues that lay in the direct path of the constituents of the injection column, due to the associated high-velocity (several hundred meters/second) ballistic pressures of, and sonic vibrations. Preliminary investigations with nanoscale entities having similar geometries and physical consistencies as envisaged nanodevices might elucidate the degree of damage, if any, that may impart to human cells and tissues via jet injection. Solid 1 μm in diameter nanomedical devices comprising of diamondoid for instance are far more likely to cause impact damage in contrast to more labile and soft bodied medical nanodevices. Another consideration is that unless sophisticated nanomedical devices are sufficiently ruggedized to withstand the G forces and pressures inherent to jet injection, they may also be subject to impact-related damage or destruction.

2.8 Transdermal Ingress

The transdermal delivery of nanomedical devices involves strategies to facilitate their transfer across the superficial 1 mm thick layer of the skin (stratum corneum) (Figure 2.21), which is comprised of flat, expired cells that are packed with keratinocytes (keratin fibers) and enveloped by lipid bilayers [238]. Directly beneath this layer reside the capillaries, which are ~5 to 10 μm in diameter that are organized as vertical loops and oriented at indiscriminate angles, having a concentration of ~10 loops/mm² [239].

An example of a strategy that might exploit this ingress pathway would involve the application of an adhesive patch that is infused with dose-directed populations of nanodevices, which would actively or passively transit through the epidermis and into the bloodstream. This conveyance strategy has a number of attractive advantages over hypodermic and jet injection techniques for nanodevice ingress that include noninvasiveness, minimal risk of infection, the capacity for accurate nanodevice loading, as well as simple and painless administration with the further ability of providing sustained release over days or even weeks. Nanomedical devices would imperceptibly progress through the various epidermal tissues facilitated by paracellular activity (e.g., fluid movement between cells) [240]. Currently (2011), there are a rapidly growing number of investigations that involve the transdermal delivery of nanocarriers and nanoparticles. These technologies include nanometric emulsions, vesicular systems, solid lipid nanoparticles, semisolid nanostructured lipid carriers, single and multiple polymeric nanoparticles, reservoir matrices, matrix diffusion-controlled devices, hydrogels, and multilayer matrix assemblies [241,242]. In addition to liposomes, which are nanoscale lipid-bilayered or multilaminar vesicles, entities

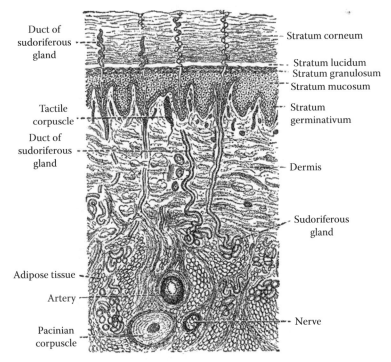

FIGURE 2.21
Artistic rendering of cross section of the skin. (From Gray, H., *Anatomy of the Human Body*, Lea & Febiger, Philadelphia, PA, 1918, Bartleby.com, 2000.)

called ethosomes, comprising phospholipid, ethanol, and water, have demonstrated efficacy for deep skin penetration for the delivery of encapsulated drugs [243].

This contemporary work will undoubtedly elucidate physiological challenges that will confront the conceptualists and designers of nanomedical devices and will influence and contribute to the development of future ingress strategies. Steady, incremental progress with these technologies will continue to ensue toward the further enhancement and sophistication of dermal permeability, and hence, may lead to increased capabilities for the successful in vivo delivery of nanoscale encapsulants, nanocrystalline drugs, targeted medical nanoparticles, and prospective autonomous nanomedical devices.

Labouta et al. are developing a "multiphoton-pixel analysis" technique for the quantification of the permeation capacities of gold nanoshells (~6 nm) within different skin layers. The luminescence of the nanoshells within a cross-sectioned segment of human skin was translated and represented as pixels via two-photon excitation fluorescence microscopy. This analytical tool, as well as inductively coupled plasma mass and atomic absorption spectroscopy, may facilitate the evolution of an optimal set of parameters, encompassing particulate morphology, dimensions, as well as surface charge and chemistry for the efficacious ingress of nanomedical compounds and nanodevices through the transdermal layers and other biological barriers [244].

2.8.1 Transfollicular Ingress

The possibility of localized and systemic nanomedical device permeation into the in vivo environment via the hair follicles (Figure 2.22) will be worthy of investigation as these pathways may be exploited as direct and relatively deep vertical ingress channels through the skin barrier. In terms of conventional drug delivery, this potential route of entry may be somewhat neglected as, comparatively speaking, hair follicle orifices offer only a small fraction (~0.1%) of the total dermal surface area that is available for the percutaneous diffusion of therapeutic entities through the stratum corneum [245]. However, they are thought to provide a significant subdermal surface area that is available for the absorption of therapeutic entities. Cumulatively, hair follicles, hair shafts, and sebaceous glands are known as pilosebaceous units, which have distinctive immune capabilities, metabolism, and biochemistry. Additionally, several species of epithelial cells, localized immune cells, and dedicated structures are involved [246]. The secretion of sebum by the sebaceous glands may also facilitate the provision of lipidic absorptive ingress routes [247].

The transfollicular, or "shunt" traversal path was initially investigated as a rapid ingress route via the transfer of charged dyes, and it was found that they could be diffused in less than an hour [248,249]. The blood vessels that surround hair follicles may indeed expedite transport progress. It was also determined that there may be an optimal dimensional range within which drug-laced particulates may best be delivered into the follicle. The 5 μm size range exhibited the highest accumulation of microbeads within the hair follicle, whereas larger sizes remained on the skin surface [246,250].

Hair follicles, which range in diameter from 10 to 70 μm, contain three main layers, which include the outer root sheath, inner root sheath, and the hair shaft itself. Of these, the outer root sheath is the most relevant to the ingress of drugs, and will be as well for the traversal of nanodevices. This is due to its continuity with the surface epidermis, thereby providing an increased surface area that is available for transfer. Nanodevices that are endowed with hydrophilic surface attributes will likely encounter significantly decreased resistance to transit in comparison to the stratum corneum, epidermis, and sebaceous duct [245]. Critical cellular interactions commence within the follicular papilla, which is

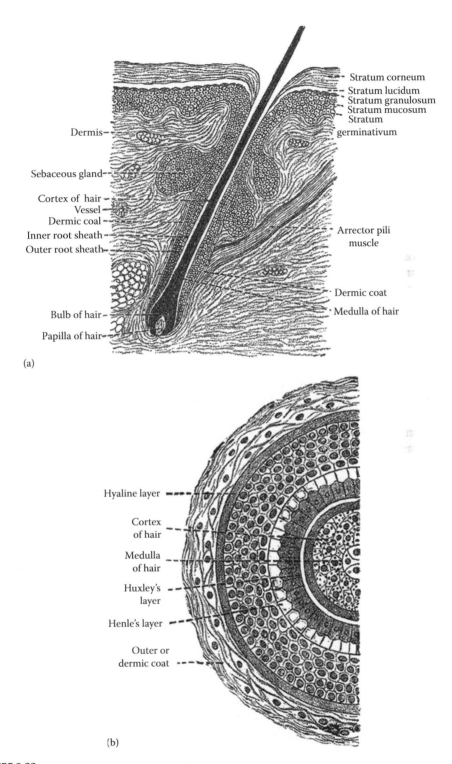

Stratum corneum
Stratum lucidum
Stratum granulosum
Stratum mucosum
Stratum germinativum

Dermis

Sebaceous gland

Cortex of hair
Vessel
Dermic coal
Inner root sheath
Outer root sheath

Arrector pili muscle

Dermic coat
Medulla of hair

Bulb of hair
Papilla of hair

(a)

Hyaline layer

Cortex of hair

Medulla of hair

Huxley's layer

Henle's layer

Outer or dermic coat

(b)

FIGURE 2.22
(a, b) Artistic rendering of the follicle with surrounding structures and lateral cross section. (From Gray, H., *Anatomy of the Human Body*, Lea & Febiger, Philadelphia, PA, 1918, Bartleby.com, 2000.)

encased by the bulb at the bottom of the hair follicle. A capillary matrix supplies the base of the follicle from the deeper subcutaneous regions, whereas the upper segment of the follicle is supplied with blood by perifollicular capillaries that are related to the shallow dermal vasculature. The sebaceous glands are also provided with an abundant complement of capillaries [247,251]. Hence, it seems plausible that nanodevices may quite straightforwardly be transferred into the systemic circulation via follicular pathways.

2.8.2 Topical Diffusive Gels and Sudoriferous Gland Ingress

Topical diffusive gels may serve as a straightforward and effective media for the transfer of nanomedical devices through the skin. Gel-infused nanodevices would be suspended as an ultrafine colloid, and hence, when applied to the skin, would diffuse into readily accessible sweat gland pores and migrate toward the deeper layers of the dermis. The soporiferous (sweat glands) populate the entire surface of the skin, and are oriented as tiny detents just below the corium, which is a deep sensitive layer under the epidermis, albeit they are typically found in the subcutaneous areola, which comprise small gaps among fibrous tissue that is enveloped by fatty milieu. Each sweat gland consists of a single tubular column having a deeper element that is configured as an oviform or spheroid, which comprises the body of the gland. The shallow duct terminates at the outermost surface of the skin as a funnel-shaped orifice [68]. On the palm of the hand reside ~370 pores/cm^2, whereas the back of the hand contains ~200 pores/cm^2, the forehead has ~175 pores/cm^2, the breast, abdomen, and forearm have ~155 pores/cm^2, and the leg and back have ~60 to 80 pores/cm^2. A typical diameter of a skin pore is ~50 μm, and an approximation of the entire pore population for the total epidermal surface of human body is ~2 million [68]. The sweat pores of the palm of the hand might serve to optimize nanodevice ingress due to the maximal potential entry points, thus facilitating expeditious device diffusion.

Several transdermal gels are on the market today, and their performance may instruct how nanodevices might be appropriately formulated within them to enable nanomedical therapeutics. In 2004, Solvay Pharmaceuticals (Marietta, GA) obtained FDA approval for a bioidentical estrogen therapy gel called EstroGel. This was the first-ever estrogen therapeutic transdermal gel in the United States for addressing moderate to severe vasomotor symptoms associated with menopause [252]. Antares Pharma (Ewing, NJ) has developed several transdermal gel products including ComiGel (testosterone for men), Elestrin (menopause), Anturol (overactive bladder), LibiGel (female sexual dysfunction), and NestraGel (contraceptive) [253].

2.8.3 Dermal Ingress Assisted by Iontophoresis, Electroporation, Sonophoresis, and Microporation

Autonomous "smart" transdermal adhesive patches may translate a low voltage into the epidermis that could enable nanodevice ingress into the patient [254]. Advances that are being made in this delivery domain include iontophoresis, electroporation, sonophoresis, and various microporation strategies [255–259]. Iontophoresis utilizes repulsive electromotive forces whereby a small voltage is applied to positively and negatively charged chambers that house solvents and active ingredients, and which carry an opposite charge. In operation, the chambers are induced to strongly repel their contents, and as a result they are jettisoned into the skin [260]. Electroporation employs microneedle electrode arrays to penetrate the stratum corneum and an applied electric field to enable feasible transdermal delivery [261].

Sonophoresis utilizes ultrasonic frequencies to increase epidermal permeation, and although high-frequency ultrasound ($\geq$0.7 MHz) was originally used to increase the permeability of the skin [262,263] it was later recognized that acoustic cavitation played a critical role in the enhancement of this phenomenon. An inverse relationship was hypothesized to exist between acoustic cavitation events (aqueous microbubble generation due to ultrasound exposure) and ultrasonic frequencies. Mitragotri et al. demonstrated that low-frequency ultrasound at 20 kHz had approximately three orders of magnitude higher efficacy for inducing skin permeability than did high-frequency ultrasound at 1 MHz [264].

Microporation entails the formation of superficial and temporary micron-scale channels within the epidermis to facilitate the delivery of water-soluble hydrophilic macromolecules that will not normally diffuse across the skin. A number of technologies may be employed in the creation of these micropores, including microneedles, radio frequencies, thermal, and laser ablation [265]. A Painless Laser Epidermal System (P.L.E.A.S.E.) has been developed by Pantec Biosolutions AG (Ruggell, Liechtenstein), which employs a pulsed diode pumped Er:YAG fractional ablative laser to create a tunable circular array of pores that are each ~200 μm in diameter and can be calibrated to depths of 20–150 μm. Because the laser is pulsed, it imparts no thermal damage to the skin surrounding the ablated pores. The result microchannel pattern, which can contain from 1 to 5000 pores within a ~5 cm² treatment area, makes available a 20–300 mm² passive diffusion zone for the conveyance of macromolecules, or for our purposes, nanomedical devices, into the capillaries below. Permeation studies with P.L.E.A.S.E. using porcine skin demonstrated that macromolecules such as triptorelin (MW ~1311.5 Da), hGH (MW ~22 kDa), and follicle-stimulating hormone (MW ~30 kDa) could be transdermally delivered [266].

2.8.4 Cascading Dermal Implant

A myriad of nanomedical devices or self-assembling nanoscale components might be sequentially administered to a patient over protracted time lines via the implementation of conceptual micron-scale cascading subdermal implants. These entities might have the capacity for self-burrowing to position themselves just below the epidermal layer at a depth of 150–200 μm in close proximity to the crests of the capillary loops, which at this depth are oriented perpendicularly to the surface of the skin [265]. These compact reservoirs may integrate hundreds or thousands of sealed nanoscale "wells" that might collectively house a diverse set of nanodevice species.

Biodegradable polymeric membranes that seal each well may be nanoengineered to vary in thickness such that local physiological conditions (e.g., pH and temperature) may be exploited as natural degradative stimuli to release specific well contents at precise times. The thinnest membranes would initially be dissolved over a predetermined time line, whereby thicker seals would degrade at increasingly slower, albeit linear, rates over time, which are synchronized with scheduled release protocols. An alternate membrane degradation strategy, utilizing seals that comprise appropriately reactive materials, might use external activation sources such as pulsed ultrasound, magnetic field frequencies, or near-infrared light [267] to mediate the cascading release sequence.

Nanomedical species ranging from drug nanoparticles to sophisticated autonomous nanodevices might be incrementally released according to a precisely programmed schedule in order to carry out complementary diagnostic, therapeutic, or monitoring tasks over a prescribed treatment cycle. This cascading release sequence may be configured to proceed for months or even years [268,269], whose administration and course of treatment would be determined and prescribed by a physician to efficaciously address a specific condition or disease state.

2.8.5 Dermal Burrowing

Freitas' envisioned nanometric telescopic manipulators, which might enable micron-sized ice-burrowing nanorobots to traverse this media at ~1 µm/s [75], may be adapted to allow the traversal of the extracellular matrix within the various skin tissue strata. This ingress strategy could have the potential for generating a degree of discomfort that is initiated by transiting nanodevices, should they have rough angular edges or extending protuberances that unwittingly mechanically perturb free nerve endings. They may also run the risk of an immune response, resulting in localized irritation [75]. Therefore, it is highly likely that rounded and smooth nanodevice surfaces will be preferable toward the prevention of any itching or rash imparted to the skin. There may, of course, be exceptions to the rule for those instances where particular nanodevice morphologies are linked to specific tasks (e.g., neurological or vascular plaque removal, or the discriminate "lancing" of cells or pathogens that are tagged with distinguishing nanometric markers for eradication). Even so, under these conditions, nanomedical designers will endeavor to integrate retractable or sheathed sharp-edged or pointed nanoscale instrumentation that would remain internalized until required for specific therapeutic assignments.

Ishiyama et al. have investigated spiral-configured magnetically driven micromachines with the aim of developing a potential application for their burrowing into tumors and subsequently eradicating them via hyperthermia. Trials were conducted with these devices whereby they were activated to spin their way through gelinatous test media under the control of a rotating magnetic field [270]. The use of a magnetic field may prove feasible as an alternative method for the actuation and ingress of augerytes through various biological barriers. This would entail an advanced capacity for the externally mediated localized manipulation of magnetic fields in multiple orientations combined with potent nanoscale superparamagnetic elements that are embedded within the augeryte helical tail sections.

2.9 Nanodevice Egress Strategies

The egress of nanomedical devices may not present as daunting a challenge as their ingress into the human body. However, this aspect of any nanomedical procedure will certainly be equivalent in importance. Egress protocols that are instituted subsequent to diagnostic or therapeutic treatments will require serious and careful contemplation, as it will be assumed that all nanodevices that are administered to the patient must be accounted for and removed, or be programmed to situate themselves at predetermined sites that will facilitate their future safe egress over a more protracted time line. A conceivable exception may be nanodevices that comprise completely of biodegradable materials. These classes of nanodevices, albeit perhaps imbued with limited capabilities, may indeed be plausible in view of the rapid progress that is being made in the areas of smart polymeric materials, artificial muscle technologies, biomimetics, advanced piezomaterials, and hybrid organic/inorganic constructs [271–281].

A theoretical, albeit long time-lined approach might involve the migration of nanodevices to the germinal matrix (*stratum corneum*) of the fingernail or toenail beds (Figure 2.23). Once situated in these areas they would implant themselves within the milieu that forms the nail material, which is comprised of proteins, keratin, and sulfur where they would be instructed to power down to static status. The encapsulated nanodevices would then slowly and naturally "grow" out of the patient within the nails at a rate ~0.05 to 1.2 mm/week. A more expeditious

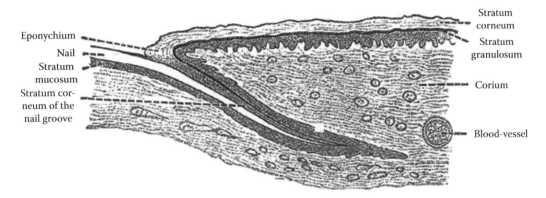

Eponychium

Nail

Stratum mucosum

Stratum corneum of the nail groove

Stratum corneum

Stratum granulosum

Corium

Blood-vessel

FIGURE 2.23
Artistic rendering of the fingernail bed wherein nanodevices may embed themselves for prolonged egress. (From Gray, H., *Anatomy of the Human Body*, Lea & Febiger, Philadelphia, PA, 1918, Bartleby.com, 2000.)

"grow-out" egress strategy would be for nanodevices to embed themselves within the biomatrix (e.g., keratin, trichohyalin granules, and melanin) of nascent hair follicles to emanate from the patient at a much more rapid ~1 cm/month. Since the diameter of hair follicles is within the ~17 to 181 μm range, there will be a considerable mass within which 1 μm in diameter nanodevices may implant themselves [282,283]. Further up the scale of egress rapidity (~24 h) for nanodevices are scenarios where they might exit from the patient via self-embedment within the biomass of the GIT, or by flushing within excretive fluids such as sweat or urine.

A hypothetical egress method that might be instituted subsequent to a nanomedical diagnostic or therapeutic task could involve the initiation of an external homing signal, perhaps generated by a dermally applied nanodevice "retrieval patch," which would trigger an auto-command for all nanodevices to immediately travel to the signal source. Once in range of the patch, nanodevices will burrow up from the deeper epidermal layers to the surface of the skin whereupon they might be adsorbed to a specifically nanoengineered undersurface of the patch for subsequent removal. Contingent on the extent of nanodevice and infrastructural sophistication, this conceptual procedure might be completed within tens of minutes.

Critical steps that are inherent to each of these egress options will be that all nanodevices are accounted for via "all-clear" verification protocols. Should any nanodevices be left behind due to a malfunction or by physical entrapment, an onboard auto-tripped signal beacon would indicate its precise location for subsequent retrieval by specialized nanodevices ("n-tugs") with enhanced propulsion systems, robust grippers, manipulator arms, and relatively large cargo holds within which the stranded nanodevices would be stowed for egress transport. The particular mode of egress should proceed in a totally discreet and innocuous manner. This process should be as innocuous and unnoticeable as the low-level perspiration that is continually emanating from the pores of the skin.

2.10 VCSN Deployment/Recovery Strategies

2.10.1 VCSN Ingress

Aside from the typical operation of the VCSN in vivo, strategies for its effective ingress and egress pose no insignificant challenges. How might these devices be introduced into the vasculature, and how they will be recovered once scanning procedures have been completed? These operations may be considered tangential, albeit essential facets of the VCSN's propulsive and navigation capabilities. Several deployment and recovery approaches might be methodically investigated in order to determine the best candidate for ingress into and egress from the human body.

VCSN deployment modes may include injection, inhalation, ingestion, or epidermal transfer as described earlier. Injection would likely be the most straightforward, though the most invasive of ingress methods, although, to reiterate, one would imagine that by the time a VCSN-caliber technology comes online for clinical use (~15 to 20 years), hypodermic injection may no longer be in regular use. The VCSN might be inhaled via an aerosolized carrier media and may enter the bloodstream via the pulmonary capillaries. Detailed permeability studies of the respiratory membrane would elucidate whether the ~1 μm VCSN might be small enough to diffuse across the lung–blood barrier, or if another method of vascular ingress from the lung may be necessary. Additional studies would aim to reveal what effects that lung-bound cilia would have on the VCSN (in that the cilia may likely attempt to "sweep" the VCSN out of the lungs, treating it as a foreign particulate), and if the VCSN might become trapped in alveolar sacs en route to vascular ingress sites.

A prescribed population of VCSNs might be swallowed in pill form and enter the bloodstream by traversing the stomach lining into the bloodstream via embedded capillaries. Issues to explore here would be toward the determination of the effects that gastric juices may have on the nanodevices. A determination of the probable impacts that this composite chemical environment would have on external VCSN surfaces/biocompatible coatings and exposed propulsive elements would be a worthwhile endeavor.

An adhesive patch or an application of a viscous gel suspension containing a predetermined number of VCSNs may provide a preferable method for administration, as the devices would unnoticeably diffuse through the various epidermal cell layers along with paracellular fluid movement (passage of water between cells) or through epidermal pores and into the bloodstream. A primary issue to explore in this area would be the ability of the devices to enter through the exterior walls of the capillaries without the initiation of biodisruption (e.g., chemical modification, elicitation of immune response).

2.10.2 VCSN Egress

Of equivalent importance to VCSN ingress would be the formulation of techniques for egress from the patient, post-scan. One hypothetical (albeit quite protracted) method, as described earlier, would be to instruct the VCSNs to migrate to the germinal matrix (behind the nail beds of the fingers and toes), where they would embed themselves in the matrix that forms the nail material (proteins, keratin, and sulfur) and permanently shut down. They would remain encapsulated there eventually and "grow" out of the body naturally.

Should prescribed protocol include that all originally deployed VCSNs are to be collected at a single location, an adhesive patch that contains a homing beacon might be applied to the stratum corneum. When the scanning procedure has been completed, all nanodevices might be instructed to lock onto the coordinates of the adhered patch and rapidly migrate from wherever they may be positioned within the patient, to bind with specially prepared "docking sites" located on the underside of the patch. This procedure might take place within minutes. Primary considerations here would be that first, all devices are accounted for via "all-clear" protocols (mentioned earlier), and second this mode of egress should proceed in a discreet and innocuous manner.

For chemically mediated adhesion, these docking sites might comprise nanotubes or nanofibers that are "decorated" with particular molecules, which have potent binding affinities (via hydrogen bonds, ionic bonds, van der Waals forces, or electrostatics) for the molecular constituents of biocompatible coatings that veil the exterior surfaces of the VCSN. Alternately, the provision of mechanical linkages may be implemented for this function, whereby dedicated telescopic docking "stalks" (similar in function to those proposed for the aggrecyte class nanodevices described earlier) may be engaged with mating orifices that are endowed with autolocking mechanisms. These docking orifices would be embedded within thin films located on the underside of the patch, to ensure stable mechanical VCSN tethering.

Much more expeditious egress methods may include commands that instruct VCSNs to implant themselves within the matrix of forming hair follicles to subsequently grow out with the hair. Even more rapid egress scenarios might include exiting the body naturally via migration and self-embedding within the biomass of the intestinal tract, or natural diffusion out of the system by bodily fluids subsequent to shutdown.

References

1. Lodish, H., Berk, A., Zipursky, S.L., Matsudaira, P., Baltimore, D., and Darnell. J., *Molecular Cell Biology*, 4th edition. New York: W.H. Freeman, 2000.
2. Anal, A.K. and Singh, H., Recent advances in microencapsulation of probiotics for industrial applications and targeted delivery. *Trends Food Sci Tech*. 18, 240–251, 2007.
3. Dalmoro, A., Enteric microparticles coated with smart polymers for controlled drug delivery applications. Dissertation, 2009.
4. Frutos, G., Prior-Cabanillas, A., París, R., and Quijada-Garrido, I., A novel controlled drug delivery system based on pH-responsive hydrogels included in soft gelatin capsules. *Acta Biomater*. 6(12), 4650–4656, 2010.
5. Bell, C.L. and Peppas, N.A., Water, solute and protein diffusion in physiologically responsive hydrogels of poly(methacrylic acid-*g*-ethylene glycol). *Biomaterials*. 17, 1203–1218, 1996.
6. Zhang, J. and Peppas, N.A., Synthesis and characterization of pH- and temperature sensitive poly(methacrylic acid)/poly(*N*-isopropylacrylamide) interpenetrating polymeric networks. *Macromolecules*. 33, 102–107, 2000.
7. Sousa, R.G., Prior-Cabanillas, A., Quijada-Garrido, I., and Barrales-Rienda, J.M., Dependence of copolymer composition, swelling history, and drug concentration on the loading of diltiazem hydrochloride (DIL_HCl) into poly[(*N*-isopropylacrylamide)-*co*-(methacrylic acid) hydrogels and its release behaviour from hydrogel slabs. *J Control Release*. 102, 595–606, 2005.
8. Ulbrich, K., Šubr, V., Seymour, L.W., and Duncan, R. Novel biodegradable hydrogels prepared using the divinylic crosslinking agent *N,O*-dimethacryloylhydroxylamine. 1. Synthesis and characterisation of rates of gel degradation, and rate of release of model drugs, in vitro and in vivo. *J Control Release*. 24(1–3), 181–190, 1993.
9. Tortora, G.J., *Principles of Human Anatomy*. Biological Sciences Textbooks, Inc., New York: Harper Collins, 1992.
10. Muller, W.A., Mechanisms of leukocyte transendothelial migration. *Annu Rev Pathol*. 28(6), 323–344, 2011.
11. Lorenzon, P., Vecile, E., Nardon, E. Ferrero, E., Harlan, J.M., Tedesco, F., and Dobrina, A., Endothelial cell E- and P selectin and vascular cell adhesion molecule 1 function as signaling receptors. *J Cell Biol*. 142, 1381–1391, 1998.
12. van Buul, J.D., Kanters, E., and Hordijk, P.L., Endothelial signaling by Ig-like cell adhesion molecules. *Arterioscler Thromb Vasc Biol*. 27, 1870–1876, 2007.
13. Huang, A.J., Manning, J.E., Bandak, T.M., Ratau, M.C., Hanser, K.R., and Silverstein, S.C., Endothelial cell cytosolic free calcium regulates neutrophil migration across monolayers of endothelial cells. *J Cell Biol*. 120, 1371–1380, 1993.

14. Hixenbaugh, E.A., Goeckeler, Z.M., Papaiya, N.N., Wysolmerski, R.B., Silverstein, S.C., and Huang, A.J., Chemoattractant-stimulated neutrophils induce regulatory myosin light chain phosphorylation and isometric tension development in endothelial cells. *Am J Physiol.* 273, H981–H988, 1997.

15. Burns, A.R., Bowden, R.A., MacDonell, S.D., Walker, D.C., Odebunmi, T.O., Donnachie, E.M., Simon, S.I., Entman, M.L., and Smith, C.W., Analysis of tight junctions during neutrophil transendothelial migration. *J Cell Sci.* 113(Pt 1), 45–57, 2000; Burns, A.R., Walker, D.C., Brown, E.S., Thurmon, L.T., Bowden, R.A., Keese, C.R., Simon, S.I., Entman, M.L., and Smith, C.W., Neutrophil transendothelial migration is independent of tight junctions and occurs preferentially at tricellular corners. *J Immunol.* 159, 2893–2903, 1997.

16. Collins, L.M. and Dawes, C., The surface area of the adult human mouth and thickness of the salivary film covering the teeth and oral mucosa. *J Dent Res.* 66(8), 1300–1302, 1987.

17. Sudhakar, Y., Kuotsu, K., and Bandyopadhyay, A.K., Buccal bioadhesive drug delivery—A promising option for orally less efficient drugs. *J Control Release.* 114, 15–40, 2006.

18. Galey, W.R., Lonsdale, H.K., and Nacht, S., The in vitro permeability of skin and buccal mucosa to selected drugs and tritiated water. *J Invest Dermat.* 67, 713–717, 1976.

19. Nicolazzo, J.A., Reed, B.L., and Finnin, B.C., Buccal penetration enhancers—How do they really work? *J Control Release.* 105(1–2), 1–15, 2005.

20. Rathbon, M.J. and Hadgraft J., Absorption of drugs from the human oral cavity. *Int J Pharm.* 74, 9–24, 1991.

21. Chen, S.Y. and Squier, C.A., The ultrastructure of the oral epithelium, in Meyer, J., Squier, C.A., and Gerson, S.J., eds., *The Structure and Function of Oral Mucosa.* Oxford: Pergamon Press, 7–30, 1984.

22. Schroeder, H.E., *Differentiation of Human Oral Stratified Epithelia.* Basel: Karger, pp. 35–152, 1981.

23. Harris, D. and Robinson, J.R., Drug delivery via the mucous membranes of the oral cavity. *J Pharm Sci.* 81, 1–10, 1992.

24. Gandhi, R.B. and Robinson, J.R., Oral cavity as a site for bioadhesive drug delivery. *Adv Drug Deliv Rev.* 13, 43–74, 1994.

25. Rathbone, M.J., Drummond, B.K., and Tucker, I.G., The oral cavity as a site for systemic drug delivery. *Adv Drug Deliv Rev.* 13, 1–22, 1994.

26. Goswami, T., Jasti, B.R., and Li, X., Estimation of the theoretical pore sizes of the porcine oral mucosa for permeation of hydrophilic permeants. *Arch Oral Biol.* 54(6), 577–582, 2009.

27. Shojaei, A.H., Buccal mucosa as a route for systemic drug delivery: A review. *J Pharm Sci.* 1, 15–30, 1998.

28. Squier, C.A., Cox, P., and Wertz, P.W., Lipid content and water permeability of skin and oral mucosa. *J Invest Dermatol.* 96, 123–126, 1991.

29. Collins, P., Laffoon, J., and Squier, C.A., Comparative study of porcine oral epithelium. *J Dent Res.* 60, 543, 1981.

30. Pozzilli, P., Manfrini, S., Costanza, F., Coppolino, G., Cavallo, M.G., Fioriti, E., and Modi, P., Biokinetics of buccal spray insulin in patients with type 1 diabetes. *Metabolism.* 54(7), 930–934, 2005.

31. Heemstra, L.B., Finnin, B.C., and Nicolazzo, J.A., The buccal mucosa as an alternative route for the systemic delivery of risperidone. *J Pharm Sci.* 99(11), 4584–4592, 2010.

32. Wang, C., Swerdloff, R., Kipnes, M., Matsumoto, A., Dobs, A., Cunningham, G., Katznelson, L., Weber, T., Friedman, T., and Snyder, P., New testosterone buccal system (Striant) delivers physiological testosterone levels: Pharmacokinetics study in hypogonadal men. *J Clin Endocrinol Metab.* 89, 3821–3829, 2004.

33. Zhang, H., Zhang, J., and Streisand, J., Oral mucosal drug delivery: Clinical pharmacokinetics and therapeutic applications. *Clin Pharmacokinet.* 41, 661–680, 2002.

34. Hoogstraate, A.J., Senel, S., Cullander, C., Verhoef, J., Junginger, H.E., and Boddé, H.E., Effects of bile salts on transport rates and routes of FITC-labelled compounds across porcine buccal epithelium in vitro. *J Control Release.* 40, 211–221, 1996.

35. Deneer, V.H.M., Drese, G.B., Roemelé, P.E.H., Verhoef, J.C., Lie-A-Huen, L., Kingma, J.H., Brouwers, J.R.B.J., and Junginger, H.E., Buccal transport of flecainide and sotalol: Effect of a bile salt and ionization state. *Int J Pharm.* 241, 127–134, 2002.

36. Senel, S., Capan, Y., Sargon, M.F., Ikinci, G., Solpan, D., Güven, O., Boddé, H.E., and Hincal, A.A., Enhancement of transbuccal permeation of morphine sulfate by sodium glycodeoxycholate in vitro. *J Control Release.* 45, 153–162, 1997.
37. Senel, S., Duchêne, D., Hincal, A.A., Capan, Y., and Ponchel, G., In vitro studies on enhancing effect of sodium glycocholate on transbuccal permeation of morphine hydrochloride. *J Control Release.* 51, 107–113, 1998.
38. Hoogstraate, A.J., Verhoef, J.C., Pijpers, A., van Leengoed, L.A.M.G., Verheijden, J.H.M., Junginger, H.E., and Boddé, H.E., In vivo buccal delivery of the peptide drug buserelin with glycodeoxycholate as an absorption enhancer in pigs. *Pharm Res.* 13 1233–1237, 1996.
39. Siegel, I.A. and Gordon, H.P., Effects of surfactants on the permeability of canine oral mucosa in vitro. *Toxicol Lett.* 26, 153–157, 1985.
40. Siegel, I.A. and Gordon, H.P., Surfactant-induced increases of permeability of rat oral mucosa to non-electrolytes in vivo. *Arch Oral Biol.* 30, 43–47, 1985.
41. Siegel, I.A. and Gordon, H.P., Surfactant-induced alterations of permeability of rabbit oral mucosa in vitro. *Exp Mol Pathol.* 44, 132–137, 1986.
42. Aungst, B.J., Rogers, N.J., and Shefter, E., Comparison of nasal, rectal, buccal, sublingual and intramuscular insulin efficacy and the effects of a bile salt absorption promoter. *J Pharmacol Exp Ther.* 244, 23–27, 1988.
43. Oh, C.K. and Ritschel, W.A., Biopharmaceutic aspects of buccal absorption of insulin. *Methods Find Exp Clin Pharmacol.* 12, 205–212, 1990.
44. Xiang, J., Fang, X., and Li, X., Transbuccal delivery of 2′,3′ dideoxycytidine: In vitro permeation study and histological investigation. *Int J Pharm.* 231, 57–66, 2002.
45. Shojaei, A.H., Buccal mucosa as a route for systemic drug delivery: A review. *J Pharm Pharm Sci.* 1, 15–30, 1998.
46. Nicolazzo, J.A., Reed, B.L., and Finnin, B.C., Assessment of the effects of sodium dodecyl sulfate on the buccal permeability of caffeine and estradiol. *J Pharm Sci.* 93, 431–440, 2004.
47. Finnin, B.C., private communication. March 25, 2011.
48. Dale, A.C., Salivary glands, in Ten Cate, A.R., ed., *Oral Histology. Development, Structure and Function.* St. Louis, MO: C.V. Mosby, 303–331, 1985.
49. Azuma, M., Tamatani, T., Kasai, Y., and Sato, M., Immortalization of normal human salivary gland cells with duct-, myoepithelial-, acinar-, or squamous phenotype by transfection with SV40 ori-mutant deoxyribonucleic acid. *Lab Invest.* 69(1), 24–42, 1993.
50. Srivastava, L.M., in Talwar, G.P. and Srivastava, L.M., eds., *Textbook of Biochemistry and Human Biology.* New Delhi, India: Prentice Hall, 2006.
51. Roussa, E., Channels and transporters in salivary glands. *Cell Tissue Res.* 343(2), 263–287, 2011.
52. Thaysen, J.H., Thorn, N.A., and Schwartz, I.L., Excretion of sodium, potassium, chloride and carbon dioxide in human parotid saliva. *Am J Physiol.* 178, 155–159, 1954.
53. Bourgery, M.J., Traité complet de l'anatomie de l'homme. Paris, France: C. Delaunay, 1831–1854.
54. Aktan, Z.A., Bilge, O., Pinar, Y.A., and Ikiz, A.O., Duplication of the parotid duct: A previously unreported anomaly. *Surg Radiol Anat.* 23(5), 353–354, 2001.
55. Williams, P.L., Bannister, L.H., Berry, M.M., Collins, P., Dyson, M., Dussek, J.E., and Ferguson, M.V.J., *Gray's Anatomy. International Student Edition*, 28th edn. London, U.K.: Churchill Livingstone, pp. 1692–1699, 1995.
56. Zenk, J. and Werner, G., Diameters of the main excretory ducts of the adult human submandibular and parotid gland. *Oral Surg Oral Med Oral Pathol.* 85, 576–580, 1998.
57. Zhang, L., Xu, H., Cai, Z.G., Mao, C., Wang, Y., Peng, X., Zhu, Z.H., and Yu, G.Y., Clinical and anatomic study on the ducts of the submandibular and sublingual glands. *J Oral Maxillofac Surg.* 68(3), 606–610, 2010.
58. Humphrey, S.P. and Williamson, R.T., A review of saliva: Normal composition, flow, and function. *J Prosthet Dent.* 85(2), 162–169, 2001.
59. Roth, G. and Calmes, R., eds., Salivary glands and saliva. in *Oral Biology.* St. Louis, MO: C.V. Mosby, pp. 196–236, 1981.

60. Segal, A. and Wong, D.T., Salivary diagnostics: Enhancing disease detection and making medicine better. *Eur J Dent Educ.* 12(Suppl. 1), 22–29, 2008.
61. Dawes, C., Effects of diet on salivary secretion and composition. *J Dent Res Suppl.* 49(6), 1263–1272, 1970.
62. Chauncey, H.H., Feller, R.P., and Hendriques, B.L., Comparative electrolyte composition of parotid, submandibular and sublingual secretions, abstracted. *J Dent Res.* 45, 1230, 1966.
63. Scarano, E., Fiorita, A., Picciotti, P.M., Passali, G.C., Calò, L., Cabras, T., Inzitari, R., Fanali, C., Messana, I., Castagnola, M., and Paludetti, G., Proteomics of saliva: Personal experience. *Acta Otorhinolaryngol Ital.* 30(3), 125–130, 2010.
64. Wood, C.M. and Dawes, C., The composition of lip mucous gland secretions, abstracted. IADR Preprinted Abstracts, 100, 1968.
65. Schneyer, L.H., Amylase content of separate salivary gland secretions of man. *J Appl Physiol.* 9(3), 453–455, 1956.
66. Dawes, C. and Wood, C.M., The composition of human lip mucous gland secretions. *Arch Oral Biol.* 18(3), 343–350, 1973.
67. Shannon, I.L., Parotid fluid flow rate as related to whole saliva volume. *Arch Oral Biol.* 7, 391–394, 1962.
68. Gray, H., *Anatomy of the Human Body*. Philadelphia, PA: Lea & Febiger, 1918, Bartleby.com, 2000. Chapter X. The Organs of the Senses and the Common Integument. (accessed 06/19/13).
69. Roussa, E., private communication, March 31, 2011.
70. Avery, J.K., *Oral Development and Histology*. New York: Thieme Medical Publishers, 309, 2002.
71. Mimura, M., Tanaka, N., Ichinose, S., Kimijima, Y., and Amagasa, T., Possible etiology of calculi formation in salivary glands: Biophysical analysis of calculus. *Med Mol Morphol.* 38(3), 189–195, 2005.
72. Iro, H., Schneider, H.T., Fodra, C., Waitz, G., Nitsche, N., Heinritz, H.H., Benninger, J., and Ell, C., Shockwave lithotripsy of salivary duct stones. *Lancet.* 339, 1333–1336, 1992.
73. Iro, H., Zenk, J., and Benzel, W., Minimally invasive therapy for sialolithiasis: The state of the art, in Myers, E.N., Bluestone, C.D., Brackmann, D.E., and Krause, C.J., eds., *Advances in Otolaryngology: Head and Neck Surgery*, Vol. 9. St. Louis, MO: C.V. Mosby, pp. 31–48, 1995.
74. Drexler, K.E., *Nanosystems: Molecular Machinery, Manufacturing, and Computation*. New York: John Wiley & Sons, 1992.
75. Freitas, R.A. Jr., *Nanomedicine, Volume I: Basic Capabilities*. Georgetown, TX: Landes Bioscience, 1999.
76. Glagolev, A.N., Proton circuits of bacterial flagella, in Skulachev, V.P. and Hinkle, P.C., eds., *Chemiosmotic Proton Circuits in Biological Membranes*. Reading, MA: Addison-Wesley, pp. 577–600, 1981.
77. Macnab, R.M. and Aizawa S.I., Bacterial motility and bacterial flagellar motor. *Annu Rev Biophys Bioeng.* 13, 51–83, 1984.
78. Yorimitsu, T. and Homma, M., Na^+-driven flagellar motor of *Vibrio*. *Biochim Biophys Acta.* 1505(1), 82–93, 2001.
79. Neidhardt, F.C., *Escherichia coli and Salmonella typhimurium: Cellular and Molecular Biology*, 2nd edition. Washington, DC: American Society for Microbiology, 123–145, 1996.
80. Manson, M.D., Tedesco, P., Berg, H.C., Harold, F.M., and Van der Drift, C., A protonmotive force drives bacterial flagella. *Proc Natl Acad Sci USA.* 74(7), 3060–3064, 1977.
81. Matsura, S., Shioi, J., and Imae, Y., Motility in *Bacillus subtilis* driven by an artificial protonmotive force. *FEBS Lett.* 82(2), 187–190, 1977.
82. Larsen, S.H., Adler, J., Gargus, J.J., and Hogg, R.W., Chemomechanical coupling without ATP: The source of energy for motility and chemotaxis in bacteria. *Proc Natl Acad Sci USA.* 71(4), 1239–1243, 1974.
83. Glagolev, A.N. and Skulachev, V.P., The proton pump is a molecular engine of motile bacteria. *Nature.* 272(5650), 280–282, 1978.
84. Chernyak, B.V., Dibrov, P.A., Glagolev, A.N., Sherman, M.Y., and Skulachev, V.P., A novel type of energetics in a marine alkali tolerant bacterium. AfNa-driven motility and sodium cycle. *FEBS Lett.* 164, 38–42, 1983.

85. Dibrov, P.A., Kostyrko, V.A., Lazarova, R.L., Skulachev, V.P., and Smirnova, I.A., The sodium cycle. 1. Na$^+$-dependent motility and modes of membrane energization in the marine alkalotolerant *Vibrio alginolyticus*. *Biochim Biophys Acta*. 850, 449–457, 1986.

86. Kitada, M., Guffanti, A.A., and Krulwich, T.A., Bioenergetic properties and viability of alkalophilic *Bacillus firnius* RAB as a function of pH and Nat contents in the incubation medium. *J Bacteriol*. 152, 1096–1104, 1982.

87. Imae, Y. and Atsumi, T., Na$^+$-driven bacterial flagellar motors. *J Bioenerg Biomembr*. 1(6), 705–716, 1989.

88. Hirota, N. and Imae, Y., Na$^+$-driven flagellar motors of an alkalophilic *Bacillus* strain YN-1. *J Biol Chem*. 258(17), 10577–10581, 1983.

89. Sugiyama, S., Matsukura, H., and Imae, Y., Relationship between Na$^+$-dependent cytoplasmic pH homeostasis and Na$^+$-dependent flagellar rotation and amino acid transport in alkalophilic *Bacillus*. *FEBS Lett*. 182(2), 265–268, 1985.

90. Imae, Y., Matsukura, H., and Kobayasi, S., Sodium-driven flagellar motors of alkalophilic *Bacillus*. *Methods Enzymol*. 125, 582–592, 1986.

91. Diez, M., Zimmermann, B., Börsch, M., König, M., Schweinberger, E., Steigmiller S, Reuter, R., Felekyan, S., Kudryavtsev, V., Seidel, C.A., and Gräber, P., Proton-powered subunit rotation in single membrane-bound F0F1-ATP synthase. *Nat Struct Mol Biol*. 11(2), 135–141, 2004.

92. Stahlberg, H., Müller, D.J., Suda, K., Fotiadis, D., Engel, A., Meier, T., Matthey, U., and Dimroth, P., Bacterial Na$^+$-ATP synthase has an undecameric rotor. *EMBO Rep*. 2(3), 229–233, 2001.

93. Edgar, M., Saliva: Its secretion, composition and functions, in Harris, M., Edgar, M., and Meghji, S., eds., *Clinical Oral Science*. Oxford, U.K.: Reed Educational and Professional Publishing, Ltd., p. 179, 1998.

94. Eliasson, L., Birkhed, D., Heyden, G., and Strömberg, N., Studies on human minor salivary gland secretions using the Periotron method. *Arch Oral Biol*. 41(12), 1179–1182, 1996.

95. Ferguson, D.B., The flow rate and composition of human labial gland saliva. *Arch Oral Biol*. 44(Suppl. 1), S11–S14, 1999.

96. Jurysta, C., Bulur, N., Oguzhan, B., Satman, I., Yilmaz, T.M., Malaisse, W.J., and Sener, A., Salivary glucose concentration and excretion in normal and diabetic subjects. *J Biomed Biotechnol*. 430426, 2009.

97. Fejerskov, O., Kidd, E., and Kidd, E.A.M., *Dental Caries: The Disease and Its Clinical Management*. Tunbridge Wells, U.K.: Gray Publishing, 2008.

98. Jiménez-Reyes, M. and Sánchez-Aguirre, F.J., Sodium and chlorine concentrations in mixed saliva of healthy and cystic fibrosis children. *Appl Radiat Isot*. 47(3), 273–277, 1996.

99. Karjalainen, S., Sewón, L., Söderling, E., Larsson, B., Johansson, I., Simell, O., Lapinleimu, H., and Seppänen, R., Salivary cholesterol of healthy adults in relation to serum cholesterol concentration and oral health. *J Dent Res*. 76(10), 1637–1643, 1997.

100. Lin, L.Y. and Chang, C.C., Determination of protein concentration in human saliva. *Gaoxiong Yi Xue Ke Xue Za Zhi*. 5(7), 389–397, 1989.

101. Arneberg, P., Quantitative determination of protein in saliva. A comparison of analytical methods. *Scand J Dent Res*. 79(1), 60–64, 1971.

102. Bortolini, M.J., De Agostini, G.G., Reis, I.T., Lamounier, R.P., Blumberg, J.B., and Espindola F.S., Total protein of whole saliva as a biomarker of anaerobic threshold. *Res Q Exerc Sport*. 80(3), 604–610, 2009.

103. Moore, K.L. and Dalley, A.F., *Clinically Oriented Anatomy*. Baltimore, MD: Lippincott Williams & Wilkins, pp. 865–872, 948, 1999.

104. Cawson, R. and Gleeson, M., Anatomy and physiology of the salivary glands, in Kerr, A.G., ed., *Scott–Brown's Otolaryngology*. Oxford, U.K.: Butterworth Heinemann, pp. 1–18, 1997.

105. Williams, P.L., *Gray's Anatomy*. Edinburgh: Churchill Livingstone, 1519, 1691–1700, 1995.

106. Martinoli, Cm, Derchi, L.E., Solbiati, L., Rizatto, G., Silvestri, E., and Giannoni, M., Color Doppler sonography of salivary glands. *AJR Am J Roentgenol*. 163, 933–941, 1994.

107. van Holten, M.J., Roesink, J.M., Terhaard, C.H., and Braam, P.M., New insights in the vascular supply of the human parotid gland—Consequences for parotid gland-sparing irradiation. *Head Neck.* 32(7), 837–843, 2010.
108. Junqueira, L.C., Carneiro, J., and Kelley, R.O., *Basic Histology*, 9th edn. New York: McGraw-Hill, 1998.
109. Rudman, R.A., in Lang, J., ed., *Clinical Anatomy of the Masticatory Apparatus and Peripharyngeal Spaces.* New York: Thieme Medical Publishers, 1995.
110. Cameron, J.R., Skofronick, J.G., and Grant, R.M., *Physics of the Body*, 2nd edition. Madison, WI: Medical Physics Publishing, p. 113, 1999.
111. Beleńkaia, I.M., Zarubina, I.L., and Spitkovskaia, L.V., Study of microcirculation of the human mouth mucosa by the method of contact microscopy. *Arkh Anat Gistol Embriol.* 72(1), 72–76, 1977.
112. Sinoway, L.I., Hendrickson, C., Davidson, W.R. Jr., Prophet, S., and Zelis, R., Characteristics of flow-mediated brachial artery vasodilation in human subjects. *Circ Res.* 64, 32–42, 1989.
113. Chuo, L.S., Mahmud, R., and Salih, Q.A., Color Doppler ultrasound examination of the main portal vein and inferior vena cava in normal Malaysian adult population: A fasting and post prandial evaluation. *Int J Cardiovasc Res.* 2(2), 2005.
114. Cohen, M.L., Cohen, B.S., Kronzon, I., Lighty, G.W., and Winer, H.E., Superior vena caval blood flow velocities in adults: A Doppler echocardiographic study. *J Appl Physiol.* 61(1), 215–219, 1986.
115. Ochs, M., Nyengaard, J.R., Jung, A., Knudsen, L., Voigt, M., Wahlers, T., Richter, J., and Gundersen, H.J., The number of alveoli in the human lung. *Am J Respir Crit Care Med.* 169(1), 120–124, 2004.
116. Shields, T.W., *General Thoracic Surgery.* Philadelphia, PA: Lippincott Williams & Wilkins, 2009.
117. Haagsman, H.P. and Diemel, R.V., Surfactant-associated proteins: Functions and structural variation. *Comp Biochem Physiol A.* 129, 91–108, 2001.
118. Schurch, S., Lee, M., and Gehr, P., Pulmonary surfactant: Surface properties and function of alveolar and airway surfactant. *Pure Appl Chem.* 64(11), 1745–1750, 1992.
119. Zhang, S., *An Atlas of Histology.* New York: Springer-Verlag, 1999.
120. Thiberville, L., Salaün, M., Lachkar, S., Dominique, S., Moreno-Swirc, S., Vever-Bizet, C., and Bourg-Heckly, G., Human in vivo fluorescence microimaging of the alveolar ducts and sacs during bronchoscopy. *Eur Respir J.* 33(5), 974–985, 2009.
121. Hyde, D.M., Tyler, N.K., Putney, L.F., Singh, P., and Gundersen, H.J., Total number and mean size of alveoli in mammalian lung estimated using fractionator sampling and unbiased estimates of the Euler characteristic of alveolar openings. *Anat Rec A Discov Mol Cell Evol Biol.* 277, 216–226, 2004.
122. Tortora, G.J., *Principals of Human Anatomy.* New York: Harper Collins, 1992.
123. Mühlfeld, C., Weibel, E.R., Hahn, U., Kummer, W., Nyengaard, J.R., and Ochs, M., Is length an appropriate estimator to characterize pulmonary alveolar capillaries? A critical evaluation in the human lung. *Anat Rec (Hoboken).* 293(7), 1270–1275, 2010.
124. Levitzky, M.G., *Pulmonary Physiology.* New York: McGraw-Hill Medical, 2007.
125. Singhal, S., Henderson, R., Horsfield, K., Harding, K., and Cumming, G., Morphometry of the human pulmonary arterial tree. *Circ Res.* 33(2), 190–197, 1973. Cited in Freitas, R.A. Jr., *Nanomedicine, Volume I: Basic Capabilities.* Georgetown, TX: Landes Bioscience, 1999.
126. Finlay, W.H., *The Mechanics of Inhaled Pharmaceutical Aerosols: An Introduction.* San Diego, CA: Academic Press, 2001.
127. Wiebert, P., Sanchez-Crespo, A., Seitz, J., Falk, R., Philipson, K., Kreyling, W.G., Moller, W., Sommerer, K., Larsson, S., and Svartengren, M., Negligible clearance of ultrafine particles retained in healthy and affected human lungs. *Eur Respir J.* 28(2), 286–290, 2006.
128. Hawkins, B.T. and Davis, T.P., The blood–brain barrier/neurovascular unit in health and disease. *Pharmacol Rev.* 57(2), 173–185, 2005.
129. Beyerle, A., Merkel, O., Stoeger, T., and Kissel, T., PEGylation affects cytotoxicity and cell compatibility of poly(ethylene imine) for lung application: Structure function relationships. *Toxicol Appl Pharmacol.* 242(2), 146–154, 2010.

130. Stoeger, T., Reinhard, C., Takenaka, S., Schroeppel, A., Karg, E., Ritter, B., Heyder, J., and Schulz, H., Instillation of six different ultrafine carbon particles indicates a surface area threshold dose for acute lung inflammation in mice. *Environ Health Perspect.* 114(3), 328–333, 2006.

131. Stoeger, T., Takenaka, S., Frankenberger, B., Ritter, B., Karg, E., Maier, K., Schulz, H., and Schmid, O., Deducing in vivo toxicity of combustion-derived nanoparticles from a cell-free oxidative potency assay and metabolic activation of organic compounds. *Environ Health Perspect.* 117, 54–60, 2009.

132. Mamdouh, Z., Chen, X., Pierini, L.M., Maxfield, F.R., and Muller, W.A., Targeted recycling of PECAM from endothelial surface-connected compartments during diapedesis. *Nature.* 421(6924), 748–753, 2003.

133. Bailey, M.M. and Berkland, C.J., Nanoparticle formulations in pulmonary drug delivery. *Med Res Rev.* 29(1), 196–212, 2009.

134. Andrade, F., Videira, M., Ferreira, D., and Sarmento, B., Nanocarriers for pulmonary administration of peptides and therapeutic proteins. *Nanomedicine (Lond).* 6(1), 123–141, 2011.

135. Mansour, H.M., Rhee, Y.S., and Wu, X., Nanomedicine in pulmonary delivery. *Int J Nanomed.* 4, 299–319, 2009.

136. Gessler, T., Inhalative pharmacotherapy in the future—Nanocarriers for pulmonary drug delivery. *Pneumologie.* 63(Suppl. 2), S113–S116, 2009.

137. Roy, I. and Vij, N., Nanodelivery in airway diseases: Challenges and therapeutic applications. *Nanomedicine.* 6(2), 237–244, 2010.

138. Buxton, D.B., Nanomedicine for the management of lung and blood diseases. *Nanomedicine (Lond).* 4(3), 331–339, 2009.

139. Pison, U, Welte, T., Giersig, M., and Groneberg, D.A., Nanomedicine for respiratory diseases. *Eur J Pharmacol.* 533(1–3), 341–350, 2006.

140. Takizawa, H., Recent development of drug delivery systems for the treatment of asthma and related disorders. *Recent Pat Inflamm Allergy Drug Discov.* 3(3), 232–239, 2009.

141. Gomez, A., The electrospray and its application to targeted drug inhalation. *Respir Care.* 47(12), 1419–1431, discussion 1431–1433, 2002.

142. Kim, S.C., Chen, D.R., Qi, C., Gelein, R.M., Finkelstein, J.N., Elder, A., Bentley, K., Oberdörster, G., and Pui, D.Y., A nanoparticle dispersion method for in vitro and in vivo nanotoxicity study. *Nanotoxicology.* 4(1), 42–51, 2010.

143. Dhand, R., Malik, S.K., Balakrishnan, M., and Verma, S.R., High speed photographic analysis of aerosols produced by metered dose inhalers. *J Pharm Pharmacol.* 40(6), 429–430, 1988.

144. Patton, J.S., Fishburn, C.S., and Weers, J.G., The lungs as a portal of entry for systemic drug delivery. *Proc Am Thorac Soc.* 1(4), 338–344, 2004.

145. Lohade, A.A., Singh, D.J., Parmar, J.J., Hegde, D.D., Menon, M.D., Soni, P.S., Samad, A., and Gaikwad, R.V., Albumin microspheres of fluticasone propionate inclusion complexes for pulmonary delivery. *Ind J Pharm Sci.* 69(5), 707–709, 2007.

146. Beyer, J., Schwartz, S., Barzen, G., Risse, G., Dullenkopf, K., Weyer, C., and Siegert, W., Use of amphotericin B aerosols for the prevention of pulmonary aspergillosis. *Infection.* 22, 143–148, 1994.

147. Brooks, A.D., Tong, W., Benedetti, F., Kaneda, Y., Miller, V., and Warrell, R.P., Inhaled aerosolization of all-trans-retinoic acid for targeted pulmonary delivery. *Cancer Chemother Pharmacol.* 46, 313–318, 2000.

148. Patton, J.S., Mechanisms of macromolecular absorption by the lungs. *Adv Drug Deliv Rev.* 19, 3–36, 1996.

149. Adjei, L.A. and Gupta, P.K., Inhalation delivery of therapeutic peptides and proteins, in Lenfant, C., executive ed., *Lung Biology in Health and Disease.* New York: Marcel Dekker, pp. 1–913, 1997.

150. Hung, O.R., Whynot, S.C., Varvel, J.R., Shafer, S.L., and Mezei, M., Pharmacokinetics of inhaled liposome-encapsulated fentanyl. *Anesthesiology.* 83, 277–284, 1995.

151 Tan, S., Hung, O., and Whynot, S.C., Sustained tissue drug concentrations following inhalation of liposome-encapsulated fentanyl in rabbits. *Drug Deliv.* 3, 251–254, 1996.

152. Masood, A.R. and Thomas, S.H.L., Systemic absorption of nebulized morphine compared with oral morphine in healthy subjects. *Br J Clin Pharmacol.* 41, 250–252, 1996.

153. Takeuchi, H., Yamamoto, H., and Kawashima, Y., Mucoadhesive nanoparticulate systems for peptide drug delivery. *Adv Drug Deliv Rev.* 47(1), 39–54, 2001.
154. Yamamoto, A., Umemori, S., and Muranishi, S., Absorption enhancement of intrapulmonary administered insulin by various absorption enhancers and protease inhibitors in rats. *J Pharm Pharmacol.* 46(1), 14–18, 1994.
155. Rudolph, C., Gleich, B., and Flemmer, A.W., Magnetic aerosol targeting of nanoparticles to cancer: Nanomagnetosols. *Methods Mol Biol.* 624, 267–280, 2010.
156. Hussain, A.A., Mechanism of nasal absorption of drugs. *Prog Clin Biol Res.* 292, 261–272, 1989.
157. Dale, O., Hjortkjaer, R., and Kharasch, E.D., Nasal administration of opioids for pain management in adults. *Acta Anaesthesiol Scand.* 46(7), 759–770, 2002.
158. Chien, Y.W., Su, K.S.E., and Chang, S.F., Chapter 1: Anatomy and physiology of the nose. *Nasal Systemic Drug Delivery.* New York: Dekker, 1–26, 1989.
159. Westin, U.E., Olfactory transfer of analgesic drugs after nasal administration. Acta Universitatis Upsaliensis. Digital comprehensive summaries of Uppsala Dissertations for the Faculty of Pharmacy 55, 64, 2007.
160. Mathison, S., Nagilla, R., and Kompella, U.B., Nasal route for direct delivery of solutes to the central nervous system: Fact or fiction? *J Drug Target.* 5(6), 415–441, 1998.
161. Illum, L., Is nose-to-brain transport of drugs in man a reality? *J Pharm Pharmacol.* 56(1), 3–17, 2004.
162. Illum, L. Nasal drug delivery-possibilities, problems and solutions. *J Control Release.* 87(1–3), 187–198, 2003.
163. Illum, L., Bioadhesive formulations for nasal peptide delivery, in Mathiowitz, E., Lehr, C.M., and Chickering, D., eds., *Drug Delivery-Issues in Fundamentals, Novel Approaches and Development.* New York: Marcel Dekker, 507–539, 1998.
164. Donald, B.R., Levey, C.G., and Paprotny, I., Planar microassembly by parallel actuation of MEMS microrobots. *J Microelectromech Syst.* 17(4), 789–808, 2008.
165. Donald, B.R., Levey, C.G., Paprotny, I., and Rus, D., Simultaneous control of multiple mems microrobots, *The Eighth International Workshop on the Algorithmic Foundations of Robotics (WAFR).* Guanajuato, Mexico, December 7–9, 2008.
166. Hall, J.S., Utility Fog: A Universal Physical Substance, Vision-21, Westlake, OH, NASAv Conference Publication, 10129, 115–126, 1993.
167. Hall, J.S., Utility fog: The stuff that dreams are made of, in Crandall, B.C., ed., *Nanotechnology: Molecular Speculations on Global Abundance.* Cambridge, MA: MIT Press, pp. 161–184, 1996.
168. Kung, M.P., Hou, C., Zhuang, Z.P., Skovronsky, D., and Kung, H.F., Binding of two potential imaging agents targeting amyloid plaques in postmortem brain tissues of patients with Alzheimer's disease. *Brain Res.* 1025(1–2), 98–105, 2004.
169. Solomon, B., Immunological approach for the treatment of Alzheimer's disease. *J Mol Neurosci.* 20(3), 283–286, 2003.
170. Talegaonkar, S. and Mishra, P.R., Intranasal delivery: An approach to bypass the blood brain barrier. *Ind J Pharmacol.* 36(3), 140–147, 2004.
171. Nowacek, A. and Gendelman, H.E., NanoART, neuroAIDS and CNS drug delivery. *Nanomedicine (Lond).* 4(5), 557–574, 2009.
172. Liu, X., Chen, C., and Smith, B.J., Progress in brain penetration evaluation in drug discovery and development. *J Pharmacol Exp Ther.* 325(2), 349–356, 2008.
173. Liu, X. and Chen, C., Strategies to optimize brain penetration in drug discovery. *Curr Opin Drug Discov Devel.* 8(4), 505–512, 2005.
174. Pardridge, W.M., Blood–brain barrier biology and methodology. *J Neurovirol.* 5(6), 556–69, 1999.
175. Weiss, N., Miller, F., Cazaubon, S., and Couraud, P.O., Biology of the blood–brain barrier: Part I. *Rev Neurol (Paris).* 165(11), 863–874, 2009.
176. Graff, C.L. and Pollack G.M., Drug transport at the blood–brain barrier and the choroid plexus. *Curr Drug Metab.* 5(1), 95–108, 2004.
177. Loscher, W. and Potschka, H., Role of drug efflux transporters in the brain for drug disposition and treatment of brain diseases. *Prog Neurobiol.* 76(1), 22–76, 2005.

178. Graff, C.L. and Pollack, G.M., Nasal drug administration: Potential for targeted central nervous system delivery. *J Pharm Sci.* 94(6), 1187–1195, 2005.

179. Thorne, R.G., Pronk, G.J., Padmanabhan V., and Frey, W.H. II., Delivery of insulin-like growth factor-I to the rat brain and spinal cord along olfactory and trigeminal pathways following intranasal administration. *Neuroscience.* 127(2), 481–496, 2004.

180. Evans, J. and Hastings, L., Accumulation of Cd(II) in the CNS depending on the route of administration: Intraperitoneal, intratracheal, or intranasal. *Fundam Appl Toxicol.* 19(2), 275–278, 1992.

181. Perlman, S., Sun, N., and Barnett, E.M., Spread of MHV-JHM from nasal cavity to white matter of spinal cord. Transneuronal movement and involvement of astrocytes. *Adv Exp Med Biol.* 380, 73–78, 1995.

182. Thorne, R.G., Emory, C.R., Ala, T.A., and Frey, W.H. II., Quantitative analysis of the olfactory pathway for drug delivery to the brain. *Brain Res.* 692(1–2), 278–282, 1995.

183. Balin, B.J., Broadwell, R.D., Salcman, M., and El-Kalliny, M., Avenues for entry of peripherally administered protein to the central nervous system in mouse, rat, and squirrel monkey. *J Comp Neurol.* 251, 260–280, 1986.

184. Vallee, R.B. and Bloom, G.S., Mechanisms of fast and slow axonal transport, in Cowan, W.M., Shooter, E.M., Stevens C.F., and Thompson, R.F., eds., *Annual Review of Neuroscience*, Vol. 14. Palo Alto, CA: Annual Reviews, Inc., pp. 59–92, 1991.

185. Oberdörster, G., Sharp, Z., Atudorei, V., Elder, A., Gelein, R., Kreyling, W., and Cox, C., Translocation of inhaled ultrafine particles to the brain. *Inhal Toxicol.* 16(6–7), 437–445, 2004.

186. Shankland, W.E., The trigeminal nerve. Part III: The maxillary division. *Cranio.* 19(2), 78–83, 2001.

187. Schaefer, M.L., Bottger, B., Silver, W.L., and Finger, T.E., Trigeminal collaterals in the nasal epithelium and olfactory bulb: A potential route for direct modulation of olfactory information by trigeminal stimuli. *J Comp Neurol.* 444(3), 221–226, 2002.

188. Hunter, D.D. and Dey, R.D., Identification and neuropeptide content of trigeminal neurons innervating the rat nasal epithelium. *Neuroscience.* 83(2):591–599, 1998.

189. Chiou, G.C., Systemic delivery of polypeptide drugs through ocular route. *J Ocul Pharmacol.* 10(1), 93–99, 1994.

190. Bartlett, J.D. and Jaanus, S.D., *Clinical Ocular Pharmacology*. St. Louis, MO: Butterworth-Heinemann/Elsevier, 2008.

191. Chiou, G.C.Y., Shen, Z.F., Zheng, Y.Q., and Chen, Y.J., Enhancement of systemic delivery of peptide drugs via ocular route with surfactants. *Drug Dev Res.* 27(2), 177–183, 1992.

192. Xuan, B., McClellan, D.A., Moore, R., and Chiou, G.C., Alternative delivery of insulin via eye drops. *Diabetes Technol Ther.* 7(5), 695–698, 2005.

193. Ahmed, I., Gokhale, R.D., Shah, M.V., and Patton, T.F., Physicochemical determinants of drug diffusion across the conjunctiva, sclera, and cornea. *J Pharm Sci.* 76, 583–586, 1987.

194. Wang, W., Sasaki, H., Chien, D.-S., and Lee, V.H.L., Lipophilicity influence on conjunctival drug penetration in the pigmented rabbit: A comparison with corneal penetration. *Curr Eye Res.* 10, 571–579, 1991.

195. Loftsson, T. and Stefánsson, E., Effect of cyclodextrins on topical drug delivery to the eye. *Drug Devel Ind Pharm.* 23, 473–481, 1997.

196. Gad, S.C., *Pharmaceutical Manufacturing Handbook: Production and Processes*, Vol. 10. Hoboken, NJ: John Wiley & Sons, 2008.

197. Loftsson, T. and Stefánsson, E., Cyclodextrins in eye drop formulations: Enhanced topical delivery of corticosteroids to the eye. *Acta Ophthalmol Scand.* 80(2), 144–150, 2002.

198. Akhter, S., Talegaonkar, S., Khan, Z.I., Jain, G.K., Khar, R.K., and Ahmad, F.J., Assessment of ocular pharmacokinetics and safety of ganciclovir loaded nanoformulations. *J Biomed Nanotechnol.* 7(1), 144–145, 2011.

199. Das, S. and Suresh, P.K., Nanosuspension: A new vehicle for the improvement of the delivery of drugs to the ocular surface. Application to amphotericin B. *Nanomedicine.* 7(2), 242–247, 2011.

200. Kaur, I.P. and Kanwar, M., Ocular preparations: The formulation approach. *Drug Devel Ind Pharm.* 28, 473–493, 2002.

201. VanSantvliet, L. and Ludwig, A., The influence of penetration enhancers on the volume instilled of eye drops. *Eur J Pharm Biopharm.* 45, 189–198, 1998.
202. Chrai, S.S., Patton, T.F., Mehta, A., and Robinson, J.R., Lacrimal and instilled fluid dynamics in the rabbit eye. *J Pharm Sci.* 62, 1112–1121, 1973.
203 Washington, N., Washington, C., and Wilson, C.G., *Physiological Pharmaceutics: Barriers to Drug Absorption.* London, UK: Taylor & Francis, 2001.
204. Prow, T.W., Toxicity of nanomaterials to the eye. *Wiley Interdiscip Rev Nanomed Nanobiotechnol.* 2(4), 317–333, 2010.
205. Calvo, P., Vila-Jato, J.L., and Alonso, M.J., Comparative in vitro evaluation of several colloidal systems, nanoparticles, nanocapsules, and nanoemulsions, as ocular drug carriers. *J Pharm Sci.* 85, 530–536, 1996.
206. Ribeiro, A., Veiga, F., Santos, D., Torres-Labandeira, J.J., Concheiro, A., and Alvarez-Lorenzo, C., Bioinspired imprinted PHEMA-hydrogels for ocular delivery of carbonic anhydrase inhibitor drugs. *Biomacromolecules.* 12(3), 701–709, 2011.
207. Kajihara, M., Sugie, T., Maeda, H., Sano, A., Fuijoka, K., Urabe, Y., Tanihara, M., and Imanishi, Y., Novel drug delivery device using silicone: Controlled release of insoluble drugs or two kinds of water-soluble drugs. *Chem Pharm Bull.* 51, 15–19, 2003.
208. Alvarez-Lorenzo, C., Hiratani, H., Gómez-Amoza, J.L., Martinez-Pacheco, R., Souto, C., and Concheiro, A., Soft contact lenses capable of sustained delivery of timolol. *J Pharm Sci.* 91, 2182–2192, 2002.
209. Alvarez-Lorenzo, C. and Concheiro, A., Molecularly imprinted polymers for drug delivery. *J Chromatogr B.* 804, 231–245, 2004.
210. Alvarez-Lorenzo, C., Yañez, F., Barreiro-Iglesias, R., and Concheiro, A., Imprinted soft contact lenses as norfloxacin delivery systems. *J Control Release.* 113, 236–244, 2006.
211. Alvarez-Lorenzo, C., Hiratani, H., and Concheiro, A., Contact lenses for drug delivery: Achieving sustained release with novel systems. *Am J Drug Deliv.* 4, 131–151, 2006.
212. Juhn, S.K. and Rybak, L.P., Labyrinthine barriers and cochlear homeostasis. *Acta Otolaryngol.* 91, 529–534, 1981.
213. Ito, J., Endo, T., Nakagawa, T., Kita, T., Kim, T.S., and Iguchi, F., A new method for drug application to the inner ear. *ORL J Otorhinolaryngol Relat Spec.* 67(5), 272–275, 2005.
214. Chen, G., Hou, S.X., Hu, P., Jin, M.Z., and Liu, J., Preliminary study on brain-targeted drug delivery via inner ear. *Yao Xue Xue Bao.* 42(10), 1102–1106, 2007.
215. Zhang, Y., Zhang, W., Löbler, M., Schmitz, K.P., Saulnier, P., Perrier, T., Pyykkö, I., and Zou, J., Inner ear biocompatibility of lipid nanocapsules after round window membrane application. *Int J Pharm.* 404(1–2), 211–219, 2011.
216. Pyykko, I. and Dalton, P., NANOEAR: 3g-nanotechnology based targeted drug delivery using the inner ear as a model target organ, 2009. http://www.nanoear.org/(accessed 06/19/13).
217. Jager, E., Venturini, C.G., Poletto, F.S., Colome, L.M., Pohlmann, J.P., Bernardi, A., Battastini, A.M., Guterres, S.S., and Pohlmann, A.R., Sustained release from lipid-core nanocapsules by varying the core viscosity and the particle surface area. *J Biomed Nanotechnol.* 5(1), 130–140, 2009.
218. Hureaux, J., Lagarce, F., Gagnadoux, F., Clavreul, A., Benoit, J.P., and Urban, T., The adaptation of lipid nano capsule formulations for blood administration in animals. *Int J Pharm.* 379(2), 266–269, 2009.
219. Huynh, N.T., Passirani, C., Saulnier, P., and Benoit, J.P., Lipid nanocapsules: A new platform for nanomedicine. *Int J Pharm.* 379, 201–209, 2009.
220. Zou, J., Saulnier, P., Perrier, T., Zhang, Y., Manninen, T., Toppila, E., and Pyykko, I., Distribution of lipid nanocapsules in different cochlear cell populations after round window membrane permeation. *J Biomed Mater Res.* 87, 10–18, 2009.
221. Tan, B.T., Foong, K.H., Lee, M.M., and Ruan, R., Polyethylenimine-mediated cochlear gene transfer in guinea pigs. *Arch Otolaryngol Head Neck Surg.* 134, 884–891, 2008.
222. Horie, R.T., Sakamoto, T., Nakagawa, T., Tabata, Y., Okamura, N., Tomiyama, N., Tachibana, M., and Ito, J., Sustained delivery of lidocaine into the cochlea using polylactic/glycolic acid microparticles. *Laryngoscope.* 120, 377–383, 2010.

223. Florea, B.I., Meaney, C., Junginger, H.E., and Borchard, G., Transfection efficiency and toxicity of polyethylenimine in differentiated Calu-3 and nondifferentiated COS-1 cell cultures. *AAPS PharmSci.* 4, E12, 2002.

224. Rosdahl, C.B. and Kowalski, M.T., *Textbook of Basic Nursing*. Philadelphia, PA: Lippincott Williams & Wilkins, 842, 2007.

225. Zubry, B., Revolution in hypodermic injection, parenteral drugs and the cost of injection. *Manag Sci Eng.* 4(3), 138–143, 2010.

226. Schramm-Baxter, J. and Mitragotri, S., Needle-free jet injections: Dependence of jet penetration and dispersion in the skin on jet power. *J Control Release.* 97(3), 527–535, 2004.

227. DERMOJET, Daniel Becker, http://www.dermojet.net/shop/technology/

228. MED-JET, Medical International Technology, http://www.mitcanada.ca/products/med.html

229. Prelude SkinPrep System, Echo Therapeutics, http://echotx.com/prelude-skinprep-system.shtml

230. Mada Medical Products Inc., publication MJ 1281, http://www.madamedical.com/pdf/MadaJet_XL_Medical.pdf

231. SQ-PEN, http://www.sqpen.nl/index.php?mid=2&lang=en

232. Hegyi, J., Hegyi, V., Messer, G., Arenberger, P., Ruzicka, T., and Berking, C., Confocal laser scanning capillaroscopy: A novel approach to the analysis of skin capillaries in vivo. *Skin Res Technol.* 15(4), 476–481, 2009.

233. Stachowiak, J.C., Li, T.H., Arora, A., Mitragotri, S., and Fletcher, D.A., Dynamic control of needle-free jet injection. *J Control Release.* 135(2), 104–112, 2009.

234. Schramm, J. and Mitragotri, S., Transdermal drug delivery by jet injectors: Energetics of jet formation and penetration. *Pharm Res.* 19, 1673–1679, 2002.

235. Mitragotri, S., Innovation—Current status and future prospects of needle-free liquid jet injectors. *Nat Rev Drug Discov.* 5, 543–548, 2006.

236. Mendosa, D. The jet injector paradox. *Diabetes Wellness Letter.* 1–3, February 1998.

237. Lamm, J., Niebyl, P., and Hood, A. Histologic artifact due to Madajet. *Arch Dermatol.* 1985, 121(7), 835–836.

238. Mitragotri, S., Blankschtein, D., and Langer, R., Ultrasound-mediated transdermal protein delivery. *Science.* 269(5225), 850, 1995.

239. Watkins, D. and Holloway, G.A. Jr., An instrument to measure cutaneous blood flow using the Doppler shift of laser light. *IEEE Trans Biomed Eng.* 25(1), 28–33, 1978.

240. Salamat-Miller, N. and Johnston, T.P., Current strategies used to enhance the paracellular transport of therapeutic polypeptides across the intestinal epithelium. *Int J Pharm.* 294(1–2), 201, 2005.

241. Hassan, A.O. and Elshafeey, A.H., Nanosized particulate systems for dermal and transdermal delivery. *J Biomed Nanotechnol.* 6(6), 621–633, 2010.

242. Doktorovova, S. and Souto, E.B., Nanostructured lipid carrier-based hydrogel formulations for drug delivery: A comprehensive review. *Exp Opin Drug Deliv.* 6(2), 165–176, 2009.

243. Ainbinder, D., Paolino, D., Fresta, M., and Touitou, E., Drug delivery applications with ethosomes. *Biomed Nanotechnol.* 6(5), 558–568, 2010.

244. Labouta, H.I., Kraus, T., El-Khordagui, L.K., and Schneider, M., Combined multiphoton imaging-pixel analysis for semiquantitation of skin penetration of gold nanoparticles. *Int J Pharm.* 413(1–2), 279–282, 2011.

245. Schaefer, H., Watts, J., Brod, J., Illel, B., Follicular penetration, in Scott, R.C., Guy, R.H., and Hadgraft, J., eds., *Prediction of Percutaneous Penetration: Methods, Measurements and Modelling*. London: IBC Technical Services, 163–173, 1990.

246. Lauer, A.C., Lieb, L.M., Ramachandran, C., Flynn, G.L., and Weiner, N.D., Transfollicular drug delivery. *Pharm Res.* 12(2), 179–186, 1995.

247. Ebling, F.J.G., Hale, P.A., and Randal, V.A., Hormones and hair growth, in Goldsmith, V.A., ed., *Physiology, Biochemistry, and Molecular Biology of the Skin*. Oxford: Oxford Press, pp. 660–696, 1991.

248. Scheuplein, R.J., Mechanism of percutaneous adsorption II. *J Invest Dermatol.* 48, 79–88, 1967.

249. Schaefer, H. and Lademann, J., The role of follicular penetration. A differential view. *Skin Pharmacol Appl Skin Physiol.* 14(Suppl. 1), 23–27, 2001.

250. Rolland, A., Wagner, N., Chatelus, B., Shroot, B., and Schaefer, H., Site specific drug delivery to pilosebaceous structures using polymeric microspheres. *Pharm Res.* 10, 1738–1744, 1988.

251. Ryan, T.J., Cutaneous circulation, in Goldsmith, V.A., ed., *Physiology, Biochemistry, and Molecular Biology of the Skin.* Oxford: Oxford Press, 1019–1084, 1991.

252. EstroGel estrogen therapy gel, http://www.estrogel.com/menopause-symptoms.htm

253. Antares Pharma product pipeline, http://www.antarespharma.com/pipeline/

254. McAllister, D.V., Wang, P.M., Davis, S.P., Park, J.H., Canatella, P.J., Allen, M.G., and Prausnitz, M.R., Microfabricated needles for transdermal delivery of macromolecules and nanoparticles: Fabrication methods and transport studies. *Proc Natl Acad Sci USA.* 100, 13755, 2003.

255. Cross, S.E. and Roberts, M.S., Physical enhancement of transdermal drug application: Is delivery technology keeping up with pharmaceutical development? *Curr Drug Deliv.* 1, 81, 2004.

256. Nanda, A., Nanda, S., and Ghilzai, N.M., Current developments using emerging transdermal technologies in physical enhancement methods. *Curr Drug Deliv.* 3, 233, 2006.

257. Banga, A.K., New technologies to allow transdermal delivery of therapeutic proteins and small water-soluble drugs. *Am J Drug Deliv.* 4, 221–302, 2006.

258. Banga, A.K., *Therapeutic Peptides and Proteins: Formulation, Processing, and Delivery Systems.* New York: Taylor & Francis Group, pp. 1–354, 2006.

259. Prausnitz, M.R., Overcoming skin's barrier: The search for effective and user-friendly drug delivery. *Diabetes Technol Ther.* 3, 233, 2001.

260. Morrow, T., Transdermal patches are more than skin deep. *Manag Care Mag.* 13(4), 50, 2004. http://www.managedcaremag.com/archives/0404/0404.biotech.html

261. Yan, K., Todo, H., and Sugibayashi, K., Transdermal drug delivery by in-skin electroporation using a microneedle array. *Int J Pharm.* 397(1–2), 77, 2010.

262. Polat, B.E., Hart, D., Langer, R., and Blankschtein, D., Ultrasound-mediated transdermal drug delivery: Mechanisms, scope, and emerging trends. *J Control Release.* 152(3), 330–348, 2011.

263. Ferrara, K.W., Driving delivery vehicles with ultrasound. *Adv Drug Deliv Rev.* 60(10), 1097, 2008.

264. Mitragotri, S., Blankschtein, D., and Langer, R., Transdermal drug delivery using low frequency sonophoresis. *Pharm Res.* 13(3), 411, 1996.

265. Banga, A.K., Microporation applications for enhancing drug delivery. *Exp Opin Drug Deliv.* 6(4), 343–354, 2009.

266. Bachhav, Y.G., Summer, S., Heinrich, A., Bragagna, T., Boehler, C., and Kalia, Y.N., Minimally invasive delivery of peptides and proteins across the skin using P.L.E.A.S.E.® technology. AAPS Annual Meeting, November 16–20, 2008, Atlanta, GE. http://www.aapsj.org/abstracts/AM_2008/AAPS2008-001168.PDF

267. Kohen, E., Santus, R., and Hirschberg, J.G., *Photobiology.* New York: Academic Press, 1995.

268. Wu, Z.J., Luo, Z., Rastogia, A., Stavchansky, S., Bowman, P.D., and Ho, P.S., Micro fabricated perforated polymer devices for long-term drug delivery. *Biomed Microdev.* 13(3), 485–491, 2011.

269. Vemula, P.K., Boilard, E., Syed, A., Campbell, N.R., Muluneh, M., Weitz, D.A., Lee, D.M., and Karp, J.M., On-demand drug delivery from self-assembled nanofibrous gels: A new approach for treatment of proteolytic disease. *J Biomed Mater Res A.* 97(2), 103–110, 2011.

270. Ishiyama, K., Arai, K.I., Sendoh, M., and Yamazaki, A., Spiral-type micro-machine for medical applications. *J Micromechatron.* 2(1), 77–86 (10), 2002.

271. Chang, J., Peng, X.F., Hijji, K., Cappello, J., Ghandehari, H., Solares, S.D., and Seog, J., Nanomechanical stimulus accelerates and directs the self-assembly of silk-elastin-like nanofibers. *J Am Chem Soc.* 133(6), 1745–1747, 2011.

272. Ahn, S.K., Deshmukh, P., Gopinadhan, M., Osuji, C.O., and Kasi, R.M., Side-chain liquid crystalline polymer networks: Exploiting nanoscale smectic polymorphism to design shape-memory polymers. *ACS Nano.* 5(4), 3085–3095, 2011.

273. Hidaka, M. and Yoshida, R., Self-oscillating gel composed of thermosensitive polymer exhibiting higher LCST. *J Control Release.* 150(2), 171–176, 2011.

274. Lee, K.M., Koerner, H., Vaia, R.A., Bunning, T.J., and White, T.J., Light-activated shape memory of glassy, azobenzene liquid crystalline polymer networks. *Soft Matter.* 7, 4318–4324, 2011.
275. Hu, Y., Chen, W., Lu, L., Liu, J., and Chang, C., Electromechanical actuation with controllable motion based on a single-walled carbon nanotube and natural biopolymer composite. *ACS Nano.* 4(6), 3498–3502, 2010.
276. Yamamoto, Y., Ito, A., Kato, M., Kawabe, Y., Shimizu, K., Fujita, H., Nagamori, E., and Kamihira, M., Preparation of artificial skeletal muscle tissues by a magnetic force-based tissue engineering technique. *J Biosci Bioeng.* 108(6), 538–543, 2009.
277. Qi, Y., Jafferis, N.T., Lyons, K. Jr., Lee, C.M., Ahmad, H., and McAlpine, M.C., Piezoelectric ribbons printed onto rubber for flexible energy conversion. *Nano Lett.* 10(2), 524–528, 2010.
278. Carbonari, R.C., Nader, G., Nishiwaki, S., and Silva, E.C.N., Experimental and numerical characterization of multi-actuated piezoelectric device designs using topology optimization. *Conference Information: Smart Structures and Materials 2005 Conference,* March 07–10, 2005, San Diego, CA. Smart Structures and Materials 2005: Smart Structures and Integrated Systems, 5764, 472–481,2005.
279. Advincula, R.C., Hybrid organic–inorganic nanomaterials based on polythiophene dendronized nanoparticles. *Dalton Trans.* (23), 2778–2784, 2006.
280. Liu, H., Xu, J., Li, Y., and Li, Y., Aggregate nanostructures of organic molecular materials. *Acc Chem Res.* 43(12), 1496–1508, 2010.
281. Shen, M. and Shi, X., Dendrimer-based organic/inorganic hybrid nanoparticles in biomedical applications. *Nanoscale.* 2(9), 1596–1610, 2010.
282. Lademanna, J., Richtera, H., Schaeferb, U.F., Blume-Peytavia, U., Teichmanna, A., Otberga, N., and Sterrya, W., Hair follicles—A long-term reservoir for drug delivery. *Skin Pharmacol Physiol.* 19(4), 232–236, 2006.
283. Alvarez-Román, R., Naik, A., Kalia, Y.N., Guy, R.H., and Fessi, H., Skin penetration and distribution of polymeric nanoparticles. *J Control Release.* 99, 53–62, 2004.

3

Design Challenges and Considerations for Nanomedical In Vivo Aqueous Propulsion, Surface Ambling, and Navigation

Frank J. Boehm

CONTENTS

3.1 Introduction: Blazing Nanomedical Trails

Two of the most daunting interlinked sets of challenges that visionists, designers, and engineers will confront in the conceptualization of advanced nanomedical devices and systems are the development of practicable and efficient nanoscale propulsive mechanisms and their associated navigational infrastructures to provide for their precise control. Robust and high-performance nanopropulsion components will have the prerequisite of being broadly adaptable under myriad in vivo physiological conditions. Navigational strategies will likely encompass and be imbued with the capacity for mediating the pace and precise orientation, in real time, of perhaps thousands or millions of autonomous nanomedical devices that perform medically beneficial functions simultaneously to address a wide range of disease states.

The accurately controlled traversal of the human in vivo environment will pose enormous, but in this author's view, not insurmountable technical design, fabrication, functionalization, and strategic challenges. The capacities of rapid and efficient motility coupled with precision navigation for negotiating the diverse repertoire of internal microstructures inherent to human physiology, which is replete with countless transitory obstacles, vascular/capillary convolutions, tortuous pathways, and hidden recesses, will require a high level of control resolution and sophisticated agility. Additional characteristics of the in vivo environment that are likely to pose significant complications for motile micronscale nanomedical devices are aqueous turbulence and shear forces.

One factor that may not be immediately considered or appreciated, though inconsequential insofar as it relates to the integrity and accuracy of nanodevice navigation, is that all activities conducted by nanomedical devices in vivo, as do all biological processes, will proceed in the complete absence of light. Thus, they will be required to perform the full spectrum of ultrahigh-resolution medical procedures autonomously while literally swimming blind. All navigational directed movements would be precisely controlled by "outbody" computers with perhaps secondary navigational bearings being provided by dedicated "repeater" nanodevices that may be transiently tethered at strategic sites within the patient for a given procedure. Additional cross verification of spatial coordinates and orientation might be provided by inter-nanodevice reference signals.

This chapter will survey an envisaged range of potential propulsive and navigation strategies that may be utilized by nanomedical devices, enabling them to access virtually any site within the human body in order to conduct useful diagnostic and therapeutic procedures. Contingent upon the particular species of nanodevice that a physician may prescribe to perform a specific medical task, dynamic modes of propulsion will be essential for the traversal of complex physiological geometries within various aqueous, gelatinous, and solid (at least from the macro perspective) media in vivo. In addition, strategies for imparting external mobility and agility for surface ambling nanomedical devices will be surveyed. Finally, approaches for conceptual navigation systems will be assessed.

3.2 Traversing the In Vivo Environment

The exemplar Vascular Cartographic Scanning Nanodevice (VCSN) nanomedical device will likely be engaged in active natation (swimming) for the duration of its cartographic spatial data acquisition tasks. The estimated time required for a nanomedical device to complete a single circuit of the human vasculature is on the order of ~60 s under resting patient conditions [1–3]. During heavy exercise, this time decreases to ~11–15 s due to vasodilation. Pulmonary-resident nanoparticulates require 1–2 s to traverse the alveolar sheet and about 5–10 s to travel through the complete pulmonary vascular structure. Transit times through various organs may be in the range of 0.7–5.0 s [1,4,5]. When transiting through the pulmonary arterial tree, for instance, nanomedical devices will be required to move through 17 bifurcations (forks), at 3.2 branches per fork [1].

Whole blood comprises myriad distinct cells and, as the latest research reveals, a complement of ~4229 blood serum compounds [1,6]. It has an average specific gravity of about 1.058 and viscosity between 4.5 and 5.5 times greater than that of water at equivalent temperature. The typical pH of blood ranges between 7.35 and 7.45, with a mean temperature of 38.0°C (100.4°F). An adult of average age and size has a complement of slightly greater than 5.7 L (6 quarts) of blood [7,8].

Biorheology concerns the movement of in vivo biological fluids, and their progress through the vasculature is described as sanguinatation. Viscosity is defined as the resistance of a fluid to shearing when the fluid is in motion [1]. Blood serum is considered to be an ideal Newtonian fluid (e.g., one that has a constant viscosity at all shear rates). High concentrations of nanodevices within the vasculature that exceed a certain threshold may radically impact blood viscosity. Although, through the implementation of multiple failsafe protocols, this condition would never be allowed to occur in nanomedical practice, it would, hypothetically, be further contingent on the shape and cumulative density of resident nanodevices.

Several dynamic forces predominate in the circulatory system, which are described as follows:

Shear rate: Velocity changes between parallel planes in fluid flow.

Shear flow: Material flow, whereby media is displaced in directions that are equivalent to one another.

Shear stress: The acting force in shear flow.

Following is a breakdown of the absolute viscosity of whole blood [1]:

Whole blood—low shear rate	*Viscosity (kg/m s)*
Hct = 45%	$\sim 100 \times 10^{-3}$
Hct = 90%	$\sim 1000 \times 10^{-3}$
Whole blood—high shear rate	*Viscosity (kg/m s)*
Hct = 45%	$\sim 10 \times 10^{-3}$
Hct = 90%	$\sim 100 \times 10^{-3}$
Human blood plasma at 310 K	$1.1–1.2 \times 10^{-3}$
Serum/interstitial fluid at 310 K	$1.0–1.1 \times 10^{-3}$

Hct = hematocrit = blood volume percentage that is comprised of red blood cells (RBCs).

At shear rates of <100 s^{-1}, weakly adhering stacked aggregates of human RBCs called rouleaux can form [9,10]. These aggregating RBCs are linked in a loose fashion via fibrinogen and globulin, which are cross-linking proteins that exist on the surfaces of cells in plasma. Rouleaux typically comprise of up to 20 RBCs, and exist as the largest of all constituents in human whole blood. When shear rates are elevated, the rouleaux tend to disperse as constituent individual red cells deform and elongate slightly. When combined, these two occurrences tend to reduce the viscosity of the blood. Interestingly, RBCs never come into contact with the vascular endothelial wall due to the plasmatic zone phenomenon. The plasmatic zone is peripheral domain of plasma, which is devoid of cells as a consequence of the axial accretion of RBCs, and serves as a lubricating element, even in the most diminutive of vessels [2].

Typical blood shear rates in the human vasculature encompass 50–700 s^{-1} in the primary arteries, to 250–2000 s^{-1} in arterioles and capillaries. For large and small veins, the shear rate is 20–200 s^{-1}. Whole blood remains in a fluid state even at 98% concentration of RBCs by volume [1,11].

Normal human male hematocrit percentages in variously sized vascular entities are

Smaller vessels	46%
100 μm	36%
30 μm	25%
8 μm	13%

Minimum hematocrit occurs at approximately ~ 15 to 20 μm, which indicates the transition from a multiple red cell flow configuration to that of a single file flow. RBC suspension viscosity approaches a minimum at about ~ 5 to 7 μm [1,12–14]. Flow conditions dictate the distribution of white cells, which are displaced (at low shear rates) toward the vascular walls by the much larger rouleaux entities [15–19]. Conversely, at high shear rates white cells travel along the central axis as they are larger than individual red cells.

In arterioles, platelet density, as well as small molecules and lipoproteins have greater abundance in close proximity to the vascular wall, as they are much smaller than either red or white cells [20–22]. The general principal that may be applied to particle distribution in blood flow is that larger particles tend to transit/flow more rapidly within the axial region of vascular entities, whereas smaller blood constituents tend to flow more slowly, and in close proximity to vessel walls [23].

By virtue of its diminutive size (~1 μm), the VCSN will naturally gravitate toward the periphery of any vascular entity. If the imaging function is to be calibrated from the central axes of dimensionally disparate vascular entities, a means must be devised to compensate for this tendency with the result, for imaging and image reconstruction purposes, of maintaining a central axial trajectory. A positional feedback loop might be implemented to apply real time corrective maneuvers to correct for lateral displacement events in vessels. Freitas estimates that a 10% maximum bloodstream concentration of nanomedical devices (for our purposes, in the size range of the VCSN) would be within safe operational limits [1].

The forces of viscous drag work to oppose micro/nanoscale locomotion in vivo, as this environment is dominated by viscosity. Inertia is negligible at the nanoscale; hence, hydrodynamic effects deviate significantly from those at the macroscale [24,25]. The design of propulsive mechanisms for nanodevices that will function within the in vivo viscous aqueous media of patients is likely to have significantly different modes of operation than their macroscale counterparts. Also of consequence at scales of ~10 nm up to several microns are entropic effects [26].

It has been thought that there exists a particular minimal dimensional threshold (~0.6 μm in diameter × 0.6 μm) below which in vivo locomotion may be deemed as virtually ineffectual. This constraint was verified in 1997 through comparative studies that involved the smallest known motile and nonmotile bacteria [27]. In contrast, an intriguing strategy for motility has been shown to be employed by a member of the smallest known free-floating and self-reproducing bacterial forms of life, known as the Mollicutes, which include the members *Spiroplasma*, *Mycoplasma*, and *Acholeplasma*. Devoid of a cell membrane, the Mollicutes are encapsulated within a quasifluid albeit rigid, cholesterol-infused casing. Interestingly, they also possess eukaryotic-like cytoskeletons. *Spiroplasmas* have a tubular diameter of ~0.2 μm and a helical morphology (Figure 3.1), which is attached to, and traced by seven parallel flat cytoskeletal fibrils that function as linear motors via the initiation of differential synchronized length variations, to sequentially toggle between

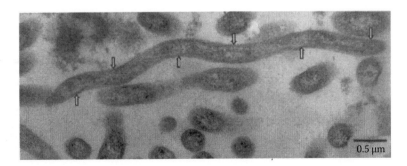

FIGURE 3.1
Chemically fixed *Spiroplasma* reveals the cytoskeleton, which traverses the innermost helical line and its attachment points. (Reproduced from Trachtenberg, S. and Gilad, R., *Mol. Microbiol.*, 41(4), 827, 2001. With permission.)

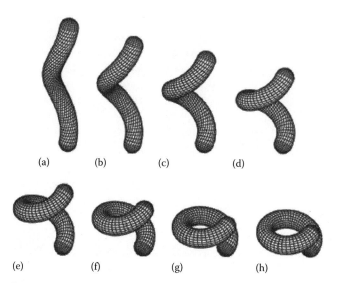

(a)   (b)   (c)   (d)

(e)   (f)   (g)   (h)

FIGURE 3.2   Three-dimensional depiction of *Spiroplasma* helical conformational sequence; from fully extended (a) to compressed (h) states, which conveys cytoskeletal based, linear motor-mediated motility. (Reproduced from Trachtenberg, S. and Gilad, R., *Mol. Microbiol.*, 41(4), 827, 2001. With permission.)

fully extended and compressed states. Hence, they mediate dynamic conformational shifts (e.g., diameter, pitch, and twist) in the cell's helical geometry (Figure 3.2) to convey motility [28,29].

An analogous biomimetic nanomedical motile strategy, similar to that which is utilized by *Spiroplasma*, may be enabled through the use of artificial muscle materials that are comprised of conductive polymers. The helical structure might be supported by multiple thin but rigid piezoelectric elements to serve as the fibrils. In vivo harvested or generated power might be conveyed to the slender yet resilient piezoelements, which would be induced to deform in response to the applied voltage to initiate similar linear motor activity and sequential conformational changes with resultant motility.

Once a nanomedical device cuts power, it will halt immediately, having no inertial "coasting" effect. Powered nanodevice natation downstream might necessitate traversing the blood flow in a somewhat erratic trajectory, as the nanodevice will be constantly seeking clear passage between the cells and other blood-resident entities that inhabit the central axis regions. A natation route counter to prevailing blood flows might follow the relatively unencumbered plasmatic zones [1].

Observations of RBC and platelet tumbling in arterioles in close proximity to vessel walls [30] indicate that onboard stabilization mechanisms will indeed be indispensable insofar as endowing nanomedical devices with the capacity to compensate for this activity. Contingent on the application, when advanced nanomedical devices are induced to undergo uncontrolled tumbling due to localized flow shear, regurgetrant eddies, complex aqueous turbulence, or as a consequence of ~direct impacts with bifurcation ridges, it would seem reasonable that they should have a means for rapidly reorienting themselves to regain positional stability [31]. Stabilization strategies that involve the integration of rapidly rotating nanoscale diamondoid disks or nanometric optical gyroscopes might serve to fulfill this critical requirement [1,32] (see Section 3.6.3).

Conversely, if the design of nanomedical propulsive mechanisms and navigational infrastructures includes externally controlled/software-based compensatory measures with a built-in expectation of relatively frequent tumbling events, it may be prudent to implement a strategy whereby nanodevices are allowed to "go with the flow" until they approach their assigned sites of operation. In these instances, propulsion might be engaged only for avoidance maneuvers and when reducing speed to prepare for passage through the endothelial wall to arrive at tissue-resident treatment sites. It is unlikely that any damage to blood constituents will be imparted by nanodevices when they transit in unison with prevailing blood flows.

This strategy, however, becomes irrelevant in cases where nanodevices must travel against the flow of blood in emergency treatment situations (e.g., to rapidly curtail the flow of blood at the site of an aneurysm or hemorrhage, or to quickly repair the damage inflicted by a serious wound). Collateral damage inflicted on RBCs and other blood-borne cells en route to an emergency repair site(s) might be regarded as an acceptable trade-off in favor of immediately addressing serious conditions or injuries. Should nanodevices some-how overshoot an exit location to access a treatment site, or miss an egress opportunity at the completion of a task, it would be a simple matter of retransiting the vasculature until the assigned destinations have been successfully engaged. Once arrived, nanodevices might be instructed to properly orient themselves in three-dimensional (3D) space rela-tive to a local (externally established) reference point, or fiducial. This may entail required velocity reduction or cessation combined with rotational maneuvers so as to align with an intended trajectory to accurately arrive at a predetermined destination for a particular diagnostic or therapeutic task.

With the advent of prospective sophisticated Compensatory Nanomedical Spatial Orientation Software (CNSOS), vascular tumbling events induced for nanodevices such as the VCSN might be deemed as inconsequential, as any shift from a referenced orientation along assigned trajectories could be autocorrected in real time. In addition, throughout the course of the VCSN spatial data acquisition process it seems unavoidable that the nanode-vices will encounter and collide with numerous free-floating cellular and proteinaceous entities. Hence, a further facet of CNSOS would correct for such collision events by draw-ing on immediate, continually refreshing positional and velocity data for the subsequent smoothing and subtraction of these anomalies from spatial data sets.

Studies have been conducted on this theme in order to elucidate and quantify the dynamics and kinetics of impacts between malleable and inflexible microspheres [33]. Other investigations have generated useful data as relates to the hydrodynamics of soli-tary natating cells; reciprocating influences of cells that swim in unison; and the altered conditions that exist at intimate proximity to solid surfaces under shear flow conditions [1,34–40].

It has been shown that flagellated bacteria such as *Escherichia coli* (K-12) experience a reduction in velocity when approaching a solid surface. Frymier et al. found that cell swimming speeds were reduced from ~15 to 5–7 μm/s when bacteria swam within 2 μm of a surface, but recovered velocity when swimming parallel to a surface [41]. Ramia et al. developed a Boundary Element Method for the determination of the motion of spheres and slender bodies in close proximity to surfaces. This model was utilized to elucidate the propulsive dynamics of a spherical bodied microorganism that is driven by a solitary rotating flagellum. It was learned that a <10% increase in velocity is expe-rienced by identical entities, which swim close to each other or that are on equivalent trajectories.

The mechanism for this speed increase is explained in terms of "the flagellar propulsive advantage derived from an increase in the ratio of the normal to tangential resistance coefficients of a slender body being offset by the apparently equally significant increase in the cell body drag." The same increment of speed increase (<10%) was noted when the model organism swam in very close proximity and parallel to a surface. However, when approaching a surface, a significant reduction in velocity was observed due to a rapid increase in drag. Ramia et al. conclude that "hydrodynamic interaction is significant only when the relevant separation distances ... are approximately equal to or smaller than the largest physical dimension of the organism in question" [36].

Micron-sized nanomedical devices that are designed to operate within the human body will have to address and surmount the viscosity of blood/plasma at low Reynolds number. The relative viscosity of human blood/plasma is ~4.5, and in one study ranged from an average of 3.28 ± 0.43 mPa in a group of 20 to 30 year old volunteers to 4.33 ± 0.73 mPa in a group of 60–70 year olds [36]. Variable levels of viscosity may also be correlated to variable vascular lumen dimensions. As Purcell points out, if a 1 μm in diameter entity is pushed through the blood and the pushing suddenly stops, it will take on the order 0.6 μs and a distance of 0.1 Å for the entity to reduce speed and stop. To propel a micron-sized entity through human blood/plasma (a highly viscous media from the perspective of a nano-medical device), Purcell illustrates that the mode of propulsion should not be reciprocal via his "scallop theorem." For example, a macroscale scallop will make progress when it rapidly closes its shell to squirt a water jet in its regular habitat. At low Reynolds number, a micron-sized scallop would move ahead a certain increment when it closes its shell. However, it would revert to its starting position on the reciprocating stroke, as it is single-hinged and has only one degree of freedom. This useful insight into the behavior of small bodies in viscous media may serve as a boon to the conceptualists and designers of the propulsive mechanisms of nanomedical devices [24].

Certain classes of nanomedical devices may employ an approach that involves ciliary beating for propulsion through the human circulatory system. Biomimetic designs that utilize polymeric, carbon nanotube or nanofiber filaments may be comparable in geometry and functionality to the cilia of *Paramecium caudatum*, which utilizes an external surface–embedded population of ~2500 cilia for motility. Alterations in the cumulative beating patterns of these cilia enable *Paramecium* to successfully traverse variably viscous aqueous environments [42–44].

When endeavoring to establish parameters for the velocity of autonomous in vivo nano-medical devices, one might consider factors such as potential impact damage that may be conveyed when there are inevitable collision events between nanodevices and RBCs or other blood-resident elements. It seems reasonable to institute a relatively conservative nanodevice speed limit that does not exceed the maximum velocity of naturally circulat-ing blood at any point within the vasculature. The speed of blood through vessels is vari-able, contingent on the location and hierarchical class of the vascular segments involved. Any changes in the cross-sectional profiles of vascular lumen or the trajectory of arteries and veins will also influence local flow velocities [45]. Hence, the velocity of blood flow may be deemed as being in a constant state of flux, which may average from 0.03 cm/s in the most diminutive of capillaries to 40–50 cm/s in the aorta. An example of absolute velocity ranges have been reported from 28.6–178.4 cm/s for the common carotid artery to 20.1–112.0 cm/s for the internal carotid artery [46].

For sophisticated autonomous nanomedical devices, appropriate velocities could be set in accordance with the particular section of the vasculature through which they are tran-siting. Hence, dynamic velocity adjustment protocols may be instituted that will spon-taneously tailor nanodevice speeds to align with real-time blood velocities, which are measured on the fly by the nanodevices themselves. Although platelet thrombosis has been shown to be activated and that platelet microparticles are generated by sustained, very high or sudden increases in shear stress (315 dynes/cm^2 at 10,500 s^{-1}) due to severe stenosis, this is not the case at a physiological shear of 420 s^{-1} [47]. Therefore, a consistent pace equivalence between nanodevices and blood flow makes it highly unlikely that platelet thrombosis will be induced. Freitas has recommended a conservatively safe and amenable nanodevice speed limit of 1 cm/s derived from RBC impact pressure data, which suggests that collisions between nanodevices and cells at greater speeds may initiate alterations in the surface areas of red cells and may inflict potential damage. RBCs may be subject to deformation at approx. >2 m/s and rupture at ~>20 m/s [1].

Additional strategies for potential in vivo nanodevice motility include those that utilize screw/corkscrew-drive elements [48]. Bacterial flagella are driven by membrane-bound self-assembled ~45 nm in diameter motors that can revolve at speeds of up to 100,000 rpm. They frequently reverse their swimming direction by abruptly toggling flagellar motor rotation from CCW to CW and back again [49–51]. A natating *E. coli* bacterium attains velocities of ~30 μm/s with a thrust energy of 0.5 pN at <1% efficiency [52,53].

Another possibility for imparting in vivo nanodevice thrust may function under the premise of volume dislocation. Fluid might be physically displaced from the leading surface of a nanodevice. The leading surface would immediately inhabit the void, prior to when it would take the surrounding fluid to do so. By inserting the originally displaced volume of fluid directly behind the nanodevice, it may make forward progress [1]. Velocity, in this scenario, would be contingent on the rate of fluid volume displacement from bow to stern of the device, proceeding either internally or externally. Several drawbacks inherent to this method of locomotion may include relatively high operating pressures and power usage coupled with the potential tendency for clogging and fouling, via the formation of biofilms, of the displacement mechanism(s).

If appropriate anti-clogging/antifouling strategies can be developed, nanometric analogs of fluidic flow-through jet drives for nanodevice propulsion may be a feasible proposition. Scaling studies and computer simulations may assist in the validation of designs to verify if such propulsion systems may be capable of sufficient thrust capacity while screening out all blood-resident elements, save for water molecules, when in transit. As human blood is comprised of ~90% water, it seems plausible that Ø ~3 Å water molecules may easily be induced to be propelled through narrow diameter (e.g., ~1 to 10 nm) nanotube jet drives, even if they are constrained to do so in single file [54]. From the nanoscale perspective, the utilization of a nanometric jet drive through blood-borne molecular constituents might be akin to using a jet ski to slide through a sea of water-filled balloons. Elucidative investigations, coupled with sophisticated computer modeling in the determination of optimal designs for the highest energy efficiencies at the micron dimensional domain at high speeds, are warranted to validate the feasibility of this approach [55,56].

A hypothetical therapeutic (~1 cm^3) dose of nanomedical devices would contain ~10^{12} entities. If these nanodevices were to be spread out as a single homogeneous layer, they would span an area of ~1 m^2 [1]. For comparison, the total surface area of the interior endothelial lining of the human vasculature is ~4000 to 7000 m^2, with a summed surface area of large veins and main arterial branches alone of ~1 m^2 (Table 3.1) [57,58]. Less concentrated doses of nanomedical devices may traverse the plasmatic zones at higher velocities, at the expense, however, of higher energy consumption. Freitas recommends a maximum "nanocrit" in the human bloodstream of approx. <10% [1].

TABLE 3.1

Estimated Surface Area of Vascular Tree in a 154 lb Male

Vascular Entity	Total Surface Area (cm²)
Aorta	156
Large arteries	3333
Small arteries	14,473
Arterioles	261,337
Total	279,299
Capillaries	1,517,295
Venules	879,989
Small veins	32,655
Large veins	6836
Vena cava	177
Total	919,657

Source: Adapted from Wolinsky, H., *Circ. Res.*, 47, 301, 1980.

3.3 Nanomedical Propulsive Mechanisms

Propulsive mechanisms will endow nanomedical devices, such as the VCSN, with complete autonomy so as to precisely navigate through the human vasculature under external computer control, coupled with (though to a lesser degree) an onboard quantum computer. The VCSN would traverse its assigned trajectories, and upon completion of its scanning tasks would gravitate (via a distinct homing signal frequency or predetermined site coordinate programming) toward an "egress" exit point (Chapter 2). The VCSN would typically navigate downstream, but would have the capacity for traveling upstream against the blood flow if required by utilizing plasmatic zones, as described earlier, which reside at blood/endothelial wall interfaces (e.g., ~0.5–12 μm thick peripheral layer within vascular entities that are >150 μm) [1,59–62].

Accurately navigating and tracking possibly thousands or conceivably millions of micron-sized devices simultaneously through the human vasculature will present immense logistical challenges. An intimate knowledge of human vascular physiology encompassing potential physiological variants thereof, whole blood and plasma elements, shear profiles, subtle and robust flow patterns in linear, arched, and bifurcated vascular domains will be critical. In addition, an in-depth knowledge of the mechanics and turbulent flows within the heart will be essential, in order to effectively guide nanomedical devices through the circulatory system with absolute control and defined purpose. A study of colloidal suspensions in solution will also be of benefit insofar as contributing to this knowledge base.

3.3.1 Biological Motile Mechanisms: Cilia and Flagella

The primary utility of centriole-based ciliated and flagellar organelles involves the transfer of fluids to impart motility to static bodies. If minute enough, ciliated and flagellated bodies will be propelled through aqueous media. Conversely, tethered bodies that are endowed with cilia and flagella will transfer fluids over their exteriors. Cilia are found in protozoan ciliates, of which there are ~10,000 species (encompassing marine and freshwater varieties), coelenterates (hydras, jellyfish, sea anemone, and corals), turbellarians (flatworms), ctenophores (comb jellies), tunicates (sea squirts), and vertebrates. The diameters of cilia range from ~0.15 to 0.3 μm and they may attain lengths from ~5 to 20 μm. When combined as compound cilia, they can extend to lengths of up to ~2000 μm. Innate functionality appears to be what primarily differentiates cilia and flagella. Whereas a cilium intermittently propels fluid in a perpendicular trajectory relative to its long axis as part of its beating stroke, a flagellum continually forces fluid along the central axis of its long helical strand, analogous to the function of a propeller. In terms of efficacy, flagella are superior as they cooperatively operate to progress the movement of any entity that they are embedded within. Their molecular motors are powered by the energy that is derived from protons as they transit through the electrically charged cell wall [63,64].

In sponge, the flagellum are oriented in such a way that water currents brought on by flagellar beating: draw water in through the ostia (water intake opening) and displace it out through the oscula (water exit opening). Cumulative flagellum action causes water currents to traverse the collar of the choanocyte (flagellated chamber) made up of a palisade (perpendicularly elongated cells) of microvilli [65]. In some species of invertebrates activated flagella, which line the internal lumen of tubular flame cells, push fluid from their base to tip, toward an external orifice [66]. This mode of action could be replicated by cilia should they be oriented perpendicular to a desired output direction.

It is not always the case that flagella are longer than cilia. It has been observed that multiple cilia may be configured such that their cumulative length is far greater than that of flagella. Flagellar length may be limited by several mechanisms. In the food-borne pathogen *Campylobacter jejuni*, the Cj1464 protein controls flagellin biosynthesis and exhibits similar attributes as the FlgM family of anti-sigma factor proteins in that it represses transcription of sigma(28)-dependent genes. The *C. jejuni* FlgM restricts the elongation of the flagellar filament by repressing the synthesis of flagellins that are sigma(28)- and sigma(54)-dependent. Constraints imposed on the length of flagella are critical as unrestrained elongation will lead to decreased motility [67].

When numerous cilia work in unison, they demonstrate a beating pattern that may be considered to be more effective and dynamic (e.g., for direction reversal) than that of flagella. Metachronically synchronized cilia beating provides a consistent aqueous flow as at any point in time individual cilia may be engaged at some increment of a power stroke, encompassing the thrusting active phase to the recovery mode preparatory to the initiation of a subsequent stroke. In the case of short cilia, only thin layers of fluid are propelled over the cell exterior. Longer compound cilia transport a comparatively significant volume of fluid and may therefore produce more extensive currents. A potent illustration of the latter instance may be provided in the comb-plates of ctenophores that comprise compound cilia. Stacks of comb-like plates successively beat through fluids in a manner that is similar to a paddle wheel [63,68,69].

The mechanical synchronization of flagellar motile sequences may enhance swimming efficiency. When fluid is displaced along the length of flagella to impart forward thrust, gyration also ensues. Hence, the design of biomimetic, synthetic flagella for nanomedical devices might incorporate stabilization or restraint mechanisms against the onset of these wayward revolving motions.

Individual flagella are self-assembled aggregates, which consist of ~30 distinct proteins. The axial segment comprises a number of secondary structures that include the rod, hook, hook–filament junction, long helical filament, and filament tip cap. The flagellar hook serves as a molecular level universal joint, which can translate the torque that is generated by the basal body–embedded rotary motor to the filament. Its structure consists of ~130 identical FlgE subunits, each of which is ~55 nm in length.

Each filament may be made of up to ~30,000 flagellin subunits. Additional elements include hook-related proteins HAP1-(FlgK), HAP2-(FliD), and HAP3-(FlgL). HAP1 and HAP3 serve to tether the hook to the filament, whereas HAP2 shapes a cap-like terminating structure (120 Å wide × 25 Å thick) at the end of the filament. Five types of rod proteins (FliE, FlgB, FlgC, FlgF, and FlgG) are also integrated into the assembly (Figure 3.3) [70,71]. The proteins that cumulatively make up the flagellar filament are synthesized within the cell and transported via a dedicated protein export mechanism in unfolded conformation and traverse a Ø 20–25 Å internal channel to the growing tip of the filament. Flagellar monomers are Ø 2 nm × 10–15 μm in length and are transported to the flagellar

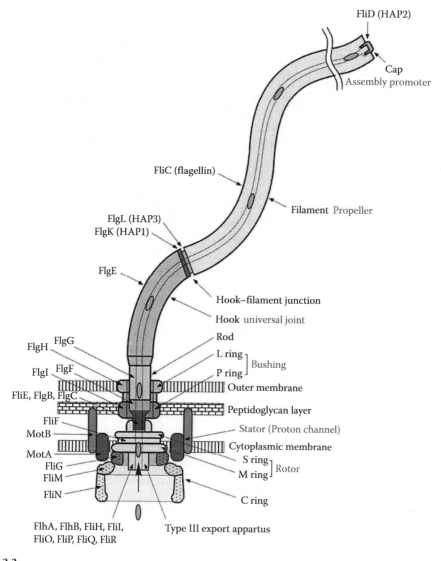

FIGURE 3.3
Anatomy of bacterial flagellum. Color differences indicate distinct protein components. (Reprinted from Yonekura, K. et al., *Res. Microbiol.*, 153, 191, 2002. With permission.)

tip via diffusion. Flagellar length can range from ~5 to 150 μm with sperm tails being the longest, at ~200 μm. The outer membrane of the main shaft is a three-layered lamination; two dense layers ~20 to 30 Å thick, which sandwich a less dense 30 Å thick layer, giving a total thickness of ~70 to 90 Å [71].

Dual tubular fibrils that sit at a distance of ~300–350 Å (center to center) are located at the core and project symmetrically for the full extent of the shaft. They have an overall diameter of ~150–250 Å and are supported by walls with a thickness of ~40–50 Å. Surrounding the central fibril pair are nine ~1600 Å in diameter longitudinal peripheral fibrils, which comprise a double set of tubules ("A" and "B") at ~200–250 Å in diameter with a wall thicknesses of ~60 Å. Tubule A is made up of 13 protofilaments and outsizes its counterpart, tubule B, which has 10. Additional strength is imparted to these tubules via a 2 nm in diameter × ~48 nm long helical protein (tektin α). This protein is oriented longitudinally, spanning the interfacial wall between A and B (Figures 3.4 and 3.5).

Tethered to the A tubule of each duplet are internal and external dynein arms that extend toward neighboring B tubules. These arms may facilitate tubule sliding during the beating sequence. Triple pairs of proteins are cross-linked to hold the axoneme together. The central pair is bound together by incrementally spaced bridges and the exterior doublet tubules are held together by pliable nexin proteins, which are positioned at 86 nm intervals and likely also support the sliding of the duplets. A third type of connecting entity emanates from the central pair as radial spokes, which bind with each A tubule of the secondary duplets, and are configured in pairs that are spaced at 96 nm intervals. Overall cilia diameters steadily decrease when proceeding from base to tip, and individual tubule

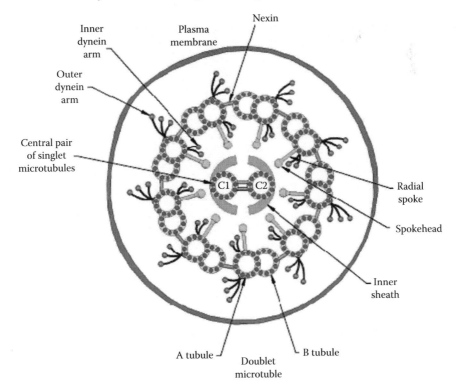

FIGURE 3.4

Flagellar doublet. (Redrawn from Huang, B. et al., *Cell*, 29, 745, 1982; Lodish, H. et al., *Molecular Cell Biology*, Scientific American Books, New York, 1998.)

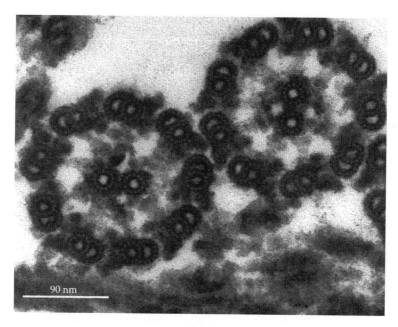

FIGURE 3.5
Cross section of isolated *Chlamydomonas* flagellar axoneme. (Courtesy of Dartmouth College E. M. Facility, image by Louisa Howard.)

length terminations are staggered as they taper. At axoneme anchoring sites, where the base of cilia interface with the cell membrane, there are nine triplets of microtubules [72].

Flagellar motors may be considered as energy translation devices that utilize and convert an electrochemical gradient to mechanical gyratory output. They are powered by gradients of protons and Na$^+$ ions that are set up across inner bacterial membranes, with more abundant populations of these elements that exist external to the cell. The rotation of these molecular motors may be driven by either the inward flow of protons, which are processed by motA–motB protein complexes, which comprise the stator of the flagellar motor, as is the case with *E. coli*, or Na$^+$ ions such as those taken up by *Vibrio cholerae*.

E. coli processes 70 H$^+$ per revolution per motA–motB complex, of which there are eight. Thus, they cumulatively process 560 protons/revolution. Flagellar motors that are H$^+$-driven may attain maximum rotational velocities of ~360 Hz (~21,600 rpm). This translates to an overall H$^+$ flow of ~200,000 protons/s. Even more impressive are Na$^+$-driven flagellar motors such as in *Vibrio*, which can reach rotational velocities of ~1700 Hz (~100,000 rpm) [73]. Very rapid flagellar rotation has been reported for *Vibrio alginolyticus* as attaining 1700 rps (~102,000 rpm) [74].

The motile pattern of bacterial entities such as *E. coli* and *Salmonella* includes straight natation for several seconds, followed by sub-second rotational movement, which may serve as a precursor to changes in direction. For linear swimming, the flagellar helical filaments group together in close proximity as a left-handed supercoiled bundle of propulsive entities at the rear of the cell body. Intermittent rotation or tumbling is initiated by the reversal in direction of the rotary motor that is located at the base of the filaments. This enables the even, albeit momentary, fragmentation of the filament bundle into an unorganized right-handed mass of separated whirling filaments and initiates a rapid change in orientation.

Interestingly, from the perspective of potentially tethering natural flagella to hybrid nanodevices for propulsion, the detachment of flagellar filaments from cells and their subsequent depolymerization may be accomplished via a facile method, which involves thermal treatment at 60°C for 10 min or immersion in an acid solution at pH 2.5. The flagellar monomers have the capacity for spontaneous reassembling into functional filaments under physiological conditions via the addition of short segments that serve as seeds or by employing a precipitant such as ammonium sulfate. Hook structures may also be reassembled in vitro under the proper conditions. It has been observed that the polymerization of axial proteins might be mediated by their randomly ordered terminal domains. The self-assembly of these proteins is contingent on the provision of a "growth template"; hence, polymerization proceeds exclusively at the tips of growing filaments [70].

3.3.2 Chemically Powered Nanomotors

A survey of strategies for the design of chemically powered nanomotors with the capacity for outpacing natural flagellar motors has been undertaken by Mirkovic et al. [75]. An initial advance in this area was accomplished in 2002 by Whitesides et al. who developed autonomous centimeter-scale "floats" that were powered through the chemical conversion of hydrogen peroxide (H_2O_2). These devices were propelled at the water/air boundary with the addition of H_2O_2 when Pt particulates were affixed to their stern sections. Oxygen bubbles, which were generated at the Pt surface as a result of the breakdown of H_2O_2, provided the recoil required to initiate thrust [76].

Initial reports of self-propelled nanoscale entities surfaced as the result of work by Mallouk et al. [77] at Pennsylvania State University, and Ozin et al. [78] at the University of Toronto. These investigators made the concomitant discovery that Pt/Au and Ni/Au bimetal nanorods, fabricated via the sequential templated electrodeposition of discrete domains of these metals within the lumen of membrane-embedded nanochannels, exhibited self-directed propulsion when immersed in aqueous H_2O_2. The kinetics involves the catalytic conversion of H_2O_2 to water and oxygen via the mechanism as follows [75]:

$$2H_2O_2 \rightarrow 2H_2O + O_2 \tag{3.1}$$

When free to move in solution, the nanorods demonstrated linear motion. When tethered to a substrate, however, they would rotate. It emerged that the orientational dynamics and speed of the nanorods are mediated by several factors, including general nanorod dimensions and those of the metallic domains, the types of metals used, the viscosity of the solvent, and concentration of the H_2O_2 fuel, surfactant additives, and parameters such as pH level and ionic potency. The quantification of these parameters enabled further advancements in the development of chemically powered nanodevices. Nanorod movement is facilitated by nanodevice geometry and chemically initiated propulsion, which prevails over hydrodynamic forces such as viscous drag and Brownian motion.

Of the potential mechanisms at work for the propulsion of nanorods, which encompass bubble recoil, cavitation, Brownian ratchet, thermal gradient, interfacial tension, and bipolar electrophoresis (electrokinetic motion), there remains some dispute as to which mechanisms are prominent in the process, although they all likely have a role. The earlier said one likely dominant candidate for nanorod propulsion is bubble recoil. Mirkovic et al. point out that oxygen gas bubbles that result from the oxidation of H_2O_2 at the Pt substrate expand to provide nanorod thrust in the opposite direction. Another plausible candidate they describe is the bipolar electrophoresis/electrokinetic model, in which the oxidation of H_2O_2, which takes place at the anodic Pt substrate, and H_2O_2 reduction, which occurs at the Au substrate, initiates the internal transfer of an electric charge that proceeds from anode to cathode. Concurrent with this process is the transfer of "charge-balancing protons and

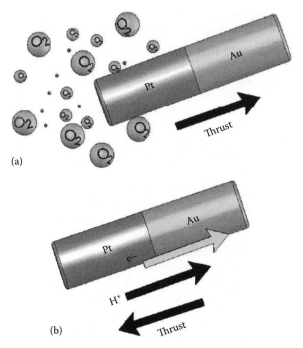

FIGURE 3.6

Potential mechanisms for nanorod propulsion: (a) bubble recoil mechanism and (b) bipolar electrophoresis/electrokinetic model. (Redrawn from Chris Wilmer in Mirkovic, T. et al., ACS Nano., 4(4), 1782–9, 2010. Copyright 2010. American Chemical Society. With permission.)

water of hydration at the nanorod-solution interface causing the nanorod to move in the other direction" (Figure 3.6) [75].

The fine control of acceleration, velocity, and deceleration for chemically powered nanodevices will be contingent on the knowledge gained in regard to the detailed kinetics of nanometric catalytic propulsion. This may facilitate the appropriate administration of future nanodevices in terms of dosages and in the calculation of timescales for the movement of variable volumes of materials in vivo (e.g., drugs, tissue, and bone rebuilding material payloads), or for the transport to egress sites of nanosurgically removed vascular or β-amyloid plaque material.

More recent investigations conducted by Zacharia et al. have revealed that there is a correlation between the surface roughness of the catalytic segment of nanorods and increased velocity. It was demonstrated that surface porosity enhanced the speed of Au/Ni nanorods (immersed in H_2O_2) of 6 µm in length, by 50% in comparison with smooth-surfaced nanorods. It was also found that shorter nanorods had higher velocities than long nanorods [79]. The integration of carbon nanotubes into the Pt component of Pt/Au nanorods served to further improve their velocity by achieving speeds of from ~20 to 50 µm/s. The inclusion of hydrazine boosted velocities even further, to 200 µm/s, which is comparable to the most rapid of flagellated microorganisms [80]. Significant increases in nanorod velocity may also be obtained when the pure Au component of Pt/Au nanorods is replaced with alloys of Au and Ag, such as $Pt–Ag_xAu_{1-x}$, which enables speeds of from ~20 to >150 µm/s to be realized. A linear enhancement in velocity was observed with increases in the atomic percentage of Ag infused within the Au/Ag alloy, for example $Ag_{25}Au_{75}$, $Ag_{50}Au_{50}$, and $Ag_{75}Au_{25}$. These improvements were ascribed to an increase in catalytic activity, superior electron transfer, and H_2O_2 decomposition in comparison to pure/isolated Au and Ag [81].

Aside from H_2O_2, other fuels such as hydrazine (H_4N_2) may be utilized as a propellant by nanorods. It is anticipated that additional potential fuels may be investigated as well, encompassing methanol, formic acid, diazomethane, azides, hydrides, and organic peroxides [75]. In the quest for biocompatible fuels, it was demonstrated by Mano and Heller that glucose oxidase (GO_x) and bilirubin oxidase (BOD) enzyme–decorated carbon fibers could be autonomously propelled when immersed in a solution that contained glucose [82]. The carbon fibers (Ø 7 μm × 0.5–1 cm long) were driven at the H_2O/O_2 interface by utilizing a glucose-oxidizing microanode and an O_2-reducing microcathode. The current that traversed the fiber flowed in conjunction with the rapid movement of ions at the interface, where viscous drag is negligible, to enable sufficient thrust to propel the fiber at a velocity of ~1 cm/s. The glucose–oxygen reaction was observed at a temperature of 37°C at pH 7 under 1 atm O_2. The composition of the coating on the fibers included centrally located hydrophobic domains, which made them buoyant at the solution/gas boundary. In contrast, the terminating ends of the fibers were coated with two types of hydrophilic bioelectrocatalysts, which enabled electrolytic contact of the fiber with the solution. One tip contained a bioelectrocatalytic thin film with the capacity for glucose oxidation (redox polymer–wired GO_x) [83], whereas the opposite tip contained a bioelectrocatalytic thin film that enabled the four-electron reduction of O_2 to water (redox polymer–wired BOD) [84]. The resulting construct was an electrically shorted biofuel cell.

The reaction at the microanode was

$$\beta\text{-D-Glucose} \rightarrow \text{D-Glucono-1, 5-lactone} + 2H^+ + 2e^- \tag{3.2}$$

The reaction at the microcathode was

$$1/2\ O_2 + 2H^+ + 2e^- \rightarrow H_2O \tag{3.3}$$

These enabled a net bioelectrochemomechanical power-generating reaction [82]:

$$\beta\text{-D-Glucose} + 1/2\ O_2 \rightarrow \text{D-Glucono-1, 5-lactone} + H_2O \tag{3.4}$$

Optimal morphological designs for nanomotors may play a considerable role in both the reduction of viscous drag and the promotion of propulsive force. Synthetic chiral geometries, akin to helical bacterial flagella, have been tested in this regard [85] as well as magnetic nanoparticles (MNP) with various geometries [86,87], angular Ni–Au nanorods that have spiraling motility [88], and a H_2O_2-driven nanospheric heterodimer that include a catalytic Pt nanosphere interfaced with a noncatalytic silica nanosphere [89]. Solovev et al. have developed a micron-scale funnel-shaped microjet engine by employing a top–down nanofabrication process and that utilizes a Pt lining and Au coating to attain excellent velocities via the formation of oxygen bubbles at the smaller diameter lead end of the funnel, and their subsequent ejection from the larger rear orifice [90]. Wang et al. utilized a facile bottom-up synthesis process that was based on the sequential deposition of Pt and Au layers onto an etched silver wire template, which produced conical microjet engines (Figures 3.7 and 3.8) with velocities that approached ~456 μm/s via the bubble recoil mechanism [91].

Solid-state microjet engines may be fabricated via the deposition of thin films of practically any material onto a sacrificial photoresist layer. Once released from their substrate via selective etching, the thin films spontaneously roll up into nanotubes with walls that can be as thin as a single atomic layer. For instance, silicon–germanium nanotubes with

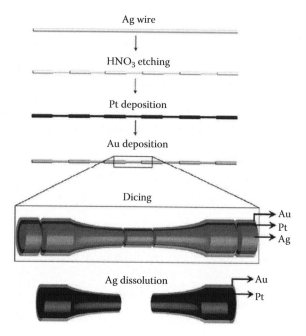

FIGURE 3.7
Depiction of template-assisted preparation of tubular microjet engine. (Reprinted with permission from Manesh, K.M. et al., *ACS Nano.*, 4, 1799–1804, 2010. Copyright 2010 American Chemical Society.)

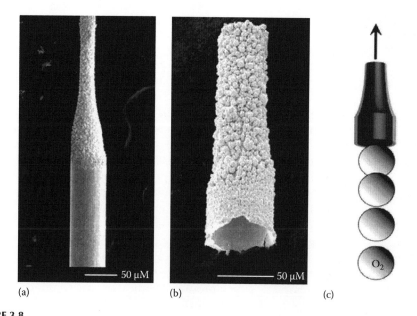

FIGURE 3.8
(a) SEM of etched Ø 50 μm Ag wire, (b) Pt–Au microjet cone subsequent to Ag dissolution, and (c) schematic of electrocatalytically generated oxygen microbubbles on the interior PT surface, which are expelled from the larger orifice of the microcone to drive the microjet. (Reprinted with permission from Manesh, K.M. et al., *ACS Nano.*, 4, 1799–1804. Copyright 2010. American Chemical Society.)

diameters of 50 and 230 nm, lengths of 12 μm, with wall thicknesses of 6 and 16 nm, respectively, were fabricated using this technique [92]. Larger microjets have also been fabricated with diameters in the 5–10 μm range and lengths of 25–100 μm.

The versatility of this process insofar as the possible range of materials that may be utilized enables myriad potential functionalities. When the inner luminal surface of the nanotubes is comprised of Pt catalyst or catalase enzymes, it has the capacity for degrading H_2O_2 fuel with the subsequent generation of oxygen that accumulates within the nanotube. These microbubbles gravitate toward the largest orifice and generate thrust via recoil action from the jet ejection of microbubbles and lumen-resident fluid.

Although the manufacture of polymer-based catalytic nanotubes has remained elusive, a method was recently developed that utilized thin film layers that were grown by molecular beam epitaxy (MBE). This process involved the heteroepitaxial growth of intrinsically strained semiconductor films to which metal layers are added to achieve what is purported to be the world's most diminutive jet engine. A composite lamination of thin films, which included InGaAs/GaAs/Cr/Pt, at respective thicknesses of 3, 3, 1, and 1 nm produced ~600 nm in diameter nanotubes weighing 1 pg. These self-propelling 5 μm long catalytic nanojet "engines" attained velocities of ~55 μm/s when they were immersed in fuel solutions comprising 18% H_2O_2 and 10% surfactant (Figure 3.9) [93]. Interestingly, when ferromagnetic constituents are introduced into the laminated structures of the nanotubes, their trajectories and conceivably velocities may be magnetically mediated [91,94]. These capabilities might be extrapolated to the finessed control of first-generation nanomedical

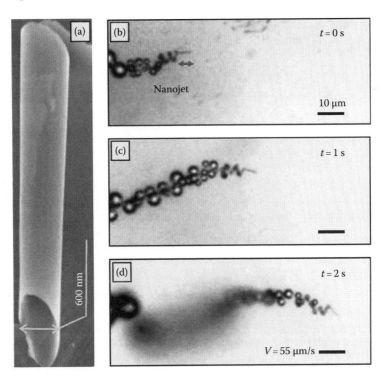

FIGURE 3.9

(a) SEM image of smallest (Ø 600 nm diameter × 5 μm long) nanojet engine to date—2011 and (b–d) nanojet trajectory over 2 s in 18% H_2O_2 fuel at 55 μm/s. (Sanchez, S., Solovev, A.A., Harazim, S.M., Deneke, C., Feng Mei, Y., and Schmidt, O.G.: The smallest man-made jet engine. *Chem Rec.* 2011. 11(6). 367–370. Copyright Wiley-VCH Verlag GmbH & Co. KGaA. Reproduced with permission.)

diagnostic and therapeutic devices via magnetic resonance imaging (MRI), for full-body procedures, or portable magnetic field–generating devices to perform more localized bio-analytical queries or to conduct nanosurgeries.

In regard to the molecular characterization and theoretical performance parameters of nanojets, atomistic molecular dynamics simulations have demonstrated that they may attain velocities of up to 400 m/s. These simulations utilized the pressurized injection of liquid propane through gold nanometric nozzles to elucidate flow attributes and stochastic lubrication at different temperatures, and when nanocoatings were applied to the external surfaces of the gold nozzles to reduce or eliminate the formation of plugging films. Factors such as nozzle opening geometries and distortions, material traits, surface tension, and nozzle orifice wettability appear to have a significant influence on the capillary flow stability of nanojets [95].

An important consideration for the use of nanojets to propel medical nanodevices in vivo concerns the reduction of the toxicity of the fuels that are proposed to power them. Researchers typically utilize high concentrations of H_2O_2 and toxic substances such as hydrazine to power catalytic micro/nanojets, which negate their utility in physiological environments. Therefore, the maximization of the efficiency of such fuels (e.g., optimal translation of chemical energy to nanomechanical force) and ideally, the discovery of potent yet biocompatible fuels are paramount. Sanchez et al. utilized thermal regulation to improve the efficacy of microjet engines and to reduce the volume of H_2O_2 required. It was learned that at temperatures in the physiological domain (~37°C) microjets could be propelled at velocities of 140 µm/s while utilizing only 0.25% H_2O_2. A surfactant was utilized to reduce surface tension and comprised "anionic tenside (5%–15%), amphoteric tenside (<5%), bronopol, benzisothiazolinone, and methylisothiazolinone." At 5% concentrations of H_2O_2, microjet velocities of up to 10 mm/s were obtained. Revealed as well was that linear trajectories, which dominate at lower speeds and temperatures and give way to those that are curvilinear at higher velocities and temperatures [94].

3.3.3 Molecular Motors

The human body encompasses a myriad of biological molecular motors that operate via the transformation of chemical energy into mechanical motion. Conceptualists and designers of molecular motors will be challenged with a complex array of issues when seeking to exploit molecular-scale movement in order to impart propulsive forces for in vivo nanomedical devices. Hundreds of different species of functional molecular motors exist within biological cells [96].

3.3.3.1 Activation of Molecular Motors

Energy for the activation of molecular motors might be derived from the temperature differentials that circulating nanodevices are exposed to as they traverse both the warmer core of patients and their cooler extremities. A single round trip through the human vasculature is generally within the range of ~60 s [1]. What is known as the Seebeck effect, involving the generation of a voltage via temperature differentials that are conveyed by two dissimilar heat-transferring materials (isolated from each other by an insulating layer), might have the capacity for harvesting sufficient thermal power to drive a range of molecular motors. The inverse of the Seebeck effect, where electric current gives rise to differences in temperature of distinct metals, is known as the Peltier or Thomson effect.

Chemical reactions, as described earlier, might be tapped to serve as ambient energy reservoirs to drive molecular motors for the actuation of nanodevices [97]. Self-governing, chemically driven molecular motors that permeate biological domains are immensely proficient in the conversion of high-energy molecular fuels into lower energy products. Chemical compounds encompassing ATP, glucose and glucosamine, lipids, proteins, and certain amino acids, as well as carbohydrates may be efficiently converted via oxidation–reduction (redox) reactions into usable voltage. In the process of conversion these molecules are subjected to structural reconfigurations, which revert to their original forms subsequent to each reduction cycle [98].

3.3.3.2 ATP Synthase

The most familiar rotary motor is ATP synthase, the enzyme that produces ATP (Table 3.2) [99–101]. This mechanism comprises a complex of a minimum of 24 proteins and actually contains two molecular rotary motors, both of which are tethered to a common shaft. Each motor attempts to rotate in a direction opposite to that of the other and each one is reversible. The F_1 motor (Figure 3.10) utilizes the free energy that is made available from ATP hydrolysis to revolve in one direction, while the F_0 motor uses

TABLE 3.2

Examples of Molecular Motor Functional Data

Molecular Motor	AD (nm)	RV (rps)	LV (μm/s)	T (pN nm)	E (%)	F
E. coli flagella	~20	300	40	~450	~100	H^+
V. alginolyticus polar flagella	~20	1700	210	~100	~100	Na^+
F_0F_1 ATPase—F_1 motor	~1	10	60	~40	~100	ATP
Myosin (skeletal muscle)	NA	NA	10	NA	~5	ATP

Source: Adapted from Yorimitsu, T. and Homma, M., *Biochim. Biophys. Acta*, 1505(1), 82, 2001.
Abbreviations: AD, Axial distance; RV, rotational velocity; LV, linear velocity; *T*, torque; *E*, efficacy; and F, fuel.

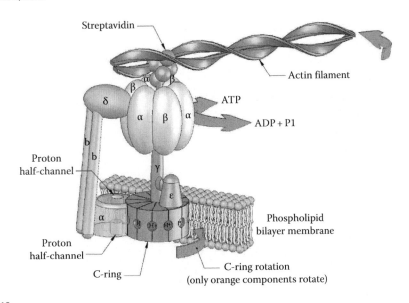

FIGURE 3.10
Nanometric ATP synthase with 2 μm long "propeller" anchored within phospholipid bilayers. (Adapted from Steinberg-Yfrach, G. et al., *Nature*, 392, 479, 1998; Bachand, G.D. et al., *Nano Lett.*, 1(1), 42, 2001.)

the energy that is stored in the transmembrane electrochemical gradient, to rotate in the opposite direction [102–109]. It is surmised that the F_0 motor is related to the bacterial flagellar motor, as they can both be activated by sodium. A difference is that the flagellar motor has eight or more stators, and hence, develops substantially greater torque than F_0 [110,111].

To activate the nanomotor, a stream of protons must travel through the membrane-bound proteins. An organized ringlike structure houses 12 copies of the c subunit. The current stream initiates ring rotation, as protons pass from one side of the membrane to the other. This rotary motion drives mechanical proteins designated as γ and ε. The γ-protein extends like a shaft into a central core formed by the chemical α- and β-proteins. The γ-protein rotation sequentially prompts each of the three β-proteins to release newly synthesized ATP.

An additional function of the γ-protein is to pry the ATP molecule loose once its synthesis is complete. To synthesize ATP at the rate of 30–50 s^{-1}, the motor must maintain a torque of 40–50 pN nm, and generate enough torque to free the ATP from F_1. This level of torque is six times greater than the highest force that is generated by kinesin or myosin, having a mechanical efficiency of almost 100%. This excludes heat engines that are restricted by the Carnot efficiency [102,111–113].

The specific function of the motor is dependent on which element manages to provide the most torque. Normally, the F_0 motor supplies the most torque, which then drives the F_1 motor in reverse, with the effect of initiating ATP synthesis. The movements involved may be characterized as quantized increments that span 120° each. When the F_1 motor manages to deliver additional torque, it will hydrolyze ATP and drive the F_0 motor in reverse. This, in effect, transforms it into an ion pump that transports ions across the membrane that it is embedded within, against the electrochemical gradient [99,114,115].

A biomimetic hybrid (natural/artificial) system that exploits photons to acquire proton-motive force and initiate ATP synthesis has been constructed, and the mechanism mimics the entire bacterial photosynthetic process [116–118]. Another nanomechanical hybrid device consisting of three subcomponents, which were powered by ATP synthase, has been developed. The substrate, serving as a base, was made of Ni with a diameter of 50–120 nm × ~200 nm in height. A specifically modified F_1-ATPase molecule was interfaced to the Ni substrate by utilizing histidine tags, which were inserted into the β-subunits. Subsequently, a nanofabricated Ni "nanopropeller" (~150 nm in diameter × 750–1000 nm in length), coated with biotinylated histidine-rich peptides, was attached to the γ-subunit tip of the F_1-ATPase via a biotin–streptavidin linkage. Rotary activation was accomplished via the addition of 2 mM ATP. The motor could be stopped through the addition of NaN_3 (sodium azide), which is a F_1-ATPase inhibitor [113,118,119].

It is conceivable that arrayed and appropriately seated banks of ATP-based rotary motors may provide sufficient propulsive force to enable VCSN travel through the human body. Single actin filaments have been tethered to the F_1 motor and have been observed rotating in classic 120° increments. High-speed imaging has elucidated that the 120° stepping is actually segmented into two increments of 90° and 30°, with each being a fraction of a millisecond in duration. The 90° increment is driven by ATP binding, whereas the 30° increment is surmised to be driven by the release of a product via hydrolysis. These two substeps are separated by two 1 ms reactions, which combined make up most of the ATP hydrolysis cycle. Rotation at full speed is ~130 revolutions/s at ATP saturation [120]. To date, several other molecular level actuating entities have been devised; one being a light-driven rotary motor [121,122].

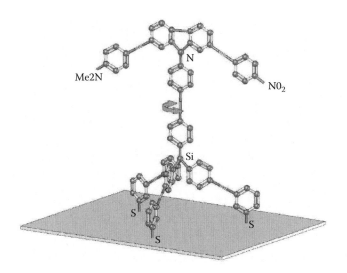

FIGURE 3.11
Electric field–driven dipole rotor. (Redrawn from Jian, H. and Tour, J.M., *J. Org. Chem.*, 68(13), 5091, 2003; Reproduced from Boehm, F., Chapter 15, Potential strategies for advanced nanomedical device ingress and egress, natation, mobility, and navigation, in Schulz, M.J. et al., eds., *Nanomedicine Design of Particles, Sensors, Motors, Implants, Robots, and Devices*, Artech House, Norwood, MA, 2009, With permission.)

3.3.3.3 Molecular Dipole Rotors

The cumulative force generated by appropriately configured molecular dipolar rotors (Figure 3.11) may be exploited to propel nanodevices within the human body to facilitate beneficial nanomedical procedures. The self-assembled synthesis of an electric field–driven dipole rotor tethered to a gold substrate was investigated by Jian and Tour. Four molecules, having caltrop geometries, consisted of two donor/acceptor arms, comprising a carbazole or oligo(phenylene ethynylene) core that possessed a potent net dipole, were mounted to a tripod base. The sulfur-terminated legs of the tripod were bonded to the Au surface via acetyl-protected benzylic thiols. The upright shaft configuration for this assemblage of molecules, which enable their utility as external field–driven molecular motors, was verified by ellipsometry [123].

Kelly et al. devised a prototype rotary molecular motor that employed phosgene as a fuel to activate 120° unidirectional clockwise rotation, and are continuing to implement modifications toward the realization of a continuously rotating device [97]. Feringa et al. constructed a photonically actuated molecular motor with the capacity for repeatable rotational motion. It comprised a chiral helical alkene, which contained an upper portion that served as a propeller, which was linked via a carbon–carbon double bond to a lower section acting as a stator. Dual thiol-functionalized legs constituted the stator and chemically tethered the motor to an Au substrate. Photonically mediated *cis–trans* isomerizations of the core double bond enabled full 360° unidirectional rotation [124]. Dahl and Branchaud achieved repeatably rotating synthetic molecular motors through the utilization of chiral biaryl molecules, which exhibited full degree unidirectional rotation about a central aryl–aryl bond [125].

3.3.3.4 Rotary Molecular Motor Using Motor Protein Pairs

A molecular motor has been constructed (Figure 3.12) that is made up of concentric cylinders, which revolve about a mutual central axis. Opposed cylinder surfaces are coated with layers of paired complementary motor proteins (e.g., actin and myosin). When ATP is injected into

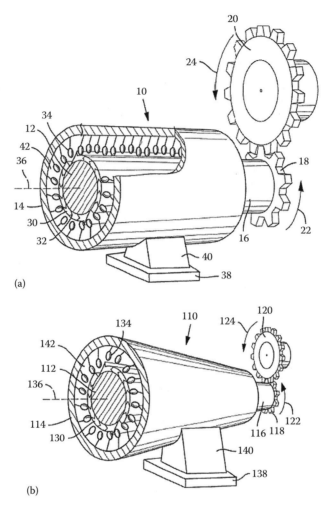

FIGURE 3.12
(a, b) Cylindrical molecular motor. (Reproduced from Schneider, T.D. and Lyakhov, I.G., Molecular motor, U.S. Patent Application P20020083710, 2002. With permission.)

the system, the actin and myosin molecules interact, consequentially inducing the cylinders to rotate in relation to one another. The resulting rotational motion might be utilized to perform useful work. When the numbers and lengths of the nested cylinders are varied, the concentration of ATP may be employed to mediate the motor's revolution rate. The length of the cylinders may also be utilized to control the energy output of the motor [126].

3.3.3.5 Brownian Motion

In the course of envisioning and engineering nanomedical device propulsion mechanisms and associated systems, researchers and nanoengineers will likely confront numerous challenges in dealing with Brownian motion. The environment at the molecular domain is governed by ubiquitous random thermal oscillations. Hence, the intensity of their effects on nanodevices at ambient in vivo temperatures is a function of scale. To reduce its influence, a decrease in temperature (from 300 to 3 K) would be necessary to diminish these fluctuations to 10% of their average ambient value of 10^{-8} W in solution. In view of this fact, it is indeed remarkable that molecular motor proteins, which process from 100 to 1000 molecules of ATP/s, which is equivalent to maximum power yields from 10^{-16} to 10^{-18} W/ molecule, have any motive control whatsoever [127–129].

It seems that useful endeavors toward the conceptualization and development of efficient molecular motors for imparting nanodevice motility might therefore be generated from the perspective of integrating strategies for the exploitation of Brownian motion in their functionality, rather than working against it. Electric potentials in biomolecular systems arise from the exchange of electrons, or through the kinetics of charge-separated domains. Equilibrium states are described by the "Principal of Detailed Balance," wherein transfers that involve any two states proceed in either direction at an equivalent rate, which negates the creation of a net flux [98]. Therefore, the design of nanometric propulsive elements that perform with efficiency under the influence of Brownian motion might be achieved only when this detailed balance is disrupted, as there is an unceasing drive toward the spontaneous reestablishment of equilibrium.

3.3.3.6 Brownian Shuttles

When ligands are combined with transition metal species, the resulting constructs are relatively stable and demonstrate redox-driven shuttling through variable oxidation states. The motive actuation of molecular shuttles may be initiated by a number of processes, including the binding and release of metal ions and the chemically mediated forging and cleavage of covalent bonds (Figure 3.13) [98]. Molecular shuttling may also be initiated when photons at particular wavelengths initiate the cleavage of chemical bonds.

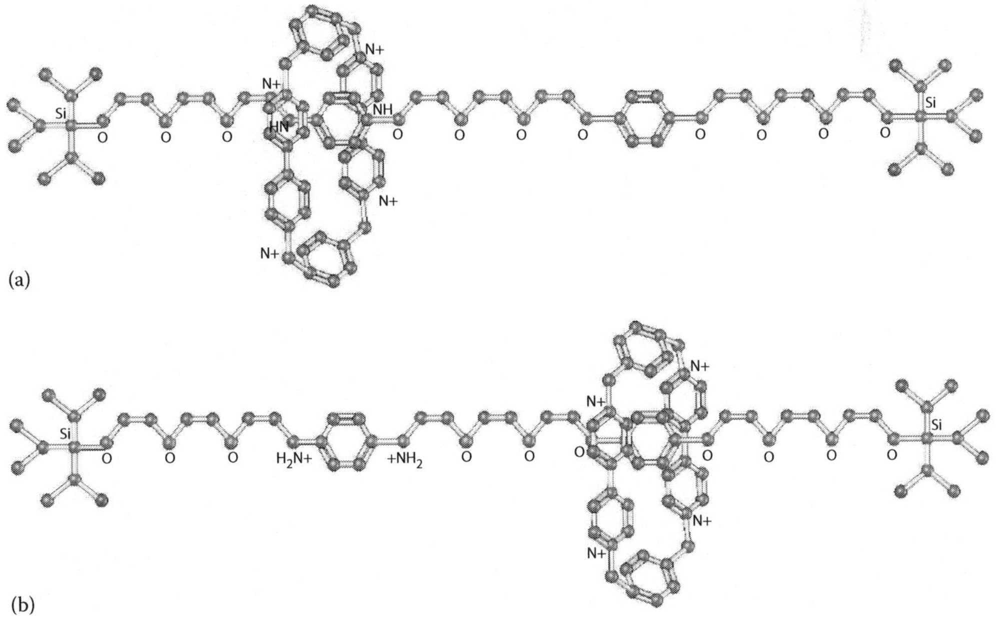

FIGURE 3.13
(a, b) Molecular shuttle. (Redrawn from Kay, E.R. et al., Angew. Chem. Int. Ed., 46(1–2), 72, 2007; Reproduced from Boehm, F., Chapter 15, Potential strategies for advanced nanomedical device ingress and egress, natation, mobility, and navigation, in Schulz, M.J. et al., *Nanomedicine Design of Particles, Sensors, Motors, Implants, Robots, and Devices*, Artech House, Norwood, MA, 2009, With permission.)

Photonically mediated shuttle activation has the advantage of running cleanly as no chemical fuels are required; thus, the process negates the generation of reaction/waste products. In addition, these virtually autonomous systems can automatically reset and might, under the appropriate parameters, operate indefinitely [130]. Speculatively, arrays of Brownian shuttles that are designed to function in a massively parallel configuration may endow nanodevices with the ability to be sequentially "pulled" through in vivo aqueous physiological media. The shuttling elements themselves might be decorated with scalloped nanoscale "petals" or "oars" to magnify the conveyed directional motive force to enable the traversal of viscous media.

3.3.3.7 Brownian Ratchet

A Brownian ratchet (Feynman–Smoluchowski ratchet) is a conceptual molecular construct that consists of an axle with a toothed ratchet and pawl attached to one end, and a paddle wheel attached to the opposite end, which may only move in one direction when molecules impact with the paddle plates. These mechanisms are proposed to operate under vacillations of thermal equilibrium and are envisioned to underlie the functionality of proteinaceous molecular motor elements.

Three primary components include

1. A randomizing element [131]
2. An energy resource that is in compliance with the second law of thermodynamics (law of increased entropy) whereby disparities in (e.g., thermal, chemical) gradients inevitably attain equilibrium, and viable energy irreversibly transitions to nonviable energy
3. The establishment of an asymmetrical state where intended movement proceeds unidirectionally

A number of Brownian ratchets under consideration encompass entropic, Hamiltonian, pulsating or tilting energy, thermally driven (e.g., Seebeck effect), and flashing. A pulsating ratchet, for instance, taps into disparate (elevated and reduced) energy states to move particulates in an intended orientation on a potential energy substrate. The creation and dissolution of chemical bonds might provide the energy reservoir necessary to drive these mechanisms and Brownian elements may be manifest as distinct molecules or intramolecular domains [98].

3.3.4 Microrobot Propulsion

Nanomedical devices will most likely have requirements for swimming at much higher velocities than their biological counterparts, for the traversal of macroscopic distances in a reasonable time. These demands will make power optimization a critical issue. An essential role might be played by a "swimming drag coefficient." This formula, presented by Avron et al., might be used to elucidate general scaling relations (e.g., that the maximum velocity of an externally powered robot is proportional to the square root of its length) [132]:

$$\delta(\gamma) = \frac{D(\gamma)\tau(\gamma)}{\eta X^2(\gamma)Ld^{-2}} \tag{3.5}$$

where

$D(\gamma)$ is the spent stroke energy
γ and $X(\gamma)$ represent the step size
$\tau(\gamma)$ is the period of the stroke
$\delta(\gamma)$ is a functional on the spacing of strokes
L is the scale

Higher swimming velocities translate to far higher energy consumption rates. A nano-medical device that swims ~100 times more quickly than a bacterium at a velocity of 1 mm/s may utilize 10^4 more energy. Optimal swimming might be considered through a more expansive perspective of control theory. "The shape of the swimmer is the control, the displacement is the output, and the dissipation is the cost function that needs to be minimized, subject to appropriate constraints" [132]. Assuming an environment domi-nated by viscosity and low Reynolds numbers [133]

$$Re = \frac{D_p \upsilon \rho}{\eta} \tag{3.6}$$

where

D_p is the particle size
υ is the velocity
ρ is the density of the media
η is the viscosity

A biological example is that a bacterium that proceeds at a velocity of 10 body lengths/s has a Reynolds number of ~10^{-5}. Nanomedical devices swimming 100 times more rap-idly might have a Reynolds number of ~10^{-3}. Drag force by itself will halt a nanowire (Ø 300 nm × 10 µm long) that is traveling at 100 µm/s in ~10^{-6} s within a distance of 1 Å. Hence, viscous drag force poses immense challenges for the controllable rotation and deter-mination of torque for nanometric elements at low Reynolds numbers [133]. Traversing the vasculature at low Reynolds numbers may indicate that fluid does not generate net forces on the swimmer [25,132]. The diminishment of the drag coefficient may lead/contribute to the development of optimal swimming action for nanomedical devices such as the VCSN.

3.3.5 Biomimetic Propulsion

A biomimetic microrobot (Figure 3.14) has been developed to enter the human ureter with the goal of noninvasively demolishing kidney stones. This mechanism device employed multiwalled carbon nanotubes that functioned as synthetic flagella that were induced to rotate helically under the power of several micromotors. Predicted natating velocities of 1 mm/s were thought feasible under 1 nW of power. With the aim of high efficiency, dual orthogonal comb drives were utilized for each motor in order to translate voltage into mechanical actuation, thus causing the nanotubes to revolve. External communications were enabled using a radio receiver or thin lead. Directed navigation was made possible via the independent motion of four abutted rotating bases, which were populated with the nanotubes [134].

The spatial volume of the microrobot was 1 mm³, with individual nanotube radii of ~30 nm. The rotating substrate was ~100 µm in length. The microrobot swam at a velocity of 0.5 mm/s with an efficiency of 2% and showed a 10 µm displacement at 100 Hz. If the

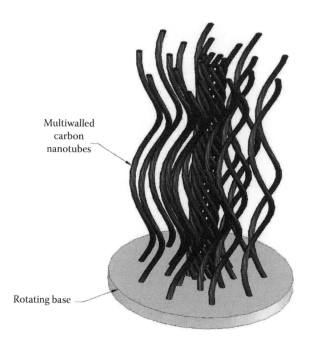

Multiwalled
carbon
nanotubes

Rotating base

FIGURE 3.14

Biomimetic flagella utilizing multiwalled carbon nanotubes attached to a rotating stage. (Redrawn from Edd, J. et al., IEEE/RSJ Intelligent Robotics and Systems Conference, Las Vegas, NV, October 2003, http://nanolab. me.cmu.edu/publications/papers/Sitti-IROS2003.pdf; Reproduced from Boehm, F., Potential strategies for advanced nanomedical device ingress and egress, natation, mobility, and navigation, in Schulz, M.J. et al., eds., *Nanomedicine Design of Particles, Sensors, Motors, Implants, Robots, and Devices*, Artech House, Norwood, MA, 2009, Chapter 15. With permission.)

rotary comb drive attained an operational torque of 130 μN·nm at an efficiency of 0.1%, it could be powered at 1 nW [134]. A several centimeter long swimming robot has also been built that utilizes a power source, sensors, and polymeric actuators [135–137].

Fan et al. reported the precisely controlled high-speed rotation of metallic (Au, Pt, Ni) nanowires (Ø 300 nm × 2–30 μm long) and multiwalled carbon nanotubes (Ø 50 nm × 5 μm long) in suspension via the application of AC voltage. The electric field was provided by four Au microelectrodes that were equidistantly spaced, which enabled "specific chirality, rotation speed, and total angle of rotation." Free-standing nanowires exhibited rotational velocities of 1803 rpm, whereas nanowires that were tethered at one end attained 445 rpm. In both instances, the nanowires could be instantaneously actuated or stopped. The solid-state microelectrode-generated electric field was demonstrated to have the capacity for overcoming variable microscale forces to initiate highly efficient linear acceleration at extremely low Reynolds numbers (10^{-5}). This group also fabricated a functional micromotor utilizing a bent gold nanowire under the power of a rotating electric field, analogous to the rotor and stator of an electric motor [133,138].

A sacrificial etching synthesis technique was used in the development of flexible multi-segmented nanomechanical nanorods comprising Pt–Au–Pt and Pt–Au–Pt–Au–Pt joined by hinges comprising a polyelectrolyte. The Au segments were etched from the polyelectrolyte-coated nanorods, which were deposited layer by layer. These nanoscale entities exhibited undulating movement through the integration of nickel elements, and when immersed in H_2O_2, were controlled by an intermittent external magnetic field, to exhibit propulsive utility as biomimetic bacterial flagellar analogs [139].

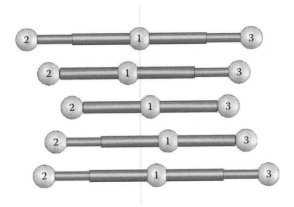

FIGURE 3.15
Biomimetic aligned sphere propulsion. (Redrawn from Najafi, A. and Golestanian, R., *Phys Rev E.* 69, 062901, 2004; Reproduced from Boehm, F., Potential strategies for advanced nanomedical device ingress and egress, natation, mobility, and navigation, in Schulz, M.J. et al., eds., *Nanomedicine Design of Particles, Sensors, Motors, Implants, Robots, and Devices*, Artech House, Norwood, MA, 2009, Chapter 15. With permission.)

Najafi and Golestanian have developed a means for propulsion that comprises three aligned spheres that are joined by two rods (Figure 3.15). The left arm is initially actuated (retracted), followed by the retraction of the right arm. Subsequently, the left arm is extended and then the right. The ensuing movement is analogous to that of an earthworm making its way through soil [140].

3.3.6 Externally Mediated Magnetic Propulsion

Early generations of nanomedical devices that are infused with ferromagnetic elements might be propelled through the human body and directed in three dimensions via MRI-generated magnetic fields. Capabilities for nanodevice tracking and the acquisition of orientation and position feedback may also be possible through MRI imaging technologies that utilize nanomagnetic entities, such as dextran-coated $Ni–Fe_2O_4$ nanoparticles as T1 and T2 contrast agents [141]. To enable this capacity, however, the force of MRI-initiated magnetic fields must prevail over the drag force of circulating blood that impacts on nanodevices, to allow for controllable nanodevice positional manipulation.

A currently significant drawback is that there exist large ferromagnetic artifacts/perturbations present that can be several times larger than the size of the nanoparticle core itself. This issue must be resolved in order to obtain, with any precision, the actual location of the ferromagnetic cores [142]. Ferromagnetic artifacts arise from MNPs as these entities have a magnetic receptiveness that is larger than that of biological tissues, and the generation of MRI images assume a homogeneous magnetic field [143].

This has implications for the acquisition of accurate spatial trajectories of MNPs, which may be initially administered to a patient for utilization as "pathway scouts" for the development and training of computer algorithms that will be used to subsequently propel and guide therapeutic magnetically endowed nanodevices through the unique courses and geometries of the vascular systems of individual patients.

The visualization of nanometric entities with conventional MRI necessitates the use of this ferromagnetic "susceptibility-based negative contrast." These artifacts must attain the dimensions of a MRI voxel, typically ($\sim$0.5 $\times$ 0.5 $\times$ 0.5 mm^3), before they may be seen.

"More precisely, the intravoxel de-phasing in the gradient echo (GE) sequence provides the most effective method to amplify the effect of a microentity that is too small to be visualized in the MR image. Experimental data demonstrated … that a single micro-entity or microrobot with a diameter as small as 15 μm relying on material with high susceptibility can indeed be detected by the intra-voxel dephasing using GE scans" [144, 145].

Martel et al. have envisioned and investigated a number of MRI-mediated propulsive and navigational techniques toward the potential enablement of precision nanomedical diagnostics and therapeutics (Chapter 14). This group conducted the first in vivo experiments to demonstrate magnetic resonance targeting via the computer-controlled propulsion and navigation of a "1.5 mm ferromagnetic bead along a planned trajectory in the carotid artery of a living swine at an average velocity of 10 cm/s" [146]. They have also exploited flagellar propulsion to track MC-1 magnetotactic bacteria (MTB), which were embedded with chains of magnetite and magnetosomes. These bacteria were induced to controllably change direction under computer-guided exposure to MRI magnetic fields and may have the capacity for the delivering drugs deep within cancerous tumors where they might traverse the interstitial space to access necrotic regions. Individual MTB have two flagellar bundles that can supply a propulsive force that is greater than 4 pN, which is 10 times higher than that supplied by archetypal bacterial flagella [144,147,148].

Ferromagnetic Ni and Ni-capped copper/tin nanowires have been induced to revolve under a rotating magnetic field, though at relatively low velocities [149,150]. Gao et al. have created flexible Au/Ag/Ni nanowires (Ø 200 nm × 6 μm long), comprising a gold head segment linked to a nickel tail segment via a flexible silver midsection. On exposure to a rotating magnetic field, the flexible midsection was induced to undulate and undergo cyclical mechanical deformations. When the Ni segment initially rotated, it was followed by the gold segment, which revolved at a dissimilar amplitude (Figure 3.16). This arrangement disrupted the Purcell symmetry and thus facilitated locomotion, in this case, through urine and highly saline samples.

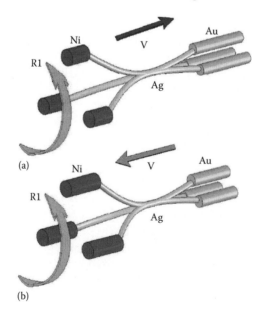

FIGURE 3.16
Schematic of magnetic Au/Ag/Ni nanowire configurations for "forward" (a) and "backward" (b) natation. (Redrawn with permission from Gao, W., Sattayasamitsathit, S., Manesh, K.M., Weihs, D., and Wang, J., Magnetically powered flexible metal nanowire motors. *J. Am. Chem. Soc.*, 132(41), 14403–14405. Copyright 2010. American Chemical Society.)

Directional movement (pushing and pulling) was accomplished by modifying the length of the Ni and Au segments (thus altering the asymmetrical geometry) and adjusting the magnetic field [151]. In the case where the Au segment was longer than the Ni segment (3 to 0.5 μm, respectively), "forward" locomotion ensued, with the Au segment in the front position. The larger rotating conical swath of the shorter Ni element (in comparison to the Au segment) induces an outward flow field in relation to the Ag midsection, and thus a larger force in the swimming direction of the Au "head." To achieve "backward" locomotion, the Au segment was shortened and the Ni segment lengthened (2 to 1 μm, respectively) enabling a velocity of 4 μm/s with the Ni "tail" in the front position. Interestingly, as earlier studies [152] have indicated, "backward" (puller) locomotion achieves higher effectiveness and repeatability than locomotion in the "forward" (pusher) direction. The stability of pulling diminutive entities through viscous aqueous media is greater than the opposite, and is "analogous to pushing a string on a frictional surface, as opposed to pulling it" [151].

A flexible artificial flagellum, comprising colloidal MNP and connected by lissom DNA fragments, was tethered to a RBC and magnetically induced to swim via controlled deformations. Dreyfus et al. utilized 1 μm in diameter superparamagnetic nanoparticles and joined them together using a number of (107 nm long) DNA duplex fragments, at 315 base pairs (bp) each to construct a 30 μm long strand. The degree of flexibility was conferred by varying the diameter of the nanoparticles and the quantity and length of the DNA linkages. The direction and velocity of the construct could be tuned by adjusting the parameters of dual oscillating magnetic fields. A linear orientation is imparted to the construct by a static homogeneous field, whereas a sinusoidal field of equal amplitude is applied perpendicularly, which results in controllable oscillation and undulation about the x-axis. When the superparamagnetic nanoparticles, which have an inclination for a particular direction of magnetization, are exposed to a magnetic field, they attain a magnetic dipole. Hence, magnetically induced torque is the result of dipolar nanoparticle interactions coupled with those between the dipole and the externally applied magnetic field [153].

Zhang et al. have devised a technique for the synthesis of a magnetic field–mediated, self-propelled artificial bacterial flagella (ABFs) (Figure 3.17), and have demonstrated the first instance of helical nanobelt propulsion in aqueous media. These artificial flagellar analogs exhibited six degrees of freedom, and might have the capacity for enabling several nanomedical applications, including as a potential tool for the nanomanipulation of cells or organelles, for sensing and transmitting information between cells and the high-resolution delivery of drugs. The ABF device comprised a trilayered helical nanobelt tail segment that consisted of a composite lamination (InGaAs—11 nm thick, GaAs—16 nm thick, and Cr—15 nm thick), which was attached to a thin square head section, made of malleable magnetic metal. The helical geometry of the tail was fabricated utilizing a self-scrolling wet etching method that resulted in a 42 nm thick × 1.8 μm wide structure with a diameter of 2.8 μm. The head section was made of a 200 nm thick × 4.5 μm (or 2.5 μm) square trilayered lamination (Cr—10 nm thick, Ni—180 nm thick, and Au—10 nm thick). A 38 μm long ABF attained a maximum velocity of ~18 μm/s at a magnetic field rotational frequency of 30 Hz and a field strength of 2.0 mT [85].

Ghosh and Fischer developed and functionalized nanostructured silicon dioxide (SiO_2) "chiral colloidal propellers" (200–300 nm wide × ~1–2 μm in length) (Figure 3.18) that could be controlled in aqueous media at micron-scale resolution under a uniform magnetic field. The fabrication process initially involved the application of a monolayer of 200–300 nm in diameter silica beads upon a 2 in. in diameter Si wafer. The helical components were synthesized en masse (~10^9 propellers/cm^2) via a shadow growth technique known as

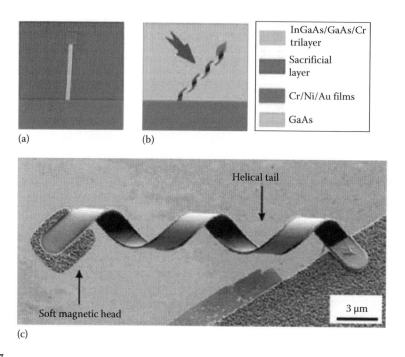

FIGURE 3.17

(a) Patterning of artificial bacterial flagella (ABF), (b) wet etching to release tail, which self-scrolls, and (c) SEM micrograph of ABF with diameter of 2.8 µm. (Reproduced with permission from Zhang, L., Abbott, J.J., Dong, L., Peyer, K.E., Kratochvil, B.E., Zhang, H., Bergeles, C., and Nelson, B.J., Characterizing the swimming properties of artificial bacterial flagella, *Nano Lett.*, 9(10), 3663–3667. Copyright 2009. American Chemical Society.)

glancing angle deposition (GLAD) whereby vapor-phase atoms are deposited on a substrate at a very oblique angle, which leads to the generation of nanostructures with unique (e.g., helical) morphologies. The atoms aggregate on the surface to form steep-angled nucleation sites upon which additional atoms adhere and grow. Hence, line-of-sight shadowing negates the condensation of atoms directly behind these nucleated structures. By increasing the tilt angle in combination with the rotation of a manipulator stage that houses the target substrate, greater distances between the columns are possible, which give rise to more porous and nanostructures [86,154].

Thermal evaporation was utilized to deposit a thin (30 nm) film of cobalt onto one half of the external surface of each device, which was subsequently magnetized via an electromagnet with the magnetic moments oriented perpendicular to the long axis. The propellers were enabled for tracking by binding a fluorophore to the helical surface by combining ~10 mg of (3-aminopropyl)dimethylethoxysilane with ~1 mg of rhodamine B isothiocyanate in 1 mL of dry ethanol at room temperature. The device was propelled over a distance of 7 µm at a velocity of 14 µm/s via a triaxial Helmholtz coil, which generated a "60 gauss (6 mT) magnetic field rotating at 66 Hz in the plane orthogonal to its direction of translation." It was calculated that every full 360° rotation could be correlated to a distance of 212 nm [86].

3.3.7 Externally Mediated Ultrasonic Propulsion

It is conceivable that nanomedical propulsion might be induced and controlled from an "outbody" ultrasonic source. An ultrasonic rotary motor drives a rotor by means of mechanical vibration that is activated in the stator by piezoelectric elements. Advantages of

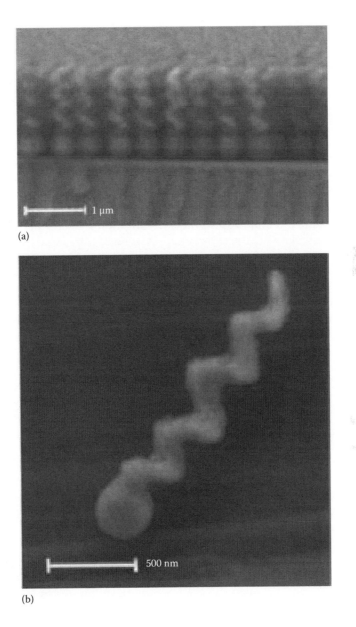

FIGURE 3.18
(a) A cross-sectioned SEM image of the GLAD nanostructured film containing ~10^9 SiO^2 helices/cm^2 and
(b) SEM image of an isolated nanopropeller depicting helical tail. (Reproduced from Ghosh, A. and Fischer, P.,
Nano Lett., 9(6), 2243, 2009. Copyright 2009. American Chemical Society. With permission.)

this class of motor, at the macroscale, include uncomplicated construction, rapid response,
positional precision, silent operation, and instantaneous cessation or resumption of operation when switched off and on, respectively. The most diminutive ultrasonic rotary motor
that has been constructed to date was reported by Morita et al. It has dimensions of 1.4 mm
outer diameter × 1.2 inner diameter × 5 mm long and functioned under frictional force.
This device comprised a PZT thin film (12 μm thick), which was synthesized via a hydrothermal method. The cylindrical stator transducer, which used a titanium base metal,
was integrated with a rotor and a preload mechanism and operated under a resonance

frequency of 227 kHz with a vibratory amplitude of 58 nm_{p-p} at a 4.0 V_{p-p} driving voltage. The highest rotational velocity and torque possible with this motor were 680 rpm and −0.67 μM m, respectively. An estimate of the output torque for an even smaller motor with an outer diameter of 0.1 mm diameter was 27 nN m. The researchers indicate that with further improvements in the chemical reaction conditions during the PZT thin film synthesis the rotational velocity/torque might be amplified sevenfold higher than its ceramic counterparts under the identical applied voltage [155].

When minimizing ultrasonic rotary motors to the micro- and nanoscale for the powering of medical nanodevices, significant but (the author surmises) not insurmountable challenges will be presented to nanomedical conceptualists and engineers toward the optimization of functional parameters, despite the dramatic reductions in scale. Prospectively, an ideal strategy for the activation of nanomedical ultrasonic rotary motors destined for operation in vivo might integrate appropriately configured arrays of piezoelements, which may be induced to oscillate via the external application of ultrasonic frequencies, thereby generating sufficient energy to operate the motor.

Piezopolymers such as polyvinylidene fluoride (PVDF) may be synthesized as thin films and can be interfaced with a variety of materials. PVDF has demonstrated generated voltages in response to mechanical deformation (g constants) that are from 10- to 20-fold higher than that of piezoceramics. This superior response arises by virtue of the tiny cross section of the film (~25 μm) upon which even slight mechanical deviations will translate to significant strains. Aside from its use in sensing applications, PVDF may find utility when integrated with nanometric propulsive components.

Interestingly, PVDF also produces electric voltage in response to exposure with near-infrared light (650–900 nm wavelength range), which can be quantified by the pyroelectric coefficient [156]. As near-infrared light may safely penetrate human tissue up to several centimeters in depth, it seems plausible that artificial flagella or other propulsive elements that are coated with thin films of PVDF might potentially assist with the provision of power to the motors that drive them, when externally activated. Speculatively, this may result in a partial (if the propulsive elements comprise nonpiezomaterials) or complete (if the propulsive elements themselves comprise piezomaterials) reciprocating loop, where some or a major portion of the power that is required by the motor is furnished by the rotating or undulating propulsive components.

An ultrasonically activated pump has been constructed that has no physically moving parts (Figure 3.19). This mechanism employs a flexural traveling wave, which synchronously displaces discrete volumes of fluid through peristaltic action. The multiple chambers that are formed between the crests of the traveling waves transfer fluid in the direction of the propagating undulation when opposed stationary stators are synchronized and activated by piezoelectric actuators. The pressure exerted between the stators is maintained at ~1 to 2 ksi (1000–2000 psi) to provide a robust seal and self-locking capability. This piezopump operated under 100 V to dispense fluid at a rate of 3.0 cc/min [157,158].

An alternate peristaltic micropump design was developed by Jang and Kan that connected three Ø 12 mm chambers, each of which was fitted with dedicated diaphragms and actuating PZT chips. The diaphragms were deflected by the PZT chips to impart an oscillating action and moved fluid perstaltically when the PZT chips were actuated sequentially. In this study the device was utilized to transfer whole blood, saline solution, and deionized water into the vein of a rat, replicating the injection of insulin for diabetes patients [159].

Hypothetically, nanoscale versions of these mechanisms might be utilized to discharge incremental aqueous "thrust packets" that may run through the entire length of

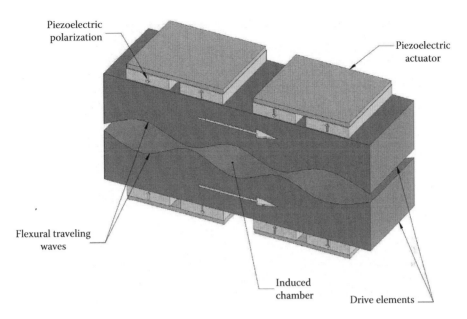

FIGURE 3.19
Miniaturized piezo-peristaltic pump. (Redrawn from Chang, Z. and Bar-Cohen, Y., Piezopumps using no physically moving parts, NDEAA Technologies, Jet Propulsion Laboratory, 1999; Chang, Z. and Bar-Cohen, Y., *Proceedings of SPIE's 7th Annual International Symposium on Smart Structures and Materials*, Newport, CA, Paper No. 3992-103 SPIE, March 1–5, 2000, http://eis.jpl.nasa.gov/ndeaa/ndeaa-pub/SPIE-2000/paper-3992-102-Piezopump.pdf. Courtesy of Yoseph Bar-Cohen, JPL/Caltech/NASA. With permission.)

nanodevices to both "pull" (when obtaining discrete volumes fluid from the leading face of the nanodevice) and "push" them (when discharging these fluid volumes from the trailing face of the nanodevice).

The smallest ultrasonic linear motor to date (SQUIGGLE) is produced by New Scale Technologies (Victor, NY). This device is 1.55 mm wide × 1.55 mm high × 6 mm long and utilizes <0.1 W of electricity to generate 20 g of force at 5 mm/s. This device incorporates a central threaded nut that mates with a threaded rod, which is surrounded by a number of piezoelectric ceramic actuators. On the application of power the ultrasonic oscillation induces the threaded nut into an orbital vibration, analogous to the motion of individual's hips when using a "Hula-Hoop." It has utility for a number of micromotion applications in the medical field, including microfluidics and implantable drug pumps [160]. If scaled down further, ultrasonic linear pumps may also serve as an alternative fluid displacement technology to potentially enable in vivo nanomedical locomotion.

The premise of utilizing ultrasonic propulsion to traverse the vasculature and other domains within the human body seems plausible; however, it will be contingent on the elucidation and implementation of safe operational protocols. Detailed studies will be warranted to elucidate the potential effects (e.g., cavitation, temperature) of the sustained generation of ultrasonic frequencies on human whole blood constituents and tissues from thousands or millions of nanodevices operating simultaneously.

3.3.8 Nanometric Piezoelectric Propulsion

Piezoelectric materials have the capacity for reversibly converting electrical energy into mechanical force via electromechanical coupling. Biocompatible piezoelectric elements are likely to play primary roles in the propulsion (as well as tracking and navigation systems) (Section 11.6) of nanomedical devices, in that they may inexhaustibly generate voltage for nanoscale propulsive components when they are mechanically strained (deformed/compressed/stretched), or are induced to oscillate through various in vivo and ex vivo stimuli (e.g., in vivo thermal gradients, fluctuations in aqueous flow, external activation via ultrasonic frequencies, and exposure to near-infrared light). Conversely, they might be activated through the application of voltage to deform, oscillate, or undulate, thereby serving as the propulsive elements themselves. A number of conventionally utilized piezomaterials include lead zirconate titanate (PZT), lead titanate (PT), and lead metaniobate ($PbNb_2O_6$). In particular, PZT-5H piezoelectric cantilevers have exhibited mechanical to electrical conversion efficiencies of >80%. Many challenges remain, however, in the synthesis of efficient PZT thin films, which have been shown to have an intrinsic decrease in the piezoelectric coefficient owing to internal defects [161,162].

Baek et al. synthesized thin films of an advanced piezoelectric material, lead magnesium niobate–lead titanate $Pb(Mg_{1/3}Nb_{2/3})O_3$–$PbTiO_3$ (PMN-PT), which showed superior "giant" piezoelectric mechanical displacement under the same applied current as conventional piezomaterials. The piezoelectric coefficients and strain levels of the material are 5–10 times higher than that of ceramic PZT, and exhibit a significant electromechanical coupling coefficient ($k_{33} \sim 0.9$). This class of piezomaterials may have strong potential in micro- and nanopropulsive applications as highly efficient oscillating drive components [163].

Piezo-activated jets based on micromachined acoustic resonators that provide considerable thrust have been investigated by Aldraihem et al. This air-based microthruster incorporated a piezoelectric diaphragm at one end, above which was an air cavity and an enclosure that contained a central orifice. When the piezoelement is activated it alters the cavity volume such that it produces a "synthetic" air jet, which may drive miniature vehicles that are biomimetically analogous to the thrust generated by a squid.

The researchers found as well that the shape of the nozzle, which extends from the orifice, is critical to the effective operation of the thrusters. A converging nozzle geometry demonstrated an increased output velocity of about 50%, which translates to a 125% improvement in the force of thrust [164]. Polsenberg investigated the use of synthetic pulsatile underwater jets for their potential in the powering of autonomous underwater vehicles (AUVs) and remotely operated vehicles (ROVs) using a speaker coil as the oscillating element [165].

Nature is replete with biomimetic inspiration for aqueous thrust. Many species of sea creatures such as salps, squid, jellyfish utilize pulsatile water jets that emanate from embedded apertures for propulsion [166–169]. On the expulsion of an internal reservoir via contraction, the forcibly ejected water forms rolling vortex rings that are known to exhibit higher thrusts than sustained jets with identical mass flux [169,170]. The creatures "inhale" subsequent volumes of water and repeat the process. The water expelled from fish gills has been considered as providing jet propulsion [171] as has the banjo catfish (*Aspredinidae*), by virtue of "opercular exhalations" [172]. The frogfish (*Histrio histrio*) of the *Antennariidae* family are also known to locomote via jet propulsion [173,174].

The microscale generation of vortex rings might be feasible using polymeric undulating reservoirs that are driven to expand and contract via artificial muscles that incorporate externally activated piezoelements. Willander et al. demonstrated a variant type of vortex ring using a 100 μm × 100 μm electrochemical microcell that operated under 3.2 V (DC), which generated microvortexes (at the anode and cathode) for the purpose of the fine mixing of solutions. Water molecules break up into negative hydroxide ions (OH^-) and protons (hydrogen ions, H^+) when an external electric field is applied and tuned between the anode and cathode of the cell. "The protons move in a spiral path in the water, and vortex rings form. Vortices with diameters ranging from 10 to 50 μm have been observed" [175]. It would be interesting to learn if a microscale vortice or multiple nanoscale vortices that are initiated at the leading faces of nanomedical devices may be exploited to "pull" them through in vivo aqueous media.

Baer et al. undertook the study of acoustic standing waves, which were manifest by a piezoelectric transducer generator that was positioned opposite a reflector to levitate aqueous droplets for applications in analytical chemistry. A concave reflector was found to significantly magnify acoustic radiation energy that favorably impacted lateral stability and reduced oscillations in the levitated sample [176]. It might be of interest to learn if the establishment of externally controllable sustained or pulsed ultrasonic standing waves, via the actuation of angularly opposed piezoelectric elements, may facilitate in vivo nanomedical device locomotion via fluctuations in the interference patterns that are generated as opposed compressions and rarefactions intersect.

A conceptual nanometric piezopropulsive mechanism might comprise an array of electrically activated thin film "piezoblades" that would oscillate laterally upon the application of current. The blades might be configured in such a way as to be alternately scalloped. If viewing a blade edge on, the upper left face might include a concave contour, whereas the lower right face would have a concave profile facing in the opposite direction giving a reversed "S"-shaped profile (Figure 3.20). Speculatively, this design might allow movement through the viscous whole blood/plasma environment, as subsequent lateral oscillations would not be reciprocal. The piezoblades would be bonded to conductive substrates (separated by an insulating barrier) that may be independently activated by current, enabling the capacity to initiate propulsive force in either direction. An extensive study of blade/fluid kinetics and overall functionality under this prospective strategy through experimentation would elucidate if in vivo nanopropulsion might be accomplished utilizing this design [177].

3.3.9 Nanofluidic Channels: Behavior and Potential for Propulsion

The environments within which nanometric propulsion-based flow-through fluidic systems would operate will be quite different in comparison to those at the micron scale. There are likely to be significant changes at this domain in that the size of nanodevices will be on equivalency with the dimensions of aqueous resident elements. Diffusion may dominate in mass/heat transfer at very rapid relative speeds as the distances at this scale are so diminutive [178].

An investigation was undertaken by Qiao and Aluru to elucidate the molecular dynamics of electroosmotic flow in nanochannels having three different widths. The applied voltage was 0.1 V and the zeta potential (electrokinetic potential in colloidal systems) at the channel wall was −10 mV. The initial channel under study was 50 nm wide, and at this width the Debye layers (electric double layers within which charges may separate considerably) did not interrelate, which revealed that flow that was close to several Debye lengths of the walls attained constancy (steady state) in a very short time, whereas flow along the center of the nanochannel was slower to achieve this state. The explanation for this is that the flow, which is intimate to the nanochannel wall, responds spontaneously to electrokinetic influence, whereas the sluggishly responding flow at the middle is dominated by viscous forces. The second channel tested was 20 nm wide and the Debye layers were found to be overlapping slightly. In this case, the electrokinetic influence pervades most of the nanochannel, thus the flow is driven by both electrokinetic and viscous components.

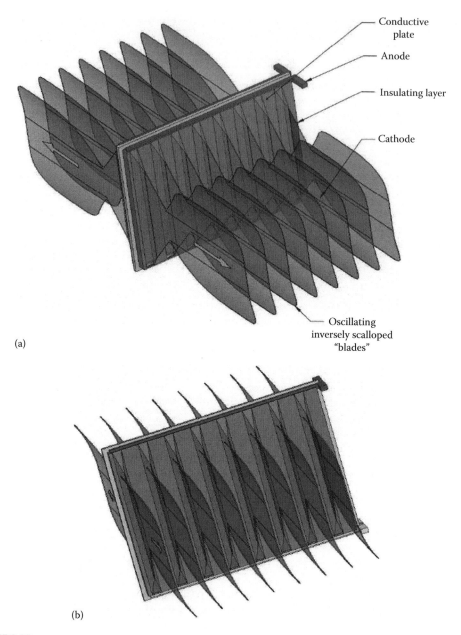

Conductive
plate

Anode

Insulating layer

Cathode

(a)

Oscillating
inversely scalloped
"blades"

(b)

FIGURE 3.20
(a, b) Artistic renderings of two views of a conceptual nanometric propulsive mechanism utilizing oscillating piezoelectric "blades."

The final channel tested was 5 nm wide, and at this dimension, the Debye layers overlap fully and the electrokinetic force is virtually homogeneous throughout the channel [179].

As to the design and nanoengineering of micro- and nanofluidic devices, Carr et al. stress the importance of visualizing the atomic level kinetics of these systems toward resolving the issue of the adsorption of solutes to microfluidic surfaces. They suggest that as surface-to-volume ratios increase, solution-borne elements have a greater propensity for diminishing the performance of devices via their binding at random sites to internal wall surfaces. These events may lead to decreases in flow efficiency, or in the worst case, cumulatively cause the complete failure of systems via clogging [180]. Atomic resolution Brownian dynamics (BD) simulations were employed to model these events in a pressure-driven, continually filled (5 nm × 5 nm × 500 nm long) "sticky" nanochannel, which was loaded with various concentrations of small solutes (dimethyl methylphosphonate) and water, over submillisecond time lines [181–184]. Adsorption models may lead to the fine-tuning of nanotube tribology and hence, enable the optimization of nanoscale fluid transport. Although these simulations were developed with the aim of optimizing lab-on-a-chip systems, they will undoubtedly have utility for the modeling of prospective nanofluidic propulsive devices within physiological fluids.

Macroscopic fluidic attributes such as surface tension, viscosity, and permittivity have completely changed values in nanometrically confined areas where most of the fluid is in close proximity to a (for the most part) charged wall. The most critical difference between macro- and nanofluidic environments is the Reynolds number (Re), where in microfluidic systems, Re <100, which translates to laminar flow. In nanofluidics, there is an increased surface/volume ratio. Surface energies become important factors in micropropulsion, and are even more significant at the nanoscale. Novel design potentials might spring from the physical effects that are apparent at this scale [178].

In fluidics, the surface free energy is required for transfer of a molecule from the interior to the surface of a fluid. The differences in energy are manifest from the interaction forces between a molecule and its neighbors in the bulk fluid and at the surface (e.g., van der Waals forces, π bonds) [178–186]. Fluids tend to adopt shapes that minimize their surface area as molecules in the bulk fluid are in a favorable energy state. Droplets are spherical in shape as geometrically, a sphere is the entity with the smallest surface/volume ratio. Pressure at the concave face of a curved surface is always greater than the pressure at the convex face (Laplace equation where γ = surface tension):

$$P_{in} = P_{out} + 2\gamma/r \qquad (3.7)$$

Proposals have been put forward for micro/nanofluidic systems that are rooted in electrical, thermal, optical, and electrochemical principals [187–197].

An electric double layer, inherent to a fluid system, has its origins from the naturally occurring surface charge and is formed as the surface charge attracts oppositely charged ions from the solution. It is made of immobile counterions close to the channel wall within the "Helmholtz layer." Excess ions in the solution side of the double layer line up in a "Helmholtz plane," which is interfaced with the electrode surface [198] with others, creating an atmosphere of ions in rapid thermal motion at the interface with the surface and is known as the diffuse electric double layer [199].

The plane dividing the inner layer of counterions with the diffuse layer is known as the Stern layer, which is close to the electrokinetic potential or zeta (ζ). The zeta potential is defined as the potential residing at the shear interface between a charged surface and an electrolyte solution [178,200].

The shear surface is the plane at which the mobile portion of the double layer can "slip" past the charged surface. Channels having diameters of several hundred nanometers or less are required to achieve total double layer overlap. Under these conditions the channel will become practically impermeable to ions that have the same charge, as the surface charge turns it into a selective barrier to the transport of either cations or anions. Conversely, when the double layer is confined to a small area near the channel wall, the central axis area is not electrically charged, allowing both cations and anions to traverse the channel [178].

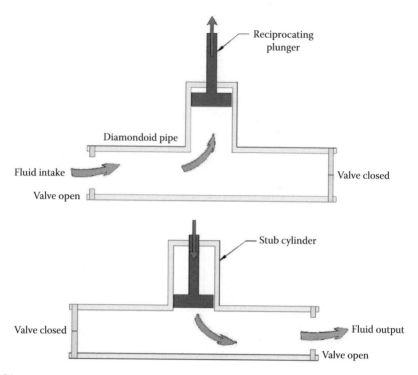

FIGURE 3.21
Single-action reciprocating positive displacement pump. (Redrawn from Freitas, R.A. Jr., *Nanomedicine, Volume I: Basic Capabilities*, Landes Bioscience, Georgetown, TX, 1999. With permission.)

3.3.10 Reciprocating Positive Displacement Pump

Nanofluidic flow may be initiated as well, through the use of mechanical energy. This can be achieved through the utilization of a side-mounted stub cylinder, which serves as a single-action reciprocating positive displacement pump (Figure 3.21). To depict a single pump cycle (derived from a description by Freitas), a valve at one end of a diamondoid tube is opened and a plunger that resides within the stub cylinder is drawn out, taking in an aqueous volume from the external environment into the lumen of the tube. The first valve is then closed, and the second valve that is seated at the opposite end of the tube is opened. The plunger is pushed into the stub cylinder, forcing an equal amount of fluid out through the open opposed end of the tube [1].

3.3.11 Aquaporin Water Channels

Water transport through aquaporins (AQP) (a family of cell membrane channel proteins, first discovered in 1992) may be very rapid in comparison to all other types of biological transport channels. In operation, a single column of water molecules traverses a 20 Å span within its channel (Figure 3.22). Water molecules and pore-lining residues interact at distinct sites, causing the molecules to change orientation and to skip from site to site, similar to saltatory conduction at the nodes of Ranvier in myelinated axons (e.g., rather than transmission as continuous waves, action potentials "hop" along the axon). The remaining portion of the channel is, for the most part, hydrophobic [202].

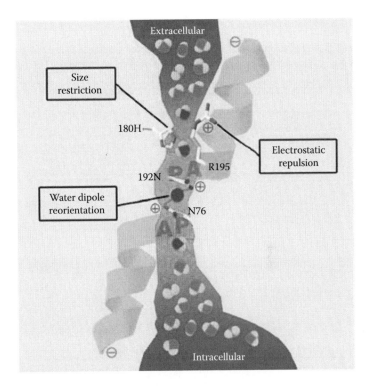

FIGURE 3.22
Cross section of AQP1 shows bulk water in extracellular and intracellular entrance/exit of the aquaporin hourglass structure. Midsection shows 20 Å channel where water molecules must pass in single file. (Reproduced from Agre, P., *Angew. Chem. Int. Ed.*, 43, 4278, 2004. With permission.)

The rate of water transport through AQP1 is ~3 × 10⁹ water molecules per subunit (two subunits total) per second [203]. This is substantially more rapid than potassium ions that permeate the KcsA channel whose rate is ~1 × 10⁸ ions/s, and among the fastest of ion channels [202,204].

Investigations into the possibility of extrapolating a biomimetic analog from one of a number of existing AQPs and their aqueous pores to artificially displace fluids may constitute a formidable task. Critical issues would involve the precise control of fluid flow and the appropriate integration of these units such that they generate sufficient thrust to serve as a viable propulsive mechanism for nanodevices such as the VCSN [205–208].

3.3.12 Potential Nanopropulsion via Superhydrophobic and Superhydrophilic Surfaces

Superhydrophobic surfaces such as those found on the upper epidermis of the leaves of the lotus flower (*Nelumbo nucifera*) possess a combination of densely populated micron and nanoscale features on their surfaces, which minimize the contact area of any entity that rests on its surface. This hierarchical structure encompasses uniquely shaped ~10 µm papillae, populated with densely clustered ~1 nm hydrophobic epicuticular crystalline wax tubules that contain high concentrations of nonacosane diols (tubule-forming compound) (Figure 3.23). These novel surface geometries induce water to bead into spheres that have contact angles (the angle at the interface of a liquid and a solid surface) of ~162° (Figure 3.24), which will roll off the leaf surface when tilted at the slightest angle (Table 3.3).

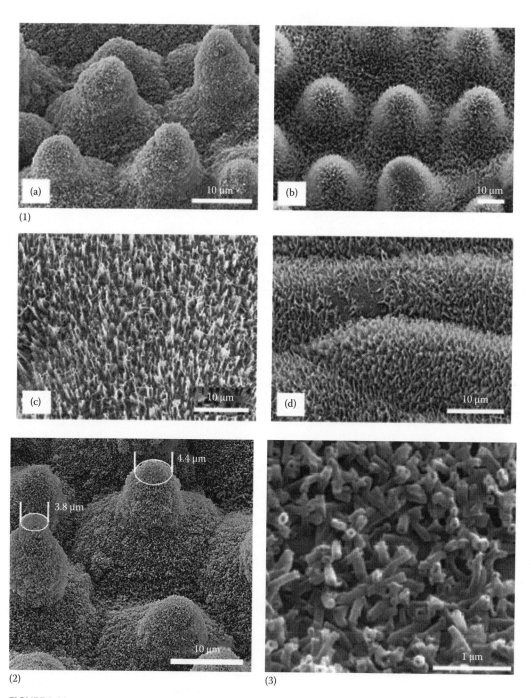

FIGURE 3.23
(1) Depiction of wax-coated superhydrophobic papillose and nonpapillose leaf surfaces: (a) *N. nucifera* (lotus), (b) *Euphorbia myrsinites*, (c) *Brassica oleracea*, and (d) *Yucca filamentosa*. (2) SEM of freeze-dried epidermis cells of the upper lotus leaf surface. (3) Lotus leaf-resident epicuticular wax crystals at a density of 200 tubules/10 μm^2. (Reproduced from Ensikat, H.J. et al., *Nanotechnology*, 2, 152, 2011. With permission.)

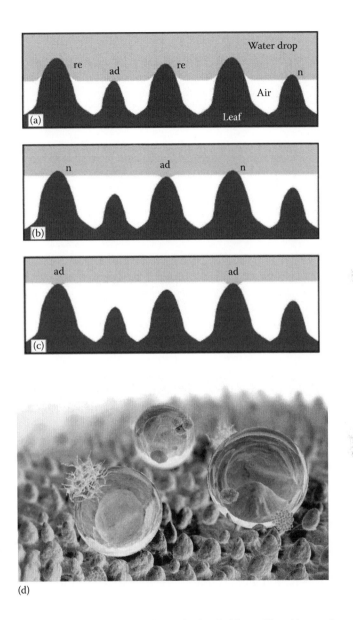

FIGURE 3.24
Schematic of contact interface of water droplet and superhydrophobic papillae: (a) at moderate pressure, there is some intrusion into the voids between papillae that meets with resistance (re) = repellent force, (b, c) as the droplet recedes interfacial contact is reduced, and when meniscus is flat, it attains equilibrium (n) = neutral force. An adhesive force = (ad) dominates just as the droplet breaks contact, (d) droplets on surface of lotus leaf demonstrating large contact angles (~160°). (a–c: Reproduced from Ensikat, H.J. et al., *Nanotechnology*, 2, 152, 2011. With permission; d: Courtesy of William Thielicke, Hamburg, Germany.)

Thus, even in the heaviest downpour, the surfaces of the leaves will remain completely dry. This "Lotus Effect" was discovered and elucidated by botanist, Dr. Wilhelm Barthlott at the University of Bonn [212]. Bhushan et al. biomimetically replicated these surface characteristics at the nanoscale to create synthetic superhydrophobic surfaces [213].

The tenebrionid desert beetle, *Stenocara* sp., found in the Namib Desert of southern Africa utilizes a unique combination of bumpy hydrophobic waxy domains and hydrophilic

TABLE 3.3

Comparative Properties and Water-Repellency of the Lotus and Other Plant Species

	Nelumbo nucifera (Lotus) (Upper Side)	*Colocasia esculenta* (Upper Side)	*Euphorbia myrsinites* (Upper Side)	*Alocasia macrorrhiza* (Lower Side)	*Brassica oleracea* (Upper Side)
Papillae density (per mm²) [209]	3431	2662	1265	2002	0
Contact angle (static) [210]	163°	165°	162°	157°	161°
Drop adhesion force (μN)[a]	8–18	28–55	30–58	80–127	7–48
Wax type	Tubules	Platelets	Platelets	Film on cuticular folds	Rodlets and tubules
Wax melting point (°C)	90–95	75–78	75–76	n.a.	65–67
Main components [211]	C_{29}^{-diols}	C_{28}^{-1-ol}	C_{26}^{-1-ol}	n.a.	C_{29} ketones C_{29} alkanes

Source: Reproduced from Ensikat, H.J. et al., *Nanotechnology*, 2, 152, 2011. With permission.
[a] Provided by D. Mohr, Nees Institute, Bonn, Germany.

waxless domains on its back to capture fog droplets (1 to 40 μm in diameter). The insect assumes a forward inclined posture, which promotes the "rolling" of the harvested water toward its mouth for drinking [214].

Speculatively, one may envision that nanoengineered superhydrophobic nanotubes, which contain arrays of water repelling domains, which line their interior surfaces at specific orientations (e.g., outward/angular) in relation to central axis of the nanotube and configured facing opposite to the intended direction of travel, might have the capacity for imparting thrust to nanodevices by virtue of continual cumulative repulsive forces that push against the surrounding water.

The linear arrangement of nanometric rows of superhydrophobic and superhydrophilic domains may theoretically convey thrust in aqueous media when water molecules are repelled (pushed) by the superhydrophobic domains, while simultaneously being attracted (pulled) by superhydrophilic domains. The intensity, and thus, the repellent/attractant forces imparted by both of these domains might be electronically controlled via electrowetting, as described later. The linear, rapidly stacottoed boosting of sequential domains along the length of the nanotube (analogous to the stadium "waves" produced by fans attending a sports event) may induce water molecules to be relayed from one domain to the next, in effect, guiding them to the exit of the nanotube and cumulatively producing a jetlike thrust.

This type of synergenistic action (asymmetric wettability) has been investigated by Chen et al., who decorated one end of a single-walled carbon nanotube with carboxyl, –COOH (hydrophilic groups) and the other with trifluoromethyl, –CF(3) (hydrophobic groups). The density of water at the hydrophobic tip of a (8,8) nanotube may be sustained at low levels, and the ends of both (6,6) and (8,8) nanotubes demonstrated the capacity for ion permeation via the existence of significant energy barriers [215].

Zuo et al. employed molecular dynamics simulations to assist in elucidating the externally mediated reversible transfer of water molecules in single file through a (6,6) carbon nanotube (Ø 8.1 Å × 23.4 Å long) that was bracketed by two (single-carbon-atom thick) graphene sheets. An electrostatic potential was initiated by an asymmetric charge distribution. It was observed that in addition to electric charge, the velocity and direction of water molecules moving through the nanotube may be heavily influenced by the interactions between internal water molecules under transport and other water molecules positioned outside of the nanotube [216].

It has been found that the adjustment of certain parameters including external chemical modification [217,218], structural manipulation [219], the smoothness of the internal surface of the nanotube [220–222], and the external electrostatic field [223,224] had significant bearings on the conduction and orientation of water molecules within the lumen of the nanotubes. Electroosmosis takes place when the channel wall is charged, which induces the creation of an electric double layer that proceeds to attract oppositely charged ions from solution. When an electric charge is applied to the surface tangentially, it will activate the mobile charges of the double layer to migrate toward the oppositely charged electrode. In very small channels, the double layer overlap inhibits electroosmotic flow velocity [178].

High-density arrays of nanofluidic channels have been fabricated utilizing nanoimprint lithography (NIL) and reactive ion etching [225,226]. Studies have been conducted that involve fluid flow through micro/nanochannels with diameters ranging between 20 nm and 20 μm, with applied voltages of −0.4 × +0.4 V. Under conditions of partial double layer overlap, asymmetrical *I–V* behavior was observed. The primary transport mechanism that moved fluid through the orifice was via electroosmosis. This illustrates the potential for the design of nanochannels that have rectified eletroosmotic flow properties [178,227]. Another interesting phenomenon is electrowetting, whereby a charged surface may be selectively toggled to exhibit alternate hydrophobic and hydrophilic states (Figure 3.25). As suggested earlier, this design might be configured to allow for the directional nanoscale manipulation of fluids at surface/solution interfaces [228,229].

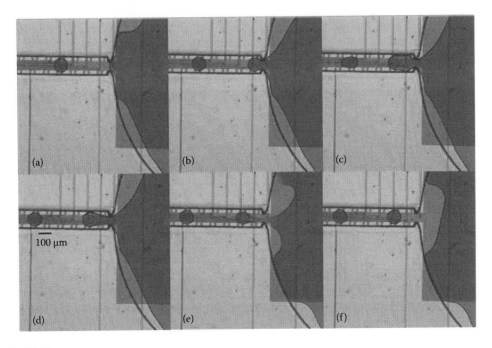

FIGURE 3.25
Dispensing of 300 pL droplets from a 140 nL reservoir on 100 μm electrodes. Channel dimensions are 150 μm wide × 20 μm high. The fluid was drawn from the reservoir by sequentially engaging the electrodes in the channel (a–f). The droplet was separated by engaging the reservoir electrode. (Reproduced from Lin, Y.Y. et al., *Sens. Actuat. B Chem.*, 150(1), 465, 2010. With permission.)

3.3.13 Thermally Mediated Nanopropulsion

A conceptual theme that might be worthy of exploration would be based on the premise of the possibility of controlled fluid displacement based on thermal differentiation [230–235] from the input port of a cylindrical- or elliptical-shaped chamber to a staggered output port. This fluid displacement might be initiated by a thermally activated medium acting on in vivo fluids residing within an appropriately configured set of internal chambers (Figure 3.26).

A substrate that laterally divides the internal chamber and runs down its length might house a tightly packed array of embedded metallic nanoshells (hollow or filled to enhance nanoshell thermal sensitivity), or a metallic grid comprising nanowires. This substrate or grid (and subsequently the chamber itself) would be further subdivided vertically by an effective thermal barrier (possibly an aerogel or hydrogel material). This barrier would enable fluid flow to be directional (forward or reverse) within the chamber, dependent on which side of the nanoshell substrate or nanowire grid is thermally activated.

The highly ordered nanoshell-impregnated substrate might be regularly interspersed with nanopores as well (or in the case of a grid, an inherent sieve-like arrangement). Enough openings should be present to allow for the free flow of fluid from lower to upper chambers via nanoconvection, a possible variation of Bénard–Marangoni convection [230–235]. The upper quadrant (or "warm" chamber) would be sealed on the input end, whereas the lower quadrant (or "cool" chamber) would be open. The reverse would be true on the "output" end, with the upper quadrant open and lower quadrant sealed. The metallic nanoshells could perhaps be activated via a carefully calibrated external near-infrared light source that would heat the nanoshells slightly, enough to possibly initiate nanofluidic convection.

The increasing temperature of the fluid within the upper chamber, in comparison with the fluid in the lower chamber, may initiate fluid expansion and its ejection from the upper output port, which would impart nanodevice thrust in the opposite direction. This displacement of warmer fluid may induce the cooler fluid within the lower chamber to be drawn up and percolated through the nanoporous/metallic grid work into the upper chamber, while being heated in transit to then be cyclically expelled through the

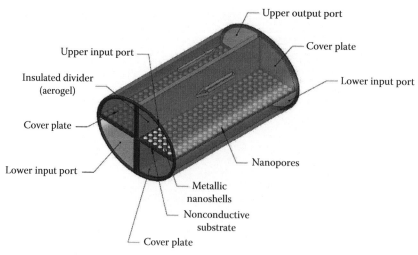

FIGURE 3.26
Conceptual thermal differential nanopropulsion system.

upper output port. Subsequently, "cooler" (ambient body temperature) fluid would enter the lower input port to replace the fluid that has been "convected" to restore the volume of the fluid that has just been ejected from the upper chamber. This intake function would apply force in the same direction as the fluid that is continually exiting the upper output port, and might cumulatively add to the overall propulsive thrust. In effect, the synergy between upper and lower chambers would result in simultaneous upper output "pushing" forces working in conjunction with lower input "pulling" forces to propel a nanodevice through aqueous media.

In another design scenario, human core temperatures might serve as the "hot" side of a nanoconvection mechanism. Perhaps the integration of an effective insulating material (possibly only nanometers thick, and having hydrogel-like attributes) might maintain, for a predetermined time period, lower temperature domains in strategic areas of the propulsive mechanism. This arrangement may sustain enough thermal differentiation to initiate convective fluidic movement and provide a nanopropulsive force. This strategy would negate the possibility of increased thermal loads on the mean core temperature of a patient, which may be impacted, albeit only temporarily, if deploying large numbers of nanodevices that are utilizing thermal convection for propulsion. This possibility might be the subject of a detailed investigative analysis and modeling.

Balsubramanian et al. have investigated pulsed high-temperature electrochemical propulsion via catalytic nanomotors utilizing Ø 25 μm Au-coated Pt wires, which served as the heat source (65°C), under 600 mA DC heat current in a fuel solution of 5 wt% H_2O_2. The enhanced distance traveled over a 2 s time line, and velocity of the thermally exposed nanowires (90 μm at 45 μm/s over those at room temperature (28 μm at 14 μm/s) was ascribed to the "thermal activation of the redox reactions of the H_2O_2 fuel at the Pt and Au segments." The incorporation of a ferromagnetic nickel element enabled the controllable "steering" of thermally activated Au–Ni–Pt nanowires [236].

3.3.14 Polymeric Nanopropulsion Engine

A polymeric nanopropulsion engine was devised by Carrillo et al., which consisted of a nozzle-like pore that incorporated catalytic domains at the capped end of a cylindrical nozzle. When submerged in a "fuel" solution of monomers, the pore was subsequently propelled by the reactions of macromolecule polymerization in a fashion analogous to a jet engine. Polymers were dispensed at a velocity that was correlated to the rate of polymerization, and movement ensued by virtue of the viscoelasticity of the polymers. The compression of the polymeric chains that were confined within the nanonozzle initiated an osmotic force that acted on the cap end, which resulted in locomotion [237].

3.3.15 Stepped Nanomagnetic Rotary Propulsion

A conceptual stepped nanomagnetic rotary mode propulsive strategy might involve a cylindrical housing that comprises entirely radially abutting electromagnetic "bars," which are arranged in alternating N/S orientations and interleaved with insulated barriers (Figure 3.27). The housing would have a hollow core, allowing for the free movement of an internal helical screw that rotates about the central axis of the housing to serve as the fluid displacing propulsive element. The screw may comprise stiff diamondoid or sapphire materials, or rigid superhydrophobic covalent organic frameworks (e.g., porous crystalline structures synthesized via the covalent binding of light elements such as H, B, C, H, and O).

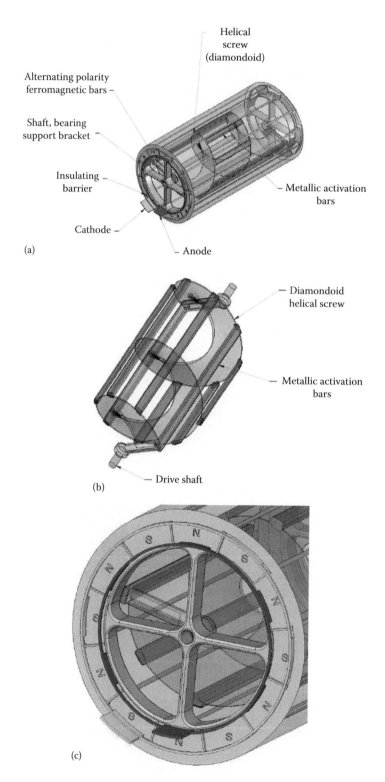

Helical
screw
(diamondoid)

Alternating polarity
ferromagnetic bars –

Shaft, bearing
support bracket ‒

Insulating –
barrier

Metallic activation
bars

Cathode –

(a)

‒ Anode

Diamondoid
helical screw

Metallic activation
bars

‒ Drive shaft

(b)

(c)

FIGURE 3.27

(a–c) Artistic representation of conceptual magnetically stepped diamondoid propulsion helical screw.

The outer diameter edges of this helical entity would be bonded to an equally spaced series of "activation bars." These entities might contain permanent magnetic and metallic elements (e.g., molecular magnets containing manganese, vanadium, iron, nickel, and cobalt clusters) [238,239], which would be configured to have their exterior faces in close physical proximity to the internal, ferromagnetic element-lined surfaces of the cylindrical housing.

In operation, the ferromagnetic bars would be sequentially electromagnetized by transiently engaged current flows, which would incrementally activate one bar at a time. These fleeting current activation events would continually "step" their way around the periphery of the housing. The rate of rotation would be contingent on velocity requirements. The induced magnetic forces would rapidly attract and then repel the activation bars, as they would also be inherently magnetized, thereby (hypothetically), initiating rotary actuation.

The helical profile and orientation would be designed such that it would have the capacity for displacing fluids reversibly, equally, and effectively in both forward and reverse directions. Both shaft ends of the propulsive component would be fitted into ultralow friction diamond bearings. The bearings themselves would be seated in open-webbed end plates, utilizing sufficient material to firmly stabilize the bearings, yet enabling maximum fluid transfer through the device.

To provide power to the unit, two donut-shaped connection rings (cathode and anode) equipped with embedded nanoelectronic interfacial connectors would abut to either end of the ferromagnetic bars. These entities would be modular, self-contained, and internally "wired" with discrete connection ports from which all connectors would draw their power. Current would be conveyed to each interfacial contact in stepped sequence, activating and magnetizing the individual bars in rapid succession.

A microscale, magnetically mediated rotation strategy was illustrated by Sacconi et al. who demonstrated the rotation of magnetic beads (2.6 μm diameter), which was initiated by a magneto-optic trap. The beads were held in place by optical tweezers and induced to rotate via a magnetic manipulator. Rotation was realized utilizing eight electromagnets having tip-pole geometry via a time orbital potential technique [240]. Effective trapping in three dimensions and the rotation of magnetic beads on three axes were demonstrated with forces up to 230 pN and force momenta of up to 10^{-16} Nm [241].

3.3.16 Undulating Wave Locomotion

A hypothetical nanometric undulating wave propulsive mechanism (Figure 3.28) might be realized by utilizing sequential ferromagnetic activation as well. Consider a hollow rectangular housing, which may be projected through the body of the VCSN. This cavity could be laterally subdivided into two or several compartments by several vertically stacked ultrathin film membranes (perhaps several nanometers thick) comprising a very pliable, yet tough polymeric material. Both side edges of the polymer membranes might be bonded to denser/thicker polymer flanges that would be doped with polarized (via giant magnetoresistance) [242] metallic/magnetic elements, making up several pairs of laterally opposed "pull nodes" along its length. Both the leading and trailing edges of the membrane would be taut and secured on either side to span the width of the housing.

The polymeric flanges would be captured (limiting vertical freedom of movement) by two sets of parallel runners, bonded to the side walls of the housing and running its length, whereby the runners would also assist in keeping the undulating membrane somewhat laterally taut. The polarized nodes in the flanges would provide "grab" points that would form the successive crests and valleys of dynamic amplitude waves along the lengths of the membranes, which would move along the z-axis in concert.

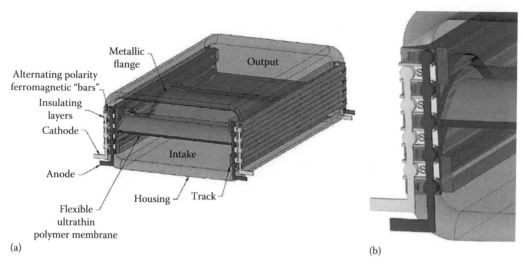

FIGURE 3.28
Conceptual undulating wave propulsion (a) with close-up (b) of magnetic "bar" arrangement.

The side walls of the housing might comprise entirely vertical stacks of laminated ferromagnetic bars running the length of the housing, and as in the rotary model, each would have individual nanoelectrical connections in order to facilitate sequential, albeit independent activation. In order to impart an undulatory motion into the membrane the pull node pairs would be sequentially activated, moving up and down in the z-axis, with each pair being in the opposite orientation to the other (e.g., when one pair is in the up position, the pair immediately following along the length of the membrane would be in the down position). This cascading sequential magnetic activation would proceed, moving incrementally in the z-axis from bar to bar and would cause the polymer membrane to undulate in a manner that may be analogous to unfurling a bed sheet via the initiation of a quick up and down motion (e.g., causing amplitude waves to ripple down the length of the sheet). The amplitude of the undulating wave might be "tuned" somewhat by modifying the ferromagnetic activation sequence and its spatial extent [243].

3.3.17 Deformative Electroactive Polymers

Deformative element nanopropulsion might be enabled through the incorporation of electroactive polymeric actuator (EPA) materials (e.g., artificial muscles) (Chapter 17), whose motion is triggered by the electrically driven mass transfer of ions or the application of electrostatic energy. The criteria for these materials as propulsive undulating membranes would be that they have the capacity for moving rapidly enough to impart sufficient force for in vivo locomotion. These classes of polymers have unique advantages over other prospective materials insofar as the possible powering of in vivo nanomedical devices as they encompass versatility, high mechanical pliability, sensitivity to applied current (~1 V), uncomplicated structural geometries, and are typically low cost, easily scalable, and devoid of acoustic noise [244].

There are a number of drawbacks, however, with present day ionically driven EPAs (e.g., polymeric gels [245], ionic polymer–metal composites [246], conjugated polymers [247], and carbon nanotubes [248]), which include limited longevity and sluggish response times [244]. These issues stem from inherent electrochemical activation and power transduction kinetics that result in (per cycle) degradation effects. Nevertheless, once these challenges are overcome it is likely that ionic EPAs will possibly find wide applicability.

Polymeric gels consist of cross-linked networks that can become swollen in a solvent. When the equilibrium between the gel and solvent is disrupted via alterations in environmental parameters, such as temperature, pH, and electric field, their volume will be changed through the expulsion of the solvent. A pH-responsive artificial muscle gel comprising polyacrylonitrile fibers exhibited sluggish contraction in an acidic solution, but a more rapid expansion in a basic solution, with a complete cycle requiring ~40 s [249]. Significantly, better response times were observed with microporous poly(vinyl alcohol) (PVA) (~10th of a second) and poly(vinyl methyl ether) (PVME) hydrogels (~1 s) [251]. A hybrid system comprising a poly(2-acrylamido-2-methylpropanesulfonic acid) (PAMPS) membrane complexed with surfactant molecules responded (in the form of reversible bending) upon the direct application of electric fields of opposite polarity [250].

Polyelectrolyte gel networks may undergo exponential deformation in water and have the capacity to absorb up to ~2000 times their own weight without dissolving themselves [252]. In view of this remarkable capability, one can envisage that appropriately configured/encased modular units of this gel might be utilized to provide propulsive thrust for nanomedical devices in a manner that is analogous to the functionality of jellyfish. Minute volumes (in relative terms) of ambient fluid could be sequentially absorbed and expelled from arrays of modular propulsive gel sacs that are incorporated into nanodevices. Voltages required to power these units might be provided by onboard piezoenergy-harvesting modules.

Otero and Sansieña have demonstrated the reversible deformation of polypyrrole/nonconducting polymer bilayers by virtue of localized stress gradients that are imposed on the materials through successive oxidation and reduction processes. They electrodeposited a polypyrrole film (~4–12 μm thick) onto a stainless steel electrode after which a nonconducting polymeric adhesive tape was applied. The resulting bilayer was subsequently peeled form the stainless steel and used as a new electrode and immersed in a LiClO$_4$ aqueous media. A Pt foil counterelectrode was employed, as well as a saturated calomel reference electrode. The bilayer was tethered to an electrical contact, whereby its free end was unconstrained and induced to move 90° in each direction (from vertical) with a 1 g weight attached. "Under a current flow of 30 mA a bilayer whose PPy film mass is 3 mg (area 3 cm^2 and thickness 6 μm) takes 3.6 s to describe a movement of 90°." It was calculated that the bilayer device was capable of carrying 1000 times its own weight with its free end. The electrochemical reaction, as well as the applied current, controlled the cumulative conformational changes of the polymeric molecular units to facilitate shrinking (compression) and swelling (expansion). Interestingly, the bilayer could be reversed at any position along its arched trajectory as well as accelerated, slowed, or halted at any point, via the manipulation of the current [253].

Electrically driven "dry" EPAs include piezoelectric polymers [254], electrostrictive polymers [255], dielectric elastomers [256], liquid crystal elastomers [257], and carbon nanotube aerogels [258]. The primary advantages of these EPAs include the potential capacity for significant actuation strains, rapid response, and extended longevity. However, they currently require considerable electrical driving fields (~100 V/μm) as a requirement for their electrostatic activation [244]. The potential utility of these EPAs as nanomedical propulsive components will necessitate a dramatic reduction of voltages from what are presently needed for activation (~1 kV). This may be enabled through the reconfiguration of these materials as thin films.

As Carpi et al. point out, field-initiated stresses and strains of electric EPA may be generally correlated to the "square of the applied electric field …" and "If the response is dominated by the field-induced reorientation of a crystalline or semicrystalline structure, then the polymer is said to be 'electrostrictive'." Additionally, "If the response is dominated by the interaction of the electrostatic charges on the electrodes (often called the Maxwell stress) then the polymer is called a 'dielectric elastomer' type of EAP." Significant electrostrictive response has been demonstrated using poly(vinylidene fluoride) (PVDF)-based materials and certain polyurethanes. The specific energy densities of (PVDF) integrated materials have been shown by Zhang et al. to surpass those of the best piezoceramics with the generation of strains that approached 5% [259–261].

Dielectric elastomers such as polydimethyl siloxane (silicone rubber) and acrylic elastomers have exhibited strains of >100%. This class of EPAs has also exceeded 10 million cycles in high humidity environments [262,263], which is critical if they are to be utilized in nanomedical in vivo applications. It was demonstrated on cadavers that an artificial muscle, comprising polytetrafluoroethylene (ePTFE), could be used as an "upper eyelid sling," and that its functionality and efficiency were comparable to a "temporalis muscle fascia sling." This work may result in a restorative blinking capability for individuals who have lost this ability due to muscular or neurological damage [264].

3.4 Potential Nanomedical Surface Ambling Strategies

Conceivably, there will be myriad requirements for nanomedical devices that are enabled with the capacity for topically negotiating a wide variety of physiological substrates to conduct medically beneficial procedures, both within and spanning the exterior surfaces of patients. There are ample strategies that operate in nature, and indeed within our own bodies, which may impart useful insights for nanomedical conceptualists, designers, and engineers toward the development of sophisticated ambulatory surface traversing nanodevices. Micro- and nanoscale "walking" will involve a power source (e.g., ATP, glucose, onboard piezogenerators) and the establishment of positional constraining mechanisms (e.g., binding with dedicated sites on molecular "tracks," cell-embedded proteins, or the lipid "heads" of externally exposed cellular phospholipid bilayers) to enable the robust and efficient traversal of micro/nanoscale surfaces.

Described later are a number of potential strategies utilized in the natural world that may serve as inspirational templates and convey insights for their synthetic replication, toward enabling first-generation microscale/nanoscale/molecular surface ambling devices to potentially facilitate precision nanomedical diagnostic and therapeutic procedures. Biomimetically derived analogs of myosin, kinesin, and dynein walking mechanisms might be utilized in the development of several classes of nanomedical surface traversing devices. These nanodevices may enable the nanomechanically mediated dissolution and removal of vascular and neurological plaques, and possibly cell clogging lipofuscin deposits, which are presumed to play a significant role in aging processes (Chapter 17).

In certain instances, arrays of surface roving nanomedical devices might be preprogrammed to penetrate through the extracellular matrix to "hand deliver" drugs; "patrol" the complete exteriors of specific organs to scan for signs of disease or potential invaders; or rapidly perform real-time molecular-scale biopsies in situ where required, and subsequently broadcast the resulting data to physician/surgeon-controlled outbody computers.

Other classes of ambling nanomedical devices may be endowed with the capacity for conducting nanosurgical procedures on individual organelles, cells, and specific sites within tissue. Applications might also include the packing of voids in bone with bone-mending compounds and/or bone-regenerating scaffolds to alleviate the damage inflicted via osteoporosis. Similar nanodevices might be administered as dedicated multicourse therapeutics for the "top dressing" of particularly fragile sites on certain bones to give them additional mass, leading to increased skeletal robustness. This capacity could conceivably be translated to the continual maintenance of bone mass for astronauts during protracted space missions as a beneficial supplement to their regular exercise regimes.

A variety of dynamic "rectifier" class nanomedical ambling devices might facilitate rapid, highly efficacious, and painless nanodental procedures and autocontinuous oral hygiene. These nanodevices might be administered via a mouthwash or oral gel to conduct a detailed survey of all tooth enamel surfaces, and associated interfaces to dislodge accumulated plaque material and bacteria, and to perform repairs on even nascent cavities. Micron-sized devices operating under the commands of external computers could be deployed for the administration of painless, yet highly efficacious anesthesia. A prescribed population of nanodevices might be administered to the oral cavity via a mouthwash, oral gel, lozenge, toothpaste, or drops, which would adhere to the inner surfaces of the mouth and proceed to rapidly ambulate into the pulp chambers of each tooth within several minutes. Once strategically placed, these devices would be externally commanded by the presiding dentist or dental surgeon to disrupt local nerve impulses to the teeth, thereby instantly numbing the nerves that are connected to any desired tooth. This capability would be reversible, and when commanded by computer, normal nerve impulse flows would be restored [265–268].

Additional rectifier species might be prescribed to ensure optimal and sustained ocular, aural, nasal, and dermal health. Within these atmosphere-exposed cavities and external human tissues, ambulatory nanomedical devices might cumulatively "walk the beat" across entire dermal surfaces and within shallow subdermal layers for signs of disease, perform in situ procedures to eradicate melanomas, or to conduct cosmetic maintenance or enhancements. Ambling nanodevices may also be deployed for protracted "personalized physiological security" tasks, wherein they might serve as in vivo "mobile stationed sentinels" to possibly enhance compromised immune systems, or to further endow normally functioning immune systems, to enable very rapid nonself responses for the immediate obliteration of any health-threatening contagion, toxin, or other suspected biochemical entity.

3.4.1 Acto-Myosin Complex

The acto-myosin complex is an actin-activated, ATPase linear molecular motor protein of the myosin superfamily, which plays essential roles in cell division, intracellular transport, the transfer, positioning and segregation of organelles, and muscle-resident contractile functions (Figure 3.29). Beyond the myosin (class II) motor, which forms the filaments that enable muscle contraction, the myosin superfamily encompasses a minimum of 34 unique classes of motors [269–272]. Myosin (class II) constituents include two identical rodlike molecular heavy chains (2–3 nm thick × 150 nm long) that are helically intertwisted. One end of each heavy-chain "tail" is endowed with a globular nodule that comprises a "head," which contains both ATP-binding sites and enzymes (~800 amino acids in size) that have the capacity to hydrolyze ATP (adenosine triphosphate) to products, adenosine diphosphate (ADP) and an orthophosphate (Pi), and to bind with actin filaments.

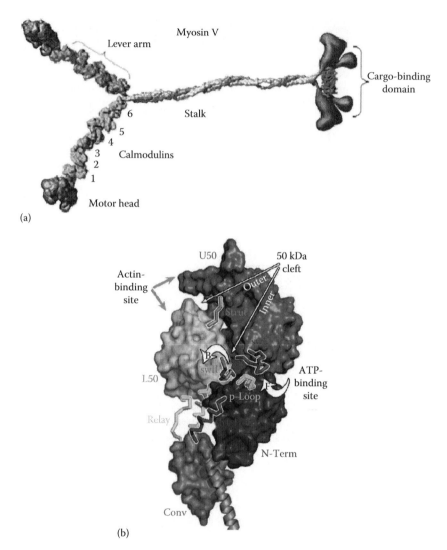

(a)

(b)

FIGURE 3.29

(a) Structure of myosin (class V) has six calmodulin (calcium-binding protein)-binding sites in its lever arm whereas myosin VI has only two. (b) Structure of myosin (class II) motor fragment depicting four subdomains including upper 50 (blue), lower 50 (light gray), N-terminal (dark gray), and converter (green), connector elements and nucleotide-binding loops. The assembly is joined by pliable links, which encompass "switch II (orange), the relay (yellow), the SH1-helix (red), and the strut (pink)." Also shown is the nucleotide-binding site, which comprises switch I (magenta), switch II (orange), and the P-loop (cyan), and the "front (F)" and "back (B)" doors (white arrows), which facilitate the entry of ATP and discharge of Pi. (a: Reproduced from Yildiz, A. and Selvin, P.R., *Acc. Chem. Res.*, 38, 572, 2005. Copyright 2005. American Chemical Society; b: Llinas, P. et al., *FEBS J.*, 279(4), 551, 2011. With permission.)

Two sets of integrated light chains are linked with the heads. Hundreds of myosin molecules self-assemble in the construction of each thick filament, wherein heavy chains overlap and the globular heads are oriented in both forward and reverse directions [273]. Myosins fleetingly employ the crossbridges that populate their surfaces to bind with and temporarily interpenetrate actin filaments. Thus, myosin filaments utilize chemomechanical transduction to exert motive force for "walking" along actin fiber filaments, cumulatively enabling muscle contraction. Conformational changes brought about by modifications in communicative pathways within the motors mediate their detachment from the actin track and repriming [269]. Myosins consume ATP at a rate of 20 s^{-1} with a step increment of ~5.5 nm, to give a velocity of ~110 nm/s.

A "swinging lever arm" hypothesis involving interactions between "lead" and "rear" heads [274] has been validated through 2 Å resolution functional studies of myosin structures to describe a series of intimate conformational changes that proceed within the motor cycle (e.g., generation of forces and movement toward the positive end of actin filaments). "The lever arm swings, thus converting the actin-coupled changes in the motor into a movement that is known as the stroke or power stroke" [269]. Kinetic data have indicated that the motor cycle is more complex than previously thought, and actually involves multiple ATP and ADP states [274]. Also, the early establishment of a "complex between actin and myosin involves salt-dependent electrostatic interactions between actin-binding loops of the motor and the actin filament" [275–277].

Myosin (class VI) motors are intriguing in that they are the only myosin species that operate in reverse. It has been elucidated that "rearrangements within the converter subdomain" are behind this myosin's capacity for large reverse strokes even though it possesses a comparatively diminutive lever arm [269]. Myosin (class V) motors are structurally configured such that they may serve as effective actin-guided cargo haulers, transporting organelles such as peroxisomes, secretory vesicles, and vacuoles. They cannot only bind organelles to actin but are active in short haul organelle transfer [278].

3.4.2 Actin Filaments

Actin filaments are long polymeric (F-actin) chains that comprise pairs of helically intertwined globular (G-actin) monomeric strands (Ø 5.6 nm). Their polymerization within the cellular cytoplasm is regulated by the interrelations of F- and G-actin sites on an actin-binding protein called cofilin I, which also induces a twist in the filament upon binding [279]. Additionally, an elongated multifunctional protein complex called Spire acts as a polymerization nucleator, the long axis core of which serves as a template for the lining up of single actin subunits that subsequently dissociates from the developing filament [280].

It was originally surmised that both actin and myosin operated exclusively within the cytoplasm. However, it has since been elucidated that they also function within the nucleus [281]. Myosin filaments may also longitudinally compress actin filaments when they slide along them. The actin filament plays several important roles in the locomotion of myosin, one of which includes the acceleration of ATPase activity through a 100-fold increase in the velocity of released hydrolysis products (which typically constitutes the slow step in the myosin motor cycle), when myosin rebinds to F-actin [269].

Elliot and Worthington posit that elemental actin–myosin contraction is an impulsive and sequential force that is conveyed by multiple myosin heads acting on a single actin filament at any instant, rather than (as formerly suggested) a simultaneous, albeit asynchronous mechanism [282]. They propose that individual myosin heads operate on single actin filaments at any given point in time in muscle contraction and that supplemental heads are recruited only "in response to a quick release of either length or tension." This strategy seems to be in alignment with a significant current body of detailed "biophysical and biochemical evidence" [283].

The median time interval between ATP hydrolyzation events on an actin filament has been experimentally found to be <2.5 ms, and the distance traveled by an individual actin filament past an individual myosin filament subsequent to individual ATP hydrolysis is ~2 nm. These results were derived from frog muscle at 0°C, and were contingent on the load that was applied to the muscle [284–287]. In other work, He et al. generated data to reveal that individual actin filaments interact with "150 myosin heads in a single half-sarcomere and each myosin head turns over ATP at a rate of around 3 s during isometric contraction." This translated to the hydrolysis of 450 ATP molecules/s on individual actin filaments. In this case, the frog muscle temperature was 5°C, thus the time interval between ATP hydrolyzation events was 2.2 ms, and the distance traveled by an individual actin filament past an individual myosin filament for every hydrolyzed ATP was 1.25 nm [287].

3.4.3 Kinesin

In humans, there exist 45 distinct kinesin species, of which the initially discovered kinesin-1 (kinesin) is deemed as the gold standard against which all subsequently revealed kinesin species are evaluated (Figure 3.30). In contrast to actin filaments that are employed by myosin to accomplish linear molecular scale transport, the kinesin motor protein has the capacity for controllably walking (at 8.3 nm increments, requiring one ATP per step) considerable distances on microtubule tracks in directed orientations, without fully releasing from the substrate (processivity). This protein comprises dual "head" motor domains that are bound to a trisegmented, 70 nm in length, double-coiled "stalk" at an amino terminus, via a hinged elastic "neck" domain, which allows the heads (spaced at ~8.3 nm) to take incremental steps in a "random walk" [288,289].

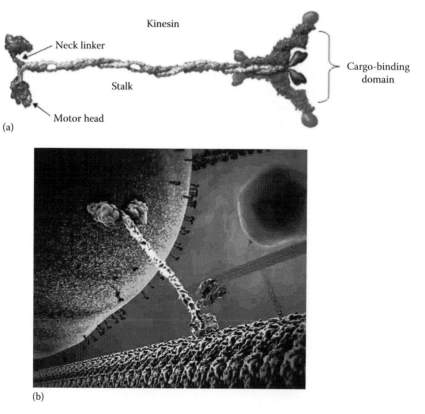

(a)

(b)

FIGURE 3.30

(a) Anatomy of conventional kinesin depicting motor head domain, mechanical amplifying legs, and cargo-binding domains. (b) Artistic representation of kinesin traversing a microtubule track. (Reproduced from Yildiz, A. and Selvin, P.R., *Acc. Chem. Res.*, 38, 572, 2005 and Harvard. With permission.)

Each of the heads contains two binding domains, which total ~350 amino acids in size. One of these binds with ATP (where it undergoes hydrolysis), whereas the other binds and interacts primarily with microtubule-embedded tubulin β-subunits. Twin globular "tail" domains, joined with the stalk at the carboxyl terminus, have selective affinities for organelles vesicles, protein assemblies, and mRNA [290–292]. Interestingly, as with what occurs in the myosin–actin filament system, the hydrolysis of ATP may ensue only when the heads are bound with the microtubule. Also, the flexible neck, its linker, and hinge cumulatively transduce and amplify the diminutive conformational change that is produced at the ATP-binding site into much more pronounced mechanical motion. Although most kinesins gravitate toward the plus ends of microtubules, which consist of polar assemblies of α/β-tubulin dimers, there is one family that moves in the opposite direction, toward the minus end of microtubules. It is thought that this is because the heads of these kinesins are located at the carboxyl terminus. For "conventional" kinesin, investigations have revealed that the neck regions mediate direction of movement [290]. The velocity of kinesin, with a "fuel" input of 20–40 ATP per second per head, is ~320 to 640 nm/s [293–295].

There has been some dispute over the exact walking mechanism that is employed by kinesin, which encompassed a hand-over-hand model, wherein the trailing head dissociates from the microtubule to take a ~8 nm step, leading its tightly bound counterpart, and an inchworm model, where a single head always takes the lead and binds to the track, while the trailing head releases to catch up. It was conclusively elucidated that hand-over-hand walking was indeed the strategy that is employed by kinesin, with both head motors hydrolyzing ATP [288,296,297].

3.4.4 Dynein

Two families of dyneins exist that include more than a dozen members each, with mammals having at least 12, which are typically involved with enabling ciliary beating, the transfer of intracellular components, and the construction mitotic spindles. The molecular body plan of dynein is quite dissimilar to those of myosins and kinesins in that the motor/head domain consists of a ring of six asymmetrically arranged units of ATPases associated with diverse cellular activities (AAA-ATPase). It is thought that ATP-mediated conformational changes that take place within the ring are translated to a 15 nm long antiparallel double-coiled stalk that emanates from between the AAA4 and AAA5 units (Figure 3.31), which houses a tip-resident site that it employs to bind with microtubules [298–300].

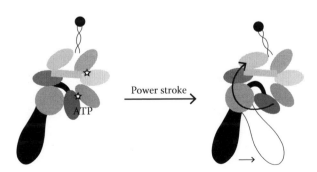

FIGURE 3.31
Dynein conformational change models. Schematic depicting how ATP may induce structural changes to the microtubule-binding domain MTBD and linker (N-terminal region) to alter binding affinities. (Reproduced from Serohijos A.W.R. et al., *PNAS*, 103(49), 18540, 2006. Copyright 2006 National Academy of Sciences, U.S.A. With permission.)

This stalk can swing in a manner that is akin to a lever arm to displace its position by ~15 nm. Hence, the power stroke of dynein is distinct from those of myosin and kinesin [301]. Cumulatively, its ATP- and microtubule-binding sites may be over 4000 amino acids in size.

Insofar as the forces generated by single dyneins, myosins, and kinesins are concerned, they have been found to be in the range of 1–10 pN [302]. Although this may indeed seem diminutive from a macroscale perspective (e.g., 10^{13} molecular motors would be required to lift a 5 kg mass), in relative terms at cellular domains, these forces are enormous. Individual motors are capable of transporting cargo that is several times their own weight through viscous cytoplasmic media while enduring Brownian buffeting, at nearly full throttle.

Yildiz et al. tracked dynein motor head stepping with nanometer precision utilizing a fluorescence imaging with one nanometer accuracy (FIONA) technique, which can locate a single fluorophore within 1 nm, in the x–y plane. This is accomplished by "taking the point spread function of a single fluorophore excited with wide field illumination and locating the center of the fluorescent spot by a 2D Gaussian fit." It was found that, as relates to dynein, individual head stepping was variable and only one head was required for processive movement. In fact, an active head exhibited the capacity for dragging along its inactive head counterpart to achieve forward advance along the microtubule. The capability of processively moving despite the lack of interhead coordination is a fundamental departure from the inherent hand-over-hand walking of kinesin and myosin [303].

3.4.5 Microtubules

Within the cytoskeleton, microtubules (24 nm outer diameter × 14 nm diameter lumen with 5 nm thick walls, and up to several micrometers in length) constitute the most rigid components, and as briefly mentioned earlier, they are stacked linear constructs (protofilaments) of molecularly polarized α/β-tubulin heterodimers, which, when assembled, have a minus end that exposes a α-subunit and a plus end that exposes a β-subunit. The dimers self-assemble in a head to tail/sheet to tube fashion integrating a staggered arrangement of 13 dimers per single complete diameter, which results in a chiral tubular structure [273,304].

Hypothetically, nanomedical ambling devices may utilize already formed microtubules to transport themselves to different sites within cells, if the binding mechanisms and kinetics of biological walkers can be replicated with a high degree of precision. Another area worthy of investigation may include whether kinesin or myosin walking along microtubules might be "shadowed" by nanodevices via some benign form of tethered attachment. Also, if nanodevices are light enough, might they "piggyback" upon the cargoes of kinesin or myosin to traverse microtubules?

3.4.6 Synthetic Nanowalkers

It is indeed intriguing that within the human body, in spite of the fact that the dual dominating influences of viscosity and Brownian motion hold sway across molecular domains, controlled nanoscale motion is possible at all [305–307]. It has been proposed in the literature that the random, molecular thermal pummelling that is experienced by molecules at ambient temperatures exceeds the average power output of motor proteins by a factor of a billion [126,308]. Yet, synthetic chemists have managed to devise ingenious systems that exhibit controlled movement at the nanoscale [98,102,309–312]. Although the modeling of both natural and synthetic molecular walking systems has been undertaken by a growing number of research groups, the actual synthesis and investigations into the real-world functionality of these entities are far less prevalent.

As illustrated via the examples described earlier of naturally evolved molecular walkers, a consistent design theme for efficient bipedal stepping along a track, in a groove or channel, or across open flat or curved surfaces is that one foot or head must always be bound to the substrate. In addition, a reliable source of ambient fuel will be required to actuate feet and heads, as sufficient onboard fuel storage within nanodevices, beyond small contingency reservoirs, is likely impractical due to extreme space constraints.

For in vivo nanomedical surface ambling applications, it seems reasonable that localized chemical fuels (e.g., lipids, cholesterol, glucose, hydrogen, carbohydrate, ATP) might be catalyzed at an as-needed rate (analogous to the kinesin hydrolysis of one ATP per step) at dedicated energy-harvesting nodes that may stud the exterior surfaces of nanodevices. Alternatively, both walking and natating classes of nanodevices may be designed to operate exclusively through the consumption of specialized synthetic biocompatible fuels that are administered concomitantly. Freitas suggests that an injected ~0.7 cm^3 dose of synthetic diamond colloid, which is purported to be extremely energy dense, "encapsulated in trillions of suitable submicron-scale biocompatible carrier devices provides an energy resource equal in size to the entire serum glucose supply," and as to fuel accessibility, "Ten trillion 0.1-micron^3 passive carriers would have a mean separation of ~10 microns in the blood" [1]. An intriguing investigation in this area might encompass an exploration of nanocarriers that might be appropriate for this application, quantification of their in vivo dwell times, and how any spent fuel by-products and intact post-procedure colloidal fuel elements may be dealt with.

Of course, insofar as nanomedical ambling devices are concerned, nanometric multipedal walking strategies may well be devised that implement three or more "feet," utilizing spider, centipede-like, conveyor belt, or Ferris wheel-type configurations to traverse physiological surfaces. There will undoubtedly be a widely diverse array of substrates across which these species of nanodevices will be expected to negotiate in the performance of diagnostic and therapeutic procedures.

Specialized nanomedical "gecks" might be endowed with the ability to transiently adhere to, and traverse the inner endothelial wall surfaces of the vasculature or lymphatic vessels without being dislodged by ambient aqueous shear forces. These devices may have the capacity for brief sequential tethering via dynamic biochemical binding or through the use of some form of physiologically compatible mechanical tethering mechanisms to enable these capabilities.

Kwon et al. demonstrated the 1D bipedal Brownian walking of 9,10-dithioanthracene (DTA) subsequent to its deposition on a copper (Cu(111)) substrate at 50–70 K. Linear walking was accomplished without the use of tracks or grooves due a mismatch between the arrangement of the surface-bound copper atoms and the spacing of the sulfur atoms in the DTA molecule. This meant that only a single sulfur atom could attain its "preferred geometry with regards to the surface at any one time. This sulfur atom then acts as an anchor for the other, which binds to the surface much less strongly making the whole molecule largely free to rotate" [288,313]. It was observed via STM imaging that the DTA molecule pivoted/stepped incrementally in alignment with a single axis and that it could make 10,000 steps unerringly [313]. Further work has demonstrated that a 9,10-dioxanthracene (anthraquinone) molecule could convey a two CO_2 molecule payload [314].

Symes (University of Edinburgh) developed a synthetic processive "hand-over-hand" molecular walker and a six station track that exploited chemical switching mechanisms. Monodentate ligand/proton exchange was utilized at the Pd(II) center of one "foot," which was stimulated via coordinating solvent/anions at elevated temperatures, and redox-driven exchange proceeded at the Cu(I)/Cu(II) center of the other foot [288].

Saffarian et al. showed the precessive movement of an activated collagenase (MMP-1) molecular ratchet on a collagen fibril that was based on the "burnt bridge" proteolysis (catalytic consumption) of collagen rather than through the action of ATP hydrolysis [315].

3.4.7 Nanoengineered DNA Walkers

DNA-based nanowalkers are attractive in that they are structurally robust and programmable. The first successful attempt in the generation of a nanoscale bipedal walker based on DNA was accomplished in 2004 by Ned Seeman's group at New York University. This nanometric automaton utilized 10 nm long single-stranded DNA oligonucleotide fragments (36 bp in length), which emanated from a DNA-duplexed body as legs with which to amble, with an inchworm gait along a track that also comprised DNA, by executing sequential attachment and detachment operations. The assembly was immersed in a nondenaturing buffer solution to negate DNA degradation.

Unpaired bases were integrated into the DNA track, which served as "footholds" that were bound in succession with obtruding complementary oligonucleotide segments at each foot of the DNA legs via "set strands." As the researchers explain, "Each set strand has an 8-base overhang, or 'toehold,' which is not complementary to any of the feet or footholds. The toehold allows the set strand to be removed by the unset strand by the method of Yurke et al." [316]. "Each unset strand is synthesized with a biotin on the 5′ end so that after an unset procedure, all the unset strands and the set strands with which they are paired can be removed from the solution by the use of streptavidin-coated magnetic beads" [317,318]. Seeman later demonstrated coordinated DNA leg movement utilizing a Brownian ratchet "burnt bridges" strategy wherein metastable track stem loops are consumed as a single-stranded DNA walker segment, which integrates a 5′ and 5′ central section makes forward progress [319,320].

Another configuration of bipedal DNA nanodevice has been investigated by Shin and Pierce who developed a DNA walker that resembles kinesin walking by taking 5 nm precessive steps along a DNA track, using attachment and detachment "fuel" strands (Figure 3.32). The length of the steps could be tuned by reconfiguring the track design. For the detection and verification of the walker movement, four different dye molecules were used to label four track–protruding oligonucleotide strands [321].

The robust biomolecular RNA polymerase (RNAP) motor may be directed via an information-based strategy to walk along DNA with nanometer resolution, wielding a linear force of 15–20 pN. This translocation is induced when RNAP proceeds to duplicate DNA-based information to RNA and is contingent on activation by ribonucleotide triphosphate (NTP). Pomerantz and coworkers demonstrated that an altered bacteriophage T7 RNAP, which had "ligand-binding motifs fused to the amino terminus of the enzyme," could be walked along DNA in a controllable manner at small increments as this reduced the number of substrates that were available for each polymerization event. It was shown earlier that binding Ni^{2+}-agarose beads to RNAP enabled incremental movement at base-pair length resolution (0.34 nm) [322,323].

3.4.8 Molecular Spiders

Alluded to earlier, it might be possible that nanoscale multipedal devices (molecular spiders) may be created to undertake certain nanomedical surface ambling tasks where more

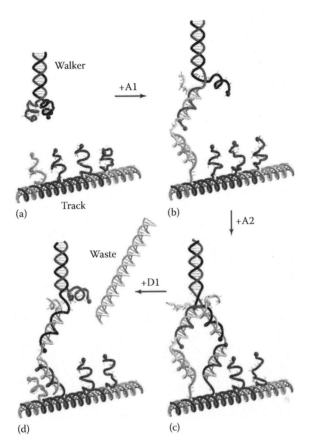

FIGURE 3.32
Depiction of DNA walking sequence: (a) walker in untethered state, (b) walker tethered to oligonucleotide 1, (c) walker tethered to oligonucleotides 1 and 2, and (d) walker released from oligonucleotide 1, generating duplex waste product. Dyes are represented by colored spheres. (Reproduced from Shin, J.S. and Pierce, N.A., *J. Am. Chem. Soc.*, 126(35), 10834, 2004. Copyright 2004. American Chemical Society. With permission.)

dynamic and higher walking velocities are required. This may be the case for nanodevices that continually patrol the oral cavity for caries, or engage in the degradation of tooth/tongue surface or peridontal pocket-resident, anaerobic gram-negative bacterial species (e.g., *Porphyromonas gingivalis*, *Campylobacter rectus*, *Fusobacterium nucleatum*, and *Eubacterium* species) and volatile sulfide compounds (VSCs) (e.g., hydrogen sulfide, methyl mercaptan, and dimethyl sulfide), which are causative agents of oral originating halitosis (oral malodour) [324]. Ideally, these nanodevices will have the capacity for progressing through an in vivo matrix and generating products (per step) without ever fully releasing from substrates.

Pei et al. have constructed hybrid polycatalytic assemblies (~25 nm in diameter) that comprised dual streptavidin molecules, which were tethered to six deoxyribozymes (nucleic acid catalysts) that initiated phosphodiesterase activity (Figure 3.33). When a population of these molecular devices were introduced into an Au-anchored (~100 to 200 nm thick) hydrogel matrix that was coated with a high-density substrate of oligonucleotides, they proceeded to diffuse through the matrix by progressively catalyzing the substrate at a pace that was equivalent to that of free catalysts in solution. The ambling velocity and processivity of these molecular spiders could be enhanced by altering the number of legs and their binding robustness, as well as increasing the number of available catalytic sites within the matrix [325].

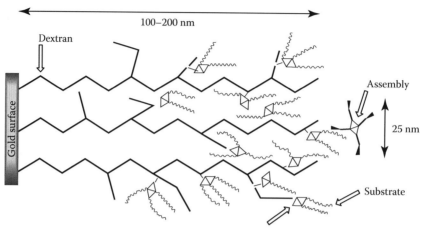

FIGURE 3.33
Schematic of multipedal walkers progressing through a hydrogel matrix asymmetrically coated with oligo-nucleotide substrates. (Reprinted from Pei, R. et al., *J. Am. Chem. Soc.*, 128(39), 12693, 2006. Copyright 2006. American Chemical Society. With permission.)

An investigation conducted by Lund et al. focused on the achievement of directionality from individual random walking three-legged molecular spiders with inert streptavidin bodies. These entities exhibited robotic-like sensing and altered their environments when autonomously guided by specifically configured pathways. In parallel trials, these entities were introduced at selected departure sites on 2D DNA origami scaffolds, and were subsequently induced to follow pathways that contained recognition element "breadcrumbs" that led to predefined destination sites. The median velocity of these molecular spiders was estimated to be (1–6 nm/min), which was more rapid than species that progressed via diffusion through all-product environments. They were directed by their immediately surrounding environments at a range of ~100 nm, for up to 50 catalytic steps [326].

Although the efficacy of the spiders was hindered by track detachments and backtracking events, and their chances of making the finish line reduced when the tracks were lengthened, this work constituted a significant advancement. As the researchers observe, "These molecular robots autonomously carry out sequences of actions such as 'start,' 'follow,' 'turn,' and 'stop,' thus laying the foundation for the synthesis of more complex robotic behaviors at the molecular level by incorporating additional layers of control mechanisms. For example, interactions between multiple molecular robots could lead to collective behavior … while the ability to read and transform secondary cues on the landscape could provide a mechanism for Turing-universal algorithmic behavior" [326–331].

Monte Carlo simulations conducted by Samii et al. to explore the optimization para-meters of bipedal and multipedal molecular spiders revealed that an increase in the number of "legs" does not contribute to their overall efficiency. A comparative study between multipedal and bipedal molecular spiders elucidated that although four-legged spiders exhibited improved efficacy and processivity, they moved more slowly than their two-legged counterparts; also that velocity and processivity may be enhanced "by tuning more than one experimental parameter simultaneously, otherwise some spider properties might improve at the expense of others" [332].

Bromley et al. synthesized a self-assembling three-legged "tumbleweed" protein complex (Figure 3.34) that performed locomotion via "cyclically ligand-gated, rectified diffusion along a DNA track, using three discrete ligand-dependent DNA-binding domains to

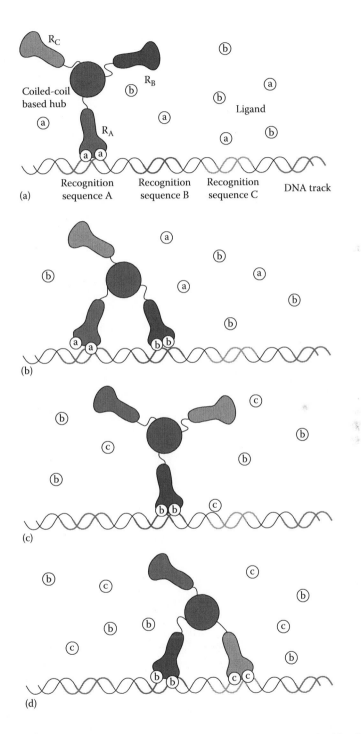

FIGURE 3.34

(a–d) Schematic of tripedal tumbleweed concept. Three protein domains RA, RB, and RC bind with DNA only when their particular ligands are present. By sequentially altering the concentrations of specific ligands, the device can cycle along the DNA track. (Reproduced from Bromley, E.H. et al., *HFSP J.*, 3(3), 204, 2009. Copyright 2009. Taylor & Francis. With permission.)

control binding and unbinding events." This motor has no power stroke hence transport along the track ensues via "stepwise-rectified diffusion" that is driven by external modifications in specific ligand concentrations [333].

3.5 Crawling, Sliding, Gliding, and Swarming Motility

Additional modes for the nanomedical traversal of physiological surfaces may include rapid centipede-like crawling, sliding, and gliding strategies. Autonomous (massively parallel) crawling nanodevices, exhibiting medically beneficial swarming motility, might be utilized to access and conduct diagnostic or therapeutic procedures on external dermal surfaces, within the lumen of sweat, oil or follicular pores, or nasal and aural passages. Sliding and gliding strategies, on the other hand, may be employed in applications for areas that have intrinsically moist or wet surfaces, such as within the oral cavity, the lumen of sex organs and elimination organs, and across ocular surfaces. Sophisticated autonomous nanomedical surface amblers would render accessible practically every domain within the human physiology.

From a purely psychological perspective, it is probable that a range of somewhat negative reactions (e.g., squeamishness to utter revulsion) might be attendant with the prospect of the in vivo and/or topical administration of large populations of microscopic, crawling sliding/gilding classes of nanodevices, as patients may naturally associate them with macroscale counterparts (e.g., spiders, centipedes, cockroaches, leeches, slugs, worms, snakes, and eels). However, some comfort may be had when one considers that there are ~100 billion individual bacteria, comprising >~1000 distinct species, that live and thrive *imperceptibly* on epidermal surfaces alone of the average healthy human individual. This does not touch on the ~10 to 100 trillion bacterial cells that are derived from thousands of species, which live within us [334]. From this perspective, humans may be thought as hybrid ultracomplex "aggregate superorganisms." Hence, the prospect of administering even several million micron scale (or smaller), equally as imperceptible and beneficial nanomedical devices, might not be caused for undue queasiness.

3.5.1 Crawling Motility

A microelectromechanical (MEM)-based device (3 cm long × 1 cm wide × 0.9 mm high with a weight of 0.5 g) was induced to crawl via "cilia-like thermal bimorph actuator arrays." The microrobot crawling elements consisted of dual actuator array chips that were populated with 64 "motion pixels," each of which contained four diagonally arranged cilia. Each set of cilia were independently controlled, which allowed for three DOF movements, gait, direction, and velocity, mediated by modifying the actuation frequency. Its capabilities included the transport of cargoes that exceeded its own weight by sevenfold, and the achievement of 250 μm/s velocities with step sizes that ranged from 1 to 4 μm [335].

It was discovered that mobile polarized T cells, which are involved in immunological migration, signaling, and receptor scanning, can perform dynamic amoeboid crawling across the surfaces antigen-presenting cells (APCs) at velocities that range from 2 to 6 μm/min by utilizing their leading edge, cell body, and uropod. Amoeboid morphological modification is also employed to enhance motility when "squeezing and gliding through narrow spaces driven by a propulsive viscoelastic cytoskeleton" [336–338].

An artificial hybrid amoeba-like cell system was devised by Yi et al., who combined nanoengineered inorganic components with biological elements, which was endowed with the ability to crawl across a glass surface by means of actin polymerization [339]. Locomotion was accomplished through the use of Ni and Au nanoparticles that were functionalized with ActA, which is a transmembrane protein from *Listeria monocytogenes*. The synthesized nanoparticles were merged with a "eukaryotic cellular actin treadmilling system containing actin nucleation factors (Arp2/3 complex and VASP) in conjunction with several ABPs [actin-binding proteins] to increase the actin recycling rate" [340]. ATP and its associated regeneration enzymes, creatine phosphate, and creatine kinase, were included in the polymerization buffer in order to sustain the biochemical power required for actin polymerization [341]. This assemblage was encapsulated, along with actin, actin-binding proteins, and ATP inside (4.52 ± 1.45 µm) diameter lipid vesicle. In effect, this hybrid construct behaved as an artificial cell, where synthetic nanobacteria and actin polymerization elements were exploited as "driving force generators" that induced movement analogous to that of natural amoeba at velocities of 0.03–0.22 µm/s.

One might ponder the idea that in vivo deployable nanomedical surface ambling devices might utilize nanometer in diameter, and thereby presumably harmless, needle-like projections or crimpons that emanate from their legs/feet to ensure a solid, albeit fleeting (microsecond) grip as they indiscernably crawl over the external surfaces of cells, tissues, and organs. Theoretically, these "nanopicks" might be temporarily inserted, interdigitating between cell membrane phospholipid heads to a several nanometer depth. This strategy would likely negate full penetration through a typical double layer (~7.5 to 10 nm thick), and facilitate the rapid reestablishment of bilayer integrity. An in-depth investigation into the kinetics and self-healing properties of cell-encapsulating phospholipid bilayers will be warranted to learn if indeed this form of traversal might be viable.

A study conducted by Doshi and Mitragotri investigated the responses of endothelial cells on exposure to nanoparticles (100 per cell) with different morphologies. They utilized spherical, elongated, and flat polystyrene nano/microparticles (500 nm–1 µm) with different polarities and found that spherical and disk-shaped particulates had no effect on endothelial cell extension and motility. In contrast, polyethyleneimine-coated, positively charged needle-shaped particulates (0.45 µm × 4.4 µm long) imparted considerable modifications in these normal cell activities in that they initiated transient cell membrane disruption, made evident via the uptake of extracellular calcein and the release of lactate dehydrogenase. The cells also underwent rapid and extensive contraction on exposure to the positively charged needles, but to a lesser degree with negatively charged needles (0.23 µm × 2.1 µm long). These effects, however, were shown to be reversible within 1 to 48 h [342].

Kim et al. have fabricated 2D superhydrophobic hexagonally packed nanoneedle arrays from honeycomb films via a "breath figures" method. The breath figures method involves the evaporation of an organic solvent in a high humidity chamber when water droplets condense into a polymer solution (e.g., polystyrene, or amphiphilic block copolymer), which then spontaneously self-organizes into a highly regular hexagonal (honeycomb) array (Figure 3.35). The top of the film is then peeled off with Scotch tape, which leaves the adhering/remaining portions of the hexagon structures on the substrate as nanoneedle arrays of sharp tips with a 10 nm radius [343]. If this process can be scaled down further, it may have utility in the synthesis of nanoneedle pads that might be employed by ambling nanodevices.

Investigations into the unique locomotive acumen of marine ragworms, such as *Nereis diversicolor* and *Nereis virens*, have inspired the possibility for the development of

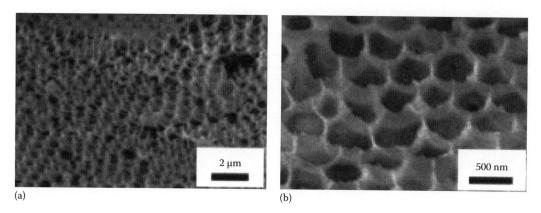

(a)   (b)

FIGURE 3.35
(a, b) SEM images of hexagonal (honeycomb) nanoneedles. (Reproduced from Kim, J. et al., *Nanoscale Res. Lett.*, 6(1), 616, 2011. With permission.)

biomimetic self-locomoting endoscopes and other crawling microdevices that might have the capacity for navigating tortuous and difficult to access cavities within the human body. These creatures are intriguing as they have the ability to move through very slippery substrates such as mud, which is similar in consistency to the mucous layer that lines the human intestinal lumen. It exhibits several modes of locomotion, including slow crawling (typical leg crawling), rapid crawling (leg crawling combined with lateral undulations), and undulatory swimming, which displaces water in a manner akin to conveyor belt. Compound, two part setae (shaft and blade) that are connected by intricate joints with integrated ligaments allow free motion of the blade independent of the shaft, albeit within a constrained freedom of movement (Figure 3.36). Fine teeth that line one side of the blades, which may serve as anchoring hooks, enable the setae to passively adapt to various slippery substrates [344].

3.5.2 Sliding Motility

Biological molecular walkers utilize only single- or dual-legged strategies. A unique single-legged kinesin (KIF1A) manages to precess along microtubules by engaging in secondary tethering interactions, whereby its movement along microtubule tracks resembles a "sliding" instead of stepping motion [345,346]. Nanoscale surface attachment mechanisms are assumed to involve van der Waals, electrostatic, capillary, and viscous forces. Since the cumulative surface areas for nanoscale attachment are very large, one can venture that aspects of all of these mechanism may come into play. Lizard species such as geckos, anoles, skinks, as well as various insects including spiders and flies employ from many thousands to millions (in the case of geckos) of adhesive setae (Figure 3.37) to negotiate vertical and even inverted surfaces.

Kellar et al. have investigated the remarkable adhesive ability of the superhydrophobic (water contact angle of 160.9°) gecko setae to adhere to even molecularly smooth surfaces (e.g., hydrophobic GaAs semiconductor) and concluded, via direct experimental evidence, that van der Waals dispersion forces were indeed the mechanism for a level of adhesion that enabled gecko vertical climbing at speeds of 1 m/s. What may be extrapolated from this finding is that the size and shape of the setae tips are primarily responsible for the robust cumulative adhesion capacities and not localized surface chemistries. Each keratinous setae (~5 μm in diameter × ~100 μm long), of which there are ~14,400 mm^{-2},

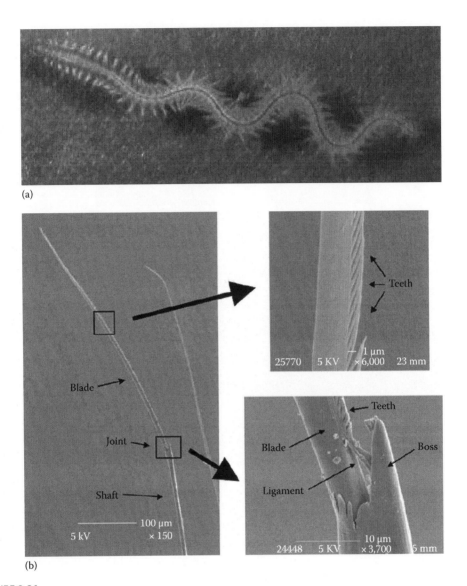

FIGURE 3.36
(a) Ragworm *N. diversicolor* in rapid crawling mode. (b) SEM of a seta depicting shaft, joint, and blade. (Reproduced from Hesselberg, T., *Naturwissenschaften*, 94(8), 613, 2007. With permission.)

further bifurcate into 100–1000 triangular spatulae (~200 nm), which are below the wavelength threshold of visible light. Under the van der Waals hypothesis, smaller spatulae will have the effect of conveying larger "adhesive force per unit area," as there will be higher interfacial surface densities [347,348].

It was revealed that the setae of Tokay geckos adhered equally well to smooth, highly hydrophobic and hydrophilic polarizable surfaces. Interestingly, the setae did not adhere to hydrophobic, weakly polarizable surfaces (e.g., PTFE). To validate the van der Waals adherence mechanism, two types of synthetic polymer hydrophobic spatulae, with similar dimensions to their natural counterparts, were made of silicone rubber and polyester resin (gecko-like synthetic adhesives [GSAs] were synthesized in more recent experiments) [347,348]. The adhesive forces of these polymeric analogs were measured using an atomic

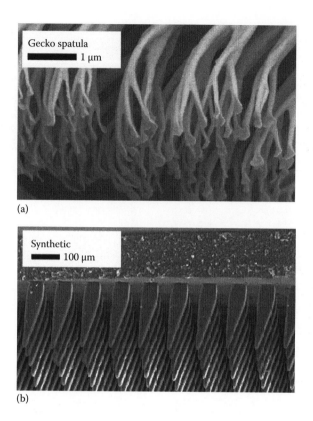

FIGURE 3.37

(a) Natural gecko spatula and (b) synthetic gecko-like synthetic adhesive (GSA). (Reproduced from Gravish, N. et al., *J. R. Soc. Interface*, 7(43), 259, 2010. The Royal Society. With permission.)

force microscope (AFM) probe and it was found that the synthetic spatulae approximated the adhesion forces of the gecko spatulae, where "47%–63% of the adhesion forces of the synthetic spatulae can be explained by van der Waals forces" [348].

It was also discovered that gecko setae are self-cleaning due to an energetic disequilibrium, which favors the adhesion of dirt particles to the substrate rather than the spatulae [349]. The adhesion of gecko spatulae are also enhanced at higher relative humidity as it "softens setae and increases viscoelastic damping" to allow equal adhesion to both smooth hydrophobic and hydrophilic surfaces [350].

Hence, it seems plausible that surface ambling nanodevices that are endowed with densely packed arrays of flexible polymeric nanofibers or nanotubes, the tips of which might serve as biomimetic setae/spatulae, might adhere to practically any physiological surface for the efficacious performance of their nanomedical procedures. This is contingent on whether they are appropriately nanoengineered to emulate the fine dynamics of gecko spatulae adhesion. In their default state, gecko setae are not adhesive. For adhesion to manifest there must be "a small vertical preload followed by a proximal shear" in a load–drag–pull, or stick–slip frictional sliding sequence, whereby a tiny perpendicular-to-substrate force is followed by a 5 μm reverse displacement [351–353]. Intriguingly, nanoscale stick–slip sliding events are quite distinct from stick–slip sliding at the macroscale [354–357]. Direct measurements have revealed that a single seta may convey 194 ± 25 μN of adhesive force. This translates to the generation of a 100 N adhesive force for a single gecko foot if all setae were to be optimally attached to a substrate [351].

Similar, but far less-dense adhesion elements functionalize the attachment pad tenant setae of the blowfly *Calliphora vicina*. Each of the 12 pulvilli (heel segments) of the blowfly contains from 4000 to 6000 (total of ~60,000) hollow secretion-filled setae that are configured as patterned rows, each of which terminate in a flat bent plate analogous to a spatula (Figure 3.38). Niederegger et al. measured the spring constant of a single setae to be 1.31 N/m via AFM. It was determined that only one-third of the total population of setae was required for the pulvillus to adhere to glass. Since the flat tips of the setae are pliable, they can increase the contact surface area so as to enhance adhesion. As with gecko setae, a brief sliding event is required to activate adhesion [358].

Pawashe et al. undertook the investigation and modeling of untethered magnetically actuated neodymium–iron–boron microscale Mag-μBots (250 μm × 130 μm × 100 μm). Activation via the alternating fields of an array of five macroscale electromagnets induced a stick–slip mode of locomotion across a silicon substrate. The microrobot attained a velocity of 2 mm/s at a frequency of 100 Hz under a maximum pulsed magnetic field strength of 2.5 mT. These researchers recently demonstrated the coupled magnetic control of three different sized submillimeter Mag-μBots, which attained top velocities of 7 mm/s at a frequency of 140 Hz under a sustained maximum magnetic field strength of 1.1 mT. These Mag-μBots that could traverse variable surfaces and function while immersed in fluid were also endowed with independent global positioning [359,360].

3.5.3 Gliding Motility

Gliding motility, as employed by *Labyrinthula*, a unicellular marine protist (eukaryotic microorganism) that lives on sea grass and marine algae, involves the initial extensile formation of filamentous netlike "tracks" along which it pulls itself, via myosin–actin complex motive force to gain access to nutrients. Preston and King reveal that *Labyrinthulids* (slime nets) utilize a specialized bothrosome organelle that secretes an external membrane, which subsequently generates numerous filamentous (above substrate) guy wire–like trackways that may be considered analogous to overhanging downward angled streetcar cables. Forward protruding filopodia utilize the addition of G-actin monomers to F-actin for outgrowth at velocities from ~50 to 200 μm/min. They also serve to anchor the suspended tracks, which allow *Labyrinthula* spindle cells (~4.6 μm wide) to glide along the 2 μm wide tracks, unaffected by substrate chemistries. The force necessary for *Labyrinthula* to surmount viscous drag in aqueous media with a ~5 μm spindle cell diameter, at a mean velocity of 1.5 μm/s was calculated to be 7×10^{-14} N (~0.1 pN). The requisite energy for a spindle cell to sustain this speed was estimated to be 5×10^{-19} J/s [361].

Cyanobacterial surface gliding motility involves the secretion of a polysaccharide gel mucilage (slime) from "nozzle-like pores" (~14 to 16 nm outer diameter × 7 nm inner diameter) embedded within their surfaces. Interactive compressive forces among nozzle-resident polymeric chains provide an expulsive gliding force, which for *Phormidium uncinatum* and *Anabaena variabilis* species attains a running velocity of ~3 μm/s, with the *Oscillatoriaceae* species reaching an even more rapid ~10 μm/s [362].

In soil-dwelling myxobacteria gliding, it has been proposed that the ejected slime (a filamentous actin gel) undergoes swelling as it clears the nozzles, thereby providing thrust, as the actin gel has a very high Young's modulus value in contrast to the comparatively weak thrust provided by polysaccharide gel swelling. Hence, the nozzles of cyanobacteria may serve as expulsive compression chambers [363,364]. It has also been observed in *P. uncinatum* that they "were either covered in a tight-fitting slime tube or had a number of thin bands of slime that wrapped in a helical fashion over the surface" [362]. This statement

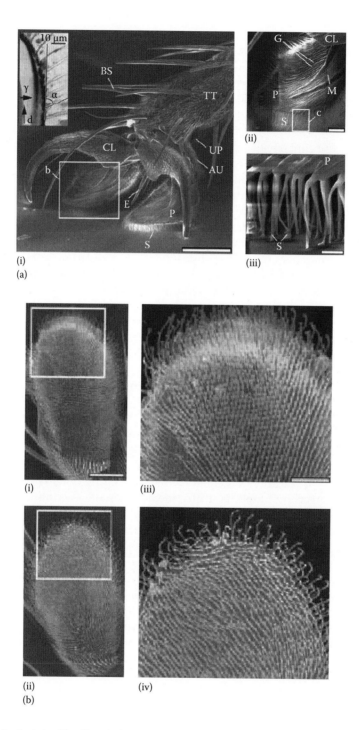

FIGURE 3.38

(a) SEM micrographs depicting blowfly pulvilli adhesion to a glass coverslip. (i) Complete pretarsus (distal segment of leg), (ii) right pulvillus, and (iii) setae of the pulvillus (scale bars—50, 20, 5 μm, respectively). AU, auxilia; BS, bristles; CL, claw; E, empodium; G, grooves on surface of pulvillus; M, midsegment of puvillus; P, pulvillus; TT, terminal tarsomere (leg segment); and UP, unguitractor plate. (b) (i–iv) SEM micrographs of right foreleg pulvilli, (i, iii) pulvillus in contact with glass, and (ii, iv) pulvillus not in contact (scale bars—50 μm (i, ii), 20 μm (iii, iv)). (Reproduced from Niederegger, S. et al., *J. Comp. Physiol. A Neuroethol. Sens. Neural Behav. Physiol.*, 187(12), 961, 2002. With permission.)

might lead one to surmise that these bacteria may also be gliding *on* the slime, which may perhaps be acting as friction-reducing lubricant. However, slime trails are typically observed as emanating from the rear of gliding cells, which strongly supports the premise that the slime is propelling the cells forward [365,366].

Plasmodium falciparum sporozoites, the causative parasite of malaria, remain rigid as they glide forward, driven by actin/myosin-based motors, to invade the secretory cells of salivary glands of the *Anopheles* mosquito vector, through molecular and cellular obstructions en route to their target hepatocyte cells in the human host, within which they initially replicate. Their modes of locomotion alternate between passive floating within the circulation and active transfer through the extracellular matrix and cell membranes. Compared to most other *Plasmodium* species, sporozoites must rapidly traverse extensive distances through various tissue types, within both their mosquito and human hosts, in order to evade annihilation from immune sentinels, in the achievement of their goal [367]. Sporozoites have been observed gliding on the surfaces of host cells, and they are thought to utilize a receptor-controlled process to finally bind with and penetrate into hepatic cells [368,369]. Circumsporozoite protein (CS), which homogeneously coats the exterior surface of a sporozoite [370], is generated and ejected from within the apical complex at its anterior end and proceeds to translocate along its outer surface to its posterior end via a "cytochalasin-sensitive process," prior to being discarded as a CS "trail" [371–375].

The dynamic motile strategies employed by *P. falciparum* sporozoites may be inspirational and instructive in the conceptualization and design of nanodevices that might initially traverse through the extracellular matrix to reach specific organs and cells, the surfaces of which they will then walk or glide across to subsequently penetrate into target cells to perform cellular diagnostic operations, or to administer cell repair or the highly localized release of drug payloads.

3.5.4 Swarm Motility

There may be instances where significant masses of nanomedical devices, comprising many millions or several billion individuals, are required to very rapidly arrive at and attend to a site or multiple sites of serious injury simultaneously, from both internal and external surfaces of the patient. They might work in a massively parallel manner to quickly neutralize ingested toxins, injected venoms, or life-threatening pathogenic microorganisms. In these cases, it may be prudent to employ strategic swarm-like motile measures to ensure the survival of the patient(s). This would involve protocols for very rapid administration, and subsequently, highly intercoordinated locomotion and navigation between constituent nanodevices to expedite and optimize treatment effectiveness.

To be clear, nanomedical device swarming would not entail any form of replication. Rather, it may constitute an alternate mode of motility comprising a purposeful externally controlled rapid movement for a prescribed nanomedical treatment in "formation." With the advent of sufficiently sophisticated fully autonomous medical nanodevices in conjunction of course, with fully informed real time or preauthorized personal consent, it may be possible in the case of high-risk patients, or as an emergency measure against an impending large-scale health crisis or biological/chemical attack, to administer nanodevices that strategically and imperceptibly self-implant in a highly distributed fashion. Once in position, these "sentinel" class nanomedical devices (Chapter 17) would immediately assume the status of being "at the ready" for any contingency while they are benignly tethered (in a dormant dwell mode) within tissues that are in close proximity to the vascular system, as well as epidermal surfaces. This approach might be analogous, in the macroworld, to having highly qualified emergency workers stationed on every block, or at every house throughout a city, who are ready to efficiently respond to any crisis at a moments notice. This strategy may allow for almost instantaneous responses to injury or other physiological insult, and might be considered as a significant immune system enhancement. However, as stated previously, these types of scenarios will only be possible if individuals are psychologically accepting these multitudes of internal miniaturized medical sentinels.

From a design perspective, the surface swarming motility in bacterial strains such as *Proteus*, *Bacillus*, and *Clostridium* (on semisolid agar plates) appears to have prerequisites, as Henrichsen suggests, of "very heavy flagellation of the cells and the fact that the translocation predominantly takes place where cells are in contact with other cells, i.e., in cell bundles, rafts, microcolonies etc." and defines the swarming of bacteria as "a kind of surface translocation produced through the action of flagella but is different from swimming. The micromorphological pattern is highly organized in (rotating) whirls and bands. The movement is continuous and regularly follows the long axis of the cells which are predominantly aggregated in bundles during the movement." Thus, cumulative propulsive force is indeed larger for cell aggregates than for individual cells and as the swarming environment becomes more difficult, the aggregate will expand [376].

Interestingly, a number of swarming bacterial spices (e.g., *Bacillus subtilis*, *Serratia liquefaciens*, and *Pseudomonas aeruginosa*) produce and release amphipathic molecular surfactants, which are excreted in such a manner as to precede the leading line of cells in the swarm, in order to diminish tension between themselves and the substrate to ease their movement across surfaces. In bacterial aggregates, the generation of surfactants is controlled via quorum sensing (cell–cell communication) presumably to make certain that their production only ensues once the appropriate numbers of individuals are available to be of benefit for the motile progress of the swarm [377].

Other examples of complex swarm behavior in nature involving coordinated interdependent group motility include communal airborne navigation in birds [378], locust swarming [379], ant networks [380], schools of fish [381], and quadruped herds [382,383]. The seeming overarching theme in swarm motility is the reliance of individual participants on their close proximity neighbors for cues on spatial orientation, directional and velocity via sensory stimuli, computation and rapid interactive adjustment. Yet, one might reasonably surmise that there must be a single or multiple cue "luminars" within the group to which other participants refer to for guidance. In the case of nanomedical devices that are moving rapidly in formation there might be multiple such cue designates who in effect are real time orchestrators of the required trajectories and velocities, which all other participants will follow to a treatment site or sites.

Vicsek et al. developed a computational "self-propelling particles" model of swarming behavior that may be applied to the clustering and migration of biological systems [384,385]. The single rule that drives the model is that "at each time step a given particle driven with a constant absolute velocity assumes the average direction of motion of the particles in its neighborhood of radius *r* with some random perturbation added." In practice, each participant's motion is influenced by the average orientation of its localized partners with the inclusion of some "noise-induced perturbation." Coherent or random collective motion was contingent on particle density and participant noise, where low noise and high density resulted in "coherent group motion" [383,386]. This model may also have utility in the determination and design of aggregate swarm motility and collision avoidance strategies for millions of nanomedical devices within the constrained confines of the human body.

3.6 Nanomedical Navigation

A robust and efficient externally computer-controlled navigational infrastructure will endow advanced nanomedical devices with the ability to locate and arrive at any point within the human body to impart beneficial medical diagnoses and/or treatments. The simultaneous and precise spatial orchestration of perhaps many millions or even billions of nanomedical devices will pose formidable challenges indeed to nanomedical device and systems developers. It may be possible, however, to reduce the perceived complexity of such a task if the problem is massively distributed among the constituent nanodevices themselves, thereby dramatically reducing the computational burden of a centralized navigation system. Utilizing a form of swarming strategy as described earlier, it might be feasible that only 1 in 100 or 1 in 1000 nanodevices would be "locked on" to single or multiple externally triangulated reference points, whereas the remaining "narray" (author's designation for nanodevice aggregate) would lock on to the homing beacons of the leading "luminar" class of nanodevices. Elements of conventional macroscale navigation systems (e.g., global positioning system [GPS] and distance measuring equipment [DME]), which are briefly described later, may serve as templates toward the realization of reliable nanomedical navigation strategies.

3.6.1 Global Positioning System

The existing commercial GPS navigation system comprises 24 satellites positioned at 12,540 miles above the earth's surface in six different orbital planes, which circumscribe the globe once every 12 h. The system is designed to supply instantaneous position, time, and velocity information to almost any site on the planet at any time, and in any weather. As relates to positional resolution, the FAA reported (subsequent to the collection of real-world data in 2011 using a number of high-quality GPS SPS receivers) that current GPS resolution (horizontal accuracy) falls within ~1 m. Enhancements that are provided by augmentation systems, such as the Wide Area Augmentation System (WAAS) and Global Differential GPS (GDGPS), enable real-time resolution that can be as high as 1 mm.

Time to first fix (TTFF) positional signal acquisition is on average <10 s, and can be as rapid as 3 s [387]. GPS satellites are precisely time-synchronized (within ~50 ns) and utilize the oscillations of cesium and rubidium atoms in four atomic clocks to keep very precise time. Coordinated Universal Time (UTC) utilizes an atomic timescale that involves numerous atomic clocks worldwide and International System of Units (SI) has updated its definition of a second as equivalent to precisely 9,192,631,770 cesium 133 atom oscillations, "at rest at a temperature of 0 K" [388].

Position is determined by triangulation using crossing radials in intersecting spheres. Half of the total transmission time is multiplied by the speed of light and then translated into distance. GPS satellites generate a one-way signal that the receiver listens for, and measures the time taken to reach the receiver. Each satellite transmits its own unique and random code that is sent with the signal. The receiver determines exactly when the signal (carrying the code) left the satellite, and matches the code at exactly the same time. When three satellites and the receiver are in synch, the three calculated spheres intersect; position is determined within the triangle formed at the intersecting area. When a forth satellite is included, a measurement of the Doppler shift of the signal can elucidate a 3D velocity and synchronize the atomic clocks as well. GPS satellites emit a very low (~50 W) power signal that spans an extensive area [389]. Lockheed Martin is currently constructing next-generation GPS III satellites, the first of which is scheduled for a 2014 launch [390].

3.6.2 Distance Measuring Equipment

DME is employed as a navigation system by which pilots can find their precise positions anywhere on the globe. In operation, an aircraft sends a 1000 MHz signal to a ground station, which replies using a different frequency. Signal linkages between ground and airborne instrumentation gives a consistent "slant range" (direct line distance from aircraft to station, not a measurement along the ground) readout by measuring time of flight for a signal transmitted from the aircraft to the station and back. Distance calculations are based on the fact that radio signals require 12.36 μs to travel 1 radar mile from a point to an object and back. The DME calculates the time needed for the signal to be received back by an aircraft, subsequent to its interrogation of a specific ground station. The total time required is translated to radar miles/distances. DMEs calculate ground speed and time-to-station information via differentiation [391].

3.6.3 Nanogyroscopes

In order to endow the VCSN and other classes of nanodevices with orientational acumen and stability, an integrated onboard nanogyroscopic capability might be devised. Considerable strides in progress have been made in this area that includes work done by Krause et al. who encased a diatomic C_2 unit within a solid endohedral $C_2Sc_2@C_{84}$ fullerene, which behaved as a rigid diatomic plane molecular rotor [392] that exhibited quantized rotation (Figure 3.39). This entity behaved as a quantum gyroscope having a cardanic (gimballed) suspension. Novel materials and molecular clusters may be grown within these carbon-shielded cages, some of which are not possible outside of this highly restricted environment [393].

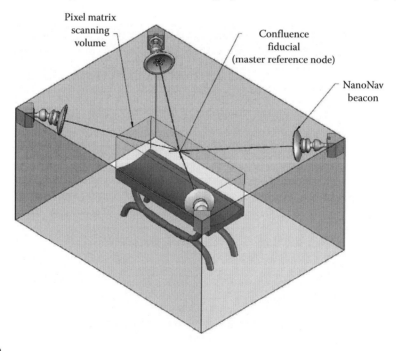

FIGURE 3.39
Artistic representation of conceptual spatial metrics room. (Reproduced from Boehm, F., Chapter 15, Potential strategies for advanced nanomedical device ingress and egress, natation, mobility, and navigation, in Schulz, M.J. et al., *Nanomedicine Design of Particles, Sensors, Motors, Implants, Robots, and Devices*, Artech House, Norwood, MA, 2009, With permission.)

A rigid cyclotriveratrylene (a macrocycle that strongly binds with metals) stator framework was utilized to support three molecular rotator groups that comprised *p*-phenylene for the study of molecular gyroscopes. The diminutive cavity dimensions in this device served to exclude gas and solvent molecules that might potentially act to hinder rotation [394]. A frictionless self-assembled heterocapsule was shown by Kitagawa et al. to behave as a supramolecular gyroscope with acetoxy, *p*-phenol, and *p*-pyridyl groups serving as the rotators. Alkoxy (carbon and hydrogen) chain elongation was observed to slow the rotation of guest molecules [395].

Freitas describes the workings and prerequisites of nanogyroscopes: "… a triaxially gimballed nanogyroscope may be regarded as having its pivot point near its centre of mass, so L_p (centre of gravity distance) becomes very small and w_{min} (critical nonwobbling nonbursting spin velocity) becomes very slow, making nanogyroscopes feasible in medical nanorobots. Taking $h = 1$ micron, $r = 0.5$ micron, $r = 3510$ kg/m^3 and $a_{min} = g$ in [1]:

$$\omega = \omega_{min} = \left(\frac{4 a_{min} L_p \left(r^2 + \frac{1}{3} h^2 \right)}{\pi h \rho r^6} \right)^{1/2} \tag{3.8}$$

then if the gimbals are aligned such that $L_p = 1$ nm between the pivot point and the effective centre of gravity along the rotation axis, then w_{min} ~400 rad/sec. If gimbal tolerances are improved to $L_p = 0.1$ nm, then w_{min} ~125 rad/sec" [1].

3.6.4 Nanomagnetic Navigation

The external steering of first-generation nanomedical devices may be accomplished through the use of MRI in conjunction with nanoscale magnetic entities (naturally occurring or artificially synthesized) that are installed onboard nanodevices or embedded within their external surfaces. Martel et al. has made significant strides in this area utilizing three species of magnetically controlled entities toward attaining access to deep tissues via the vascular system. It is suggested that several classes of nanodevices might be employed to compensate for the changing physiological conditions that arise within the smaller vascular domains. The first were therapeutic magnetic microcarriers (TMMC) (Ø ~50 µm), comprised of poly(D,L-lactic-*co*-glycolic acid) PLGA microparticles that encapsulated therapeutics along with FeCo MNP (Ø ~180 nm). A second strategy integrated Ø ~20 nm superparamagnetic iron oxide nanoparticles (SPIONs) within a thermosensitive biocompatible N-isopropylacrylamide (PNIPA) hydrogel. In this case, the MNP were activated by magnetic frequencies to enable hyperthermia and thermally mediated "computer-triggered" drug delivery. The MNP were also employed as propulsive and tracking agents. A third unique approach involved the tracking and directional control of MC-1 MTB (Ø ~1–2 µm), which exhibited propulsive forces of >4 pN (10 times higher than those of common bacterial counterparts) that were provided by dual flagellar bundles [144,396,397]. It was shown that MTB cell-embedded single-domain magnetosome chains enabled computer-mediated directional control and tracking.

Insofar as the actual detection of micron-scale entities using MRI is concerned, Martel explains "… susceptibility-based negative contrast in MRI can provide a mean to detect these microentities. When such artifact reaches the size of a typical MRI voxel (~0.5 × 0.5 × 0.5 mm^3), the micro-entity becomes visible by MRI in the form of a susceptibility artifact."

His team has demonstrated that individual micron-scale (Ø ~15 μm) particulates comprised of high susceptibility materials may be detected via "the intra-voxel dephasing using GE scans" [144].

An autothrusting tubular microjet, in the form of a concave hyperbolic-shaped cone, was externally controlled in this manner when a magnetic Ni layer was interspersed between an interior catalytic Pt layer and an exterior noncatalytic Au layer. Optimal performance was attained with a 150 μm long microjet with an inlet diameter of 30 μm and an outlet diameter of 50 μm. The microjet was induced by an external magnetic field to retrieve and transport a 100 μm magnetic microspheric payload [75].

Ghosh and Fischer described the use of a triaxial Helmholtz coil, which generated a uniform ~50 gauss rotating magnetic field at frequencies reaching 170 Hz, to enable the 3D directional control of colloidal SiO_2 helical propellers (200–300 nm wide × 1–2 μm long), which rotated around their long axes as they were coated on one side of their helical surfaces with a 30 nm thin film of cobalt. In the absence of a magnetic field, the nanodevices exhibited random trajectories within a 5 × 5 μm area, which were driven by Brownian motion. The propellers were tracked via the adherence of a fluorophore, comprised of (3-aminopropyl)dimethylethoxysilane, rhodamine B isothiocyanate, and dry ethanol, to the SiO_2 surface [86].

3.6.5 Conceptual VCSN Navigation System

In view of the rapid pace of advancements in nanotechnology and nanomedicine, one may envision that in the not too distant future (~20 years), a compact nanomedical navigational system might be devised for clinical use by which in vivo nanodevices, such as the VCSN, may be spatially directed (under computer control) and tracked to ensure, in the case of the VCSN, precise and robust scanning procedure efficacy. It could also assist with the controlled and orderly nanodevice egress from the body once the scanning procedure is complete; to verify that upon the scan completion phase, all devices have indeed been accounted for and have vacated the patient. Essential navigational system requirements would include safe and reliable operation, with multiple redundant systems, the precursors of which we now see in onboard aircraft controls. Full operability within confined areas (e.g., clinical settings) would be required, with enough flexibility engineered into the system so that it may convey equivalent efficacy in rugged and remote environments. Therefore, such a system would ideally embody inherent high-portability attributes, as well as relatively simple user-friendly setup and calibration interface.

The following suggestions may assist with the development of potential capacities for the completely automated control of internalized VCSN, to orchestrate the vascular system mapping procedure. Of course, this system would be equipped with embedded intervention protocols whereby physicians and/or qualified medical imaging technicians could halt the imaging process for any reason, at any point during the scanning procedure. Individual VCSN devices, perhaps numbering in the thousands, would each be tracked and accounted for, and finally, safely dispersed from the patient at predetermined egress locations upon completion of spatial data acquisition.

Touching on a potentially feasible VCSN navigation system in a future formal clinical setting, a small-scale (analogous to) GPS system might utilize spatial triangulation in conjunction with a fine-scale Cartesian coordinate system to accurately navigate and track nanodevices. This system might potentially operate via the use of multiple pulsed, range-finding near-infrared lasers that are generated from three or four wireless positioning "NanoNav" beacons, with the fourth, possibly employed for time synchronization.

Cumulatively, the beacons would establish a spatial "confluence fiducial" Master Reference Node (MRN) (Figure 3.39) within a smaller beam dispersal device that is positioned just above the patient. All navigation and tracking of nanomedical entities would be extrapolated relative to this spatially demarcated point in 3D space via dedicated computer algorithms. In space-constrained areas, in rough terrain, or in remote environments, portable and ruggedized versions of this system could be set up in closer proximity to the patient, under the proviso that a well-defined separation between the beacons can be established, which will allow for precise triangulation.

Directed nanodevice locomotion in vivo may likely involve positional feedback loops to enable self-centering trajectories within the lumen of myriad vascular entities that nanodevices will encounter (although there may be an alternative to this strategy as described as follows). Several issues for consideration here are

1. When several thousand VCSN entities are deployed in order to minimize the scanning time line (~5 min may be deemed as acceptable), individual nanodevices will require tagging and tracking, which may entail for example, the integration of metallic nanoshells each of which possesses a distinct identifying signature encrypted into a nanobarcode. This might be accomplished by synthesizing nanoshells with specific diameters and metallic (e.g., Ag, Au) "skin" thicknesses. The nanoshells could conceivably be nanoengineered to have distinct plasmon surface resonance responses when interrogated with near-infrared photonic wavelengths, or perhaps ultrasonic pulses.

   Encoded nanowires have been demonstrated in the application of a particles-based universal array for high-throughput single-nucleotide polymorphisms (SNP) genotyping. Adjacent nanometer-sized stripes of Au and Ag were applied by electroplating and encoded via their variable reflectivity. A 13-stripe multiplexed format was calculated to facilitate the creation of a library of 4160 unique nanowires [398]. Quantum dots (Ø <10 nm) have excellent potential as well in serving as nanobarcodes as they fluoresce over an extensive range of colors, contingent on their physical dimensions when interrogated under specific wavelengths of light. The composition of an exemplar core of a quantum dot may include cadmium selenide that is coated with a thin shell of zinc sulfide [399].

2. Ideally, the VCSN would traverse along the central luminal axes of vascular entities, so as to reliably gather accurate spatial scanning data from this position. However, as previously described, there is a tendency for smaller particles to be displaced toward the periphery of the arteries, veins, etc., by red cells and white cells, by virtue of their being much larger (≥ ~20 μm). Consequently, they tend to dominate in the blood flow and travel along the central axis. A self-centering mechanism might be coupled with the imaging/scanning apparatus, in that nanodevice feedback loops would consistently recalculate and adjust position to maintain the central location in relation to their proximity to vascular walls. However, as stated earlier, there may be an option to this scenario that might eliminate its requirement. This may involve the development of a specialized algorithm that would use individual scanning target-hit sites as reference points during the image reconstruction process. Each targeted spatial data acquisition event (most likely in milliseconds and possibly initiated by directed ultrasonics or miniaturized LIDAR technology) may reference all end-point target-hit coordinates relative to the position of the VCSN, in subsequent nanometer-thick "slices"

to potentially result in a corrective "smoothing" effect using a coordinate-based "pixel matrix" imaging and display system (Chapter 1), giving spatially accurate outcomes. This might allow the VCSN to proceed at any position within the vascular lumen while in transit without affecting spatial precision or the resulting image quality.

3. As each VCSN approaches vascular or lymphatic branch points (bifurcations), an approach that may assist with ensuring full scanning coverage might be to pre-program half of the nanodevices to always stay to the right (or top) when encountering bifurcations, and the other half to always stay to the left (or bottom) while in transit. Top and bottom are mentioned, as some branch points may indeed be oriented in this way, as well as diagonally. The VCSN will undoubtedly encounter angular and/or curved bifurcation configurations that are oriented anywhere between vertical z-axis and horizontal (x- and y-axis) planes.

3.6.6 VCSN Navigation and Tracking: Conceptual NanoNav System

Investigations into the potential for precise VCSN positional determination and effective guidance via triangulation in a clinical setting may be a worthy endeavor. Navigational control of singular and multiple in vivo VCSNs from external sources may perhaps be accomplished by utilizing beacons having functionality that is analogous to the satellites employed for the commercial/military GPS systems, described earlier. Hypothetically, it may be feasible to employ wide-scanning programmable near-infrared laser light, which can safely penetrate human tissues, to precisely orchestrate and follow numerous ~1 μm in diameter nanodevices in vivo. It is also possible that directed ultrasound might be utilized in combination with certain species of laser for nanomedical navigation. Conventional GPS frequencies and employed wavelengths (L1 frequency 1575.42 MHz, wavelength 19.05 cm) (L2 frequency 1227.60 MHz, wavelength 24.45 cm) would most likely be ineffective for in vivo nanomedical operations.

Initially, it had not been feasible to operate nanoelectromechanical (NEMs) systems at microwave frequencies (0.3–300 GHz) as femtometer displacements could not be detected. Dual advances, which were achieved in 2003, allowed access to this domain. The first was the introduction of silicon carbide epilayers, which demonstrated a higher stiffness than typical silicon, enabling high frequencies to be generated [400]. Second was the realization of high-frequency displacement transducers that enabled "the ubiquitous passive embedding impedances that arise from electrical connections to the macroworld to be nulled" (if uncontrolled, these parasitic impedances overwhelm the electromechanical impedance of interest—the "signal"—in ultrasmall NEMS) [401,402]. To achieve the appropriate resolution, a conceptual nanonav system (NNS) might utilize wavelengths in the terahertz domain (30–1000 μm) [403,404], within which displacements of down to 100 fm have been shown to be measurable [405].

A NNS strategy, described earlier, may utilize three or four interferenced beacons that operate within a clinical vibrationless "spatial metrics" room (Figure 3.39). Beacon self-referencing might be achieved when at least three beacons transmit specific signals that intersect at precise spatial coordinates in relationship to the location of the patient, possibly being facilitated by a compact photonic collimating device. This sequence would establish a highly accurate and stable confluence fudicial set point (MRN), which would be recorded and maintained within a dedicated external computer system with multiple redundant backups. The primary NNS would subsequently home in on and autocalibrate to this fiducial. All subsequent in vivo spatial measurements acquired by the VCSN,

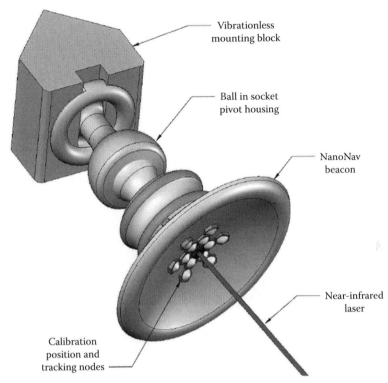

Vibrationless
mounting block

Ball in socket
pivot housing

NanoNav
beacon

Near-infrared
laser

Calibration
position and
tracking nodes

FIGURE 3.40
Artistic representation of conceptual NanoNav beacon.

as well as the image reconstruction process enabled by the Pixel Matrix system, would be correlated to this known reference node.

Each NNS beacon (Figure 3.40) would send out a continual stream of pulsed interrogation signals that would be received by all in vivo VCSNs, and as described earlier, each nanodevice would be tagged and tracked. The NNS would compute the time of flight of signals sent from the beacons to each of possibly thousands of VCSN devices to quantify their exact locations in 3D space in relation to the fiducial. A fourth beacon might be utilized for the determination of velocity. The NNS may incorporate multiple cesium atomic clocks to make certain that time/distance calculations are accurate and correct. Hence, the global positions of all VCSNs would be triangulated within a predetermined pixelated volume in 3D space.

The actual "steering" of individual VCSNs through the vasculature or lymphatic system will present significant and complex challenges. Not only will each nanodevice be required to constantly gather spatial measurements on the fly as relates to its local environment (e.g., registering distances from itself to target points on vascular walls), but would be required to be endowed with the capacity for traveling in specific directions (ideally following the axes of all vascular entities) at prescribed velocities. Theoretically, VCSN onboard navigation equipment may include a number of "look-ahead" distance quantifying ultrasonic pulsed beam emitters/receivers, which would function in a manner analogous to automobile headlights moving through a dark tunnel.

Look-ahead interrogation signals, originating from each VCSN, would rapidly (approximately nanoseconds) map upcoming trajectories within vascular or lymphatic lumen at forward projected micron or millimeter distances. These streaming data should provide a sufficient heads up to inform the nanodevices as to what specific trajectories they should be following. This near-range look-ahead data may be transmitted to external computers, which would almost instantaneously calculate and issue navigational commands to the VCSN in a form of synchronized data-exchange loop, under which an onboard quantum computer would continually refresh/modify direction and velocity.

Modularly configured and highly portable NNS systems are envisioned that may be developed for use in remote locations and in aerospace and space travel applications (Chapter 16). In these cases, scaled-down NNS beacons would be positioned at as close as possible proximity to the patient. Also, the establishment of the MRN will likely not need to be directly positioned above the patient as it is apt to be in a formal clinical setting. Rather, as long as it is located within range of the beacons, it could be offset and still operate with equal effectiveness. Hence, the fundamental requirement would be for setting a stable "reference point against which all subsequently acquired VCSN spatial data would be calibrated" [406].

3.6.7 VCSN Propulsion and Navigation Testing

Concurrent with, and in addition to extensive computer modeling and simulations to discern the best strategic routes for the optimal approach for addressing VCSN navigation challenges, an experimental test bed might be designed and fabricated to investigate various micro-, and subsequently, nanopropulsive devices and navigation strategies.

Preliminary experimentation with tissue-engineered vascular entities, including all physiological geometries and orientations that might be expected to be encountered in vivo, may indicate and further elucidate which approach would be most appropriate for attempting to precisely control the navigation of ~1 µm nanomedical devices in vivo. These benchtop "vascular test beds" might be initially infused with a transparent fluid that has similar viscous properties to whole blood to potentially simplify observations of VCSN behavior within these environments [407–411].

This testing system may include tissue-engineered elements, and function as a hybrid closed-loop fluid circulation system. It could be designed with inherent capacities for the introduction of adjustable pressure, flow rates, turbulence profiles, bifurcations, blockage/pinch point capabilities, etc. At more advanced stages, real whole blood (safety-certified and provided by volunteers), or appropriate blood substitutes might be used in these studies to further refine VCSN navigation, tagging, and tracking technologies. The aim would be to evolve and refine these models, techniques, and strategies to potentially move them closer to "real-world" safe and robust operation and application.

3.7 Proposed Research Tasking List: VCSN Propulsion Component and Navigation System

Following is a list of preliminary suggestions, considerations, and relevant questions as relates to perceived areas of investigation for exemplar VCSN propulsion components and navigation systems.

3.7.1 Propulsion Component

1. Identify the most promising in vivo locomotive technologies that might be scaled down to the nanoscale while maintaining required functionality (e.g., molecular motors ATP, flagella-like motive entities, nanofluidic jets, ultrasonic [piezo] propulsion, and biomimetic entities).

2. Create conceptual designs for these potential candidates and their perceived subcomponents.

3. Conduct an in-depth investigation into the structure and function of the ATP synthase molecular motor with the aim of possibly constructing an inorganic analog that follows the same principals of operation.

4. Might there be enough propulsive force generated by an optimally configured "nanopropeller" tethered to this ATP synthase analog to displace sufficient fluid to impart a usable thrust?

5. How may this device behave in a fluid having the same viscosity as human whole blood?

6. Might there be any means of increasing the torque of this (analogous to ATP synthase) motor?

7. Quantify/model what the cumulative propulsive force imparted by multiple modular units, operating in unison might be.

8. Investigate the precise physics involved with selected nanopropulsive entities. Develop computer models and simulations to reflect envisaged function set against a simulated in vivo environment.

9. Narrow down selection process to one or two preferred technologies that hold the greatest potential for enabling in vivo motility for a nanomedical device. Optimize designs to demonstrate evidence of reliable and robust propulsive operation in an aqueous environment.

10. Investigate and verify the functionality of these propulsive entities, and attempt to fabricate these components, initially at the microscale and then toward size reduction to the nanoscale.

11. Conduct and assess the appropriate materials and identify the most promising fabrication techniques. Design conceptual power controls and nanoelectronic infrastructure for selected propulsion components.

12. Investigate and quantify in intimate detail, the viscosity levels, shear rates, shear flows, and shear stress parameters that exist within the human vasculature.

13. Will different blood types and individuals exhibiting various blood-borne-disease states have an effect on whole blood viscosity, shear rates, flows, and stresses, and to what extent?

14. Determine what motive forces will be required to propel a ~1 μm diameter nanodevice through the vascular system, cognizant of the potentially substantial overdesign that may be necessary to reliably surmount maximum upstream blood flow rates.

15. Study and model projected collision profiles between a 1 μm in diameter entity and the various classes of whole blood constituents it would encounter while in vivo (e.g., red and white cells, platelets, aggregates of red cells, lipoproteins, and plasma molecules).

16. Investigate and model potential strategies for evasive maneuvers that might be implemented to reduce or avoid VCSN collisions with whole blood constituents.

17. Explore (via computer models and simulations) propulsive tactics that a nanomedical device might employ while traversing the human vasculature when displaced from the central luminal axis to still retain the capacity for accurate spatial data acquisition, and subsequent image reconstruction.

18. Investigate (via computer models and simulations) how a nanomedical device might compensate for the tendency for peripheral displacement (being pushed toward the vascular wall) brought on by the presence of much larger red and white cells in the vascular lumen.

3.7.2 Navigation System

1. Investigate whether an analog to GPS system utilizing triangulation might be scaled down to function within the confines of a "spatial metrics" room in a clinical setting.

2. Explore alternative signal emitting (e.g., near-infrared light, RF signals, directed ultrasound) beacons (analogous to the satellites used in commercial GPS configurations) that might be used in such a system to precisely locate and track singular and multiple micron-sized entities traveling within the human body.

3. Might there be differences between the effectiveness of sustained and pulsed interrogation signals when used in conjunction with in vivo nanoshells for VCSN tracking?

4. What other possibilities/strategies exist that might accomplish the goal of navigating and tracking micron-sized VCSNs within the human body?

5. Explore conceptual possibilities (e.g., via device programming, positional feedback loop) for implementing a self-centering capability for a nanomedical device to maintain central axis transit status when traversing the vascular lumen. Rapidly calculable central axis positions may play critical roles in navigation and as a reference for spatial data-based image reconstruction.

6. Investigate and model potential strategies for externally controlled evasive maneuvers that might be implemented to reduce or avoid VCSN collisions with whole blood constituents.

7. Systematically investigate, model, and catalog a comprehensive array of potential dimensional and material combinations for nanoshells (e.g., various skin thickness and core sizes) appropriate for application to nanomedical device navigation and tracking capabilities.

8. Explore how nanoshells might be embedded within and functionalized for use with a VCSN, serving as precise reference nodes for navigation and tracking.

9. Explore the possibility of hollow-core nanoshell fabrication, and set up experimentation to determine and document various signature resonances and reflectance that might be elicited from these entities by incrementally varying overall dimensions, skin thickness, and core materials.

10. Explore thermal profiles inherent to various nanoshells when exposed to particular types of activation signals.

11. Might there be any significant variances in the thermal/resonance/reflectance characteristics of nanoshells with hollow centers in response to variable interrogating signals if they were to be filled with various inert gases?

12. Explore possibilities for how C_{60} fullerenes that contain encapsulated metal atoms of various types may be utilized as tracking nodes for VCSN navigation.

13. What changes in thermal response might be elicited from a metallic nanoshell if the core were to be filled with hydrogel materials? Might thermal responses be "tuned" using this combination?

14. What navigation protocols would be activated in the event of VCSN failure, physical trapping, or other modes of incapacitation?

15. Investigate, conceptualize, and test (using a tissue-engineered benchtop vascular test bed) the safest and most effective strategies for VCSN deployment and recovery.

16. Explore how VCSNs might be rapidly activated to initiate "egress," and what strategies may be employed to guide perhaps thousands of devices to predetermined "outbody" exit locations.

17. How would optimal sites for post-scan device egress be selected? Would all devices exit at a defined location or at several locations simultaneously, contingent with where in the system they happen to be positioned when egress commands are issued?

18. Consideration will have to be given to whether egressing VCSNs may pose any risk through the possibility of becoming airborne once they have vacated the patient (e.g., through the epidermis).

19. Might it possible for airborne devices to be reinternalized by the patient and/or other individuals (e.g., medical workers) who are positioned in relative proximity to the patient through inhalation, and what propulsive/navigational protocols might be instituted in these (albeit presumably rare) cases.

20. Explore what strategy for nanodevice egress might prove to be the simplest, safest, and most effective. Perhaps, they may be directed to accumulate in locations having mucous membrane environments to minimize airborne release events. Conversely, they could be programmed to embed themselves in the biomass of the gastrointestinal tract to be naturally eliminated.

References

1. Freitas Jr., R.A., *Nanomedicine, Volume I: Basic Capabilities*, Landes Bioscience, Georgetown, TX, 1999.
2. Fung, Y.C., *Biomechanics: Mechanical Properties of Living Tissues*, 2nd edn., Springer-Verlag, New York, 1993.
3. Devlin, T.M., *Textbook of Biochemistry with Clinical Correlations*, 3rd edn., Wiley-Liss, New York, 1992.
4. Fung, Y.C., *Biodynamics: Circulation*, Springer-Verlag, New York, 1984.
5. Nunn, J.F., *Nunn's Applied Respiratory Physiology*, 4th edn., Butterworth Heinemann Ltd., London, U.K., 1993.

6. Psychogios, N., Hau, D.D., and Peng, J., The human serum metabolome. *PLoS One.* 6(2), e16957, 2011.

7. Lawrence, C.D., The Virtual Cardiac Cath Lab, 1996. http://user.sfcc.net/clawrence/vccl/cath.htm. Blood chemistry, http://user.gru.net/clawrence/vccl/chpt7/human.htm

8. Berkow, R., Beers, M.H., and Fletcher, A.J., eds., *The Merck Manual of Medical Information*, Merck Research Laboratories, Whitehouse Station, NJ, 1997.

9. Wang, T., Pan, T.W., Xing, Z.W., and Glowinski, R., Numerical simulation of rheology of red blood cell rouleaux in microchannels. *Phys Rev E Stat Nonlin Soft Matter Phys.* 79(4 Pt 1), 041916, 2009.

10. Borhan, A. and Gupta, N.R., Single-file motion of red blood cells in capillaries, p. 170, in Pozrikidis, C., ed., *Modeling and Simulation of Capsules and Biological Cells*, Chapman & Hall/CRC, Boca Raton, FL, 2003.

11. Mason, S.G. and Goldsmith, H.L., The flow behavior of particulate suspensions, in Wolstenholme, G.E.W. and Knight, J., eds., *Circulatory and Respiratory Mass Transport*, Little, Brown & Co., Boston, MA, 105–129, 1969.

12. Cokelet, G.R., Blood rheology interpreted through the flow properties of the red cell, in Grayson, J. and Zingg, W., eds., *Microcirculation*, Vol. I, Plenum Press, New York, 9–32, 1976.

13. Gaehtgens, P., In vitro studies of blood rheology in microscopic tubes, in Gross, D.R. and Hwang, N.H.C., eds., *The Rheology of Blood, Blood Vessels, and Associated Tissues*, Sijthoff & Noordhoff, Amsterdam, the Netherlands, pp. 257–275, 1981.

14. Gaehtgens, P., Flow of blood through narrow capillaries: Rheological mechanisms determining capillary hematocrit and apparent viscosity. *Biorheology.* 17(1–2), 183–189, 1980.

15. Chien, S., Biophysical behavior of red cells in suspensions, Chapter 26, in Surgenor, D. and Mac, N., eds., *The Red Blood Cell*, 2nd edn., Vol. II, Academic Press, New York, 1031–1133, 1975.

16. Vejlens, G., The distribution of leukocytes in the vascular system. *Acta Pathol Microbiol Scand.* 33, 159–190, 1938.

17. Nobis, U., Pries, A.R., and Gaehtgens, P., Rheological mechanisms contributing to WBC-margination, in Bagge, U., Born, G.V.R., and Gaehtgens, P. eds., *White Blood Cells: Morphology and Rheology as Related to Function*, Martinus Nijhoff, the Hague, pp. 57–65, 1982.

18 Goldsmith, H.L. and Spain, S., Margination of leukocytes in blood flow through small tubes. *Microvasc Res.* 27(2), 204–222, 1984.

19. Nobis, U., Pries, A.R., Cokelet, G.R., and Gaehtgens, P., Radial distribution of white cells during blood flow in small tubes. *Microvasc Res.* 29(3), 295–304, 1985.

20. Palmer, A.A., Platelet and leukocyte skimming. *Bibl Anat.* 9, 300–393, 1967.

21. Beck, M.R. and Eckstein, E.C., Preliminary reports on platelet concentration in capillary tube flows of whole blood. *Biorheology.* 17(5–6), 455–464, 1980.

22. Tangelder, G.J., Slaaf, D.W., Teirlinck, H.C., and Reneman, R.S., Distribution of blood platelets flowing in arterioles. *Am J Physiol.* 248(3 Pt 2), H318–H323, 1985.

23. Cokelet, G.R., The rheology and tube flow of blood, Chapter 14, in Richard Skalak, R. and Chien, S., eds., *Handbook of Bioengineering*, McGraw-Hill, New York, 1987.

24. Purcell, E.M., Life at low Reynolds numbers. *Am J Phys.* 45, 3–11, 1977.

25. Berg, H.C., *Random Walks in Biology*, Princeton University Press, Princeton, NJ, 1983.

26. Weiss, P., Another face of entropy. *Sci News.* 154, 108–109, 1998.

27. Dusenbery, D.B., Minimum size limit for useful locomotion by free-swimming microbes. *Proc Natl Acad Sci USA.* 94, 10949–10954, 1997.

28. Trachtenberg, S. and Gilad, R., A bacterial linear motor: Cellular and molecular organization of the contractile cytoskeleton of the helical bacterium *Spiroplasma melliferum* BC3. *Mol Microbiol.* 41(4), 827–848, 2001.

29. Trachtenberg, S., Shaping and moving a spiroplasma. *J Mol Microbiol Biotechnol.* 7(1–2), 78–87, 2004.

30. Crowl, L.M. and Fogelson, A.L., Computational model of whole blood exhibiting lateral platelet motion induced by red blood cells. *Int J Numer Method Biomed Eng.* 26(3–4), 471–487, 2010.

31. Shapere, A. and Wilczek, F., Self-propulsion at low Reynolds number. *Phys Rev Lett.* 58(20), 2051–2054, 1987.

32. Scheuer, J., Fiber microcoil optical gyroscope. *Opt Lett.* 34(11), 1630–1632, 2009.
33. Goldsmith, H.L. and Mason, S.G., The flow of suspensions through tubes. III. Collisions of small uniform spheres. *Proc R Soc A.* 282(1391), 569–591, 1964.
34. Lighthill, J., Flagellar hydrodynamics. *SIAM Rev.* 18, 161–230, 1976.
35. Higdon, J.J.L., The hydrodynamics of flagellar propulsion: Helical waves. *J Fluid Mech.* 94, 331–351, 1979.
36. Ramia, M., Tullock, D.L., and Phan-Thien, N., The role of hydrodynamic interaction in the locomotion of microorganisms. *Biophys J.* 65(2), 755–778, 1993.
37. Winet, H., Wall drag on free-moving ciliated micro-organisms. *J Exp Biol.* 59, 753–766, 1973.
38. Levin, M.D., Morton-Firth, C.J., Abouhamad, W.N., Bourret, R.B., and Bray, D., Origins of individual swimming behavior in bacteria. *Biophys J.* 74, 175–181, 1998.
39. Drescher, K., Dunkel, J., Cisneros, L.H., Ganguly, S., and Goldstein, R.E., Fluid dynamics and noise in bacterial cell-cell and cell-surface scattering. *Proc Natl Acad Sci USA.* 108(27), 10940–10945, 2011.
40. Janssen, P.J. and Graham, M.D., Coexistence of tight and loose bundled states in a model of bacterial flagellar dynamics. *Phys Rev E Stat Nonlin Soft Matter Phys.* 84(1 Pt 1), 011910, 2011.
41. Frymier, P.D., Ford, R.M., Berg, H.C., and Cummings, P.T., Three-dimensional tracking of motile bacteria near a solid planar surface. *Proc Natl Acad Sci USA.* 92(13), 6195–6199, 1995.
42. Khaderi, S.N., Baltussen, M.G., Anderson, P.D., den Toonder, J.M., and Onck, P.R., Breaking of symmetry in microfluidic propulsion driven by artificial cilia. *Phys Rev E Stat Nonlin Soft Matter Phys.* 82(2 Pt 2), 027302, 2010.
43. Hamel, A., Fisch, C., Combettes, L., Dupuis-Williams, P., and Baroud, C.N., Transitions between three swimming gaits in Paramecium escape. *Proc Natl Acad Sci USA.* 108(18), 7290–7295, 2011.
44. Osterman, N. and Vilfan, A., Finding the ciliary beating pattern with optimal efficiency. *Proc Natl Acad Sci USA.* 108(38), 15727–15732, 2011.
45. Anderson, C.M., Turski, P.A., and Edelman, R.R., Flow quantification, in Anderson, C.M., Edelman, R.R., and Turski, P.A., eds., *Clinical Magnetic Resonance Angiography*, Raven, New York, 127–128, 1993.
46. Blackshear, W.M., Phillips, D.J., Chikos, P.M., Harley, J.D., Thiele, B.L., and Strandness, D.E. Jr., Carotid artery velocity patterns in normal and stenotic vessels. *Stroke.* 11(1), 67–71, 1980.
47. Holme, P.A., Orvim, U., Hamers, M.J., Solum, N.O., Brosstad, F.R., Barstad, R.M., and Sakariassenm, K.S., Shear-induced platelet activation and platelet microparticle formation at blood flow conditions as in arteries with a severe stenosis. *Arterioscler Thromb Vasc Biol.* 17(4), 646–653, 1997.
48. Goldstein, S.F. and Charon, N.W., Motility of the spirochete *Leptospira. Cell Motil Cytoskeleton.* 9, 101–110, 1988.
49. Baker, M.A.B. and Berry, R.M., An introduction to the physics of the bacterial flagellar motor: A nanoscale rotary electric motor. *Contemp Phys.* 50(6), 617–632, 2009.
50. Paul, K., Brunstetter, D., Titen, S., and Blair, D.F., A molecular mechanism of direction switching in the flagellar motor of *Escherichia coli. Proc Natl Acad Sci USA.* 108(41), 17171–17176, 2011.
51. Naber, H., Two alternative models for spontaneous flagellar motor switching in *Halobacterium salinarium. J Theor Biol.* 181(4), 343–358, 1996.
52. Kim, M., Bird, J.C., Van Parys, A.J., Breuer, K.S., and Powers, T.R., A macroscopic scale model of bacterial flagellar bundling. *Proc Natl Acad Sci USA.* 100(26), 15481–15485, 2003.
53. Chattopadhyay, S., Moldovan, R., Yeung, C., and Wu, X.L., Swimming efficiency of bacterium *Escherichia coli. Proc Natl Acad Sci USA.* 103, 13712–13717, 2006.
54. Hanasaki, I., Yonebayashi, T., and Kawano, S., Molecular dynamics of a water jet from a carbon nanotube. *Phys Rev E Stat Nonlin Soft Matter Phys.* 79(4 Pt 2), 046307, 2009.
55. Darbandi, M. and Roohi, E., Study of subsonic–supersonic gas flow through micro/nanoscale nozzles using unstructured DSMC solver. *Microfluid Nanofluid.* 10(2), 321–335, 2011.
56. Murad, S. and Puri, I.K., Dynamics of nanoscale jet formation and impingement on flat surfaces. *Phys Fluids.* 19, 128102, 2007.
57. Aird, W.C., Spatial and temporal dynamics of the endothelium. *J Thromb Haemost.* 3(7), 1392–1406, 2005.

58. Wolinsky, H., A proposal linking clearance of circulating lipoproteins to tissue metabolic activity as a basis for understanding atherogenesis. *Circ Res.* 47, 301–311, 1980.

59. Pries, A.R., Secomb, T.W., Sperandio, M., and Gaehtgens, P., Blood flow resistance during hemodilution: Effect of plasma composition. *Cardiovasc Res.* 37(1), 225–235, 1998.

60. Copley, A.L., Adherence and viscosity of blood contacting foreign surfaces, and the plasmatic zone in blood circulation. *Nature.* 181(4608), 551–552, 1958.

61. Bulpitt, C.J., Dollery, C.T., and Kohner, E.M., The marginal plasma zone in the retinal microcirculation. *Cardiovasc Res.* 4(2), 207–212, 1970.

62. Vink, H. and Duling, B.R., Identification of distinct luminal domains for macromolecules, erythrocytes, and leukocytes within mammalian capillaries. *Circ Res.* 79(3), 581–589, 1996.

63. Pitelka, D.R. and Schooley, C.N., The fine structure of the flagellar apparatus in *Trichonympha.* *J Morphol.* 102, 199–246, 1958.

64. Bray, D., *Cell Movements*, 2nd edn., Garland Publishing, New York, 259–261, 2001.

65. Fjerdingstad, E.J., The ultrastructure of choanocyte collars in *Spongilla lacustris. Z Zellforsch.* 53, 645057, 1961.

66. von Bonsdorff, C.H. and Telkkä, A., The flagellar structure of the flame cell in fish tapeworm (*Diphyllobothrium latum*). *Z Zellforsch Mikrosk Anat.* 70(2), 169–179, 1966.

67. Wösten, M.M., van Dijk, L., Veenendaal, A.K., de Zoete, M.R., Bleumink-Pluijm, N.M., and van Putten, J.P., Temperature-dependent FlgM/FliA complex formation regulates *Campylobacter jejuni* flagella length. *Mol Microbiol.* 75(6), 1577–1591, 2010.

68. Tamm, S.L., Regeneration of ciliary comb plates in the ctenophore *Mnemiopsis leidyi. i.* morphology. *J Morphol.* 273(1), 109–120, 2012.

69. Tamm, S.L., Mechanical synchronization of ciliary beating within comb plates of ctenophores. *J Exp Biol.* 113, 401–408, 1984.

70. Vonderviszt, F. and Namba, K., Structure, function and assembly of flagellar axial proteins, in Scheibel, T., ed., *Fibrous Proteins*, Landes Bioscience, Georgetown, TX, 2008.

71. Yonekura, K., Maki-Yonekura, S., and Namba, K., Growth mechanism of the bacterial flagellar filament. *Res Microbiol.* 153, 191–197, 2002.

72. Lodish, H., Baltimore, D., Berk, A., Zipursky, S.L., Matsudaira, P., and Darnell, J., *Molecular Cell Biology*, Scientific American Books, New York, 1998.

73. Garrett, R. and Grisham, C.M., *Biochemistry*, Brooks/Cole, Boston, MA, Chapter 16, 504, 2008.

74. Magariyama, Y., Sugiyama, S., Muramoto, K., Maekawa, Y., Kawagishi, I., Imae, Y., and Kudo, S., Very fast flagellar rotation. *Nature.* 371(6500), 752, 1994.

75. Mirkovic, T., Zacharia, N.S., Scholes, G.D., and Ozin, G.A., Fuel for thought: Chemically powered nanomotors out-swim nature's flagellated bacteria. *ACS Nano.* 4(4), 1782–1789, 2010.

76. Ismagilov, R.F. Schwartz, A., Bowden, N., and Whitesides, G.M., Autonomous movement and self-assembly. *Angew Chem Int Ed.* 41, 652–654, 2002.

77. Paxton, W.F., Kistler, K.C., Olmeda, C.C., Sen, A., St. Angelo, S.K., Cao, Y., Mallouk, T.E., Lammert, P.E., and Crespi, V.H., Catalytic nanomotors: Autonomous movement of striped nanorods. *J Am Chem Soc.* 126, 13424–13431, 2004.

78. Fournier-Bidoz, S., Arsenault, A.C., Manners, I., and Ozin, G.A., Synthetic self-propelled nanomotors. *Chem Commun.* (4), 441–443, 2005.

79. Zacharia, N.S., Sadeq, Z.S., and Ozin, G.A., Enhanced speed of bimetallic nanorod motors by surface roughening. *Chem Commun.* 39, 5856–5858, 2009.

80. Laocharoensuk, R., Burdick, J., and Wang, J., CNT-induced acceleration of catalytic nanomotors. *ACS Nano.* 2, 1069–1075, 2008.

81. Demirok, U.K., Laocharoensuk, R., Manesh, K.M., and Wang, J., Ultrafast catalytic alloy nanomotors. *Angew Chem.* 47, 9349–9351, 2008.

82. Mano, N. and Heller, A., Bioelectrochemical propulsion. *J Am Chem Soc.* 127, 11574–11575, 2005.

83. Mao, F., Mano, N., and Heller, A., Long tethers binding redox centers to polymer backbones enhance electron transport in enzyme "wiring" hydrogels. *J Am Chem Soc.* 125(16), 4951–4957, 2003.

84. Mano, N., Kim, H.H., Zhang, Y., and Heller, A., An oxygen cathode operating in a physiological solution. *J Am Chem Soc.* 124(22), 6480–6486, 2002.

85. Zhang, L., Abbott, J.J., Dong, L., Peyer, K.E., Kratochvil, B.E., Zhang, H., Bergeles, C., and Nelson, B.J., Characterizing the swimming properties of artificial bacterial flagella. *Nano Lett.* 9(10), 3663–3667, 2009.

86. Ghosh, A. and Fischer, P., Controlled propulsion of artificial magnetic nanostructured propellers. *Nano Lett.* 9(6), 2243–2245, 2009.

87. Nunes, J., Herlihy, K.P., Mair, L., Superfine, R., and DeSimone, J.M., Multifunctional shape and size specific magneto-polymer composite polymers. *Nano Lett.* 10(4), 1113–1119, 2010.

88. Ozin, G.A., Manners, I., Fournier-Bidoz, S., and Arsenault, A., Dream nanomachines. *Adv Mater.* 17, 3011–3018, 2005.

89. Valadares, L.F., Tao, Y.G., Zacharia, N.S., Kitaev, V., Galembeck, F., Kapral, R., and Ozin, G.A., Catalytic nanomotors: Self-propelled sphere dimers. *Small.* 4, 565–572, 2010.

90. Solovev, A.A., Mei, Y., Urena, E.B., Huang, G., and Schmidt, O.G., Catalytic microtubular jet engines self-propelled by accumulated gas bubbles. *Small.* 5, 1688–1692, 2009.

91. Manesh, K.M., Yuan, R., Clark, M., Kagan, D., Balasubramanian, S., and Wang, J., Template-assisted fabrication of salt-independent catalytic tubular microengines. *ACS Nano.* 4, 1799–1804, 2010.

92. Schmidt, O.G. and Eberl, K., Nanotechnology. Thin solid films roll up into nanotubes. *Nature.* 410(6825), 168, 2001.

93. Sanchez, S., Solovev, A.A., Harazim, S.M., Deneke, C., Feng Mei, Y., and Schmidt, O.G., The smallest man-made jet engine. *Chem Rec.* 11(6), 367–370, 2011.

94. Sanchez, S., Ananth, A.N., Fomin, V., Viehrig, M., and Schmidt, O.G., Superfast motion of catalytic microjet engines at physiological temperature. *J Am Chem Soc.* 133(38), 14860–14863, 2011.

95. Moseler, M. and Landman, U., Formation, stability, and breakup of nanojets. *Science.* 289(5482), 1165–1170, 2000.

96. Vale, R.D. and Milligan, R.A., The way things move: Looking under the hood of molecular motor proteins. *Science.* 288(5463), 88–95, 2000.

97. Kelly, T.R., Cai, X., Damkaci, F., Panicker, S.B., Tu, B., Bushell, S.M., Cornella, I., Piggott, M.J., Salives, R., Cavero, M., Zhao, Y., and Jasmin, S., Progress toward a rationally designed, chemically powered rotary molecular motor. *J Am Chem Soc.* 129(2), 376–386, 2007.

98. Kay, E.R., Leigh, D.A., and Zerbetto, F., Synthetic molecular motors and mechanical machines. *Angew Chem Int Ed.* 46(1–2), 72–191, 2007.

99. (a) Boyer, P.D., The binding change mechanism for ATP synthase—Some probabilities and possibilities. *Biochim Biophys Acta.* 1140(3), 215–250, 1993. (b) Boyer, P.D., Energy, life, and ATP (nobel lecture). *Angew Chem Int Ed.* 37(17), 2296–2307, 1998.

100. (a) Walker, J.E., ATP synthesis by rotary catalysis. *Angew Chem Int Ed.* 37, 2308, 1998. (b) Stock, D., Leslie, A.G.W., and Walker, J.E., *Science.* 286, 1700–1705, 1999.

101. Yorimitsu, T. and Homma, M., Na(+)-driven flagellar motor of *Vibrio. Biochim Biophys Acta.* 1505(1), 82–93, 2001.

102. Balzani, V., Venturi, M., and Credi, A., *Molecular Devices and Machines—A Journey into the Nanoworld,* Wiley-VCH, Weinheim, Germany, 2003.

103. Oster, G., Wang, H., and Grabe, M., How Fo-ATPase generates rotary torque. *Phil Trans R Soc Lond B.* 2000.

104. Elston, T., Wang H., and Oster, G., Energy transduction in ATP synthase. *Nature.* 391, 510–513, 1998.

105. Wang, H. and Oster, G., Energy transduction in the F1 motor of ATP synthase. *Nature.* 396, 279–282, 1998.

106. Dimroth, P., Wang, H., Grabe M., and Oster, G., Energy transduction in the sodium F-ATPase of *Propionigenium modestum. Proc Natl Acad Sci USA.* 96, 4924–4929, 1999.

107. Oster, G. and Wang, H., ATP synthase: Two motors, two fuels. *Structure.* 7, R67–R72, 1999.

108. Oster, G. and Wang, H., Reverse engineering a protein: The mechanochemistry of ATP synthase. *Biochim Biophys Acta.* 1458, 482–510, 2000.

109. Oster, G. and Wang, H., Why is the efficiency of the F1 ATPase so high? *Bioenerg Biomembr.* 32, 459–469, 2000.

110. Berg, H.C., Torque generation by the flagellar rotary motor. *Biophys J.* 68(4 Suppl.), 163S–166S, discussion 166S–167S, 1995.
111. Muramoto, K., Kawagishi, I., Kudo, S., Magariyama, Y., Imae, Y., and Homma, M., High-speed rotation and speed stability of the sodium-driven flagellar motor in *Vibrio alginolyticus*. *J Mol Biol.* 251(1), 50–58, 1995.
112. Smirnov, A.Y., Savel'ev, S., Mourokh, L.G., and Nori, F., Proton transport and torque generation in rotary biomotors. *Phys Rev E Stat Nonlin Soft Matter Phys.* 78(3 Pt 1), 031921, 2008.
113. Soong, R.K., Bachand, G.D., Neves, H.P., Olkhovets, A.G., Craighead, H.G., and Montemagno, C.D., Powering an inorganic nanodevice with a biomolecular motor. *Science.* 5496, 1555–1558, 2000.
114. Kinosita, K. Jr., Yasuda, R., Noji, H., Ishiwata, S., and Yoshida, M., F1-ATPase: A rotary motor made of a single molecule. *Cell.* 93(1), 21–24, 1998.
115. (a) Rastogi, V.K. and Girvin, M.E., Structural changes linked to proton translocation by subunit c of the ATP synthase. *Nature.* 402(6759), 263–268, 1999. (b) Seelert, H., Poetsch, A., Dencher, N.A., Engel, A., Stahlberg, H., and Müller, D.J., Structural biology. Proton-powered turbine of a plant motor. *Nature.* 405(6785), 418–419, 2000.
116. Gust, D., Moore, T.A., and Moore, A.L., Mimicking photosynthetic solar energy transduction. *Acc Chem Res.* 34(1), 40–48, 2001.
117. Steinberg-Yfrach, G., Liddell, P.A., Hung, S.C., Moore, A.L., Gust, D., and Moore, T.A., Artificial photosynthetic reaction centers in liposomes: Photochemical generation of transmembrane proton potential. *Nature.* 385, 239–241, 1997.
118. Steinberg-Yfrach, G., Rigaud, J.L., Durantini, E.N., Moore, A.L., Gust, D., and Moore, T.A., Light-driven production at ATP catalyzed by F0F1-ATP synthase in an artificial photosynthetic membrane. *Nature.* 392, 479–482, 1998.
119. Bachand, G.D., Soong, R.K., Neeves, H.P., Olkhovets, A., Craighead, H.G., and Montemagno, C.D., Precision attachment of individual F1-ATPase biomolecular motors on nanofabricated substrates. *Nano Lett.* 1(1), 42–44, 2001.
120. Yasuda, R., Noji, H., Yoshida, M., Kinosita, K. Jr., and Itoh, H., Resolution of distinct rotational substeps by submillisecond kinetic analysis of F1-ATPase. *Nature.* 410(6831), 898–904, 2001.
121. Balzani, V.V., Credi, A., Raymo, F.M., and Stoddart, J.F., Artificial molecular machines. *Angew Chem Int Ed Engl.* 39(19), 3348–3391, 2000.
122. Koumura, N., Zijlstra, R.W.J., van Delden, R.A., Harada, N., and Feringa, B.L., Light-driven monodirectional molecular rotor. *Nature.* 401, 152–155, 1999.
123. Jian, H. and Tour, J.M., En route to surface-bound electric field-driven molecular motors. *J Org Chem.* 68(13), 5091–5103, 2003.
124. van Delden, R.A., ter Wiel, M.K., Pollard, M.M., Vicario, J., Koumura, N., and Feringa, B.L., Unidirectional molecular motor on a gold surface. *Nature.* 437(7063), 1337–1340, 2005.
125. (a) Dahl, B.J. and Branchaud, B.P., Synthesis and characterization of a functionalized chiral biaryl capable of exhibiting unidirectional bond rotation. *Tetrahedron Lett.* 45(52), 9599–9602, 2004. (b) Dahl, B.J. and Branchaud, B.P., 180 degree unidirectional bond rotation in a biaryl lactone artificial molecular motor prototype. *Org Lett.* 8(25), 5841–5844, 2006.
126. Schneider, T.D. and Lyakhov, I.G., Molecular motor. US Patent Application P20020083710, 2002.
127. Schliwa, M., ed., *Molecular Motors*, Wiley-VCH, Weinheim, Germany, 2003.
128. Astumian, R.D. and Hanggi, P., Brownian motors. *Phys Today.* 55(11), 33–39, 2002.
129. Jones, R.A.L., *Soft Machines: Nanotechnology and Life*, Oxford University Press, Oxford, U.K., 2004.
130. Leigh, D.A. and Perez, E.M., Shuttling through reversible covalent chemistry. *Chem Commun.* (20), 2262–2263, 2004.
131. Linke, H., Humphrey, T.E., Lindelof, P.E., Lofgren, A., Newbury, R., Omling, P., Sushkov, A.O., Taylor, R.P., and Xu, H., Quantum ratchets and quantum heat pumps. *Appl Phys A Mater Sci Process.* 75(2), 237–246, 2002.
132. Avron, J.E., Gat, O., and Kenneth, O., Swimming microbots: Dissipation, optimal stroke and scaling. Department of Physics, Department of Electrical Engineering, Technion, Haifa, 32000, Israel, March 25, 2004. http://physics.technion.ac.il/~avron/files/pdf/optimal-swim-12.pdf

178. Mela, P., Tas, N.R., ten Elshof, J.E., and van den Berg, A., Nanofluidics, in *Encyclopedia of Nanoscience and Nanotechnology*, American Scientific Publishers, Valencia, CA, 2004.
179. Qiao, R., and Aluru, N.R., Transient Analysis of Electroosmotic Flow in Nano-diameter Channels, p. 28–31. *Technical Proceedings of the 2002 International Conference on Modeling and Simulation of Microsystems, Nanotech 2002*, Vol. 1, Chapter 2: Micro and Nano Fluidic Systems. http://www.nsti.org/publications/MSM/2002/pdf/196.pdf (accessed July 20, 13)
180. Carr, R., Comer, J., Ginsberg, M.D., and Aksimentiev, A., Atoms-to-microns model for small solute transport through sticky nanochannels. *Lab Chip.* 11(22), 3766–3773, 2011.
181. Im, W., Seefeld, S., and Roux, B., A grand canonical Monte Carlo–Brownian dynamics algorithm for simulating ion channels. *Biophys J.* 79(2), 788–801, 2000.
182. Fayad, G.N. and Hadjiconstantinou, N.G., Realistic Brownian dynamics simulations of biological molecule separation in nanofluidic devices. *Microfluid Nanofluid.* 8, 521–529, 2010.
183. Li, Y., Xu, J., and Li, D., Molecular dynamics simulation of nanoscale liquid flows. *Microfluid Nanofluid.* 9, 1011–1031, 2010.
184. Ermak, D.L. and McCammon, J.A., Brownian dynamics with hydrodynamic interactions. *J Chem Phys.* 69(4), 1352–1360, 1978.
185. Liu, Y., Liu, M., Lau, W.M., and Yang, J., Ion size and image effect on electrokinetic flows. *Langmuir.* 24(6), 2884–2891, 2008.
186. Reyes, Y., Paulis, M., and Leiza, J.R., Modeling the equilibrium morphology of nanodroplets in the presence of nanofillers. *J Colloid Interface Sci.* 352(2), 359–365, 2010.
187. Tuzun, R.E., Noid, D.W., Sumpter, B.G., and Merkle, R.C., Dynamics of fluid flow inside carbon nanotubes. *Nanotechnology.* 7, 241–246, 1996.
188. Tuzun, R.E., Noid, D.W., Sumpter, B.G., and Merkle, R.C., Dynamics of He/C_{60} flow inside carbon nanotubes. *Nanotechnology.* 8,112–118, 1997.
189. Gelb, L.D. and Hopkins, A.C., Dynamics of the capillary rise in nanocylinders. *Nano Lett.* 2, 1281–1285, 2002.
190. Sokhan, V.P., Nicholson, D., and Quirke, N.J., Fluid flow in nanopores: Accurate boundary conditions for carbon nanotubes. *J Chem Phys.* 117, 8531–8539, 2002.
191. De Groot, B.L. and Grubmüller, H., Water permeation across biological membranes: Mechanism and dynamics of aquaporin-1 and GlpF. *Science.* 294, 2353–2357, 2001.
192. Hummer, G., Rasaiah, J.C., and Noworyta, J.P., Water conduction through the hydrophobic channel of a carbon nanotube. *Nature.* 414, 188–190, 2001.
193. Siwy, Z. and Fulinski, A., Fabrication of a synthetic nanopore ion pump. *Phys Rev Lett.* 89, 198103, 2002.
194. Gao, Y. and Bando, Y., Carbon nanothermometer containing gallium—Gallium's macroscopic properties are retained on a miniature scale in this nanodevice. *Nature.* 415, 599, 2002.
195. Dujardin, E., Ebbesen, T.W., Hiura, H., and Tanigaki, H.K., Capillarity and wetting of carbon nanotubes. *Science.* 265, 1850–1852, 1994.
196. Sun, L. and Crooks, R.M., Single carbon nanotube membranes: A well-defined model for studying mass transport through nanoporous materials. *J Am Chem Soc.* 122, 12340–12345, 2000.
197. Kim, W.S., Lee, J., and Ruoff, R.S., Nanofluidic channel fabrication and characterization by micromachining, in *Proceedings of IMECE'03 2003 ASME International Mechanical Engineering Congress*, Washington, DC, Paper no. IMECE2003-41588, pp. 841–846, November 15–21, 2003.
198. Nakamura, M., Sato, N., Hoshi, N., and Sakata, O., Outer Helmholtz plane of the electrical double layer formed at the solid electrode–liquid interface. *Chemphyschem.* 12(8), 1430–1434, 2011.
199. Etchenique, R. and Buhse, T., Viscoelasticity in the diffuse electric double layer. *Analyst.* 127(10), 1347–1352, 2002.
200. Giupponi, G. and Pagonabarraga, I., Determination of the zeta potential for highly charged colloidal suspensions. *Philos Transact A Math Phys Eng Sci.* 369(1945), 2546–2554, 2011.
201. Kozono, D., Yasui, M., King, L.S., and Agre, P., Aquaporin water channels: Atomic structure molecular dynamics meet clinical medicine. *J Clin Invest.* 109(11), 1395–1399, 2002.

202. Zeidel, M.L., Ambudkar, S.V., Smith, B.L., and Agre, P., Reconstitution of functional water channels in liposomes containing purified red cell CHIP28 protein. *Biochemistry*. 31, 7436–7440, 1992.
203. Iwamoto, M. and Oiki, S., Counting ion and water molecules in a streaming file through the open-filter structure of the K channel. *J Neurosci*. 31(34), 12180–12188, 2011.
204. Krane, C.M. and Kishor, B.K., Aquaporins: The membrane water channels of the biological world. *Biologist*. 50(2), 81–86, 2003.
205. Morais-Cabral, J.H., Zhou, Y., and MacKinnon, R., Energetic optimization of ion conduction rate by the K+ selectivity filter. *Nature*. 414, 37–42, 2001.
206. Preston, G.M., Carroll, T.P., Guggino, W.B., and Agre, P., Appearance of water channels in *Xenopus* oocytes expressing red cell CHIP28 protein. *Science*. 256, 385–387, 1992.
207. Ibata, K., Takimoto, S., Morisaku, T., Miyawaki, A., and Yasui, M., Analysis of aquaporin-mediated diffusional water permeability by coherent anti-stokes Raman scattering microscopy. *Biophys J*. 101(9), 2277–2283, 2011.
208. Agre, P., Aquaporin water channels (nobel lecture). *Angew Chem Int Ed*. 43, 4278–4290, 2004.
209. Ensikat, H.J., Ditsche-Kuru, P., Neinhuis, C., Barthlott, W., and Beilstein, J., Superhydrophobicity in perfection: The outstanding properties of the lotus leaf. *Nanotechnology*. 2, 152–161, 2011.
210. Bhushan, B., Jung, C.J., and Nosonovsky, M., Lotus Effect: Surfaces with roughness-induced superhydrophobicity, self-cleaning, and low adhesion, in Bhushan, B., ed., *Handbook of Nanotechnology*, 3rd edn., Springer, New York, pp. 1437–1524, 2010.
211. Wagner, P., Fürstner, R., Barthlott, W., and Neinhuis, C., Quantitative assessment to the structural basis of water repellency in natural and technical surfaces. *J Exp Bot*. 54(385), 1295–1303, 2003.
212. Neinhuis, C. and Barthlott, W., Characterization and distribution of water-repellent, self-cleaning plant surfaces. *Ann Bot*. 79, 667–677, 1997.
213. Ensikat, H.J., Boese, M., Mader, W., Barthlott, W., and Koch, K., Crystallinity of plant epicuticular waxes: Electron and X-ray diffraction studies. *Chem Phys Lipids*. 144(1), 45–59, 2006.
214. Parker, A.R. and Lawrence, C.R., Water capture by a desert beetle. *Nature*. 414(6859), 33–34, 2001.
215. Chen, Q., Meng, L., Li, Q., Wang, D., Guo, W., Shuai, Z., and Jiang, L., Water transport and purification in nanochannels controlled by asymmetric wettability. *Small*. 7(15), 2225–2231, 2011.
216. Zuo, G., Shen, R., Ma, S., and Guo, W., Transport properties of single-file water molecules inside a carbon nanotube biomimicking water channel. *ACS Nano*. 4(1), 205–210, 2010.
217. Joseph, S., Mashl, R.J., Jakobsson, E., and Aluru, N.R., Electrolytic transport in modified carbon nanotubes. *Nano Lett*. 3, 1399–1403, 2003.
218. Striolo, A., Water self-diffusion through narrow oxygenated carbon nanotubes. *Nanotechnology*. 18, 475704, 2007.
219. Wan, R.Z., Li, J.Y., Lu, H.J., and Fang, H.P., Controllable water channel gating of nanometer dimensions. *J Am Chem Soc*. 127, 7166–7170, 2005.
220. Majumder, M., Chopra, N., Andrews, R., and Hinds, B.J., Nanoscale hydrodynamics: Enhanced flow in carbon nanotubes. *Nature*. 438, 44, 2005.
221. Leung, K. and Rempe, S.B., Ion rejection by nanoporous membranes in pressure-driven molecular dynamics simulations. *J Comput Theor Nanosci*. 6(8), 1948–1955, 2009.
222. Zheng, Y.G., Ye, H.F., Zhang, Z.Q., and Zhang, H.W., Water diffusion inside carbon nanotubes: Mutual effects of surface and confinement. *Phys Chem Chem Phys*. 14(2), 964–967, 2012.
223. Li, J.Y., Gong, X.J., Lu, H.J., Li, D., Fang, H.P., and Zhou, R.H., Electrostatic gating of a nanometer water channel. *Proc Natl Acad Sci USA*. 104, 3687–3692, 2007.
224. Meng, X.W., Wang, Y., Zhao, Y.J., and Huang, J.P., Gating of a water nanochannel driven by dipolar molecules. *J Phys Chem B*. 115(16), 4768–4773, 2011.
225. Ahn, S., Choi, J., Kim, E., Dong, K.Y., Jeon, H., Ju, B.K., and Lee, K.B., Combined laser interference and photolithography patterning of a hybrid mask mold for nanoimprint lithography. *J Nanosci Nanotechnol*. 11(7), 6039–6043, 2011.
226. Harms, Z.D., Mogensen, K.B., Nunes, P.S., Zhou, K., Hildenbrand, B.W., Mitra, I., Tan, Z., Zlotnick, A., Kutter, J.P., and Jacobson, S.C., Nanofluidic devices with two pores in series for resistive-pulse sensing of single virus capsids. *Anal Chem*. 83(24), 9573–9578, 2011.

227. Alam, J. and Bowman, J.C., Energy-conserving simulation of incompressible electro-osmotic and pressure-driven flow. *Theoret Comput Fluid Dyn.* 16, 133–150, 2002.
228. Wheeler, A.R., Moon, H., Kim, C.J., Loo, J.A., and Garrell, R.L., Electrowetting-based microfluidics for analysis of peptides and proteins by matrix-assisted laser desorption/ionization mass spectrometry. *Anal Chem.* 76(16), 4833–4838, 2004.
229. Lin, Y.Y., Evans, R.D., Welch, E., Hsu, B.N., Madison, A.C., and Fair, R.B., Low voltage electrowetting-on-dielectric platform using multi-layer insulators. *Sens Actuat B Chem.* 150(1), 465–470, 2010.
230. Rayleigh–Bénard and Bénard–Marangoni convection, The Experimental Nonlinear Physics Group, Department of Physics, University of Toronto, Toronto, Ontario, Canada, 2004. http://www.physics.utoronto.ca/nonlinear/thermal.html
231. Zeng, Z., Mizuseki, H., Higashino, K., and Kawazoe, Y., Direct numerical simulation of oscillatory Marangoni convection in cylindrical liquid bridges. *J Cryst Growth.* 204, 395–404, 1999.
232. Zeng, Z., Mizuseki, H., Ichinoseki, K., Higashino, K., and Kawazoe, Y., Marangoni convection in half-zone liquid bridge. *Mater Trans JIM.* 40, 1331–1336, 1999.
233. Aa, Y., Cao, Z.H., Tang, Z.M., Sun, Z.W., and Hu, W.R., Experimental study on the transition process to the oscillatory thermocapillary convections in a floating half zone. *Microgravity Sci Technol.* 17(4), 5–13, 2005,
234. Shevtsova, V.M., Melnikov, D.E., and Legros, J.C., Multistability of oscillatory thermocapillary convection in a liquid bridge. *Phys Rev E Stat Nonlin Soft Matter Phys.* 68(6 Pt 2), 066311, 2003.
235. Maksimović, A., Lugomer, S., Geretovszky, Zs., and Szörényi, T., Laser-induced convection nanostructures on SiON/Si interface. *J Appl Phys.* 104, 124905, 2008.
236. Balsubramanian, S., Kagan, D., Manesh, K.M., Calvo-Marzal, P., Flechsig, G.U., and Wang, J., Thermal modulation of nanomotor movement. *Small.* 13, 1569–1574, 2009.
237. Carrillo, J.M.Y., Jeon, J.H., and Dobrynin, A.V., A model of polymeric nanopropulsion engine. *Macromolecules.* 40(14), 5171–5175, 2007.
238. Postnikov, A.V., Kortus, J., and Pederson, M.R., Density functional studies of molecular magnets, Institute of Metal Physics, Russian Academy of Sciences, Moscow, Russia, 2003. http://psi-k.dl.ac.uk/newsletters/News_61/Highlight_61.pdf
239. van Slageren, J., Introduction to molecular magnetism, Universität Stuttgart, Germany, 2004. http://www.pi1.physik.uni-stuttgart.de/Praesentationen/Daten/123/123.pdf
240. Petrich, W., Anderson, M.H., Ensher, J.R., and Cornell, E.A., Stable, tightly confining magnetic trap for evaporative cooling of neutral cooling. *Phys Rev Lett.* 74, 3352, 1995.
241. Sacconi, L., Romano, G., Ballerini, R., Capitanio, M., De Pas, M., Giuntini, M., Dunlap, D., Finzi, L., and Pavone, F.S., Three-dimensional magneto-optic trap for micro-object manipulation. *Optics Lett.* 26(17), 1359–1361, 2001.
242. Hickey, B.J., Marrows, C.H., Greig, D., and Morgan, G.J., Giant magnetoresistance, condensed matter research, magnetism and superconductivity, University of Leeds, England, U.K., 2004. http://www.stoner.leeds.ac.uk/research/gmr.htm
243. Chen, Z. and Doi, Y., Numerical study on propulsion by undulating motion in laminar-turbulent flow, in *24th Symposium on Naval Hydrodynamics*, Fukuoka, Japan, July 8–13, 2002.
244. Carpi, F., Kornbluh, R., Sommer-Larsen, P., and Alici, G., Electroactive polymer actuators as artificial muscles: Are they ready for bioinspired applications? *Bioinspir Biomim.* 6(4), 045006, 2011.
245. Otero, T.F., Reactive conducting polymers as actuating sensors and tactile muscles. *Bioinspir Biomim.* 3(3), 035004, 2008.
246. Yun, J.S., Yang, K.S., Choi, N.J., Lee, H.K., Moon, S.E., and Kim do, H., Microvalves based on ionic polymer-metal composites for microfluidic application. *J Nanosci Nanotechnol.* 11(7), 5975–5979, 2011.
247. Baughman, R.H., Conducting polymer artificial muscles. *Synth Metals.* 78(3), 339–353, 1996.
248. Li. J., Ma, W., Song, L., Niu, Z., Cai, L., Zeng, Q., Zhang, X., Dong, H., Zhao, D., Zhou, W., and Xie, S., Superfast-response and ultrahigh-power-density electromechanical actuators based on hierarchal carbon nanotube electrodes and chitosan. *Nano Lett.* 11(11), 4636–4641, 2011.

249. Brock, D., Lee, W., Segalman, D., and Witkowski, W., A dynamic model of a linear actuator based on polymer hydrogel. *J Intell Mater Syst Struct*. 5(6), 764–771, 1994.
250. Osada, Y. and Gong, J., Stimuli-responsive polymer gels and their application to chemomechanical systems. *Prog Polym Sci*. 18(2), 187–226, 1993.
251. Okuzaki, H. and Osada, Y., Electro-driven chemomechanical polymer gel as an intelligent soft material. *J Biomater Sci Polym Ed*. 5(5), 485–496, 1994.
252. Osada, Y. and Gong, J.P., Soft and wet materials: Polymer gels. *Adv Mater*. 10(11), 827–837, 1998.
253. Otero, T.F. and Sansieña, J.M., Soft and wet conducting polymers for artificial muscles. *Adv Mater*. 10(6), 491–494, 1998.
254. Kappel, M., Abel, M., and Gerhard, R., Characterization and calibration of piezoelectric polymers: In situ measurements of body vibrations. *Rev Sci Instrum*. 82(7), 075110, 2011.
255. Cianchetti, M., Mattoli, V., Mazzolai, B., Laschi, C., and Dario, P., A new design methodology of electrostrictive actuators for bioinspired robotics. *Sens Actuat Pt B*. 142(1), 288–297, 2009.
256. Brochu, P. and Pei, Q., Advances in dielectric elastomers for actuators and artificial muscles. *Macromol Rapid Commun*. 31(1), 10–36, 2010.
257. Na, Y.H., Aburaya, Y., Orihara, H., and Hiraoka, K., Measurement of electrically induced shear strain in a chiral smectic liquid-crystal elastomer. *Phys Rev E Stat Nonlin Soft Matter Phys*. 83(6 Pt 1), 061709, 2011.
258. Aliev, A.E., Oh, J., Kozlov, M.E., Kuznetsov, A.A., Fang, S., Fonseca, A.F., Ovalle, R., Lima, M.D., Haque, M.H., Gartstein, Y.N., Zhang, M., Zakhidov, A.A., and Baughman, R.H., Giant-stroke, superelastic carbon nanotube aerogel muscles. *Science*. 323(5921), 1575–1578, 2009.
259. Zhang, Q.M., Bharti, V.V., and Zhao, X., Giant electrostriction and relaxor ferroelectric behavior in electron-irradiated poly(vinylidene fluoride–trifluoroethylene) copolymer. *Science*. 280(5372), 2101–2104, 1998.
260. Cheng, Z.Y., Bharti, V., Xu, T.B., Xu, H., Mai, T., and Zhang, Q.M., Electrostrictive poly(vinylidene fluoride-trifluoroethylene) copolymers. *Sens Actuat A Phys*. 90(1–2), 138–147, 2001.
261. Zhang, Q.M., Li, H., Poh, M., Xia, F., Cheng, Z.Y., Xu, H., and Huang, C., An all-organic composite actuator material with a high dielectric constant. *Nature*. 419(6904), 284–287, 2002.
262. Kornbluh, R. and Pelrine, R., Chapter 4 - High-performance acrylic and silicone elastomers, p. 33–42, in Carpi, F., DeRossi, D., Kornbluh, R., Pelrine, R., and Sommer - Larsen, P., eds., *Dielectric Elastomers as Electromechanical Transducers*, Elsevier, Amsterdam, 2008.
263. Kornbluh, R., Wong-Foy, A., Pelrine, R., Prahlad, H., and McCoy, B., Long-lifetime all-polymer artificial muscle transducers. *MRS Proc*. 1271-JJ03-01, 2010.
264. Senders, C.W., Tollefson, T.T., Curtiss, S., Wong-Foy, A., and Prahlad, H., Force requirements for artificial muscle to create an eyelid blink with eyelid sling. *Arch Facial Plast Surg*. 12, 30–36, 2010.
265. Freitas, R.A. Jr., Nanodentistry. *J Am Dent Assoc*. 131(11), 1559–1565, 2000.
266. Schleyer, T.L., Nanodentistry. Fact or fiction? *J Am Dent Assoc*. 131(11), 1567–1568, 2000.
267. Sharma, S., Cross, S.E., Hsueh, C., Wali, R.P., Stieg, A.Z., and Gimzewski, J.K., Nanocharacterization in dentistry. *Int J Mol Sci*. 11(6), 2523–2545, 2010.
268. Kanaparthy, R. and Kanaparthy, A., The changing face of dentistry: Nanotechnology. *Int J Nanomed*. 6(2), 799–804, 2011.
269. Llinas, P., Pylypenko, O., Isabet, T., Mukherjea, M., Sweeney, H.L., and Houdusse, A.M., How myosin motors power cellular functions: An exciting journey from structure to function. *FEBS J*. 279(4), 551–562, 2011.
270. Odronitz, F. and Kollmar, M., Drawing the tree of eukaryotic life based on the analysis of 2,269 manually annotated myosins from 328 species. *Genome Biol*. 8, R196, 2007.
271. (No authors listed), Fifty important papers in the history of muscle contraction and myosin motility. *J Muscle Res Cell Motil*. 25, 483–487, 2004.
272. De La Cruz, E.M. and Ostap, E.M., Relating biochemistry and function in the myosin superfamily. *Curr Opin Cell Biol*. 16, 61–67, 2004.
273. Junqueira, L.C., Carneiro, J., and Kelley, R.O., *Basic Histology*, 9th edn., McGraw-Hill, New York, 1998.

274. Geeves, M.A. and Holmes, K.C., Structural mechanism of muscle contraction. *Ann Rev Biochem.* 68, 687–728, 1999.

275. Bagshaw, C.R. and Trentham, D.R., The characterization of myosin-product complexes and of product-release steps during the magnesium ion dependent adenosine triphosphatase reaction. *Biochem J.* 141, 331–349, 1974.

276. Geeves, M.A. and Conibear, P.B., The role of three-state docking of myosin S1 with actin in force generation. *Biophys J.* 68, 194S–199S, 1995.

277. Furch, M., Geeves, M.A., and Manstein, D.J., Modulation of actin affinity and actomyosin adenosine triphosphatase by charge changes in the myosin motor domain. *Biochemistry.* 37, 6317–6326, 1998.

278. Hammer, J.A. 3rd and Sellers, J.R., Walking to work: Roles for class V myosins as cargo transporters. *Nat Rev Mol Cell Biol.* 13(1), 13–26, 2011.

279. Wong, D.Y. and Sept, D., The interaction of cofilin with the actin filament. *J Mol Biol.* 413(1), 97–105, 2011.

280. Sitar, T., Gallinger, J., Ducka, A.M., Ikonen, T.P., Wohlhoefler, M., Schmoller, K.M., Bausch, A.R., Joel, P., Trybus, K.M., Noegel, A.A., Schleicher, M., Huber, R., and Holak, T.A., Molecular architecture of the Spire-actin nucleus and its implication for actin filament assembly. *Proc Natl Acad Sci USA.* 108(49), 19575–19580, 2011.

281. de Lanerolle, P. and Serebryannyy, L., Nuclear actin and myosins: Life without filaments. *Nat Cell Biol.* 13(11), 1282–1288, 2011.

282. Higuchi, H. and Goldman, Y.E., Sliding distance per ATP molecule hydrolysed during isotonic shortening of skinned muscle fibres. *Biophys J.* 69, 1491–1507, 1995.

283. Elliott, G.F. and Worthington, C.R., Along the road not taken: How many myosin heads act on a single actin filament at any instant in working muscle? *Prog Biophys Mol Biol.* 108(1–2), 82–92, 2012.

284. Worthington, C.R. and Elliott, G.F., Muscle-contraction: The step-size distance and the impulse-time per ATP. *Int J Biol Macromol.* 18, 123–131, 1996.

285. Hill, A.V., The heat of shortening and the dynamic constants of muscle. *Proc R Soc B.* 126, 136–195, 1938.

286. Hill, A.V., The effect of load on the heat of shortening of a muscle. *Proc R Soc B.* 159, 297–324, 1964.

287. He, Z.H., Chillingworth, R.K., Brune, M., Corrie, J.E., Trentham, D.R., Webb, M.R., and Ferenczi, M.A., ATPase kinetics on activation of rabbit and frog permeabilized isometric muscle fibres: A real time phosphate assay. *J Physiol.* 501(Pt 1), 125–148, 1997.

288. Symes, M.D., Walking molecules, PhD thesis, School of Chemistry, University of Edinburgh, Edinburgh, April 2009. http://www.era.lib.ed.ac.uk/bitstream/1842/3195/1/MD%20Symes%20PhD%20thesis%2009.pdf

289. Astumian, R.D., Biasing the random walk of a molecular motor. *J Phys Condens Matter.* 17(47), S3753–S3766, 2005.

290. Woehlke, G. and Schliwa, M., Walking on two heads: The many talents of kinesin. *Nat Rev Mol Cell Biol.* 1(1), 50–58, 2000.

291. Yildiz, A. and Selvin, P.R., Kinesin: Walking, crawling or sliding along? *Trends Cell Biol.* 15(2), 112–120, 2005.

292. Vale, R.D., The molecular motor toolbox for intracellular transport. *Cell.* 112(4), 467–480, 2003.

293. Hackney, D., Evidence for alternating head catalysis by kinesin during microtubule-stimulated ATP hydrolysis. *Proc Natl Acad Sci USA.* 91, 6865–6869, 1994.

294. Ma, Y.Z. and Taylor, E.W., Interacting head mechanism of microtubule-kinesin ATPase. *J Biol Chem.* 272, 724–730, 1997.

295. Gilbert, S.P., Moyer, M.L., and Johnson, K.A., Alternating site mechanism of the kinesin ATPase. *Biochemistry.* 37, 792–799, 1998.

296. Kaseda, K., Higuchi, H., and Hirose, K., Alternate fast and slow stepping of a heterodimeric kinesin molecule. *Nat Cell Biol.* 5(12), 1079–1082, 2003.

297. Yildiz, A. and Selvin, P.R., Fluorescence imaging with one nanometer accuracy (FIONA): Application to molecular motors. *Acc Chem Res.* 38, 572, 2005.

298. Schliwa, M. and Woehlke, G. Molecular motors. *Nature.* 422(6933), 759–765, 2003.

299. Koonce, M.P. and Tikhonenko, I., Functional elements within the dynein microtubule-binding domain. *Mol Biol Cell.* 11, 5230–5529, 2000.

300. Carter, A.P., Cho, C., Jin, L., and Vale, R.D., Crystal structure of the dynein motor domain. *Science.* 331(6021), 1159–1165, 2011.

301. Burgess, S.A., Walker, M.L., Sakakibara, H., Knight, P.J., and Oiwa, K., Dynein structure and power stroke. *Nature.* 421, 715–718, 2003.

302. Howard, J., *Mechanics of Motor Proteins and the Cytoskeleton,* Sinauer, Sunderland, MA, 2001.

303. Dewitt, M.A., Chang, A.Y., Combs, P.A., and Yildiz, A., Cytoplasmic dynein moves through uncoordinated stepping of the AAA+ ring domains. *Science.* 335, 221–225, 2012.

304. Ji, X.Y. and Feng, X.Q., Mechanochemical modeling of dynamic microtubule growth involving sheet-to-tube transition. *PLoS One.* 6(12), e29049, 2011.

305. Brown, R., A Brief Account of Microscopical Observations - On the Particles Contained in the Pollen of Plants and On the General Existence of Active Molecules, p. 463–486, in Bennett, J.J., ed., The Miscellaneous Botanical Works of Robert Brown, Ray Society, London, 1866.

306. Einstein, A., Die von der Molekularkinetischen Theorie der Wärme Gefordete Bewegung von in ruhenden Flüssigkeiten Suspendierten Teilchen (The molecular kinetic theory of heat required by the movement of suspended particles in stationary liquids). *Ann Phys.* 17, 549–560, 1905.

307. Ye, H., Zhang, H., Zhang, Z., and Zheng, Y., Size and temperature effects on the viscosity of water inside carbon nanotubes. *Nanoscale Res Lett.* 6(1), 87, 2011.

308. Reimann, P. and Hanggi, P., Introduction to the physics of Brownian motors. *Appl Phys A.* 75, 169–178, 2002.

309. Nasiri, M., Moradian, A., and Miri, M., Dynamics of noncontact rack-and-pinion device: Periodic back-and-forth motion of the rack. *Phys Rev E Stat Nonlin Soft Matter Phys.* 82(3 Pt 2), 037101, 2010.

310. Hess, H. and Dumont, E.L., Fatigue failure and molecular machine design. *Small.* 7(12), 1619–1623, 2011.

311. Wang, J. and Manesh, K.M., Motion control at the nanoscale. *Small.* 6(3), 338–345, 2010.

312. Mirkovic, T., Zacharia, N.S., Scholes, G.D., and Ozin, G.A., Nanolocomotion—Catalytic nano-motors and nanorotors. *Small.* 6(2), 159–167, 2010.

313. Kwon, K.Y., Wong, K.L., Pawin, G., Bartels, L., Stolbov, S., and Rahman, T.S., Unidirectional adsorbate motion on a high-symmetry surface: "Walking" molecules can stay the course. *Phys Rev Lett.* 95(16), 166101, 2005.

314. Wong, K.L., Pawin, G., Kwon, K.Y., Lin, X., Jiao, T., Solanki, U., Fawcett, R.H., Bartels, L., Stolbov, S., and Rahman, T.S., A molecule carrier. *Science.* 315(5817), 1391–1393, 2007.

315. Saffarian, S., Collier, I.E., Marmer, B.L., Elson, E.L., and Goldberg, G., Interstitial collagenase is a Brownian ratchet driven by proteolysis of collagen. *Science.* 306(5693), 108–111, 2004.

316. Yurke, B., Turberfield, A.J., Mills, A.P. Jr., Simmel, F.C., and Neumann, J.L., A DNA-fuelled molecular machine made of DNA. *Nature.* 406(6796), 605–608, 2000.

317. Yan, H., Zhang, X., Shen, Z., and Seeman, N.C., A robust DNA mechanical device controlled by hybridization topology. *Nature.* 415(6867), 62–65, 2002.

318. Sherman, W.B. and Seeman, N.C., A precisely controlled DNA biped walking device. *Nano Lett.* 4(7), 1203–1207, 2004.

319. Omabegho, T., Sha, R., and Seeman, N.C., A bipedal DNA Brownian motor with coordinated legs. *Science.* 324(5923), 67–71, 2009.

320. Mai, J., Sokolov, I.M., and Blumen, A., Directed particle diffusion under "burnt bridges" conditions. *Phys Rev E Stat Nonlin Soft Matter Phys.* 64(1 Pt 1), 011102, 2001.

321. Shin, J.S. and Pierce, N.A., A synthetic DNA walker for molecular transport. *J Am Chem Soc.* 126(35), 10834–10835, 2004.

322. Pomerantz, R.T., Anikin, M., Zlatanova, J., and McAllister, W.T., RNA polymerase as an information-dependant molecular motor, in *11th Foresight Conference on Molecular Nanotechnology,* Palo Alto, CA, October 9–12, 2003.

323. Kashlev, M., Martin, E., Polyakov, A., Severinov, K., Nikiforov, V., and Goldfarb, A., Histidine-tagged RNA polymerase: Dissection of the transcription cycle using immobilized enzyme. *Gene.* 130(1), 9–14, 1993.

324. Quirynen, M., Management of oral malodour. *J Clin Periodontol.* 30(Suppl. 5), 17–18, 2003.

325. Pei, R., Taylor, S.K., Stefanovic, D., Rudchenko, S., Mitchell, T.E., and Stojanovic, M.N., Behavior of polycatalytic assemblies in a substrate-displaying matrix. *J Am Chem Soc.* 128(39), 12693–12699, 2006.

326. Lund, K., Manzo, A.J., Dabby, N., Michelotti, N., Johnson-Buck, A., Nangreave, J., Taylor, S., Pei, R., Stojanovic, M.N., Walter, N.G., Winfree, E., and Yan, H., Molecular robots guided by prescriptive landscapes. *Nature.* 465(7295), 206–210, 2010.

327. Turing, A.M., On computable numbers, with an application to the Entscheidungs problem. *Proc London Math Soc Series.* 2, 230–265, 1936.

328. Bonabeau, E., Dorigo, M., and Theraulaz, G., *Swarm Intelligence: From Natural to Artificial Systems.* Oxford University Press, New York, 1999.

329. Rus, D., Butler, Z., Kotay, K., and Vona, M., Self-reconfiguring robots. *Commun ACM.* 45, 3945, 2002.

330. Von Neumann, J., in Burks, A.W., ed., *Theory of Self-Reproducing Automata*, University of Illinois Press, Urbana, IL, 1966.

331. Bennett, C.H., The thermodynamics of computation—A review. *Int J Theor Phys.* 21, 905–940, 1982.

332. Samii, L., Blab, G.A., Bromley, E.H., Linke, H., Curmi, P.M., Zuckermann, M.J., and Forde, N.R., Time-dependent motor properties of multipedal molecular spiders. *Phys Rev E Stat Nonlin Soft Matter Phys.* 84(3–1), 031111, 2011.

333. Bromley, E.H., Kuwada, N.J., Zuckermann, M.J., Donadini, R., Samii, L., Blab, G.A., Gemmen, G.J., Lopez, B.J., Curmi, P.M., Forde, N.R., Woolfson, D.N., and Linke, H., The tumbleweed: Towards a synthetic protein motor. *HFSP J.* 3(3), 204–212, 2009.

334. Proctor, L.M., The Human Microbiome Project in 2011 and beyond. *Cell Host Microbe.* 10(4), 287–291, 2011.

335. Erdem, E.Y., Yu-Ming Chen, Mohebbi, M., Suh, J.W., Kovacs, G., Darling, R.B., and Böhringer, K.F., Thermally actuated omnidirectional walking microrobot. *J Microelectromech Syst.* 19(3), 433, 2010.

336. Friedl, P. and Bröcker, E.B., TCR triggering on the move: Diversity of T-cell interactions with antigen-presenting cells. *Immunol Rev.* 186, 83–89, 2002.

337. Friedl, P., Borgmann, S., and Brocker, E.B., Leukocyte crawling through extracellular matrix and the *Dictyostelium* paradigm of movement—Lessons from a social amoeba. *J Leukoc Biol.* 70, 491–509, 2001.

338. Friedl, P., Entschladen, F., Conrad, C., Niggemann, B., and Zanker, K.S., CD4+ T lymphocytes migrating in three-dimensional collagen lattices lack focal adhesions and utilize β1 integrin-independent strategies for polarization, interaction with collagen fibers and locomotion. *Eur J Immunol.* 28, 2331–2343, 1998.

339. Yi, J., Schmidt, J., Chien, A., Montemagno, C.D., Engineering an artificial amoeba propelled by nanoparticle-triggered actin polymerization. *Nanotechnology.* 20(8), 085101, 2009.

340. Mogilner, A. and Edelstein-Keshet, L., Regulation of actin dynamics in rapidly moving cells: A quantitative analysis. *Biophys J.* 83(3), 1237–1258, 2002.

341. Wallimann, T. and Hemmer, W., Creatine kinase in non-muscle tissues and cells. *Mol Cell Biochem.* 133–134, 193–220, 1994.

342. Doshi, N. and Mitragotri, S., Needle-shaped polymeric particles induce transient disruption of cell membranes. *J R Soc Interface.* 7(Suppl. 4), S403–S410, 2010.

343. Kim, J., Lew, B., and Kim, W.S., Facile fabrication of super-hydrophobic nano-needle arrays via breath figures method. *Nanoscale Res Lett.* 6(1), 616, 2011.

344. Hesselberg, T., Biomimetics and the case of the remarkable ragworms. *Naturwissenschaften.* 94(8), 613–621, 2007.

345. von Delius, M. and Leigh, D.A., Walking molecules. *Chem Soc Rev.* 40(7), 3656–3676, 2011.

346. Hirokawa, N., Nitta, R., and Okada, Y., The mechanisms of kinesin motor motility: Lessons from the monomeric motor KIF1A. *Nat Rev Mol Cell Biol.* 10(12), 877–884, 2009.

347. Gravish, N., Wilkinson, M., Sponberg, S., Parness, A., Esparza, N., Soto, D., Yamaguchi, T., Broide, M., Cutkosky, M., Creton, C., and Autumn, K., Rate-dependent frictional adhesion in natural and synthetic gecko setae. *J R Soc Interface.* 7(43), 259–269, 2010.

348. Autumn, K., Sitti, M., Liang, Y.A., Peattie, A.M., Hansen, W.R., Sponberg, S., Kenny, T.W., Fearing, R., Israelachvili, J.N., and Full, R.J., Evidence for van der Waals adhesion in gecko setae. *Proc Natl Acad Sci USA.* 99(19), 12252–12256, 2002.

349. Hansen, W.R. and Autumn, K., Evidence for self-cleaning in gecko setae. *Proc Natl Acad Sci USA.* 102(2), 385–389, 2005.

350. Puthoff, J.B., Prowse, M.S., Wilkinson, M., and Autumn, K., Changes in materials properties explain the effects of humidity on gecko adhesion. *J Exp Biol.* 213(Pt 21), 3699–3704, 2010.

351. Autumn, K., Liang, Y.A., Hsieh, S.T., Zesch, W., Chan, W.-P., Kenny, W.T., Fearing, R., and Full, R.J., Adhesive force of a single gecko foot-hair. *Nature.* 405, 681–685, 2000.

352. Autumn, K. and Hansen, W. Ultrahydrophobicity indicates a nonadhesive default state in gecko setae. *J Comp Physiol A: Sens Neural Behav Physiol.* 192, 1205–1212, 2006.

353. Autumn, K. and Gravish, N., Gecko adhesion: Evolutionary nanotechnology. *Philos Transact A Math Phys Eng Sci.* 366(1870), 1575–1590, 2008.

354. Gnecco, E., Bennewitz, R., Gyalog, T., Loppacher, C., Bammerlin, M., Meyer, E., and Guntherodt, H.J., Velocity dependence of atomic friction. *Phys Rev Lett.* 84, 1172–1175, 2000.

355. Richetti, P., Drummond, C., Israelachvili, J., In, M., and Zana, R., Inverted stick–slip friction. *Europhys Lett.* 55, 653–659, 2001.

356. Riedo, E., Gnecco, E., Bennewitz, R., Meyer, E., Brune, H., Interaction potential and hopping dynamics governing sliding friction. *Phys Rev Lett.* 91, 084502, 2003.

357. Tambe, N.S. and Bhushan, B., Friction model for the velocity dependence of nanoscale friction. *Nanotechnology.* 16, 2309–2324, 2005.

358. Niederegger, S., Gorb, S., and Jiao, Y., Contact behaviour of tenent setae in attachment pads of the blowfly *Calliphora vicina* (Diptera, Calliphoridae). *J Comp Physiol A Neuroethol Sens Neural Behav Physiol.* 187(12), 961–970, 2002.

359. Floyd, S., Pawashe, C., and Sitti, M., Dynamic modeling of stick slip motion in an untethered magnetic micro-robot. In *proceeding of: Robotics: Science and Systems IV*, Eidgenössische Technische Hochschule Zürich, Zurich, Switzerland, June 25–28, 2008.

360. Diller, E.D., Floyd, S., Pawashe, C., and Sitti, M., Control of multiple heterogeneous magnetic micro-robots on non-specialized surfaces. *ICRA.* 115–120, 2011.

361. Preston, T.M. and King, C.A., Actin-based motility in the net slime mould *Labyrinthula*: Evidence for the role of myosin in gliding movement. *J Eukaryot Microbiol.* 52(6), 461–475, 2005.

362. Wolgemuth, C.W. and Oster, G., The junctional pore complex and the propulsion of bacterial cells. *J Mol Microbiol Biotechnol.* 7(1–2), 72–77, 2004.

363. Jeon, J. and Dobrynin, A.V., Polymer confinement and bacterial gliding motility. *Eur Phys J E Soft Matter.* 17(3), 361–372, 2005.

364. Wolgemuth, C., Hoiczyk, E., Kaiser, D., and Oster, G., How myxobacteria glide. *Curr Biol.* 12(5), 369–377, 2002.

365. Hoiczyk, E., Gliding motility in cyanobacterial: Observations and possible explanations. *Arch Microbiol.* 174, 11–17, 2000.

366. Hoiczyk, E. and Baumeister, W., The junctional pore complex, a prokaryotic secretion organelle, is the molecular motor underlying gliding motility in cyanobacteria. *Curr Biol.* 8, 1161–1168, 1998.

367. Montagna, G.N., Matuschewski, K., and Buscaglia, C.A., *Plasmodium* sporozoite motility: An update. *Front Biosci.* 17, 726–744, 2012.

368. Vanderberg, J., Chew, S., and Stewart, M.J., *Plasmodium* sporozoite interactions with macrophages in vitro: A video microscopic analysis. *J Protozool.* 37, 528–536, 1990.

369. Sinnis, P., Willnow, T.E., Briones, M.R.S., Herz, J., and Nussenzweig, V., Remnant lipoproteins inhibit malaria sporozoite invasion of hepatocytes. *J Exp Med.* 184, 945–954, 1996.

370. Yoshida, N., Potocnjak, P., Nussenzweig, V., and Nussenzweig, R.S., Biosynthesis of Pb44, the protective antigen of sporozoites of *Plasmodium berghei*. *J Exp Med*. 154, 1225–1236, 1981.

371. Fine, E., Aikawa, M., Cochrane, A.H., and Nussenzweig, R.S., Immuno-electron microscopic observations on *Plasmodium knowlesi* sporozoites: Localization of protective antigen and its precursors. *Am J Trop Med Hyg*. 33, 220–226, 1984.

372. Nagasawa, H., Aikawa, M., Procell, P.M., Campbell, G.H., Collins, W.E., and Campbell, C.C., *Plasmodium malariae*: Distribution of circumsporozoite protein in midgut oocysts and salivary gland sporozoites. *Exp Parasitol*. 66, 27–34, 1988.

373. Stewart, M.J. and Vanderberg, J.P., Malaria sporozoites release circumsporozoite protein from their apical end and translocate it along their surface. *J Protozool*. 38, 411–421, 1991.

374. Stewart, M.J. and Vanderberg, J.P., Malaria sporozoites leave behind trails of Circumsporozoite protein during gliding motility. *J Protozool*. 35, 389–393, 1988.

375. Stewart, M.J. and Vanderberg, J.P., Electron microscopic analysis of circumsporozoite protein trail formation by gliding malaria sporozoites. *J Protozool*. 39, 663–671, 1992.

376. Henrichsen, J., Bacterial surface translocation: A survey and a classification. *Bacteriol Rev*. 36(4), 478–503, 1972.

377. Kearns, D.B., A field guide to bacterial swarming motility. *Nat Rev Microbiol*. 8(9), 634–644, 2010.

378. Nagy, M., Akos, Z., Biro, D., and Vicsek, T. Hierarchical group dynamics in pigeon flocks. *Nature*. 464, 890–893, 2010.

379. Harrington, M., Serotonin triggers swarming in locusts. *Lab Anim (NY)*. 38(3), 72, 2009.

380. Latty, T., Ramsch, K., Ito, K., Nakagaki, T., Sumpter, D.J., Middendorf, M., and Beekman, M., Structure and formation of ant transportation networks. *J R Soc Interface*. 8(62), 1298–1306, 2011.

381. Capello, M., Soria, M., Cotel, P., Deneubourg, J.L., and Dagorn, L., Quantifying the interplay between environmental and social effects on aggregated-fish dynamics. *PLoS One*. 6(12), e28109, 2011.

382. Cressman, R. and Garay, J., The effects of opportunistic and intentional predators on the herding behavior of prey. *Ecology*. 92(2), 432–440, 2011.

383. Shklarsh, A., Ariel, G., Schneidman, E., and Ben-Jacob, E., Smart swarms of bacteria-inspired agents with performance adaptable interactions. *PLoS Comput Biol*. 7(9), e1002177, 2011.

384. Couzin, I.D., Krause, J., James, R., Ruxton, G.D., and Franks, N.R., Collective memory and spatial sorting in animal groups. *J Theor Biol*. 218, 1–11, 2002.

385. Couzin, I.D., Krause, J., Franks, N.R., and Levin, S.A., Effective leadership and decision-making in animal groups on the move. *Nature*. 433, 513–516, 2005.

386. Vicsek, T., Czirok, A., Ben-Jacob, E., Cohen, I., and Shochet, O., Novel type of phase transition in a system of self-driven particles. *Phys Rev Lett*. 75, 1226, 1995.

387. Li, B., Zhang, J., Mumford, P., and Dempster, A.G., How good is assisted GPS?, in *International Global Navigation Satellite Systems Society IGNSS Symposium 2011*, University of New South Wales, Sydney, NSW, Australia, November 15–17, 2011.

388. The World Time System, National Physical Laboratory, Middlesex, U.K., March 25, 2010. http://www.npl.co.uk/science-technology/time-frequency/time/research/the-world-time-system

389. Position Determination with GPS. April 19, 2009. http://www.kowoma.de/en/gps/positioning.htm

390. GPS Status Updates. http://www.lockheedmartin.com/products/GPS/gpsstatusupdates.html

391. Rogers, T., Distance measuring equipment (DME), June 11, 2011. http://allaboutairplanes.wordpress.com/2011/06/11/distance-measuring-equipment-dme/

392. Krause, M., Hulman, M., Kuzmany, H., Dubay, O., Kresse, G., Vietze, K., Seifert, G., Wang, C., and Shinohara, H., Fullerene quantum gyroscope. *Phys Rev Lett*. 93(13), 137403, 2004.

393. Stevenson, S. Rice, G., Burbank, P., Craft, J., Glass, T., Harich, K., Cromer, F., Jordan, M.R., Hadju, E., Bible, R., Olmstead, M.M., Maitrap, K., Fischer, A.J., Balch, A.L., and Dorn, H.C., Small-bandgap endohedral metallofullerenes in high yield and purity. *Nature*. 401, 55–57, 1999.

394. Khan, N.S., Perez-Aguilar, J.M., Kaufmann, T., Hill, P.A., Taratula, O., Lee, O.S., Carroll, P.J., Saven, J.G., and Dmochowski, I.J., Multiple hindered rotators in a gyroscope-inspired tribenzylamine hemicryptophane. *J Org Chem.* 76(5), 1418–1424, 2011.

395. Kitagawa, H., Kobori, Y., Yamanaka, M., Yoza, K., and Kobayashi, K., Molecular recognition and self-assembly special feature: Encapsulated-guest rotation in a self-assembled heterocapsule directed toward a supramolecular gyroscope. *Proc Natl Acad Sci USA.* 106(26), 10444–10448, 2009.

396. Frankel, R.B. and Blakemore, R.P., Navigational compass in magnetic bacteria. *J Magn. Magn. Mater.* 15–18(3), 1562–1564, 1980.

397. Debarros, H., Esquivel, D.M.S., and Farina, M., Magnetotaxis. *Sci Progr.* 74, 347–359, 1990.

398. Sha, M.Y., Walton, I.D., Norton, S.M., Taylor, M., Yamanaka, M., Natan, M.J., Xu, C., Drmanac, S., Huang, S., Borcherding, A., Drmanac, R., and Penn, S.G., Multiplexed SNP genotyping using nanobarcode particle technology. *Anal Bioanal Chem.* 384(3), 658–666, 2006.

399. Andrews, R.J., Neuroprotection at the nanolevel—Part I: Introduction to nanoneurosurgery. *Ann NY Acad Sci.* 1122, 169–184, 2007.

400. Yang, Y.T., Ekinci, K.L., Huang, X.M.H., Schiavone, L.M., Roukes, M.L., Zorman, C.A., and Mehregany, M., Monocrystalline silicon carbide nanoelectromechanical systems. *Appl Phys Lett.* 78(2), 162–164, 2001.

401. Ekinci, K.L., Yang, Y.T., Huang, X.M.H., and Roukes, M.L., Balanced electronic detection of displacement in nanoelectromechanical systems. *Appl Phys Lett.* 81, 2253–2255, 2002.

402. Huang, X.M.H., Zorman, C.A., Mehregany, M., and Roukes, M.L., Nanoelectromechanical systems: Nanodevice motion at microwave frequencies. *Nature.* 421(6922), 496, 2003.

403. Huber, A.J., Keilmann, F., Wittborn, J., Aizpurua, J., and Hillenbrand, R., Terahertz near-field nanoscopy of mobile carriers in single semiconductor nanodevices. *Nano Lett.* 8(11), 3766–3770, 2008.

404. Kienle, D. and Léonard, F., Terahertz response of carbon nanotube transistors. *Phys Rev Lett.* 103(2), 026601, 2009.

405. Dagher, G., Hole, S., and Lewiner, J., A preliminary study of space charge distribution measurements at nanometer spatial resolution. *IEEE Trans Dielectr Electr Insul.* 13(5), 1036–1041, 2006.

406. Boehm, F., Potential strategies for advanced nanomedical device ingress and egress, natation, mobility, and navigation, Chapter 15, in Schulz, M.J., Shanov, V.N., and Yun, Y., eds., *Nanomedicine Design of Particles, Sensors, Motors, Implants, Robots, and Devices*, Artech House, Norwood, MA, 2009.

407. Moulin, V., Goulet, F., Berthod, F., Germain, L., and Auger, F.A., Tissue engineering: A tool to understand the physiological mechanisms. *Med Sci (Paris).* 19(10), 1003–1010, 2003.

408. Black, A.F., Berthoda, F., L'heureux, N., Germaina, L., and Auger, F.A., In vitro reconstruction of a human capillary-like network in a tissue-engineered skin equivalent. *FASEB J.* 12(13), 1331–1340, 1998.

409. Stoclet, J.C., Laflamme, K., Auger, F.A., and Germain, L., Human tissue engineered blood vessels: A novel support for vascular biology and pharmacology research. *Med Sci (Paris).* 20(6–7), 675–678, 2004.

410. Auger, F.A., Berthod, F., Moulin, V., Pouliot, R., and Germain, L., Tissue-engineered skin substitutes: From in vitro constructs to in vivo applications. *Biotechnol Appl Biochem.* 39(Pt 3), 263–275, 2004.

411. Additional papers by Auger F.A. on tissue engineering. http://www.ncbi.nlm.nih.gov/sites/entrez?cmd=search&db=pubmed&term=Auger%20FA%5Bau%5D&dispmax=50

412. Serohijos, A.W.R., Chen, Y., Ding, F., Elston, T.C., and Dokholyan, N.V., A structural model reveals energy transduction in dynein, *PNAS* 103(49), 18540–18545, 2006.

4

Design Challenges and Considerations for Nanomedical Energy Harvesting and Generation

Frank J. Boehm

CONTENTS

4.1 Provision of Power for Autonomous Nanomedical Devices

Advanced autonomous nanomedical devices of all classes will have the requirement of sources of energy that will enable them to dependably transit and navigate through the human body; establish and maintain communications with "outbody" control computers as well as companion nanodevices; conduct internal computation; and most importantly, successfully perform the specific medical procedures that they are tasked with accomplishing. This chapter will explore what may constitute one of the more challenging aspects of nanomedical design, as the onboard provision of robust and reliable energy harvesting or generation will be essential for the operation of most species of medical nanodevices. A range of potential designs and strategies will be investigated which might facilitate the efficient conversion of energy that is harvested from in vivo biofluids (primarily blood/plasma resident) that permeate the patient's "inbody" environment. Additional design considerations that must be taken into account will be associated with the cumulative dissipation of heat that will be generated as a consequence of nanodevice energy sources, which are converted and expended as useful work. This will be especially critical when perhaps millions of nanodevices work concurrently in vivo to perform massively parallel procedures, such as chromatin replacement or cell repair operations, at millions of distinct "treatment" sites within the patient. The conceptual exemplar VCSN device design will serve as a model template to elucidate the characteristics of particular envisioned energy-harvesting and energy-generating components, which might be utilized as modular onboard mechanisms for the powering of nanomedical devices.

4.2 Energy Sources Inherent to Living Systems

Energy is an indispensable prerequisite resource that is necessary before biological cells may perform useful work. Many energy-harvesting/generating mechanisms in living systems are interconvertible. The two primary types of energy are potential and kinetic. Potential energies might be viewed as analogous to storage batteries in biological systems, whereas kinetic energy is manifest in all forms of biological actuation [1]. In order for thermal energy to be effective in enabling work, it must initially be transferred from a region of higher temperature (characterized by rapid molecular motions) to a lower temperature domain.

Interestingly, temperature differentials exist, and indeed are common, between the internal and external environments of biological cells. In 1971, Mercer [2] calculated a temperature gradient of $0.4°C/cm^2$ between the interior and exterior of the bacteria *Streptococcus faecalis*, which was derived from data by Forrest and Walker [3]. Yang et al. recently (2011) utilized quantum dot (QD) "nanothermometers" to measure the temperatures of individual living cells and observed that heterogeneous temperatures exist between specific organelles. Mitochondria, for instance, initiate thermogenesis as they generate biochemical energy. It was found that temperature differences of several degrees Fahrenheit existed between certain areas of mouse cells. Nanometric CdSe (cadmium and selenium) QDs were utilized that emit specific wavelengths of light associated with particular temperatures, which were interrogated by external instrumentation [4]. Maestro et al. measured externally induced temperature changes within HeLa cervical cancer cells subsequent to the incorporation of CdSe-QD nanothermometers. Intracellular temperatures ranging from 25°C to about 50°C were measured in real time by two photon–excited emission shifts in the QDs [5].

These developing capabilities may enable the precise temperature mapping of various human cell types under ambient physiological conditions to determine whether nanomedical devices might potentially tap into intracellular thermal gradients for the extraction of energy while performing diagnostic or therapeutic tasks in vivo. Though an intriguing potential source of energy for autonomous nanomedical devices, cells themselves are not equipped to tap into this particular reservoir of available power [1,6].

The kinetic energy of photons is termed radiant energy, and is critical for all living systems. Photonic energy is translated into thermal energy (e.g., when molecules absorb photons and transform them into molecular motion). In photosynthesis, the photonic energy that is taken up by chlorophyll is converted into other forms of energy, which is stored in chemical covalent bonds. The movement of electrons and other charged particles is also a form of kinetic energy. Most biochemical reactions involve the formation or dissolution covalent bonds. This energy is apparent when chemicals are engaged in energy-releasing reactions. Glucose has a high potential energy that cells degrade on a continuous basis. Energy released from glucose provides energy for many types of cellular activities [1].

Concentration gradients constitute a second important biological form of potential energy. For instance, when a concentration of a particular substance is present on one side of a permeable membrane that is dissimilar from a substance that is present on the other side, a concentration gradient is initiated. Concentration gradients are formed between internal and external regions of cells, which selectively exchange nutrients, waste products, and ions with their environments. Compartments within cells often contain varying concentrations of ions and other molecules (e.g., the concentrations of protons that reside within a lysosome are ~500-fold higher than those which inhabit the cytosol). A third form of potential energy in cells involves the energy of charge separation and is known as an electric potential. Intriguingly, there exists a gradient of electric charge across the plasma membrane of practically all cells, with a value of 0.07 V per 3.5×10^{-7} cm, or 200,000 V/cm [1].

4.3 Energy-Harvesting Strategies for Autonomous Nanomedical Devices

The envisaged functionality of energy-harvesting/generating components relates to the provision of robust, reliable, precisely controllable, and sustainable electron flow to all onboard VCSN components and systems. Ideally, these components will be modular, stand-alone mechanisms that operate in unison with hundreds or thousands of identical units to extract raw power in vivo from human whole blood glucose or other sufficiently available biofuels. They might utilize enzymatic catalytic processes (e.g., redox reactions) to acquire and transmit the required electron flows. A limited energy storage capability (ultrathin film battery) that serves as a buffer might be integrated into the VCSN in order to enable an additional window of normal device operation should a malfunction occur with the energy-harvesting component. An important issue to explore and address will pertain to the elimination of any possible of "biofouling" events, whereby in vivo proteins or macrophages may accumulate and clog the catalytic surfaces of the component, rendering it useless. Assistance in solving this potentially critical problem may arise via the development of a feasible biocompatible nanoporous coating.

There are a number of potential (free-electron) harvesting and generating technologies that might be down scalable for use in nanometric applications and operations. These may encompass varied geometric configurations, and innovative uses of ultrathin film materials. Unique biomimetically derived extrapolations of natural systems may also lead to the development of nanoscale power-harvesting or -generating mechanisms. Each of these entities includes their own set of inherent prompts for investigation and experimentation.

4.3.1 Ultrathin Film Membrane Lamination for Glucose Conversion

A proposed configuration for a nanoscale power-harvesting component for in vivo applications might incorporate nanoporous laminated ultrathin film electrodes (anode and cathode), which are separated by insulating barriers, effectively isolating positive and negative charges. Anodic and cathodic membranes will be distinct from one another in that the anode functions to electrooxidize glucose, whereas the cathode functions to electroreduce oxygen [7]. The controlled release of electrons that reside in both the anode and cathode might be mediated through the incorporation of electronic gates that are activated externally by either pulsed radio frequencies, ultrasonic signals, or via magnetic or photonic means. Ultrathin film laminations would be configured in such a way as to convey electric current through an embedded nanoelectronic infrastructure, to power all components of the VCSN. Electrons may be extracted from in vivo biofuels through the enzymatic catalysis of molecules such as glucose. Glucose is selected as a first choice for anode biofuel due to its abundance in whole blood. However, it is conceivable that other molecules, which demonstrate potential as viable biofuels and provide sufficient whole blood concentrations, might be investigated. These alternate species include carboxylic acid, carbohydrates, starches, and lactate molecules. The cathode might utilize either complexed or dissolved oxygen that is inherent to hemoglobin or myoglobin [8]. Appropriate enzymes would be embedded and immobilized within the ultrathin film layers in a manner such that the enzyme reaction centers are intimately interfaced with specific conductive layers of the laminated membrane. These task-specific enzymes might be further functionalized when combined with a redox polymer (RP) in the formation of an electronically active layer [7].

As a sustained and reliable current flow will be required for the optimum operation of all VCSN components and systems, biofouling countermeasures will have a considerable impact, and will pose significant challenges. Any anti-biofouling agent that is applied as a coating to the outer surface of the VCSN must possess attributes of noninterference with energy supplies, scanning entities, communications, or propulsion.

The envisaged timeline for the VCSN scanning procedure would be about 5 min. All engineered ultrathin film coatings would act as an interface between the external device surfaces and whole blood components. These coatings would be selected for their inert properties in vivo, discrete permeability, along with the capacity to stave off unwanted molecular species for long periods, allowing for an extensive remedial/recovery window should functional issues arise involving motility, navigation, or communications. Accessibility to reliable power will be essential for nanodevices in facilitating their reception of recovery commands, and for the elicitation of device response by external communication beacons. In the rare event that no communication is possible, a tagging protocol could be initiated for tracking to enable nanodevice retrieval or to ensure that they will diffuse from the body through natural processes.

Controlled molecular adherence and dissociation rates are highlighted as important parameters for the characterization of overall stability and sustainability of a viable working electric current. The endowment of appropriately configured electrode surfaces with the ability for enabling dynamic binding affinities with particular molecular species illustrates another area of importance for the optimization and continuity of electron flow.

Innovative studies on the extraction of electricity from glucose via enzymatic action have been conducted by Heller et al., who synthesized enzyme films that were comprised of immobilized redox enzymes and redox hydrogels (Figures 4.1 and 4.2). Their reaction

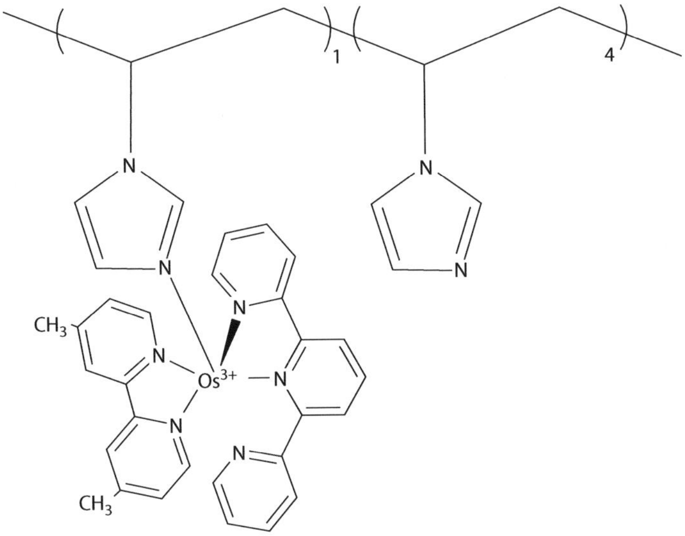

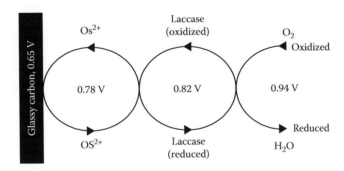

FIGURE 4.1
Structure of laccase "wiring" redox polymer. (Reproduced from Calabrese, B.S. et al., *J. Am. Chem. Soc.*, 123(24), 5802, 2001. Copyright 2001. American Chemical Society. With permission.)

FIGURE 4.2
The electrocatalytic cascade. (Reproduced from Calabrese, B.S. et al., *J. Am. Chem. Soc.*, 123(24), 5802, 2001. Copyright 2001. American Chemical Society. With permission.)

centers were "wired" to carbon fiber electrodes [9]. In an experimental setup, two carbon fibers (Ø 7 μm) were utilized as electrodes and were coated with an electrocatalyst. One electrode was a glucose-oxidizing anode, while the other was an oxygen-reducing cathode. The anode was coated with an electrocatalyzing thin film that comprised a cross-linked electrostatic adduct of glucose oxidase (from *Aspergillus niger*). This film was covalently bonded to a reducing-potential copolymer (poly(*N*-vinylimidazole)) with osmium complexes tethered to its backbone, which catalyzed the electrooxidation of glucose to gluconolactone. This electrically connected the reaction center of the glucose oxidase to the carbon fiber of the anode [10]. The cathode was similar, but was also coated with the electrostatic adduct of laccase (from *Coriolus hirsutus*) and an oxidizing-potential copolymer. The laccase cathode facilitated the four-electron reduction of O_2 to water (near neutral pH 5) at body temperature (37°C) [11].

As Heller points out,

> When a redox enzyme is adsorbed on the surface of an electrode, its electroactivity is orientation-dependent. Only ~1% of the molecules, oriented with their redox centers proximal to the surface, are electroactive. In contrast, when the enzyme is immobilized in an electron-conducting redox polymer hydrogel, electrons are transferred through colliding mobile polymer-bound redox functions. As a result, all enzyme molecules are electroactive, irrespective of their orientation. Furthermore, because multiple layers of enzyme molecules are "wired" in the film, the current density is ~10^3-fold greater than that of an absorbed, randomly oriented, enzyme monolayer directly adsorbed on an electrode [9,10].

RPs are thought to facilitate the diffusion of electrons via a number of routes, which encompass "percolation" among immobilized redox centers; transient reduced and oxidized redox center collisions; and electron or hole conduction via conjugated backbones. In addition, electron-transporting impacts are amplified in conjunction with increasingly mobile-tethered redox centers [11]. Hence, it would appear to follow that the maximization of electron transferral may be facilitated by optimizing the mobility of the redox centers within the polymer.

According to Heller and coworkers, their biofuel cell unit could produce 1 µW with both electrodes working at 0.5 mA/cm^2, which is more than sufficient for powering an autonomous implanted sensor–transmitter system [7,10,12]. To quote a prescient observation by Dr. Robert Nowak [13] of DARPA as per Heller's achievement at the time (2001): "After many years of research by groups world-wide, Heller's group has achieved record current densities, which allow for extreme miniaturisation."

Gallaway and Barton studied the performance of oxygen-reducing enzymatic electrodes that comprised RPs and laccase from *Trametes versicolor* ("turkey tail" mushroom) on rotating glassy carbon disks, and achieved current densities of ~2.1 mA/cm^2 at 0.65 V at 900 rpm in a 0.1 M pH 4 citrate buffer under 40°C. When composite electrodes, having high surface areas were employed, a current density of 13 ± 0.8 mA/cm^2 was achieved at 900 rpm. It was also found that when restrictions on mass transport were further reduced, current densities surpassed 20 mA/cm^2 [14].

A micron-scale bioelectrode devised by Wen et al. integrated a coating of carboxylated carbon nanotubes onto carbon microfiber electrodes. This high surface area electrode was suitable for the immobilization of glucose oxidase enzymes. A carbon nanotube coating concentration of 13 µg/cm produced a coating depth of 17 µm enabling a 2000-fold increase in surface capacitance. The coated electrode was modified further via the addition of a cross-linked biocatalytic hydrogel comprised of glucose oxidase in conjunction with a conductive RP. Upon the oxidation of glucose in an oxygen-free glucose solution, the current density attained was 16.6 mA/cm^2 at 0.5 V (vs. Ag/AgCl) [15].

4.3.2 Enzymatically Active Thin Films

Investigations have been conducted with nanocomposite hydrogel thin films that comprised alternating layers of organometallic RP and oxidoreductase enzymes. These thin film layers, composed of oppositely charged molecules, were sequentially deposited on a gold substrate via electrostatic assembly. This mode of electrostatic bonding between cationic RPs and anionic oxidoreductase enzymes facilitated the transfer of electrons from the enzymes, by way of the RP to the electrode surface [12,16,17] (Figure 4.3).

Pishko et al. demonstrated biosensing monolayers (~100 Å thick) for the detection of glucose, lactate, and other analytes, which contained single RP/enzyme layers. The synthesis

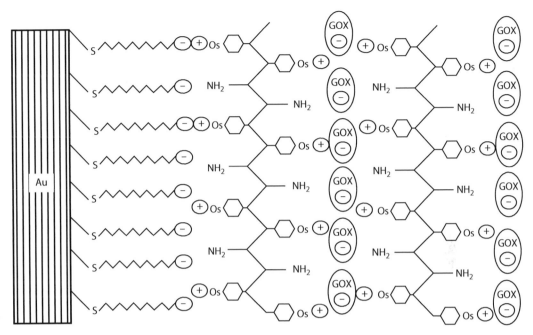

FIGURE 4.3
Depiction of multilayered polycationic/polyanionic structure where positive redox polymers have an electrostatic affinity for negatively charged enzymes and the Au substrate. (Reproduced from Sirkar, K. et al., *Anal. Chem.*, 72(13), 2930, 2000. With permission.)

of these nanocomposite films was based on the electrostatic attraction between poly-cationic osmium RP, and a polyanionic enzyme glucose oxidase (GOX), lactate oxidase (LAX), or pyruvate oxidase (PYX). The gold electrode substrate was functionalized with ll-mercaptoundecanoic acid (MUA), where the thiol end group was chemisorbed. The carboxylic acid end group of MUA set up a net negative charge at the solution/electrode interface, as at a pK_a of 6.5, the acid group is somewhat deprotonated at a pH of 7.4 [12].

Modified polymers of organometallic osmium complexes are polycationic and may be electrostatically bound to negatively functionalized substrates. The electrostatic bonding of anionic GOX or LAX is made possible by utilizing positively charged RP layers. This process may be repeated as required for the deposition of multiple layers in the creation of nanocomposite structures (e.g., alternating polyanionic/polycationic films), and the RPs are physically stabilized by multivalent contacts. Although these highly charged multi-layered films did not dissociate when continually exposed to water for 3 weeks, indicating structural stability, a degree of water penetration, and hence hydrogel film swelling, is necessary to sustain state of electroneutrality. As Pishko et al. observe, "As RP is oxidized, the oxidation state of Os changes from +2 to +3 and thus the charge on the complex changes from +1 to +2. Electroneutrality must be maintained and thus counter ions must move into the film along with associated water molecules of hydration" [12,18–23].

Polyelectrolyte layer-based nanocomposite films are thought to be nanoporous, and the expansion and collapse of the film potential may be representative of the pore structure and volume changes at the nanometer level [21]. It is possible that pore structural changes may arise from changes in salt concentrations. The oxidoreductase-catalyzed reaction with Os sites within a RP acts as an electron relay between embedded enzymes and the electrode surface. Electrons are transferred between redox sites in a self-exchange reaction until they are shuttled to the (positive) electrode surface. Hence, a linear current density/glucose concentration relationship is created. As observed in a Pishko et al. study, a glucose concentration of 20 mM generated a current density of approximately +0.3 µA/cm², whereas an anticipated current density of +0.4 µA/cm² could be possible when mass transfer limitation are removed [23].

4.3.3 ATP Conversion

Adenosine triphosphate (ATP) liberates 7.3 kcal/mol of energy when one of three phosphate groups is cleaved from its structure and the energy is subsequently transferred to energy-absorbing (endergonic) reactions inside a cell. The structure of ATP consists of the adenine nucleotide (ribose sugar, adenine base, and phosphate group) in addition to two other phosphate groups [24] (Figure 4.4). The ATPase enzyme catalyzes the hydrolysis of ATP to adenosine diphosphate (ADP) and releases free energy in the process. Hypothetically, a strategy might be devised to facilitate the attraction and isolation of ATP molecules (e.g., via the immobilization of ATPase arrays within specialized energy-harvesting substrates) on a nanomedical device for a sufficient duration, such that the embedded ATPase units may initiate the cleavage of the third phosphate group from transient ATP and direct the resulting free energy into an onboard power conduit. This may constitute an intriguing area for investigation. Montemagno and Bachand have harnessed ATP to create a biomolecular motor that might be used to propel a nanomedical device [25–27]. Mobility component technologies for nanodevices will be another critical area to be addressed (Chapter 3).

4.3.4 Nanometric Biofuel Cells

A nanoscale proton-exchange membrane (PEM) utilizing an appropriate assemblage of nanoporous ultrathin films may demonstrate capacity for the generation of enough electron-flow output for use as a power source [8]. In-depth studies of the specific configurations and kinetics of fuel cells and PEMs at atomic and molecular levels may be a suitable prerequisite for exploring this possibility. Hydrogen (along with its isotopes deuterium, tritium, and muonium) is the simplest element of the periodic table, having one electron. Although a quantum gas, it also exists in liquid and solid forms, such as the hydrocarbon CH_4. The dissociation of H_2O or CH_4 utilizing an appropriate primary energy might produce a future synthetic fuel. Metal hydride–filled nanotubes could possibly be employed as electrodes for the reversible storage of electricity [28], in that nickel serves as an excellent catalyst for the dissociation of molecular hydrogen [29]. It may be possible to store hydrogen in

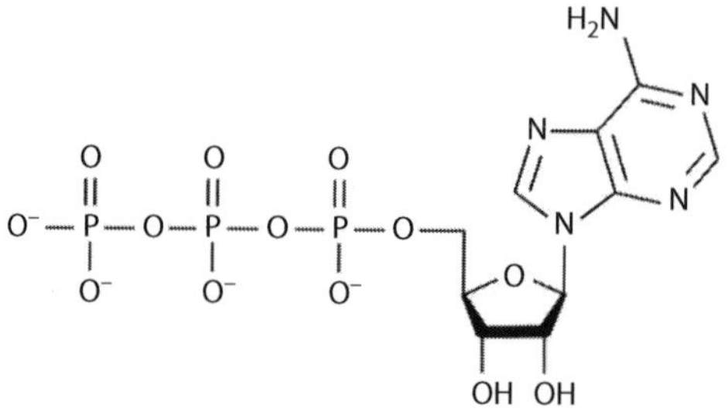

FIGURE 4.4
Chemical structure of ATP molecule depicting three phosphate groups, the last of which is cleaved by ATPase to release 7.3 kcal/mol of energy, thereby transitioning to ADP. (Image freely licensed from Wikimedia Commons.)

nanotube or nanoscroll arrays with high packing density. Investigations into the potential powering a VCSN with a nanoscale version of a PEM that would strip the electrons from hydrogen atoms bound up in H_2O might be a worthwhile endeavor.

A supramolecular complex has been devised that produces pure hydrogen, which is activated by light. It uses two light-absorbing ruthenium subunits on either end of the molecule, and connector subunits that link them to a central reactive rhodium subunit, which collects electrons and transfers them to water. The water molecules are subsequently split as sufficient energy (e.g., light generates more than two electrons at a time) is produced by this complex to release the hydrogen from the oxygen [30]. It may be plausible that this type of supramolecular complex could power a nanomedical device when activated by near-infrared photons to potentially catalyze water molecules in the bloodstream for the extraction of usable hydrogen fuel.

Biffinger et al. have shown that conventional PEMs may be replaced by nanoporous polymeric filters (with 0.2 μm in diameter pores × 20–50 μm thick) comprising cellulose, nylon, or polycarbonate materials in small microbial biofuel cells (MFCs) with active areas of 2 cm^2 and had comparable robustness and energy outputs to Nafion-117 membranes. When combined with an oxygen-reducing cathode (graphite felt), the biofuel cell produced a power density output of 16 W/m^3. The group also investigated larger (5 cm^3) and smaller (0.025 cm^3) active surface area MFCs with respective produced power densities of 0.6 and 10 W/m^3. The anodes were also isolated from naturally occurring bacteria, which serve to hinder the formation of biofilms. The power generated by these "mini-MFCs" ranged from a low of 9 μW, utilizing a cellulose nitrate membrane (physical degradation after 20 h use), to maxima of 17 and 19 μW for nylon and polycarbonate membranes, respectively. The amplified power outputs of the latter two membranes are surmised to be the result of their open porous structures, which augment diffusion in contrast to the osmotic flow inherent to membranes comprised of cellulose and Nafion. The polycarbonate demonstrated sustained operation over 500 h with a negligible decrease in power production [31].

MFCs are of interest as they may operate under variable conditions, including at room temperature and under neutral pH, and can utilize an array of unconventional complex organic substances as fuels, including proteins, fats, and carbohydrates [32,33]. This functionality is possible due to the interception of electrons from "exoelectrogen" microorganism electron transport pathways that are transferred to electrodes. The versatility of these MFCs is facilitated by microbes such as *Shewanella oneidensis* DSP10, which have metabolic capacities in both aerobic and anaerobic environments [31,34]. Intriguingly, electrons may transit along conductive hairlike nanowires that are extruded by *S. oneidensis* and other microbes, which form electrical connections between the cell and electrode [35–37] (Figure 4.5).

4.3.5 Biomimetic Microorganism Functionality

It was revealed by Chaudhuri and Lovley that the microorganism *Rhodoferax ferrireducens* has a substantial sustained capacity for the almost complete (83%) catalyzation of glucose directly into electricity. This was accomplished without the requirement of a mediator to assist in the transfer of electrons when it was adhered to a graphite anode (which served as the electron receptor) for extended periods. In addition to glucose, *R. ferrireducens* also generated current from sugars such as fructose, sucrose, and xylose [38]. If a biomimetic extrapolation of the functional unit of *R. ferrireducens* could be designed to emulate this functionality, it might demonstrate the potential for the generation of viable electric current from available in vivo glucose for nanodevices.

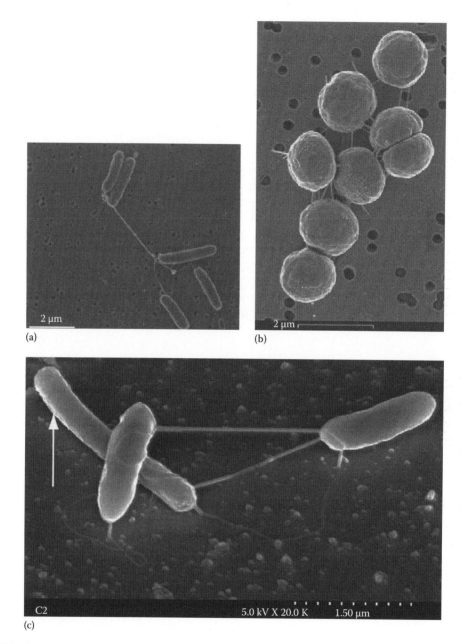

(a)

(b)

(c)

FIGURE 4.5

(a) SEM image of *S. oneidensis* MR-1. (b) SEM image of *Synechocystis* sp. PCC 6803. (c) SEM image of *Pelotomaculum thermopropionicum* and *Methnobacterium thermoautotrophicus* (arrow) depicting inter-genera nanowire connectivity. (Reproduced from Gorby, Y.A. et al., *Proc. Natl. Acad. Sci. U S A*, 103(30), 11358, 2006. Copyright 2006. National Academy of Sciences, U.S.A. With permission.)

Under controlled laboratory conditions in an optimized fuel cell, *R. ferrireducens* generated a sustained current density of ~31 mA/m^2 (0.20 mA; 265 mV), with the application of 1000 Ω of resistance to mediate the anode → cathode electron flow. The power output could be significantly enhanced by increasing the surface area of the electrodes. When the graphite rod anode (6.5 × 10^{-3} m^2 surface area) was replaced with graphite felt (20.0 × 10^{-3} m^2 surface area),

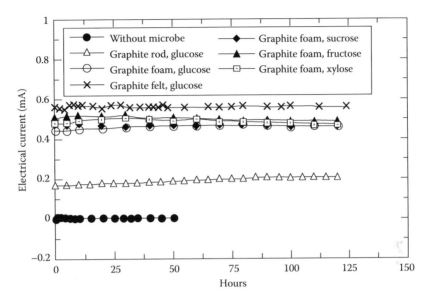

FIGURE 4.6
Comparison of the electrical current generated by *R. ferrireducens* in a fuel cell at 25°C, illustrating the effects of three different types of graphite electrodes and sugars. (Reproduced from Chaudhuri, S.K. and Lovley, D.R., *Nat. Biotechnol.*, 21(10), 1229, 2003.)

the generated current almost tripled to (~0.57 mA; 620 mV), and interestingly, was increased by 2.4 times (~74 mA/m²; 445 mV) utilizing a porous graphite foam electrode (6.1 × 10⁻³ m² surface area) (Figure 4.6). The higher current exhibited by the graphite foam was thought to be due to an increased concentration of cells (0.086 mg protein/cm²) that adhered to the foam electrodes, in contrast to the graphite rods (0.032 mg protein/cm²) [38].

4.4 Energy-Generating Strategies for Advanced Nanomedical Devices

Prospective nanoscale power could also be realized through the generation of energy via the assistance of outbody sources (e.g., near-infrared laser light, ultrasonics, magnetics), which might activate dedicated arrays of receptor elements that are embedded within the external "skin" of the VCSN. Although this mode of power generation might circumvent some forms of biofouling potential plasma protein and biofilm adherence, ingestion by macrophages or white cells and possible activation of other immune responses will remain of concern. Additional robust and reliable methods for the nanometric generation of free electron flow might include piezoelectronics, thermopiles, and the incorporation of biomimetic entities such as electroplax stacks, photosynthetic entities, energy-generating microorganisms, and hydrostatics.

4.4.1 Laminated Ultrathin Film Nanoscale Thermopiles

Energy generation via laminated ultrathin film nanoscale thermopiles comprising appropriately configured thermodynamic materials or embedded entities such as gold nanoshells, for example, might be configured to initiate and maintain temperature differentials within nanodevices [39]. This might result in electron generation via the Seebeck effect, which involves the extraction of current by the effects of temperature differences between thermally resistant materials. If a disparate enough thermal contrast can be achieved and sustained to allow free electron flow, it may hold promise for powering a nanomedical device. This alternative may require an external photon source (near-infrared range—λ ~650 to 900 nm, with capacity for ~12 cm tissue depth) for emitting the proper photonic frequency for the purpose of inducing localized excitation within a thermally sensitive material that is interfaced with an appropriately thermally resistive material. Nanowires could be arranged in such a way as to tap into the interface between the two materials in order to transfer the current that is generated in this manner [40].

Efficiency would be contingent on the thermal/nonthermal conductivity of the materials employed. An investigation into potential materials that might maintain the temperature differential required in vivo to generate current via this method would be required. One class of thermoelectric materials that exhibit the best potential might be semiconductors that contain multiple quantum wells (MQWs or superlattices). MQW structures may only conduct electrons in two dimensions (2D), and this flow has been shown to increase with smaller well widths [40].

4.4.2 Piezoelectric Materials

A further possible option for in vivo energy production may be through the innovative use of piezoelectric materials. Various piezonanogenerator elements have been investigated, including nanowires comprising zinc oxide (ZnO), indium nitride (InN), cadmium sulfide (CdS) and sodium niobate ($NaNbO_3$), lead zirconate titanate (PZT), and polyvinylidene fluoride (PVDF) [41–46]. Modular nanoscale units comprising piezoelectric elements may be induced to flex mechanically via an external ultrasonic frequency source. It is well known that these materials will generate a voltage when they are mechanically stressed. If this functionality can be scaled down to the nanometric domain and appropriately integrated, piezomaterials may hold strong potential as a viable and reliable nanomedical energy-generating mechanism [47,48].

Single crystal ZnO nanosprings (~500 to 800 nm diameter with ribbons ~10 to 60 nm wide × ~5 to 20 nm thick) were fabricated for the first time in 2003 by Zhang et al. [48]. This technology may exhibit potential for the fabrication of very sensitive piezoelectric transducers. When adsorbed in appropriate densities on a conductive substrate, nanosprings may show the capacity for generating electron flow when they are mechanically induced to oscillate via an external source. Qi et al. have developed a technique for the transferral of nanometer-thick crystalline piezoelectric ribbons, comprising the single crystal perovskite, zirconate titanate (PZT), from host substrates (e.g., MgO or $SrTiO_3$) onto flexible macroscopic rubber substrates. PZT cantilevers have exhibited efficient mechanical to electrical energy conversions of over 80% [49,50]. It might be possible that such piezoribbons adhered to ultrathin flexible films might comprise interconnected power-generating "fins" that populate the exterior surfaces of nanodevices, which are induced to movement by fluid flow turbulence and shear forces.

Park et al. have developed a piezoelectric nanocomposite generator (NCG) via the integration of (Ø ~100 nm) piezoelectric barium titanate ($BaTiO_3$) nanoparticles with reduced graphene oxide, as well as single-walled carbon nanotubes (SWCNTs) (Ø ~5 to 20 nm × ~10 μm) and double-walled carbon nanotubes (MWCNTs) (Ø ~3 nm), which were diffused within polydimethylsiloxane (PDMS) (a nontoxic silicon-based organic polymer) and spin-cast onto

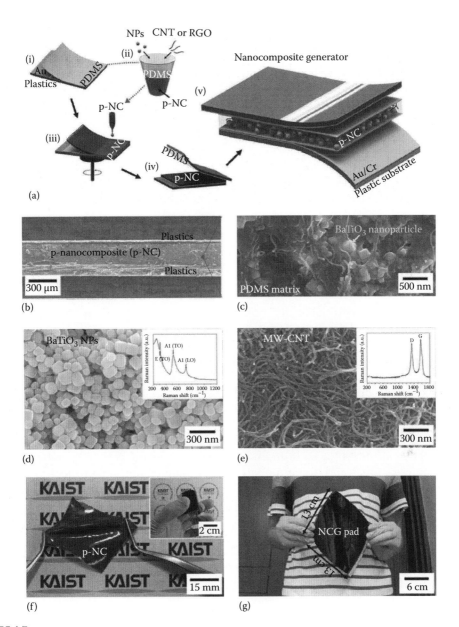

FIGURE 4.7

(a) Graphic representation of NCG fabrication. (b) SEM of NCG cross section. (c) Magnification of piezoelectric nanocomposite. (d) SEM of BaTiO₃ nanoparticles with inset Raman spectrum. (e) Magnification of MWCNTs with inset Raman spectrum. (f) Piezoelectric energy is also generated via stretching, inset depicts 3 cm wide × 4 cm long sample. (g) Larger NCGs may be fabricated via spin-casting or Mylar bar-coating. (Reproduced by Park, K.I. et al., *Adv. Mater.*, 24(22), 2999, 2012. With permission.)

flexible metal-coated plastic substrates (Figure 4.7). Piezoelectric energy is generated by the BaTiO₃ nanoparticles when they are mechanically stressed, whereas the carbon nanotubes serve as dispersed stress-reinforcing agents and conductive elements. A sample NCG device (3 cm wide × 4 cm long) consistently produced an open circuit voltage of ~3.2 V and a short-circuited current signal of 250–350 nA. The current output was virtually unchanged after 1200 bending cycles and the device exhibited excellent mechanical stability [51].

4.4.3 Biomimetic Electrocytes/Electroplax

The electric organs of the South American freshwater electric eel (*Electrophorus electricus*), Mediterranean seawater electric ray (*Torpedo nobiliana*), African and Chinese catfish (*Malopterurus electricus* and *Parasilurus asota*), respectively, are termed electroplax and are comprised of excitable cells, with flattened morphology, called electrocytes [52,53]. Electrocytes are arranged in series as stacks and a single electrocyte produces pulses in the range of ~0.14 V, with pulse durations ranging from under a millisecond to ~10 ms. These pulses can be repetitively generated from 10 to 100 times/s. A typical stack comprising 5500 electrocytes that discharge simultaneously can generate potentials of over 600 V [54]. Investigations into the development of a modular biomimetic version of the electrocyte subunit might lead to a viable source of power in vivo, if such an entity could be developed and subsequently configured in stacked arrays. The primary elements/mechanisms that drive electrocyte cell electrical discharge are sodium and potassium ion-exchange channels [55]. Both of these elements are available in usable amounts within human plasma and whole blood (sodium: 3.1–3.4×10^{-3}, potassium: 1.6–2.4×10^{-3}) (g/cm^3) [8]. Explorations into the specific electronic properties of other species of ion channels may also be a worthwhile endeavor.

With the advent of controllable advanced self-assembly processes and molecular manufacturing, nanoscale energy-harvesting strategies that are based on the functionality of electrocytes and electroplax stacks might be realized. Networks of carbon nanotubes with applications as ion-to-electron transducers in ion-selective electrodes have been demonstrated by Crespo et al. [56,57], as has their use on various other substrates by other groups [58–60]. As Crespo et al. observe, "The extraordinary capacity of carbon nanotubes to promote electron transfer between heterogeneous phases made the presence of electroactive polymers or any other ion-to-electron transfer promoter unnecessary" [56]. When coupled with electroactive polymer layers/membranes that are nanoengineered to have highly selective affinities for sodium and potassium ions, the carbon nanotubes (due to their high surface areas and accommodation of populations of mobile electrons on their surfaces) may have the capacity for extracting and transmission of electrons from these ions to onboard nanodevice electronic infrastructures and energy storage modules. Self-assembled metallomacrocycle ionophores (e.g., redox-responsive organometallic analog of 12-crown-3) contain rigid receptors that have demonstrated high affinities for both lithium and sodium ions. A cavity is formed by arene ligands, within which a sodium ion may fit perfectly [61,62] (Figure 4.8). Conductive heterocycle-based conjugated polymers, such as polypyrrole, when doped with tetrasulfonated dibenzo-18-crown-6, exhibit an attraction for potassium ions [63].

A conceptual biomimetic electroplax stack might comprise solid-state nanotube-based ion-to-electron transducers that operate in conjunction with conductive polymeric ion recognition membranes, which convert available sodium and potassium ions in the bloodstream to useful electron flow for in vivo nanodevices (Figure 4.9). Similar to the functionality of an individual electroplax in *E. electricus*, which generate an action potential that is on par with typical nerve and muscle fibers [55], the envisaged modular nanometric transducers would be stacked in series and configured as voltaic piles of perhaps hundreds or thousands of elements. This stacked arrangement is what enables the large cumulative electrical discharges that are possible in *E. electricus*. For in vivo nanodevices, however, appropriately scaled down (in both physical dimensions and electric potential) ion-to-electron transducers might supply the required ~10^9 W/m^3, which is estimated to be the upper limit for whole nanorobot operational power density [8]. Voltage gates that

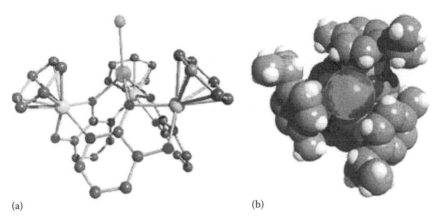

(a)   (b)

FIGURE 4.8
Molecular structure of 3, resident in the analog 12-crown-3 crystal. (a) Side view, devoid of cymene (aromatic compound) side chains and hydrogen atoms, for clarity. (b) A sodium ion fits snugly within the cavity provided by aromatic hydrocarbon (arene) ligands. (Reproduced from Piotrowski, H. et al., *J. Am. Chem. Soc.*, 123(11), 2699, 2001. Copyright 2001. American Chemical Society. With permission.)

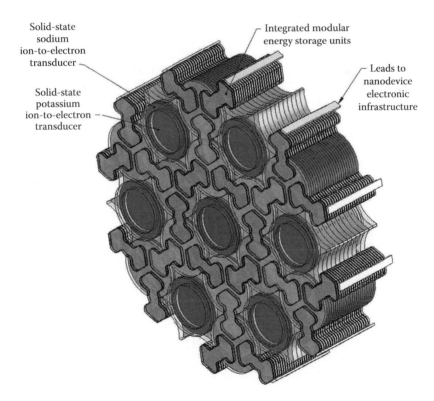

FIGURE 4.9
Conceptual tessellated biomimetic analog of electroplax stack.

are strategically positioned along stacks of integrated modular energy storage units (that run alongside the transducers) might be utilized to control the variable currents that are required for particular nanodevice components, such as quantum computers, scanning elements, propulsion, and communication systems.

4.4.4 Biomimetic Photosynthetic Reactive Structures

Nanomedical energy-generating alternatives may reside in the development of biomimetic photosynthetic reactive structures, perhaps through the incorporation of photon-activated substructures that are analogous to chlorophyll and carotenoid pigments. If this class of mechanism can be designed and configured in such a manner that they will elicit membrane potential when activated by a photonic source, they may exhibit the possibility for producing enough output electron flow to power a nanomedical device [64,65]. Laminated ultrathin film materials can exhibit exceptional characteristics in regard to electron-transfer processes by virtue of the nanometric scales involved [66].

As assembly comprises light-harvesting and redox-active layers, in effect, an artificial "leaf" has been fabricated by Kaschak and coworkers via the sequential deposition of approximately nanometer-thick ultrathin films. The resulting product consisted of a five-component lamination, which enabled incremental electron charge transfer. The light-harvesting element of the assembly contained coumarin (C), and fluorescein (F)-derivatized poly(allylamine hydrochloride), C-PAH and F-PAH, palladium (II)-tetrakis(4-N,N,N-trimethylanilinium)porphyrin (PdTAPP^{4+}), or palladium (II)-tetrakis(4-sulfonatophenyl)porphyrin (P) (PdTSPP^{4-}) layers, which were interleaved with anionic $Zr(HPO_4)_2 \cdot H_2O$ (R-ZrP) layers. Films of R-ZrP or $HTiNbO_5$ separated the porphyrin electron donor from a polyviologen electron acceptor layer [67,68]. The layers C, F, and P (chromophoric units) function to collect a significant portion of the visible light spectrum. The direct excitation of the P layer, or a C → F → P transfer of energy, generates in the P layer, a long-lived triplet excited state. Electron transfer from the excited P layer to the viologen gives rise to a long-lived charge separated state that has a ~50% efficiency. Zeolites inherently comprises regular microporous frameworks, which may serve well as hosts in organized supramolecular assemblies for photon-induced charge separation mechanisms [67–72]. Atomic force microscopy (AFM) and ellipsometry on planar supports may be utilized to verify the characterization of the layer-by-layer growth of these thin film constructs, as well as elemental analysis, measurements of surface areas, and transmission electron microscopy (TEM). The appropriate spacing of approximately nanometer-thick inorganic sheets that comprise these sandwiched assemblies serves to inhibit the interpenetration of the redox-active layers, thus preventing back electron-transfer reactions [67].

Simulated photosynthetic reaction centers combined with light-harvesting antenna and hybrid constructs that fuse biological light-harvesting complexes have also been explored and may lead to feasible strategies for the conversion of photons from outbody near-infrared lasers to available electrons for in vivo nanodevices. Ghosh et al. have investigated two theoretical models involving the transfer of electrons from accessory light-harvesting antenna pigments to an artificial reaction center (e.g., a molecular triad consisting of donor, photosensitive unit, and acceptor elements). One configuration allowed for direct energy transfer to the reaction center from the surrounding pigments, whereas the other employed a cascading strategy that transferred energy via a linear chain of light-harvesting chromophores, in which case only a single chromophore was interfaced with the reaction center (Figure 4.10). It was revealed that the latter cascading system absorbed photons over a more extensive wavelength range and demonstrated a higher efficacy for their conversion into electrons than the direct multiplexed connection system.

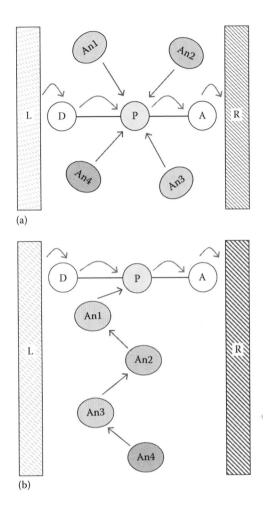

FIGURE 4.10
Schematic depicting two theoretical configurations of an artificial photosystem, which include a molecular triad comprised of (D) donor, (P) photosensitive porphyrin, (A) acceptor, and four light-harvesting complexes (An1, An2, An3, An4) inset between two electrodes (L/R). Straight red arrows indicate energy-exchange processes; curved green arrows indicate electron routing. (a) P is circumscribed by the four accessory light-harvesting antenna complexes that are directly linked to the reaction center. (b) P is interfaced to the reaction center via a single antenna complex at the end of a linear chain in a cascading energy-exchange arrangement. (Reproduced from Ghosh, P.K. et al., *Phys. Rev. E Stat. Nonlin. Soft Matter Phys.*, 84(6 Pt 1), 061138, 2011. http://pre.aps.org/abstract/PRE/v84/i6/e061138 Copyright 2011. American Physical Society. With permission.)

The light-harvesting antenna complex comprised two blue photon (λ 450 nm)-absorbing molecules (bis(phenylethynyl)anthracene) and two green photon (λ 513 nm)-absorbing molecules (boron dipyrromethene) with a quantum yield (i.e., number of reactions per photon) of 30% over a broad wavelength spectrum. The molecular triad reaction center, comprising ferrocene–porphyrin–fullerene (Fc-P-C_{60}), absorbed red photons (λ 620 nm) with a quantum yield of 90%. Intimate (~10 Å) positional proximities of the light-harvesting antenna chromophores in relation to the reaction center will result in stable/strong excitonic (Förster) coupling [73].

Werwie et al. have developed a hybrid system that coupled biological light-harvesting complexes (recombinant chlorophyll *a/b* complex II (LHCII) containing ~50 pigments) with type II core-shell CdTe/CdSe/ZnS QDs (Ø 6.2 nm), which increased the photonic utilization of the QDs considerably, particularly in the red and far-red regions of the spectrum. The addition of a dye to the biological pigment served to further enhance/expand the spectral absorptive range. The minimum donor–acceptor distance was ~5.6 nm and the maximum attainable energy transfer efficiency from the light-harvesting complex to the QD in this study was 68% [74]. In view of the possibility of an efficient nanometric hybrid organic/inorganic light-harvesting and charge separation system, it may be hypothetically feasible, for instance, that particular species of purple bacteria [75], or the unique chlorophyll *f*, found in stromatolites [76] (ancient layered structures comprised of sediment-sequestering cyanobacteria), which absorb in the near infrared/infrared might be interfaced with biocompatible near-infrared QDs (e.g., $Ag(2)S$) [77] or possibly SWCNTs, both of which have the capacity of fluorescence in the 1000–1320 nm second near-infrared region (NIR-II). These hybrid constructs might supply energy to in vivo nanodevices when irradiated by external near-infrared laser light.

Chen et al. have devised photovoltaic cells that are activated by 980 nm wavelength laser light. These films comprised "rare-earth up-converting nanophosphors" and integrated into conventional dye-sensitized solar cells. The luminescence of the nanophosphors was effectively absorbed by the dyes to produce 0.47 mW of output power. The researchers covered the photovoltaic cells with one to six layers of porcine intestinal tissue (~1 mm thickness per layer) to emulate their utility in subdermal applications. Subsequent power outputs ranging from 0.02 to 0.28 mW were achieved, which was deemed to be sufficient for the powering of in vivo medical devices. This strategy, if sufficiently downward scalable, might be plausible as an energy-generating mechanism for nanomedical devices as well [78].

Stacked TiO_2/graphene nanosheet units were studied by Yang et al. to learn if they might serve as a biomimetic analog of stacked granum structures. Granum comprises the core element in photosynthesis and contains stacks of ~10 to 100 thylakoids, which house electron acceptors and pigments. It was found that the photoelectronic kinetics of graphene was 20-fold higher in comparison to pristine TiO_2 in thin films that contained 25 stacked units. Interestingly, when these films are thicker, photocathode current is transformed to photoanode current. The functionality of the graphene is akin to that of the granum b6f complex (links Photosystem II to Photosystem I) in that it separates charges and transits electrons through the stacked layers [79]. Photonically activated power-generating modules that are configured similarly to that of the conceptual electroplax stack, described earlier, might employ ultrathin-stacked layers of TiO_2 and graphene to provide usable electron flow and power storage for the VCSN and other autonomous nanomedical devices.

4.4.5 Nanoscale Photonic Antenna

A visible light antenna, analogous to dipole antennas that receive radio waves, has been fashioned from multiwalled carbon nanotube arrays by Wang et al., which demonstrated two primary antenna effects:

1. "The polarization effect suppresses the response of an antenna when the electric field of the incoming radiation is polarized perpendicular to the dipole antenna axis."
2. "The antenna length effect maximizes the antenna response when the antenna length is a multiple of half-wavelength of the radiation" [80].

It has been found that biological entities may guide the organized configuration of light-harvesting pigments through chemically mediated linkages and/or electrostatics. Nanoscale light-harvesting antennae, investigated by Nam et al., comprised porphyrins (deep red photosensitive pigments), which were assembled on a structural template that was furnished by the M13 virus. The advantage of using viruses as templates for this application resides in the highly structured order of their protein coats. The filamentous M13 virus geometry consists of ~2700 identical α-helical coat proteins (pVIII) that are evenly arranged along its DNA, providing a coat assembly that is 6.5 nm in diameter × 880 nm in length. The researchers selected Zn(II) deuteroporphyrin IX 2,4-bis(ethylene glycol) (ZnDPEG) as the porphyrin for this study because of its well-defined optical attributes. Roughly, ~1500 to 3000 zinc porphyrins were bound to pVIII samples utilizing a carbodiimide (dehydration agent employed for carboxylic acid activation)-coupling reaction [81]. This template strategy will likely prove very useful for the self-assembly of various species of light-sensitive nanoscale antennae, as well as other energy-harvesting and -generating components, to facilitate the design of precision controls. The earlier findings may have relevance for the powering of in vivo nanodevices in that if ultrasensitive photon-harvesting/current-transferring devices can be developed they may potentially be modified to accept photons that are delivered by physiologically safe near-infrared wavelengths for conversion to electrons.

4.4.6 Graphene

Monocrystalline graphitic films (graphene) are a class of materials (2D semimetals) that may be exploited for promising applications when incorporated into nanomedical energy-harvesting/generating mechanisms. Graphene films comprise carbon atoms that are arranged in honeycomb geometry and are typically a single or a few atoms thick that can be synthesized to be of very high quality. They are metallic and stable under ambient conditions and exhibit a tiny overlap between valence and conductance bands. Novoselov et al. found that through the application of a gate voltage, mobilities of ~10,000 cm^2/Vs may be induced at room temperature. A strong ambipolar electric field effect is exhibited and electrons and holes at concentrations of up to 10^{13} cm^2 may be observed. In multilayered graphene, mobilities approaching ~15,000 cm^2/Vs at 300 K and ~60,000 cm^2/Vs at 4 K were demonstrated. By virtue of its atomic thickness, capacity for ballistic transport, and maintenance of significant currents (>10^8 A/cm^2), graphene may serve as a versatile and dynamic element in myriad advanced nanomedical energy-harvesting and -generating strategies [82].

The selective doping of atomic layered graphene with various atomic elements (Figure 4.11) can impart tunable piezoelectric attributes to the nanomaterial, which are comparable to 3D piezomaterials, through the disruption of inversion symmetry. Thus, graphene may be nanoengineered to enable dynamic control over the perhaps dedicated generation of electronic energy to various nanodevice components, which have different power requirements [83]. Ong and Reed calculated the d31 and e31 piezoelectric coefficients of graphene. These coefficients correlate in-plane strain and electrical polarization that is normal to the plane.

4.4.7 Graphene Oxide Acoustic Energy Harvesting

A highly efficient and flexible nanogenerator based on graphene derivative, graphene oxide (GO), was developed by Que et al., which utilized functional groups that included oxygen to endow GO with the capacities of harvesting acoustic energy and sequestering charge. The structure of GO encompasses carbonaceous hexagonal rings that house both sp^2- and sp^3-hybridized carbon atoms that contain functional hydroxyl and epoxide groups

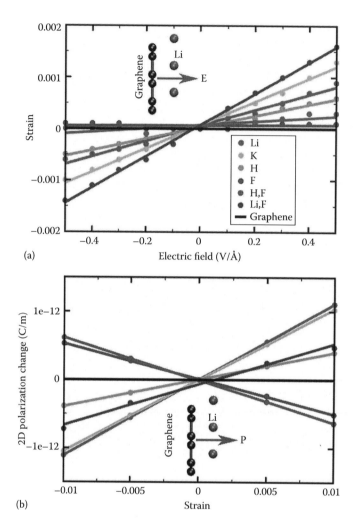

FIGURE 4.11

(a) A perpendicularly applied electric field induces an equibiaxial strain in the normal plane of the graphene sheet, resulting in a linear association between low field strain and the electric field. The d31 piezoelectric coefficient is derived from this slope. Inset depicts positive electric field direction. (b) The application to graphene of equibiaxial in-plane strain initiates the modification of the perpendicular-to-sheet polarization. The relative linear e31 piezoelectric coefficient slope × 2 is found at low strains. (Reprinted with permission from Ong, M.T. and Reed, E.J., *ACS Nano.*, 6(2), 1387. Copyright 2012 American Chemical Society.)

on basal planes. In addition, carbonyl and carboxyl groups reside at sheet edges. The electronic and chemical attributes of the GO can be altered considerably by virtue of its integrated functional groups [84,85]. The efficiency of the nanogenerator in the conversion of acoustic energy to electricity was 12.1%. This value was intimately related to the pH of the suspension that was employed in the synthesis of the GO films.

The GO film sample was induced to oscillate on exposure of the acoustic vibrations that were supplied by a tuning fork, which produced a sustained absolute alternating current of ~3.23 nA with a signal-to-noise ratio of over 1000. A clear indicator of the sensitivity of the film to acoustic activation was that ambient background noise generated a detectable current of ~2.9 pA. Further experimentation revealed that no current was generated in a reference device, or an identical device that comprised graphene; hence, it was the charged GO film that initiated current flow. Also, current was generated, no matter whether the GO film was negatively or positively charged [86].

4.4.8 Hydrostatic Streaming Currents/Nanofluidics

An intriguing discovery involved the production of a streaming electric current via hydrostatic pressure when a liquid, in this case water, was forced through micropores (Ø 10–16 μm) within a 3 mm thick glass filter, imparting opposite charge properties to each end of the pores. Yang et al. achieved an external current of 1–2 μA under a 30 cm pressure drop. The current output could be increased via the configuration of an array of micropores that are connected to a load and the use of solutions that contain higher concentrations of sodium [87].

If nanotubes might be utilized as the nanopore entities and arranged as ordered monolayers, a directed and pressurized liquid input might emulate these phenomena to perhaps generate enough electron flow to power a nanomedical device. It was confirmed experimentally by Ghosh et al. that an electric current could be generated by the fluid that flows past a bundle of SWCNTs that had a median diameter of 1.5 nm. The magnitude of the current was dependent on the ionic conductivity and polar nature of the liquid. The investigators found that in water at a flow rate of 0.3 m/s, the voltage generated was 3.2 mV. They explain that the primary mechanism for this capability may involve "a direct forcing of the free charge carriers in the nanotubes by the fluctuating coulombic field of the liquid flowing past the nanotubes." The basis proposed is that of "pulsating asymmetric ratchets," where charge fluctuations are generated by the flow at the surfaces of the nanotubes, as well as the presence of an electric double layer at the interface of the electrolyte and microchannel walls [88]. Potential power generated in this way would be worthy of exploration when the nanotubes are immersed within biological fluids.

4.5 Proposed Research Tasking List: VCSN Power-Harvesting/Generating Component

Following is a list of preliminary suggestions, considerations, and relevant questions as relates to perceived areas of investigation toward the design of exemplar VCSN energy-harvesting and -generating mechanisms.

4.5.1 Glucose Conversion Membrane

1. Create a molecular database for the purposes of elucidating the specific properties (e.g., location of reaction center(s), electronic profile, spatial configuration) of potential in vivo biofuel candidates, along with the candidate enzymes that might catalyze these molecules for the extraction of electrons.

2. Source and configure an appropriate molecular simulation software program toward the investigation, and visualization of proposed in vivo energy-harvesting and/or -generating mechanisms and strategies.

3. Develop a materials library/database that is specific to this task (e.g., list and define specific properties and model molecular structures of materials that exhibit both biocompatibility and either conductive, semiconductive, or insulating electronic attributes).

4. Generate a blood chemistry and blood type reference library/database complete with specific 3D graphics representations of all whole blood/plasma constituents (e.g., every species of cell and molecular entity that nanodevices are likely to encounter in vivo, for use in investigative computer modeling and simulations). Note: this work will be relevant and applicable to the visualization of the functionality of various aspects of many VCSN components and systems, as well as the study of any future in vivo nanomedical device components.

5. Calculate current density estimates for the optimal and sustained operation of each potential VCSN component and cumulative systems to arrive at a projected total current density requirement for the nanodevice. Extrapolations of values from macro/microscale models and simulations of these entities may assist in the determination of these estimates.

6. Investigate projected energy storage capacities for the VCSN device. Develop preliminary conceptual designs for efficient nanometric energy storage.

7. Conceptualize and design monolayer layouts, integrating various nanopore geometries and distributions, as well as topographical configurations that might provide large surface areas (enabling increased molecular biofuel turnover) on ultrathin film laminations.

8. Conceptualize and design layouts that would integrate the constituents of ultrathin film layer laminations and their specific configurations with a focus to optimizing electron/current flow in the system. This task might include the elucidation of individual monolayer dynamics (e.g., conductive, semiconductive, and insulating); strategies for integrated monolayer operation (electron conveyance from layer to layer); routing required for interlayer connectivity; potential nanopore geometries to potentially enhance functionality; and the strategic placement of electrical contacts (in the context of overall device design schemes).

9. Design conceptual layout of an integrated nanoelectronic insulating barrier that would separate anode and cathode to ensure the prevention of electron tunneling. Elucidate the minimum material thickness that may be attainable using different materials, while still maintaining optimal operating conditions.

10. Investigate materials that would be best suited for use as a nanoelectronic insulating barrier to isolate anode and cathode ultrathin film layers. Possibilities might include hydrogels, aerogels, band insulators such as crystalline Si, C, etc., due to the Pauli's exclusion principle [89], or Mott insulators [90] due to coulomb blockade [91].

11. Design conceptual layout of an integrated nanoelectronic voltage-gate junction. This gate might serve as a toggle for the initiation and suspension of electron flow to the spatial data acquisition mechanisms and other integrated VCSN components.

12. Investigate materials that may be appropriate for utilization as a nanoelectronic voltage gate. Calculate the required voltage threshold obtainable prior to the initialization of robust electron release through ultrathin film layers.

13. Explore external signal source candidates (e.g., radio frequencies, ultrasonics, magnetics, photonics) that might be employed to specifically toggle nanometric voltage-gate mechanisms.

14. Investigate and catalog the molecular geometries, and elucidate the sustained structural integrity of biocompatible materials with electronic functionality,

when they are synthesized as ultrathin films and are immersed in biological fluids (e.g., whole blood) for a 24 h period.

15. Identify and simulate potential fabrication strategies that may be best employed for the synthesis of ultrathin film configurations using these materials.

16. Conduct computer simulations to elucidate the optimal number and geometric configurations (e.g., specific topography, nanopore distribution) of ultrathin film layers that might be required to immobilize various enzymes while exhibiting the capacity for robust electron/current flow at the nanoscale.

17. Quantify the minimum thickness that may be attained with ultrathin film monolayers while retaining mechanical stability and exhibiting attributes as reliable conductors, semiconductors, and insulators.

18. Identify the full range of nanopore sizes, morphological parameters, and molecular scale coatings (e.g., silane-coupling agents) that may accommodate selected enzymes for immobilization within ultrathin film laminations.

19. Investigate the current density output of a 1000 μm × 1000 μm × 10 μm thick membranous test strip utilizing selected enzymes and biocompatible ultrathin film material combinations. Extrapolate the resulting data as relates to the estimated external real estate that might be dedicated to the generation of energy for the VCSN.

20. Fabricate trial samples of diamondoid, carbon mesh, sapphire, various polymers, and other selected ultrathin film materials (solid and nanoporous). These samples could incorporate gradated thicknesses and an appropriate range of nanopore diameters and might facilitate the discovery of intimate molecular properties and the overall potential viability of these thin films as both viable electron conveyance entities and biocompatible interfacial organic/inorganic materials.

21. Develop variously doped configurations of these thin films for specific investigations into their "tunable" electronic properties and optimal electron flow/dispersion rates.

22. Identify specific synthesis techniques that will result in the highest quality ultrathin films achievable at angstrom level thicknesses.

23. Investigate the most effective techniques for creating ultrathin films with controllable geometries and configurations of nanopores (e.g., laser, electron beam, ion beam sculpting, self-assembly of distinct nanoporous entities).

24. Study electron current flow pathways and patterns in solid and nanoporous ultrathin film monolayers (pure and doped) and multiple laminated thin films. Explore possible methods by which to enhance, diminish, direct, and otherwise manipulate a usable electron flow.

25. Investigate possible molecular coating chemistries for both anode and cathode electrodes that might have affinities for targeted biofuel molecules. Explore the means for potentially enhancing the adherence qualities between conductive thin film layers and enzymatic reaction centers. This molecular coating should be completely nontoxic and exhibit no potential for negative bioreactivity.

26. Isolate optimum chemistries of these bioattractant coatings for both anode and cathode.

27. Identify specific enzymes and any other relevant molecular species that might exhibit the most favorable capacity for attracting and effectively catalyzing glucose molecules. Explore these attributes as relates to carboxylic acid, carbohydrates, starch, and lactate molecules as well.

28. Investigate and define the precise location, orientation, and configuration of the reaction centers of selected enzyme species, and model these geometries for 3D simulation studies.

29. Investigate potential molecular docking/undocking modes (e.g., adherence, reaction, and release) and inherent reaction center kinetics to develop possible strategies for controlled physical access to these reactive sites.

30. Evolve optimal operational methodologies and the design of nanometric tool tips/contacts for tapping into these molecular reaction centers toward the achievement of the highest possible rate of electron extraction/power output.

31. Measure and chart the energy flow produced by a single glucose molecule (and other isolated molecular biofuel candidates) as they adhere to and are catalyzed by each of the selected enzyme species.

32. Explore the precise mechanisms by which glucose molecules (and other potential biofuel molecules) adsorb to, are catalyzed by, and dissociate from various selected enzyme species and functionalized surfaces. Elucidate individual and cumulative throughput times for these sequential events.

33. Investigate strategies for organizing, introducing, guiding, interfacing (e.g., self-assembly techniques), and immobilizing the reaction centers of selected enzymes within the nanopores embedded in ultrathin film monolayers, as well as multiple nanopores within various laminated ultrathin film substrates.

34. Investigate and generate possible concepts and strategies for energy-harvesting/generating membrane biofouling countermeasures.

35. Investigate methods for attracting targeted biofuel molecules, while keeping other blood-borne constituents (biofilms) from adsorbing to and congesting/degrading the functional efficiency of the catalyzing surface.

36. Devise potential strategies for increasing the transitory population density of biofuel molecules (e.g., larger surface area, varied/stacked nanopore arrangements, etc.) on the catalyzing surface.

37. Investigate and quantify the concentration of glucose molecules that adhere to various catalytic surfaces while immersed in normal human whole blood per defined surface areas.

38. Investigate what the maximum population densities of enzymes or synthetic nanoscale catalysts might be (for selected species) when they are nested as arrays on the surfaces of thin films/membranes with a test area of 1 cm² in the determination of optimal configurations and concentrations that may enable robust catalytic capabilities, with the aim of producing optimal free electron flow.

39. Study how the distribution/spacing of enzymes or synthetic nanoscale catalysts affects catalytic efficiencies when they are exposed to selected biofuels.

40. Investigate interfacial behaviors and molecular kinetics when a single nanotube, nanohorn, or nanowire tip/probe is brought into contact (at selected docking points)

with a glucose molecule? Will simple contact initiate any level of electron transition into and through these entities?

41. Quantify similar attributes when isolated nanotubes, nanohorns, or nanowire tips are contacted with other selected enzymes and biofuel molecules.

42. Discover whether selected catalytic enzymes or nanoparticle catalysts might be immobilized within carbon nanotubes.

43. Might nanotubes comprised of other materials facilitate the extraction of electrons from glucose, or other potential biofuel molecules?

44. If so, may these nanotubes be aligned and aggregated so as to form a monolayer?

45. Investigate whether C_{60} or any other members of the fullerene family might be useful in facilitating the immobilization or encapsulation of selected catalytic enzymes or nanoparticles, while allowing accessibility and the retention of their catalytic attributes.

46. Investigate whether nanotubes, nanohorns, nanowires, or a species of fullerene might be utilized as enzymatic reaction center "conduits" for the potential elicitation and initiation of electron conveyance.

4.5.2 Nanoscale Thermodynamic Mechanisms

1. Compile a materials library/database that is specific to this task (e.g., define specific properties and model molecular geometries of all known thermodynamic materials that exhibit the potential for thermal conductivity and insulating functionality, which may be fabricated as ultrathin films). This might prove to be a useful resource in the elucidation of specific molecular interactions between these materials via 3D computer simulations.

2. Investigate and record all possible and plausible thermodynamic conducting and insulating combinations with the aim of finding the best candidates for the possible generation of robust, reliable, and controllable electron flow at the nanoscale, via the Seebeck effect.

3. Develop computer algorithms to facilitate investigations of molecular bonding kinetics, thermal properties, and free energy profiles at selected material interfaces.

4. Select thermodynamic materials, based on preliminary investigations, which will retain their functionality when they are scaled down to the nanometric domain.

5. Investigate the behavior of nanoshells with spherical and other geometries, comprised of metallic (e.g., Au, Ag, Pt, Pd) skins, and solid or hollow cores consisting of various materials (e.g., silica, conductive polymers), when they are embedded within selected heat-resistant materials, and connected to an output electrode. When the nanoshells are activated into plasmon resonance via near-infrared light, quantify the temperature differential between the two materials, whether the Seebeck effect might be initiated, and to what extent.

6. Continue this line of investigation while methodically varying nanoshell metallic wall thicknesses and core dimensions. Substitute nanoshell skin materials, cores, and insulating substrates, and test novel configurations of single-sandwiched and multi-stratified nanoshell/insulator layers, as well as various nanoshell packing densities. Investigate optimal dimensions/geometries and material combinations

that might contribute to a robust, sustainable, and potentially controllable electron flow output.

7. Investigate the hyperthermic behavior of various magnetic nanoparticles with different compositions (e.g., Fe_3O_4, $CoFe_2O_4$, SPIONs) and morphologies toward the identification of optimal candidates that may be embedded within thermoresistant materials to potentially generate voltage via the Seebeck effect.

8. Explore by what means the resulting electron flow might be tapped into and extracted via nanowires, nanotubes, etc., to potentially convey and route power to VCSN components.

9. Investigate the most effective and least invasive methods for external "outbody" activation and control of thermally conductive and insulating nanomaterials when they are immersed in trial biofluids (whole blood/plasma) and activated by ultrasound, near-infrared photonics, and magnetic fields.

10. Investigate and define preliminary safe operating parameters for proposed in vivo thermally activated power-generating mechanisms.

11. Source and investigate potential extremophilic and thermophilic organisms and microorganisms with the aim of incorporating biomimetically analogous attributes that may be of utility in the potential development of viable nanoscale thermoelectric conversion mechanisms.

12. Might the Seebeck effect be initiated by employing the nominal human core temperature as the high end (hot-side) thermal base that would transfer heat to an extremely "thermophilic" nanomaterial, which is interfaced with a very "thermophobic" (cold-side) nanomaterial?

13. Through experimentation with several of the most promising strategies for the thermal generation of electron flow, find optimal electron outputs for a 100 μm^2 test surface area for each. Subsequently, attempt to further reduce the dimensions of the test area down to 1 μm^2.

14. Quantify the minimal thickness of optimized aerogel material that might be possible while still maintaining its unique thermal insulating properties. Might a thin aerogel membrane be utilized as a potent enough barrier between two thermally disparate materials to maintain the required differentiation for the initiation of the Seebeck effect? Could the aerogel itself serve as the cold side of such a system?

4.5.3 Piezoelectric Entities

1. Assemble a complete molecular structural library of all known piezonanomaterials that exhibit electron generation via mechanical flexing with potential for power generation at the nanoscale.

2. Apply a selection process to these materials (e.g., lead zirconium titanate, lithium miobate, ZnO, metalized silicon nitride) to discern which materials might have the best potential for robust and reliable power generation via externally activated flexing.

3. Investigate potential activation signals (ultrasound, photonics, magnetic fields, etc.) that exhibit the strongest capacity for the instantaneous and robust activation of mechanical flexure in the generation of electron flow using these piezonanomaterials.

4. Select the best potential candidate combinations of activation signals and piezonanomaterials.

5. Devise a benchtop test bed apparatus that emulates the in vivo conditions of the human vasculature, with an internalized testing stage, to elucidate how signal propagation and material responses are affected when piezonanomaterials are immersed within an opaque aqueous environment (whole blood), and observe their potential effectiveness for the generation of usable electron flow under these conditions.

6. Investigate, via computer modeling, how signal conveyance might be affected between external activation sources and internalized mobile piezonanomaterials (e.g., nominal status of the VCSN as it traverses the human vasculature), and if they may have possible thermal influence, contingent on piezoelement concentrations, on simulated human core temperature. Develop a perceived safe operating range, estimated signal envelopes, and signal intensity parameters for various signal activation and piezonanomaterial combinations.

7. Develop in vitro experimentation to discover if any deleterious effects may be caused by selected (pulsed vs. sustained) signals, within estimated safe operating parameters, on blood-borne cells, tissue cells, proteins, etc., and if these bio-entities might initiate signal distortion or diminishment.

8. Investigate what the maximum operating parameters and ultrasonic outputs are for selected piezomaterials and determine what the potential maximum voltage output per μm^2 might be for each material within these parameters.

4.5.4 Biomimetic Electrocytes and Electroplax Stacks

1. Investigate the molecular configurations, electron flow kinetics, and specific functionality of electrocyte cells from the freshwater electric eel (*E. electricus*) and the seawater (*T. nobiliana*) electric ray. The aim would be for the potential development of a biomimetic electroplax stack that might utilize the manipulation and control of sodium and potassium ion concentrations to chemically generate free electron flow.

2. Create highly detailed computer graphic renderings (molecular models) of electrocyte cell active subunits, as well as fully assembled electroplax stacks, for applications in functional kinetics studies and for use as a design aid.

3. Investigate materials that might possibly be utilized as active substrates and study potential optimal geometries (e.g., nanopore configurations, nanomeshes, embedded subunit entities) in an attempt to replicate the functionality of the reactive elements of an electrocyte cell.

4. Create a structure/function library that encompasses ion channel configurations, nuclear pores, blood/brain barrier molecular transit sites, cell membrane bilayers, and similar biological entities. Develop molecular models of these mechanisms to facilitate detailed investigations into the specific functions of these natural systems toward the conceptualization of potential bio-inspired energy extraction designs.

5. Study the neuron, synapse, and other constituents of human and animal nervous systems to gain an intimate knowledge of the biological signal propagation processes and self-refreshing mechanisms that might be applicable to and further enhance the development of a functional biomimetic electroplax stack.

6. Generate several conceptual designs for arrays of energy-producing units that are analogous to natural electroplax stack systems, and study how voltage/current might be generated, conveyed, and directed from these systems.

4.5.5 Biomimetic Photosynthetic Mechanisms

1. Create a structure/function library that includes molecular models of natural photosynthetic reaction centers, pigments, and accessory pigments to facilitate the design of a biomimetic photonic energy-harvesting mechanism. Investigate how electrons are generated and propagated in these natural systems with the aim of creating an analogous entity that might mimic these structures and their electron-generating activity.

2. Investigate and select inorganic material analogs that might exhibit equivalencies in functionality to natural photosynthetic reaction centers, pigments, and accessory pigments.

3. Investigate photosynthetic processes and associated molecular mechanisms in diatomic species.

4. Generate conceptual designs for potential modular test unit cells (beginning with ~1 cm^2 and reducing to ~100 μm^2) that integrate substrate, photon-harvesting mechanism, photosynthetic reactive entity, and electron conveyance infrastructure, which when combined might constitute a prototype energy-generating mechanism for the VCSN.

5. Develop strategies for channeling and intensifying the propagation of photons to a biomimetic photosynthetic unit cell, perhaps by employing an integrated light source (quantum laser activated by an "outbody" signal to potentially trigger a self-sustaining energy loop). In this scenario, arrays of photonic reaction centers might generate enough energy to power all VCSN components, as well as to provide a predetermined amount of surplus energy, which might be utilized to enable the sustained or pulsed firing of the quantum lasers into the reaction centers, thereby (hypothetically) enhancing power generation.

6. Develop a strategy whereby photonically reactive sites may be induced to sustainably generate energy, solely through activation by an external photon source (e.g., near infrared), which is deemed as safe when propagating through human tissues.

7. Investigate the most potent fluorochromes for peak emission wavelengths and sustainability of photon emission. Might these fluorochromes generate enough photonic energy to be harvested and converted into electron flow?

8. Study QDs and details of their fluorescence attributes. Might QDs be "tuned" such that they may be utilized as photon sources, when activated to fluoresce by external sources, and robust enough to engage photonic reaction centers to generate electron flow?

9. Investigate the specifics of in vivo biophotonic processes and how this particular photon-generating phenomenon might be utilized to potentially initiate electron mobility in nanomedical devices, via sequestration by nanoscale photonically sensitive entities or photomultipliers.

10. By methodically exploring the full range of photonic wavelengths, isolate the best candidates that will safely propagate through human tissues while simultaneously exhibiting robust photonic distribution in vivo, which may effectively activate photosynthetically reactive surfaces on a ~1 μm in diameter nanodevice.

4.5.6 Nanoscale PEM

1. Investigate the specific kinetics of existing fuel cell technologies to potentially extrapolate the functionality of these mechanisms at the nanometric scale.

2. Compile a library that depicts selected PEM materials and processes at the molecular level for use in computer modeling and simulation studies.

3. Investigate and fabricate PEM test strips ($\sim$1 cm^2 and $\sim$100 μm^2) that incorporate perceived optimal nanopore sizes employing, for example, nanoporous membranes, nanotube monolayers, and polymer–zeolite nanocomposites [92–95]. Quantify flow rates and electron-harvesting efficiencies that might be accomplished at the nanoscale.

4. Conceptualize and design possible mechanisms for conveying subsequently generated electrons to nanowires or other nanoelectronic component inputs.

References

1. Lodish, H., Berk, A., Zipursky, S.L., Matsudaira, P., Baltimore, D., and Darnell, J., *Molecular Cell Biology*, 4th edn. New York: W.H. Freeman, 2000.
2. Mercer, W.B., The living cell as an open thermodynamic system: Bacteria and irreversible thermodynamics, Technical Manuscript 640, Project 1B061102B71A. U.S. Army Biological Defense Research Center, May 1971.
3. Forrest, W.W. and Walker, D.S., Thermodynamics of biological growth. *Nature*. 196, 990–991, 1962.
4. Yang, J.M., Yang, H., and Lin, L., Quantum dot nano thermometers reveal heterogeneous local thermogenesis in living cells. *ACS Nano*. 5(6), 5067–5071, 2011.
5. Maestro, L.M., Rodríguez, E.M., Rodríguez, F.S., la Cruz, M.C., Juarranz, A., Naccache, R., Vetrone, F., Jaque, D., Capobianco, J.A., and Solé, J.G., CdSe quantum dots for two-photon fluorescence thermal imaging. *Nano Lett*. 10(12), 5109–5115, 2010.
6. Muller, A.W. and Schulze-Makuch, D., Thermal energy and the origin of life. *Orig Life Evol Biosph*. 36(2), 177–189, 2006.
7. Chen, T., Barton, S.C., Binyamin, G., Gao, Z., Zhang, Y., Kim, H.H., and Heller, A., A miniature biofuel cell. *J Am Chem Soc*. 123(35), 8630–8631, 2001.
8. Robert A.F. Jr., *Nanomedicine, Volume I: Basic Capabilities*. Georgetown, TX: Landes Bioscience, 1999. http://www.nanomedicine.com/NMI.htm
9. Mano, N., Mao, F., and Heller, A., A miniature biofuel cell operating in a physiological buffer. *J Am Chem Soc*. 124(44), 12962–12963, 2002.
10. Calabrese, B.S., Kim, H.H., Binyamin, G., Zhang, Y., and Heller, A., The "wired" laccase cathode: High current density electroreduction of O(2) to water at +0.7 V (NHE) at pH 5. *J Am Chem Soc*. 123(24), 5802–5803, 2001.
11. Rajagopalan, R. and Heller, A., Electrical "wiring" of glucose oxidase in electrons conducting hydrogels, *Molecular Electronics: A Chemistry for the 21st Century*, Monograph, Jortner, J. and Ratner, M. London, U.K.: Blackwell Science, 1997.
12. Sirkar, K., Revzin, A., and Pishko, M.V., Glucose and lactate biosensors based on redox polymer/oxidoreductase nanocomposite thin films. *Anal Chem*. 72(13), 2930–2936, 2000.
13. Ritter, S., Biofuel cells get smaller. *Chem Eng News*. 79(36), 10, 2001.
14. Gallaway, J.W. and Barton, S.A.C., Effect of redox polymer synthesis on the performance of a mediated laccase oxygen cathode. *J Electroanal Chem*. 626(1–2), 149–155, 2009.

15. Wen, H., Nallathambi, V., Chakraborty, D., and Barton, S.C., Carbon fiber microelectrodes modified with carbon nanotubes as a new support for immobilization of glucose oxidase. *Microchim Acta*. 175(3–4), 283–289, 2011.

16. Laurent, D. and Schlenoff, J., Multilayer assemblies of redox polyelectrolytes. *Langmuir*. 13(6), 1552–1557, 1997.

17. Pishko, M.V., Katakis, I., Lindquist, S.I., Ling Ye, Gregg, B.A., and Heller A., Direct electrical communication between graphite electrodes and surface adsorbed glucose oxidase/redox polymer complexes. *Angew Chem Int Ed Engl*. 29, 82–84, 1990.

18. Hou, S.F., Yang, K.S., Fang, H.Q., and Chen, H.Y., Amperometric glucose enzyme electrode by immobilizing glucose oxidase in multilayers on self-assembled monolayers surface. *Talanta*. 47(3), 561–567, 1998.

19. Dubas, S.T. and Schlenoff, J.B., Swelling and smoothing of polyelectrolyte multilayers by salt. *Langmuir*. 17(25), 7725–7727, 2001.

20. Fery, A., Scholer, B., Cassagneau, T., and Caruso, F., Nanoporous thin films formed by salt-induced structural changes in multilayers of poly(acrylic acid) and poly(allylamine). *Langmuir*. 17(13), 3779–3783, 2001.

21. Hammond, P.T. and Whitesides, G.M., Formation of polymer microstructures by selective deposition of polyion multilayers using patterned self-assembled monolayers as a template. *Macromolecules*. 28(22), 7569–7571, 1995.

22. Sukhorikov, G.B., Schmitt, J., and Decher, G., Reversible swelling of polyanion/polycation multilayer films in solutions of different ionic strength. *Ber Bunsenges Phys Chem*. 100(6), 948–953, 1996.

23. Pishko, M.V., Revzin, A., and Simonian, A.L., Mass transfer in amperometric biosensors based on nanocomposite thin films of redox polymers and oxidoreductases. *Sensors*. 2(3), 79–90, 2002.

24. Farabee, M.J., ATP and biological energy. http://www.emc.maricopa.edu/faculty/farabee/BIOBK/BioBookATP.html (accessed April 16, 2012).

25. Montemagno, C.D., Nanomachines: A roadmap for realizing the vision. *J Nanoparticle Res*. 3(1), 1–3, 2001.

26. Montemagno, C.D. and Bachand, G.D., Constructing nanomechanical devices powered by biomolecular motors. *Nanotechnology*. 10(3), 225–331, 1999.

27. Bachand, G.D. and Montemagno, C.D., Constructing organic/inorganic NEMS devices powered by biomolecular motors. *Biomed Microdev*. 2(3), 179–184, 2000.

28. Sakai, T., Matsuoka, M., and Iwakura, C., Rare earth metallics for metal-hydrogen batteries. *Handbook on the Physics and Chemistry of Rare Earths*, Gschneider, K.A. Jr. and Eyring, L., eds. New York: Elsevier, Vol. 21, p. 133, 1995.

29. Schlapbach, L., Zuttel, A., Gröning, P., Gröning, O., and Aebi, P., Hydrogen for novel materials and devices. *Appl Phys A*. 72(2), 245–253, 2001.

30. Brewer, K.J., Elvington, M., and Miao, R., Photochemical reactivity of mixed-metal supramolecular complexes: Applications as photochemical molecular devices, *228th American Chemical Society National Meeting*. Philadelphia, PA, August 21–26, 2004.

31. Biffinger, J.C., Ray, R., Little, B., and Ringeisen, B.R., Diversifying biological fuel cell designs by use of nanoporous filters. *Environ Sci Technol*. 41(4), 1444–1449, 2007.

32. Bullen, R.A., Arnot, T.C., Lakeman, J.B., and Walsh, F.C., Biofuel cells and their development. *Biosens Bioelectron*. 21(11), 2015–2045, 2006.

33. Palmore, G.T.R. and Whitesides, G.M., Microbial and enzymic biofuel cells. *ACS Symp Ser*. 566, 271–290, 1994.

34. Nealson, K.H., Belz, A., and McKee, B., Breathing metals as a way of life: Geobiology in action. *Antonie Van Leeuwenhoek*. 81, 215–222, 2002.

35. Xie, X., Hu, L., Pasta, M., Wells, G.F., Kong, D., Criddle, C.S., and Cui, Y., Three-dimensional carbon nanotube-textile anode for high-performance microbial fuel cells. *Nano Lett*. 11(1), 291–296, 2011.

36. Logan, B.E., Exoelectrogenic bacteria that power microbial fuel cells. *Nat Rev Microbiol*. 7(5), 375–381, 2009.

37. Gorby, Y.A., Yanina, S., McLean, J.S., Rosso, K.M., Moyles, D., Dohnalkova, A., Beveridge, T.J., Chang, I.S., Kim, B.H., Kim, K.S., Culley, D.E., Reed, S.B., Romine, M.F., Saffarini, D.A., Hill, E.A., Shi, L., Elias, D.A., Kennedy, D.W., Pinchuk, G., Watanabe, K., Ishii, S., Logan, B., Nealson, K.H., and Fredrickson, J.K., Electrically conductive bacterial nanowires produced by *Shewanella oneidensis* strain MR-1 and other microorganisms. *Proc Natl Acad Sci USA*. 103(30), 11358–11363, 2006.

38. Chaudhuri, S.K. and Lovley, D.R., Electricity generation by direct oxidation of glucose in mediatorless microbial fuel cells. *Nat Biotechnol*. 21(10), 1229–1232, 2003.

39. Pham, T., Jackson, J.B., Halas, N.J., and Lee, T.R., Preparation and characterization of gold nanoshells coated with self-assembled monolayers. *Langmuir*. 18(12), 4915, 2002.

40. Kimmel, J., Thermoelectric materials. Physics, Special Topics Paper, 152, 1999.

41. Wang, Z.L. and Song, J., Piezoelectric nanogenerators based on zinc oxide nanowire arrays. *Science*. 312(5771), 242–246, 2006.

42. Huang, C.T., Song, J., Tsai, C.M., Lee, W.F., Lien, D.H., Gao, Z., Hao, Y., Chen, L.J., and Wang, Z.L., Single-InN-nanowire nanogenerator with up to 1 V output voltage. *Adv Mater*. 22(36), 4008–4013, 2010.

43. Lin Y.F., Song, J.H., Ding, Y., Lu, S.H., and Wang, Z.L., Piezoelectric using CdS nanowires. *Appl Phys Lett*. 92, 022105, 2008.

44. Hoon, J.J., Lee, M., Hong, J.I., Ding Y., Chen, C.Y., Chou, L.J., and Wang, Z.L., Lead-free NaNbO$_3$ nanowires for a high output piezoelectric nanogenerator. *ACS Nano*. 5(12), 10041–10046, 2011.

45. Tang, H., Lin, Y., Andrews, C., and Sodano, H.A., Nanocomposites with increased energy density through high aspect ratio PZT nanowires. *Nanotechnology*. 22(1), 015702, 2011.

46. Cha, S., Kim, S.M., Kim, H., Ku, J., Sohn, J.I., Park, Y.J., Song, B.G., Jung, M.H., Lee, E.K., Choi, B.L., Park, J.J., Wang, Z.L., Kim, J.M., and Kim, K., Porous PVDF as effective sonic wave driven nanogenerators. *Nano Lett*. 11(12), 5142–5147, 2011.

47. Perçin, G. and Khuri-Yakub, B.T., Piezoelectrically actuated flex tensional micromachined ultrasound transducers. *Ultrasonics*. 40(1–8), 441–448, 2002.

48. Zhang, H.F., Wang, C.M., Buck, E.C., and Wang, L.S., Synthesis, characterization, and manipulation of helical SiO$_2$ nanosprings Zhang. *Nano Lett (Commun)*. 3(5), 577–580, 2003.

49. Qi, Y., Jafferis, N.T., Lyons, K. Jr., Lee, C.M., Ahmad, H., and McAlpine, M.C., Piezoelectric ribbons printed onto rubber for flexible energy conversion. *Nano Lett*. 10(2), 524–528, 2010.

50. Flynn, A.M. and Sanders, S.R., Fundamental limits on energy transfer and circuit considerations for piezoelectric transformers. *IEEE Trans Power Electron*. 17(1), 8–14, 2002.

51. Park, K.I., Lee, M., Liu, Y., Moon, S., Hwang, G.T., Zhu, G., Kim, J.E., Kim, S.O., Kim, D.K., Wang, Z.L., and Lee, K.J., Flexible Nanocomposite generator made of BaTiO(3) nanoparticles and graphitic carbons. *Adv Mater*. 24(22), 2999–3004, 2012.

52. Noda, M., Shimizu, S., Tanabe, T., Takai, T., Kayano, T., Ikeda, T., Takahashi, H., Nakayama, H., Kanaoka, Y., and Minamino, N., Primary structure of *Electrophorus electricus* sodium channel deduced from cDNA sequence. *Nature*. 312(5990), 121–127, 1984.

53. Miller, C. and White, M.M., Dimeric structure of single chloride channels from Torpedo electroplax. *Proc Natl Acad Sci USA*. 81(9), 2772–2775, 1984.

54. Gotter, A.L., Kaetzel, M.A., and Dedman, J.R., *Electrophorus electricus* as a model system for the study of membrane excitability. *Comp Biochem Physiol A Mol Integr Physiol*. 119(1), 225–241, 1998.

55. Nachmansohn, D., *Chemical and Molecular Basis of Nerve Activity*. New York: Academic Press, 1959.

56. Crespo, G.A., Macho, S., and Rius, F.X., Ion-selective electrodes using carbon nanotubes as ion-to-electron transducers. *Anal Chem*. 80(4), 1316–1322, 2008.

57. Crespo, G.A., Macho, S., Bobacka, J., and Rius, F.X., Transduction mechanism of carbon nanotubes in solid-contact ion-selective electrodes. *Anal Chem*. 81(2), 676–681, 2009.

58. Bobacka, J., Ivaska, A., and Lewenstam, A., Potentiometric ion sensors. *Chem Rev*. 108(2), 329–351, 2008.

59. Xu, J. and Lavan, D.A., Designing artificial cells to harness the biological ion concentration gradient. *Nat Nanotechnol*. 3(11), 666–670, 2008.

60. Novell, M., Parilla, M., Crespo, G.A., Rius, F.X., and Andrade, F.J., Paper based ion-selective potentiometric sensors. *Anal Chem.* 84(11), 4695–4702, 2012.
61. Piotrowski, H., Polborn, K., Hilt, G., and Severin, K., A self-assembled metallomacrocyclic iono-phore with high affinity and selectivity for Li+ and Na+. *J Am Chem Soc.* 123(11), 2699–2700, 2001.
62. Piotrowski, H., Hilt, G., Schulz, A., Mayer, P., Polborn, K., and Severin, K., Self-assembled organometallic [12] metallacrown-3 complexes. *Chemistry.* 7(15), 3196–3208, 2001.
63. Walton, D.J. and Hall C.E., Functional dopants in conducting polymers. *Synth Metals.* 45(3), 363–371, 1991.
64. Blankenship, R.E., *Molecular Mechanisms of Photosynthesis.* Oxford: Blackwell Science, 2001.
65. Gust, D., Moore, T.A., and Moore, A.L., Mimicking photosynthetic solar energy transduction. *Acc Chem Res.* 34(1), 40–48, 2001.
66. Bhat, V. and Domen, K., *Electron Transfer in Chemistry*, Balzani, V., ed. Weinheim, Germany: Wiley-VCH, Vol. 4, 487, 2001.
67. (a) Kaschak, D.M., Lean, J.T., Waraksa, C.C., Saupe, G.B., Usami, H., and Mallouk, T.E., Photoinduced energy and electron transfer reactions in lamellar polyanion/polycation thin films: Toward an inorganic "leaf." *J Am Chem Soc.* 121, 3435–3445, 1999. (b) Kaschak, D.M., Johnson, S.A., Waraksa, C.C., Pogue, J., and Mallouk, T.E., Artificial photosynthesis in lamellar assemblies of metal poly(pyridyl) complexes and metalloporphyrins. *Coord Chem Rev.* 185–186, 403–416, 1999.
68. Balzani, V., Venturi, M., and Credi, A., *Molecular Devices and Machines, A Journey into the Nanoworld.* Weinheim, Germany: Wiley-VCH, 2003.
69. Vaidyalingam, A.S., Coutant, M.A., and Dutta, P.K., *Electron Transfer in Chemistry*, Balzani, V., ed. Weinheim, Germany: Wiley-VCH, Vol. 4, 412, 2001.
70. (a) Fukuzumi, S., Urano, T., and Suenobu, T., Photoinduced charge-separation using 10-meth-ylacridinium ion loaded in Zeolite Y as a photocatalyst with negligible back electron transfer across the zeolite-solution interface. *J Chem Soc Chem Commun.* 213–214, 1996. (b) Sykora, M. and Kinkaid, J.R., Photochemical energy storage in a spatially organized zeolite-based photore-dox system. *Nature.* 387, 162–164, 1997.
71. Corma, A., Fornés, V., Galletero, M.S., García, H., and Scaiano, J.C., Evidence for through-framework electron transfer in intrazeolite photochemistry. Case of Ru(bpy)3(2+) and methyl-viologen in novel delaminated ITQ-2 zeolite. *Chem Commun (Camb).* 4, 334–335, 2002.
72. Ranjit, K.T. and Kevan, L., Photoreduction of methylviologen in Zeolite X. *J Phys Chem B.* 106, 1104–1109, 2002.
73. Ghosh, P.K., Smirnov, A.Y., and Nori, F., Artificial photosynthetic reaction centers coupled to light-harvesting antennas. *Phys Rev E Stat Nonlin Soft Matter Phys.* 84(6 Pt 1), 061138, 2011.
74. Werwie, M., Xu, X., Haase, M., Basché, T., and Paulsen, H., Bio serves nano: Biological light-harvesting complex as energy donor for semiconductor quantum dots. *Langmuir.* 28(13), 5810–5818, 2012.
75. McLuskey, K., Prince, S.M., Cogdell, R.J., and Isaacs, N.W., The crystallographic structure of the B800-820 LH3 light-harvesting complex from the purple bacteria *Rhodopseudomonas acidophila* strain 7050. *Biochemistry.* 40(30), 8783–8789, 2001.
76. Chen, M., Schliep, M., Willows, R.D., Cai, Z.L., Neilan, B.A., and Scheer, H., A red-shifted chlorophyll. *Science.* 329(5997), 1318–1319, 2010.
77. Zhang, Y., Hong, G., Zhang, Y., Chen, G., Li, F., Dai, H., and Wang, Q., Ag(2)S quantum dot: A bright and biocompatible fluorescent nanoprobe in the second near-infrared window. *ACS Nano.* 6(5), 3695–3702, 2012.
78. Chen, Z., Zhang, L., Sun, Y., Hu, J., and Wang, D., 980-nm laser-driven photovoltaic cells based on rare-earth up-converting phosphors for biomedical applications. *Adv Funct Mater.* 19(23), 3815–3820, 2009.
79. Yang, N., Zhang, Y., Halpert, J.E., Zhai, J., Wang, D., and Jiang, L., Granum-like stacking struc-tures with TiO(2)-graphene nanosheets for improving photo-electric conversion. *Small.* 8(11), 1762–1770, 2012.

80. Wang, Y., Kempa, K., Kimball, B., Carlson, J.B., Benham, G., Li, W.Z., Kempa, T., Rybczynski, J., Herczynski, A., and Ren, Z.F., Receiving and transmitting light-like radio waves antenna effect in arrays of aligned carbon nanotubes. *Appl Phys Lett.* 85(13), 2607–2609, 2004.
81. Nam, Y.S., Shin, T., Park, H., Magyar, A.P., Choi, K., Fantner, G., Nelson, K.A., and Belcher, A.M., Virus-templated assembly of porphyrins into light-harvesting nanoantennae. *J Am Chem Soc.* 132(5), 1462–1463, 2010.
82. Novoselov, K.S., Geim, A.K., Morozov, S.V., Jiang, D., Zhang, Y., Dubonos, S.V., Grigorieva, I.V., and Firsov, A.A., Electric field effect in atomically thin carbon films. *Science.* 306(5696), 666–669, 2004.
83. Ong, M.T. and Reed, E.J., Engineered piezoelectricity in graphene. *ACS Nano.* 6(2), 1387–1394, 2012.
84. Jung, I., Dikin, D.A., Piner, R.D., and Ruoff, R.S., Tunable electrical conductivity of individual graphene oxide sheets reduced at "low" temperatures. *Nano Lett.* 8(12), 4283–4287, 2008.
85. Johari, P. and Shenoy, V.B., Modulating optical properties of graphene oxide: Role of prominent functional groups. *ACS Nano.* 5(9), 7640–7647, 2011.
86. Que, R., Shao, Q., Li, Q., Shao, M., Cai, S., Wang, S., and Lee, S.T., Flexible nanogenerators based on graphene oxide films for acoustic energy harvesting. *Angew Chem Int Ed Engl.* 51(22), 5418–5422, 2012.
87. Yang, J., Lu, F., Kostiuk, L.W., and Kwok, D.Y., Electrokinetic microchannel battery by means of electrokinetic and microfluidic phenomena. *J Micromech Microeng.* 13, 963–970, 2003.
88. Ghosh, S., Sood, A.K., and Kumar, N., Carbon nanotube flow sensors. *Science.* 299(5609), 1042–1044, 2003.
89. Freire, J.A. and Voss, G., Master equation approach to charge injection and transport in organic insulators. *J Chem Phys.* 122(12), 124705, 2005.
90. Sabeth, F., Iimori, T., and Ohta, N., Insulator–metal transitions induced by electric field and photoirradiation in organic Mott insulator deuterated κ-(BEDT-TTF)(2)Cu[N(CN)(2)]Br. *J Am Chem Soc.* 134(16), 6984–6986, 2012.
91. Cho, S., Kim, D., Syers, P., Butch, N.P., Paglione, J., and Fuhrer, M.S., Topological insulator quantum dot with tunable barriers. *Nano Lett.* 12(1), 469–472, 2012.
92. Biffinger, J.C., Ray, R., Little, B., and Ringeisen, B.R., Diversifying biological fuel cell designs by use of nanoporous filters. *Environ Sci Technol.* 41(4), 1444–1449, 2007.
93. Wang, C., Waje, M., Wang, X., Tang, J.M., Haddon, R.C., and Yan, Y., Proton exchange membrane fuel cells with carbon nanotube based electrodes. *Nano Lett.* 4, 345–348, 2004.
94. Girishkumar, G., Rettker, M., Underhile, R., Binz, D., Vinodgopal, K., McGinn, P., and Kamat, P., Single-wall carbon nanotube-based proton exchange membrane assembly for hydrogen fuel cells. *Langmuir.* 21(18), 8487–8494, 2005.
95. Yan, Y., *Polymer–Zeolite Nanocomposite High Temperature Proton Exchange Membrane for Fuel Cells.* Sacramento, CA: California Energy Commission (CEC), 1999.

5

Design Challenges and Considerations for Nanomedical Electronic Entities and Infrastructure

Frank J. Boehm

CONTENTS

5.1 Nanoelectronic Infrastructure

Nanoelectronic infrastructures for nanomedical devices such as the vascular cartographic scanning nanodevice (VCSN) might comprise various nanoscale electronic elements, analogous in functionality to counterpart components that are utilized in macroscale electronic devices. This embedded nanometric circuitry would consist of nanoparticles, nanowires, transistors, resistors, voltage gates, capacitors, switches, amplifiers, along with standardized connection formats. This nanocircuitry will organize and convey harvested or generated electron flow to and from all VCSN components and subcomponents. A solid-state quantum computing entity (Chapter 7) would reside as the heart of the VCSN, serve as a secondary control mechanism for the nanodevice, and play a vital role in the management of onboard nanoelectronics. Primary control will reside within "outbody" computers. Several layers of redundancy might be designed into the nanoelectronic infrastructure to ensure reliable and robust operational integrity. Additional attributes will include integrated safety parameter protocols, self-diagnostic elements, and (dormant until activated) circuit rerouting capabilities.

The spatial data acquisition units will rapidly convert harvested or generated electron flow into appropriately pulsed signals (e.g., ultrasonic). These signals will traverse turbid in vivo media (whole blood) to impact and reflect back from the interior luminal surfaces of the vascular endothelial wall. The return signals will subsequently be translated into electrical signals of varying intensity and when correlated with time-of-flight algorithms, will provide accurate three-dimensional (3D) spatial measurements and Cartesian coordinates for registered target contact points. These return electrical signals will be conveyed directly to the quantum computer for preprocessing and subsequent transfer via the communications/data transfer beacon (Chapter 6) to "outbody" computers housing the Pixel Matrix image reconstruction system, for final processing and display.

All nanoelectronic components will likely be embedded in appropriate and effective insulating materials in order to prevent electron tunneling and for the elimination of any potential electrical shorting events. Primary structures comprising the nanoelectronic system, including junctions and connectors, will ideally be designed to take modular form, and as much as possible, adhere to a set of standardized configurations, once developed, to facilitate fabrication processes, as well as to simplify the organization of hierarchical assembly procedures. Self-assembly will serve as a powerful and cost-effective strategy for interfacing myriad nanoelectronic components into functional nanocircuitry. Nanoparticles have been self-assembled to form light-emitting devices [1] and self-assembled aggregates of colloidal entities served as a substitute for single crystalline photovoltaic elements in dye/nanoparticle-enhanced solar cells [2,3]. Customized DNA oligonucleotides, tethered to dynamic multilevel and movable substrates, may be exploited via their precision complementary base pairing to orient nanometric elements that are attached to their ends, into intimate proximity to facilitate the construction of nanoelectronic circuits [4].

5.2 Nanoelectronic Infrastructure: Potential Research Aims for Exemplar VCSN

1. To thoroughly investigate, methodically design, develop, and stringently test (to verify and quantify reliable and robust functionality) a full range (e.g., nanowires, transistors, resistors, voltage gates, capacitors, switches, amplifiers, and standardized connectors) of complementary modular nanoscale electronic components and circuitry. The aim for the development of these entities would be their integration to enable full functionality for every component of the VCSN. Note: these entities, once developed, will not be exclusive to the VCSN nanomedical technology, but may have potentially extensive and possibly ubiquitous applications in

many diverse areas. These sectors would include, but are not limited to consumer products, scientific instrumentation, military electronics, advanced (quantum) computers, enhancement of existing medical implants and devices, other species of micro/nanorobotics, miniaturized homeland security technologies, advanced nanosensing in myriad applications, energy harvesting and generation, renewable energy, aerospace/aircraft enhancement, microsatellites and reconnaissance spacecraft, planetary and deep space exploration, as well as applications in MEMS, NEMS, bioMEMS, and cross-disciplinary scientific research, to "any" class of future nanomedical devices/systems, and to nanotechnologies in general.

2. Develop integration and interconnectivity strategies for each of these elements aimed at specific VCSN components and subcomponents.

3. Elucidate strategies and designs for the nanometric "wiring" of a complete VCSN device. Devise conceptual nanoelectronic infrastructure possibilities, taking into account overall thermal effects, electron tunneling issues, shielding strategies for protection against external/ambient electromagnetic interference, redundant subsystems, and automated rerouting capacities.

4. Development of a dedicated nanocomponent connection standard (to be utilized throughout the VCSN device) to facilitate ease of design and manufacture.

5. Conceptualization, design, and characterization of potential fabrication processes (e.g., massively parallel nanofabrication [5], nanolithography [6], nanopantography [7], ion-beam sculpting [8], laser-guided deposition [9], self-assembly [10], DNA-based manufacturing [4]) for the realization of nanoelectronic components.

6. Proof of principal, and subsequent demonstration (stand-alone, as well as when combined with other elements) of envisaged nanoelectronic component capabilities within projected operating parameters.

5.3 Nanowires: A Brief History

1997 First successful fabrication of GaN nanorods by reaction of Ga_2O with NH_3. Rods are between 4 and 5 nm inside nanotubes [11].

1998 Morales and Lieber synthesize Si and Ge nanowires with a combination of laser ablation, cluster formation, and vapor–liquid–solid (VLS) growth [12].

1999 Zhu and Fan demonstrate that GaN nanorods are in fact single crystal GaN structures. It is shown that GaN can be grown in alumina membranes [13].

2000 Cheng et al. demonstrate ordered GaN nanowire growth in a honeycomb structure of anodic alumina [14].

2001

1. Chen et al. report high-purity, high-quality GaN nanowires via application of catalysts [15].

2. Lauhon et al. synthesizes nanowires 50 nm in diameter having germanium core and silicon shell, also multi-shell wires of silicon, silicon oxide, and germanium [16].

3. Cui et al. synthesize boron-doped silicon nanowires are enabled as highly selective and sensitive biochemical nanosensors [17].

2002 Development of single gallium nitride nanowire lasers [18].

2003 Lee and colleagues fabricate smallest (Ø 1 nm) nanowires to date, comprising silicon [19].

2004

1. Lauhon et al. review the integration of functional heterojunctions within semiconductor nanowires during synthesis, with possibilities of increasing their inherent complexity as nanoscale components in nanotechnological systems [20].

2. Katz and Willner describe methods for the segregation of semiconducting from metallic carbon nanotubes and the molecular/biomolecular functionalization of their side walls and ends giving rise to new classes of nanowires [21].

3. Nanowire arrays decorated with specific antibodies detect influenza A. Patolsky et al. envision that "The possibility of large-scale integration of these nanowire devices suggests potential for simultaneous detection of a large number of distinct viral threats at the single virus level" [22].

2005

1. Shi et al. reveal that the thermal and thermoelectric attributes of single semiconducting nanowires (e.g., bismuth telluride) are influenced primarily by their crystalline structure (e.g., crystal quality, chemical makeup, and surface characteristics) [23].

2. Reguera et al. discover microbial conductive nanowires (pili) [24].

3. Yang et al. prepare nanowires via a nanomolding process for the first time and utilize molecular imprinting to create molecular recognition sites on nanowire surfaces [25,26].

2006 Hayden et al. demonstrate avalanche multiplication of photocurrent in nanometric photodiodes comprising silicon–cadmium sulfide (Cds) nanowires with high detection sensitivity (<100) photons and subwavelength spatial resolution (~250 nm) [27].

2007 Field-effect transistors (FETs) and photodetectors based on nanowires are reported [28,29].

2008 Yuan et al. synthesize rigid hybrid water-soluble liquid crystal-like nanowires comprising a silsesquioxane core encompassed by oligo(ethylene glycol) methacrylate units. The radial and linear dimensions of these nanowires were tunable through the polymerization of their backbones and side chains and they could be transformed to silica nanowires via pyrolyzation [30].

2009 Cui et al. review various atomic scale diffusion techniques and lead-free nanosoldering toward enabling the interconnectivity of nanowires and nanotubes in the fabrication of functional and complex nanoelectronic circuitry [31].

2010

1. Singh reviews the use of biodegradable and lipid-based nanomaterials, including nanowires, which might be chemically functionalized to target specific organs in enabling advanced nanomedical drug delivery [32].

2. Guo reviews various techniques for the creation of nanowire and nanotube nanojunctions [33].

3. Takei et al. demonstrate the integration of highly ordered nanowire arrays into a flexible "artificial electronic skin" pressure sensor [34].

2011

1. Noy discusses the possibility of utilizing nanowires and nanotubes as intimate interfacial conduits to facilitate data exchange between biological and synthetic constructs in "bionanoelectronics" [35].
2. Nanowires comprising single crystalline porous silicon are synthesized that accept a wide range of dopants that are both electronically and optically active [36].
3. Chen et al. synthesize linear and branched heteronanostructures of silicon nanotubes and gold nanowires with both linear and branched configurations with potential for the construction of nanocircuitry [37].
4. Xu et al. synthesize coiled silicon nanowires on pre-strained poly(dimethylsiloxane) (PDMS) substrates, which were induced to buckle once the pre-strain was released. The resulting coiled nanowires could be stretched to twice their default length [38].

2012

1. Espinosa et al. review progress, via experimental and computational methods, toward the quantification of the electromechanical and mechanical attributes of piezoelectric nanowires [39].
2. Long et al. [40] and Liu et al. [41] survey advances in the area of macroscale semiconducting inorganic nanowire assembly technologies and their applications in advanced electronics.
3. Wilner et al. describe the dynamic and diverse capacities of DNA nanowires, including their electrochemical attributes [42].
4. Lim et al. develop an in situ synthesis technique that allows for the fine control of (In,Ga)N (and other materials) nanowire dimensions and the composition of discreet domains along their lengths to enable the fabrication of complex nanowire structures that will lead to significantly enhanced functionality [43].

5.3.1 Description of Nanowires

Multiple integrated systems that comprise the proposed exemplar VCSN will require an enormous population of nanoscale interconnects to enable their optimal functionality. These connecting entities may comprise myriad nanomaterials with properties that are tailored to their designated functionality, many of which might serve as highly conductive nanometric power transmission cables and high capacity optical data transfer conduits. Nanowires or quantum wires are anisotropic nanocrystals with a high aspect ratio (length/diameter) having diameters from 1 to 200 nm and lengths up to several centimeters [44]. These entities may be synthesized by various techniques (see Section 5.3.2) resulting in the generation of different compositions, cross-sectional profiles [43], and morphologies [38]. One can envision that tightly packed laminations of flat single dimensional nanowires, which are interleaved and isolated by insulating nanowire layers to prevent cross talk and electron tunneling, may indeed have the capacity for conveying sufficient electrical power to all onboard nanodevice systems (e.g., core quantum computer, communications, propulsion, navigation) and associated subsystems and components at the required levels of complexity. If nanodevices such as the VCSN are fabricated via atomic level "printing" or other types of nanomanufacturing systems, complex, 3D circuitry may be laid down layer-by-layer under pre-programmed computer control.

5.3.2 Nanowire Synthesis

Following is a brief summative survey (by no means comprehensive) of various techniques that may be employed for the synthesis of nanowires, which might be utilized as nanomedical electronic components. A Web of Science "nanowire" search term returned 6985 results (May 27, 2012).

Criteria for the synthesis of high-quality nanowires that serve as the intricate, albeit robust, "nervous systems" of sophisticated autonomous nanomedical devices will include finely tuned chemical composition, consistent morphology, tightly controlled dimensions, well-defined and reliable electronic, thermal, and mechanical properties, and the capacity for being rapidly produced in large volumes.

Semiconducting, copper oxide (cuprous oxide [Cu_2O] and cupric oxide [CuO]) high surface area nanowires possess bandgaps of 2.0 and 1.2 eV, respectively, which endows them with good photovoltaic properties. These nanowires may be grown in aqueous solutions via chemical mixing techniques to generate a variety of single-, bi-, or polycrystalline nanowires that range in diameter from 5 to 50 nm and in length from 200 nm to 20 μm [45]. Electrochemical cells that incorporate nanoporous templates comprising anodic aluminum oxide [46] or polycarbonate membrane [47] may also be employed to expedite their fabrication. In addition, shaping agents such as surfactants hexadecyl trimethyl ammonium bromide (CTAB) or sodium dodecylbenzenesulfonate (SDS), or polymers including polyethylene glycol (PEG) or polyvinyl pyrrolidone (PVP) can be used. Precursor nanowires of copper hydroxide and copper oxalate may be synthesized via a hydrothermal process using heated chemical solutions to produce CuO nanowires through subsequent annealing in an oxygen atmosphere. Direct thermal oxidation may be utilized to grow copper oxide nanowires from clean bulk copper substrates including thin films, foils, and nanoparticles, at temperatures from 400°C to 600°C in a high oxygen milieu [45].

To describe template-directed synthesis further, in this method, a template serves as a scaffold against which other types of materials are synthesized. The templates may consist of nanoscale channels in mesoporous materials such as silica, porous alumina, and polycarbonate membranes. These nanoscale channels can be filled using chemical conversion, colloidal sol–gel capillary forces, electrochemical methods, and centrifugation. The nanowires are subsequently released through the selective removal of the host matrix. The template method is quite versatile and has been employed in the fabrication of nanowires, tubules, and fibrils of electrically conductive metals, polymers, semiconductors, carbon, and other materials, which are typically of polycrystalline nature. Porous alumina membranes are excellent host materials with pores that are arranged in a regular hexagonal lattice with pore densities of ~10^{11} pores/cm². Various inorganic materials such as Au, Ag, Pt, TiO_2, MnO_2, ZnO, SnO_2, electronically conductive polymers, polypyrrole, poly(3-methylthiophene), polyaniline, and carbon nanotubules may also be utilized [48–50].

Nanowires that are allowed to react with specific chemicals or are exposed, for example, to electron beam irradiation under carefully controlled conditions may be transformed to other phases or into another substance without losing their inherent nanowire attributes. This provides a technique for producing nanowire compositions that would otherwise be very challenging to fabricate directly [51,52]. Semiconductor nanofibers have been fabricated using a solvothermal method. A solvent is combined with metal precursors and crystal growth agents such as amines, after which this solution is placed in an autoclave under high pressure and temperature, which leads to crystal growth and assembly [53,54].

Germanium nanowires were grown in a low-pressure chemical vapor deposition reactor using a VLS method at different temperatures. Several types of gold (Au) nanoparticles, ranging in size and thickness $\varnothing$ 3–14 nm × 0.1–3 nm, respectively, served as catalysts and it was found that at 300°C the resulting nanowires had tapered structures, whereas straight and longer nanowires with smaller diameters (~3 nm) were produced at 260°C–280°C. These nanowires might be applied as p-type ballistic Ge transistors [55].

Oxide-assisted laser ablation, by which a bulk target is irradiated by a laser, resulting in material vaporization, produced $\varnothing$ ~60 nm gallium arsenide and silicon nanowires [56]. Silicon oxide (SiO_x) nanowires with minimum diameters of ~10 nm × several tens of micrometers in length were generated through the laser ablation of a silicon-containing target [57]. No catalyst or template is required for this technique.

Nanobelts/ribbons have been grown through the simple evaporation of metal oxide powders (ZnO, SnO_2, Ga_2O_3) at high temperatures. When ZnO powders on the surface of an alumina plate were thermally evaporated at 1400°C for 2 h, long (~20 μm to mm) high-purity nanobelts with rectangular cross-sectional profiles were produced, having widths ranging from 50 to 300 nm, thicknesses from 10 to 30 nm, and a width-to-thickness ratio of ~5 to 10 [58–60]. These structures may be used as scaffolds, or if nanowires are sandwiched and sealed between them, they could serve as insulating elements for "nanocable" conduits. InGaAs nanowires have been grown in V grooves within an InP substrate (~7 μm deep), which were made by photolithography followed by chemical etching. The resulting nanowire diameters were ~10 nm × ~20 nm [61]. Platinum nanowires ~2 to 3 nm diameter and ~1000 nm long have been fabricated via chemical synthesis. This process used platinum chloride (H_2PtCl_6) in a mesoporous honeycomb silicate material (FSM-16) containing $\varnothing$ ~3.0 nm pores, which served as a template. Platinum nanowires were formed via photoreduction when a vapor of alcohol and water was adsorbed to the substrate surface [62].

Coaxial heterostructures in the form of multiple semiconductor shells wrapped around crystalline silicon and germanium nanowires have also been synthesized. These nanowires are grown by catalysis from a nanoparticle of gold using a VLS growth technique. Multiple coaxial shells of doped silicon, germanium, and silicon oxide are formed by gas-phase CVD. These multi-shell devices represent a high-quality single crystal material that may have potentially diverse functionality (e.g., serving as gated FETs) due to high compositional control [63].

Gold nanowires (4 nm wide × 1 nm thick × 7 μm long) have been "written" by a gold-coated piezoresistive cantilever that was mounted to an atomic force microscope, in contact mode, under high vacuum conditions. The cantilever tip was coated with 50 nm of gold using an electron beam evaporation technique. By bringing the tip into contact with a Si (111) surface, and moving the tip (acting as a quill) across the surface, the nanowires were literally drawn. At room temperature, the Au will migrate from the tip at an average speed of 10 nm/s with the line width being determined by the cantilever tip profile. Writing velocities of higher than 50 nm/s resulted in disconnected wires or dots. The volume of gold that is deposited may be controlled by resistively heating the cantilever; however, this can exhibit thermal drift. Electron transport has been measured across the gold nanowire and the electrical resistivity is 1.5×10^{-4} Ω m compared with bulk Au at 2.2×10^{-10} Ω m. These nanowires may have utility as interconnects. Arrays of cantilevers would facilitate the parallel fabrication of these entities [64].

It was demonstrated by Wang et al. that the electrical conductivity of silica nanowires could be altered by the number of Au nanoparticles that are embedded or "peapodded" within them (Figure 5.1). These nanometric entities were synthesized via microwave plasma-enhanced chemical vapor deposition (MWPECVD). The electron transport kinetics within these nanostructures, elucidated by thermally dependent conductivity quantification, was found to involve a band-tail hopping process (a model wherein multiple trap states extend from a high-density domain, in close proximity to band edges, to a low-density domain deeper into the bandgap and electron transfer is envisioned as a sequence of trap and release events) [65]. Higher conductivities were correlated with "the higher density of hopping states and shorter hopping distance." The researchers postulate that these hybrid entities might be integrated into semiconductor circuits and optoelectronic devices [66].

Pure crystalline silver nanowires with diameters of 0.4 nm (four atoms per unit cell) and lengths in the micron range have been synthesized within the nanopores of organic templates [67]. When the radii of nanowires approach the electron Fermi wavelength, conductivity becomes quantized, where the number of conductive pathways is function

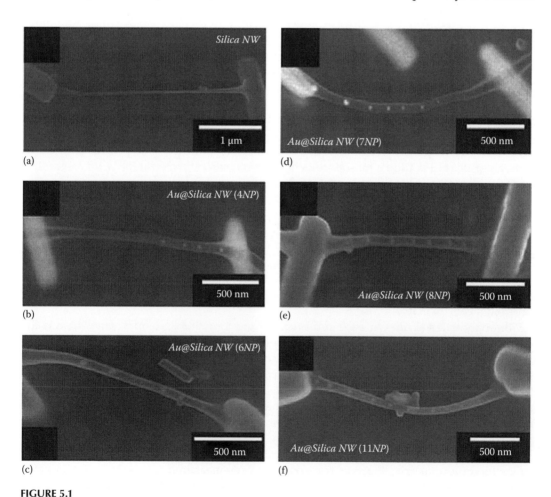

FIGURE 5.1
(a–f) Scanning electron microscope (SEM) depiction of single silica nanowires containing different numbers of embedded Au nanoparticles.

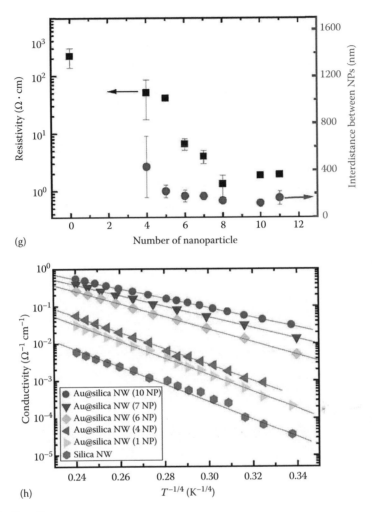

(g)

(h)

FIGURE 5.1 (Continued)

(g) Particle to particle and resistivity of individual silica nanowires as associated with Au nanoparticle residency. (h) Altered conductivity of individual silica nanowires as relates to the number of embedded Au nanoparticles under a temperature range of 77 to 300 K. (Wang, S.B. et al., *Nanoscale*, 4(12), 3660, 2012. Repeoduced by permission of The Royal Society of Chemistry.)

of the geometries of the nanowires. Silver nanowires may also be produced within the lumen of nanotubes, incorporating silver halides in solution chemistry techniques. They have been shown to have 50% filling rates via capillary action. SWNTs are better suited than MWNTs for continuous filling with a wide variety of materials because they are much more uniform and defect-free structures [68]. Additionally, Ag nanowire aggregates with an urchin-like geometries (Figure 5.2) were synthesized at room temperature through the reaction of $AgNO_3$(aq) with copper when combined with cetyltrimethylammonium chloride and HNO_3(aq) on screen-printed carbon (SPC) electrodes. The dimensions of the resulting nanowires were Ø 100 nm × ~10 µm in length. This technique might serve as an alternate fabrication strategy as an initial step in the production of large quantities of nanowires (if done in massively parallel fashion), which might be followed by an appropriate dissociation technique to separate nanowire aggregates into individual entities [69].

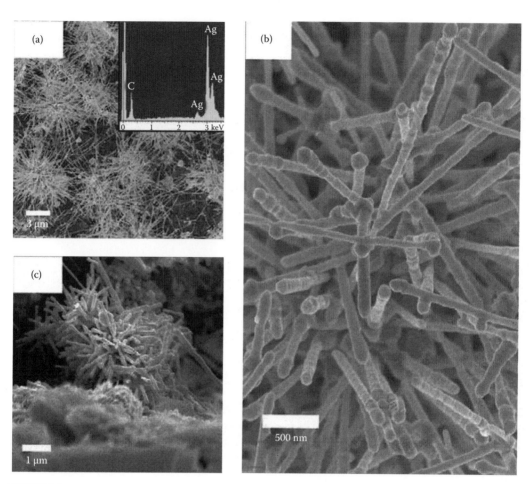

FIGURE 5.2
(a) SEM image of urchin-resembling Ag nanowire aggregates on a screen-printed carbon (SPC) electrode (inset is result of energy-dispersive spectroscopy [EDS]). (b, c) Increasing magnifications of Ag nanowire morphology. (Reproduced with permission from Hsiao, W.H. et al., *ACS Appl. Mater. Interfaces*, 3(9), 3280. Copyright 2011 American Chemical Society.)

Recently, a method has been developed for the conformal shaping, lateral compression, bending, cutting, or periodic straining of prefabricated silver nanowires (Figure 5.3) using a laser shock technique to facilitate the generation of diverse morphologies. A laser pulse is employed to vaporize an ablative coating that is confined along with a metal foil to which aligned nanowires are adhered, which is positioned above a silicon mold that is formed to a desired nanowire geometry. A potent (localized) plasmatic shock wave is produced as a result of the rapid expansion of the ablative coating, which is induced by the laser pulse to subsequently pressure-shape the metal foil and the underlying nanowires to the contours of the mold [70].

Zhang et al. utilized a sol–gel process called "micro-casting" by which a pure aluminum substrate was etched with nanochannels and employed as a template to grow zinc oxide (ZnO) with potential for the synthesis of other types of semiconductor nanowires. The uniform hexagonal nanowire geometries (Ø ~60 nm) were physically constrained along

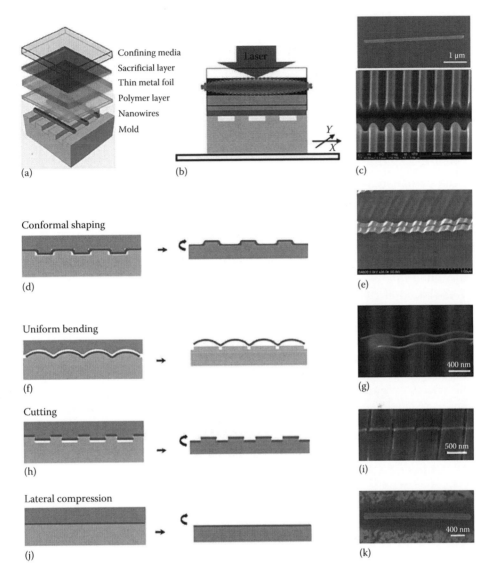

FIGURE 5.3
Schematic of laser shock-based process for the controllable modification of Ag nanowires. (a) Exploded depiction of forming assembly. (b) Laser shock procedure. (c) SEM of unmodified Ag nanowires and channeled silicon mold. (d, f, h, j) Schematics of nanowire conformal shaping, bending, cutting, and compression processes. (e, g, i, k) SEMs of resulting Ag nanowires post-laser shock modification. (Reproduced with permission from Li, J. et al., *Nano Lett.*, 12, 3224. Copyright 2012 American Chemical Society.)

the nanochannels during growth, and the fabrication of smaller nanowires is possible via a reduction in the nanochannel dimensions [71].

Nanorods composed of Cu were synthesized via a novel biotemplating strategy that exploits the morphological surface structures of viruses. Bacteriophages, fd and M13 (Ø 6.6 nm × 880 nm long) [72], and the plant virus tobacco mosaic virus (TMV) (Ø 18 nm × 300 nm long) [73] may be utilized as nanorod-like templates, as they possess functional groups on their surfaces that have affinities with metal atoms in the formation of nucleation sites to facilitate the growth of nanoparticles. The nanorods were achieved with the TMV via a two-phase electroless deposition process, where the virus template was initially activated by the seeding of Pd nanoparticles followed by their utilization as catalysts in the reduction of Cu^{2+}, which induces continuous nanocrystalline growth to coat the template surface [74].

There are many additional strategies for the synthesis of nanowires, which have recently been reviewed by Long et al. [40] and Lapierre and Sunkara [75]. Table 5.1 provides a sampling of various nanowires and methods for their synthesis.

5.3.3 Nanowire Networks and Arrays

Within the extremely constrained interiors of nanomedical devices, a critical design challenge will involve the optimal spatial arrangement of myriad electronic components and nanowire-based interconnects. The maximization of (available) surface area-to-volume ratio may be facilitated by the integration of highly ordered (densely packed and short) nanowire array modules that serve as electronic "manifolds" from which longer nanowires might be routed to interface with various onboard components. Hiralal et al. calculated that in comparison to a 1 cm² × 5 µm thick layer, an array of Ø 20 nm nanowires spaced at 20 nm will increase the surface area by 300% while reducing the material that is required by four-fifths, and "The increased ratio of electronically and coordinatively unsaturated surface atoms to internal atoms increases, resulting in higher reactivity" [104].

When epitaxial (geometric alignment of layered crystalline structures) growth conditions are not satisfied, nanowires will "crawl" parallel to a substrate. This is a critical factor in the growth of potential nanowire electronics [105,106]. Nanowires may be aligned by microfluidic assisted nanowire integration [107] whereby a droplet of the nanowire solution is placed at the open end of a microchannel that is formed between a PDMS micromold and a Si/glass substrate, which subsequently filled via the capillary effect. After solvent evaporation and liftoff of the micromold, bundles of Ø ~10 to 100 nm diameter nanowires are aligned at the edges of the microchannels to form a parallel array. By rotating the microchannel 90° and repeating the process, it is possible to fabricate arrays of nanowire cross junctions [108]. Another strategy involves the alignment of nanowires through the application of a strong electromagnetic field during the growth process [109]. Drawbacks to these methods include potentially large pitches between the nanowires and limited yield.

Highly dense and well-aligned nanowires will be required for the integration of these networks into nanodevices. A Langmuir–Blodgett technique (organized monolayers that are formed on the surface of water) has been developed for the purpose of assembling high-density nanowire arrays [40,110]. Liu et al. have demonstrated the synthesis of highly ordered, ultrathin (~4 to 9 nm) and super long (several hundred micrometers) arrays of tellurium (Te) and silver telluride (Ag_2Te) nanowires that spanned areas of ~100 µm², using a Langmuir–Blodgett process [111].

Regular and uniform arrays of nanowires may be created with diameters from ~5 nm to several 100 nm by direct electrodeposition into porous anodic aluminum oxide templates. Single electron tunneling can occur when interwire coupling is present. This leads to spontaneous electrostatic polarization of the nanowires. This non-lithographic method has advantages as it grows nanostructures directly rather than obtaining them through the removal of material. It is possible to write the structure on a semiconductor surface via a focused ion beam or scanning probe microscope; however, this only applies to the fabrication of small batches. For larger throughput, the approach of self-organizing island

TABLE 5.1

Examples of Various Nanowire (nw)/Nanorod (nr) Materials and Associated Synthesis Techniques

Material (nw/nr)	Dimensions—Ø × length	Synthesis Technique	Reference
Ag (silver) nw	100 nm × 5–10 μm	Printing	[76]
Ag (silver) nw	100 nm × 20 μm	Colloidal synthesis	[77]
Ag (silver) nw	70 nm × ~8 μm	Bubble template	[78]
Ag (silver) nw	nw: ~35 nm × ~15 nm	Electrostatics and electrospinning	[79]
Au (gold) nr (composite)	nr: 19 nm × 77 nm		
Al (aluminum) nw	20–120 nm × 300 nm	Chemical vapor deposition	[80]
BaWO$_4$ (barium tungstate) nr	100–200 nm × ~>2 μm	Nanoporous alumina templating	[81]
BaCrO$_4$ (barium chromate) nr	100–200 nm × ~>2 μm	Nanoporous alumina templating	[81]
Bi (bismuth) nw	30–200 nm × ~mm	Extrusion	[82]
BiSb (bismuth–antimony) nw	~100 nm × ~60 μm	Anodized aluminum oxide template	[83]
Bi$_2$Te$_3$ (bismuth telluride) nw	~65 nm × ~150 nm	On-film formation of nanowires	[84]
CdS (cadmium sulfide) nw	30–60 nm × ~20–30 μm	Chemical vapor deposition	[85]
CdSe (cadmium selenide) nw	50 nm × 10 μm	Chemical vapor deposition	[85]
Cu (Copper) nr	~35 nm × 300 mm	Biotemplating	[74]
CuO (copper oxide) nr	20–30 nm × 150–200 nm	Hydrothermal method	[86]
Cu:Ni (cupronickel) nw	~116 nm × ~28 μm	Hydrothermal method	[87]
α-Fe$_2$O$_3$ (iron oxide) nw	20–70 nm × 10–20 μm	Thermal oxidation method	[88]
GaAs (gallium arsenide) nw	150–450 nm × 130 nm	Nanosphere lithography (NSL) and selected area metal organic chemical vapor deposition (SA-MOCVD)	[89]
Ge (germanium) nw	10–25 nm × 10 μm	Thermal decomposition	[90]
InAs (indium arsenide) nw	~30–120 nm × 2.5 μm	Molecular beam epitaxy	[91]
MgO (magnesium oxide) nw	40–50 nm × 200 nm	Thermal evaporation (w/o catalyst)	[92]
MgO (magnesium oxide) nw	20–30 nm × ~2 μm	Thermal evaporation (with catalyst)	[92]
Mo (molybdenum) nw	0.6–0.8 nm × ~20 nm	Encapsulation within double-walled carbon nanotubes	[93]
Ni (nickel) nw	50 nm × 50 μm	Nanoporous alumina templating	[94]
PbS (lead sulfide) nw	9–15 nm × 4–10 μm	Solution–liquid–solid growth	[95]
PbSe (lead selenide) nw			
Se (selenium) nw	51–208 nm × ~3 μm	Morphology-directing agent growth	[96]
Si (silicon) nw	20–300 nm × 5–150 μm	Aqueous electroless etching	[97]
SnO$_2$ (tin dioxide) nw	40–80 nm × 2–3 μm	Vapor–liquid–solid growth	[98]
Pd (palladium) nw	~4 nm × 50–200 nm	Solvent-based one-pot method	[99]
Pt (platinum) nw	10 nm × 200 nm	Thermally assisted photoreduction	[100]
TiO$_2$ (titanium) nw	80–150 nm × 2–3 μm	Thermal reactive evaporation	[101]
W (tungsten) nw	10–100 nm × 2–3 μm	Thermal evaporation	[102]
Zn (zinc) nw	5–5 nm × 1–4 μm	Solution phase deposition	[103]

development by lattice-mismatched semiconductor systems is employed. Examples of templates that might be employed for the synthesis of nanowire arrays are zeolites, molecular sieves, polymer nuclear track membranes, or porous anodic aluminum oxide films. Average nanowire dimensions from this technology range from ~4 to ~200 nm diameter with 1 to 50 μm long, with pore densities of 10^9 to 10^{11} cm^{-2}.

AC electrolysis is used to deposit metals and semiconductors into the pores resulting in the formation of nanowire arrays. The sandwiching of a 10 nm nanowire array between metal contact layers forms a capacitance tunnel junction where the bottom junction is a barrier oxide layer (~10 to 20 nm) and the top junction (~8 Å) nickel oxide film grown on the tips of nickel nanowires constitutes the source and drain. The exciton energies quantified by Raman spectroscopy polarized along the linear axis are 2.376 eV for larger diameter nanowires and 2.417 eV for small diameter nanowires [112].

A blown bubble strategy has been developed for the fabrication of well-aligned nanowire arrays over large areas with tunable densities. This three-step procedure involves the initial preparation of a homogeneous polymeric suspension of nanowires, which is subsequently expanded from a circular die to form a bubble at controlled rates of expansion and pressure. The nanowires that permeate the suspension auto-align with the expansion of the host film by virtue of the generated shear force. The resulting film can then transferred to substrates with variable geometries. In the study that was conducted by Yu et al., a bubble film with dimensions of Ø 35 cm × 50 cm in height uniformly coated two Ø 150 mm Si wafers with negligible angular deviation [113].

Transparent electrodes comprising silver nanowire networks with nanowire diameters ranging from 45 to 110 nm at pitches of 500, 700, and 1000 nm were fabricated by van de Groep et al. via electron beam lithography. The optimal light transmittance attained was 91%, while a low resistance was observed at 6.5 Ω/sq. The researchers point out that "due to the two-dimensional (2D) periodic structure, our networks can also function as a scattering layer, thereby combining the functionality of an electrical contact and a light trapping scheme in one design" [114]. This dual functionality may have significant utility in the capture and transfer of energy from an external near-infrared laser light source in the powering of multiple autonomous nanomedical devices.

The higher diamondoids (0.5–2 nm) comprise the tiniest naturally occurring (from raw petroleum) hydrogen-terminated cubic isomeric form of diamond. Although lower diamondoids such as adamantane [115], diamantane [116], and triamantane [117] may be chemically synthesized, higher diamondoids, including tetramantane, pentamantane, hexamantane, heptamantane, octamantane, nonamantane, decamantane, undecamantane [118], have been recalcitrant in this regard (Figure 5.4). However, progress continues to be made [120]. The face fused cages of diamondoids exist in myriad 3D geometries that are highly stable, rigid, and strong, which may enable the potential incremental construction of nanorods [121]. Tetramantane is the shortest (1 nm long) of a class of rod-shaped diamondoids where the long axes is oriented at 90° to the (110) diamond lattice plane. Additional cuboidal cages may be added, thereby increasing the rod length by 0.10 to 0.15 nm increments. Other classes of diamondoids have helical and disk-shaped morphologies. In terms of their electronic attributes, H-terminated diamondoids, like diamond, are the only semiconductor that exhibits electron affinity, and may emit electrons spontaneously [122]. Diamond crystallites are under study as cold-cathode field emitter tips.

It is conceivable that with the advent of molecular assemblers and nanomanufacturing [123–127] that these novel diamondoid building blocks might be utilized in the construction of sophisticated nanorod networks to serve as electronic interconnects, or as structural

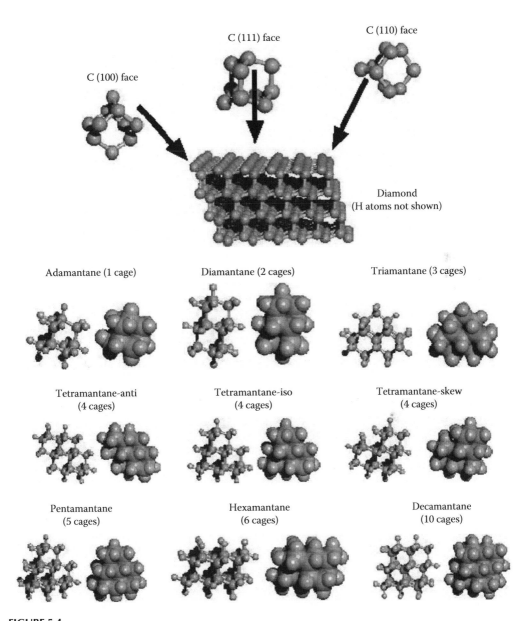

FIGURE 5.4
Lower and higher diamondoids discovered by ChevronTexaco (2002). (Reproduced from Freitas, R., *First Symposium on Molecular Machine Systems, First Foresight Conference on Advanced Nanotechnology*, October 22, 2004. http://www.molecularassembler.com/Papers/PathDiamMolMfg.htm. With permission.)

elements of electronic components themselves. Since these subnanometer entities may lend themselves to precise manipulation and controlled orientation in facilitating the assembly of nanomedical device circuitry, it seems plausible that if they are presentable/dispensed as distinct, highly constrained feedstocks that they might be built up element-by-element via massively parallel DNA-based nanofabrication [4], laid down as layer-by-layer laminations using programmable molecular/nanometric 3D printing [128], or perhaps configured by self-directed capillary forming [129]. As with all nanocircuitry that integrates nanowires, nanotubes, nanorods, nanobelts, etc., it will be imperative that appropriate, highly efficient insulating materials (e.g., carbon aerogel) are utilized for shielding, to ensure that electron tunneling or shorting events are negated.

Paraschiv et al. have devised a self-assembly process that exploits the chemistries of alkoxo-bridged copper(II), which serve as nodes in the design of interpenetrating diamondoid complexes (Figure 5.5) that employ anionic cyano complexes as linkers. This solid-state supramolecular construct employs heterocubane (Cu_4O_4) nodes that are joined by aurocyanide ($Au(CN)_2$) rods [130].

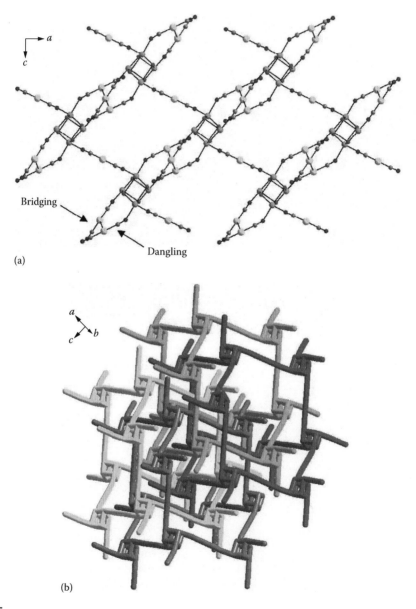

FIGURE 5.5
(a) Isomeric view of an isolated diamondoid net. (b) Depiction of fourfold diamondoid packing. Deprotonated monoethanolamine and water molecules are removed for clarity. (Paraschiv, C. et al., *Dalton Trans.*, 7, 1195, 2005. Reproduced by permission of The Royal Society of Chemistry.)

5.3.4 Mechanical Properties of Nanowires

Nanowires that are integrated into laminated nanoscale circuitry should be highly mechanically stable as length requirements of more than 1 μm (optimal nanodevice diameter) will be unlikely. However, when designed for incorporation into 3D nanocircuitry, it is possible that flexible ultrathin nanowires or nanobelts will be required to follow tortuous routing, which will necessitate bending or twisting at multiple sites. Hence, to ensure optimal and safe nanodevice operation, nanowires and similar nanomaterials, which enable the interconnectivity of nanoscale electronic entities, should undergo an extensive regimen of testing to ensure that they possess the highest level of mechanical integrity.

It was shown that diminutive nanorod whiskers can exhibit higher strength than what is observed in macroscopic single crystals. This is due to a reduction in the number of defects per unit length of the material and the physical robustness of the nanowire can be influenced by its crystalline orientation. Atomic force microscopy was used to test the mechanical strength of a single SiC nanowire (Ø 21.5 nm), and it was found that the Young's modulus was 660 Gpa [131]. In comparison, germanium (Ge) nanowires (Ø 40–160 nm) [132], ZnO nanowires (Ø ~17 nm) [133], and tin oxide (SnO_2) nanowires (Ø ~90 nm) [134] exhibited Young's moduli of ~112, ~220, and ~100 Gpa, respectively.

Gold nanowires that were fabricated by the electron beam irradiation of a gold thin film had diameters that ranged from 0.5 to 3 nm. Below Ø 0.6 nm, the structures showed stability and helical packing and comprised several identical spiral strands. Above Ø 0.6 nm, a multiwalled morphology was prevalent that exhibited several closely packed curved layers, which is a common structural trait in metallic nanowires [135,136]. From Ø 0.6 to 1.0 nm, a double wall existed and from Ø 1.10 to 1.66 nm, a triple wall configuration was evident. Larger wires (up to 3 nm in diameter) have a face-centered-cubic (fcc) crystalline structure that is formed within the core region, surrounded by noncrystalline curved surfaces. At diameters above 3 nm the nanowire was almost completely crystalline, and in an Au nanowire the atomic structure and symmetry has a bearing on conductance. A Ø 1.76 nm nanowire exhibited good stability and was shown to be mechanically more resilient than other diameters [137].

5.3.5 Optical Properties of Nanowires

Advanced autonomous nanomedical devices will likely integrate photonic and electronic circuitry, as nanophotonic circuits might possess the advantages of high speeds and greater flexibility in device design. The combination of nanowire-based light sources with pliable subwavelength nanowire/nanotube/nanoribbon waveguides may form the basis of diverse and sophisticated photonic circuitry with the capacity for powering and fine controlling the required highly precise functionality of medical nanodevices. As semiconducting oxide nanoribbons have the capacity for transmitting both electrons and photons simultaneously, they may facilitate optimal circuit compactness [138].

ZnO nanowires were grown to form natural wide bandgap ultraviolet laser (green, blue) cavities at room temperature. Their diameters ranged from 20 to 150 nm with lengths of up to 10 μm. Under optical excitation, surface-emitting lasing was observed at 385 nm, with an emission line width of less than 0.3 nm. To achieve lasing at room temperature, the binding energy of the exciton must be greater than the thermal energy (26 meV). In ZnO nanowires, the exciton binding energy is ~60 meV [139]. Lasing devoid of fabricated mirrors enables nanowires to function as natural resonant cavities. By creating p–n junctions within the nanowires, the possibility exists for the creation of electron ejection UV/blue lasers [140].

These nanowires are excited with <ps (picosecond) pulses of 4.35 eV photons (285 nm) to induce photoluminescence and lasing. Tunability, by virtue of nanowire lattice orientation, can produce varying optical properties [141] and polarization-sensitive nanoscale photodetectors have been created utilizing intrinsic anisotropy. This property may prove useful in the development of photonic circuitry, optical switches, interconnects, near-field imagery, and high-resolution detectors.

Nanowire-based lasers comprised of pure ZnO crystals (Ø ~100 nm) emit, as mentioned earlier, in the ultraviolet region. They can be grown vertically via epitaxy and when formed appear similar to the bristles of a brush, with an average length of ~10 μm. They may be made longer if the growth process is allowed to continue. Sapphire crystals, coated in patterns with a thin film of Au, are submerged in a hot gas of ZnO. The gold film acts as the catalyst and within ~10 min, millions of ZnO wires form above the pattern on the sapphire seeds. At room temperature, a visible light laser optically pumps the nanowires, which excites the ZnO molecules to initiate photon emission. Cross sections of the nanowires reveal hexagonal geometries with perfectly flat caps at their ends, as are the interfaces between the bottom of the nanowires and the substrate. These surfaces behave as nanometric reflective mirrors that cause the photons that are emitted by the excited ZnO molecules to bounce back and forth between them. This reflected light incites the ZnO molecules to emit additional photons until the light is amplified to a particular threshold, beyond which a burst of UV light is emitted from the end cap. A method for the electrical pumping these nanowires might be to attach electrodes to either end to subsequently stimulate photon emission via electrons [139].

A single crystal nanowire can behave as an efficient electrically driven laser. Investigators believe that these nanoscale lasers might be manipulated to emit over a wide range of wavelengths (ultraviolet to the near infrared). Single crystals of CdS (Ø 80–100 nm) assembled on a substrate of heavily doped silicon were shown to be defect-free, and exhibited excellent electron transport properties. When current is slowly increased through the nanowire, a rapid increase in light intensity emits more than ~200 mA, which is the threshold of lasing. Gallium nitride and indium phosphide may also serve as excellent nanowire laser materials [142].

5.3.6 Electronic Properties of Nanowires

In contrast to nanotubes, nanowires are amenable to being assembled in a predictable manner as their dimensions and electronic properties can be precisely controlled during synthesis, and they may be assembled in parallel [143,144]. They are also cold-cathode field emitters. There are a number of critical criteria that influence electron transfer through one-dimensional (1D) nanowires, including composition, diameter, surface properties, axial crystalline orientation, and quality. Two primary types of electron transfer through nanowires encompass diffusive and ballistic modes. In the diffusive mode, where nanowire lengths (several micrometers) are beyond the carrier mean free path (mean distance that an electron may travel freely without colliding with an obstruction and diverging from its initial path), electrons/holes experience multiple scattering events due to crystalline lattice mismatches, embedded impurities, and other structural imperfections. In contrast, electrons in very short nanowires undergo ballistic transport without scattering, as the nanowire length is significantly shorter than the carrier mean free path and there is negligible resistance. In these nanowires, when the diameter of nanowire approaches the Fermi wavelength, which in the majority of metallic materials is ~0.5 nm, conductivity becomes quantized. For Ø ~1 μm nanomedical devices, an estimate of practical nanowire lengths may fall in the range from ~5 (in nanowire manifolds) to ~100 nm (for long distance, relatively speaking, component interconnects); hence, electron transport will likely remain in the ballistic domain [145].

A silicon carbide nanowire was shown to exhibit a high electron field emission with high stability. The turn-on fields for Si and SiC nanowires are 15 and 20 V/μm with a current density of 0.01 mA/cm^2, comparable to nanotubes and diamond [146,147]. A significant current gain was observed in a simple Si nanowire-based bipolar transistor, suggesting high-efficiency electron injection and electron mobility within the nanowires. Logic gates have been produced to allow computation with a half-adder using p-type silicon and n-type gallium nitride wires to form crossed nanoscale p–n junctions [148]. A gold nanowire with a 1.76 nm diameter, as a special case, exhibits enhanced conductivity due to its particular molecular structure [137].

5.3.7 Thermal Properties of Nanowires

The thermal stability of semiconductor nanowires will be critical when considering their potential integration with nanomedical electronics. A significant challenge is to retain or enhance the electrical conductivity of nanowires, and other nanoelectronic components, while minimizing thermal conductivity. This will be especially important in regard to the highly compact nanoelectronics that are housed in perhaps millions of nanodevices, which might be administered for a given nanomedical procedure. The cumulative thermal dissipation from these nanodevices could impart undesired negative impacts such as raising the core temperature of the patient. Hence, the minimization of generated heat in nanosystems will be paramount. Lee et al. developed Si–Ge alloy nanowires and particular nanowire geometries that exhibited reduced thermal conductivity and acted to optimize the depletion of thermal phonons, and a low thermal conductivity in the range of ~1.2 W/m K at 450 K was reported. For nanowires of over Ø ~100 nm, surface boundary scattering is dominant, whereas the suppression of phonon (cumulative excitatory state of atoms/molecules in condensed materials) mobility is evident in alloyed nanowires with smaller dimensions.

The thermal conductivity of silicon nanowires, for example, is >2 orders of magnitude smaller than that of bulk silicon [149]. When phonon lengths are shorter than the diameters of nanowires (several nanometers—which may indeed be the required dimensional domain of nanowires that are packed into Ø ~1 μm nanodevices), they are suppressed. Phonon mobility may be modified considerably at this size domain via increased boundary scattering, altered phonon dispersion (due to confinement), and phonon transport quantification [149]. However, a similar effect may be induced in larger diameter nanowires through the introduction of crystalline structural defects or impurities, albeit these modifications may also have an impact on electronic properties. It is therefore imperative that all elements of the thermoelectric figure of merit (ZT) (interpreted as ZT $\equiv S^2\sigma T/\kappa$, where S is the Seebeck coefficient, σ the electrical conductivity, and κ the thermal conductivity comprising a lattice or phonon component [κ_l] and electron component [κ_e]) are accounted for in order to compensate for the influences of nanowire diameter, impurities, and structural defects on thermoelectronic mobility [150,151].

Zhou et al. investigated the Seebeck coefficients, thermal and electrical conductivities of semiconducting silicide (chromium disilicide [CrSi$_2$]) nanowires (Ø 78–103 nm × 2.8–5.8 μm long) and correlated these values with their crystalline structures [151]. The S of bulk CrSi$_2$ at room temperature is ~96 μV/K, with an electrical resistivity of 10^{-3} Ω cm and thermal conductivity of ~10 W/m k [152,153], and the ZT of nanowires in this study had equivalent values. However, as the authors state, "the capability demonstrated here for the growth and combined TE structure characterization of individual CrSi$_2$ NWs will enable us to employ the synthesis and characterization methods to further investigate NW structures of other silicides with high bulk ZT values." These higher ZT silicides include β-FeSi$_2$ (ZT 0.4), MnSi$_{1.8}$ (ZT 0.7), and ReSi$_{1.8}$ (ZT 0.8) with the last two at 500–900 K [154,155]. These types of in-depth studies are likely to facilitate the functional optimization of nanowire structures, which may be applied to the design of stable high-performance nanoelectronics with minimized heat dissipation.

The thermal and electrical shielding of individual nanowires has been enabled by melting and encapsulating Ø ~10 to 100 nm Ge nanowires within a carbon sheath (1–5 nm wall thickness) to confine the molten Ge and demonstrated capabilities for in situ cutting, interconnection, and welding [156,157]. Deng et al. have synthesized Ø 30–400 nm × 40 μm long coaxial copper-core/carbon-sheath nanocables (Figure 5.6) in solution via a single-step hydrothermal method [158]. The Cu may be etched away to produce amorphous carbon nanotubes, which might be utilized as standardized sheaths for housing other species of metallic nanowires. This class of nanomaterials may provide sufficient insulating

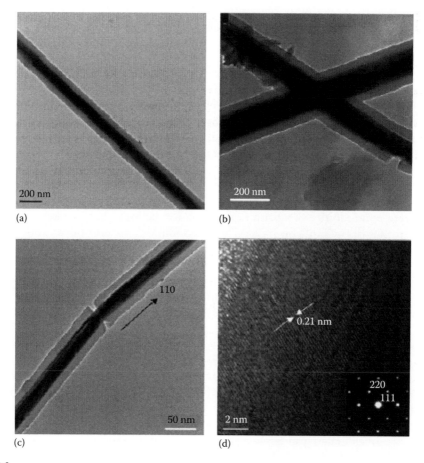

FIGURE 5.6
(a–c) TEM images and (d) HRTEM image of coaxial copper-core/carbon-sheath nanocables (inset in d is SAED pattern taken from (–110) zone axis). (Reprinted with permission from Deng, B. et al., *J. Phys. Chem. B*, 110(24), 11711. Copyright 2006 American Chemical Society.)

protection for closely abutted nanowires in the prevention of electron tunneling to facilitate their integration into nanomedical electronic circuitry.

5.3.8 Magnetic Properties of Nanowires

Magnetic nanowires might be integrated with electronics in nanomedical devices to assist, for instance, with navigation (Chapter 3). When interfaced with nanoelectronics, superparamagnetic iron oxide nanowires or magnetic nanoparticle/nanowire composites may be employed as analogs of the internal compasses that are utilized by magnetotactic bacteria (e.g., *Magnetospirillum gryphiswaldense* MSR-1 and *Magnetospirillum magneticum* AMB-1) [159,160] as directional reference indicators. Osterloh et al. synthesized $LiMo_3Se_3$–Fe_3O_4 nanowire–nanoparticle composites through a reaction (in tetrahydrofuran), between 3-iodopropionic acid–treated $LiMo_3Se_3$ nanowire bundles (4–6 nm thick) and Fe_3O_4 nanoparticles (Ø 2.8, 5.3, 12.5 nm) that were stabilized with oleic acid. It was deduced that the Fe_3O_4 nanoparticles were bonded to the nanowires by carboxylate groups from propionic acid linkers. Ultrasonication of the composites resulted in the formation of fragmented clusters (~340 nm long × ~20 nm thick), which had the capacity for being aligned via a (900 Oe) magnetic field [161].

An AC electrolysis technique was utilized by Routkevitch et al. to synthesize arrays of tightly spaced ferromagnetic nanowires employing Fe, Ni, and Co to create very high levels of saturation magnetism. Metal oxides were used in place of metallic nanoparticles, as nanoparticles tend to oxidize rapidly. The metal wires within the matrix were thereby chemically sealed, which keeps the metal in its unoxidized state. Magnetic properties may be widely varied through the use of this system [112]. Tulchinsky et al. produced highly uniform arrays of magnetic nanowires non-lithographically via a molecular beam epitaxial evaporation/shadowing technique on a nanometric corrugated surface. The corrugated surface was generated by the laser-focused Cr atom deposition in lines, which were formed by a standing wave directed along the gradient of the light intensity. Fe was subsequently evaporated perpendicularly to the Cr lines and the dimensions of the resulting nanowires were ~100 nm in width × ~0.15 mm in length. The Fe wires were then removed by immersion in an iron etch. By superimposing dual standing waves oriented at 90° to each other, iron islands may be fabricated, forming a 2D grid with a spacing of 213 nm. If each island stores one bit of information, the dots in this configuration have an information density close to 16 Gbits/in.^{2} [162].

The magnetic properties of as-synthesized Fe(1–x)Mn(x)Si nanowires at room temperature were reported by Hung et al. who measured strong ferromagnetism and a high magnetoresistance (−41.6% at 25 K under 9 T) in an individual nanowire [163]. In another interesting study, Mandal et al. found that spontaneous magnetism was initiated in PbS and Mn-doped PbS nanowires (Ø 30 nm), which were embedded in a polymer, at temperatures between 5 and 300 K. The source of ferromagnetism of the undoped PbS sample was thought to be the result "anionic defects arising out of nonstoichiometric growth" as PbS has an inherent concentration (1×10^{17}–1×10^{21} cm^{-3}) of defects. In the Mn-doped samples, the magnetism was construed to arise from the interactions of free carrier spins with Mn^{2+} magnetic moments [164].

5.3.9 Binary Wire Utilizing Quantum Dots

A binary wire comprises capacitively coupled double quantum dot (QD) cells that are charged with single electrons. Metal islands created by electrobeam lithography are connected in series by tunnel junctions with a capacitance of ~2.5 e/mV. Polarization switching is initiated by an applied input signal in one cell that leads to a change in polarization in an adjacent cell, analogous to falling dominoes. This arrangement is termed quantum dot cellular automata (QCA), a transistorless computational paradigm that offers solutions to issues such as device density, interconnect problems, and power dissipation [165–167]. The coulomb interaction is exploited in this architecture, which employs arrays of basic cells to execute digital logic functions. Digital data are encoded in the arrangements of individual electrons within the cells.

In a four-dot system, a typical cell consists of four dots located at the vertices of a square. When the cell is charged with two excess electrons, they occupy diagonal sites because of mutual electrostatic repulsion. They constitute energetically equivalent ground states of the cell. In a binary wire, a linear array of cells capacitively connected in series has the same functionality as a four-dot system. If the polarization of a double-dot cell is forced from −1 to +1, the neighboring cell will flip from +1 to −1. A QCA wire exploits this principal. The polarization at the input of the wire leads in succession to polarization changes in all the cells along the wire, and the system will relax in its new ground state. No current is flowing down the wire; therefore, power dissipation is very small [166]. Simulations have been made of various imperfections in the wire, including variations in the sizes of the cells, inconsistencies in intercellular spacing, and the presence of extra electrons [166,167]. The results indicate that the wire still functioned properly as the highly nonlinear response function acts to correct mistakes and restore the signal level [168].

5.3.10 Spider Silk–Templated Optical Fibers

Hollow optical silica fibers with Ø ~1 μm were fabricated by coating the silk thread from a *Nephila madagascariensis* spider with a glassy solution, and through subsequent extraction via baking at 420°C, which removes the silk by calcination. The silk was dipped repeatedly (as a wick into wax) into a solution of tetraethyl orthosilicate and when dried and subsequently baked, the coating was observed to shrink fivefold (from 5 to ~1 μm) [169]. Utilizing the silk from spider (*Stegodyphus pacificus*), with the thinnest known silk at Ø ~10 nm, it is conceivable that Ø ~2 nm fibers might be attainable when shrinkage is factored in. These diminutive hollow fibers might be employed as optical interconnects for data conveyance, or serve as waveguides for QD lasers in highly compact 3D nanoelectrophotonic circuitry (see Section 5.14).

5.3.11 DNA Nanowires

Nanowire diameters of ~2 nm have been realized through the adsorption of gold QDs along DNA templates. The free ends of the DNA nanowire may be configured with sequences that attach to complementary sequences, which are tethered to connection pads via hybridization. The two free ends will spontaneously seek each other out through chemical/electronic affinities and bind together correctly in solution. This method might be adapted to the construction of 3D wiring in aqueous media, as Au QDs can also catalyze subsequently deposited metal to build up continuous metallic nanowires. DNA is an excellent candidate as a nanowire template due to its flexibility, narrow diameter, and free-end targeting. The length of the templated nanowires can be controlled, as a DNA synthesizer could produce the DNA or enzymes following a template. The "wiring" within a nanodevice will be extremely dense and, hence, will require appropriate insulation.

Insulating options could include surface oxidation, the formation of a glass coating via reactions with salines or coating with alkane thiols. The average spacing of Au clusters adhered to the DNA duplex segments was ~2 nm. Interestingly, this is nearly equivalent to the electron tunneling distance between metal particles. There are several strategies for binding gold clusters to DNA, including covalent attachment, photoreaction, intercalation, or the electrostatic binding of positively charged gold particles to negatively charged DNA. Silver and other metals have also been nested within the duplex structure [170].

There are two primary categories of metal ion binding sites that are inherent to DNA, which include nucleobases and anionic phosphate groups [171].

An alternate strategy for the engineering of DNA molecules in the demonstration of metallic conduction involves the replacement of the imino proton of each base pair with a metal ion [172,173]. Both metallic-like conduction (M-DNA) and semiconducting properties (B-DNA) with a bandgap of several hundred meV at room temperature have been shown. Molecular devices based completely on DNA might be enabled via this engineered variance of conductance [174]. Hassanien et al. utilized 6 μm long λ-DNA as a template in the self-assembly of cuprous oxide (Cu_2O) nanowires (Ø 12–23 nm—among the smallest reported to date 2012) and observed that they comprised individual DNA-bound Cu_2O crystallites that fused over a period of time via a process akin to Ostwald ripening, whereby inhomogeneous smaller particulates dissolve and redeposit onto larger particles. This process was surmised to be driven by surface tension, as well as the "free energy of interaction with the template." The resulting nanowires exhibited a conductivity of 2.2–3.3 S/cm and indicated strong quantum confinement properties [171].

5.3.12 Molecular Wires

Molecular wires are fundamental conductive molecular entities (Ø ~3 nm) comprising organic molecules or conjugated assemblies thereof, which straddle two reservoirs of electrons. The molecular orbitals, when coupled to leads, enable pathways for electrons [175,176]. A class of semiconducting oligothiophene organic molecules have found extensive application as molecular wires. In what is referred to as a M-B-M molecular system, two equivalent redox centers (M), albeit in different oxidative conditions, contend for the charge through a "mediating molecular bridge (B)," which serves as the mediating conduit for electron transfer. Rodríguez González et al. prepared a set of oligothiophene–vinylene oligomers of variable lengths that served as spacers and which were terminated on both ends by ferrocenes (an organometallic "sandwich" compound—dual cyclopentadienyl rings bound on either side of a metal core atom), which was constructed analogously to a M-B-M system. Subsequent to analysis of these constructs, the researchers concluded that this molecular wire was an excellent contender to "unimolecularly transport electronic stimuli between distant electrogenerating centers (i.e., metallic electrodes or nanoparticles)." They were also impressed with the "ability to transmit the interferrocene coupling over distances near 40 Å, which is an outstanding wirelike feature" [177].

Reed et al. studied a benzene molecule with two sulfur atoms on either end of the benzene ring (1,4-benzene dithiolate) at room temperature, which was positioned between opposing Au contacts that were spaced at 8 Å. The benzene-1,4-dithiolate molecule was a component of a self-assembled monolayer (SAM) and a highly reproducible current of ~0.7 V was measured [178].

5.4 Electronic Properties of Carbon Nanotubes

In terms of the electrical conductance of carbon nanotubes, they may be either metallic (free-flowing ballistic current) or semiconducting (containing energy gaps that slow the current). The position of electrons (n) and holes (p) or a combination of the two are dependent on the nanotube chirality, diameter, and synthesis method. These nanometric entities have shown to be excellent electron field emitters (via electrons that tunnel through the surface potential barrier), with tremendous current densities for such diminutive structures [179–182]. Interestingly, it was observed by Wang et al. that nanotube tip geometries, which included open-ended samples with variously oriented graphene fragments, play a considerable role in field emission attributes in comparison to the nanotube length [183].

Bonard et al. investigated the field emissive properties of various carbon nanotube films, comprising closed SWNTs (Ø ~1.4 nm), as well as closed (Ø ~14 nm), opened (Ø ~15 nm), and catalytic (Ø ~22 nm) MWNTs (Figure 5.7) with a typical nanotube density of $10^9/cm^2$. The highest emission voltages were observed with the catalytic and opened MWNTs, at >5 V/μm E_{to} (turn-on field) and >15 V/μm E_{thr} (threshold field). In contrast, the emission voltages of the

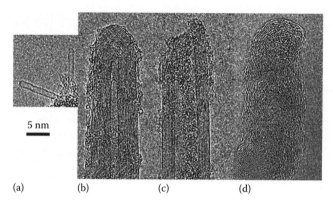

(a)   (b)   (c)   (d)

FIGURE 5.7
TEM images of various carbon nanotube tips: (a) SWNT (Ø ~1.4 nm), (b) closed MWNT (Ø ~14 nm), (c) opened MWNT (Ø ~15 nm), and (d) catalytic MWNT (Ø ~22 nm). (Reproduced from Bonard, J.M. et al., *Appl. Phys. A*, 69(3), 245, 1999. With kind permission from Springer Science and Business Media.)

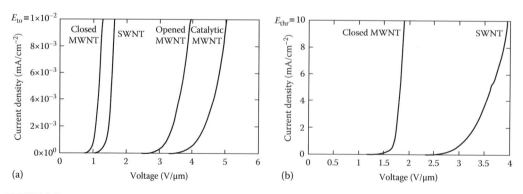

FIGURE 5.8
Current–voltage characteristics of various carbon nanotube films: (a) turn-on field (E_{to}) and (b) threshold field E_{thr} (Reproduced from Bonard, J.M. et al., *Appl. Phys. A*, 69(3), 245, 1999. With kind permission from Springer Science and Business Media.)

closed SWNT and MWNT films were <2.7 V/µm E_{to} and <5 V/µm E_{thr} (Figure 5.8). It was also learned that when the nanotubes were oriented perpendicularly to the substrate it resulted in "higher field amplification at the nanotube tips and thus in lower operating voltages." The state of the nanotube tips in this case as well was surmised to contribute in a significant way to the overall emissive quality [184].

Nanotubes may also be doped with various materials that will alter their electrical properties. For example, when a SWNT is doped with bromine or potassium, its conductivity will increase by a factor of 30 (at 300 K). A potassium-doped nanotube (1.5 µm in length) was demonstrated to electrostatically form a QD at its tip, and thereby induced the entire nanotube to behave as a QD with tunnel barriers for ingress and egress [185]. This characteristic has also been observed in longer metal nanotubes [186,187]. Li et al. investigated ZnO-coated carbon nanotubes that exhibited current density stability and improved homogeneous emission, which were due to an increase in emission sites that were provided by the adsorbed ZnO nanostructures [188]. Shorter nanotubes have different electrical properties than longer ones due to quantum size effects. These unique electronic properties are due to quantum confinement of electrons normal to the central nanotube axis. In the radial direction, electrons are confined by the monolayer thickness of the graphene sheet. Because of this quantum confinement, electrons may propagate along the tube axis and standing waves are set up around the circumference of the tube.

The field emission current for a SWNT is ~1 µA per tube [189] while the maximum current that can be drawn is ~2 mA. Rather than a DC bias, the emission can be pulsed and may serve to protect the tube from ionic bombardment [190]. The current that is transferrable through a MWNT is equivalent to a current density of over 10^7 A/cm^2 [191]. The local electric field directly above the emitting surface required for field emission is ~3 V/nm and electron emission emanates from the entire cap (not from a few local atoms that are positioned there) and flows through the outermost layer of the tube [192]. Local density states are attributed to the presence of pentagonal defects [193] and density states may attain values that are 30-fold higher at the nanotube tip in contrast to its body [194]. Interestingly, adsorbates on the nanotube cap can have the effect of enhancing emission and with the cap removed, the emission emanates from the graphene edges [195]. Although several deeper energy levels participate in carbon nanotube field emission, the occupied level that is closest to the Fermi point will supply most of the emitted electrons. The position of this level is contingent on localized atomic configurations. Hence, differences may be anticipated when comparing one nanotube to the next, unless they are highly uniform. The resistance of a nanotube, regardless of length, has been predicted to be a minimum of ~6500 Ω [191].

It was found through calculations that a configuration of two disparate concentric nanotubes, with the inner one being metallic and the outer one being semiconducting or insulating, has inherent stability. This arrangement constitutes a nanoscale-shielded cable, and serves to eliminate the need for doping [196]. Fink et al. utilized a single nanotube in a high-resolution electron beam instrument (low-energy electron projection microscope) wherein electrons were extracted via the application of voltage between the MWNT and the sample. The nanotube produced a highly coherent beam that allowed the acquisition of in-line electron holograms of the observed objects, and had the same quality as atom-sized W emitters [197,198].

Emissive functionality has been observed over a very large current range (~10 pA to ~0.2 mA) through the testing of a variety of nanotube species as single emitters and in film form. It was found that as-synthesized capped nanotubes were far more efficient than open nanotubes. When the nanotube ends are open, there is a serious degradation of emission characteristics, and the voltage that is required to initiate emissive current is found to be a factor of two higher than that needed for closed nanotubes. For a closed MWNT, the field amplification factor (e.g., the electric field lines that are concentrated around the cap curvature) was found to be 40,000 at a 1 mm interelectrode distance and 10,800 for an opened MWNT [194].

In semiconducting (zig-zag type) nanotubes, electrons and positive holes (their charge opposites) constitute energy bandgaps that inhabit particular orbitals around an atom, which are interleaved regions between these orbitals where charges are forbidden to flow. The bandgap of a semiconducting nanotube is inversely proportional to the nanotube diameter. For a 0.6–1.6 diameter SWNT, the band gaps are 0.4–1 eV; at larger diameters the bandgap gets close to zero. For a 1 nm diameter × 3 um long nanotube, ~2.6 meV is required to add an electron and overcome the Coulomb repulsion between electrons. Armchair nanotubes are metallic and thereby, may serve as good electrical interconnects. This quality can be optimized if they are isolated. Controlling the environment around these nanotubes is critical, as chemical binding events will degrade their conductive abilities. One method for maintaining armchair nanotube separation is to grow them in place [199].

De Heer et al. observed that a MWNT under 0.4 mA at 10−9 mbar for more than two months, suffered no degradation and that current densities of ~1 mA/cm2 produced stable emission rates in MWNT films [200]. Diagnostic x-ray radiation has been generated utilizing nanotube based cold cathode field emission in pulsed and continuous mode. A 50 nm diameter bundle of purified SWNTs (each 1.4 nm in diameter) was used and the emission current was 28 mA , which emanated from a 0.2 cm2 area. High frequency, high intensity pulsed x-rays (at 100 KHz) were used for this application, demonstrating that nanotube based cathodes may provide focused electron beams to obtain high-resolution medical imaging [201].

5.5 Inorganic Nanotubes

There exist a number of inorganic compounds that possess inherent structures that are analogous to graphene and hence have very similar or identical morphologies to carbon nanotubes [202]. These include metal dichalcogenides, which encompass sulfides, selenides, and tellurides; halides, inclusive of chlorides, bromides, and iodides; as well as various ternary/quaternary compounds, oxides, and hydroxides [203]. Bismuth nanotubes are semiconducting regardless of diameter, chirality, or number of walls and can act as insulators. Their bandgaps typically decrease with increases in diameter, and at Ø approx. >18 Å both Bi(n, 0) and Bi(n, n) type of nanotubes have a forbidden bandgap of 0.63 eV, which is equivalent to that of single "puckered" Bi sheets. When these nanotubes form, the bismuth atoms form a trigonal pyramid sheet, whereby Bi atoms bind with three of its neighbors [204,205].

Hexagonal boron nitride (BN) sheets also exhibit a crystalline structure that is similar to graphene, where C–C pairs may be visualized as being replaced by B–N pairs to construct nanotubes and other fullerene-like geometries. BN nanotubes with diameters larger than 1 nm are shown to have bandgaps of 4–5 eV [206]. Semiconducting zigzag boron monoxide (B_2O) and titanium diboride (TiB_2) nanotubes were found to have bandgaps of 1.63 and 1.32 eV, respectively, whereas a boron carbide (B_4C) nanotube bandgap is 2.32 eV. The bandgaps of titanium dioxide (TiO_2) nanotubes were found to decrease in step with the decrease in diameter [203].

Elias et al. demonstrated a technique for the transformation of hexagonal ZnO nanowire arrays into ZnO nanotube arrays via a three-step chemical and electrochemical procedure.

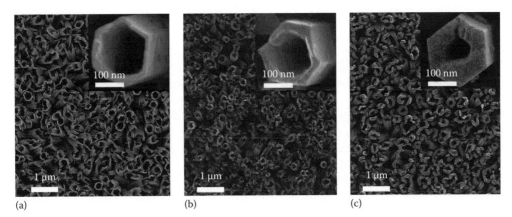

(a)   (b)   (c)

FIGURE 5.9
Scanning electron microscopy images of ZnO nanotube arrays: (a) following initial dissolution of the core and (b, c) thickening of the ZnO nanotube walls via subsequent electrochemical deposition. (Reproduced with permission from Elias, J. et al., *Chem. Mater.*, 20, 6633. Copyright 2008 American Chemical Society.)

The initial step involved the O_2 reduction of zinc chloride ($ZnCl_2$) and potassium chloride (KCl) to enable the electrodeposition of nanowire arrays. Second, the cores of the ZnO nanowires were discriminately etched in a solution of KCl to produce ZnO nanotubes ($\emptyset$ ~200–500 nm × 1–5 μm long). Subsequently, in a third deposition step, the wall thicknesses of the nanotubes could be tuned (~20 to 45 nm) [207] (Figure 5.9).

Ye et al. developed two methods for increasing the field emission properties of ZnO nanorods, including the narrowing of their tip radius to $\emptyset$ ~5 nm, or decorating them with platinum (Pt) or silver (Ag) nanoparticles. The researchers determined that similar modifications might be utilized to augment the field emission of ZnO nanotubes. A turn-on field of as low as 2 V/μm and a current density as high as 1 mA/cm² was accomplished through these methods. It was postulated that the enhanced geometry of the nanotube tip and the additional infusion of electrons from the adhered metallic nanoparticles facilitated this dramatic improvement [208].

These types of inorganic semiconducting nanotubes may be electronically tuned by controlling the number of layers within their structures and/or functionalizing their external surfaces with various types of nanoparticles, thus they may have utility for the gating of nanoelectronic connections in medical nanodevices.

5.6 Y-Junction Nanotubes

Three-terminal Y-junction carbon nanotubes might be integrated into ultradense nanoelectronics to function as branched in situ control gates to enable "electronic switching and differential current gain" [209,210]. Bandaru et al. demonstrated electrical switching in a carbon nanotube Y-junction for the first time (2005). When ~4.6 V was applied to the stem of a MWNT Y-junction, the voltage in both bifurcated branches was stepped down to ~2 V. This effect was surmised to be due to several factors, including reduced branch diameters, as well as varied morphology and defects within the branches [211].

A nanochannel alumina template-based method involving the pyrolysis of acetylene using a cobalt catalyst was developed by Li et al. for the fabrication of tunable, reproducible, and high-yield Y-junction carbon nanotubes (Ø ~90 to 100 nm stems with Ø ~50 to 60 nm branches × ~20 to 30 μm long) at a density of 10^9 cm^{-2} [212]. These nanotubes have been classified as p–p isotype semiconductor heterojunctions that can be connected in parallel arrays, and it has been proposed that they might serve as three-terminal nanoscale transistors through the application of different voltages to each branch of the Y-junction [213].

Contacts were added to Y-junctions via the sputtering of a silver or gold island-like film to their exteriors. Subsequent to the application of a bias of 10–20 V over several hours, metal particulates migrated to the tips of the junctions, thereby producing low resistance contacts. The bandgap is observed to change as the current is transferred from the larger diameter stem to the smaller diameter branches, and exhibits reproducible rectification at room temperature. At equilibrium, the Fermi level is constant across the junction, which occurs via the transfer of holes from the large bandgap side to the small bandgap side to initiate band "bending." When forward bias is applied, the Fermi level shifts and lowers the barrier to the holes, thereby enabling the current to increase dramatically. The negatively applied voltage "pulls" the positively charged holes across the junction [214]. This class of nanoscale junction might find utility when incorporated into the nanoelectrical interconnects for nanomedical devices where rectification functions are required.

AuBuchon et al. developed multi-branched carbon nanotube structures via the initial synthesis of primary carbon nanotube (Ø ~30 to 60 nm) arrays (using a Ni growth catalyst) with a density of ~2 × 10^9 cm^2. Subsequently, the perpendicular growth of smaller diameter (Ø ~5 to 10 nm) nanotube branches along the lengths of the primary nanotube "backbones" was induced by field-guided bidirectional growth (Figure 5.10). This growth was facilitated by a self-seeding process, whereby material from the original Ni catalyst nanoparticles is utilized in the sputtering of Ni onto the exterior sidewalls of the primary nanotubes to initiate the growth of the branches.

The researchers envision that these types of structures may hold promise in the evolution of highly dense nanoelectronics arrays of transistors and switches [209].

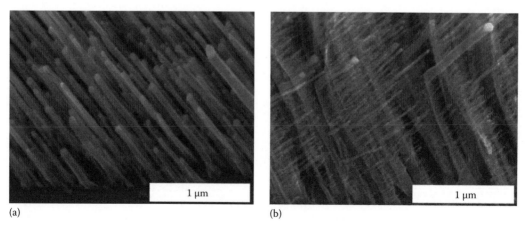

(a)   (b)

FIGURE 5.10
SEM images depicting (a) primary nanotube array and (b) perpendicularly oriented nanotube branches. (Reproduced with permission from Aubuchon, J.F. et al., *Nano Lett.*, 6(2), 324. Copyright 2006 American Chemical Society.)

5.7 Electronic Properties of QDs

A quantum well provides a confining potential along the growth direction, while an electrostatically induced potential barrier accomplishes lateral confinement. Coulomb forces (the electrostatic interaction of charged particles) between carriers direct the charging of QDs and their recombination dynamics. Cavity quantum electrodynamics (a field involving atomic physics and quantum optics) shows that spontaneous radiative emission from excited atoms may be strongly enhanced or diminished through the confinement of atoms within a specially designed cavity, or between mirrors [215]. The Purcell effect pertains to the modification of emission due to the manipulation of the local environment.

QDs are Ø ~2 to 10 nm semiconducting nanoparticles that have been referred to as "artificial atoms," as the electrons contained within these systems exhibit both quantized charge and energy. In nanomedical devices these intriguing diminutive entities might enable multiple functionalities when designed into nanoelectronic/photonic circuit architectures, serving as transistors, onboard lasing devices, cellular automata in enabling computation (Chapter 7), and facilitate the specific control of electron flow between components. A remarkable feature of a QD when it is interfaced with electronic terminals is that its capacitance, or the current that flows through it may be altered by "many orders of magnitude when its charge is changed by a single electron" [216,217].

In a QD transistor, electrons must initially tunnel into the dot in order to traverse the distance from source to drain. A self-assembled semiconducting QD (~30 nm × 5 nm high) may house approximately a million atoms, wherein the majority of electrons are bound to the nuclei of the material. However, unbound electrons may number from one to several hundred. The de Broglie wavelength of these electrons is similar to the dimensions of the dot; hence, they can express themselves as waves. The electrons occupy discrete quantum levels and possess a distinct excitation spectrum [218].

The energy scales involved in QDs are on par with the ionization energies of atoms. This is the energy required for the addition or removal of an electron from the dot (typically called the charging energy), which is dominated by the coulomb interaction. Single electron transport can occur up to room temperature, and the dimension of the QD in this case should be ~20 nm in diameter. The electron tunneling times through barriers (some gate oxides can be as thin as ~9 Å) can range from pico- (10^{-12}) to femto- (10^{-15}) seconds [219–222]. In a multi-dot array, a charge from one dot is capable of shifting the electrostatic potential of another, or an electron may coherently tunnel back and forth between various dots [223].

When a charge is progressively more confined, its energy will increase; hence, coulomb and self-charging energies are elevated with decreasing QD size. In a QD with a radius of 1–6 nm, the electronic spacing can be greater than ~100 meV and spectral tunability might span a range as wide as 1 eV. For instance, the coulomb charging energies for InAs QDs (Ø 20.4 and 10.2 nm) on GaAs were 17.8 and 24.8 meV, respectively [224], whereas for cadmium selenide (CdSe) QDs, with dimensions of Ø less than ~10 nm, charging energies of >100 meV were observed [225].

5.8 Single Electron Transistor

Single electron transistors (SETs) are based on nanoscale metallic "Coulomb islands" that contain approximately a million mobile electrons, which may be switched off and on by virtue of extremely subtle charge differences (initiated by single electrons) on connecting electronic gates. An SET has three terminals (e.g., gate, source, and drain) as does a FET. When the gate voltage attains half the charge of an electron on the gate capacitor, the tunneling current can increase dramatically. Electrons that reside beyond the confines of an island must exceed a particular thermal energy threshold in order to overcome the Coulomb blockade to access them [226–228]. Through the fine control of external gate voltages, electrons may be induced to ingress into these nanometric islands one by one, creating in effect an "electron turnstile." This is facilitated by nanoscale phenomenon wherein electric charges, rather than exhibiting continuous flow, are conveyed as quantized packets. Principally, a typical SET comprises two-tunnel junctions that share a common electrode. The tunnel junction consists of two metal elements that are separated by a very thin (~1 nm) insulating barrier. Electrons can only move from one electrode to the other by tunneling through this insulator [229,230].

In 1994, Nakajima et al. demonstrated the modulation of a source/drain current in a Ø ~30 nm SET with a Coulomb blockade at 150 K [231], which contributed to the development of such devices that operated at room temperature (300 K) [232]. Karrea and Bergstrom stipulated in 2007 that "For room temperature operation, which is a critical requirement for practical applications, the capacitance of the SET device needs to be of the order of attofarads, thus limiting the dimension of the quantum confining islands below 10 nm" [233]. In 2011, Cheng et al. created a Ø 1.5 nm metal oxide SET, interfaced with 1–1.2 nm thick nanowires, which accommodated only two, one, or zero electrons, thereby enabling a clear demarcation of its quantum states [234].

As we can see clear progress in the development of these devices, one may surmise that in the not too distant future, SETs might play a considerable role in the nanoelectronic circuitry designs of medical nanodevices. When incorporated into well-configured electronic architectures, SETs may be utilized for precisely controlling the activation and deactivation of multiple operations for in vivo nanomedical devices, possibly from outbody sources. An inherent threshold voltage may engineered into electrodes that are linked to components, albeit separated by ultrathin tunnel junctions, and might remain queued until the gate is selectively activated by perhaps a particular pulsed radio frequency signal or via photonic means, to allow the current to flow and trigger, for instance, the scanning mechanisms of the VCSN.

5.9 Nanometric Supercapacitors

Nanometric supercapacitors may have significant utility as potential energy storage devices when employed as power reservoirs within nanomedical devices, as they demonstrate rapid charging/discharging performance in comparison to batteries, highly stable operational longevity; may comprise relatively environmentally compatible (and potentially biocompatible) nonreactive materials; and demonstrate steadily improving energy densities. Charge in supercapacitors is stored in electrochemical double layers (EDLs) and resident energy density levels are contingent on the extent of the cumulative available surface area and conductivity of its constituent elements. Carbon nanotubes make for excellent supercapacitive elements due to a number of attractive features, encompassing high conductivity and power density, large surface area, chemical stability, and low mass density. A supercapacitor has been developed from two carbon nanotube-based active electrodes that were submerged in an electrolyte and separated by an ion-permeable membrane, which negated electron transfer. The increased surface area inherent to carbon nanotubes exponentially augments the level of potential capacitance. One of the primary challenges is the control of the physical dimensions of the nanotubes, as their electronic properties are intimately influenced by their length, diameter, and chirality [235,236].

Kim et al. fabricated high-performance supercapacitors that consisted of vertical arrays of carbon nanotubes, which worked in conjunction with nonaqueous electrolytes (e.g., ionic liquids and organic electrolytes). When combined with ionic liquid, the supercapacitor demonstrated excellent power performance in specific capacitance (~75 F/g), energy density (~27 Wh/kg), and maximum power (~987 kW/kg). Moreover, when the nanotubes were electrochemically oxidized and induced tip opening, the specific capacitance and energy density increased further to ~158 F/g and ~53 Wh/kg, respectively. This remarkable performance was attributed to several factors, including a rapid relaxation time constant (0.2 s), rapid ion transport (facilitated by nanotube alignment), and a wide, ionic liquid-enabled, operational voltage [237].

A flexible supercapacitor comprising graphene films was fabricated by El-Kady et al. through the direct laser reduction of graphite oxide films using a standard LightScribe DVD optical drive. The resulting films showed high electrical conductivity (1738 S/m^2) and a specific surface area of 1520 m^2/g. These electrodes demonstrated "ultrahigh energy density values in different electrolytes while maintaining the high power density and excellent cycle stability" [236]. The innate maximum capacitance of a single layer of graphene has been observed to be ~21 µF/cm^2 [238]. When immersed in aqueous potassium hydroxide and organic electrolyte, the specific capacitance was observed to be 130 and 99 F/g, respectively [239]. If the entire surface area (individual graphene sheet surface area is 2630 m^2/g) was to be utilized, it has been calculated as theoretically possible that the EDL capacitance of graphene-based supercapacitors might attain ~550 F/g [236].

Interestingly, in the prospective biomimetic domain, Type IV Pili (T4P)-based networks of microbial nanowires embedded in *Geobacter sulfurreducens* biofilms have exhibited supercapacitor-like traits. These highly porous biofilms consist of ~95% electrolyte, which enables "high electrolytic accessibility for the movement of ions," which is required for sustaining the electroneutrality as a prerequisite to capacitor formation [240,241]. T4P are pliable follicle-like entities (Ø 6 nm × ~2 to 3 µm long) that have demonstrated long-range conductivity that is similar to that of metals [242]. It had been suggested that peptide-based and proteinaceous (e.g., flagella, amyloid, and amyloid-like fibrils) nanotubes might be incorporated into nanoelectronic circuitry. These self-assembling nanosystems possess inherent advantages such as biocompatibility, structural diversity, and the potential for tunable adaptability via genetic engineering [243].

It may be plausible that biocompatible macroscale supercapacitors could be designed that once administered, in perhaps contingents of thousands, might autoimplant themselves in a more or less evenly distributed fashion throughout the tissues of a patient to serve as long-term resident "charging stations." These rapid recharge nodes could contain standardized docking/plug in ports to accommodate the recharging of most primary species of transitory nanomedical devices.

5.10 Spin Electronics Using Nanotubes

Ferromagnetic contacts have been employed to inject and detect spin-polarized electrons within multiwalled nanotubes (MWNTs). Due to the small diameters involved, individual magnet domains can be probed. As the alignment of magnetization within the contacts transitions from parallel to antiparallel, the nanotube resistance status may be flipped from low to high. In addition, spin-polarized electrons can be injected from ferromagnetic to non-ferromagnetic materials [244,245] and through oxide tunnel barriers [246–248]. Spin coherent effects improve the nanotube ferromagnetic interface and resistance will drop dramatically as the magnetic field is increased [244,249]. These phenomena may usher in nanotube-based spin electronics, whereby in vivo nanodevices might be specifically activated and deactivated via the application of focused, externally generated magnetic fields.

Wei et al. undertook to investigate the properties of individual magnetic nickelocene molecule adherence to single-walled carbon nanotubes in order to determine what species of linker group might prove optimal in facilitating spin-polarized electron transfer from the molecule to nanotube. The linker candidates included an amide group, as well as aziridine and pyrrolidine rings. It was discovered that only the aziridine permitted spin polarization transfer from the nickelocene to the nanotube with "efficient spin-filtering functionality." As all of the atoms of a single-walled carbon nanotube are present at the surface, it can be anticipated that even seemingly subtle surface alterations may result in significant impacts on the conveyance of electrons [250]. Therefore, the attachment of magnetic molecules to nanotubes with functional linkers such as aziridine may lead to addressable/switchable supramolecular spintronic devices that allow for the precise manipulation of electron transmission, and hence, potentially magnetically controlled in vivo medical nanodevices.

5.11 Nanostructured Conductive Polymers

Nanostructured conductive polymers are unique materials in that they are as electrically conductive as metals, but can retain their mechanical properties (Figure 5.11). This attribute may have important utility in the design and routing capacity of circuitry for advanced nanomedical devices such as the VCSN. The primary classes of conductive polymers include polypyrrole, polyaniline, polyacetylene, and polythiophene. When these

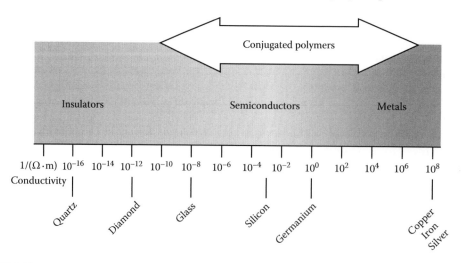

FIGURE 5.11
Conductivity of conjugated polymers. (Reproduced from Korzhov, M. et al., *PhysicaPlus, Online Magazine of the Israel Physical Society (IPS)*, 10, 2008. With permission.)

types of polymers are doped with electron acceptors or donors, their conductivity may be induced to increase by many orders of magnitude [251,252].

The majority of conjugated polymers possess hole mobilities that span from 10^{-7} to 10^{-5} cm^2/V/s. In contrast, self-assembling regioregular poly(3-alkylthiophene)s (rrP3ATs) exhibit considerably higher mobilities (10^{-2} cm^2/V/s) [252,253]. This is made possible due to 3D organizational scheme that encompasses backbone conformational ordering, the π-stacking of planar polymer chains, and interchain lamellar stacking [254]. The "capping" of each conductive polymeric unit allows them to link with chemical groups that are receptive to binding with structured polymers, metals, silicon, and other material substrates. Their material characteristics may be varied to a much greater extent than any other conductive polymer, as subtle conformational variations may translate into significant changes in conductivity [255,256].

Ravichandran et al. have reviewed the use of conductive polymers in biomedical engineering (constituting one of the multiple facets of nanomedical endeavor), where they might be utilized as artificial muscles [257], to initiate nerve regeneration [258,259], enable precision drug release [260] and neural recording [259], and to serve as synergistic body/machine interfaces by enabling the fusion of electronic devices with human tissues (Figure 5.12) [261].

Electron transfer in conductive polymers is attributed to the effects of monomeric polymerization or doping, which create nonlinear imperfections (e.g., bipolarons, polarons, or solitons) [262]. The conjugated bonds between carbon atoms are alternating single and double bonds that reside along the backbone of an otherwise insulated construct, giving rise to polymeric conductivity. Further, "Every bond in the backbone contains a localized 'sigma' (s) bond, which forms a strong chemical bond and every double bond also contains a less strongly localized 'pi' (p) bond" [263,264]. These polymers transfer current via doped ions that must be integral elements within the structure, in that they translate charge as excess electrons. "The dopant neutralizes the unstable backbone when the polymer is in the oxidized form. On application of a potential across the film, a flux of ions either in or out of the film, dependent on dopant charge and motility, disrupts the stable backbone, resulting in the passage of charge through the polymer film" [265].

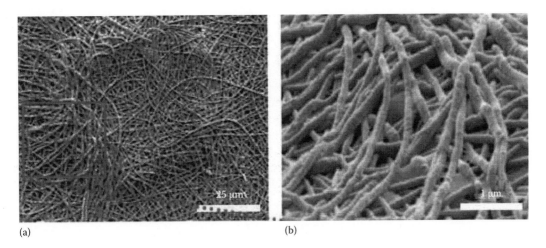

(a)   (b)

FIGURE 5.12
(a) Top view of poly(3,4-ethylenedioxythiophene) (PEDOT) nanotubes and (b) three-dimensional view of PEDOT nanotubes. (Reproduced from Heeger, A.J. et al., *The Nobel Prize in Chemistry, 2000: Conductive Polymers*, Royal Swedish Academy of Sciences, Stockholm, Sweden, 2000; Abidian, M.R. and Martin, D.C., *Biomaterials*, 29(9), 1273, 2008. With permission.)

One of the primary issues that have limited the utilization of conductive polymers for the stimulation of cells in tissue engineering is that they do not inherently biodegrade. Zelikin et al. have endeavored to address this shortcoming through the development of a conductive polymer (polypyrrole) that was erodable via the chemical and electrochemical polymerization of β-substituted pyrrole monomers, which included ionizable and/or hydrolyzable side groups [266]. Shi et al. has combined biodegradable elements such as polylactide, polyglycolide, and associated copolymers or ester linkages with conductive polymers [267]. Guimard et al. took an alternate approach through the synthesis of a conductive polymer that contained both conductive and degradable backbone units, which may offer improved control of conductivity and degradation [268]. In nanomedical devices, adjunctive conductive polymer nanoparticles or protrusile nanowires might serve as potential interfacial conduits between advanced synthetic nanodevices and a variety of human cell and tissue types. They might provide selective therapeutic electrical stimulation to facilitate muscle or nerve regeneration at specific sites within the heart or the brain, respectively, or for the repair of other organs and tissues.

5.12 Electronic Properties of Thin Films

Thin magnetic ceramic films of lanthanum, strontium, manganese, and oxygen (LSMO) that are several angstroms thick and magnetoresistive can be fabricated by pulsed laser ablation. These thin films demonstrated giant magnetoresistance (GMR) and colossal magnetoresistance (CMR) under a magnetic field of 5–10 T. Their electrical resistance may be decreased by more than 1000% in comparison to <20% in conventional thin films [270]. Transparent conducting oxides (TCOs) have a tunable optical gap and electrical conductivity via extended solid-solution phases. Oxides of cations in these films are Zn^{2+}, Cd^{2+}, In^{3+}, Ga^{3+}, and Sn^{4+}. Indium oxide doped with Sn, forming indium tin oxide (ITO), is a commonly used TCO due to its excellent conductivity and transparency. Its conductivity is facilitated by octahedrally coordinated In layers. Cubic Cd_2SnO_4 shows high electron mobility and good transparency [271]. However, ITO has drawbacks, such as cracking, when used on flexible substrates, is expensive, and necessitates the use of high temperatures during fabrication. Liu and Yu have developed a transparent Ag nanowire–based thin film on a plastic substrate that is a strong contender for flexible electronics as it exhibited excellent pliability. Ag also has the highest conductivity (6.3×10^7 S/m) of all the metals [272].

In diminutive nanomedical devices, it seems obvious that the requirement for macroscale flexibility will be negated. However, spatial flex allowances will likely be necessary in some designs in order to accommodate movement, albeit on the order of angstroms or nanometers, for the flexing of integrated ultrathin film piezoelectric elements that are assigned for power generation or are used as onboard cantilevered sensors. It is envisaged by the author that contingent on the class and species of nanodevice, modular components (e.g., 1–10 nm^2) might be self-assembled using DNA-based manufacturing affinities [4], built up atom by atom utilizing diamond mechanosynthesis [273], or other prospective forms of nanomanufacturing [274] (e.g., nanoscale 3D printing).

The ultimate in ultrathin films for potentially enabling nanomedical device electronics might be (one atomic layer thick) graphene sheets. The fabrication of extremely dense circuitry with these elements seems plausible as graphene is highly conductive (~298 S/cm)

[275] and individual graphene sheets might be laminated/interdigitated within alternating sheets of ultrathin insulating materials in conjunction with selective patterning via nanoscale etching. The edges of graphene might interface with other graphene sheets, nanowires, or nanotubes that are positioned in appropriate orientations to facilitate circuit routing.

Organic thin films investigated by Centurion et al. exhibited high electrically conductive affinity/sensitivity for water vapor, which may be useful as onboard moisture/perspiration sensors to perhaps facilitate diagnostics or the guidance of surface-ambling nanomedical devices. A layer-by-layer technique was employed to fabricate nanostructured thin films comprising linear poly(allylamine hydrochloride) (PAH) and poly(amidoamine) dendrimer (PAMAM) polyelectrolytes, which was infused with cobalt-tetrasulfonated phthalocyanine (CoTsPc) [276].

5.13 Nanoscale Antenna

Nanoscale antennae will play essential roles as communications conduits that serve as the vital interface between nanodevice resident nanoelectronic/computing infrastructures and outbody computers. They will be responsible for the receipt of critical real-time commands from physicians and the conveyance of large volumes of data acquired in vivo, through highly compressed data streams. Hence, their designs should aim to optimize robustness and reliability to enable their efficient functionality within the challenging in vivo environment of patients. Advanced autonomous nanomedical devices may be endowed with a combination of a number of dedicated stand-alone antennae, and those that are integrated as arrays within communications and data transfer beacons (Chapter 6).

Halas et al. fabricated an integrated "plasmonic antenna-graphene photodetector" that comprised plasmonic clusters (gold heptamers consisting of Ø 130 nm disks at 15 nm interdisk spacing), which were interdigitated between two single layers of graphene (Figure 5.13). This nanoantenna device demonstrated an increased photocurrent efficacy of 800% in the conversion of both near-infrared and visible light photons, in contrast to graphene by itself. The photocurrent was enhanced through the transport of hot electrons that were produced in the antennae via the degradation of plasmons, as well as the "direct plasmon-enhanced excitation of intrinsic graphene electrons." The internal quantum efficiency of this device, encompassing near-infrared and visible photons, was observed to be ~20% with approximated mobilities in the range from 350 to 1300 cm^2 V/s. The sensitivity of the antenna to particular wavelengths may be tuned by virtue of altering the diameters of the constituent heptamer disks. For example, when the disk diameters were changed from 80 to 180 nm, the Fano resonance (resonant scattering) was correspondingly modified from 650 to 950 nm along with associated shifts in the resulting photocurrents [277].

An optical Yagi-Uda (directional element) nanoantenna array was investigated by Dregely et al. that may pave the way for future, highly efficient nanometric detection and emission in three dimensions. In effect, the researchers have demonstrated an optical antenna array that is analogous in functionality to radiofrequency antenna arrays with the potential for beam steering. The nanoantenna array was fabricated on a glass substrate via electron beam lithography employing a layer-by-layer stacking technique, which resulted

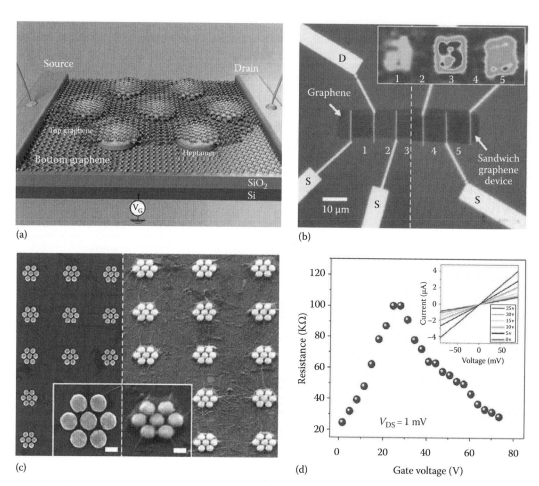

(a)   (b)   (c)   (d)

FIGURE 5.13
Depiction of nanoantenna photodetector. (a) Illustration of single gold heptamer encapsulated between two graphene monolayers. (b) Image (optical microscope) of the device prior to (left) and following (right) application of top graphene layer. Inset: G mode Raman mapping of device segments exposed to 785 nm wavelength. (c) SEM image of heptamer array in segment 3 of (b). (d) Electrical transport at 1 mV drain bias. Inset: gate voltage (*I–V* plots: 0–25 V). (Reproduced with permission from Fang, Z. et al., *Nano Lett.*, 12(7), 3808. Copyright 2012 American Chemical Society.)

in a three-tiered construct consisting of gold elements and nanorods that were embedded within a photopolymer. Individual nanoantennae comprised three layers, each spaced at 100 nm from one another, which included a central feed element (250 nm) that was bracketed by a front director (230 nm) and back reflector (300 nm). The overall dimensions of the nanoantenna array were 90 × 90 μm.

The researchers suggest that the 3D Yagi-Uda nanoantenna array might be employed for beam steering applications at near-infrared wavelengths (e.g., ~λ = 1500 nm) (near-infrared range is from 800 to 2500 nm), which will be amenable for use with in vivo nanomedical devices as near-infrared light may pass harmlessly through human tissues. The capacity for directivity of these arrays may facilitate the acquisition of externally generated pulsed near-infrared laser light communications by in vivo nanomedical devices [278].

5.14 Integrated 3D Nanoelectronics

The strategy of fabricating bottom-up 3D integrated circuits layer by layer may provide multiple advantages for nanomedical devices, including extremely high density (e.g., employing ultrathin nanowires or nanoribbons), high-speed performance, and frugal power use.

Ahn et al. have developed a straightforward technique to enable the combination of a wide range of disparate materials in the fabrication of heterogeneous integrated electronic circuitry in two or three dimensions. An additive transfer printing technique was employed, utilizing soft stamps, to repeatedly interface layers of semiconducting nanomaterials (e.g., SWNTs) with single crystalline nanowires, and silicon, gallium nitride, and gallium arsenide nanoribbons on rigid or flexible substrates. Electronic connectivity between multiple layers was accomplished by the simple evaporation of metals into photopatterned openings in the interlayers. The deposition and configuration of electrodes, gates, and device interconnects followed by the addition of a spin-coated prepolymer (e.g., polyamic acid) interlayer and repeated transfer printing enabled the construction of highly novel and versatile electronic systems that "would be impossible to achieve with other techniques" [279].

Javey et al. demonstrated the construction of a multifunctional 3D electronic system by employing the layer-by-layer assembly of germanium/silicon (Ge/Si) core/shell nanowires to build up a vertical, 10-layered stack of multi-nanowire FETs. Transport quantification studies verified that the high performance of the devices in each layer was reproducible and uniform from layer to layer. The researchers also showed that when inverter logical gates and nanowire floating gate memory elements were layered on plastic substrates, they exhibited stable write and erase functions [280].

The exploitation of DNA oligonucleotide complementary base pairing may provide a powerful approach for the bottom-up fabrication of complex nanoelectronic systems in three dimensions [4]. Top-down nanoelectronic systems are currently restricted by lithographic resolution (albeit a new quantum optical lithography technique presented by Pavel of Storex Technologies in July 2012, at SPIE Advanced Lithography 2012, touted a 2 nm half-pitch line resolution) [281], and the dimensions of nanowires. Nanowires are also constrained insofar as the volume of digital data that they may convey in comparison to digitized optical fiber strategies [282,283]. Another issue related to the conveyance of current at the nanoscale is that when interconnects approach smaller dimensions (e.g., >10 nm) their electrical resistance increases, as does heating. Conventional chip manufacturers currently employ copper for interconnects, which is applied by vapor deposition, to fill vertical holes that run through layers of circuits. Any defects, including diminutive bubbles that may occur in the cooling process, along any length of the cumulative 100 km copper wiring interconnects in today's (2012) chips will cause failures and force the rejection of the chip. In fact, interconnects are now the primary cause of signal delay, heating, and power drain in state-of-the-art integrated circuits. Due to the enormous scale of present semiconductor chip manufacturing infrastructures, it can take up to a decade to incorporate a new material, such as carbon nanotubes, into chips [284].

New and dynamic nanomanufacturing strategies may likely alleviate the problems described earlier, especially in regard to the introduction of new materials, through the capacity of being rapidly reconfigurable. An inherent advantage of nanoscale circuits in medical nanodevices would seem to be that as the distances that current/signals must traverse are minimized to the nanometer range, the heat that is manifest through resistance should decrease significantly. Cumulatively, however, localized waste heat from nanodevice power generation will emanate from nanodevices, though it will most likely be dissipated rapidly. Freitas calculates that the power generation for a nanodevice with a volume of 1 μm³ "corresponds with power densities around 10^7 W/m³, several orders of magnitude larger than power densities in tissue." Due to rapid local heat dissipation, however, he estimates that there will be a "negligible maximum temperature elevation of about 10^{-4}°C" [285]. One may surmise that resistance will be further minimized through the utilization of ultralow defect materials, such as carbon nanotubes, graphene, thin films, and nanowires that are synthesized as atomic layer laminations.

Nucleic acid scaffolding may enable the precision placement of plasmonically active nanoparticles (e.g., Au, Ag), which may be regarded as custom reconfigurable modular nanoelectronic elements, contingent on their composition and geometric assemblage. Michelotti et al. suggest that positive synergies may result from the assembly of nanoelectronic components (synthesized by nucleic acid nanomanufacturing) using top-down nanolithography, in the fabrication of intricate solid-state nanocircuits [286]. Wang et al. undertook to review the emerging field of dynamic self-assembling 3D nanoparticle superstructures, which may contain variable architectures including discrete artificial molecules, 1D spaced chains, 2D sheets, and 3D helical entities (nanoparticle-decorated nanoribbons) and superlattices [3]. The spatial positioning of nanoparticles into geometries such as triangles and rectangles has been demonstrated through the use of cyclic DNA oligonucleotide templates [287], and these assemblies could be reconfigurated via the addition of specifically altered oligonucleotides [288]. Hypothetically, precision nanoparticle placement/assembly strategies might enable the capacity to fabricate highly complex nanoelectronics in three dimensions within which conductive, semiconducting, and insulating nanoparticles are logically arranged (along with various other classes of nanomaterials) in specific patterns to form integrated sheathed nanowires, transistors, capacitors, and gates. These constructs would be interfaced with energy-harvesting/generating components to subsequently supply current to all onboard nanodevice components.

5.15 Proposed Research Tasking List: VCSN Nanoelectronic Infrastructure

Following is a list of preliminary suggestions, considerations, and relevant questions as relates to perceived areas of investigation for the exemplar VCSN nanoelectronic infrastructure:

1. Select materials that possess appropriate electronic attributes (conducting, semiconducting, insulating) for the potential development of the nanoelectronic infrastructure for a Ø ~1 μm scale nanodevice.

2. Create a materials library/database, and molecular/electronic structural models for these materials (for use in simulations).

3. Investigate whether selected materials might preserve their electronic attributes and exhibit stable functionality when scaled to nanometric levels.

4. Explore the electronic profiles of pure, in contrast to doped nanomaterials, to discern what enhancements or advantages might be garnered as relates to their electronic reliability and robustness when doped with various elements.

5. Investigate and conceptualize designs and models with the purpose of developing nanometrically functional analogs of interconnects, transistors, resistors, voltage gates, capacitors, switches, amplifiers, and a nanometric connection standard that may be applicable to all of the aforementioned elements.

6. Generate concepts and designs for possible modular nanometric "circuitry," which might integrate several embedded electronic components into one modular unit (e.g., embedded within, or integrated onto the surface of specifically configured ultrathin film substrates). This might be a desirable alternative to the combination of multiple distinct subunits (perhaps cumulatively complicating assembly processes) especially when resultant collective functionality and outputs are shown to be similar.

7. Investigate optimal fabrication techniques that may be extrapolated from the semiconductor industry, MEMS, NEMS, thin film deposition (also explore potential DNA-based assembly) that might be applicable to massively parallel manufacturing processes for nanoelectronic elements.

8. Explore the possible use of single-walled nanotubes (SWNTs), MWNTs that possess various chiralities, as well as nanowires, C_{60}, and other potential entities from the fullerene family, as potential integral components for the construction of a nanoelectronic infrastructure.

9. Investigate the electronic characteristics of selected metals grown by vapor deposition and other fabrication methods to specific dimensions and geometries.

10. Study and catalog the electronic properties and parameters of metallic nanoshells. Conduct systematic trials using varied metallic skin thicknesses and core dimensions of nanoshells to elucidate their optimal electronic profiles, and identify their potential roles in nanoelectronic circuitry.

11. Continue with this line of investigation by utilizing various material combinations, nanoshell clusters, embedded and encapsulated nanoshells, and various packing density strategies.

12. How might electrical energy be stored at the nanoscale (e.g., nanoscale batteries, supercapacitors, laminated thin film architectures/substrates, hydrogen filled nanotubes, nanoscrolls)? What strategies might enhance storage capacity, stability, and longevity?

13. Prepare experiments to explore the specific field emission parameters of SWNTs, double-walled nanotubes (DWNTs), MWNTs, and a selected range of nanowires comprising selected materials. Develop a means for immobilizing these entities perpendicularly between two conductive ultrathin films, which would serve as electrodes. The bottom electrode would serve as the negative cathode, whereas the upper film electrode would serve as the positive anode. The gap between them, straddled by the sample(s), might be test filled with a range of insulating materials, including aerogels and hydrogels.

Conceptually, the tip segments of the samples would protrude beyond the external surfaces of the top and bottom thin films. Apply varying voltages to the thin film electrodes to discern whether the samples might be induced to initiate field emission. Determine what threshold voltages might be accommodated by various nanotube or nanowire configurations and elucidate their field emission output energies. Quantify electron emission distances and plume profiles, which emanate from the tips of nanotubes and/or nanowires in correspondence to various voltage intensities in a vacuum-encapsulated cavity. The aim here might be to determine if electrons will traverse a gap of specific distance beyond the tips of nanotubes or nanowires, to electronically activate a separate component (e.g., nanometric capacitive ultrasonic transducer) without a physical–mechanical interface.

14. If it is revealed that field emission is possible by means of the earlier trials, attempt to encapsulate the assembly in a vacuum cavity within various hydrophobic housings, utilizing materials that have been selected as possible candidates for the fabrication of the VCSN. Determine if this assembly might function within a sealed encasement when immersed in an aqueous environment over a several hour time period, in view of the envisaged VCSN requirement for sustained deployment within human whole blood for the duration (~5 min) of the scanning task.

References

1. Zhang, Q., Atay, T., Tischler, J.R., Bradley, M.S., Bulovic, V., and Nurmikko, A.V., Highly efficient resonant coupling of optical excitations in hybrid organic/inorganic semiconductor nanostructures. *Nat Nanotechnol.* 2(9), 555–559, 2007.
2. Kamat, P.V., Tvrdy, K., Baker, D.R., and Radich, J.G., Beyond photovoltaics: Semiconductor nanoarchitectures for liquid-junction solar cells. *Chem Rev.* 110(11), 6664–6688, 2010.
3. Wang, L., Xu, L., Kuang, H., Xu, C., and Kotov, N.A., Dynamic nanoparticle assemblies. *Acc Chem Res.* 45(11), 1916–1926, 2012.
4. Boehm, F.J., *An Investigation of Nucleic Acid/DNA-Based Manufacturing.* Center for Responsible Nanotechnology, Menlo Park, CA, August 2004. http://wise-nano.org/w/Boehm_DNA_Study
5. Luttge, R., Massively parallel fabrication of repetitive nanostructures: Nanolithography for nanoarrays. *J Phys D Appl Phys.* 42(12), 123001, 2009.
6. Haaheim, J. and Nafday, O.A., Dip pen nanolithography: A "Desktop Nanofab" approach using high-throughput flexible nanopatterning. *Scanning.* 30(2), 137–150, 2008.
7. Xu, L., Vemula, S.C., Jain, M., Nam, S.K., Donnelly, V.M., Economou, D.J., and Ruchhoeft, P., Nanopantography: A new method for massively parallel nanopatterning over large areas. *Nano Lett.* 5(12), 2563–2568, 2005.
8. Li, J., Stein, D., McMullan, C., Branton, D., Aziz, M.J., and Golovchenko, J.A., Ion-beam sculpting at nanometre length scales. *Nature.* 412(6843), 166–169, 2001.
9. Li, Q., Gao, K., Hu Z.,Yu, W., Xu, N., Sun, J., and Wu, J., Photoluminescence and lasing properties of catalyst-free ZnO nanorod arrays fabricated by pulsed laser deposition. *J Phys Chem C.* 116(3), 2330–2335, 2012.
10. Park, J. and Lu, W., Self-assembly of nanoparticles into heterogeneous structures with gradient material properties. *Phys Rev E Stat Nonlin Soft Matter Phys.* 83(3 Pt 1), 031402, 2011.
11. Han, W., Fan, S., Li, Q., and Hu, Y., Synthesis of gallium nitride nanorods through a carbon nanotube confined reaction. *Science.* 277(5330), 1287–1289, 1997.
12. Morales, A.M. and Lieber, C.M., A laser ablation method for the synthesis of crystalline semiconductor nanowires. *Science.* 279(5348), 208–211, 1998.
13. Zhu, J. and Fan, S., Nanostructure of GaN and SiC nanowires based on carbon nanotubes. *J Mater Res.* 14, 1175–1177, 1999.
14. Cheng, G.S., Zhang, L.D., Chen, S.H., Li, Y., Li, L., Zhu, X.G., Zhu, Y., Fei, G.T., and Mao, Y.Q., Ordered nanostructure of single-crystalline GaN nanowires in a honeycomb structure of anodic alumina. *J Mater Res.* 15(2), 347–350, 2000.
15. Chen, C.C., Yeh, C.C., Chen, C.H., Yu, M.Y., Liu, H.L., Wu, J.J., Chen, K.H., Chen, L.C., Peng, J.Y., and Chen, Y.F., Catalytic growth and characterization of gallium nitride nanowires. *J Am Chem Soc.* 123(12), 2791–2798, 2001.

16. Lauhon, L.J., Gudiksen, M.S., Wang, D., and Lieber, C.M., Epitaxial core-shell and core-multi-shell nanowire heterostructure. *Nature*. 420(6911), 57–61, 2002.
17. Cui, Y., Wei, Q., Park, H., and Lieber, C.M., Nanowire nanosensors for highly sensitive and selective detection of biological and chemical species. *Science*. 293(5533), 1289–1292, 2001.
18. Johnson, J.C., Choi, H.J., Knutsen, K.P., Schaller, R.D., Yang, P., and Saykally, R.J., Single gallium nitride nanowire lasers. *Nat Mater*. 1(2), 106–110, 2002.
19. Ma, D.D., Lee, C.S., Au, F.C., Tong, S.Y., and Lee, S.T., Small-diameter silicon nanowire surfaces. *Science*. 299(5614), 1874–1877, 2003.
20. Lauhon, L.J., Gudiksen, M.S., and Lieber, C.M., Semiconductor nanowire heterostructures. *Philos Transact A Math Phys Eng Sci*. 362(1819), 1247–1260, 2004.
21. Katz, E. and Willner, I., Biomolecule-functionalized carbon nanotubes: Applications in nano-bioelectronics. *Chemphyschem*. 5(8), 1084–1104, 2004.
22. Patolsky, F., Zheng, G., Hayden, O., Lakadamyali, M., Zhuang, X., and Lieber, C.M., Electrical detection of single viruses. *Proc Natl Acad Sci USA*. 101(39), 14017–14022, 2004.
23. Shi, L., Yu, C., and Zhou, J., Thermal characterization and sensor applications of one-dimensional nanostructures employing microelectromechanical systems. *J Phys Chem B*. 109(47), 22102–22111, 2005.
24. Reguera, G., McCarthy, K.D., Mehta, T., Nicoll, J.S., Tuominen, M.T., and Lovley, D.R., Extracellular electron transfer via microbial nanowires. *Nature*. 435(7045), 1098–1101, 2005.
25. Yang, H.H., Zhang, S.Q., Tan, F., Zhuang, Z.X., and Wang, X.R., Surface molecularly imprinted nanowires for biorecognition. *J Am Chem Soc*. 127(5), 1378–1379, 2005.
26. Flavin, K. and Resmini, M., Imprinted nanomaterials: A new class of synthetic receptors. *Anal Bioanal Chem*. 393(2), 437–444, 2009.
27. Hayden, O., Agarwal, R., and Lieber, C.M., Nanoscale avalanche photodiodes for highly sensitive and spatially resolved photon detection. *Nat Mater*. 5(5), 352–356, 2006.
28. Ju, S., Facchetti, A., Xuan, Y., Liu, J., Ishikawa, F., Ye, P., Zhou, C., Marks, T.J., and Janes, D.B., Fabrication of fully transparent nanowire transistors for transparent and flexible electronics. *Nat Nanotechnol*. 2(6), 378–384, 2007.
29. Soci, C., Zhang, A., Xiang, B., Dayeh, S.A., Aplin, D.P., Park, J., Bao, X.Y., Lo, Y.H., and Wang, D., ZnO nanowire UV photodetectors with high internal gain. *Nano Lett*. 7(4):1003–1009, 2007.
30. Yuan, J., Xu, Y., Walther, A., Bolisetty, S., Schumacher, M., Schmalz, H., Ballauff, M., and Müller, A.H., Water-soluble organo-silica hybrid nanowires. *Nat Mater*. 7(9), 718–722, 2008.
31. Cui, Q., Gao, F., Mukherjee, S., and Gu, Z., Joining and interconnect formation of nanowires and carbon nanotubes for nanoelectronics and nanosystems. *Small*. 5(11):1246–1257, 2009.
32. Singh, S., Nanomedicine-nanoscale drugs and delivery systems. *J Nanosci Nanotechnol*. 10(12), 7906–7918, 2010.
33. Guo, S., The creation of nanojunctions. *Nanoscale*. 2(12), 2521–2529, 2010.
34. Takei, K., Takahashi, T., Ho, J.C., Ko, H., Gillies, A.G., Leu, P.W., Fearing, R.S., and Javey, A., Nanowire active-matrix circuitry for low-voltage macroscale artificial skin. *Nat Mater*. 9(10), 821–826, 2010.
35. Noy, A., Bionanoelectronics. *Adv Mater*. 23(7), 807–820, 2011.
36. Qu, Y., Zhou, H., and Duan, X., Porous silicon nanowires. *Nanoscale*. 3(10), 4060–4068, 2011.
37. Chen, B., Meng, G., Xu, Q., Zhu, X., Kong, M., Chu, Z., Han, F., and Zhang, Z., Crystalline silicon nanotubes and their connections with gold nanowires in both linear and branched topologies. *ACS Nano*. 4(12), 7105–7112, 2010.
38. Xu, F., Lu, W., and Zhu, Y., Controlled 3D buckling of silicon nanowires for stretchable electronics. *ACS Nano*. 5(1), 672–678, 2011.
39. Espinosa, H.D., Bernal, R.A., and Minary-Jolandan, M., A review of mechanical and electromechanical properties of piezoelectric nanowires. *Adv Mater*. 24(34), 4656–4675, 2012.
40. Long, Y.Z., Yu, M., Sun, B., Gu, C.Z., and Fan, Z., Recent advances in large-scale assembly of semiconducting inorganic nanowires and nanofibers for electronics, sensors and photovoltaics. *Chem Soc Rev*. 41(12), 4560–4580, 2012.

41. Liu, X., Long, Y.Z., Liao, L., Duan, X., and Fan, Z., Large-scale integration of semiconductor nanowires for high-performance flexible electronics. *ACS Nano.* 6(3), 1888–1900, 2012.
42. Wilner, O.I., Willner, B., and Willner, I., DNA nanotechnology. *Adv Exp Med Biol.* 733, 97–114, 2012.
43. Lim, S.K., Crawford, S., Haberfehlner, G., and Gradečak, S., Controlled modulation of diameter and composition along individual III–V nitride nanowires. *Nano Lett.* 13(2), 331–336, 2013.
44. Shui, J. and Li, J.C., Platinum nanowires produced by electrospinning. *Nano Lett.* 9(4), 1307–1314, 2009.
45. Filipič, G. and Cvelbar, U., Copper oxide nanowires: A review of growth. *Nanotechnology.* 23(19), 194001, 2012.
46. Shin, H.S., Song, J.Y., and Yu, J., Template-assisted electrochemical synthesis of cuprous oxide nanowires. *Mater Lett.* 63(3–4), 397–399, 2009.
47. Hsieh, C.T., Chen, J.M., Lin, H.H., and Shih, H.C., Synthesis of well-ordered CuO nanofibers by a self-catalytic growth mechanism. *Appl Phys Lett.* 82, 3316, 2003.
48. Wu, Y., Yan, H., Huang, M., Messer, B., Song, J.H., and Yang, P., Inorganic semiconductor nanowires: Rational growth, assembly, and novel properties. *Chemistry.* 8(6), 1260–1268, 2002.
49. Huczko, A., Template-based synthesis of nanomaterials. *Appl Phys A Mater Sci Process.* 70(4), 365–366, 2000.
50. Cao, G. and Liu, D., Template-based synthesis of nanorod, nanowire, and nanotube arrays. *Adv Colloid Interface Sci.* 136(1–2), 45–64, 2008.
51. Dai, H.J., Wong, E.W., Lu, Y.Z., Fan, S.S., and Lieber, C.M., Synthesis and characterization of carbide nanorods. *Nature.* 375(6534), 69–772, 1995.
52. Pan, Z., Dai, Z.R., and Wng, Z.L., Lead oxide nanobelts and phase transformation induced by electron beam irradiation. *Appl Phys Lett.* 80, 309–311, 2002.
53. Fan, L., Song, H., Zhao, H., Pan, G., Liu, L., Dong, B., Wang, F., Bai, X., Qin, R., Kong, X., and Ren, X., CdS/Cyclohexylamine inorganic–organic hybrid semiconductor nanofibers with strong quantum confinement effect. *J Nanosci Nanotechnol.* 8(8), 3914–3920, 2008.
54. Liu, Y.F., Zeng, J.H., Zhang, W.X., Yu, W.C., Qian, Y.T., Cao, J.B., and Zhang, W.Q., Solvothermal route to Bi$_3$Se$_4$ nanorods at low temperature *J Mater Res.* 16(12), 3361–3365, 2001.
55. Simanullang, M., Usami, K., Kodera, T., Uchida, K., and Oda, S., Germanium nanowires with 3-nm-diameter prepared by low temperature vapour–liquid–solid chemical vapour deposition. *J Nanosci Nanotechnol.* 11(9), 8163–8168, 2011.
56. Lee, S.T., Wang, N., Zhang, Y.F., and Tang, Y.H., Oxide-assisted semiconductor nanowire growth. *MRS Bull.* 24(8), 36–42, 1999.
57. Aharonovich, I., Tamir, S., and Lifshitz, Y., Growth of SiO(x) nanowires by laser ablation. *Nanotechnology.* 19(6), 065608, 2008.
58. Pan, Z.W., Dai, Z.R., and Wang, Z.L., Nanobelts of semiconducting oxides. *Science.* 291(5510), 1947–1949, 2001.
59. Berta, Y., Ma, C., and Wang, Z.L., Measuring the aspect ratios of ZnO nanobelts. *Micron.* 33(78), 687–691, 2002.
60. Mcguire, K., Pan, Z.W., Wang, Z.L., Milkie, D., Menéndez, J., and Rao, A.M., Raman studies of semiconducting oxide nanobelts. *J Nanosci Nanotechnol.* 2(5), 499–502, 2002.
61. Sugaya, T., Ogura, M., Sugiyama, Y., Matsumoto, K., Yonei, K., and Sekiguchi, T., Trench-type narrow InGaAs quantum wires fabricated on a (311) A InP substrate. *Appl Phys Lett.* 78(1), 76–78, 2001.
62. Sakamoto, Y., Fukuoka, A., Higuchi, T., Shimomura, N., Inagaki, S., and Ichikawa, M., Synthesis of platinum nanowires in organic–inorganic mesoporous silica templates by photoreduction: Formation mechanism and isolation. *J Phys Chem B.* 108, 853–858, 2004.
63. Lauhon, L.J., Gudiksen, M.S., Wang, D., and Lieber, C.M., Epitaxial core-shell and core-multi-shell nanowire heterostructures. *Nature.* 420(6911), 57–61, 2002.
64. Ramsperger, U., Uchihashi, T., and Nejoh, H., Fabrication and lateral electronic transport measurements of gold nanowires. *Appl Phys Lett.* 78(1), 85–87, 2001.
65. Haug, F.J., Band tails. http://www.superstrate.net/pv/amorphous/band-tails.html (accessed May 27, 2012).

66. Wang, S.B., Hu, M.S., Chang, S.J., Chong, C.W., Han, H.C., Huang, B.R., Chen, L.C., and Chen, K.H., Gold nanoparticle-modulated conductivity in gold peapodded silica nanowires. *Nanoscale*. 4(12), 3660–3664, 2012.

67. Zhao, J., Calin, B., Han, J., and Lu, J.P., Quantum transport properties of ultrathin silver nanowires. *Cond Mat*. 0209535(1), 1–4, 2002.

68. Sloan, J., Wright, D.M., Woo, H.G., Bailey, S., Brown, G., York, A.P.E., Coleman, K.S., Hutchison, J.L., and Green, M.L.H., Capillarity and silver nanowire formation in single walled carbon nanotubes. *Chem Commun*. 8, 699–700, 1999.

69. Hsiao, W.H., Chen, H.Y., Yang, Y.C., Chen, Y.L., Lee, C.Y., and Chiu, H.T., Surface-enhanced Raman scattering imaging of a single molecule on urchin-like silver nanowires. *ACS Appl Mater Interfaces*. 3(9), 3280–3284, 2011.

70. Li, J., Liao, Y., Suslov, S., and Cheng, G.J., Laser shock-based platform for controllable forming of nanowires. *Nano Lett*. 12, 3224, 2012.

71. Zhang, H., Ma, X., Xu, J., Niu, J., and Yang, D., Arrays of ZnO nanowires fabricated by a simple chemical solution route. *Nanotechnology*. 14, 423, 2003.

72. Glucksman, M.J., Bhattacharjee, S., and Makowski, L., 3-Dimensional structure of a cloning vector-X-ray-diffraction studies of filamentous bacteriophage-M13 at 7-Angstrom resolution. *J Mol Biol*. 226, 455–470, 1992.

73. Namba, K., Pattanayek, R., and Stubbs, G., Visualization of protein–nucleic acid interactions in a virus refined structure of intact tobacco mosaic virus at 2.9 Å resolution by X-ray fiber diffraction. *J Mol Biol*. 208, 307–325, 1989.

74. Zhou, J.C., Soto, C.M., Chen, M.S., Bruckman, M.A., Moore, M.H., Barry, E., Ratna, B.R., Pehrsson, P.E., Spies, B.R., and Confer, T.S., Biotemplating rod-like viruses for the synthesis of copper nanorods and nanowires. *J Nanobiotechnol*. 10(1), 18, 2012.

75. Lapierre, R. and Sunkara, M. Nanowires for energy. *Nanotechnology*. 23(19), 190201, 2012.

76. Komoda, N., Nogi, M., Suganuma, K., Kohno, K., Akiyama, Y., and Otsuka, K. Printed silver nanowire antennas with low signal loss at high-frequency radio. *Nanoscale*. 4(10), 3148–3153, 2012.

77. Ditlbacher, H., Hohenau, A., Wagner, D., Kreibig, U., Rogers, M., Hofer, F., Aussenegg, F.R., and Krenn, J.R., Silver nanowires as surface plasmon resonators. *Phys Rev Lett*. 95(25), 257403, 2005.

78. Tokuno, T., Nogi, M., Jiu, J., Sugahara, T., and Suganuma, K., Transparent electrodes fabricated via the self-assembly of silver nanowires using a bubble template. *Langmuir*. 28(25), 9298–9302, 2012.

79. Zhang, C.L., Lv, K.P., Huang, H.T., Cong, H.P., and Yu, S.H., Co-assembly of Au nanorods with Ag nanowires within polymer nanofiber matrix for enhanced SERS property by electrospinning. *Nanoscale*. 4(17), 5348–5355, 2012.

80. Benson, J., Boukhalfa, S., Magasinski, A., Kvit, A., and Yushin, G., Chemical vapor deposition of aluminum nanowires on metal substrates for electrical energy storage applications. *ACS Nano*. 6(1), 118–125, 2012.

81. Mao, Y. and Wong, S.S., General, room-temperature method for the synthesis of isolated as well as arrays of single-crystalline ABO4-type nanorods. *J Am Chem Soc*. 126(46), 15245–15252, 2004.

82. Cheng, Y.T., Weiner, A.M., and Wong, C.A., Stress-induced growth of bismuth nanowires. *Appl Phys Lett*. 81(17), 3248–3250, 2002.

83. Siegal, M.P., Overmyer, D.L., Yelton, W.G., and Webb, E.B. III, Electroforming of Bi(1−x)Sb(x) nanowires for high-efficiency micro-thermoelectric cooling devices on a chip. Final LDRD Report SAND2006-6940, November 2006.

84. Ham, J., Shim, W., Kim do, H., Lee, S., Roh, J., Sohn, S.W., Oh, K.H., Voorhees, P.W., and Lee, W., Direct growth of compound semiconductor nanowires by on-film formation of nanowires: Bismuth telluride. *Nano Lett*. 9(8), 2867–2872, 2009.

85. Wu, H., Meng, F., Li, L., Jin, S., and Zheng, G., Dislocation-driven CdS and CdSe nanowire growth. *ACS Nano*. 6(5), 4461–4468, 2012.

86. Cheng, G., Synthesis and characterisation of CuO nanorods via a hydrothermal method. *Micro Nano Lett*. 6, 774–776, 2011.

87. Rathmell, A.R., Nguyen, M., Chi, M., and Wiley, B.J., Synthesis of oxidation-resistant cupronickel nanowires for transparent conducting nanowire networks. *Nano Lett.* 12(6), 3193–3199, 2012.

88. Xu, Y., Yun, G., Dong, Z., Kashkarov, P., Narlikar, A., and Zhang, H., Effect of surface pressurization on the growth of α-Fe_2O_3 nanostructures. *Nanoscale.* 4(1), 257–260, 2012.

89. Madaria, A.R., Yao, M., Chi, C., Huang, N., Lin, C., Li, R., Povinelli, M.L., Dapkus, P.D., and Zhou, C., Toward optimized light utilization in nanowire arrays using scalable nanosphere lithography and selected area growth. *Nano Lett.* 12(6), 2839–2845, 2012.

90. Mullane, E., Geaney, H., and Ryan, K.M., Size controlled growth of germanium nanorods and nanowires by solution pyrolysis directly on a substrate. *Chem Commun (Camb).* 48(44), 5446–5448, 2012.

91. Hertenberger, S., Rudolph, D., Becker, J., Bichler, M., Finley, J.J., Abstreiter, G., and Koblmüller, G., Rate-limiting mechanisms in high-temperature growth of catalyst-free InAs nanowires with large thermal stability. *Nanotechnology.* 23(23), 235602, 2012.

92. Kar, S. and Chaudhuri, S., Synthesis and characterization of one-dimensional MgO nanostructures. *J Nanosci Nanotechnol.* 6(5), 1447–1452, 2006.

93. Muramatsu, H., Hayashi, T., Kim, Y.A., Shimamoto, D., Endo, M., Terrones, M., and Dresselhaus, M.S., Synthesis and isolation of molybdenum atomic wires. *Nano Lett.* 8(1), 237–240, 2008.

94. Proenca, M.P., Sousa, C.T., Ventura, J., Vazquez, M., and Araujo, J.P., Distinguishing nanowire and nanotube formation by the deposition current transients. *Nanoscale Res Lett.* 7(1), 280, 2012.

95. Onicha, A.C., Petchsang, N., Kosel, T.H., and Kuno, M., Controlled synthesis of compositionally tunable ternary PbSe(x)S(1−x) as well as binary PbSe and PbS nanowires. *ACS Nano.* 6(3), 2833–2843, 2012.

96. Lee, S., Hong, S., Park, B., Paik, S.R., and Jung, S., Agarose and gellan as morphology-directing agents for the preparation of selenium nanowires in water. *Carbohydr Res.* 344(2), 260–262, 2009.

97. Hochbaum, A.I., Chen, R., Delgado, R.D., Liang, W., Garnett, E.C., Najarian, M., Majumdar A., and Yang, P., Enhanced thermoelectric performance of rough silicon nanowires. *Nature.* 451(7175), 163–167, 2008.

98. Luo, L.B., Liang, F.X., and Jie, J.S., Sn-catalyzed synthesis of SnO_2 nanowires and their optoelectronic characteristics. *Nanotechnology.* 22(48), 485701, 2011.

99. Zhang, Z.C., Zhang, X., Yu, Q.Y., Liu, Z.C., Xu, C.M., Gao, J.S., Zhuang, J., and Wang, X., Pd cluster nanowires as highly efficient catalysts for selective hydrogenation reactions. *Chemistry.* 18(9), 2639–2645, 2012.

100. Shen, Y.L., Chen, S.Y., Song, J.M., and Chen, I.G., Ultra-long Pt nanolawns supported on TiO_2 coated carbon fibers as 3D hybrid catalyst for methanol oxidation. *Nanoscale Res Lett.* 7(1), 237, 2012.

101. Wu, J.M., Tin-doped rutile titanium dioxide nanowires: Luminescence, gas sensor, and field emission properties. *J Nanosci Nanotechnol.* 12(2), 1434–1439, 2012.

102. Hong, K., Xie, M., Hu, R., and Wu, H., Diameter control of tungsten oxide nanowires as grown by thermal evaporation. *Nanotechnology.* 19(8), 085604, 2008.

103. Kao, M.C., Chen, H.Z., Young, S.L., Lin, C.C., and Kung, C.Y., Structure and photovoltaic properties of ZnO nanowire for dye-sensitized solar cells. *Nanoscale Res Lett.* 7(1), 260, 2012.

104. Hiralal, P., Unalan, H.E., and Amaratunga, G.A., Nanowires for energy generation. *Nanotechnology.* 23(19), 194002, 2012.

105. Wu, Y., Yan, H., Huang, M., Messer, B., Song, J.H., and Yang, P., Inorganic semiconductor nanowires: Rational growth, assembly, and novel properties. *Chemistry.* 8(6), 1260–1268, 2002.

106. Wu, Y., Yan, H., and Yang, P., Semiconductor nanowire array: Potential substrates for photocatalysis and photovoltaics. *Topics Catal.* 19(2), 197, 2002.

107. Messer, B., Song, J.H., and Yang, P., Microchannel networks for nanowire patterning. *J Am Chem Soc.* 122, 10232–10233, 2000.

108. Huang, Y., Duan, X.F., Wei, Q.Q., and Lieber, C.M., Directed assembly of one-dimensional nanostructures into functional networks. *Science.* 291(5504), 630–633, 2001.

109. Duan, X.F., Huang, Y., Cui, Y., Wang, J.F., and Lieber, C.M., Indium phosphide nanowires as building blocks for nanoscale electronic and optoelectronic devices. *Nature.* 409(6816), 66–69, 2001.

110. Kim, F., Kwan, S., Akana, J., and Yang, P., Langmuir–Blodgett nanorod assembly. *J Am Chem Soc.* 123(18), 4360–4361, 2001.
111. Liu, J.W., Zhu, J.H., Zhang, C.L., Liang, H.W., and Yu, S.H., Mesostructured assemblies of ultrathin superlong tellurium nanowires and their photoconductivity. *J Am Chem Soc.* 132(26), 8945–8952, 2010.
112. Routkevitch, D., Tager, A.A., Haruyama, J., Almawlawi, D., Moskovits, M., and Xu, J.M., Nonlithographic nano-wire arrays: Fabrication, physics, and device applications. *IEEE Trans Electron Devices.* 43(10), 1646–1658, 1996.
113. Yu, G., Cao, A., and Lieber, C.M., Large-area blown bubble films of aligned nanowires and carbon nanotubes. *Nat Nanotechnol.* 2(6), 372–377, 2007.
114. van de Groep, J., Spinelli, P., and Polman, A., Transparent conducting silver nanowire network. *Nano Lett.* 12(6), 3138–3144, 2012.
115. von Schleyer, P.R., A simple preparation of adamantane. *J Am Chem Soc.* 79(12), 3292, 1957.
116. Cupas, C., Schleyer, P.v.R., and Trecker D.J., Congressane. *J Am Chem Soc.* 87(4), 917–918, 1965.
117. Williams, V.Z. Jr., Schleyer, P.v.R., Gleicher, G.J., and Rodewald, L.B., Triamantane. *J Am Chem Soc.* 88(16), 3862–3863, 1966.
118. Dahl, J.E., Carlson, R.M., and Liu, S., Diamondoid-containing thermally conductive materials. U.S. Patent 7, 276, 222, 2004.
119. Freitas, R., Pathway to diamond-based molecular manufacturing. *First Symposium on Molecular Machine Systems, First Foresight Conference on Advanced Nanotechnology*, October 22, 2004. http://www.molecularassembler.com/Papers/PathDiamMolMfg.htm
120. Dahl, J.E., Moldowan, J.M., Wei, Z., Lipton, P.A., Denisevich, P., Gat, R., Liu, S., Schreiner, P.R., and Carlson, R.M., Synthesis of higher diamondoids and implications for their formation in petroleum. *Angew Chem Int Ed Engl.* 49(51), 9881–9885, 2010.
121. Schreiner, P.R., Fokin, A.A., Reisenauer, H.P., Tkachenko, B.A., Vass, E., Olmstead, M.M., Bläser, D., Boese, R., Dahl, J.E., and Carlson, R.M., Tetramantane: Parent of a new family of sigma-helicenes. *J Am Chem Soc.* 131(32), 11292–11293, 2009.
122. Dahl, J.E., Liu, S.G., and Carlson, R.M.K., Isolation and structure of higher diamondoids, nanometer-sized diamond molecules. *Science.* 299, 96, 2002.
123. Drexler, K.E., *Nanosystems—Molecular Machinery, Manufacturing, and Computation*. John Wiley & Sons, New York, 1992.
124. Phoenix, C., Studying molecular manufacturing. *IEEE Technol Soc Mag.* 23(4), 41–47, 2004.
125. Seker, U.O. and Demir, H.V., Material binding peptides for nanotechnology. *Molecules.* 16(2), 1426–1451, 2011.
126. Freitas, R.A. Jr. and Merkle, R.C., *Kinematic Self-Replicating Machines*. Landes Bioscience, Georgetown, TX, 2004.
127. Henderson, J., Shi, S., Cakmaktepe, S., and Crawford, T.M., Pattern transfer nanomanufacturing using magnetic recording for programmed nanoparticle assembly. *Nanotechnology.* 223(18), 185304, 2012.
128. Zhang, Z., Zhang, X., Xin, Z., Deng, M., Wen, Y., and Song, Y., Synthesis of monodisperse silver nanoparticles for ink-jet printed flexible electronics. *Nanotechnology.* 22(42), 425601, 2011.
129. De Volder, M., Tawfick, S.H., Park, S.J., Copic, D., Zhao, Z., Lu, W., and Hart, A.J., Diverse 3D microarchitectures made by capillary forming of carbon nanotubes. *Adv Mater.* 22(39), 4384–4389, 2010.
130. Paraschiv, C., Andruh, M., Ferlay, S., Hosseini, M.W., Kyritsakas, N., Planeix, J.M., and Stanica, N., Alkoxo-bridged copper II complexes as nodes in designing solid-state architectures. The interplay of coordinative and d10–d10 metal–metal interactions in sustaining supramolecular solid-state architectures. *Dalton Trans.* (7), 1195–1202, 2005.
131. Wong, E.W., Sheehan, P.E., and Lieber, C.M., Nanobeam mechanics: Elasticity, strength and toughness of nanorods and nanotubes. *Science.* 277(5334), 1971–1975, 1997.
132. Ngo, L.T., Almécija, D., Sader, J.E., Daly, B., Petkov, N., Holmes, J.D., Erts, D., and Boland, J.J., Ultimate-strength germanium nanowires. *Nano Lett.* 6(12), 2964–2968, 2006.
133. Wen, B., Sader, J.E., and Boland, J.J., Mechanical properties of ZnO nanowires. *Phys Rev Lett.* 101(17), 175502, 2008.

134. Barth, S., Harnagea, C., Mathur, S., and Rosei, F., The elastic moduli of oriented tin oxide nanowires. *Nanotechnology.* 20(11), 115705, 2009.
135. Gulseren, O., Ercolessi, F., and Tosatti, E., Noncrystalline structures of ultrathin unsupported nanowires. *Phys Rev Lett.* 80(17), 3775–3778, 1998.
136. Bilalbegović, G., Structure and stability of finite gold nanowires. *Phys Rev B.* 58, 15412, 1998.
137. Wang, B., Yin, S., Wang, G., Buldum, A., and Zhao, J., Novel structures and properties of gold nanowires. *Phys Rev Lett.* 86(10), 2046–2049, 2001.
138. Law, M., Sirbuly, D.J., Johnson, J.C., Goldberger, J., Saykally, R.J., and Yang, P., Nanoribbon waveguides for subwavelength photonics integration. *Science.* 305(5688), 1269–1273, 2004.
139. Huang, M.H., Mao, S., Feick, H., Yan, H., Wu, Y., Kind, H., Weber, E., Russo, R., and Yang P., Room-temperature ultraviolet nanowire nanolasers. *Science.* 292(5523), 1897–1899, 2001.
140. Johnson, J.C., Yan, H., Schaller, R.D., Haber, L., Saykally, R.J., and Yang, P., Single nanowire lasers. *J Phys Chem B.* 105, 11387–11390, 2001.
141. Wang, J., Gudiksen, M.S., Duan, X., Cui, Y., and Lieber, C.M., Highly polarized photoluminescence and photodetection from single indium phosphide nanowires. *Science.* 293(5534), 1455–1457, 2001.
142. Duan, X., Huang, Y., Agarwal, R., and Lieber, C.M., Single-nanowire electrically driven lasers. *Nature.* 421(6920), 241–245, 2003.
143. Cui, Y., Duan, X.F., Hu, J.T., and Lieber, C.M., Doping and electrical transport in SiNWs. *J Phys Chem B.* 104, 5213–5215, 2000.
144. Chung, S.W., Yu, J.Y., and Heath, J.R., Silicon nanowire devices. *Appl Phys Lett.* 76, 2068–2070, 2000.
145. Bhushan, B., *Springer Handbook of Nanotechnology*, 2nd edn. Springer, New York, 2007.
146. Pan, Z.W., Lai, H.L., Au, F.C.K., Duan, X.F., Zhou, W.Y., Shi, W.S. et al., Oriented silicon carbide nanowires: Synthesis and field emission properties. *Adv Mater.* 12, 1186–1190, 2000.
147. Zhou, X.T., Lai, H.L., Peng, H.Y., Au, F.C.K., Liao, L.S., Wang, N., Bello, I., Lee, C.S., and Lee, S.T., Thin beta-SiC nanorods and their field emission properties. *Chem Phys Lett.* 318, 58–62, 2000.
148. Huang, Y., Duan, X.F., Cui, Y., Lauhon, L.J., Kim, K.H., and Lieber, C.M., Logic gates and computation from assembled nanowire building blocks. *Science.* 294, 1313–1317, 2001.
149. Li, D., Wu, Y., Kim, P., Shi, L., Yang, P., and Majumdar, A., Thermal conductivity of individual silicon nanowires. *Appl Phys Lett.* 83, 2934, 2003.
150. Lee, E.K., Yin, L., Lee, Y., Lee, J.W., Lee, S.J., Lee, J., Cha, S.N., Whang, D., Hwang, G.S., Hippalgaonkar, K., Majumdar, A., Yu, C., Choi, B.L., Kim, J.M., and Kim, K., Large thermoelectric figure-of-merits from SiGe nanowires by simultaneously measuring electrical and thermal transport properties. *Nano Lett.* 12(6), 2918–2923, 2012.
151. Zhou, F., Szczech, J., Pettes, M.T., Moore, A.L., Jin, S., and Shi, L., Determination of transport properties in chromium disilicide nanowires via combined thermoelectric and structural characterizations. *Nano Lett.* 7(6), 1649–1654, 2007.
152. Dasgupta, T., Etourneau, J., Chevalier, B., Matar, S.F., and Umarji A.M., Structural, thermal, and electrical properties of $CrSi_2$. *J Appl Phys.* 103(11), 113516–113517, 2008.
153. Abd El Qader, M., Structural, electrical and thermoelectric properties of chromium silicate thin films. MSc thesis, University of Nevada, Las Vegas, NV, August 2011.
154. Rowe, D.M., *CRC Handbook of Thermoelectrics*, Chapters 23–25. CRC Press, Boca Raton, FL, 1994.
155. Sakamaki Y., Kuwabara K., Jiajun G., Inui H., Yamaguchi M., Yamamoto A., Obara H. Crystal structure and thermoelectric properties of ReSi1.75 based silicides. *Mater Sci Forum.* 426–432, 1777, 2003.
156. Wu, Y. and Yang, P.D., Germanium/carbon core-sheath nanostructures. *Appl Phys Lett.* 77, 43, 2000.
157. Wu, Y. and Yang, P., Melting and welding semiconductor nanowires in nanotubes. *Adv Mater.* 13(7), 520–523, 2001.
158. Deng, B., Xu, A.W., Chen, G.Y., Song, R.Q., and Chen, L., Synthesis of copper-core/carbon-sheath nanocables by a surfactant-assisted hydrothermal reduction/carbonization process. *J Phys Chem B.* 110(24), 11711–11716, 2006.

159. Oestreicher, Z., Valverde-Tercedor, C., Chen, L., Jimenez-Lopez, C., Bazylinski, D.A., Casillas-Ituarte, N.N., Lower, S.K., and Lower, B.H., Magnetosomes and magnetite crystals produced by magneto-tactic bacteria as resolved by atomic force microscopy and transmission electron microscopy. *Micron.* 43(12), 1331–1335, 2012.

160. Zeytuni, N., Ozyamak, E., Ben-Harush, K., Davidov, G., Levin, M., Gat, Y., Moyal, T., Brik, A., Komeili, A., and Zarivach, R., Self-recognition mechanism of MamA, a magnetosome-associated TPR-containing protein, promotes complex assembly. *Proc Natl Acad Sci USA.* 108(33), E480-7, 2011.

161. Osterloh, F.E., Hiramatsu, H., Dumas, R.K., and Liu, K., Fe_3O_4–$LiMo_3Se_3$ nanoparticle clusters as superparamagnetic nanocompasses. *Langmuir.* 21(21), 9709–9713, 2005.

162. Tulchinsky, D.A., Kelley, M.H., McClelland, J.J., Gupta, R., and Celotta, R.J., Fabrication and domain imaging of iron magnetic nanowire arrays. *J Vac Sci Tech A.* 16(3), 1817–1819, 1998.

163. Hung, M.H., Wang, C.Y., Tang, J., Lin, C.C., Hou, T.C., Jiang, X., Wang, K.L., and Chen, L.J., Free-standing and single crystalline $Fe(1-x)Mn(x)Si$ nanowires with room-temperature ferromagnetism and excellent magnetic response. *ACS Nano.* 6(6), 4884–4891, 2012.

164. Mandal, S.K., Mandal, A.R., and Banerjee, S., High ferromagnetic transition temperature in PbS and PbS:Mn nanowires. *ACS Appl Mater Interfaces.* 4(1), 205–209, 2012.

165. Lent, C.S. and Tougaw, P.D., A device architecture for computing with quantum dots. *Proc IEEE.* 85(4), 541–557, 1997.

166. Tougaw, P.D. and Lent, C.S., Dynamic behavior of quantum cellular automata. *J Appl Phys.* 80(8), 4722–4737, 1996.

167. Lent, C.S., Tougaw, P.D., Porod, W., and Berstein, G.H., Quantum cellular automata. *Nanotechnology.* 4, 49–57, 1993.

168. Orlov, A.O., Amlani, I., Toth, G., Lent, C.S., Berstein, G.H., and Snider, G.L., Experimental demonstration of a binary wire for quantum-dot cellular automata. *Appl Phys Lett.* 74(19), 2875–2877, 1999.

169. Huang, L., Wang, H., Hayashi, C.Y., Tian, B., Zhao, D., and Yan, Y., Single-strand spider silk templating for the formation of hierarchically ordered hollow mesoporous silical fibers. *J Mater Chem.* 13, 666–668, 2003.

170. Hainfeld, J.F., Furuya, F.R., Powell, R.D., and Liu, W., DNA nanowires. *Microsc. Microanal.* 7 (Suppl. 2: Proceedings) (*Proceedings of the Fifty-Ninth Annual Meeting*, Microscopy Society of America), Bailey, G.W., Price, R.L., Voelkl, E., and Musselman, I.H., eds. Springer-Verlag, New York, 1034–1035, 2001.

171. Hassanien, R., Al-Said, S.A., Siller, L., Little, R., Wright, N.G., Houlton, A., and Horrocks, B.R., Smooth and conductive DNA-templated Cu_2O nanowires: Growth morphology, spectroscopic and electrical characterization. *Nanotechnology.* 23(7), 075601, 2012.

172. Aich, P., Labiuk, S.L., Tari, L.W., Delbaere, L.J., Roesler, W.J., Falk, K.J., Steer, R.P., and Lee, J.S., M-DNA: A complex between divalent metal ions and DNA which behaves as a molecular wire. *J Mol Biol.* 294(2), 477–485, 1999.

173. Lee, J.S., Latimer, L.J., and Reid, R.S., A cooperative conformational change in duplex DNA induced by Zn^{2+} and other divalent metal ions. *Biochem Cell Biol.* 71(3–4), 162–168, 1993.

174. Rakitin, A., Aich, P., Papadopoulos, C., Kobzar, Y., Vedeneev, A.S., Lee, J.S., and Xu, J.M. Metallic conduction through engineered DNA: DNA nanoelectronic building blocks. *Phys Rev Lett.* 86(16), 3670–3673, 2001.

175. Aviram, A. and Ratner, M.A., Molecular rectifiers. *Chem Phys Lett.* 29(2), 257, 1974.

176. Aviram, A., eds., *Proceedings of the Conference on Molecular Electronics: Science and Technology, December 1997.* Humacao, Puerto Rico (*Ann NY Acad Sci.*), June 1998.

177. Rodríguez González, S., Ruiz Delgado, M.C., Caballero, R., De la Cruz, P., Langa, F., López, N.J.T., and Casado, J., Delocalization-to-localization charge transition in diferrocenyl-oligothienylene-vinylene molecular wires as a function of the size by Raman spectroscopy. *J Am Chem Soc.* 134(12), 5675–5681, 2012.

178. Reed, M.A., Zhou, C., Muller, C.J., Burgin, T.P., and Tour, J.M., Conductance of a molecular junction. *Science.* 278, 252, 1997.

179. Zou, R., Hu, J., Song, Y., Wang, N., Chen, H., Chen, H., Wu, J., Sun, Y., and Chen, Z., Carbon nanotubes as field emitter. *J Nanosci Nanotechnol.* 10(12), 7876–7896, 2010.
180. Heo, S.H., Kim, H.J., Ha, J.M., and Cho, S.O., A vacuum-sealed miniature X-ray tube based on carbon nanotube field emitters. *Nanoscale Res Lett.* 7(1), 258, 2012.
181. Li, Y. and Cheng, H.W., Field emission stability of anodic aluminum oxide carbon nanotube field emitter in the triode structure. *J Nanosci Nanotechnol.* 9(5), 3301–3307, 2009.
182. Li, C., Zhang, Y., Cole, M.T., Shivareddy, S.G., Barnard, J.S., Lei, W., Wang, B., Pribat, D., Amaratunga, G.A., and Milne, W.I., Hot electron field emission via individually transistor-ballasted carbon nanotube arrays. *ACS Nano.* 6(4), 3236–3242, 2012.
183. Wang, M.S., Peng, L.M., Wang, J.Y., and Chen, Q., Electron field emission characteristics and field evaporation of a single carbon nanotube. *J Phys Chem B.* 109(1), 110–113, 2005.
184. Bonard, J.M., Salvetat, J.P., Stöckli, T., Forró, L., and Châtelain, A., Field emission from carbon nanotubes: Perspectives for applications and clues to the emission mechanism. *Appl Phys A.* 69(3), 245–254, 1999.
185. Park, J. and McEuen, P.L., Formation of a p-type quantum dot at the end of an n-type carbon nanotube. *Appl Phys Lett.* 79(9), 1363–1366, 2001.
186. Bockrath, M., Cobden, D.H., McEuen, P.L., Chopra, N.G., Zettl, A., Thess, A., and Smalley, R.E., Single electron transport in ropes of carbon nanotubes. *Science.* 275(5308), 1922–1925, 1997.
187. Tans, S.J., Devoret, M.H., Dai, H., Thess, A., Smalley, R.E., Geerligs, L.J., and Dekker, C., Individual single-wall carbon nanotubes as quantum wires. *Nature.* 386(6624), 474–477, 1997.
188. Li, K.W., Lian, H.B., Cai, J.H., Wang, Y.T., and Lee, K.Y., Electron field emission characteristics of different surface morphologies of ZnO nanostructures coated on carbon nanotubes. *J Nanosci Nanotechnol.* 11(12), 11019–11022, 2011.
189. Dean, K.A. and Chalamala, B.R., Current saturation mechanisms in carbon nanotube field emitters. *Appl Phys Lett.* 76, 375–377, 2000.
190. Lim, S.C., Lee, K., Lee, I.H., and Lee, Y.H., Field emission and application of carbon nanotubes. *Nano.* 2(2), 69–89, 2007.
191. Schonenberger, C., Multiwall carbon nanotubes. *PhysicsWeb Phys World Mag.* 13(6), 1–5, 2000.
192. Krishna, A., Factors effecting field emission from multiwalled carbon nanotubes. M.Sc. Thesis, Department of Electrical and Computer Engineering, Louisiana State University, Baton Rouge, LA, 2005.
193. Carroll, D.L., Redlich, P., Ajayan, P.M., Charlier, J.C., Blase, X., De Vita, A., and Car, R., Electronic structure and localized states at carbon nanotube tips. *Phys Rev Lett.* 78, 2811–2814, 1997.
194. Bonard, J.M., Salvetat, J.P., Stockli, T., Forro, L., and Chatelain, A., Why are carbon nanotubes such excellent field emitters. *Sixth Foresight Conference on Molecular Nanotechnology*, 1998.
195. Saito, Y., Hamaguchi, K., Hata, K., Tohji, K., Kasuya, A., Nishina, Y., Uchida, K., Tasaka. Y., Ikazaki, F., Yumura, M., Field emission from carbon nanotubes: Purified single-walled and multi-walled tubes. *Ultramicroscopy.* 73(1–4), 1–6, 1998.
196. Dresselhaus, M., Dresselhaus, G., Eklund, P., and Saito, R., Carbon nanotubes. *Phys World.* 33–38, January 1998.
197. Schmid, H. and Fink, H.-W., Carbon nanotubes are coherent electron sources. *Appl Phys Lett.* 70, 2679–2680, 1997.
198. Fink, H.W., Stocker, W., and Schmid, H., Holography with low-energy electrons. *Phys Rev Lett.* 65(10), 1204–1206, 1990.
199. Lieber, C., Ouyang, M., Huang, J.L., and Chang, C.L., Energy gaps in "metallic" single walled carbon nanotubes. *Science.* 292(5517), 702–705, 2001.
200. De Heer, W.A., Chatelain, A., and Ugarte, D., A carbon nanotube field-emission electron source. *Science.* 270(5239), 1179–1180, 1995.
201. Yue, G.Z., Qiu, Q., Gao, B., Chang, S., Lu, J.P., and Zhou, O., Generation of continuous and pulsed diagnostic imaging x-ray radiation using a carbon-nanotube-based field emission cathode. *Appl Phys Lett.* 81(2), 355–357, 2002.
202. Boldt, R., Kaiser, M., Kohler, D., Krumeich, F., and Ruck, M., High yield synthesis and structure of double-walled bismuth nanotubes. *Nano Lett.* 10, 208–210, 2010.

203. Tenne, R. and Rao, C.N., Inorganic nanotubes. *Philos Transact A Math Phys Eng Sci.* 362(1823), 2099–2125, 2004.
204. Kharissova, O.V., Osorio, M., Vázquez, M.S., and Kharisov, B.I., Computational chemistry calculations of stability for bismuth nanotubes, fullerene-like structures and hydrogen-containing nanostructures. *J Mol Model.* 18(8), 3981–3992, 2012.
205. Su, C., Liu, H.T., and Li, J.M., Bismuth nanotubes: Potential semiconducting nanomaterials. *Nanotechnology.* 13(6), 746–749, 2002.
206. Ishigami, M., Sau, J.D., Aloni, S., Cohen, M.L., and Zettl, A., Observation of the giant stark effect in boron-nitride nanotubes. *Phys Rev Lett.* 94(5), 056804, 2005.
207. Elias, J., Tena-Zaera, R., Wang, G.Y., and Lévy-Clément, C., Conversion of ZnO nanowires into nanotubes with tailored dimensions. *Chem Mater.* 20, 6633–6637, 2008.
208. Ye, C.H., Bando, Y., Fang, X.S., Shen, G.Z., and Golberg, D., Enhanced field-emission performance of ZnO nanorods by two alternative approaches. *J Phys Chem C.* 111(34), 12673–12676, 2007.
209. Aubuchon, J.F., Chen, L.H., Daraio, C., and Jin, S., Multi-branching carbon nanotubes via self-seeded catalysts. *Nano Lett.* 6(2), 324–328, 2006.
210. Perkins, B.R., Wang, D.P., Soltman, D., Yin, A.J., Xu, J.M., and Zaslavsky, A., Differential current amplification in three-terminal Y-junction carbon nanotube devices. *Appl Phys Lett.* 87, 123504, 2005.
211. Bandaru, P.R., Daraio, C., Jin, S., and Rao, A.M., Novel electrical switching behaviour and logic in carbon nanotube Y-junctions. *Nat Mater.* 4(9), 663–666, 2005.
212. Li, C. Papadopoulos, J.M., and Xu, J., Nanoelectronics: Growing Y-junction carbon nanotubes. *Nature.* 402, 253–254, 1999.
213. Popov, V.N., Carbon nanotubes: Properties and application. *Mater Sci Eng R.* 43, 61–102, 2004.
214. Papadopoulos, C., Rakitin, A., Li, J., Vedeneev, A.S., and Xu, J.M., Electronic transport in Y-junction carbon nanotubes. *Phys Rev Lett.* 85(16), 3476–3479, 2000.
215. Petroff, P.M., Lorke, A., and Imamoglu, A., Epitaxially self-assembled quantum dots. *Phys Today.* 54(5), 46–52, 2001.
216. Kastner, M.A., Artificial atoms, Part I. *Phys Today.* 46(1), 24–27, 1993.
217. Foxman, E.B., Meirav, U., McEuen, P.L., Kastner, M.A., Klein, O., Belk, P.A., Abusch, D.M., and Wind, S.J., Crossover from single-level to multilevel transport in artificial atoms. *Phys Rev B Condens Matter.* 50(19), 14193–14199, 1994.
218. Williamson, A.J., Energy states of quantum dots. *Int J High Speed Electron Syst.* 12(1), 15–43, 2002.
219. Kouwenhoven, L.P. and McEuen, P.L., Single electron transport through a quantum dot, Chapter 13. *Nanotechnology*, Timp, G., ed. Springer-Verlag, New York, Inc. 1999.
220. Krishnan, M., Chang, L., King, T.-J., Bokor, J., and Hu, C., MOSFETs with 9 to 13 Å thick gate oxides. *IEDM Tech Dig.* 241–244, 1999.
221. Momose, H.S., Ono, M., Yoshitomi, T., Ohguro, T., Nakamura, S.-I., Saito, M., and Iwai, H., 1.5 nm direct-tunneling gate oxide Si MOSFETs. *IEEE Trans Electron Devices.* 43(8), 1233–1242, 1996.
222. Ge, N., Wong, C.M., Lingle, R.L. Jr., McNeill, J.D., Gaffney, K.J., and Harris, C.B., Femtosecond dynamics of electron localization at interfaces. *Science.* 279(5348), 202–205, 1998.
223. Kouwenhoven, L.P., Marcus, C.M., McEuen, P.L., Tarucha, S., Westervelt, R.M., and Wingreen, N.S., Electron transport in quantum dots. *Proceedings of the NATO Advanced Study Institute on Mesoscopic Electron Transport*, Sohn, L.L., Kouwenhoven, L.P., and Schön G., eds. Kluwer Series E345, 105–214, 1997.
224. Stier, O., Grundmann, M., and Bimberg, D., Electronic and optical properties of strained quantum dots modeled by 8-band k.p theory. *Phys Rev B Condens Matter Mater Phys.* 59(8), 5688–5701, 1999.
225. Leatherdale, C.A., Photophysics of cadmium selenide quantum dot solids. Ph.D. Thesis, Massachusetts Institute of Technology, Cambridge, MA, 2000.
226. Kastner, M.A., The single-electron transistor. *Rev Modern Phys.* 64, 849–858, 1992.
227. Likharev, K.K. and Claeson, T., Single electronics. *Sci Am.* 266(6), 80–85, 1992.
228. Devoret, M.H., Esteve, D., and Urbina, C., Single-electron transfer in metallic nanostructures. *Nature.* 360, 547, 1992.

229. Hadley, P., Single-electron tunneling devices. *Lectures on Superconductivity in Networks and Mesoscopicsystems*, Giovannella, C. and Lambert, C.J., eds. AIP Conference Proceedings 427. Woodbury, New York, 256–270, 1998.

230. Goldhaber-Gordon, D., Montemerlo, M.S., Love, J.C., Opiteck, G.J., and Ellenbogen, J.C., Overview of nanoelectronic devices, *The Proceedings of the IEEE*. The MITRE Corporation, MP97W0000136, April 1997.

231. Nakajima Y., Fabrication of a silicon quantum wire surrounded by silicon dioxide and its transport properties. *Appl Phys Lett*. 65, 2833–2835, 1994.

232. Takahashi, Y., Fabrication techniques for a single-electron transistor operating at room temperature. *Electron Lett*. 31, 136–137, 1995.

233. Karrea, P.S.K. and Bergstrom, P.L., Room temperature operational single electron transistor fabricated by focused ion beam deposition. *J Appl Phys*. 102, 024316, 2007.

234. Cheng, G., Siles, P.F., Bi, F., Cen, C., Bogorin, D.F., Bark, C.W., Folkman, C.M., Park, J.W., Eom, C.B., Medeiros-Ribeiro, G., and Levy, J., Sketched oxide single-electron transistor. *Nat Nanotechnol*. 6(6), 343–347, 2011.

235. Lee, Y.H., An, K.H., Lee, J.Y., and Lim, S.C., Carbon nanotube-based supercapacitors. *Encyclopedia of Nanoscience and Nanotechnology*. American Scientific Publishers, Stevenson Ranch, CA, pp. 625–634, 2004.

236. El-Kady, M.F., Strong, V., Dubin, S., and Kaner, R.B., Laser scribing of high-performance and flexible graphene-based electrochemical capacitors. *Science*. 335(6074), 1326–1330, 2012.

237. Kim, B., Chung, H., and Kim, W., High-performance supercapacitors based on vertically aligned carbon nanotubes and nonaqueous electrolytes. *Nanotechnology*. 23(15), 155401, 2012.

238. Xia, J., Chen, F., Li, J., and Tao, N., Measurement of the quantum capacitance of graphene. *Nat Nanotechnol*. 4(8), 505–509, 2009.

239. Stoller, M.D., Park, S., Zhu, Y., An, J., and Ruoff, R.S., Graphene-based ultracapacitors. *Nano Lett*. 8(10), 3498–3502, 2008.

240. Malvankar, N.S., Metser, T., Tuominen, M.T., and Lovley, D.R., Supercapacitors based on *c*-type cytochromes using conductive nanostructured networks of living bacteria. *Chemphyschem*. 13, 463–468, 2012.

241. Lovley, D.R., Electromicrobiology. *Annu Rev Microbiol*. 66, 391–409, 2012.

242. Malvankar, N.S., Vargas, M., Nevin, K.P., Franks, A.E., Leang, C., Kim, B.C., Inoue, K., Mester, T., Covalla, S.F., Johnson, J.P., Rotello, V.M., Tuominen, M.T., and Lovley, D.R., Tunable metallic-like conductivity in microbial nanowire networks. *Nat Nanotechnol*. 6, 573–579, 2011.

243. Petrov, A. and Audette, G.F., Peptide and protein-based nanotubes for nanobiotechnology. *Wiley Interdiscip Rev Nanomed Nanobiotechnol*. 4(5), 575–585, 2012.

244. Alphenaar, B.W., Tsukagoshi, K., and Ago, H., Spin electronics using carbon nanotubes. *Phys E*. 6, 848–851, 2000.

245. Tsukagoshi, K., Alphenaar, B.W., and Ago, H., Coherent transport of electron spin in a ferromagnetically contacted carbon nanotube. *Nature*. 401, 572–574, 1999.

246. Aronov, A.G., Spin injection in metals and polarization of nuclei. *JETP Lett*. 24, 32, 1976.

247. Julliere, M., Tunneling between ferromagnetic films. *Phys Lett*. 54A, 225–226, 1975.

248. Moodera, J.S., Kinder, L.R., Wong, T.M., and Meservey, R., Large magnetoresistance at room temperature in ferromagnetic thin film tunnel junctions. *Phys Rev Lett*. 74(16), 3273–3276, 1995.

249. Hueso, L.E., Pruneda, J.M., Ferrari, V., Burnell, G., Valdes-Herrera, J.P., Simons, B.D., Littlewood, P.B., Artacho, E., Fert, A., and Mathur, N.D., Transformation of spin information into large electrical signals using carbon nanotubes. *Nature*. 445(7126), 410–413, 2007.

250. Wei, P., Sun, L., Benassi, E., Shen, Z., Sanvito, S., and Hou, S., Effects of the covalent linker groups on the spin transport properties of single nickelocene molecules attached to single-walled carbon nanotubes. *J Chem Phys*. 136(19), 194707, 2012.

251. Korzhov, M., Shikler, R., and Andelman, D., Plastic which conducts electricity? *PhysicaPlus, Online Magazine of the Israel Physical Society (IPS)*, 10, 2008.

252. Saafan, S.A., Ayad, M.M., and El-Ghazzawy, E.H., The effect of preparation conditions on the growth rate of films, the yield of precipitated powder and the DC conductivity of polypyrrole. *Turk J Phys.* 29, 363–370, 2005.

253. Kline, J., McGehee, D., Kadnikova, E.N., Liu, J., and Fréchet, J.M.J., Controlling the field-effect mobility of regioregular polythiophene by changing the molecular weight. *Adv Mater.* 15(18), 1519–1522, 2003.

254. Osaka, I. and McCullough, R.D., Advances in molecular design and synthesis of regioregular polythiophenes. *Acc Chem Res.* 41(9), 1202–1214, 2008.

255. McCullough, R.D., Sauvea, G., Lia, B., Jeffries-Ela, M., Santhanama, S., and Schultza, L., Regioregular polythiophene nanowires and sensors. Bao, Z. and Gundlach, D.J., eds., *Proceedings of SPIE, 5940, 594005-1-7 Organic Field-Effect Transistors IV*, SPIE, Bellingham, WA, 2005.

256. Zhai, L. and McCullough, R.D., Regioregular polythiophene/gold nanoparticle hybrid material. *J Mater Chem.* 14, 141–143, 2004.

257. Otero, T.F. and Sansinena, J.M., Soft and wet conducting polymers for artificial muscles. *Adv Mater.* 10, 491–494, 1998.

258. Schmidt, C.E., Shastri, V.R., Vacanti, J.P., and Langer, R., Stimulation of neurite outgrowth using an electrically conducting polymer. *Proc Natl Acad Sci USA.* 94, 8948–8953, 1997.

259. Abidian, M.R. and Martin, D.C., Multifunctional nanobiomaterials for neural interfaces. *Adv Funct Mater.* 19, 573–585, 2009.

260. Abidian, M.R., Kim, D.H., and Martin, D.C., Conducting polymer nanotubes for controlled drug release. *Adv Mater.* 18, 405–409, 2006.

261. Warren, L.F., Walker, J.A., Anderson, D.P., Rhodes, C.G., and Buckley, L.J., A study of conducting polymer morphology. *J Electrochem Soc.* 136, 2286–2295, 1989.

262. Saxena, V. and Malhotra, B.D., *Handbook of Polymers in Electronics.* Rapra Technology, Shrewsbury, U.K., 3, 2002.

263. Wise, D.L., Wnek, G.E., Trantolo, D.J., Cooper, T.M., Gresser, J.D., and Marcel, D., *Electrical and Optical Polymer Systems: Fundamentals, Methods and Application.* Marcel Dekker, New York, 1031, 1998.

264. Heeger, A.J., MacDiarmid, A.G., and Shirakawa, H., *The Nobel Prize in Chemistry, 2000: Conductive Polymers.* Royal Swedish Academy of Sciences, Stockholm, Sweden, 2000.

265. Ravichandran, R., Sundarrajan, S., Venugopal, J.R., Mukherjee, S., and Ramakrishna, S., Applications of conducting polymers and their issues in biomedical engineering. *J R Soc Interface.* 7(Suppl. 5), S559–S579, 2010.

266. Zelikin, A.N., Lynn, D.M., Farhadi, J., Martin, I., Shastri, V., and Langer, R., Erodible conducting polymers for potential biomedical applications. *Angew Chem Int Ed.* 41(1), 141–144, 2002.

267. Shi, G., Rouabhia, M., Wang, Z., Dao, L.H., and Zhang, Z., A novel electrically conductive and biodegradable composite made of polypyrrole nanoparticles and polylactide. *Biomaterials.* 25, 2477–2488, 2004.

268. Guimard, N.K., Sessler, J.L., and Schmidt, C.E., Design of a novel electrically conducting biocompatible polymer with degradable linkages for biomedical applications. *Mater Res Soc Symp Proc.* 950, 99–104, 2007.

269. Abidian, M.R. and Martin, D.C., Experimental and theoretical characterization of implantable neural microelectrodes modified with conducting polymer nanotubes. *Biomaterials.* 29(9), 1273–1283, 2008.

270. Yarris, L., New technique produces magnetic thin films at a fraction of the current cost. *Science Beat*, Berkley Lab, November 17, 1995.

271. Freeman, A.J., Poeppelmeier, K.R., Mason, T.O., Chang, R.P.H., and Marks, T.J., Chemical and thin-film strategies for new transparent conducting oxides. *MRS Bulletin*, 25(8), 45–51, 2000.

272. Liu, C.H. and Yu, X., Silver nanowire-based transparent, flexible, and conductive thin film. *Nanoscale Res Lett.* 6(1), 75, 2011.

273. Merkle, R.C. and Freitas, R.A. Jr., Theoretical analysis of a carbon–carbon dimer placement tool for diamond mechanosynthesis. *J Nanosci Nanotechnol.* 3(4), 319–324, 2003.

274. Liddle, J.A. and Gallatin, G.M., Lithography, metrology and nanomanufacturing. *Nanoscale.* 3(7), 2679–2688, 2011.
275. Pei, S., Zhao, J., Du, J., Ren, W., and Cheng, H.M., Direct reduction of graphene oxide films into highly conductive and flexible graphene films by hydrohalic acids. *Carbon.* 48, 4466–4474, 2010.
276. Centurion, L.M., Moreira, W.C., and Zucolotto, V., Tailoring molecular architectures with cobalt tetrasulfonated phthalocyanine: Immobilization in layer-by-layer films and sensing applications. *J Nanosci Nanotechnol.* 12(3), 2399–2405, 2012.
277. Fang, Z., Liu, Z., Wang, Y., Ajayan, P.M., Nordlander, P., and Halas, N.J., Graphene-antenna sandwich photodetector. *Nano Lett.* 12(7), 3808–3813, 2012.
278. Dregely, D., Taubert, R., Dorfmüller, J., Vogelgesang, R., Kern, K., and Giessen, H., 3D optical Yagi-Uda nanoantenna array. *Nat Commun.* 2, 267, 2011.
279. Ahn, J.H., Kim, H.S., Lee, K.J., Jeon, S., Kang, S.J., Sun, Y., Nuzzo, R.G., and Rogers, J.A., Heterogeneous three-dimensional electronics by use of printed semiconductor nanomaterials. *Science.* 314(5806), 1754–1757, 2006.
280. Javey, A., Nam, S., Friedman, R.S., Yan, H., and Lieber, C.M., Layer-by-layer assembly of nanowires for three-dimensional, multifunctional electronics. *Nano Lett.* 7(3), 773–777, 2007.
281. Pavel, E., 2 nm quantum optical lithography. Storex Technologies Inc. (Romania) SPIE Advanced Lithography 2012, Paper 8323-63, February 12–16, 2012.
282. Lu, W. and Lieber, C.M., Nanoelectronics from the bottom up. *Nat Mater.* 6, 841–850, 2007.
283. Engheta, N., Circuits with light at nanoscales: Optical nanocircuits inspired by metamaterials. *Science.* 317, 1698–1702, 2007.
284. Bourzac, K., Making wiring that doesn't trip up computer chips. *MIT Technol Rev.*, July 10, 2012. http://www.technologyreview.com/news/428466/making-wiring-that-doesnt-trip-up-computer-chips/ (accessed 06/23/13)
285. Freitas, R.A. Jr., *Nanomedicine, Volume I: Basic Capabilities.* Landes Bioscience, Georgetown, TX, 1999.
286. Michelotti, N., Johnson-Buck, A., Manzo, A.J., and Walter, N.G., Beyond DNA origami: The unfolding prospects of nucleic acid nanotechnology. *Wiley Interdiscip Rev Nanomed Nanobiotechnol.* 4(2), 139–152, 2012.
287. Aldaye, F.A. and Sleiman, H.F., Dynamic DNA templates for discrete gold nanoparticle assemblies: Control of geometry, modularity, write/erase and structural switching. *J Am Chem Soc.* 129(14), 4130–4131, 2007.
288. Maye, M.M., Kumara, M.T., Nykypanchuk, D., Sherman, W.B., and Gang, O., Switching binary states of nanoparticle superlattices and dimer clusters by DNA strands. *Nat Nanotechnol.* 5(2), 116–120, 2010.

6

Design Challenges and Considerations for Nanomedical Device Signal Acquisition and Propagation

Frank J. Boehm

CONTENTS

6.1 VCSN Spatial Data Acquisition Component

Spatial data acquisition elements are envisaged to serve as the primary imaging units for the vascular cartographic scanning nanodevice (VCSN). These densely arrayed components would carry out the actual in vivo digital cartographic tasks in order to provide unprecedented ultrahigh-resolution three-dimensional (3D) maps of the vascular or lymphatic systems. The means by which this spatial data might be acquired in vivo at the nanoscale and subsequently conveyed to an external computer will undoubtedly present major technological challenges. The endowment of spatial data acquisition components with spectrographic capabilities (Chapter 1) might greatly enhance the diagnostic value of the obtained cartographic information, enabling, for example, the capacity for differentiating the chemistries of vascular and neurological plaque materials from that of healthy vascular endothelial wall surfaces.

Several suggestions for potential pathways toward the development of this component might initially include detailed investigations into nanometric capacitive ultrasonic transducers, and thin film bulk acoustic resonators (FBARs). Hypothetically, nested nanomagnetic entities might exhibit the possibility of inducing localized Larmor precession (as in magnetic resonance imaging [MRI]) through the generation of transient magnetic standing waves. Quantum dot/wire lasers may potentially be utilized for the generation of nanoscale LIDAR-like topographies, or might be employed to initiate detectable sonic echoes when they impact the surface of the blood vessel walls. Lasers might be utilized in conjunction with ultrasound to achieve elucidation of vascular wall topographies.

Biophotonic emission, which is inherent in all biosystems, may allow the gathering of spatial data through the development of ultrasensitive nanoscale photon detectors/multipliers. Another novel method may involve the measurement of very subtle temperature differentials that may exist between circulating whole blood and the relatively static endothelial walls of the vascular system. This information may present a means of isolating and defining the interface between the two, thereby generating a topographical profile. The possibility of devising nanometric thermocouples might also be investigated to learn if they may have the ability to discern minute temperature differentials as low as $0.093°C \pm 0.032°C$, which in one study has been shown to be the maximum variance in temperature between vessel wall-resident vascular plaque (which is thought to emanate higher temperatures due to the heat released by constituent inflamed cells) and the circulating blood [1].

Shear flow friction or localized interfacial sonic vibration may also provide a means by which to define inner vascular surface topography, if a technique could be developed for detecting the mobile/static interface between transiting fluid (blood) and luminal endothelial walls in vivo. Speculatively, slight deviations in electrical charge profiles between the two tissue species at their interface [2] might be detected by an in vivo nanomedical device that is properly equipped for such a task.

The conceptualization and development of a nanomedical spatial data acquisition component might encompass some of the criteria set out as follows:

1. Sequential and systematic investigation into and subsequent development of a nanoscale spatial data acquisition component for application in vivo (e.g., for high-resolution 3D mapping of vascular, lymphatic, and gastrointestinal systems). This device would have the inherent further purpose of eventual integration and utilization as the primary spatial data-gathering mechanism for the VCSN, which would be used to obtain and disseminate all cartographic information.

2. Generation of designs, proof-of-principal concepts, and demonstration of a robust, accurate (~<1 µm resolution), and reliable mechanism for mapping inner endothelial vascular wall surfaces, including all bifurcated vessels down to capillary level. Further capabilities will include elucidation of vascular wall thickness via the isolation of secondary echo signatures, and ability to differentiate between plaque material, lesions, and healthy endothelial wall surfaces.

3. The preferred mechanism for gathering spatial data might incorporate nanoscale capacitive ultrasonic transducers, or other piezoelectronic ultrasound emanating entities. The requirement would be for the acquisition and conveyance (for subsequent display) of a very finely detailed topography of inner endothelial wall surfaces by scanning through turbid media (e.g., consisting of human whole blood in the vascular system, and to a lesser extent, lymph for lymphatic system mapping), and semisolid materials (such would be the case for gastrointestinal tract scanning).

4. Alternately, the generation of proof-of-principal concepts and demonstration of robust and reliable in vivo spatial data acquisition by other potential means. For example, quantum dot laser or nanoscale LIDAR type technology; nanomagnetics for potential initiation of localized atomic precession in H atoms embedded within the endothelial wall; thermal differentiation at the interface between the solid endothelial walls and flowing blood.

5. Demonstration of component resistance to biofouling (e.g., via proteins and other whole blood constituents) for a reasonable duration (note: envisioned VCSN scanning time = ~5 min).

6. Elucidation of potential fabrication/synthesis processes (e.g., massively parallel fabrication via molecular assemblers or DNA-based nanomanufacturing capabilities) for the modular manufacture of this component.

6.2 Nanoscale Ultrasonic Transducers

Macroscale ultrasonic transducers utilize the piezoelectric effect. Certain materials (Table 6.1) will exhibit a charge on their surface when they are mechanically stressed. Conversely, there is a reverse effect of physical deformation in these materials when an electrical charge is applied. Ultrasonic sensors typically utilize a single transducer to both transmit and receive high-frequency sound that is beyond the range of human hearing (>20 kHz). They may be employed to measure distance by means of transmitting a short

TABLE 6.1

Examples of Piezoelectric Materials with Potential Utility in the Development
of Nanomedical Ultrasonic Transducers

Materials with Piezoelectric Attributes		
Crystals	**Ceramics**	**Other Materials**
Aluminum orthophosphate ($AlPO_4$)	Barium titanate ($BaTiO_3$)	Aluminum nitride (AlN)
Gallium orthophosphate ($GaPO_4$)	Barium sodium niobate ($Ba_2NaNb_5O_5$)	Lanthanum gallium silicate ($La_3Ga_5SiO_{14}$)
Langasite ($La_3Ga_5SiO_{14}$)		
Lithium tetraborate ($Li_2B_2O_3$)	Bismuth ferrite ($BiFeO_3$)	Polyvinylidene fluoride (PVDF)
Tourmaline ((Na^{1+}, Ca^{2+})(Li^{1+}, Mg^{2+}, Al^{3+})$\cdot$(Al^{3+}, Fe^{3+}, Mn^{3+})$6(BO_3)^3(Si_6O_{18})(OH)_4$)	Lead metaniobate ($Pb(NbO_3)$)	Potassium sodium tartrate ($C_4H_4KNaO_6$)
	Lead zirconate titanate (PZT) ($Pb(ZrTi)O_3$)	Zinc oxide (ZnO)
Trigonal crystallized silica quartz (SiO_2)	Lithium niobate ($LiNbO_3$)	
	Lead potassium niobate ($Pb_2KNb_5O_{15}$)	
	Potassium niobate ($KNbO_3$)	
	Sodium tungsten bronze ($NaxWO_3$)	
	Strontium titanate ($SrTiO_3$)	

ultrasonic burst to a target, which is then reflected back to the sensor. Based on time-of-flight calculations and the speed of sound in the medium of interest, a distance is deduced. The speed of sound in blood is 1570 m/s, and in soft tissue 1540 m/s [3,4].

6.2.1 Description of Ultrasonic Transducers

There exist many different types of ultrasonic transducers that are fabricated for specific applications. The species of interest most appropriate for the VCSN will likely consist of those that retain robust functionality when they are immersed in fluids (e.g., within human whole blood/plasma). Scaling is a critical factor, as the intention will be to fabricate and operate these types of mechanisms at the nanoscale level and to incorporate them into nanomedical imaging devices. When immersed in fluids, piezoelectric transducers tend to be inefficient due to the impedance (ratio of pressure to flow) mismatch between the piezoelectric and the fluid. For instance, in water a piezoceramic has an impedance of ~30 × 10⁶ kg/m² s versus 1 × 10⁶ kg/m² s for water itself. The geometries of piezoelectric devices will have an impact on their electrical impedance. They are limited to strain levels of about 10^{-4} and a surface displacement of ~0.5 μm, which transmits in the lower MHz range [5].

6.2.2 Capacitive Micromachined Ultrasonic Transducers

One of the smallest functional ultrasonic transducers that have been fabricated to date are called capacitive micromachined ultrasonic transducers (CMUTs). This technology has been evolving over the last 20 years and has recently been introduced to the medical marketplace for applications such as endoscopic and intracardiac imaging. These transducers are fabricated lithographically as two-dimensional (2D) wafer-resident arrays that may contain as many as several thousand discrete units to provide real-time 3D imagery.

Individual elements are accessible electronically via interconnects that run through the wafer from behind [6]. The latest CMUTs are fabricated by utilizing current MEMS and integrated circuit technologies. From the nanomedical perspective, when prospectively administering thousands of VCSN units, CMUTs would have an advantage in that their operation is not impeded by the self-heating effects that their piezoelectric counterparts are prone to. Generated heat would be dissipated via the highly thermally conductive silicon from which they are constructed. This allows CMUT operation in high power and continuous wave applications such as high intensity–focused ultrasound. It has been demonstrated by Khuri-Yakub and coworkers that CMUTs may tolerate >90 min of continuous operation while generating acoustic pressures of "2 MPa peak to peak on the surface" [6–8]. As the VCSN scanning procedure is envisioned to be completed within a 5 min window, it may be speculated that nanoscale CMUTs, should they be possible to fabricate in the future, might serve as suitable candidates for VCSN-integrated imaging elements.

6.2.2.1 CMUT Fabrication

To illustrate one of the numerous possible CMUT fabrication techniques (Figure 6.1), a p-type (100) silicon wafer (heavily doped with a phosphorous gas for good conductivity) is coated with a 1 μm oxide layer, grown with a wet oxidation process. A 3500 Å layer of LPCVD (low-pressure chemical deposition) nitride is then deposited. A sacrificial layer is deposited and dry-etched into octagonal islands, defining the transducer cavity areas. Membrane material is then deposited (residual stress used is ~80 Mpa = 800 atm). For this technique, a silicon nitride membrane (0.53 μm thick) with a polysilicon sacrificial layer provides the best results [9]. Electron beam lithography is used to form the pattern of holes. Their small size allows for efficient vacuum sealing of the cavity (0.09 μm gap height). A 0.16 μm layer of insulating material is located directly above the bottom electrode.

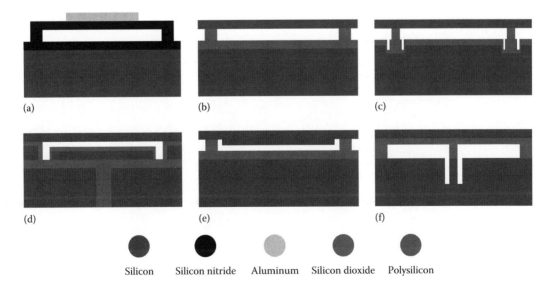

FIGURE 6.1
Cross-sectioned schematics of various CMUT geometries fabricated by different techniques: (a) sacrificial release process, (b) simple wafer-bonding process, (c) local oxidation of silicon (LOCOS) process, (d) thick buried oxide process, (e) added plate mass, and (f) compliant post structure. (Adapted and redrawn from Khuri-Yakub, B.T. and Oralkan, O., *J Micromech Microeng.* 21(5), 54004, 2011. With permission.)

In a final step, aluminum is sputtered and wet etch–patterned to serve as the top electrode. The same aluminum deposition also defines the bonding contacts to the bottom electrode through a lithographically etched trench. The wafer is cut and the CMUTs are mounted to a circuit board [5,9].

Individual transducers are connected in parallel to others via an electrode that is positioned directly above the cavity region, which links the cells together. Parasitic capacitance is reduced when narrow interconnects are employed; however, resistance will be higher between the cells. The optimum dimensions at this scale were found to be ~3 μm wide and 0.2 μm thick [9].

6.2.2.2 CMUT Mechanical and Electronic Properties

CMUT unit cell diameters can be in the range of ~30 μm with about 2500 connected in parallel to make up a device. The CMUTs are fabricated with current microelectromechanical systems (MEMS) technology and e-beam lithography, and appear to have the potential for further miniaturization with these techniques [9,10]. The CMUTs can be octagonal in shape or may be fabricated to have different geometries in ordered arrays to comprise a transducer (Figure 6.2).

The first immersion capacitive transducer was developed in 1979 [11]. In the last decade, micromachining techniques were reported, which described the manufacture of transducers with a suspended membrane over a back plate [12]. More advanced fabrication technologies and procedures have evolved and have sparked several simultaneous developments [10,13–15]. Capacitive ultrasonic transducers may have many advantages over piezoelectric transducers. These transducers have a concave membrane (to focus the signal) made of metallized silicon nitride suspended above a heavily doped silicon base. There is a sealed vacuum cavity between the two surfaces. When DC voltage (35 V—DC bias voltage for both transmitter and receiver) is applied between the metallized membrane and the silicon base, coulomb forces attract the membrane toward the base. Residual stress inside the membrane will resist the attraction. When AC voltage activates the membrane, robust

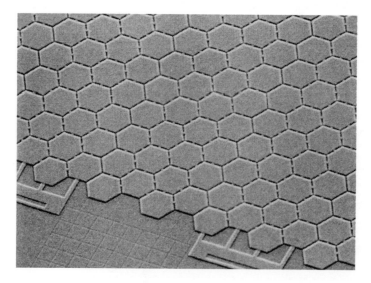

FIGURE 6.2
Depiction of CMUT array. (Reproduced from Machida, S. et al., Capacitive Micromachined Ultrasonic Transducer with Driving Voltage over 100V and Vibration Durability over 10^{11} Cycles, in Proc. IEEE Transducers '09, 2218–2221, 2009. Copyright, Hitachi Medical Corporation.)

ultrasound generation will be emanated. If the membrane has an appropriate bias and it is impacted by an ultrasonic wave, a significant detection current is created [5].

The dimensions of the membrane will determine the operating frequency of the ultrasonic signal. The dynamic range for these transducers is >100 dB at 4.5 MHz. More than 100% bandwidth is exhibited for an untuned transducer when interfaced with electronics having 50 Ω input impedance. The bandwidth in immersion is determined by the transformer ratio (e.g., where mechanical impedance of the immersion medium is greater than the membrane impedance). For wideband operation the membrane thickness and the void from the membrane to base should be as low as possible, whereas the DC bias voltage should be as high as possible. It is necessary that the gap between the membrane and base should be vacuum-sealed in order to reduce the loss caused by water hydrolyzation under the high electric field within the cavity [9]. The detection of an echoed ultrasonic wave is measured by the fractional change of the CMUT capacitance when it is impacted by ultrasonic waves. Therefore, it is desirable that the gap between membrane and base be as narrow as possible to enable high sensitivity. In an optimized system, dual CMUTs might be used, where emitter possesses a thick gap (for robust emission) and the receiver has a thin gap for optimum receiving sensitivity.

6.3 Optoacoustics

Ultrasonic excitation and detection can occur via laser light. An ultrasonic transducer can be induced to produce signals via heating and mechanical deformation through the use of a laser [16,17]. An additional scheme employs the absorption of laser light by tissue to create pressure waves that are detected by a transducer. The tissue is exposed to a pulsed laser and the photons are absorbed into the tissue, which results in a subtle temperature increase. This thermal increase causes a slight expansion in the tissue that produces a pressure wave that can be detected by the transducer. A time-resolved measurement may be ascertained through the use of a digital oscilloscope. Several signal traces are averaged and transferred to a computer for analysis [18].

6.4 Thermoacoustics

High-intensity ultrasonic waves may also result from the conduction of heat, from porous silicon to air, without the requirement of any mechanical vibrational system. The concept of a "thermaphone" was developed ~95 years ago, which consisted of an acoustic entity that was a simple self-supporting thin metal film [19]. A current version of this device comprises a patterned 30 nm thick aluminum film, a microporous silicon layer (10 μm thick), and a p-type crystalline silicon (c-SI) wafer. Within the porous silicon reside numerous confined nanocrystallites that contain 3D nanopores [20]. These devices have a broad frequency range; however, they consume more power than a conventional resonant device. It remains to be seen if this type of system might lend itself to downscaling and be amenable with the immersion criteria that is required for integration and operation with in vivo deployed nanodevices.

6.5 Surface Acoustic Wave Devices

Surface acoustic wave (SAW) devices comprise piezoelectric ceramic lead–zirconate–titanate (PZT) or quartz–homeotype gallium–orthophosphate crystals, which are purported to be more efficient piezoelectric materials than quartz [21]. The piezoelectric material is electrically activated by components called interdigital transducers, which are a photolithographically fabricated pattern of interdigitated metallic electrodes on a piezoelectric substrate. When an electric field is injected between the interdigitated combs it initiates the deformation of the surface, due to the piezoelectric nature of the substrate, and creates a standing wave.

Several problems, however, may plague the downscaling of a SAW-configured device and prevent its proper functionality. One such issue is the occurrence of corrupting second-order effects such as electromagnetic feed-through, ohmic losses, and diffraction. Another concern lies in the lithographic fabrication processes for these devices, which are also affected by second-order degradation. The size of these devices is almost at inverse proportion to frequency; however, when narrow-gap SAW configurations are combined with near-field phase-shift lithography (utilizing phase-shifting masks to modify the amplitude and phase, which results in higher resolution) low-cost SAW devices may be produced that operate above 5 GHz [22].

6.6 Thin Film Bulk Acoustic Resonator

This type of resonator has advantages over SAW devices. It is made using thin film semiconductor process to construct a laminated sandwich (e.g., metal–aluminum–nitride–metal), or ZnO piezoelectric stack [23]. When an AC current is applied to this structure the various layers expand and contract, which generate a vibration. The resonance takes place in the body of the device as opposed to only on the surface, as in a SAW device. An advantage of FBAR technology is that it can utilize power more efficiently at higher frequencies than with SAWs interdigitated structures. The vibrating membrane creates a high Q resonance and can operate at frequencies above 10 GHz [24]. Possibilities for miniaturization are also more viable for these types of resonators.

6.7 Biocompatibility and Safety of Ultrasonic Transducers

For appropriately designed nanodevices, nanometric ultrasonic transducers will likely be situated on peripheral surfaces. Dependent on the materials required for fabricating these devices at the nanoscale, biocompatibility might be accomplished via the application of ultrathin coatings of polyethylene glycol (PEG) or its derivatives [25], perfluorinated surfactant compounds [26], thermoplastic vulcanizate (TPV), or olefinic-based thermoplastic elastomer (TEO), and other styrenic-based thermoplastic elastomer (TPE) compounds, such as those that are produced by RTP Company [27]. Alternately, ceramic mixtures (e.g., Al_2O_3, CaO, TiO_2, SiO_2, Fe_2O_3, ZrO_2) might be employed [28].

It may be possible that an ultrathin film of diamondoid or equally inert substance may be utilized to coat the entire external surface of nanodevices.

The America Institute of Ultrasound in Medicine states that no significant biological effects have been reliably observed in mammalian tissue exposed in vivo to unfocused ~MHz ultrasound with intensities of 1000 W/m^2 or less [29]. The onset of continuous wave ultrasound-induced lysis of human erythrocytes has occasionally been detected experimentally at intensities of as low as 60 W/m at 1.6 MHz when micron size gas bubbles are also present [30]. Exposures of any duration >500 kW/m^2 may cause cavitation (transient microbubbles implode and produce temperature spikes of ~10^3 K and pressure spikes of ~10^3 atm within a few microns radius of implosion sites) and other harmful effects in biological tissue [31].

6.8 Carbon Nanotubes for Potential In Vivo Spatial Data Acquisition Device

Carbon nanotubes (CNTs) have a multitude of attractive qualities that might be exploited should they be incorporated as elements of a nanomedical spatial data acquisition component. They are chemically inert, biocompatible, and have many exceptional and desirable mechanical, electronic, thermal, and optical properties (Figure 6.3). As they are quite flexible and potentially tunable to a given application, CNTs may be amenable for integration into the scanning components of nanodevices such as the VCSN.

If one is considering drawing on the electron field-emitting capabilities of CNTs, a means must be devised for reliably delivering enough energy to them for attaining and sustaining the field-emitting threshold. In turn, achieved electron emission must have a practical function in the scheme of the scanning component design. It seems obvious that attempts to acquire any meaningful in vivo spatial data by somehow utilizing exposed CNT field-emitted electron flow, by itself, are likely to be unsuccessful. Although it has been demonstrated that one or several water molecules, which are adsorbed to the tip of a

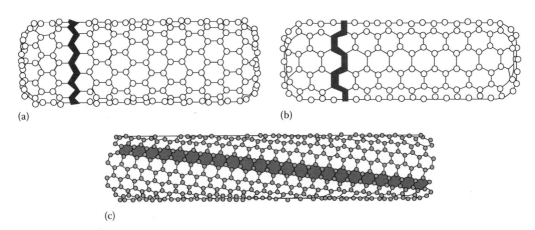

(a) (b)

(c)

FIGURE 6.3
(a–c) Three configurations of carbon nanotubes. (Reproduced from Yildirim, T., NIST, http://www.ncnr.nist.gov/staff/taner/nanotube/, accessed March 25, 2012. With permission.)

CNT, may actually enhance field emission [32], this is likely to not be the case when CNTs are fully immersed in aqueous media (e.g., blood/plasma). Free CNT field-emitted electrons in vivo would quickly dissipate into solution and almost instantaneously recombine with the closest molecular entity, most likely with water molecules. Therefore, electrons would be negated from ever reaching a target to convey useful information. Hence, to have utility, CNT field-emitted electrons might be contained and guided within miniaturized vacuum-sealed cavities [33] that are positioned directly above CNT tips to potentially activate additional integrated functional entities, such as arrays of nanoscale ultrasonic transducers.

6.9 Nanometric Fibers for Near-Field Optics

Optical micro/nanofibers comprising tellurite (Ø 250 nm) and silica (Ø 400 nm) fibers have been developed for use in near-field optics [35,36]. Near-field scanning optical microscopes have overcome the optical anomaly known as diffraction, which tends to distort the resolution of a sample. Bringing an optical fiber to within 10 nm (the near field) of the sample surface eliminates the normal effects of diffraction. The result is a clear 3D image that will resolve even individual molecules [37]. Near-field optics might play an important role in the acquisition of cellular chemical and topographical data to enable noninvasive in vivo biopsies, and potentially working as an element of a VCSN nanospectroscopic capability (Chapter 1).

6.10 MRI: Spatial Data Acquisition at the Atomic Level

MRI acquires spatial data information from which to derive medical imagery through the detection of the relative spin states of certain atoms with an odd number of electrons (1H, 7Li, 13C, 17O, 19F, 23Na) under an applied magnetic field and radio frequency (RF) pulses. The atom of choice for this type of imaging is hydrogen. One cubic centimeter of tissue contains 6.7×10^{22} H atoms. Electrons create a magnetic field much greater than the nuclear field and protons exhibit quantization in a magnetic field. The strength of a magnetic field is measured in gauss or tesla (T) (1 T = 10,000 gauss). For comparison, the magnetic field of the earth is 0.5 gauss. When protons are exposed to a 1.5 T (15,000 gauss) magnetic field, the energy difference between the high- and low-energy states is ~63 MHz, and for every million protons, 10 additional protons will be in the negative state compared to those in the higher-energy state. In MRI, ~1000 collection repetitions are utilized to obtain a reasonable image quality due to the fleeting nature of the signal [38].

Spin angular momentum in atoms has both magnitude and direction. A spinning particle generates a magnetic field and a "magnetic moment," behaving like an atomic bar magnet with both north and south poles. When placed in a magnetic field of sufficient strength, the magnetic moment of an atoms nucleus tends to align itself parallel or antiparallel in relation to the applied field. Parallel alignment has a lower-energy state (N-S-N-S) and antiparallel alignment a higher state (N-N-S-S). In a magnetic field, an atomic particle also spins with oscillation and its axis is on an angle relative to the direction of the magnetic field (precession). There is a characteristic frequency (Larmor constant = ~42.58 MHz/T for hydrogen) to the wobble of the atomic nucleus, depending on the species and its environment/temperature. Increasing the magnetic field strength increases the frequency, and decreasing the field strength will lower it. When tissue is placed in a strong magnetic field, the net magnetic vector is established in a matter of seconds. Spin exists in multiples of ½, and is either plus or minus. Individual unpaired electrons, protons, and neutrons possess a spin of ½. A particle with a net spin when placed in a magnetic field can absorb a photon of a certain frequency. This frequency depends on the gyromagnetic ratio of the particle [39].

When RF waves (10–100 MHz) are also applied perpendicular to the magnetic field, the atomic magnetic moment of an atom can be induced to flip. This happens when the frequency of the radio signal matches the nuclei characteristic precessional frequency that lies within the RF range. When this match occurs, the resonance frequency is attained. A nucleus absorbs energy from the radio signal that is precisely equal to the difference between the two energy states and hence, it jumps into the higher state. Flipping also occurs when a nucleus reemits this energy when it reverts back to the lower-energy state, which will happen spontaneously but not instantaneously. This transition may be detected regardless of whether the nucleus is being excited to the higher state or is falling to the lower one. To image hydrogen clinically, the frequency employed is ~15 to 80 MHz [39].

When applied to molecules, a series of resonances (packets) can distinguish a single atom's bonding properties and how individual nuclei are affected by other atoms residing in the molecule. By keeping the magnetic field constant and varying the RF, the signals can be spread out over a spectrum that is analogous to a prism spreading visible light. This is called RF spectroscopy and is used for chemical analysis [40].

The human body comprises mostly water and fat. These two constituents contain many hydrogen atoms, which are mainly bound up in H_2O, as well as in several isotopes, making up ~63% of total body volume. A hydrogen atom, having only one proton for its nucleus, has a significant magnetic moment. This is why it is the most important element for use in MRI. Thermal and magnetic equilibrium is a magnetized state attained when slightly more nuclei are aligned in parallel rather than antiparallel in relation to the applied field. Subsequently, a RF is applied so as to induce the flipping of the nuclei, by absorbing or reradiating energy to the RF field. The electromagnetic spectrum of the human body is opaque to the RF range up into the high end of the spectrum. Body images may be formed as it is semitransparent to RF radiation. However, the RF wavelength is longer than the required resolution for imaging the body; therefore, it cannot be used directly, in its place a magnetic coding system is used [40].

The RF signal released by a proton is called the "free induction decay" signal. The more tightly bound a water molecule is, the shorter its relaxation time. Quantities called relaxation times (T1 and T2) are critical for producing the contrast required for imaging tissues in the human body. The T1 and T2 times vary considerably in the different structures and fluids within the human body and are strongly influenced by viscosity and the rigidity of tissues. The T1 time for water in a magnetic field (0.2–2.0 T) is 2 s. The T1 time for fat is in the tens of milliseconds as fat magnetizes more quickly than does water. The T1 relaxation energy is transferred to neighboring molecules in the local environment and is called spin–lattice relaxation. Energy may also be given up to nearby nuclei and is called spin–spin relaxation [40].

Placing a sample in a homogeneous magnetic field will not produce tomographic MR images, as all protons experience virtually the same magnetic field; thus, all emitted signals will be identical. A second gradient field is required so that protons within the sample will emit different frequency signals that are dependent on their spatial position. The magnetic field varies across a scanned area and the resonance frequencies of spins also vary. The spins resonance frequencies are determined, therefore, by their location along the gradient axis. The number of spins that resonate at a particular frequency determines the amplitude of that frequency within the spectrum of detectable resonance frequencies. For each frequency constituent of the measured signal, the strength and direction of the applied gradient may be used to calculate the spectral coordinates of that signal [40].

By combining a frequency gradient with a pulse having the proper frequency and bandwidth a small slice of a sample can be excited, which allows for slice-by-slice image acquisition. To produce a 2D image of spin densities in a sample, the locations in the first axis are encoded by frequencies, and locations in the second axis are encoded by phase. A typical imaging procedure begins with a selection-slice excitation by application of a temporary gradient. Frequency encoding is determined by applying the frequency-encoding gradient in the x-axis during acquisition. The next step is phase encoding along the y-axis. Both frequency and pulse of the detected signal encode spatial coordinates. Stepwise increases in both gradients segment the sample into small cubes (voxels). The signal of any given voxel is the sum of all spin contributions, which makes the resolution of an image dependent on the size of the voxels. The cumulative spins within a voxel may not be distinguished from one another [40].

6.11 Localized Magnetic Resonance for Potential In Vivo Spatial Data Acquisition

Consider an in vivo nanodevice containing laminated ultrathin ferroelectric films, or coiled ferromagnetic cylinders, comprising its scanning apparatus. A transient (standing wave) magnetic field might be generated from this nanomagnetic scanning strip/array to hypothetically initiate highly localized precession in the hydrogen atoms that are embedded within endothelial lined vascular walls as it passes by. Magnetic field strength studies aimed at the determination of the exact intensity of a magnetic field that might be required for the initiation of localized and precession states may constitute an intriguing topic of research to this end.

Classical MRI employs potent magnetic fields to accomplish atomic nuclei precession. A much reduced (in strength) and highly localized magnetic field that emanates from an in vivo nanodevice may be able to initiate some degree of precession (albeit fleeting as the nanodevice(s) will be in transit) for a time period that is sufficiently long to detect reemission energy from nuclei. The required transverse RF waves may emanate "inbody" from a patch that is adhered to the skin of the patient. They might also be generated from an external localized beacon that is a component of a nanomedical "spatial metrics" room (Chapter 3).

Considering that there may be thousands of nanodevices traversing the vasculature simultaneously, small, robust, and highly portable RF-emitting/detecting mechanisms might be implemented. These devices would both transmit the pulsed RF signals into the patient and receive the voluminous signal streams coming from the internalized nuclei, which are reemitting RF energy.

6.12 Quantum Lasers for In Vivo Spatial Data Acquisition

Sufficiently powerful quantum dot laser light may have the potential for serving as a very powerful tool in the acquisition of nanomedical spatial data in vivo. Quantum dots (Ø 3–60 nm) are very efficient light transmitters that might provide enough photonic energy to reach the endothelial wall of vascular or lymphatic vessels and reflect back to a photomultiplying sensor to convey highly accurate distance measurement information.

In biosystems, a single photon of red light at $\lambda = 700$ nm has energy of 280 zJ, blue photon at $\lambda = 500$ nm has 500 zJ, and ultraviolet at $\lambda = 200$ nm has 1000 zJ. These energies may be detected by an appropriate photosensitive nanosensor. The optical sensor need not be the size of a given wavelength as demonstrated by a 1 nm chlorophyll molecule, which has the capacity for absorbing 660 nm photons. A further example is provided by cyanine–quinone chromophore molecules (artificial bioelectronic entities) that are ~1 nm in size, which can detect optical photons of $\lambda = 580–630$ nm. They can also trigger and reset in 1–3 ps influenced by tunneling transit times linked with the redevelopment of zwitter-ionic (macromolecules with oppositely charged groups on its chain ends) states of inputs [31,41,42].

6.13 Brief Survey of Laser-Based Spatial Data Acquisition Technologies

A number of laser technologies are presented later, including several that are not presently utilized in the biomedical realm, to illustrate how a laser operates when employed as a spatial information-gathering device. Extrapolations may be made from these examples to possibly inspire methods by which in vivo spatial data may be captured and conveyed using lasing mechanisms based on these system concepts.

6.13.1 Light Detection and Ranging

A conventional laser system that is used for gathering topographic spatial data is called light detection and ranging (LIDAR) (Figure 6.4). It can be considered as the optical equivalent of radar and uses near-infrared laser light, which is completely safe for humans [43]. There are three types of LIDAR:

1. Range finders: Used to measure distances to a solid target.
2. Differential absorption LIDAR (DIAL): Used to measure chemical concentrations. It employs two different laser wavelengths. One wavelength is absorbed by the molecule of interest and the other is not. The intensity difference between the two return signals can be applied to ascertain the concentration of the molecular species under study.
3. Doppler LIDAR: Used to measure the velocity of a target. When the laser light hits a moving target, the wavelength of the reflected light changes minutely. If the target moves away from the LIDAR, the return light will have a longer wavelength "red shift," if coming toward the LIDAR it will exhibit a shorter wavelength "blue shift." It can be used to measure dust particles in the air, and hence, wind velocity [44].

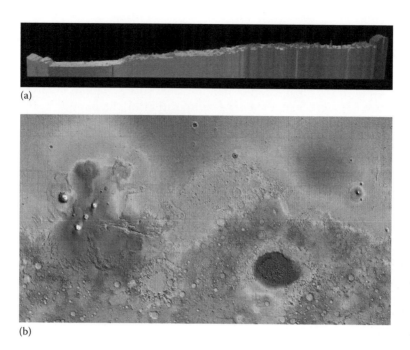

(a)

(b)

FIGURE 6.4
LIDAR images from Mars Orbiter Laser Altimeter (MOLA), onboard the Mars Global Surveyor (MGS) spacecraft [50]. (a) Cross section of Mars topography running from the North (left) to South poles. (b) Topographic map of the Martian surface. The instrument transmitted infrared laser pulses toward Mars at a rate of 10 Hz and measured the time of flight to determine the range of the MGS spacecraft to the Martian surface. It completed its mission of mapping the entire surface of Mars in 2001. (Images courtesy of the MOLA Science Team and NASA).

6.13.2 Laser Altimetry

Laser altimetry can rapidly generate accurate, dense, digital models of topography and vertical structure of a target surface. Two techniques that are in use are called "small footprint," which is time-of-flight laser altimetry, and "large footprint," which is a waveform-digitizing technique that can analyze a complete elevation profile at once [45].

6.13.3 Time-of-Flight LIDAR

The distance between the sensor and any reflective surface in the target area is calculated by measuring the time between the generation and return of each laser pulse (pulsing is accomplished by using a rotating mirror) [46]. It typically has a 1 m diameter sampling area, and records the distance to the first reflective surface it encounters. The laser ranges are combined with sensor position and orientation information (utilizing GPS) to generate a geo-referenced point cloud that is in effect a 3D representation of the scanned area [45].

6.13.4 Scanning LIDAR Imager of Canopies by Echo Recovery

An instrument called scanning LIDAR imager of canopies by echo recovery (SLICER) is used to capture entire waveforms. It does this by digitizing an entire height-varying return signal and generates a waveform that records the reflection of light from multiple height-varied elements in a 5–25 m diameter sampling area. Detailed information of the vertical structures within the footprint can be obtained, and can determine the ground surface beneath a very dense canopy [46]. Higher-density data can be obtained by achieving a higher laser repetition rate. This rate stands at about 50 kHz today, and expected to reach 100 kHz by 2005. NASA is developing waveform-digitizing sensors that have been tested in NASA's Laser Vegetation Imaging Sensor [47]. LIDAR systems were first deployed in space in 1971 when flown onboard Apollo missions 15–17. In 1994, an instrument called Lidar In-Space Technology Experiment (LITE) flew aboard the Space Shuttle Discovery, and there have since been many LIDAR-endowed space missions (Figure 6.4). Airborne LIDAR technology was first introduced commercially around 1995 and there are currently ~200 LIDAR systems in operation worldwide, with top-of-the-line systems providing 400,000 laser pulses per second. Leica Geosystems (Norcross, GE) has released a new 500 kHz pulse rate city-mapping LIDAR that is endowed with a "point density multiplier" technology that allows for the emission of half a billion points per second [48,49].

The Mars Orbiter Laser Altimeter (MOLA) flew onboard NASA's Mars Global Surveyor (MGS) spacecraft. The distance from the MGS to the surface of Mars was quantified by MOLA via the calculation of the time of flight of its emitted laser pulses. "The topographic height of the planet's surface at the laser footprint is then determined through the geometry of the planet radius, the spacecraft orbit altitude, and the pointing angle of the instrument [50]."

6.13.5 Laser-Induced Fluorescence and Near-Infrared Spectroscopy

Laser-induced fluorescence (LIF) has the capacity for differentiating between healthy and diseased tissue. It was demonstrated that fibrous and fatty heart tissue could be distinguished from healthy myocardium spectroscopically when these techniques were used in conjunction with a robust analysis method such as principal component analysis (PCA), which is a mathematical procedure for reducing a dataset and defining meaningful variables [51,52]. Noninvasive near-infrared spectroscopy (NIS) can be utilized in the determination of the chemical composition of coronary plaques [53,54] and allows for the sustained real-time quantification of localized oxygen saturation in tissues. More timely, rapid, and precise medical evaluations, as well as post-therapeutic observations, make NIS a potentially important tool for the improvement of patient outcomes [55].

6.14 Discussion of Nanomedical Laser-Based In Vivo Spatial Data Acquisition

If a laser-based spatial data acquisition system such as LIDAR could be extremely miniaturized to the micro- or nanoscale and applied to the biological realm, there would undoubtedly be formidable technical challenges involved in its realization. Not the least of these would be the development of the capability for generating and sustaining an appropriately robust signal such that it may propagate through turbid media (e.g., whole blood) and return back from a target of interest, such as a blood vessel wall. A quantum dot laser might provide the required photon stream to reach the target, and single-photon detectors may have the ability to sense incoming return signals. A critical prerequisite will include an in-depth investigation into the mechanism/kinetics of light scattering in human tissue (e.g., human blood and vascular walls) to gain a better understanding of the potential problems that may be involved with gathering in vivo spatial data in this manner.

6.14.1 Description of Laser Light/Photonic Absorption and Scattering in Tissue

Whole blood is problematic as relates to the measurement of optical properties due to its attribute of being a highly absorptive substance. It is important to discern how the microstructure of this dynamic multicomponent tissue influences light transmission in vivo and what the actual dimensions of these light dispersing entities might be. Results of experiments on typical human tissues have shown that the average scattering size is <0.5 μm, which is in the same dimensional range as cellular organelles. Red blood cells (RBCs), however, have no nucleus and hence the entire cell itself is the scattering medium. Blood cells are ~5 to 15 μm in diameter, making the scattering qualities of blood quite distinct from those of other tissue types [56].

Blood cell morphology plays a critical role as well. The biconcave shape of the RBC in the circulation generates a forward scattering profile that is quite distinct from spherical geometries [57]. Due to their discoid morphology and relatively large surface area, RBCs can form single file (rouleaux) configurations, thus giving rise to the generation of variable signals and imaging artifacts under different flow modes. Scattering is a very pronounced property of light interaction with tissues; therefore, an intimate grasp of photonic scattering mechanisms is essential toward the development of any laser-based in vivo nanomedical diagnostic modality. The optical characteristics of a tissue may be derived from time-resolved measurements of diffuse reflectance. Fitting a theoretical model to the data recorded does this, and a specific Monte Carlo (statistical simulation method) model has evolved for this purpose [56].

When we imagine a stream of photons traversing the blood, subsequently to being emanated from a quantum dot laser, individual photons will invariably cascade and scatter (seemingly chaotically) among resident RBCs and other blood constituents. However, it may be the case that by conducting repeated trials in order to study the detailed propagation of laser light through the blood at various flow rates within different vascular vessel diameters, a discernable profile or scattering signature may emerge. Although quite random due to nonlinear scattering, a certain percentage of photons may indeed manage to impact the endothelial walls and reflect back to interrogating nanodevices such as the VCSN. It seems plausible that an algorithm may be gleaned from this information and applied to the interpretation of reflected photonic spatial data, whereby the whole blood component scattering signatures or "noise," now specifically defined, might be identified and deleted from the dataset. What remains may contain useful target-hit "signals" from which to construct very specific spatial data coordinate maps of particular slices of vascular/lymphatic/gastrointestinal entities of interest. Perhaps patterns of photons that are reflected back from vascular vessel walls (comprising tessellated endothelial cells and the intracellular matrix that holds them together) might be fitted to depict specific profiles, imparting further physiological information via the interpretation of parameters encompassing wavelength, spectrographic signatures, or return-photon intensity ratios.

Another method of tissue characterization might entail the use of harmonically modulated light sources, rather than short pulses, to take measurements. Experiments have been conducted with diffuse reflection measurements at several wavelengths and modulated frequencies up to 1 GHz. Fitting a diffusion model to the recorded data had the capacity for revealing an optical profile [58]. Blood cells moving inside tissues generate Doppler shifts that may be measured via the analysis of frequency components of diffuse and scattered laser light with higher resolution. This is known as the laser Doppler perfusion imaging system, and it has been utilized in the determination of vascular damage from photodynamic therapy [59].

Lasers can generate monochromatic and nonionizing light that may be absorbed by and targeted to specific biomolecules, and can be focused to different spot sizes for specific areas. When considering nanomedical lasers as future imaging modalities, light/tissue interactions must be nondestructive, in that they must not induce any form of damaging chemical or thermal reactions. Useful features for laser-based tissue diagnostics are scattering and reemission. By studying wavelengths associated with scattered and reemitted light, as well as temporal and spatial/angular distributions, information (albeit indirect) might be derived from multiple scattering events in tissues. These data may facilitate distinguishing between essential and characteristic tissue-resident molecules, define average cell size, and elucidate the existence of domains embedded within the tissue that have optically divergent properties. Methods of tissue characterization include resonant light absorption coupled with reemission, LIF, and nonresonant inelastic scattering (e.g., diffuse reflection spectroscopy, absorption spectroscopy, time-resolved transmittance, or reflectance spectroscopy) [51] (Chapter 6). Optimal light/tissue interaction data may be acquired by defining the appropriate parameters such as light intensity, irradiation, geometry, wavelength, exposure time, and pulsed or continuous signals. The average transport of photons, along with their energy through a turbid aqueous medium, can be mathematically derived by the radiative transport equation [60,61]. This formula weighs the energy balance of incoming, outgoing, absorbed, and emitted photons of a very small volume of the sample medium. The tissue characterized is that of a homogeneous matrix, having randomly distributed absorption and scattering centers [51,61,62].

A photon in tissue has an average ~5 mm path length prior to absorption, ~0.04 mm between two scattering events, and generally exhibits forward directed scattering [63–65]. When the focus is on spatial light distribution and the target is complex tissue geometry, then a probabilistic method that is based on the Monte Carlo concept has the minimal quantity of restrictions in regard to optical properties, detection geometries, and illumination [66–69]. Monte Carlo simulations are required for detailed information of the spatial distribution of light flux in tissue with a complex geometry, having high accuracy [51]. Tissue is not a homogeneous material, but rather it is infused with many random elements. A spatial dependence on permittivity (proportion existing between electrical displacement and electric field intensity) exists. In atmospheric optics, dual values are implemented, including an average value coupled with a random component. The refractive index of tissue is variable due to the morphology of the targeted area. To find geometrical solutions, boundary conditions based on electromagnetic fields within a cell and scattering fields outside the cell must be defined. Electrical and magnetic surface currents may facilitate the expression of boundary conditions for a cell or particle [51].

6.14.2 Nanomedical Laser Safety

The potential for the conveyance of detrimental thermal or photonic effects that might be induced by quantum laser-based nanomedical imaging procedures to the patient will constitute imperative issues to investigate and resolve. Rigorous testing should be undertaken to verify that no degradation or instigation of unanticipated biological activity is imparted by their use. An important facet of investigation will entail the quantification of an optimal frequency/wavelength range that might be appropriate for this advanced diagnostic application. The identification of specific tissue and cellular tolerances for laser light, and pulse durations thereof, would serve to facilitate the development of safe operating parameters.

6.15 Potential Concepts for VCSN Spatial Data Acquisition Component

Described later are a number of conceptual nanomedical spatial data acquisition mechanisms for prospective nanodevices in the same functional class as the exemplar VCSN, which may have the ability to obtain high-resolution 3D scanning data for the imaging of human vascular, lymphatic, and gastrointestinal systems.

6.15.1 Spatial Data Acquisition Design Concept #1

What follows is a proposed conceptual hybrid design that would integrate nanotubes or nanowires in conjunction with two additional functional components working in unison. To encapsulate, this spatial data acquisition component subunit would generate ultrasonic pulses via an ultrathin piezoelectric membrane, in the 0.75–3.0 MHz range, reflect from the target (e.g., endothelial wall), and return as an echo to generate a detectable voltage when the membrane is again mechanically deformed, this time by the reflective incoming pressure wave (Figure 6.5).

The configuration of individual, albeit interconnected units embedded within an array of identical counterparts would consist of nanotubes/nanowires that are positioned directly beneath nanometric capacitive ultrasonic transducers, while being adhered to a conductive plate. When electrically actuated, the membrane surface would emit a pulsed ultrasonic wave. The nanoscale ultrasonic transducer might be based on similar principles as the CMUT [5,9], and would serve as the primary functional spatial data acquisition component.

Following is a hypothetical determination of the population of scanning units that might be required to enable the scanning capabilities of the VCSN. The circumference

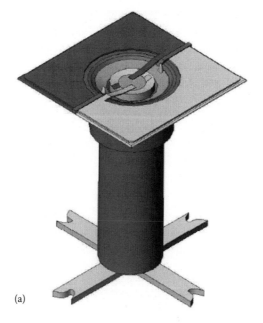

(a)

FIGURE 6.5
Artistic rendering of embedded multiwalled carbon nanotube field emission units for the activation of nanoscale capacitive ultrasonic transducers for spatial data acquisition. (a) Individual modular unit.

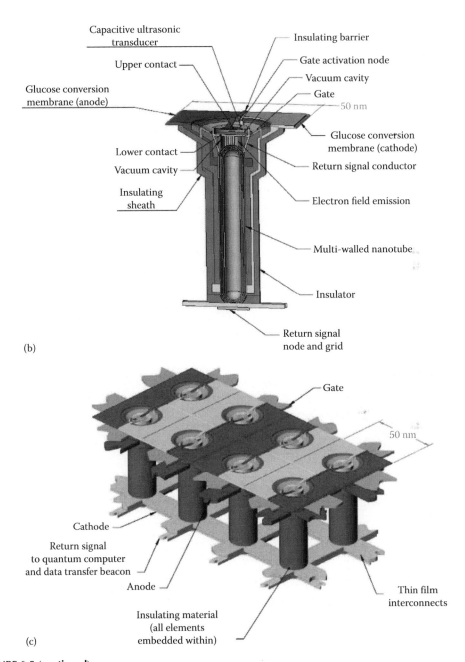

FIGURE 6.5 (continued)
Artistic rendering of embedded multiwalled carbon nanotube field emission units for the activation of nanoscale capacitive ultrasonic transducers for spatial data acquisition. (b) Cross section of individual unit. (c) Potential scanning array configuration.

of a ~1 μm in diameter VCSN device is Ø ~1000 nm × π = 3140 nm. The arrayed sensing area comprises a ~200 nm wide band that circumscribes the perimeter of the nanodevice. This raised scanning band houses tessellated arrays of transducer cells (described later). These abutted hexagonal scanning cells might measure ~10 nm linearly, which gives ~314 cells per row that extend around the girth of the VCSN. The cell size, as mentioned earlier, will give a width of ~20 rows, to fill the ~200 nm wide scanning band for a total of ~6280 cells. This figure is speculative and may vary (e.g., in practice a far reduced concentration of cells may be required) in accordance with the results of per cell resolution parameter trials and the design of interconnects that may have the capacity for single voxel return signal-current differentiation.

In regard to the shrinking dimensions of CMUT transducer cells, a 2003 study by Hutchins et al. discussed lateral dimensions of hexagonal micromachined CMUTs that ranged from ~25 to 100 μm [70]. In a 2011 work, Khuri-Yakub and coworkers revealed the achievement of a 40 nm gap height (between the base of the cell and the resonating membrane) and ~12 to 40 μm plate diameters [71].

A further advance by Khuri-Yakub and coworkers in 2012 described the first in vivo testing of a 24 CMUT forward looking transducer cell array, which enabled an imaging/ablation catheter to provide high-resolution 2D imagery at >8 MHz with a 30 mm imaging depth penetration [72]. This development is indeed prescient, in that further advances may be anticipated that will further enhance and miniaturize CMUT technologies to the point (in ~10 to 15 years) that they may be translated to the nanomedical domain and integrated into sophisticated diagnostic and therapeutic nanodevices.

The current design would incorporate a conductive surface that surrounds the capacitive ultrasonic transducer. This area (perhaps a nanoporous, ultrathin film membrane separated by a vertical insulating divider that is thick enough to prevent tunneling) may act as the glucose-catalyzing electrode, coated with the appropriate enzymes (e.g., glucose oxidase). The conductive membrane could incorporate protruding nano-fibers/tubes into its design to serve as coupling interconnects with enzyme channels in order to interface with, and be "wired" to their reaction centers so as to produce current. Freitas has suggested a maximum current density of ~1000 pW for 1 μm^3 nanomedical devices [31].

The harvested current may be transferred via conductive nanowires through an insulating (perhaps vacuum-sealed) sheath that encases a multiwalled nanotube, which terminates within electrode layers that mechanically support it. These electrodes would send current along the length of the nanotube, from bottom (cathode) to top (anode), hypothetically inducing a field emission state (cold cathode), and in turn activating the ultrasonic transducer. The viability and workable parameters of these functions would necessitate verification via stringent investigation. As various localized environmental and materials-based factors are likely to influence current flow along the nanotubes, this would be an important subject of inquiry.

In this scenario, individual emit/receive (E/R) units might draw energy from localized power sources, however, would be connected in parallel to evenly distribute current via the nesting of conductive membranes at the top portion of the module. The return signal layer would mechanically stabilize the nanotube at its lower tip, in addition to its function as a return signal conduit. There has been successful experimentation with gating nanotubes [73] and this concept may lead to strategies for the external control of the E/R units. It may be advantageous to provide a centralized power source/battery reservoir that is fueled by arrays of glucose electrodes, so as to feed power to all E/R units simultaneously via the nanotubes. This may serve to simplify the external control of signal initiation.

Of course, it will be desirable to have a major portion of the fabrication of this type of array conducted via self-assembly. Perhaps, a monolayer of pure nanotubes could be embedded within a thin film of insulating material at the appropriate location along its vertical axis. The orientation of this initial layer might allow for the subsequent, carefully designed layer-by-layer construction of conductive, semiconductive, and insulating materials to be added as required, to develop the local nanoelectronic infrastructure.

Ultrasonic signals that emanate from the E/R units would reflect from inner vascular walls, for example, and back to their source. This echo transit time would facilitate the calculation of distance through variations in the derived return signal, which may be directed through a dedicated return signal conductor through the length of the nanotube/nanowire, and into a return signal grid at the base of the nanotube. This grid would then guide the signal to the data transfer beacon (Section 6.19) and "outbody" to an external receiver/computer.

An additional significant issue, which will require investigation and experimental verification, are component/current matching configurations (e.g., particular components may have varying operational energy requirements to enable optimal operation), so as to ensure robust and sustained scanning operations. The surface area of the glucose electrode membranes, for example, should be optimized to generate sufficient current to initiate field emission in the embedded nanotubes. Field-emitted electrons will be required to deliver enough current to power the capacitive transducer so that it may in turn launch an ultrasonic pulse.

Glucose molecule attachment and dissociation turnover values will also be a critical variable to quantify. Once glucose molecules bind with the enzymatically activated membrane/electrode and its catalyzed electrons are spent, a method of molecular ejection might be necessary in order to ensure that an appropriate amount of physical real estate is available for the next wave of "electron donors" to make solid contact.

6.15.2 Spatial Data Acquisition Design Concept #2

This concept derives from the possibility of using banks of quantum dot lasers embedded within a laminated thin film structure to act as a relatively intense and focused photon source. These quantum lasers may be powered by a glucose-catalyzing membrane electrode component, or by a range of other potential body power-harvesting mechanisms (Chapter 4). The core component enabling this spatial data acquisition entity would be a capacitive ultrasonic transducer, as referred to in concept #1. This particular transducer, however, would integrate walls that comprise nanophotovoltaic cell structures, which convert incoming photons into the current that is required to initiate device operation (Figure 6.6).

Consideration has been given to the idea of having the current generated by the glucose membrane electrode or other power-generating mechanisms, controllably conveyed directly to the component from the source of generation in order to circumvent the necessity of incorporating intermediate subcomponents that might be required to power the ultrasonic capacitive transducer. However, it might be advantageous to employ a condition by which there is a concentration of energy that accumulates at the gate junctions. Contingent on the type and thickness of the gate junction barrier material, higher queued voltages may be realized. This could conceivably enable the generation of more robust pulsed voltages when "current packets" are released by a specific gate triggering frequency and in turn create the possibility of emanating stronger acquisition signals.

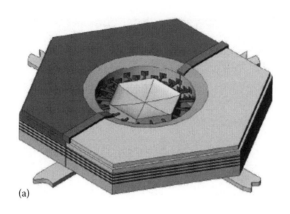

(a)

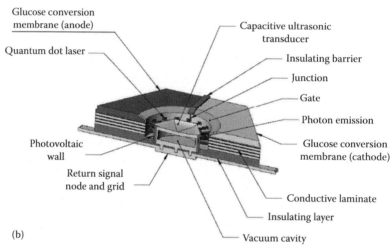

Glucose conversion
membrane (anode)

Capacitive ultrasonic
transducer

Quantum dot laser

Insulating barrier

Junction

Gate

Photon emission

Photovoltaic
wall

Glucose conversion
membrane (cathode)

Return signal
node and grid

Conductive laminate

Insulating layer

(b)

Vacuum cavity

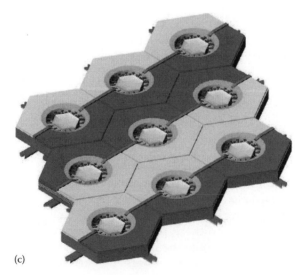

(c)

FIGURE 6.6
Artistic rendering of quantum dot laser activation of nanoscale capacitive ultrasonic transducers, with nanophotovoltaic walls for spatial data acquisition. (a) Individual modular unit. (b) Cross section of individual unit.
(c) Potential scanning array configuration.

This configuration may have some advantages such as a more direct current flow path by virtue of utilizing a more straightforward and compact linear thin film lamination design. This would also free up a substantial amount of real estate (always at a premium in the design of nanomedical devices) leaving space for the integration of additional components and capabilities. The pulsed ultrasonic signals that emanate from the ultrasonic capacitive transducer would have equivalent intensity along with an inherent "signal-out" signature or profile. This profile may be, thus, easily differentiated from (reflective ultrasonic) "signal-in" signatures, as these would most likely be weaker and staggered in intensity. These data might then be referenced and prorated against precalibrated baseline values.

6.15.3 Spatial Data Acquisition Design Concept #3

This concept would utilize an alternate type of ultrasonic wave propagation in the form of tightly nested FBARs. As described earlier, in contrast to the incorporation of vibrating membranes that are voltage responsive, the bulk material of these resonators undergoes expansion and retraction, thereby initiating ultrasonic emission. The FBARs might be fabricated as Ø ~5 nm cylindrical geometries via nanolithography. Should these entities be arrayed at 5–10 per row, and embedded and isolated somewhat (sufficiently to avoid crosstalk interference) within an insulating material, they would form a band that circumscribes the girth of the VCSN to comprise a compact 360° scanning component array (Figure 6.7).

To facilitate the differentiation of ultrasonic response echo signals (conveying high-resolution spatial coordinate data), subsequent rows of FBARs could contain elements with gradated lengths, which translate to predetermined variations in physical volumes, hence enabling distinctive response signatures per row. In addition, individual FBAR elements of each radial row might themselves be further sequentially length gradated. This arrangement would assign every individual FBAR element with its own unique response signature, thereby tagging each unit of distance that it measures as a spatial coordinate in 3D space, which could be correlated to a particular tracked VCSN spatial coordinate position and orientation for a given point in time (e.g., real-time positional feedback loops would monitor the exact locations and orientations of every VCSN in vivo, at microsecond refresh rates) (Chapter 3). This might enable the generation of very high (<~micrometers)-resolution in vivo topographic imagery.

6.15.4 Spatial Data Acquisition Design Concept #4

The modular configuration employed for this spatial data acquisition concept would entail the integration of a bowtie laser that is adhered to an appropriately electronically contacted substrate. The bowtie laser would have a stadium-shaped geometry, working on the principal of a whispering gallery mode diffusion of photons, in the form of laser emission through its mass. When charged, it would evolve four primary emission sites between its *x*- and *y*-axes. The idea here would be to harness these four emission sites to project streams of photons toward the photovoltaic walls (described earlier) of four strategically placed capacitive ultrasonic transducers (Figure 6.8).

Photonic conversion to electron flow within the photovoltaic walls would provide the electronic pulse required by the transducers to launch ultrasonic pulses to the target. The return signal would vibrate the transducer membrane, thereby generating a

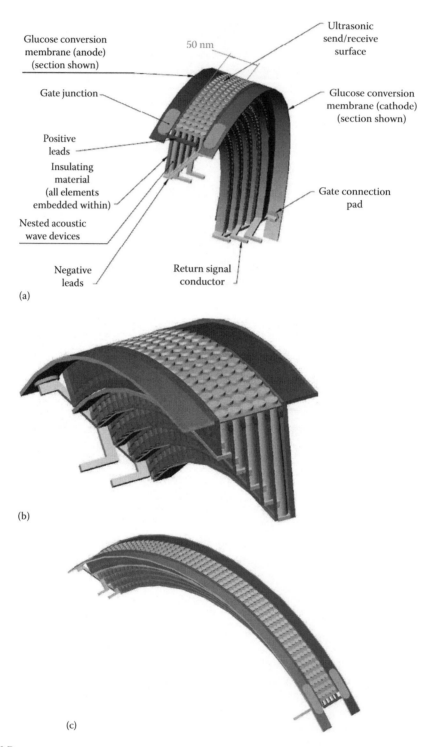

FIGURE 6.7
Artistic rendering of nested cylindrical FBAR elements with sequential gradated lengths for spatial data acquisition: (a) depiction of underside of quadrant, (b, c) alternate views of quadrant.

current and transiting downward through the structure to convey its return signal current through contacts at the base of the transducer. These interconnected contacts would be tethered to the data transfer beacon, which would transmit the acquired spatial data to a pixel matrix display system (Chapter 1). The cavity that houses the bowtie laser and transducers might be vacuum-sealed and protected by an ultrathin, albeit highly resilient top cover to facilitate efficient laser operation. This cover may comprise diamondoid or sapphire nanomaterials due to their inherent rigidity and relative biological inertness when they are immersed within the aqueous environment of human blood. It will be prudent, however, to investigate and verify whether the exposure of these materials to continual ultrasonic traversal will impart degradative effects over time.

Individual units of the quad-transducer package, along with the bowtie laser-activating component, might be powered by one of the various possible energy-harvesting mechanisms explored earlier (Chapter 4). These modular units might have dimensions of

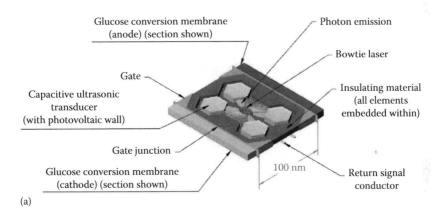

(a)

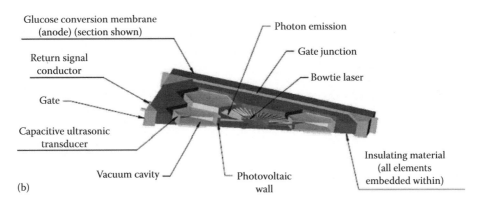

(b)

FIGURE 6.8
Artistic rendering of core bowtie laser activation of four surrounding nanoscale capacitive ultrasonic transducers, containing nanophotovoltaic walls for spatial data acquisition. (a) Individual modular unit, (b) cross section of individual unit.

(continued)

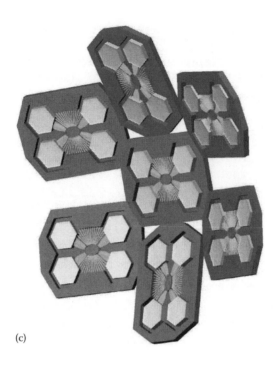

(c)

FIGURE 6.8 (continued)
Artistic rendering of core bowtie laser activation of four surrounding nanoscale capacitive ultrasonic transducers, containing nanophotovoltaic walls for spatial data acquisition. (c) potential scanning array configuration.

~100 nm, which would be joined in parallel to laterally span the 200 nm wide scanning band that circumscribes the VCSN.

6.15.5 Spatial Data Acquisition Design Concept #5

This concept would integrate the FBAR technology (described earlier) as well, however, in a different configuration. Leads attached to both top and bottom (on opposite ends) would convey current to rectangular thin film FBAR strips. These strips, separated by thin insulating materials to isolate them, would form the ~200 nm wide scanning band that circumscribes the VCSN, which will emit ultrasonic pulses when activated (Figure 6.9). Target reflected ultrasonic pulses would return to the FBAR surfaces, thereby distorting them mechanically and generating a detectable voltage, which would transit through conductive nanowires embedded within the base of each FBAR element (for data differentiation) and leading to the data transfer beacon.

6.15.6 Spatial Data Acquisition Design Concept #6

This concept would utilize either embedded permanent magnetic nanoparticles (e.g., neodymium [$Nd_2Fe_{14}B$]) or magnetic fields that are produced by a current being passed through metallic nanocoils, which are wrapped around nested ferromagnetic cylinders (Figure 6.10). Although these nanoparticles or nanocoils would be isolated entities, they would serve as constituents of an array, and thus would be appropriately shielded from their neighboring counterparts. The nanocoils themselves would not be separate entities, but rather would be fabricated in situ. This might be accomplished by applying a thin film of the desired conductive material to the external surfaces of bundled nanoscale ferromagnetic cylinders via masked Molecular Beam Epitaxy (ordered single crystal deposition technique).

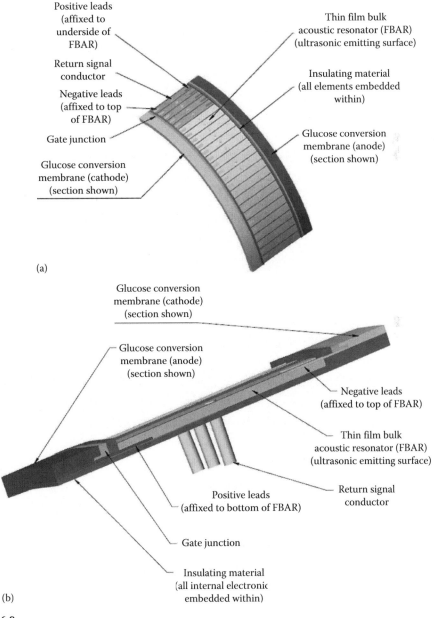

(a)

(b)

FIGURE 6.9
Artistic rendering of alternate FBAR strip array of scanning elements for spatial data acquisition. (a) Top isometric view of quadrant. (b) Cross section of FBAR strip element.

(*continued*)

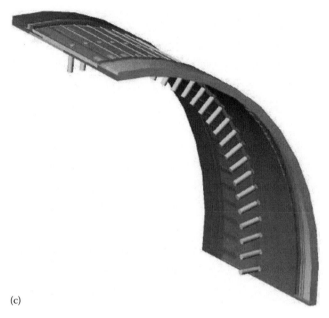

(c)

FIGURE 6.9 (continued)
Artistic rendering of alternate FBAR strip array of scanning elements for spatial data acquisition. (c) Underside isometric view of quadrant.

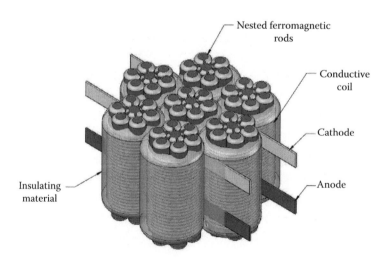

FIGURE 6.10
Artistic rendering of nanoscale ferromagnetic bundled rods with externally etched nanocoils that may serve as nanoelectromagnets to potentially induce low-level proton precession for spatial data acquisition.

As relates to the potential fabrication of the nanocoil subassemblies, a laser of appropriate frequency might be mounted to a very precise positioning stage. The laser would advance along the length of the nested cylinders (individual subassemblies might be held in place by a magnetic field and caused to rotate by a separate laser) and scribe the previously applied conductive film through to the surface of the nested cylinder material, resulting in a helical pattern. This may be analogous to the bundled cylinders being encased by a coil of conductive material through which current can travel and possibly creating a nanoscale electromagnet. When the system is completely assembled, linear thin film anode and cathode strips would be contacted with the upper and lower regions of the coils to be subsequently embedded within an insulating material to negate the possibility of shorting the system.

As an alternate strategy to the use nanocoil electromagnets, an appropriate species of robustly magnetic nanoparticles, possibly comprising neodymium iron boron ($Nd_2Fe_{14}B$) or samarium–cobalt (Sm-Co), may be encased within nested or laminated thin film layers to cumulatively function as modular magnetic units.

The premise of this concept is based on the hypothetical possibility that highly localized, low magnetic field strength induced precession events involving the proton spins of hydrogen atoms, which are embedded within the membranes of endothelial cells that tessellate the luminal walls of the entire vasculature (as well as lymphatic and gastrointestinal systems), might be initiated by nanocoil electromagnets or embedded aggregates of magnetically active neodymium iron boron or samarium cobalt nanoparticles.

In one configuration, a magnetic field would emanate from the VCSN to serve as an initial reference-axis magnetic field, motivating the precession and alignment of proton spins to assume a "spin-up" or "spin-down" state, or any increment toward the direction of "up" or "down" contingent on possible magnetic field strength. The effect envisaged here would be the production of a magnetic standing wave that radiates outward from the VCSN that is traversing the vascular pathways and creating a 360° ring of momentarily magnetically "misaligned" protons within the vessel walls of the vasculature. A continuous and rapidly pulsed RF signal of the appropriate strength and orientation, orthogonal to the VCSN emanated field, might be launched externally, either from an adhered patch that is affixed to the patient or from a stand-alone RF-emitting grid in relative position to the patient. Protons might be induced to "flip" and revert back to the aligned direction to emit a signal in the process that may be detected by the same RF device that generated the initial flip-inducing signal. Even slight angular variations in the precession of protons may provide sufficient signal integrity for the conveyance of precise spatial coordinate data with which to reconstruct a vascular topographic image.

Due to the intimate proximity of the magnetic sources within a nanomedical device to the vessel walls, it seems conceivable that even very low magnetic fields, in the nanotesla range, might be sufficient to induce a slight "deviation from ambient" proton spins that might be exploited to compile imaging data. The effects of ultralow magnetic fields on proton precession have been investigated. When exposed to a 100 μT magnetic field, the proton of a hydrogen atom requires ~10 s to relax to equilibrium from a Larmor frequency of 4 kHz, which is assisted primarily by thermal oscillations. Under a 100 μT magnetic field, the proton relaxation time is reduced to ~7.5 s and the Larmor frequency is correspondingly decreased to ~400 Hz. At a field strength of >~1 μT, the Larmor frequency was found to be only a few hertz, and further down, a very weakly polarized proton generates a magnetic field that resides in the several picotesla domain [74].

6.15.7 Spatial Data Acquisition Design Concept #7

This concept integrates a module that consists of vertical cavity surface-emitting lasers, which are nested in close proximity to an ultrasensitive photon detection/multiplier

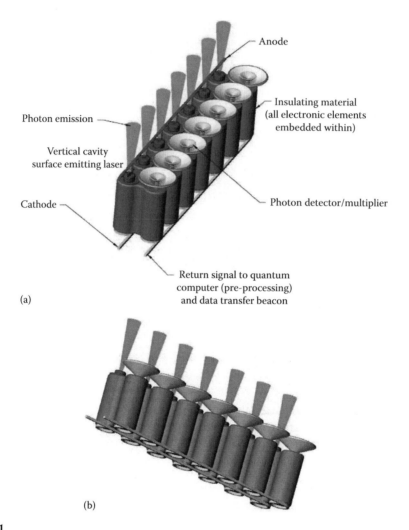

FIGURE 6.11

Artistic rendering of vertical cavity surface-emitting lasers working in conjunction with ultrasensitive photon detection/multiplier elements. (a) Top isometric view depicting modular paired units and (b) underside isometric view depicting electronic coupling of paired units.

device (Figure 6.11). This system would be derived from a LIDAR-type strategy in the gathering of spatial data coordinates. The emanating laser pulses would be extremely rapid in order to facilitate full coverage of targeted areas while in transit. Although a certain percentage of the photonic stream would be lost to scattering and absorption by whole blood elements, there may be an adequate volume of photons that reach the endothelial wall and reflect back to the photon detector/multiplier. These returning photons might be translated into a variable current that may be deciphered to infer distances that are traversed at given points and times.

The VCSN itself would be constantly tracked and clocked as relates to its precise location and orientation in 3D space. These data would serve as positional reference coordinates against which the emitted and received signal positions could be tabulated.

Studies of the biological effects of quantum dot lasing in vivo will be an important topic for investigation. The wavelengths employed will most likely be in the near-infrared region of the spectrum.

6.16 VCSN Communications and Data Transfer Beacon

The communications and data transfer component will serve as the primary link between individual VCSN entities (allowing for communicative exchange between devices) and "outbody" computers. This component will be designed to convey all preprocessed spatial data that are stored in the onboard quantum computer to the Pixel Matrix software, which is housed in external computers. It will also seamlessly communicate with the NanoNav system (Chapter 3) from the onset of the scanning procedure. This link will ensure the transferral of real-time accurate bearings and orientation for the VCSN while it is engaged in scanning/imaging procedures in vivo. Of equivalent importance will be internalized nanomedical device communications that will allocate, convey, execute, and verify myriad externally issued commands.

The data transfer component might be designed to incorporate nanometric entities that exhibit the capability for acting as nanoscale antennae for reliable transmission of commands and acquired spatial data. The data transfer beacon itself may be configured in a concave geometry to serve as a nanoscale "dish" that assigns incoming signals to specific focal points, thereby potentially intensifying received signals. This strategy may also function in reverse, as an array of antennae would transmit data streams to a single convergent output signal of sufficient intensity to reach outbody receivers. In addition to receiving commands and conveying spatial data, the data transfer beacon may also transmit acquired physiological spectrographic information, perhaps carried on a dedicated frequency so as to isolate and ensure data stream integrity.

The VCSN might integrate four data transfer beacons—two on the bow and stern of the upper deck, and two on the bow and stern of the lower deck—to provide an enhanced surface area for the reception of incoming and the transmittal of outgoing signals. While multiple VCSN devices (perhaps administered as a complement of thousands to reduce scanning times) are traversing through vessels at various locations throughout the human body, inter-nanodevice and external communications are likely to be very rapid. Outbody transmitters and receivers would have the signal conveyance capacity to transmit and receive data from within a full 360° spherical coverage envelope, which has the patient at its core. In some instances, the four VCSN data transfer beacons may simultaneously transmit identical data to potentially amplify the signal. Alternatively, as alluded to earlier, the data may be subdivided by dedicating particular beacon segments for the transmission of specific types of information (e.g., inter-nanodevice communications, incoming operational commands, outgoing command acknowledgement and task verification messages, conveyance of spectral data, and spatial data transmission).

All communications would be highly encrypted to ensure security and conducted under external computer control by an attending physician. Onboard VCSN quantum computers would play a secondary and complementary role in communication tasks by overseeing inter-VCSN communications and "self-speak" internal communications. All VCSN data transmissions would be monitored and recorded at all times, primarily for patient-specific archiving, but also to serve as a reference archive of the exact sequence of events should there be some type of error or deviation during the scanning procedure.

6.17 Molecular Communications Theory

Successful nanomedical communications will require multiple elements that function seamlessly as a system. Shannon defines a communication system as comprising five elements:

1. An *information source* that generates a message for conveyance to the receiver
2. A *transmitter* that translates the message into some form of signal that makes it amenable for transfer
3. A *channel* that will serve as the conveyance conduit for delivering the message via the signal
4. A *receiver* that obtains the signal and reconstructs it to convey the message
5. A *destination* is the entity to which the message is intended [75]

The signal is comprises a series of symbols that convey an average quantity of information, measured in bits or symbols [75]. A receiver is a device whose state is established by an external signal, and a particular amount of signal power (in J/s) is necessary to differentiate the signals from each other in the presence of thermal noise (also in J/s). One cannot send information at a rate faster than the channel capacity. If attempted, a measure of noise will be received that limits the rate to the value of the channel capacity. If the transmission is less than or equal to the channel capacity, it follows that information conveyance is possible with a controllable error rate [76].

Criteria for molecular communications include that signals must be meticulously encoded before the transmission of information and then carefully decoded upon reception. Although both of these steps require delays, the overall transmission may approach channel capacity levels, or in the case of molecular machines, the "machine capacity." Encoding and decoding a communication signal requires a memory element to record signals as they are being processed. A time-encoded message might be received, recorded, and processed by a complex of simple molecular machines and a molecular receiver may decode a message [76].

6.18 Photonic Antennae

A visible light antenna, analogous to the antennae that receive radio waves, has been fashioned from CNTs. When the size of a radio antenna is equal to or is fractional with respect to the incoming wavelength, the RF wave will excite electrons into usable currents. This is a much more difficult task when dealing with optical wavelengths at hundreds of nanometers. This antenna effect has been observed by Wang et al., utilizing an array of CNTs where the incoming light excited microelectrical currents. Precise measurement of this current will require nanodiodes that can process electrical pulses at optical frequencies (1015 Hz). The nanotubes involved were ~50 nm in diameter with several hundred nanometers long. Exhibiting the behavior of dipole radio antennas, nanotubes have the capacity for responding to light. Interestingly, they also have a polarizing effect as the response will vanish if incoming light is polarized at right angles in relation to the orientation of the nanotube [77].

To optimize the antenna effect, the nanotube length should be close to the multiple of a half wavelength; although, it would still function at quarter wavelengths if a metallic ground was implemented. It is apparently possible to activate nanotubes under the infrared frequency. However, longer tubes would be necessary to compensate for the longer wavelength as compared to visible light. Wavelengths of 1.2–1.5 μm are commonly employed in contemporary communication systems [78] and for wireless applications the visible to near-infrared optical range wavelengths are utilized [79].

A high-performance nanometric semiconducting germanium (Ge) nanowire antenna has been developed as a tunable photodetector that operates within the optical communication band at near-infrared wavelengths (e.g., 1550 nm). Cao et al. synthesized the Ge nanowire antenna via a chemical deposition process and added metallic electrical contacts "(2 nm of Ti/400 nm of Al and 5 nm of Cr/400 nm of Pt)" to either end of the Ø 250 nm × 1–2 μm long nanowires via e-beam lithography techniques. Significantly, the antenna photoresponse was improved by ~25-fold, enabling wavelength and polarization tunability. The device could also operate at high speeds (>100 GHz) while enabling ultralow dark currents (~20 pA) at a low power draw [80].

Conceivably, arrays of strategically integrated nanoantenna, as described earlier, that are "wired" into the VCSN might provide the required communication interface between the in vivo environment and outbody computer systems. Near-infrared light may be a prudent choice for transmission signals as it can safely travel through human tissues and has been observed, in one study, to achieve tissue penetration depths of ~23 cm, or ~9 in. at 630–800 nm wavelengths [81].

6.19 Data Transfer Beacon

The entire surface area of the VCSN data transfer beacon might consist of a tessellated configuration of isolated (via shielding) ultrathin film piezoresonators whose "tuned" constituents would oscillate only when initiated by specifically calibrated incoming frequencies from external command transmitters (Figure 6.12). These piezoresonators, once activated by a particular frequency, might in turn translate its unique oscillation into an explicit voltage value to trigger dedicated circuitry that is "hard-wired" for the execution of specific commands. In regard to VCSN data transmission, a convergence signal node may serve as a focal point for outbody signals from multiple resonators to transmit data by means of an enhanced amplified primary signal.

A low-cost, flexible, highly integrated, and low-voltage (±3.3 V) reconfigurable piezoelectric array was developed by Triger et al. that incorporated multiple tessellated elements that were used to construct 2D arrays with different geometries, enabling 3D beam forming on a single modular platform. Each "tile" housed 16 piezotransmission and reception channels, where each channel was integrated with its own adjustable preamplifier. One of the goals of this work was to realize the close coupling of transducers and electronics,

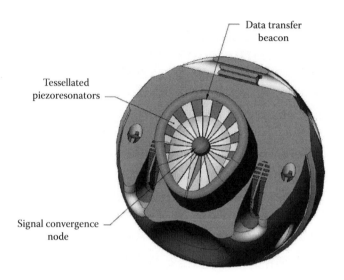

FIGURE 6.12
Artistic rendering of cutaway section of VCSN data transfer beacon comprising specifically tuned tessellated thin film piezoelectric resonators.

which filled a footprint of 16 × 16 mm. An advantage of this system in comparison to CMUT arrays is that the dead space between active transducer elements can be significantly decreased [82].

6.20 Proposed Research Tasking List: VCSN Spatial Data Acquisition Component/Communications and Data Transfer Component

Following is a list of preliminary suggestions, considerations, and relevant questions as relates to perceived areas of investigation for the exemplar VCSN spatial data acquisition component.

6.20.1 Spatial Data Acquisition Component

1. Develop a technical database for capacitive ultrasonic transducers, FBARs, single crystal zinc oxide nanosprings, and other piezoelectronic technologies that might potentially be fabricated and functionalized as a nanoscale in vivo spatial data acquisition component.

2. Design conceptual layouts for each of the proposed methods for these perceived technologies.

3. Investigate the specific physics of each proposed technology to discern which one might be best suited for the task as a nanoscale in vivo spatial data acquisition component.

4. Source the appropriate materials/composites (e.g., must be biocompatible and chemically inert) and design potentially optimal configurations for the selected technology.

5. Estimate ultrasonic distance ranges, target-hit dimensional specificity, and return signal integrity/resolution for each of the selected technologies, initially working with microscale entities with aim of eventual scale down to nanoscale levels.

6. Investigate and identify the best potential methods and geometries for generating ultrasonic signals at the nanoscale that might be applied to in vivo spatial data acquisition.

7. Source an engineering design software program best suited for investigative simulations for this task. Model all conceptual mechanisms to be used in investigations that will reflect inherent molecular kinetics as well.

8. Study various fabrication methods for the manufacture of nanoscale ultrasonic generating entities and select best of these for each technology.

9. Investigate a method for creating the vacuum cavity required for a capacitive ultrasonic transducer at the nanoscale.

10. Determine the minimal vacuum cavity possible that will allow for proper functionality of the flexing membrane for a nanometric capacitive ultrasonic transducer.

11. Develop concepts/designs for nanoelectronic interfaces with the energy-harvesting component, as well as electrical contact/signal conveyance strategies for the nanometric capacitive ultrasonic transducer.

12. Investigate various mechanisms/signals for the activation and termination of signal generation and retrieval for the spatial data acquisition component.

13. Investigate the specific physics of how ultrasonic signals of varying frequencies emanating from a single unit and from nested arrays of piezotransducer units will behave when immersed within the in vivo whole blood environment.

14. Determine the optimum ultrasonic signal frequency and strength required to obtain ultrahigh-resolution spatial data from the in vivo environment.

15. Explore ultrasonic signal propagation parameters and profiles when it transits through whole blood constituents, and reflects back from the vascular endothelial wall (e.g., initial ultrasonic signal strength required for this task, percentage of signal scattering and loss, return signal integrity, resolution, return signal interpretation and translation via algorithms into digital spatial data display format).

16. Investigate the possible utilization of secondary ultrasonic signal echoes that might be differentiated and isolated from primary return signal data sets, to be employed for discerning vessel wall thickness and external surface profiles of vascular, lymphatic, and gastrointestinal entities.

17. Explore biocompatibility and chemical stability issues related to the installation and operation of a nanoscale ultrasonic element array. Will the ultrasonic signal propagating surface require coating with a biocompatible polymer? What effect will pulsed ultrasonic emissions have on this coating? Will such a coating mechanically degrade via vibration over a certain time line?

18. Single crystal zinc oxide nanosprings [83] may have the potential to serve as very sensitive piezoelectric transducers (dimensions of ~500 to 800 nm with ribbons ~10 to 60 nm wide and ~5 to 20 nm thick). Investigate the spatial data acquisition potential of these entities in terms of their capability for emanating and receiving ultrasonic signals. May one distinguish a voltage differential when an ultrasonic

burst is launched, and reflected back from a target surface? Can correlated values be established between return voltage intensity and the distance from a target?

19. Investigate the principals governing electrolocation in *Apteronotus albifrons* (black ghost knife fish) [84] to gather any insights that may be applied to the development of biomimetically inspired neural-like mechanisms. These studies might also offer potential elucidation into spatial information-gathering principles regarding data manipulation involved with the acquisition of such information.

20. The body of *A. albifrons* is studded with ~15,000 dedicated tube-shaped receptor organs. Study the physiological kinetics and specific geometries of these organs with an aim to the possible development of biomimetic designs and fabrication techniques for the manufacture of nested, modular spatial data acquisition units.

21. Conduct studies into the physiological and molecular functional aspects of arthropod ommatidia (individual visual receptor units) [85] and the compound eye as an entire mechanism to elucidate optical organization, photon flows patterns and rates, acquired spatial data distribution and conveyance systems, and image construction modalities. How might this knowledge apply to and possibly enhance the design and fabrication of a nanoscale spatial data acquisition component and to perhaps inspire element-nesting configurations thereof?

22. Investigate the principals of echolocation inherent in dolphin and bat species with the goal of their potential extrapolated application for the development of possible nanoscale analogous constructs of these spatial information systems.

23. Utilize known molecular physiology and functionality of rod and cone structures in the human retina to elucidate and possibly develop a template/model for simulation studies to investigate how photons are manipulated, translated, dispersed to and along the optic nerves of the visual system. Attempt to biomimetically emulate constituent components of these systems and inherent mechanisms (e.g., photonic conveyance, image reconstruction, signal processing modalities, geometric nesting configurations) for possible application to the creation of designs for analogous nanoscale spatial data acquisition entities.

24. Determine whether quantum dots might be fused to the open ends of a CNT (either SWNT or MWNT) [86] and be activated by nanotube field emission to possibly initiate lasing. If this might be accomplished, then quantum dots having various dimensions (therefore, emitting photons at varying optical frequencies) might be used to assist in spectroscopic determinations. It might be far more efficient (from a component design perspective) to potentially integrate a nanospectrometer to work in conjunction with the spatial data acquisition component, whose data may be intertwined with the spatial data signal.

6.20.2 Communications and Data Transfer Component

1. Systematically investigate what materials and potential subcomponents might be utilized to construct a nanoscale communication node.

2. Explore whether singular or differently arrayed banks of nanotubes might be used to send and receive optical signals (ideally in the near-infrared frequency range) for possible translation into electronic/communication signals. Determine the optimum nanotube length and specific frequency that might impart the most robust and stable signal transfer.

3. From the earlier results, investigate whether this signal might (in a preliminary experimental setup) propagate through engineered tissues and aqueous environments, analogous to the whole blood. What effects will these materials have on signal efficiency?

4. Develop and construct an experimental mock-up whereby a single nanotube or array of nanotubes (test both SWNT and MWNT) might be induced to receive a signal (e.g., external source computer command) and respond in a manner that would indicate that the message was indeed received and the information embedded therein was correctly translated.

5. Investigate methods by which transmitted/translated information might be monitored within such a mock-up to verify appropriate and robust signal propagation and intact message integrity post-transmission.

6. Explore various signal modes (e.g., photonic, ultrasonic, RF) to quantify which species of signal will exhibit the potential capacity for conveying large amounts of data safely and effectively from an in vivo location to "outbody" and vice versa.

7. Develop a means for testing whether selected signal modes might be utilized to robustly convey data to a range of nanoscale entities (e.g., nanotubes, nanowires, piezoentities, quantum entities).

8. Systematically explore the full range of fullerenes (e.g., C_{60}, C_{70}, C_{80}, nanotubes, nanohorns, nanotorus, nano-onions) to determine whether they might have the capability of receiving and sending communication signals.

9. Determine if ultrathin films made of C_{60} might be configured in such a way that the electrons that populate their exterior surfaces might be excited by a particular incoming signal (verify efficacy of the full range of candidate signals) giving rise to the potentiality for sending and receiving encoded information laden signals.

10. Discover if there might be a technique to enable the oscillation of quantum dots in such a way as to enable their receptivity for an information-embedded signal.

11. Study, model, and simulate prospective data flow rates, times, and capacities to elucidate what communication links might be possible from the interior of the human body to external computers.

12. Investigate potential nanoscale mechanism variants for use in exploratory operation simulations of envisaged in vivo communication send/receive concepts, signal species, and various candidates for external broadcast and reception antennae.

13. Investigate and simulate problems that might be encountered during transmission and reception processes to a mobile in vivo entity while in transit through the human vasculature.

14. Explore whether there might be a method for "locking on" to a fiducial embedded into the external surface of a roving in vivo nanoscale entity that would ensure uninterrupted tracking of the device, coupled with "com-signal" source identification.

15. Incoming signals may excite electrons in the nanotubes to the point where a level of field emission may be activated. A portion of the field-emitted electrons may be transferred to the quantum dot, affecting it electronically. This even subtle change might be measured externally and would indicate that the signal has indeed been transferred. Iterative and varied test-signal transmissions might be correlated with concurrent changes observed in the quantum dot electronic profile to verify the precise degree of signal reception.

16. Investigate whether there might be a means of linking the lock-on capability to the communication signal.

17. Explore the problem of, and devise strategies for how nanodevice communication signals (e.g., commands from external sources) and acquired spatial data, along with spectral data, might be transmitted from a multitude (perhaps thousands) of VCSN units that are simultaneously traversing the human vasculature and be subsequently and coherently received externally.

18. Develop a communication organizational model (algorithms) of how one might identify and convey specific signals to perhaps thousands of in vivo nanomedical devices.

19. Might it be more efficient to command the VCSN to transmit spatial data at regular intervals rather than emanating real-time streams of acquired data while "on the fly" through the vasculature?

20. Quantify what the maximum amount of data is which might be temporarily stored within an onboard quantum computer prior to a data stream launch.

21. Investigate and design several different conceptual configurations for a nanometric communication node for integration into the VCSN.

22. What might the signal-reactive entities residing within the VCSN communication beacon consist of? Should the VCSN tracking fiducial be integrated into the communication beacon itself?

23. What amount of energy might be required to power the communication node and what nanoelectronic connections would be appropriate? Should the beacon be shielded from the other VCSN components to ensure clean signal conveyance?

24. Explore what level of signal-to-noise ratio may be achieved for a nanometric (estimated $\varnothing$ ~300 to 400 nm) communication beacon. How will this ratio translate and be affected by the presence of four identical beacons?

25. Model and run simulations employing selected nanometric antennae and potential information bearing signals to elucidate optimal signal-to-noise ratios for several antennae/signal combinations.

26. Investigate and catalog any potential com-signal distortions and/or artifacts that might be anticipated when attempting to convey a signal from within the human body to "outbody" receivers and vice versa.

27. What human physiological factors and processes might impact the integrity of "multi-location source" signals being transmitted to and from within the in vivo vasculature?

28. Explore whether it might make sense to demarcate the communication beacons themselves into dedicated domains (e.g., procedural scanning commands, spatial data conveyance, and navigation-related communications).

29. Might a single "global" form of com-signal encapsulate and convey both external computer commands to in vivo nanodevices and carry transmitted spatial/spectral data from the patient?

30. If so, how would the different aspects of these signals be classified and differentiated so as to translate them into the desired resultant form?

31. Investigate whether two different nanoscale entities (e.g., nanotubes, quantum dots) might be integrated into the same communication node mechanism, each responding differently to the same signal species. Might this arrangement facilitate the differentiation of conveyed signals?

32. Explore what protocols, testing mechanisms, and signal calibrations might be necessary as a prerequisite to the initiation of nanodevice (in vivo and outbody) communications?

33. Quantify the appropriate signal intensity and frequency required to robustly propagate a com-signal from in vivo, through aqueous environments and tissues of various densities to outbody that would ensure a smooth transfer of information while maintaining signal integrity, strength, and clarity.

34. Explore specific effects on a com-signal when propagating through tissues that have variable densities (e.g., a VCSN-emitting signals from behind a bone mass in relative position to an outbody receiver). In what ways may the com-signal be affected and how might these effects be compensated for?

35. Explore, model, and simulate any perceived tissue-related com-signal scattering effects, diffraction, or "reflectance" in this model. Reflectance may occur when the VCSN is transmitting from close to or behind a bone mass or dense tissue. May a quantifiable scattering pattern be derived from these studies? If so, might there be a technique developed for identifying and eradicating (or muting) these defined scattering pattern anomalies (inherent to the signal) from the data set?

36. Test this com-signal model using a maximum reference parameter that will represent signal propagation through the equivalent of ~4 ft of tissue. This suggested thickness is an overcompensated parameter and it is quite unlikely that signals will traverse a thicker layer of tissue than this for any given patient.

37. What is the specific mechanism that would initiate the launch of a data stream from the VCSN?

38. Explore to what extent VCSN internal communications would be required, and what infrastructure might be needed to facilitate this capability.

39. Explore to what extent VCSN inter-device (collective) communications would be required, and what mechanisms might be utilized to enable this capability. Attempt to define instances and purposes that will necessitate the implementation of inter-device "chatter" and devise strategies for its initiation and organization.

40. Should there be a com-protocol in place whereby able and fully functional VCSNs would (upon notification) come to the rescue of nanodevices that have failed; have been trapped; or are otherwise incapacitated? Hypothetically, they may locate these nanodevices and "chaperone" them to a suitable egress site.

41. If a nanodevice should run into trouble, a distress "ping" might automatically be engaged to signal its requirement for assistance. How might this function be woven into inter-device communications and how may other nanodevices be programmed to react and respond to this?

42. Investigate how one would ensure that all VCSNs have egressed from the patient post-scan. Perhaps, a specialized interrogating signal might be employed for this process. If no responses are elicited from the nanodevices (inherent VCSN programming might include an auto-response to this particular interrogating signal), then an "all-clear" status would be implemented.

43. To cross-reference this status (to locate any residual and still internalized nanodevices whose power/communication capabilities have failed), an additional signal (e.g., infrared light) might be used to detect the fiducials that are embedded within these nanodevices. This protocol may give final verification of all-clear status.

44. Conceptualize, design, and fabricate a prototype nanometric communication node that would incorporate a tessellated array of precisely tuned ultrathin film piezoresonator elements. Individual elements would oscillate in response to a very specific frequency, subsequently emitting specific output voltages and activating task-dedicated circuitry. For example, an isolated element that is caused to oscillate via a particular incoming frequency might initiate and execute a "propulsion stop" command by virtue of the "hard-wired" circuitry that is interfaced with this particular resonator. The element would oscillate at a predetermined activation frequency and generate the voltage required to engage the propulsion stop circuit.

45. A strategy for a "global" resonant element "nonresponse" status (possibly by precise frequency calibration) might be developed to ensure that no other piezoelements (save the one being specifically activated) will oscillate in response to any other frequency except its own. Incoming frequencies may, however, initiate the generation of certain signal "harmonics" that are manifest in the oscillations of a particular piezoelement. These peripheral artifacts would have to be accounted for and muted, or ideally negated.

References

1. Rzeszutko, Ł., Legutko, J., Kałuza, G.L., Wizimirski, M., Richter, A., Chyrchel, M., Heba, G., Dubiel, J.S., and Dudek, D., Assessment of culprit plaque temperature by intracoronary thermography appears inconclusive in patients with acute coronary syndromes. *Arterioscler Thromb Vasc Biol.* 26(8), 1889–1894, 2006.

2. Godin, C. and Caprani, A., Interactions of erythrocytes with an artificial wall: Influence of the electrical surface charge. *Eur Biophys J.* 25(1), 25–30, 1996.

3. Fung, Y.C., *Biomechanics: Motion, Flow, Stress, and Growth.* Springer-Verlag, New York, 1990.

4. Hussey, M., *Basic Physics and Technology of Medical Diagnostics Ultrasound.* Elsevier, New York, 1985.

5. Ladabaum, I., Jin, X., Soh, H.T., Atalar, A., and Khuri-Yakub, B.T., Surface micromachined capacitive ultrasonic transducers. *IEEE Trans Ultrason Ferroelectr Freq Control.* 45(3), 678–690, 1998.

6. Khuri-Yakub, B.T. and Oralkan, O., Capacitive micromachined ultrasonic transducers for medical imaging and therapy. *J Micromech Microeng.* 21(5), 54004–54014, 2011.

7. Wong, S.H., Watkins, R.D., Kupnik, M., Butts-Pauly, K., and Khuri-Yakub, B.T., Feasibility of MR-temperature mapping of ultrasonic heating from a CMUT. *IEEE Trans. Ultrason Ferroelectr Freq Control.* 55, 811–818, 2008.

8. Wong, S.H., Kupnik, M., Watkins, R.D., Butts-Pauly, K.B., and Khuri-Yakub, B.T., Capacitive micromachined ultrasonic transducers for therapeutic ultrasound applications. *IEEE Trans Biomed Eng.* 57, 114–123, 2010.

9. Jin, X., Ladabaum, I., Degertekin, F.L., Calmes, S., and Khuri-Yakub, B.T., Fabrication and characterization of surface micromachined capacitive ultrasonic immersion transducers. *IEEE J Microelectromech Syst.* 8(1), 100–114, 1999.

10. Haller, M.I., Micromachined ultrasonic devices and materials. PhD dissertation, Stanford University, Stanford, CA, 1997.

11. Cantrell, J.H., Heyman, J.S., Yost, W.T., Torbett, M.A., and Breazeale, M.A., Broadband electrostatic acoustic transducer for ultrasonic measurement in liquids. *Rev Sci Instrum.* 50(1), 31–33, 1979.

12. Hohm, D. and Hess, G., A subminiature condensor microphone with silicon-nitride membrane and silicon backplate. *J Acoust Soc Amer.* 85(1), 476–480, 1989.

13. Haller, M.I. and Khuri-Yakub, B.T., A surface micromachined electrostatic ultrasonic air transducer. *Ultrasonics Symposium.* Cannes, France, 1241–1244, 1994.
14. Eccardt, P., Niederer, K., Scheiter, T., and Hierold, C., Surface micromachined ultrasound transducers in CMOS technology. *Ultrasonics Symposium.* San Antonio, TX, 959–962, 1996.
15. Eccardt, P.C. and Niederer, K., Micromachined ultrasound transducers with improved coupling factors from a CMOS compatible process. *Ultrasonics.* 38(1–8), 774–780, 2000.
16. White, R.M., Generation of elastic waves by transient surface heating. *J Appl Phys.* 34(12), 3559–3567, 1963.
17. Noroy, M.H., Royer, D., and Fink, M., The laser-generated ultra-sonic phased array: Analysis and experiments. *J Acoust Soc Am.* 94(4), 1934–1943, 1993.
18. Jacques, S.L. and Paltauf, G., *What is Optoacoustic Imaging?* Oregon Medical Laser Center, Portland, OR, 2000. http://omlc.ogi.edu/news/oct00/saratov2000/intro.html
19. Arnold, H.D. and Crandall, I.B., The thermaphone as a precision source of sound. *Phys Rev.* 10(1), 22–38, 1917.
20. Cullis, A.G., Canham, L.T., and Calcott, P.D.J., The structural and luminescence properties of porous silicon. *J Appl Phys.* 82(3), 909, 1997.
21. Benes, E., Groschl, M., Seifert, F., and Pohl, A., Comparision between BAW and SAW sensor principals. *IEEE Trans Ultrason Ferroelect Freq Contr.* 45(5), 1314–1330, 1998.
22. Hesjedal, T. and Seidel, W., Near-field elastomeric mask photolithography fabrication of high-frequency surface acoustic wave transducers. *Nanotechnology.* 14(1), 91, 2003.
23. Chen, D., Wang, J., Liu, Q., Xu, Y., Li, D., and Liu, Y., Highly sensitive ZnO thin film bulk acoustic resonator for hydrogen detection. *J Micromech Microeng.* 21(11), 5018, 2011.
24. Farina, M. and Rozzi, T., Electromagnetic modeling of thin-film bulk acoustic resonators. *IEEE Trans Microwave Theory Tech.* 52(11), 2496–2502, 2004.
25. Creative PEGWorks, Winston Salem, NC. (provides custom biopolymer synthesis) http://www.creativepegworks.com/(accessed 06/23/13).
26. HPV Robust Summaries and Test Plan-CAS# 86508-42-1, Perflouro compounds, 2003. http://www.epa.gov/hpv/pubs/summaries/perfluro/c13244rt2.pdf (accessed 06/23/13).
27. RTP Company Introduces Biocompatible Thermoplastic Elastomers For Medical Devices, PRWEB. Winona, MN, June 11, 2010. http://www.prweb.com/releases/2010/06/prweb4114454.htm
28. Biocompatible Ceramics, Sigma-Aldrich Co. LLC, 2011. http://www.sigmaaldrich.com/materials-science/material-science-products.html?TablePage=21071121 (accessed 06/23/13).
29. Miller, D.L., Safety assurance in obstetrical ultrasound. *Semin Ultrasound CT MR.* 29(2), 156–164, 2008.
30. Williams, A.R., Effects of ultrasound on blood and the circulation, in Nyborg, W.L. and Ziskin, M.C., eds., *Biological Effects of Ultrasound.* Churchill Livingstone, New York, 49–65, 1985.
31. Freitas, R.A. Jr., *Nanomedicine Vol 1: Basic Capabilities.* Landes Bioscience, Georgetown, TX, 1999.
32. Yildirim, T., NIST. http://www.ncnr.nist.gov/staff/taner/nanotube/ (accessed March 25, 2012).
33. Maiti, A., Andzelm, J., Tanpipat, N., and von Allmen, P., Effect of adsorbates on field emission from carbon nanotubes. *Phys Rev Lett.* 87(15), 155502, 2001.
34. Filip, L.D., Smith, R.C., Carey, J.D., and Silva, S.R., Electron transfer from a carbon nanotube into vacuum under high electric fields. *J Phys Condens Matter.* 21(19), 195302, 2009.
35. Wang, S.S., Fu, J., Qiu, M., Huang, K.J., Ma, Z., and Tong, L.M., Modeling endface output patterns of optical micro/nanofibers. *Opt Express.* 16(12), 8887–8895, 2008.
36. Ma, Z., Wang, S.S., Yang, Q., and Tong, L.M., Near-field optical imaging of evanescent waves guided by micro/nanofibers. *Chin Phys Lett.* 24(10), 3006–3008, 2007.
37. Hinterdorfer, P., Garcia-Parajo, M.F., and Dufrêne, Y.F., Single-molecule imaging of cell surfaces using near-field nanoscopy. *Acc Chem Res.* 45(3), 327–336, 2012.
38. Cohen, M.S., *Basic Magnetization Physics.* Ahmanson Lovelace Brain Mapping Center (UCLA), Los Angeles, CA, 1992.
39. Hornak, J.P., The basics of MRI, 2011. http://www.cis.rit.edu/htbooks/mri/(accessed 06/23/13).

40. Strange, B.A., Imaging the functions of human hippocampus. Ph.D. Thesis, Wellcome Department of Cognitive Neurology, Institute of Neurology, University College London, London, U.K., 1998.

41. Birge, R.R., Introduction to molecular and biomolecular electronics, in Birge, R.R., ed., *Molecular and Biomolecular Electronics*. Advances in Chemistry Series 240, American Chemical Society, Washington DC, Chapter 1, 1–14, 1994.

42. Birge, R.R., Molecular electronics, in Crandall, B.C. and Lewis, J., eds., *Nanotechnology: Research and Perspectives*. MIT Press, Cambridge, MA, 149–170, 1992.

43. Harding, D., *Principles of Airborne Laser Altimeter Terrain Mapping*. NASA's Goddard Space Flight Center, Greenbelt, MD, March 2000.

44. Center for LIDAR Information Coordination and Knowledge. http://lidar.cr.usgs.gov/ (accessed March 25, 2012).

45. Flood, M., Laser altimetry: From science to commercial Lidar mapping. *Photogram Eng Remote Sens.* 67(11), 2001.

46. Antonarakis, A.S., Saatchi, S.S., Chazdon, R.L., and Moorcroft, P.R., Using Lidar and Radar measurements to constrain predictions of forest ecosystem structure and function. *Ecol Appl.* 21(4), 1120–1137, 2011.

47. Blair, J.B., Rabine, D.L., and Hofton, M.A., The Laser Vegetation Imaging Sensor: A medium altitude, digitization only, airborne laser altimeter for mapping vegetation and topography. *ISPRS J Photogram Remote Sensing.* 54, 115–122, 1999.

48. Lemmens, M., Airborne Lidar scanners, status and developments. *GIM Int.* 25(2), 2011. http://www.gim-international.com/issues/articles/id1667 Airborne_Lidar_Scanners.html

49. Leica ALS70 Airborne Laser Scanner. http://www.leica-geosystems.com/en/Leica-ALS70-Airborne-Laser-Scanner_94516.htm (accessed 06/23/13).

50. Abshire, J.B., Sun, X., and Afzal, R.S., Mars orbiter laser altimeter: receiver model and performance analysis. *Appl Opt.* 39(15), 2449–60, 2000. The Mars Orbiter Laser Altimeter. http://mola.gsfc.nasa.gov/ (accessed 06/23/13).

51. Enejder, A.M.K., Light scattering and absorption in tissue models and measurements. Thesis, Lund Institute of Technology, Sweden, 1997.

52. Nilsson, A.M., Heinrich, D., Olajos, J., and Andersson-Engels, S., Near infrared diffuse reflection and laser-induced fluorescence spectroscopy for myocardial tissue characterisation. *Spectrochim Acta A Mol Biomol Spectrosc.* 53A(11), 1901–1912, 1997.

53. Rieber J., Intravascular imaging and its integration into coronary angiography (Article in German). *Dtsch Med Wochenschr.* 137(14), 726–731, 2012.

54. Madder, R.D., Smith, J.L., Dixon, S.R., Goldstein, J.A., Composition of target lesions by near-infrared spectroscopy in patients with acute coronary syndrome versus stable angina. *Circ Cardiovasc Interv.* 5(1), 55–61, 2012.

55. Hirsch, J.C., Charpie, J.R., Gurney, J.G., and Ohye, R.G., Role of near infrared spectroscopy in pediatric cardiac surgery. *Prog Pediatr Cardiol.* 29(2), 93–96, 2010.

56. Pifferi, A., Taroni, P., Valentini, G., and Engels, S.A., Real time methods for fitting time-resolved reflectance and transmittance measurements with a Monte-Carlo model. *Appl Opt.* 37, 2774–2780, 1998.

57. Nilsson, A.M.K., Alsholm, P., Karlsson, A., and Engels, S.A., T-matrix computations of light scattering by red blood cells. *Appl Opt.* 37, 2735–2748, 1998.

58. Shah, N., Eker, C., Espinoza, J., Fishkin, J., Hornung, R., Tromberg, B., and Butler, J., Multi-wavelength, in vivo measurements of human breast tissue optical properties reveal hormonal-dependent absorption and scattering variations. *Proc Natl Acad Sci USA.* 1999.

59. Liu, D.L., Svanberg, K., Wang, I., Engles, S.A., and Svanberg, S., Laser Doppler perfusion imaging: New technique for determination of perfusion of splanchic organs and tumor tissue. *Lasers Surg Med.* 20, 473–479, 1997.

60. Ishumaru, A., *Wave Propagation and Scattering in Random Media*. Academic Press, New York, 1978.

61. Swanson, N.L., Gehman, V.M., Billard, B.D., and Gennaro, T.L., Limits of the small-angle approximation to the radiative transport equation. *J Opt Soc Am A Opt Image Sci Vis.* 18(2), 385–391, 2001.

62. Kim, A.D. and Keller, J.B., Light propagation in biological tissue. *J Opt Soc Am A Opt Image Sci Vis.* 20(1), 92–98, 2003.
63. Jacques, S.L., Alter, C.A., and Prahl, S.A., Angular dependence of HeNe laser light scattering by human dermis. *Lasers Life Sci.* 1, 309–333, 1987.
64. Yoon, G., Welch, A.J., Motamedi, M., and van Gemert, M.J.C., Development and application of three-dimensional light distribution model for laser irradiated tissue. *IEEE J Quant Electr.* 23(10), 1721–1733, 1987.
65. Arnfield, M.R., Tulip, J., and McPhee, M.S., Optical propagation in tissue with anisotropic scattering. *IEEE Trans Biomed Eng.* 35(5), 372–381, 1988.
66. Graaff, R., Koelink, M.H., de Mul, F.F., Zijistra, W.G., Dassel, A.C., and Aarnoudse, J.G., Condensed Monte Carlo simulations for the description of light transport. *Appl Opt.* 32(4), 426–434, 1993.
67. Flock, S.T., Wilson, B.C., and Patterson, M.S., Hybrid Monte Carlo-diffusion theory modelling of light distributions in tissue, in Berns, M.W., ed., *Laser Interaction with Tissue. Proc Soc Photo-Opt Instrum Eng.* 908, 20–28, 1998.
68. Wang, L. and Jacques, S.L., Hybrid model of Monte Carlo simulation and diffusion theory for light reflectance by turbid media. *J Opt Soc Am A Opt Image Sci Vis.* 10(8), 1746–1752, 1993.
69. Kienle, A. and Patterson, M.S., Determination of the optical properties of turbid media from a single Monte Carlo simulation. *Phys Med Biol.* 41(10), 2221–2227, 1996.
70. Hutchins, D.A., McIntosh, J.S., Neild, A., Billson, D.R., and Noble, R.A., Radiated fields of capacitive micromachined ultrasonic transducers in air. *J Acoust Soc Am.* 114(3), 1435–1449, 2003.
71. Park, K.K., Lee, H., Kupnik, M., and Khuri-Yakub, B.T., Fabrication of capacitive micromachined ultrasonic transducers via local oxidation and direct wafer bonding. *J MEMS.* 20(1), 95–103, 2011.
72. Stephens, D.N., Truong, U.T., Nikoozadeh, A., Oralkan, O., Seo, C.H., Cannata, J., Dentinger, A., Thomenius, K., de la Rama, A., Nguyen, T., Lin, F., Khuri-Yakub, P., Mahajan, A., Shivkumar, K., O'Donnell, M., and Sahn, D.J., First in vivo use of a capacitive micromachined ultrasound transducer array-based imaging and ablation. *J Ultrasound Med.* 31(2), 247–256, 2012.
73. Javey, A., Shim, M., and Dai, H., Electrical properties and devices of large-diameter single-walled carbon nanotubes. *Appl Phys Lett.* 80, 1064, 2001.
74. Smart, A.G., Ultralow magnetic fields elicit unexplained spin dynamics in water. *Phys Today.* 14, 2011.
75. Shannon, C.E., A mathematical theory of communication. *Bell System Tech J.* 27, 379–423, 623–656, 1948.
76. Schneider, T.D., Theory of molecular machines. I. Channel capacity of molecular machines. *J Theor Biol.* 148, 83–123, 1991.
77. Wang, Y., Kempa, K., Kimball, B., Carlson, J.B., Benham, G., Li, W.Z., Kempa, T., Rybczynski, J., Herczynski, A., and Ren, Z.F., Receiving and transmitting light-like radio waves: Antenna effect in arrays of aligned carbon nanotubes. *Appl Phys Lett.* 85(13), 2607–2609, 2004.
78. Lourenço, M.A. and Homewood, K.P., Dislocation-engineered silicon light emitters for photonic integration. *Semicond Sci Technol.* 23(6), 064005, 2008.
79. Langer, K.D. and Grubor, J., Recent developments in optical wireless communications using infrared and visible light. *9th International Conference on Transparent Optical Networks. ICTON.'07*, Rome, Italy, Vol. 3, pp. 146–151, July 1–5, 2007.
80. Cao, L., Park, J.S., Fan, P., Clemens, B., and Brongersma, M.L., Resonant germanium nanoantenna photodetectors. *Nano Lett.* 10(4), 1229–1233, 2010.
81. Whelan, H.T., Buchmann, E.V., Dhokalia, A., Kane, M.P., Whelan, N.T., Wong-Riley, M.T.T., Eells, J.T., Gould, L.J., Hammamieh, R., Das, R., and Jett, M., Effect of NASA light-emitting diode irradiation on molecular changes for wound healing in diabetic mice. *J Clin Laser Med Surg.* 21(2), 67–74, 2003.
82. Triger, S., Saillant, J.F., Demore, C.E., Cochran, S., and Cumming, D.R., Low-voltage coded excitation utilizing a miniaturized integrated ultrasound system employing piezoelectric 2-D arrays. *IEEE Trans Ultrason Ferroelectr Freq Control.* 57(2), 353–362, 2010.

83. Gao, P.X. and Wang, Z.L., High-yield synthesis of single-crystal nanosprings of ZnO. *Small.* 1(10), 945–949, 2005.
84. Chen, L., House, J.L., Krahe, R., and Nelson, M.E., Modeling signal and background components of electrosensory scenes. *J Comp Physiol A Neuroethol Sens Neural Behav Physiol.* 191(4), 331–345, 2005.
85. Paterson, J.R., García-Bellido, D.C., Lee, M.S., Brock, G.A., Jago, J.B., and Edgecombe, G.D., Acute vision in the giant Cambrian predator *Anomalocaris* and the origin of compound eyes. *Nature.* 480(7376), 237–240, 2011.
86. Banerjee, S. and Wong, S.S., In situ quantum dot growth on multiwalled carbon nanotubes. *J Am Chem Soc.* 125(34), 10342–10350, 2003.

7

Design Challenges and Considerations for Nanomedical Computation

Frank J. Boehm

CONTENTS

7.1 Nanomedical Computation

The most energy-intensive elements of nanomedical devices will be those that undertake enormous computational loads to control virtually every onboard system, concomitant with outbody and inter-nanodevice communications.

A quantum computer, which exploits the entanglement of electron and nuclear spins to process information [1], might comprise the core enabler of the exemplar vascular cartographic scanning nanodevice (VCSN) via the control of all components and systems.

In the case of the VCSN, this entity will preprocess all acquired spatial data, facilitate the transmission of the resulting data sets, and ensure that all operational protocols are being adhered to within predetermined parameters. With the advent of molecular manufacturing, it is conceivable that a VCSN-resident quantum computer might be integrated by potentially assembling the physical structure of the VCSN, complete with nanoelectronic "wiring" and interface incorporation throughout the process, around this "quantum seed."

Quantum computers could handle all internal, inter-device, and "outbody" communications, oversee regular internal diagnostics checks, and utilize fail-safe strategies (e.g., engaging and activating redundant systems), if deemed necessary. These components will exist ideally as solid-state entities under the external control of a dedicated computer that is administered by medical personnel. They will also have the intrinsic capacity to be reprogrammed, if required, from external computers.

The development of a quantum computer for nanodevices such as the VCSN will be particularly challenging in view of

1. The requirement for the compression of robust computing power into a very constrained physical space (e.g., a 10,000 element logic system that occupies $<\sim100$ nm^3) [2]

2. Integration/hard wiring and extensive testing with all other VCSN components (e.g., continual operation in the gigahertz range at $\sim10^{-9}$ W) [2]

3. The design and development of intricate three-dimensional (3D) designs and elemental organization, which will be required in order to guide its nanofabrication

The unique core feature of quantum computers is that in addition to having qubits (where a qubit comprises a single unit of quantum information), which are in either binary "on" or "off" states, they can be in superpositional (all) states simultaneously. Hence, numerous calculations can proceed in parallel, engaging multiple qubits at the same time. To illustrate the unprecedented computational power of a quantum computer, it is estimated that such a device comprises only 250 qubits, with each qubit being encoded by an atom "would require a classical computer built from all the atoms in the visible universe to encode the same information" [3]. This degree of computational horsepower, coupled with atomic scale compactness, will likely provide a viable platform with which to functionalize sophisticated autonomous nanomedical devices.

Although many researchers have estimated that practical quantum computers may be several decades away, rapid progress is being made on this front [4–9]. When one peers through the Kurzweil lens and examines his law of accelerating returns, which postulates that technological change is increasingly exponential, the advent of the quantum computer may be closer than we imagine [10,11]. Kurzweil also poses an intriguing strategy for evolving an artificial intelligence (AI) that might inspire a strategy for endowing autonomous nanomedical devices with a form of "synthetic sentience" [12]. "Intelligence as an association of lesser intelligences is both a theory of natural intelligence and a paradigm for the organisation of machine intelligence. As our computer systems become more complicated, one way to organise them is to develop smaller systems, each of which is relatively complete with its own structural integrity, and then define languages and processes that let these lesser 'experts' interact" [13].

7.2 Perceived Research Goals for VCSN Quantum Computer

1. Methodical investigation into current quantum computing advances to discern what might be the most appropriate path/mechanism to follow toward the eventual development of a viable core quantum computing device for the VCSN.

2. Exploration of various solid-state quantum computing entities (qubits) and elucidation of their data processing capabilities to assess their suitability in translating significant volumes of spatial data acquired by the VCSN scanning components.

3. Discern what the smallest possible physical footprint of a self-contained quantum computer might be, and how it may be interfaced with myriad VCSN elements in enabling robust and precisely controllable/reliable data inputs and outputs.

4. Identify the best signal conveyance strategies for stable reciprocating signal transfer between a VCSN-embedded quantum computer that traverses the in vivo environment and external control computers.

5. Explore what specific and most efficient quantum computing algorithms might be developed to appropriately cope with the enormous flow of information in the form of acquired spatial/spectral data, assimilation of commands from outbody computers, additional communications (e.g., internal, inter-device), and the fine control of all onboard components and systems.

6. Survey the optimum materials and logic elements that might be employed to construct a quantum computing device with prospective dimensions of $<{\sim}500$ nm^3.

7. Elucidate what the optimum qubit model might be for quantum computation (e.g., photon polarization, magnetic precession, electron orbital states) and how this data may be physically programmed, transferred, and translated.

7.3 Nanometric Computation

Following is a survey of potential nanometric scale computing technologies that might be utilized or the control of nanomedical devices with myriad capabilities.

7.3.1 Quantum Computation

As briefly described earlier, quantum computation involves the processing of information by employing quantum mechanical systems. Quantum mechanics is the mathematical set of rules for the creation of physical theories. There has been much effort applied in the attempt to gain complete control over single quantum systems. One indication of progress in this area came with the development of the "atom trap" where a single atom is isolated, and different aspects of its behavior can be observed with great precision. Electronic devices that operate using only single electrons have also been devised and demonstrated. One of the challenges facing the development of quantum computing is the writing of superior quantum algorithms. This is proving difficult, as some parts of the process are very counterintuitive. The fundamental concept of classical computation and information is the "bit." Quantum computation is built on an analogous concept, the quantum bit, or qubit, as described earlier. Qubits are realized as actual physical entities, but are also described in terms of mathematical objects with specific characteristics. An advantage to treating qubits as abstract entities is that it allows a greater freedom to construct a general theory of quantum computation and information without having to rely on a specific system for its materialization [14].

Qubits are states of 0 and 1 just as a classical bit, and two possible states are $|0\rangle$ and $|1\rangle$. The Dirac notation ($|\rangle$) is a standard notation for states in quantum mechanics. The difference between classical bits and qubits is that qubits can also dwell in states other than $|0\rangle$ and $|1\rangle$. It is also possible to form linear combinations of states or superpositions. As Nielson and Chuang articulate, the state of a qubit is defined as a "vector in a two-dimensional (2D) complex vector space. The special states $|0\rangle$ and $|1\rangle$ are known as computational basis states, and form an orthonormal basis for this vector space." When measuring a qubit, the basic states are observed as well as the probability of another state. The divide between the "hidden" state of a qubit and the observable states constitutes the core of quantum computation and information. There is an associative deficit between these hidden and abstract qubit states and reality. A simple analogy might be that a musical note comprises many inherent albeit subtle harmonics. There is, however, "an indirect correspondence, for qubit states can be manipulated and transformed in ways which lead to measurement outcomes which depend distinctly on the different properties of the state." Hence, "these quantum states have real and experimentally verifiable consequences," which are critical to quantum computational power. The capacity for qubits to encompass superposition goes against rational perception as they can reside in a continuum of states between $|0\rangle$ and $|1\rangle$ (and in both) until scrutinized [14].

Physical entities that are suitable as qubits can take the form of photonic polarizations; nuclear spin positions in a homogeneous magnetic field and the two states that electrons may inhabit as they revolve about an atom. Within atoms, electrons can be present in either "ground" or "excited" states ($|0\rangle$ and $|1\rangle$), which can be reversibly switched via the application of light that possesses the appropriate level of energy and duration. By reducing the photonic exposure time, an electron can be induced to be positioned midway between $|0\rangle$ and $|1\rangle$ states to reside in the $|+\rangle$ or superposition state. Flip states can take place on the order of nanoseconds where the energy of an electron is typically about 10 eV, corresponding to a linear velocity of 2×10^8 cm/s, and the nuclear velocity is 10^5 cm/s [14].

An abstract entity called a Bloch sphere (Figure 7.1) is employed to visualize the state of a single qubit. In reality, the mere act of measurement alters the state of a qubit, and for reasons that remain unknown, it will break from its superpositional states to either $|0\rangle$ or $|1\rangle$. A substantial reservoir of "concealed" data is retained in the state of a qubit, and the potential quantity of this supplemental data rises exponentially with the number of qubits. These unobservable data represent the core potency of quantum mechanics as relate to their use in information processing [14].

In a quantum computer a superposition of N qubits may store 2^N binary digits, as an operation performs numerous calculations simultaneously in a massively parallel manner. An example of this can be illustrated in the case of a photon that interacts with an atom, which is engaged in a superposition of states. The photon will drive all states into superposition, in effect, generating yet another superposition that corresponds to all solutions of the original states. Thus, the quantum computational advantage over

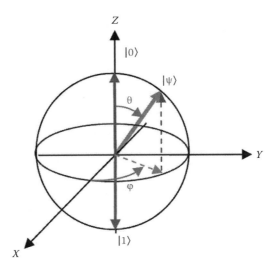

FIGURE 7.1
A Bloch sphere: geometrically depicted qubit, as a "pure state" bilevel quantum mechanical system. (From Amri, T., Wikimedia Commons.)

conventional computers is exponential [15]. Current processors function sequentially on 64 bit numbers whereas a 64-bit quantum computer would concurrently operate on the entire set of 2^{64} (10^{19}) binary values. Theories relating to quantum computing have been accumulating at a rapid pace [15–20], and a variety of elemental quantum computational entities have been investigated:

1. A NOT gate comprising two qubits from cooled beryllium ion in a radio-frequency trap [21]
2. Single photons trapped in quantum cavities to cesium atom states [22]
3. Analog quantum computer utilizing electrons afloat on liquid helium [23]
4. NMR methods for storing data in nuclear spins (less vulnerable to distortion) as opposed to electron states [15,24]
5. Nanoscale superinductors comprising Josephson junction ladders [25]
6. Double quantum dot spin and valley degrees of freedom in graphene, carbon nanotubes, and silicon [26]
7. Open system optically pumped trapped ions [27]
8. Spin–orbit qubits in indium arsenide nanowires [28]
9. Deep center defects in diamond (nitrogen vacancy [NV(–1)] deep center), 4H silicon carbide (SiC), and other tetrahedrally coordinated compound semiconductors (e.g., AlP, AlAs, AlSb, GaP, GaAs, GaSb, InP, InAs, InSb, ZnS, ZnSe, ZnTe, and CdTe [29,30]

NAND gates (AND and NOT gates—fundamental elements of all Boolean computers) can be realized utilizing the resonance effects between proton and electron spins within H atoms [15]. Another significant advance is the discovery of error-correcting procedures. In quantum computers, it is not possible to verify that a qubit is in a certain state, as the act of measuring will demolish coherence. It has been proven, however, that data may be reliably preserved and read from a several qubit system even if there is a corrupt element and error correction can be applied on the fly during the computation function itself [31–33].

The maximum population threshold of potential quantum states that can reside within an enclosed domain is called the Bekenstein-bound and the optimal processing speed is constrained by the minimum quantum state transition time, which must not be shorter than the time it takes for light to traverse a defined distance [14,15,34]. It has been proposed that by programming of several thousand superpositional electron states, significant volumes of data could conceivably be packed into an individual atom (e.g., Si atom memory at 250 Tbit/in.^{2}) [35]. Freitas calculates that "in theory, a single carbon atom of mass $m = 2 \times 10^{-26}$ kg and radius $R \sim 0.15$ nm could be impressed with up to $I_{Bek} \sim 10^8$ bits and could process information up to $I_{Bek} \sim 10^{26}$ bits/s in an optimally designed quantum computer." For a 1 µm^3 computer of mass $\sim 10^{-15}$ kg, $I_{Bek} \sim 10^{22}$ bits the maximum storage capacity and $I_{Bek} \sim 10^{37}$ bits/s maximum processing capacity [15]. He also suggests that dedicated nanometric computational "organs" might someday be implanted [36–40] within the body for service over the lifetime of the patient. These organs could serve as data repositories (library nodes), perhaps including personal archived medical/anatomical data and record, and communications encryption [15]. They may assist with nanomedical device computation in that nanodevices might intermittently dock with these nodes in order to transfer their data loads, and possibly replenish energy supplies. If a nanodevice should experience damage or a malfunction, it might seek refuge at one of these nodes until the appropriate nanodevice egress protocols are engaged.

Advanced autonomous nanomedical devices such as the VCSN will require considerable computational storage capacity using nanometric scale elements that are designed at the atomic level to facilitate the acquisition and preprocessing of spatial and spectrographic data relating to the mapping of the entire vascular or lymphatic systems. Quantum data storage technologies will likely align well with this requirement. One mode of quantum computation involves a two-electron semiconducting quantum dot qubit device. This configuration involves two electrons that are trapped within an 800 nm square quantum dot, which reside in a gallium arsenide substrate. In this arrangement there are only two positional states possible, as the negatively charged electrons repel each other to secure the furthest separation distance possible and end up diagonally opposed as either upper right/lower left or lower right/upper left, due to coulomb forces. These electron states then would represent 1s and 0s and could be manipulated by pulsed voltages and magnetic fields to enable computation [41].

Zhou et al. have achieved the high-fidelity reversible storage and retrieval of single polarization-encoded photons utilizing a solid-state atomic frequency comb in rare earth ion-doped crystals. Neodymium-doped yttrium vanadate (Nd^{3+}:YVO_4) crystals (10 ppm dopant level) posses a unique electronic structure that can be regarded as an atomic frozen gas with exemplary coherence, as relates to optical and spin transitions [42]. They also exhibit the capacity for the highly efficacious [43] "storage" of light for extended durations (several seconds) in praseodymium-doped yttrium orthosilicate (Pr^{3+}:Y_2SiO_5) [44] over a wide bandwidth [45]. Similar work has also been done with europium-doped yttrium orthosilicate ($^{153}Eu^{3+}$:Y_2SiO_5) [46]. These accomplishments represent significant advances in the development of reliable quantum data storage and networks. Under the Heisenberg uncertainty principle, the "Classical measurement and reconstruction strategies for storing light must necessarily destroy quantum information …" as the effect of the act of measurement. However, recent advances in quantum memory devices are making incremental progress in circumventing this consequence [43].

7.3.2 Reversible Computing

Recurring queries attempt to answer the question: What is the maximum amount of information that might be stored in a defined unit of physical matter? Some considerations to keep in mind when attempting to design a quantum computer for a nanomedical device might include

1. Minimization of onboard computation requirements
2. Maximization of algorithmic efficiency (e.g., super-Turing computers) [47,48]
3. Minimization of power/heat dissipation per computation [15]

Fredkin and Toffoli, in articulating a conservative logic strategy for computation, have postulated that "it is ideally possible to build sequential circuits with zero internal power dissipation," in enabling universal computation capacities at finite speeds with zero errors. A mechanistic model based on (e.g., hard spheres and flat pates) would determine a "ballistic trajectory isomorphic with the desired computation." Albeit, a trajectory that would be unknown to the computer designer. Bennett postulates that "ballistic models are unrealistic because they require the parts to be assembled with perfect precision and isolated from thermal noise, which would eventually randomize the trajectory and lead to errors. Possible quantum effects could be exploited to prevent this undesired equipartition of the kinetic energy" [49,50]. Under microphysics, the design of idealized "computing primitives," intended for high-performance computation, should extend beyond the abstract realm of mathematical constructs to reflect plausible physical effects that occur in natural systems. Further, "in the world of microscopic physics interactions are dissipationless; also, predictable interactions can take place in a much shorter space and time, since the accuracy of the interaction laws does not depend on averages taken over many particles. Thus, microphysics appears to have many attractions for the efficiency-minded designer" [49].

Another computational model is the Brownian computer, which permits thermal noise to so strongly mediate the trajectory that it becomes a "random walk through the entire accessible (low-potential-energy) portion of a computer's configuration space." In contrast to the ballistic model, the Brownian model involves higher dissipation, thus reversibility occurs "in the limit of zero speed." Both of these representations are based on the requirement, in terms of programming, that all computations should be logically reversible, and that output exclusively specifies input [15,50,51].

The closest natural analogy to a Brownian computer resides in the intrinsic replication, transcription, and translation processes of DNA, which dissipates 20–100 kT per step (kT is the characteristic thermal energy necessary to elevate the thermodynamic entropy of a system). In 1949, von Neumann stated that at room temperature, the operation a computer must dissipate approximately 3×10^{-22} J "per elementary act of information that is per elementary decision of a two-way alternative and per elementary transmittal of one unit of information" [50,52]. It was later suggested by Landauer that it was not computation itself but rather the process of data erasure that produced thermal dissipation [53]. It has since been recognized, in theory, that a considerable amount of computation may be accomplished per generated kT of waste heat [50].

A straightforward form of reversible computing is called a "retractile cascade" during which all inputs and intermediate states that culminate in results are preserved throughout a given computation. Subsequent to arriving at the final result, it is copied to an output register, whereupon the original input data are erased. This procedure may be cascaded in multiple steps and consequently removed in reverse [15].

Hall envisions that nanocomputer constituents such as gates and latches, including adders, shifters, and other logical elements, will be nanofabricated and operate within nanoscale domains. He articulates a number of reversible computing strategies, why they are required, and stipulates that "in a reversible electronic computer, there must never be a point where a switch is closed between two wires at different voltages. The current flow across such a switch could theoretically be harnessed to do useful work, but is instead dissipated as heat." Also, in the design of electronic reversible logic, "we must assume wires and switches with no resistance at all. Remarkably, however, we need assume nothing else" [54].

Reversible processors based on a Reduced Instruction Set Computer (RISC) architecture utilize small highly optimized series of instructions rather than more specialized sets of commands, which are typically employed in other computational architectures. The advantages of RISC architectures in enhancing performance include

1. Enabling vacated chip real estate to be employed in increasing the throughput velocity of frequently utilized commands, which far outweighs the unavoidable shortfalls in performance of rarely utilized instructions
2. Facilitation of design optimization
3. Allowance for the endowment of microprocessors with procedures that are typically reserved for larger more powerful computers
4. Translational simplification of high-level language, which results in higher program efficiencies [55]

Frank and Knight have proposed a reversible 3D "mesh of processors" as an "optimal physically realistic model for scalable computers." They state that "any physical architecture based on irreversible logic devices would be asymptotically slower than realizations of our model, and we argue that no physical realization of computation aside from quantum computation could be asymptotically faster." They predict that as computer technologies continue to shrink that an intimate understanding of reversible computing and the physics of computation will be invaluable in the "creation of the most powerful nanosupercomputers of the coming century" [56].

Drexler has proposed a design for a rod logic system that might utilize nanoscale rods that are decorated with "gate" and "probe" knobs (Figure 7.2), where the positional shift of one rod is dependent on the other. This construct is analogous to the functionality of a transistor in that "the ability of current to flow in one conducting path is dependent on the voltage of another conducting path." Using this strategy, mechanical nanocomputers (Table 7.1) may be possible that imbue the identical logic systems as contemporary electronic computers. However, the shifting elements must be encased within a matrix that contains tight intersecting channels to ensure constrained rod movement, yet with the ability to be blocked. Each logic gate would be comprised of several hundred atoms.

7.3.3 Helical Logic

A hypothetical helical logic computation strategy proposed by Merkle and Drexler would utilize the presence or vacancies of individual electrons, or holes, to facilitate the encoding of 1s and 0s. Electrons within the circuit, which is completely embedded in a revolving

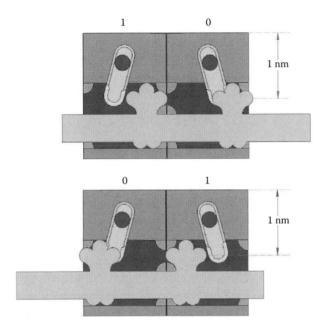

FIGURE 7.2
Dual nanocomputers (cross-section) gate mechanisms in starting position possess one control rod and two gate knobs viewed laterally. A pair of rods with affixed knobs is viewed end on, where each constitutes a single molecule. During computation, the lateral rod is drawn to the left. One of the end-on rods is now blocked while the other is free (e.g., mechanical analogy of transistor operation). (Adapted from design by Drexler, K.E., *NanoCon Proceedings*, 1989. http://www.halcyon.com/nanojbl/NanoConProc/nanocon2.html, accessed October 22, 2012.)

TABLE 7.1

Drexler's Mechanical Nanocomputer Design Specifications

Nanocomputer Element	Description
Interlock gates	10^6
Logic rods	10^5
Registers	10^4
Mass	$\sim 10^{-16}$ kg
Operations/s pW	$\sim 2 \times 10^4$
Processing speed (assuming 1 bit per register)	$\sim 10^9$ operations/s (~ 1 gigaflop)
	($\sim 10^{28}$ operations/s m^3)
	$\sim 10^{13}$ bits/s
	($\sim 10^{32}$ bits/s m^3)
Total power	~ 0.013 zJ (per gate per cycle)
Total cubic volume	~ 400 nm^3 (includes energy-buffering flywheel and other elements)

Sources: Freitas, R.A. Jr., *Nanomedicine, Volume I: Basic Capabilities*, Landes Bioscience, Georgetown, TX, 1999; Drexler, K.E., *Nanosystems: Molecular Machinery, Manufacturing, and Computation*, John Wiley & Sons, New York, 1992.

electric field, would be induced to traverse along helical trajectories and restricted to sections of single turns of the helix, analogous to water being transported via an Archimedes screw. Each helical turn could conceivably host an independent carrier; thus, allowing for a high data concentration [58].

A particular universal logic process might employ dual helices; one of which separates into two "descendant" helices. At the deviation point, electrostatic alterations in the potential as a consequence of a present or vacant carrier in the adjoining helix would mediate the path followed by a carrier in the dividing helix. The inverse of this process might be exploited to meld a pair of formerly disparate helical trajectories into a solitary outgoing trajectory without imposing a dissipative conversion. As these functions are reversible in terms of thermodynamics and logic, energy dissipation may be maintained at minimal levels. The combination of thermodynamic reversibility through the utilization of single charge carriers "permits a single electron to trigger another single electron." Hence, the requirement of numerous electrons to switch a single electron is negated, and the energy dissipated per logic operation might be lowered to approx. $<10^{-27}$ J at 1 K and a speed of 10 GHz [58].

In conventional computation, the erasure of a bit of data or the combination of two computation paths results in energy dissipation, adding to entropy, which may for the most part be circumvented utilizing reversible logic, albeit at the expense of speed. Helical logic evades many of the issues related to conventional clock distribution as well. With the implementation of double helical logic, it is possible that further reductions in energy dissipation might be realized. In terms of advancing nanomedical device computation, additional explorations of single electron, atomically precise logic devices that demonstrate thermodynamic reversibility, will be a worthy endeavor [58].

The elucidation of the specific thermodynamics of electron-based computation [59,60] will be critical in the design of future, highly dense nanomedical "intelligences," as cumulative thermal dissipation from perhaps millions of in vivo nanodevices must be kept within a range of safety that will not induce "clinically significant effects." Freitas calculates that as relates to passive thermal transfer via thermophysical conductivity, "in the case of a ~1 cm³ dose of spherical diamond nanorobots (~10^{12} devices at ~1 μm³ each) infused into the 5400 cm³ adult human male blood volume ..." that their presence at this loading may be considered as "clinically insignificant. Blood heat capacity similarly is virtually unchanged." At the upper threshold of 10% nanocrit (Nct), he deduces that in the instance of diamondoid nanorobots transiting through the circulation; they "will not significantly alter the heat capacity of the blood, hence the active conduction mechanism in human thermoregulation should be largely unaffected" [61].

7.3.4 Quantum Spintronics

As envisaged by Awschalom et al., spintronics might provide a potential path for realizing solid-state quantum computers made of diamond that operate at room temperature. This facet of electronics exploits not only an electron's charge but also its spin, or magnetic dipole moment. An early application of spintronics (1998) was employed in the read heads of computer hard drives, wherein giant magnetoresistance was utilized to recognize data in hard disk–embedded magnetic domains. Spin transfer nano-oscillators are currently (2012) being investigated to potentially enhance wireless communications [62]. Quantum spintronics engages the manipulation of the quantum attributes of electron spins to effectively substitute typical 0s and 1s used in conventional computing with qubits, as described earlier (Section 7.1), which can concurrently inhabit superpositions of 0 and 1 [63].

The distinguishing traits of an electron, in addition to its spin, are mass and charge. Individual electrons innately exhibit an identical level of spin, which is equivalent to one half the fundamental quantum unit of angular momentum. The magnetic to mechanical moment ratio of a spinning electron is equal to twice the corresponding ratio for electron orbital motion [64]. In endeavoring to build a quantum computer whose foundation is exclusively reliant on electron spins, an important question might relate to the quantification of spin polarization decay rates. This would require a strict command over quantum coherence (the pure quantum character of all data-conveying elements in the device). Quantum data derived from electron charges has the propensity to lose coherence or is apt to vanish in picoseconds, even under cryogenic temperatures. Hence, quantum data that relies on spin may be inherently more robust [65]. An investigation to elucidate the lowest energy that is necessary to flip a single manganese atom was conducted. It was found that under a 1.4 T magnetic field, in a vacuum at close to absolute 0°C, it took 0.0005 eV to flip the atom between up/down states, which is 10,000 times lower than the energy of an isolated hydrogen bond. For comparison, a single photon of visible light possesses ~2 e/V of energy, equivalent to 4000 times that was necessary to flip the atom [66].

Molecular metal oxides (polyoxometalates [POMs]), which are shown to possess advantageous structural, electronic, and chemical attributes, have been studied by Clemente-Juan et al. toward possible applications in nanomagnetics, molecular spintronics, and quantum computing [67]. This group proposes that mixed valence POMs might serve as optimal magnetic molecules with which to scrutinize the electrical manipulation of spin states, and may be integrated as quantum spintronics elements (e.g., gates/switches) via the enablement of unique effects:

1. Capacity to mediate atomic populations (oxidation states) in the system. Utilizing the mixed valence POM species $[PMo_{12}O_{40}(VO)_2]^{q-}$, two localized spins may be attached to a redox-active unit.

2. Unimolecular spintronics, where charge may be distributed in the system by means of an electric field, thereby initiating a "position-dependent chemical potential." In effect, the external control of the magnetic properties of POM may be possible when the molecule is interfaced with an electronic circuit.

3. The highly reproducible diminishment of quantum decoherence. The principal sources of decoherence in POMs, namely "hyperfine couplings and dipolar spin–spin interactions," may be reduced through the preparation of "nuclear-spin-free compounds and by diluting the magnetic centers, while conserving the crystallinity." POMs can host rare earth lanthanoids with unusual (e.g., C5 axial) symmetries [68] to allow for the tuning of nanomagnetic anisotropies, while simultaneously maintaining their magnetic segregation.

4. The synthesis of quantum gates (as extensions of switching devices) where "coherent quantum manipulation" may occur in enabling transient OFF–ON–OFF sequences as the result of extended duration coherence in POM qubits.

Thus, POMs may provide unprecedented opportunities for the fine control of molecular quantum spins in facilitating the development of molecular spintronics to drive quantum computing [67].

7.3.5 Molecular Computation

The minimal quantity of energy that must be dissipated by molecular computation in obtaining 1 bit of information may be represented by

$$E_{min} = k_B T \ln(2) \, \text{J/bit} \tag{7.1}$$

This equation is derived/related to the second law of thermodynamics. There is a specific upper threshold, which limits the number of "decisions" that a molecular computer may make in relation to the energy dissipated in doing so. This constraint will be a critical factor in molecular computer design and fabrication. Theoretically, bits at the molecular level may be considered as equivalent to their counterparts at the macroscopic scale, hence, the premise that molecular machines may conduct accurate logical operations. The implication being that molecular computation might be possible while dissipating minimal energy [69].

Shannon's channel capacity theorem leads to the notion that single molecular computation can be exact, virtually free of errors [70,71] and may be possible, as described earlier (Section 7.3.4), without energy dissipation. An illustration of this from molecular biology comes in the form of the restriction enzyme, *Eco*RI endonuclease, which carries out Boolean logic with high efficacy whenever it binds to DNA. Nevertheless, when the molecule is "escorted" via Brownian motion to its particular DNA-resident sequence (5'-GAATTC-3'), heat is released upon binding [72]. Resultant output operations conducted via molecular computation, which are "disturbed" by thermal noise, must concurrently dissipate energy (second law of thermodynamics). Although there is no energetic stricture for computation [73], it is a prerequisite for data output [74].

7.3.6 DNA Computation

Intuitively, the suggestion that massively parallel DNA-based computation might direct nanomedical devices seems untenable, as we envision typical DNA functionality as being exclusive to operating in aqueous milieu. Although it is likely that the ideal and most robust configuration of nanocomputers for autonomous medical nanodevices would be in the solid state, there may be instances where subsequent to dedicated and brief diagnostic or therapeutic tasks, nanodevices controlled by DNA computers might be imbued with encoded instructions for the initiation of self-disassembly and biodegradability. Hypothetically, in these cases, pliable nanodevices might contain fluid-filled cores that encapsulate DNA-based self-repairable "computers," perhaps serving as a "hybridic" species of artificial cell [75]. Instructions could conceivably be conveyed to external nanomedical instrumentation (e.g., nanogrippers [76], cellular lances [77], nanobiopsy [77], nanosyringes [78,79]—also comprised of biodegradable nanomaterials) when core-resident oligonucleotide fragments are induced to bind with specific synthetic (inner-wall protruding) receptors that are embedded within the membrane, which encases the nanodevice core. Modifications of chemical or electronic properties in wall-embedded molecules that ensue as a result of this oligonucleotide fragment binding might directly initiate the activation of dedicated diagnostic or therapeutic operations.

In an alternate configuration, stacks of nanoporous ultrathin films (e.g., graphene-based) fixed within the nanodevice core may serve as instruction routing/transmitting grids when specifically encoded single DNA strands transit through either single, or a sequential series of nanopores to "flip" computational switches, in initiating specific commands. Precursors to this concept might be illustrated via the single nanopore DNA assays that are currently (2012) being developed [80–82]. Individual nanopores could be interfaced with nanowires that penetrate through the core membrane to activate/manipulate specific nanoinstrument "stations" as directed by the core DNA/grid computer.

It has been demonstrated that solid-state (surface-mediated) DNA computing may be accomplished [83,84]. Liu et al. utilized the "immobilization and manipulation of combinatorial mixtures" of DNA on a gold substrate. In this investigation, all potential solutions to a computation problem were encoded in a set of DNA molecules that were tethered to a maleimide-functionalized gold surface, whereupon a consecutive series of "hybridization operations and exonuclease digestion" were employed to recognize and eradicate those DNA sequences that were not involved in the resolution of the problem. Subsequent to multiple cycles, the problem was resolved via identification utilizing a polymerase chain reaction, which amplified the remaining oligonucleotides for hybridization to an addressed array. The authors of this study point out that this approach is amenable with automation and scalability, and that "the use of solid-phase formats simplifies the complex repetitive chemical processes, as has been demonstrated in DNA and protein synthesis" [85].

The morphological aspects of DNA computation may be configured beyond typical duplexes or single-stranded oligonucleotides. Topological reconfigurations of DNA may, for example, produce Borromean rings, which are comprised of three or more interlocking rings. When any single ring is severed, the remaining interring connections will collapse. The validation of logical statements can be embodied by the integrity of linkages [15,86–88]. Adleman synthesized the first DNA computational device and revealed the power it held in the resolution of complex problems. He surmised it likely that "a single molecule of DNA can be used to encode the 'instantaneous description' of a Turing machine," and "the eventual emergence of a general purpose computer consisting of nothing more than a single macromolecule conjugated to a ribosome like collection of enzymes that act on it" [89,90].

DNA-based computational speed has been estimated at ~1.014 operations/s, or 100 teraflops (100 trillion floating-point operations per second) [91]. For perspective, IBM's Sequoia, one of the world's fastest supercomputers to date (2012), has the capacity for performing at a top speed of 20 petaflops = 20,000 teraflops [92]. DNA's parallelism has definite advantages for computation, as within the human body the transfer of information in the generation of molecules is swift and quite efficient. Hemoglobin molecules (comprised of 500 amino acids) are generated 500 trillion times per second. This translates to $\sim(15 \times 10^{18})$ "read" functions by ribosomes per minute [13]. In terms of storage capacity, DNA requires only 1 nm^3 to store a bit of information [91].

The contrast between in silico and DNA-based computation is that in silicon-based computation, each possibility must be independently analyzed until the correct answer is arrived at, whereas with DNA, all possibilities may be tested concurrently. However, DNA computation output is much more sluggish due to inherent inaccuracies, pair mismatches, and the integrity of enzymatic precision. "These difficulties will escalate exponentially as calculations necessary to solve a problem become more complex. Also, the cost of versatility can translate to instability, and a built-in redundancy that accommodates fault tolerance might culminate in an enormous slowdown in DNA reactivity" [93]. It is likely that DNA computation will never keep pace with silicon-based counterparts. Nevertheless, its utility in nanomedicine in vivo may be useful as relates to computation and highly localized control at molecular and cellular domains [91].

7.4 Nanometric Data Storage

7.4.1 Molecular Magnets

Molecular magnetism has made it feasible to store magnetic data in single molecules and could exponentially increase computer capacities. The controlled behavior of dimers of molecular magnets that interact according to the laws of quantum mechanics may lead to their application for the quantum processing of information. It has been demonstrated that isolated nanoscale magnetic molecules, whose behavior may be likened to that of a compass, might be blocked in a desired direction by a magnetic field, below its "blocking temperature." This level of stability gives assurance that information encoded by the magnetic field will be stored and can be retrieved at a later point in time [94].

At the molecular level, the "tunneling effect" can alter molecular magnetization, which is a drawback for the storage of information as it can culminate in the loss of element orientation, which are intended for blockage and in turn, to information loss. This effect might have utility when controlled with the aim of developing quantum devices that could operate using different principles. Investigators have demonstrated an example of two molecular magnets that are antiferromagnetically coupled, which orients them in opposite directions. Hence, each magnet influences its adjacent partner; therefore, the quantum attributes of the single-molecule magnet dimer are different from that of an individual single-molecule magnet [94].

The encapsulation of disk-shaped molecular magnets ($Mn_{12}Ac$) within multiwalled carbon nanotubes (MWNTs) (Ø ~6.5 ± 1.8 nm interior × 10–50 μm long) (Figure 7.3) has been

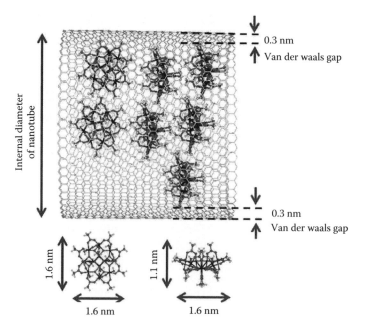

FIGURE 7.3
Molecular magnets ($Mn_{12}Ac$) encapsulated within the innermost layer of a MWNT as a potential nanoscale data storage device. Top and side views and dimensions of $Mn_{12}Ac$ are shown at bottom. (Image provided from Giménez-López, M. del C. et al., *Nat. Commun.*, 2, 407, 2011. With permission.)

investigated by Giménez-López et al., which may lead to the realization of magnetic data storage devices with ultrahigh density. In addition to the $Mn_{12}Ac$ structures and magnetic properties remaining unaltered once encapsulated, the molecules underwent significant "orientational ordering," which is beneficial for both data addressing and the control of nanotube electronic attributes. The $Mn_{12}Ac$ were also mobile within the MWNTs, which indicated that they were under the influence of van der Waals forces, and not covalently bound. The smallest nanotube diameter that can accommodate the $Mn_{12}Ac$ molecules (1.1 nm × 1.6 nm × 1.6 nm) is Ø 2.2 nm. This is inclusive of requisite 0.3 nm van der Waals gap that resides between the surfaces of the encapsulated molecule and the inner-wall faces of the nanotube [95].

7.4.2 Buckyballs (C_{60})

A potential tunable dual-level carbon nanotube-based system for information storage may be possible. A nanotube memory would exhibit high switching speeds, high packing density, and stability with nonvolatile data storage. Under specific conditions, a "bucky shuttle" will self-assemble from elemental carbon. This hybrid nanocapsule was synthesized by Kwon et al. via the thermal annealing of diamond powder (Ø ~4 to 6 nm) and heating in a graphite crucible in an inert argon atmosphere at 1800°C for 1 h. This forms multiwalled nanocapsules and smaller internalized fullerenes with diameters indicative of C_{60} (0.7 nm). In some instances, the enclosed fullerenes can transit relatively freely within the nanocapsule, with movement similar to a shuttle. Typically, however, the C_{60} is found at either end of the nanocapsule due to the concentrated attractive interwall interactions at these locations in contrast to those over the length (1.5 nm) of the nanocapsule. A $C_{60}@C_{480}$ system was fabricated as an optimized structure to encase a C_{60} molecule with an interwall distance of 3.4 Å. To transfer the C_{60} from one end of the nanocapsule to the other while effectively determining its location, the C_{60} should carry a net charge. This is accomplished via a $K@C_{60}$ complex, which forms naturally during synthesis in the presence of potassium. The valence electron of the encapsulated K atom is initially shifted to the C_{60} shell and then further transited to the outer graphitic nanocapsule. The enclosed K^+ ion does not alter the chemical makeup of the C_{60} [96].

For the write function, the C_{60} changes position from "bit 1" to "bit 0" via the application of an electric field (~1.5 V) between the C_{480} end caps, corresponding to the energetics of the switching field for C_{60} (Es = ±0.1 V/Å). The data, which is physically stored in the position of the C_{60}, is read noninvasively by distinguishing the polarity of the nanocapsule. Connecting nanocapsules in parallel serves to augment the total charge transfer (in this case, a single electron) as relates to the current pulse. The highest density can be realized by packing these memory elements in a form analogous to a carton of eggs. Rows of nanocapsules may be joined at either ends by nanowire electrodes such that a distinct memory node is defined at their crossing points. When a switching voltage is applied amid two crossing electrodes, a nonzero field will be generated in a single memory component. Manifold nanocapsule memory units may be addressed in parallel for the reading and writing of multiple bits. The switching (transit) interval for the C_{60} was found to be 4 ps at a 0.1 THz access rate, with a data throughput rate estimated to be ~10 Gb/s. Additionally, a 0.5 ps pulse of a 0.1–0.5 V/Å field was found to be adequate for the detachment of the C_{60}^+ ion from its end location to alter the memory state [96].

Cho et al. exploited charge variations in C_{60} molecules that were embedded within an insulating poly(4-vinyl phenol) layer. The voltage shift in this device was strongly dependent on the type of electrode used (e.g., Au, Al). The memory lifetime of this device at 300 K was calculated to be 10 years [97]. Along similar lines, Ling et al. synthesized a hybrid nonvolatile rewritable flash memory, which comprised carbazole electron donors and C_{60} electron acceptors, which were covalently bonded to a polymeric film of poly(N-vinylcarbazole) (PVK). Write, read, and erase states were available in a device that consisted of a core thin film of PVK-C_{60} laminated on either face by indium tin oxide and Al electrodes [98].

7.4.3 Multi-Quantum Dot Systems

It has been shown experimentally that multi-quantum dot systems may be employed as static single-electron memory devices with retention times of several hours [99]. The entrapment of carriers in quantum dots acts to negate their diffusion and dramatically decreases the rate of their recombination with ionized impurities, leading to decoherence. This feature can also be useful for information storage, and might be used as the basis for the development of devices with enhanced memory densities. The manipulation of charge storage in quantum dots can thus enable the rapid inscription and retrieval of data [100,101] with quantum dot switches and logic gates operating at >15 Tb/s. These systems may serve as key components in quantum computation that might be utilized for the storage, translation, and conveyance of large volumes of spatial nanomedical imaging data that is simultaneously collected by the scanning elements of the exemplar VCSN. This data would subsequently be conveyed to "outbody" computers.

A double-layered construct of self-aligned silicon quantum dots (upper layer—Ø 5 nm, lower layer—Ø 3 nm) with a high nanocrystal density (approx. >10^{12} dots/cm²) was demonstrated by Nassiopoulou and Salonidou to improve memory retention when compared to a single quantum dot layer. The researchers integrated two individual layers of "silicon nanocrystals within the gate dielectric of a MOS [metal–oxide–semiconductor] structure ...." Further improvements were seen in a double layer comprising vertically aligned nanocrystals of equal size (Ø 3 nm) with significantly larger dot-to-dot distances. It was learned that the "relative distance of the layers and their position from the silicon substrate and the gate metal are critical for optimum memory operation." The loss of charge in these systems over a projected 10 years of operation was ~12% [102].

Insights into electron transport through multiple quantum dots were conveyed by Gong et al. who noted that "mutually coupled multi-QD systems, in comparison with a single-QD structure, exhibit more intricate electron transport behaviors because these systems provide more Feynman paths for electron transmission" [103]. In quantum theory, the Feynman path integral formalism refers to the *probability* of a given particle being detected at a certain location and time between a hypothetical point A and point B, as in the quantum domain there are infinite space–time possibilities for its trajectory. As Feynman himself alluded

> In quantum mechanics the probability of an event which can happen in several different ways is the absolute square of a sum of complex contributions, one from each alternative way. The probability that a particle will be found to have a path $x(t)$ lying somewhere within a region of space time is the square of a sum of contributions, one from each path in the region [104].

Under a suitable magnetic fluctuations or spin–orbit interactions, a parallel-coupled quantum dot system, for instance, has additional parameters available with which to manipulate electronic transport. As such, the molecular conditions of the coupled quantum dots and electrical contacts may be regulated. In certain instances the full decoupling of molecular states and electrical contacts can occur, which gives rise to the "formation of remarkable bound states in the continuum" [103].

7.4.4 Ion Traps

Quantum data storage may involve qubits that reside within large arrays of interconnected ion traps wherein a qubit of data is encoded in the sustained dual electronic states of each ion [105]. To perform one or two qubit logic, the relevant ions are transited to accumulator regions where they interact with lasers that drive gates. An encoding method was demonstrated by Kielpinski et al. that stored a qubit of quantum information in the "decoherence-free subspace" (environmentally decoupled qubit isolating domain) of $^9Be^+$ (beryllium) ions. This strategy protected the qubit from storage-limiting dephasing, which typically occurs through "random fluctuations of the energy difference" of qubits, via their interaction with the environment [106,107].

A Penning trap (capable of containing charged particles within an electromagnetic field) was employed for the study of quantum control in modeling 2D $^9Be^+$ ion crystal arrays, which are created through mutual coulomb repulsion under cooling via a Doppler laser. The morphology of $^9Be^+$ ion crystals, representing a "spatial ensemble of qubits," was controlled via the application of external potentials and a laser. Stored under a 4.5 T magnetic field and activated by microwaves, the $^9Be^+$ ion ground-state qubits (at 124 GHz electron spin-flip transition and ~300 MHz nuclear spin-flip transition) are useful in elucidating strategies for "single ion addressing useful for the realization of complex entangled states" [108–110]. This work presents a further possibility, which may culminate in the development of a highly dense, solid-state quantum data storage strategy.

7.4.5 Quantum Dot Cellular Automata

Nanomedical information may be stored by means of electronic and magnetic interactions in molecular quantum dot cellular automata (MQCA), which may comprise grid-like arrays of quantum dot cells (localized regions of charge contained within semiconductors, molecules, magnetic nanoparticles, or metallic islands), analogous to von Neumann's cellular automata [111]. These systems can enable computation at an ultralow power draw with extremely rapid switching, where charge/magnetic configurations between molecular redox-active sites are exploited to encode binary information. Cell-to-cell coupling is achieved through coulomb interactions between proximal molecules, where electrons are held in antipodal sites via repulsion. This system negates the requirement of electrical current flow and transistors, yet has the capacity for moving signals across multiple cells. Lent et al. explain that the molecular constituents of these systems may be considered "not as current switches but as structured charge containers" [112].

Digital logic gates, based on the location of two electrons in a four-dot cell, coupled by tunnel junctions in a ring of four cells that surround a central cell (configured as a cruciform), may be utilized to encode binary information. The cell is charged by two excess electrons that occupy a diagonal polarization representing "0" and "1." Quantum dot cells do not communicate through the transfer of electrons but rather by the electric fields of their electrons. A high-energy state exists when electrons are in close proximity to each other due to their repulsive force. When the electrons are distanced from each other, they relax and the system transitions to a lower-energy state. The fundamental logic device is a three-input majority logic gate comprising five cells: a central logic cell, three inputs, and an output cell. The central dot serves to improve the activities of each cell. In operation, the polarization of the logic cell becomes that of the majority of the three input cells [113]. These devices can be cascaded such that three inputs of a subsequent cell are triggered by the outputs of previous gates. The resulting output can then be interfaced to drive subsequent logic gates [114]. A 2D self-assembly of DNA crystal tiles of a cellular automaton was shown to fabricate a fractal pattern (Sierpinski triangle) as it grew [115].

Arima et al. revealed a new category of engineered organometallic molecule (6-3,6-bis(1-ethylferrocen)-9H-carbazol-9-yl-6-hexan-1-thiols), also referred to as "bisferrocene," that exhibited the simultaneous capacity to meet all essential structural and functional prerequisites of cells to comprise quantum cellular automata, namely, the ability to effectively retain charge in different quantum dots for the strict encoding of Boolean states, allowing for the clocking deletion of a state when an external signal is applied and to maintain stable solid-state geometries to facilitate electrostatic interactions [116]. In another development, Wang and Ma studied double-caged fluorinated fullerene molecules $(e(-)@C_{20}F_{18}(XH)2C_{20}F_{18}$ $(X = N, B))$, which can serve as binary encoding electron switches that possess bistable charge configurations, as a potential novel contender for MQCA. They suggest that room temperature operation may be achieved by shrinking MQCA elements to ~2 nm, which will act to "increase the state energy difference." At this scale, densities in MQCA may contain 10^{11}–10^{12} cells with an energy dissipation that approaches the lowest level dictated by physics [117].

Wang and Liu have proposed a conceptual nanopatterned graphene quantum dot cellular automata (GQD-QCA) (Figure 7.4) for the transmission of binary data and to conduct logic operations that would utilize single graphene sheets as planar substrates to accommodate complete device architectures and be amenable with conventional (2012) electronics [118]. It was suggested that semiconductor–metal–semiconductor graphene nanoribbon (GNR) junctions [119] (Figure 7.5) might serve as GQDs to facilitate the construction of highly dense QCAs with ultrafast operation. It was calculated that, due to their shapes and structures, Z-shaped GNR junctions have the capacity to fully confine electronic states. Further, this spatial confinement may be altered by modifying the length of the junction and,

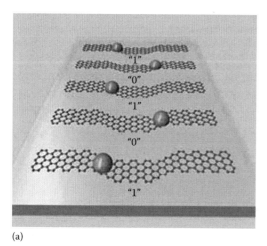

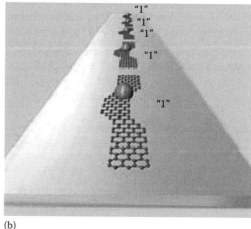

(a)   (b)

FIGURE 7.4
Depiction of five QCA cells oriented (a) vertically—5 nm intercell distance and (b) horizontally—8 nm intercell distance. Spheres represent the presence of electrons within bits 1 and 0. (Reproduced from Wang, Z.F. and Liu, F., *Nanoscale*, 3(10), 4201, 2011. With permission.)

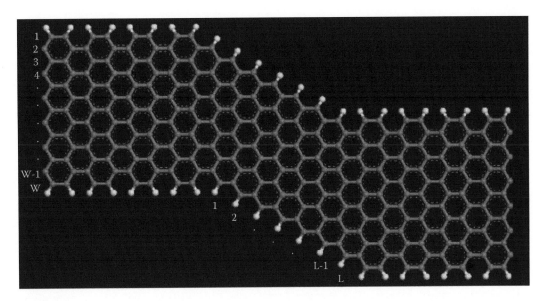

FIGURE 7.5
Z-shaped graphene nanoribbon junction comprised of left lead, middle junction, and right lead. (Reproduced from Wang, Z.F. et al., *Appl. Phys. Lett.*, 91, 053109-1-3, 2007. With permission.)

interestingly, the confined states remain stable despite the presence of significant anomalies at the edges of the junction. The researchers note that additional graphene nanostructures, such as graphene nanoflakes, might be employed to form QCA cells [120,121].

A binary wire comprises capacitively coupled double (quantum) dot cells that are charged with single electrons. Metal islands fabricated by electron beam lithography are connected in series via tunnel junctions with a capacitance of ~2.5 e/mV. Polarization switching is initiated by an applied input signal in one cell that incites a change in polarization in an adjacent cell, analogous to a falling cascade of dominoes. This arrangement constitutes an alternate form of QCA [122,123]. If the polarization of a double-dot cell is forced from −1 to +1, its neighboring cell will flip from +1 to −1. A QCA wire exploits this principal, in that the polarization at the input of the wire leads in succession to polarization changes in all of the cells along the wire, with a subsequent system relaxation in its new ground state. Since no current flows through the wire, power dissipation is minimal [124]. Simulations have been conducted through the insertion of various imperfections within the wire, including variations in the dimensions of the cells that comprise it, errors in intercellular spacing, and the presence of extra electrons [124,125]. Results have indicated that the wire maintained proper functionality. The highly nonlinear response function acts to correct mistakes and restore the signal level [123].

7.4.6 Magnetic Nanowires

Highly uniform arrays of magnetic nanowires were non-lithographically produced by Tulchinsky et al. via a molecular beam epitaxial evaporation/shadowing technique on a nanoscopically corrugated surface. The corrugated surface was produced by the laser-focused deposition of Cr atoms in lines that were formed by a standing wave, directed along the gradient of the light intensity. Iron was subsequently evaporated at a perpendicular orientation to the Cr lines and the ferromagnetic nanowire dimensions acquired

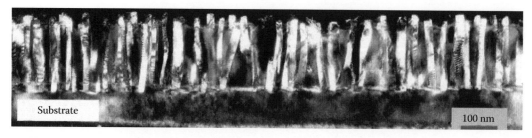

FIGURE 7.6
Side-view depiction of single crystalline α-Fe nanowires on a SrTiO$_3$ (001) substrate via the decomposition of La$_{0.5}$Sr$_{0.5}$FeO$_3$ perovskite. (Reproduced from Mohaddes-Ardabili, L. et al., *Nat. Mater.*, 3(8), 533, 2004. With permission.)

were ~100 nm wide and ~0.15 mm long. These nanowires could be removed from the substrate by immersion into an iron etch. By superimposing two standing waves at 90° to each other, iron island domains with an average length of ~16 μm were produced, forming a 2D grid with a spacing of 213 nm. If each domain were to store 1 bit of information, this configuration might enable a data storage density of ~15 Gbits/in.^{2} [126].

The synthesis of Co$_x$Ni$_{1-x}$ alloy nanowires (Ø 130 nm × 20 μm long) was accomplished by electrochemical deposition utilizing a nanoporous hard anodic aluminum oxide membrane template. The resulting Co–Ni nanowires were sheltered from oxidation subsequent to their release from the alumina template by a 10 nm thick SiO$_2$ coating that was initially applied to the template by atomic layer deposition. It was discovered that a high Co content (51–71 at%) facilitated the manipulation of the magnetic performance of the nanowires, allowing for the control of their magnetocrystalline anisotropy, which is amenable for applications in data storage and the development of unique spintronic devices [127].

Kou et al. demonstrated for the first time an analog memory effect in an array of Ni$_{90}$Fe$_{10}$ nanowires (Ø 35 nm × 20 μm long) with a 60 nm center-to-center spacing. It was surmised that the memory effect had its source in a "strong magnetic dipole interaction among the nanowires." A capacity for passively retaining the peak magnetic field in multiple magnetic field pulses was exhibited in the array, which could later be read by a magnetic field sensor (Gauss meter). This very low cost system withstood and measured electromagnetic pulses as high as several hundred Oe (Oersted) without degradation [128].

Self-assembled arrays of single crystalline α-Fe nanowires (Figure 7.6) have been synthesized through the phase decomposition of a single-phase La0.5Sr0.5FeO3 perovskite target during thin film growth on a single crystalline SrTiO$_3$ (001) substrate, via pulsed laser deposition. Interestingly, the magnetic properties (e.g., coercivity and remanence) of these nanowires, and hence their efficacy in data storage, may be tuned as the result of the various diameters and cross-sectional geometries that are produced at different temperatures. The diameters of the nanowires were decreased under lower deposition temperatures (Ø 40–50 nm at 840°C, Ø 15–20 nm at 760°C, and Ø 4–6 nm at 560°C) and their cross-sectional geometries transitioned from square, octagonal, to circular at 840°C, 760°C, and 560°C, respectively (Figure 7.7) [129].

7.4.7 "Millipede" Data Storage

The "Millipede" data storage strategy, devised by Vettiger et al., utilized a thermomechanical local-probe technique to read, write, and delete data in ultrathin polymeric

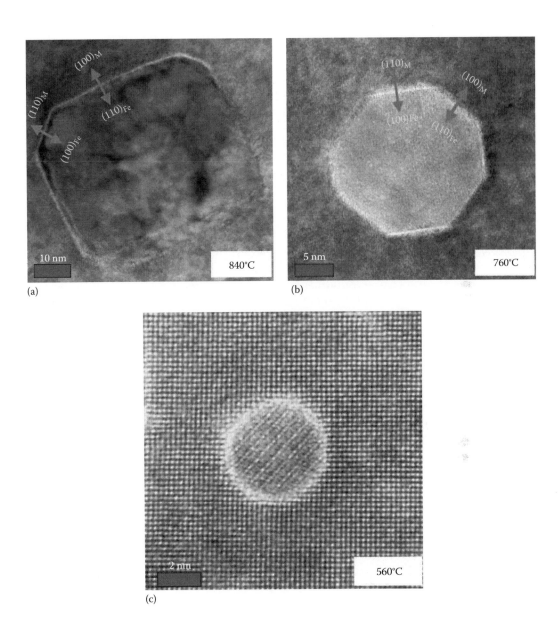

FIGURE 7.7
(a–c) Distinct alterations in cross-sectional geometries of single crystalline α-Fe nanowires under different temperatures. (Reproduced from Mohaddes-Ardabili, L. et al., *Nat. Mater.*, 3(8), 533, 2004. With permission.)

(polymethylmethacrylate [PMMA]) films. Silicon substrates were coated with 40 nm thick PMMA layer to achieve obtain data storage densities of up to 1 Tb/in.[2] by utilizing bit (indentation) sizes in the range of 10–50 nm. Indentations with dimensions of 40 nm were scribed at a 120 nm pitch (translating to a density of 400 Gb/in.[2]) using parallel arrays of atomic force microscope (AFM) cantilever tips. These nanometrically sharp tips are dependable implements that provide a critical purpose, namely, "the ultimate local confinement of interaction" [130].

This 2D-cantilever array data storage approach operates via the mechanical x/y scanning of storage media in massively parallel fashion [131,132]. A sensor-controlled feedback loop mediates z-axis actuator motion and thus the orientation of the cantilever array, which might conceivably contain >1000 cantilever tips to enable simultaneous contact with, and bit reading from the storage media. To significantly simplify the system, the feedback control is configured for the total chip rather than its individual constituent cantilevers, which necessitates a high level of uniformity insofar as cantilever tip lengths and flexing profiles. An anti-vibratory function is integrated as well to facilitate precision leveling during read/write events [133]. The storage function involves magnetic raster scanning of the storage media by the chip, where individual cantilevers inscribe and retrieve data in dedicated storage fields [134]. This strategy negates lateral positioning requirements, which would compensate for deviations in tip tolerances [130].

One drawback of this system was that to ensure proper functionality, the temperature between the chip array and the medium substrate could not deviate beyond 1°C of the nominal operating temperature. Four integrated heat sensors were utilized to control dedicated heaters to maintain thermal stability [134]. Hypothetically, an analogous derivative of the Millipede system might be scaled down and designed as modular nanometric units to provide a substantial data storage capacity for nanomedical devices. Nanofibers, nanowires, or C_{60} molecules could potentially serve as nanocantilevers to operate in conjunction with magnetically functionalized ultrathin film monolayer storage media.

7.4.8 Optical Crystals

Silicon nanocrystal-based nonvolatile memory devices that were fabricated via ion implantation have been investigated by Walters et al., which operate via the optical detection of variable intensities of photoluminescence, enabling the deciphering of programmed logic states. Data were shown to be electronically and optically inscribed and deleted through charge injection and internal photoemission, respectively. This device used gate oxide–integrated silicon nanocrystals to replace typically utilized polysilicon floating gates. The retention of data was maintained for 100 s at room temperature [135]. Ng et al. studied the stability and performance of a silicon nanocrystal (~4 nm)-based flash memory that contained 7 and 3 nm thick tunnel oxides, which both accommodated 10^5 write/erase cycles at 85°C. This translated to projected charge losses over 10 years of 20% for the 7 nm thick tunnel oxide, and 70% for the 3 nm thick tunnel oxide [136].

A completely optical memory based on injection-locking bistability [137] and comprising an embedded InGaAsP/InP heterostructure photonic crystal laser ($4 \times 0.3 \times 0.16\ \mu m^3$ active region) was demonstrated by Chen et al. This robust device operated under low power (25 µW) at high switching speeds (~60 ps). Active memory functions were enabled under 100 µW pump power and a waveguide switching power of 22 and 71 µW. This device executed continuous wave operations at room temperature in an "InP air-bridge structure," where the InP was highly thermally conductive and thus could dissipate heat from the cavity with a 10-fold improvement over InGaAsP [138].

Clausen et al. employed a rare earth ion-doped biaxial yttrium orthosilicate (Y_2SiO_5) crystal in the development of an optical solid-state quantum memory with a polarization state retrieval reliability of ~97.5%. Data were encoded into what are known as "heralded" single-photon qubits, where the detection of an idler photon of a photon pair "heralds" the emergence/presence of its signal photon, which serves as the polarization qubit [139]. In another investigation of photon quantum storage in solids, Gündoğan et al. demonstrated single-photon solid-state quantum storage and retrieval in a praseodymium-doped crystal. The duration of qubit storage duration in this instance was 500 ns, while the storage and retrieval efficiency was determined to be 10% with qubit fidelity of 95% [140].

7.4.9 DNA Data Storage

Data storage for nanomedical devices may be possible utilizing binary DNA substrates. There are a number of attractive advantages for the implementation of DNA as a nanomedical data storage medium, encompassing

1. *Capacity for high-density data storage.* Church et al. note that "At theoretical maximum, DNA can encode 2 bits per nucleotide (nt) or 455 exabytes per gram of single-stranded DNA" [141]. For reference, one terabyte = 10^{12} bytes, whereas one exabyte = 10^{18} bytes.

2. *Inherent biocompatibility.* Nanomedical data storage modules may likely be derived from the patient's own DNA.

3. *Prolonged viability.* DNA has the capacity for remaining viable in terms of stable data preservation, for hundreds of years [142,143].

4. *Relatively straightforward data accessibility and retrieval.* Nanomedical data might be retrieved via compact high-throughput sequencing, utilizing solid-state nanoporous arrays [144].

The practical use of DNA for data storage in nanomedical devices will be contingent; however, on significant technological advances in the synthesis of oligonucleotides and sequencing of DNA. Sennels and Bentin estimate that as a prerequisite for realistic large-scale DNA storage "an increase in scale of synthesis on the order of 7-orders-of-magnitude, and a corresponding 6-order-of-magnitude increase of scale of sequenced features would be necessary to reach storage-capacities in the exabyte-range" [141,143]. Strategic issues to be explored when considering the prospective use of DNA computation and/or storage to enable nanomedical devices might include investigations into the limits of their packing density and feasible operation within the tight spatial constraints ($\sim$300–400 nm^3) at the cores of nanodevices (at nominal external nanodevice dimensions of $\sim$1 μm). Hypothetically, highly dense stacks of ultrathin ($\sim$2 nm) self-assembling solid-state (crystalline) DNA tiles [145,146] might have the capacity for retaining binary data that can be rapidly optically encoded and read by onboard nanowire or quantum dot–based lasers.

7.4.10 Atomic Data Storage

In conventional electronics (2012), $\sim$1 million atoms are required to magnetically store a single bit of data. An idealistic data storage device that would reside at the core of an advanced autonomous nanomedical device might require an atomically engineered solid-state entity with a data retention capacity in the range of 10^9–10^{10} bits [15].

Loth et al. have managed to store one nonvolatile bit of data within a group of only 12 antiferromagnetic Fe atoms, and a byte (8 bits) within 96 atoms, on a Cu_2N substrate at 1 K (-272.15°C), where each bit occupied an area of 9 nm^2. At room temperature (293 K/20°C), a bit could be stored on 150 such atoms. Antiferromagnetic atoms are devoid of intrinsic magnetic moments and thus are not susceptible to magnetic fields. Adjacent antiferromagnetic atoms possess oppositely aligned magnetic moments; hence, the character of these bits allowed for independent switching, which occurred at $>\sim$7 mV (via an AFM tip), without disturbing the states of adjoining bits. In contrast, ferromagnetic inter-atom state perturbation does occur in switching as the atomic magnetic moments are aligned [147].

A single-atom quantum memory was devised by Specht et al. who discerned the photonic polarization qubit states of an isolated ^{87}Rb atom, which was trapped in a high-finesse optical cavity (midway between two conical mirrors). The atom exhibited a fidelity of 93% with minimal decoherence, which enabled >180 μs coherence times [148]. In another such study, Hétet et al. employed a single ^{138}Ba$^+$ ion that might be utilized in a prospective quantum memory application [149]. Quaade et al. utilized a scanning tunneling microscope (STM) to demonstrate reversible binary data storage at room temperature using a single hydrogen atom on a silicon dimer at a Si(100) surface. The electron-induced directional switching of the H atom occurred at a negative sample bias at –2.7 V, which was employed rather than a positive bias, which would likely desorb the H atom from the surface. The state of the H atom switch could be read using a bias voltage of –1.5 V via a STM single line scan at 3 Å to one side of the switch, and could be set by a –2.7 V pulse. A 4-bit desorbed H atom memory node array was also fabricated [150].

An electron-spin qubit tethered to a donated phosphorus atom in natural silicon was shown by Pla et al. to have a coherence time of over 200 μs, making it amenable for scalable longer-term quantum memory. Spin coherence times may be extended even further with the use of "isotopically enriched" ^{28}Si [151,152]. Subsequent to suppressing the interactions of other donor electron spins with a magnetic field, Tyryshkin et al. observed a donor $T2$ electron spin coherence of 10 s at 1.8 K in pristine ^{28}Si crystals. The $T1$ value for shallow phosphorous donors has been reported to be close to an hour at 1.2 K and 0.35 T [153].

7.4.11 Cortical Memristive Memory

An alternate pathway in the quest for dense nonvolatile nanoscale data storage for nanomedical devices may involve the biomimetic emulation of synapses of the brain. Within the human cortex the concentration of synapses numbers ~10^{10}/cm^2, whereas in today's microprocessors the transistor density is close to 10^9/cm^2. A basic electronic memristive nanodevice comprised of a several nanometer-thick memristive material (e.g., titanium oxide and other transition metal oxides), which is interfaced on either side by two metallic nanowires, creates an entity that can vary its resistance over a certain timeline in association with the intensity of the current that transits through it. Hence, akin to a diminutive analog memory, it "remembers" how to respond to variable current flows and varies its resistance state accordingly. Neuromorphic crossbar (grid-like) constructs have been fabricated in an attempt to emulate, albeit with stacked/linear architectures, the organization of neurons and synapses [154–156]. Kim et al. observed in their study of flexible resistive random access memory that "By integration of a high-performance single crystal silicon transistor with a titanium oxide based memristor, random access to memory cells on flexible substrates was achieved without any electrical interference from adjacent cells" [155].

7.5 Nanomedical Computation: Safety and Security

Concurrent with the evolution of sophisticated nanomedical devices that function to enable myriad benefits for patients will be the responsibility to ensure that computational devices embedded within them are sufficiently protected by robust quantum security protocols.

These measures will serve to negate infection by advanced computer viruses (which will undoubtedly also evolve), or unscrupulous hacking, which might otherwise have potentially devastating consequences.

A proof of principal to evidence the possibility of transmission of a virus from a hand-embedded computer chip was conducted by Mark Gasson (University of Reading's School of Systems Engineering). During the course of trials, Gasson demonstrated that his implanted chip, which was purposefully infected with a computer virus, was subsequently able to transmit the virus to external control systems [157]. This research has pertinent implications for future patients who opt for therapies that are enabled by nanomedical devices. Nanomedical software could conceivably be infected or disabled by other classes of nanodevices or AI-controlled implants that reside within their own bodies. Disruptive code might also conceivably be unwittingly conveyed by other implanted patients who are within transmission range or surreptitiously transmitted wirelessly from external sources over great distances. It will be prudent, if not critical, to establish international standardized software protocols for the protection of nanomedical quantum computation devices and other nanocomputers to certify that they will be compatible when in operation within patients, and rendered "immune" to external online corruption.

7.6 Proposed Research Tasking List: VCSN Quantum Computing Component

Following is a list of preliminary suggestions, considerations, and relevant questions as relates to perceived areas of investigation toward the development of the exemplar VCSN quantum computing component:

1. Initiate a preliminary survey to discern the state-of-the-art work being done toward the development of quantum computation technologies.

2. Based on this research, select the quantum computation modality that might best be suited to control the functionalities of the VCSN.

3. Investigate what materials may exhibit the most robust and stable environment for qubit manipulation.

4. Explore what methodologies, materials, and fabrication techniques might be best suited for the construction of quantum computing circuitry.

5. Research, design, and fabricate a prototype quantum circuit on an appropriate ultrathin film substrate.

6. Investigate how a quantum computer would transmit commands to specific VCSN components. What mode of signal conveyance might be appropriate and optimal? Assuming that a global language would be established for internalized commands, how will command domains be partitioned within the quantum computer itself? Would distinct computational domains be dedicated to and programmed with component control-specific data? Would the components themselves be equipped with embedded command translation nodes to derive specific instruction sets from the data that is sent from the quantum computer? Perhaps dedicated command codes might be developed to differentiate simultaneous

command streams in order to avoid any confusion as to what signal is destined for which component. Feedback loops could verify that specific commands have been carried out successfully.

7. Investigate IBM's "Millipede" technology (see Section 7.4.7) to discern if an analogous method of computation might be designed that would be appropriate for the VCSN.

8. Investigate the plausibility of allocating a portion of a quantum data storage node to be utilized as a transient cache for acquired spatial data, which would intermittently be purged and refreshed with new incoming data.

9. In view of the many demands that would be made on a VCSN-resident quantum computer (e.g., direction/control of all navigational, propulsive, and scanning components, preprocessing of acquired spatial data, and real-time translation of all communications), investigate what the maximum capacity requirements of temporary spatial data storage might be. Speculatively, there may be several hundreds to thousands of modular scanning units onboard the VCSN.

10. How would a hypothetical VCSN quantum computer be physically organized? How and where would its functional domains be allocated?

11. What routing strategy might be implemented to physically interface the quantum computer to all VCSN elements and how would each of these connections be tested and verified?

12. Might a quantum computer be fabricated as a lamination of layer-by-layer ultrathin film circuitry to incrementally build up a functional entity? (e.g., each layer might be comprised of precisely synthesized quantum circuitry)

13. Conceptualize and design, once an optimal quantum computer design is achieved, preliminary manufacturing techniques (e.g., large-scale ultrathin film lamination techniques, self-assembly, or nucleic acid–based manufacturing), which may be applied to their massively parallel fabrication.

14. Might it be feasible, and what strategy might be employed, to fabricate the VCSN structure around a solid-state or aqueously immersed/encased quantum computer "seed" by building up layer by layer, precisely configured laminations while laying down all nanoelectronic connections in the process?

15. What strategies may be employed to physically shield and isolate a quantum computer from potentially damaging aberrations that might result from background radiation, peripheral electromagnetic fields, etc.?

16. Determine the best approach (based on the survey of current quantum computer research) for the optimal configuration of qubit computing that might have specific application to the VCSN and its requirement for processing enormous volumes of spatial data.

17. Determine the physical and electronic constraints that emerge as the result of increasing qubit density.

18. What quantum effects might impinge on the robust functionality and integrity of input/output data within a quantum computer?

19. Investigate scenarios by which a quantum computer might be spontaneously activated and deactivated from an external source during normal operations, and internally, in the event of external control infrastructure failure.

20. Develop fail-safe protocols that could be instituted to address issues such as specific component failure, total device failure, power interruption, device entrapment, loss of propulsion, navigational, or communications control.

21. Subsequent to a survey of existing quantum computation modalities, investigate what entity might be most appropriate in representing a qubit (e.g., atom, electron, photon, etc.).

22. Assess the strategic efficiencies of preprocessing acquired spatial data prior to the transmission of data streams, in contrast to transmitting acquired data in real time, to be fully processed by more powerful external quantum computers.

23. Investigate and simulate a scenario in which perhaps thousands of VCSNs might be deployed simultaneously. Determine the level of independent activity that would be appropriate for quantum computers embedded within each VCSN, and what levels of interconnectivity and collective computation may be required to rapidly (5 min) accomplish the scanning of the entire human vasculature or lymphatic system.

24. What echelon of redundancy (e.g., multiple standby layers of identical quantum circuitry that may be activated in the event of original circuit failures) should be integrated into a VCSN-resident quantum computer so as to ensure optimum reliability of operation?

25. Estimate what operational computing power and memory capacity should be incorporated into the quantum computer of the VCSN toward discerning an appropriate level of supplemental computing ability that could be made available if required.

26. What emergency backup protocols might be engaged to negate events where data are inadvertently lost or corrupted in some way?

27. What type of encoding might be utilized to protect the VCSN against any software "infectant" (either accidental or malicious) that could deleteriously affect the optimal functionality of its quantum computer?

28. Should all VCSN quantum computers be "factory" programmed in an identical manner, or might a certain percentage be endowed with specialized "mission executive" status programming? (e.g., these VCSNs may be endowed with enhanced status so as to coordinate and possibly issue commands "in the field" contingent on local conditions, and to deal with unanticipated situations).

29. Investigate how external primary and backup quantum computer systems might be configured and designed. Perhaps an external "backup array" would receive signals that are broadcast from in vivo VCSNs and would replicate exactly, all nanodevice internal computations, as well as all received and transmitted data streams that have occurred during the entire scanning procedure. Each of the quantum computers residing in the backup array "rack" would be assigned and dedicated to the replication of all data from its particular internalized VCSN quantum computer "twin." These data backup/storage strategy may serve as a reliable permanent record of all computations that are executed by each VCSN during the course of the scanning process. It might also be utilized in error tracing, the recovery of corrupted or lost data and serve as an accurate patient archive. In the future, when quantum technologies are sufficiently advanced, instantaneous backup might be accomplished via quantum entanglement.

References

1. Simmons, S., Brown, R.M., Riemann, H., Abrosimov, N.V., Becker, P., Pohl, H.J., Thewalt, M.L., Itoh, K.M., and Morton, J.J., Entanglement in a solid-state spin ensemble. *Nature.* 470(7332), 69–72, 2011.
2. Merkle, R.C., Nanotechnology and medicine, in *Advances in Anti-Aging Medicine*, Klatz, R.M., ed. Liebert Press, Palo Alto, CA, Vol. I, 277–286, 1996.
3. Forshaw, J., Jeff Forshaw: Quantum computers are leaping ahead. The Observer, May 6, 2012. http://www.guardian.co.uk/science/2012/may/06/quantum-computing-physics-jeff-forshaw (accessed October 15, 2012).
4. Demming, A., Opposites attract: Nanomagnetism in theory and practice. *Nanotechnology.* 23(39), 390201, 2012.
5. Pouthier, V., Vibrons in finite size molecular lattices: A route for high-fidelity quantum state transfer at room temperature. *J Phys Condens Matter.* 24(44), 445401, 2012.
6. Fitzsimons, J. and Twamley, J., Globally controlled quantum wires for perfect qubit transport, mirroring, and computing. *Phys Rev Lett.* 97(9), 090502, 2006.
7. Szumniak, P., Bednarek, S., Partoens, B., and Peeters, F.M., Spin-orbit-mediated manipulation of heavy-hole spin qubits in gated semiconductor nanodevices. *Phys Rev Lett.* 109(10), 107201, 2012.
8. Pla, J.J., Tan, K.Y., Dehollain, J.P., Lim, W.H., Morton, J.J., Jamieson, D.N., Dzurak, A.S., and Morello, A., A single-atom electron spin qubit in silicon. *Nature.* 489(7417), 541–545, 2012.
9. Morello, A., Pla, J.J., Zwanenburg, F.A., Chan, K.W., Tan, K.Y., Huebl, H., Möttönen, M., Nugroho, C.D., Yang, C., van Donkelaar, J.A., Alves, A.D., Jamieson, D.N., Escott, C.C., Hollenberg, L.C., Clark, R.G., and Dzurak, A.S., Single-shot readout of an electron spin in silicon. *Nature.* 467(7316), 687–691, 2010.
10. Kurzweil, R., The law of accelerating returns. Kurzweil AI Network, March 7, 2001. http://www.kurzweilai.net/the-law-of-accelerating-returns (accessed October 15, 2012).
11. Kurzweil, R., *The Age of Spiritual Machines When Computers Exceed Human Intelligence.* Penguin, New York, 1999. http://www.penguinputnam.com/static/packages/us/kurzweil/excerpts/exmain.htm (accessed October 15, 2012).
12. Ostman, C., Synthetic sentience on demand, 1998. http://project.cyberpunk.ru/idb/synthetic_sentience.html (accessed October 15, 2012).
13. Kurzweil, R., *The Age of Intelligent Machines.* MIT Press, Cambridge, MA, 1990.
14. Nielson, M.A. and Chuang, I.L., *Quantum Computation and Quantum Information.* Cambridge University Press, Cambridge, 2010.
15. Freitas, R.A. Jr., *Nanomedicine, Volume I: Basic Capabilities.* Landes Bioscience, Georgetown, TX, 1999.
16. Sun, J., Wu, X., Palade, V., Fang, W., Lai, C.H., and Xu, W., Convergence analysis and improvements of quantum-behaved particle swarm optimization. *Inf Sci.* 193, 81–103, 2012.
17. Terhal, B.M., Hassler, F., and Divincenzo, D.P., From Majorana fermions to topological order. *Phys Rev Lett.* 108(26), 260504, 2012.
18. Morimae, T. and Fujii, K., Blind topological measurement-based quantum computation. *Nat Commun.* 3, 1036, 2012.
19. Raussendorf, R., Key ideas in quantum error correction. *Philos Transact A Math Phys Eng Sci.* 370(1975), 4541–4565, 2012.
20. Tempel, D.G. and Aspuru-Guzik, A., Quantum computing without wavefunctions: Time-dependent density functional theory for universal quantum computation. *Sci Rep.* 2, 391, 2012.
21. Monroe, C., Meekhof, D.M., King, B.E., Itano, W.M., and Wineland, D.J., Demonstration of a fundamental quantum logic gate. *Phys Rev Lett.* 75(25), 4714–4717, 1995.
22. Turchette, Q.A., Hood, C.J., Lange, W., Mabuchi, H., and Kimble, H.J., Measurement of conditional phase shifts for quantum logic. *Phys Rev Lett.* 75(25), 4710–4713, 1995.
23. Platzman, P.M. and Dykman, M.I., Quantum computing with electrons floating on liquid helium. *Science.* 284(5422), 1967–1969, 1999.

24. Criger, B., Passante, G., Park, D., and Laflamme, R., Recent advances in nuclear magnetic resonance quantum information processing. *Philos Transact A Math Phys Eng Sci.* 370(1976), 4620–4635, 2012.

25. Bell, M.T., Sadovskyy, I.A., Ioffe, L.B., Kitaev, A.Y., and Gershenson, M.E., Quantum superinductor with tunable nonlinearity. *Phys Rev Lett.* 109(13), 137003, 2012.

26. Rohling, N. and Burkard, G., Universal quantum computing with spin and valley arXiv:1203.5041v1 [cond-mat.mes-hall] March 22, 2012. http://arxiv.org/pdf/1203.5041v1.pdf (accessed 06/23/13).

27. Barreiro, J.T., Müller, M., Schindler, P., Nigg, D., Monz, T., Chwalla, M., Hennrich, M., Roos, C.F., Zoller, P., and Blatt, R., An open-system quantum simulator with trapped ions. *Nature.* 470(7335), 486–491, 2011.

28. Nadj-Perge, S., Frolov, S.M., Bakkers, E.P., and Kouwenhoven, L.P., Spin-orbit qubit in a semiconductor nanowire. *Nature.* 468(7327), 1084–1087, 2010.

29. Weber, J.R., Koehl, W.F., Varley, J.B., Janotti, A., Buckley, B.B., Van de Walle, C.G., and Awschalom, D.D., Quantum computing with defects. *Proc Natl Acad Sci USA.* 107(19), 8513–8518, 2010.

30. Duke, C.B., Atomic and electronic structure of tetrahedrally coordinated compound semiconductor interfaces. *J Vac Sci Technol A.* 6(3), 1957–1963, 1988.

31. Zhang, J., Laflamme, R., and Suter, D., Experimental implementation of encoded logical qubit operations in a perfect quantum error correcting code. *Phys Rev Lett.* 109(10), 100503, 2012.

32. Reed, M.D., DiCarlo, L., Nigg, S.E., Sun, L., Frunzio, L., Girvin, S.M., and Schoelkopf, R.J., Realization of three-qubit quantum error correction with superconducting circuits. *Nature.* 482(7385), 382–385, 2012.

33. Vijay, R., Slichter, D.H., and Siddiqi, I., Observation of quantum jumps in a superconducting artificial atom. *Phys Rev Lett.* 106(11), 110502, 2011.

34. Fujiwara, M., Tanaka, A., Takahashi, S., Yoshino, K., Nambu, Y., Tajima, A., Miki, S., Yamashita, T., Wang, Z., Tomita, A., and Sasaki, M., After pulselike phenomenon of superconducting single photon detector in high speed quantum key distribution system. *Opt Express.* 19(20), 19562–19571, 2011.

35. Bennewitz, R., Crain, J.N., Kirakosian, A., Lin, J.L., McChesney, J.L., Petrovykh, D.Y., and Himpsel, F.J., Atomic scale memory at a silicon surface. *Nanotechnology.* 13, 499, 2002.

36. Farra, R., Sheppard, N.F. Jr., McCabe, L., Neer, R.M., Anderson, J.M., Santini, J.T. Jr., Cima, M.J., and Langer, R., First-in-human testing of a wirelessly controlled drug delivery microchip. *Sci Transl Med.* 4(122), 122ra21, 2012.

37. Rapoport, B.I., Kedzierski, J.T., and Sarpeshkar, R., A glucose fuel cell for implantable brain-machine interfaces. *PLoS One.* 7(6), e38436, 2012.

38. Theunisse, H.J., Gotthardt, M., and Mylanus, E.A., Surgical planning and evaluation of implanting a penetrating cochlear nerve implant in human temporal bones using microcomputed tomography. *Otol Neurotol.* 33(6), 1027–1033, 2012.

39. Warwick, K., Gasson, M., Hutt, B., Goodhew, I., Kyberd, P., Andrews, B., Teddy, P., and Shad, A., The application of implant technology for cybernetic systems. *Arch Neurol.* 60(10), 1369–1373, 2003.

40. Jung, L.H., Shany, N., Lehmann, T., Preston, P., Lovell, N.H., and Suaning, G.J., Towards a chip scale neurostimulator: System architecture of a current-driven 98 channel neurostimulator via a two-wire interface. *Conf Proc IEEE Eng Med Biol Soc.* 2011, 6737–6740, 2011.

41. Jefferson, J., Fearn, M., Tipton, D.L.J., and Spiller, T.S., Two-electron quantum dots as scalable qubits. Technical Report, Hewlett-Packard Laboratories, Bristol, U.K., July 30, 2002. http://www.hpl.hp.com/techreports/2002/HPL-2002-175R1.pdf

42. Zhou, Z.Q., Lin, W.B., Yang, M., Li, C.F., and Guo, G.C., Realization of reliable solid-state quantum memory for photonic polarization qubit. *Phys Rev Lett.* 108(19), 190505, 2012.

43. Hedges, M.P., Longdell, J.J., Li, Y., and Sellars, M.J., Efficient quantum memory for light. *Nature.* 465(7301), 1052–1056, 2010.

44. Longdell, J.J., Fraval, E., Sellars, M.J., and Manson, N.B., Stopped light with storage times greater than one second using electromagnetically induced transparency in a solid. *Phys Rev Lett.* 95(6), 063601, 2005.

45. Saglamyurek, E., Sinclair, N., Jin, J., Slater, J.A., Oblak, D., Bussiéres, F., George, M., Ricken, R., Sohler, W., and Tittel, W., Broadband waveguide quantum memory for entangled photons. *Nature*. 469(7331), 512–515, 2011.

46. Timoney, N., Lauritzen, B., Usmani, I., Afzelius, M., and Gisin, N., Atomic frequency comb memory with spin-wave storage in $^{153}Eu^{3+}$:Y_2SiO_5. *J Phys B At Mol Opt Phys*. 45, 124001, 2012.

47. Hodges, A., Computer science. Beyond Turing's machines. *Science*. 336(6078), 163–164, 2012.

48. Larger, L., Soriano, M.C., Brunner, D., Appeltant, L., Gutierrez, J.M., Pesquera, L., Mirasso, C.R., and Fischer, I., Photonic information processing beyond Turing: An optoelectronic implementation of reservoir computing. *Opt Express*. 20(3), 3241–3249, 2012.

49. Fredkin, E. and Toffoli, T., Conservative logic. *Int J Theor Phys*. 21, 219–253, 1982.

50. Bennett, C., The thermodynamics of computation—A review. *Int J Theor Phys*. 21, 905–940, 1981.

51. Drexler, K.E., *Nanosystems: Molecular Machinery, Manufacturing, and Computation*. John Wiley & Sons, New York, 1992.

52. von Neumann, J., Fourth University of Illinois lecture, in *Theory of Self-Reproducing Automata*, Burks, A.W., ed. University of Illinois Press, Urbana, Champaign, IL, 66, 1966.

53. Landauer, R., Irreversibility and heat generation in the computing process. *IBM J Res Develop*. 3, 183–191, 1961.

54. Hall, J.S., Nanocomputers and reversible logic. *Nanotechnology*. 5,157–167, 1994.

55. Joy, W.N., Reduced Instruction Set Computers (RISC). Academic/Industrial Interplay Drives Computer Performance Forward, 1997. http://www.cs.washington.edu/homes/lazowska/cra/risc.html (accessed October 22, 2012).

56. Frank, M.P. and Knight, T.F. Jr., Ultimate theoretical models of nanocomputers. *Nanotechnology*. 9, 162–176, 1998.

57. Drexler, K.E., Rod logic for molecular computing. *NanoCon Proceedings*, 1989. http://www.halcyon.com/nanojbl/NanoConProc/nanocon2.html (accessed October 22, 2012).

58. Merkle, R.C. and Drexler, K.E., Helical logic. *Nanotechnology*. 7(4), 325–339, 1992. http://www.zyvex.com/nanotech/helical/helical.html (accessed October 22, 2012).

59. Wang, K.L., Issues of nanoelectronics: A possible roadmap. *J Nanosci Nanotechnol*. 2(3–4), 235–266, 2002.

60. Landauer, R., Dissipation and noise immunity in computation, measurement, and communication. *J Stat Phys*. 54(5–6), 1509–1517, 1989.

61. Freitas, R.A. Jr., *Nanomedicine, Volume IIA: Biocompatibility*. Landes Bioscience, Georgetown, TX, 2003.

62. Georges, B., Grollier, J., Darques, M., Cros, V., Deranlot, C., Marcilhac, B., Faini, G., and Fert, A., Coupling efficiency for phase locking of a spin transfer nano-oscillator to a microwave current. *Phys Rev Lett*. 101(1), 017201, 2008.

63. Awschalom, D.D., Epstein, R., and Hanson, R., The diamond age of spintronics. *Sci Am*. 297(4), 84–91, 2007.

64. Muralidhar, K., Classical origin of quantum spin. *Apeiron*. 18(2), 146–160, 2011.

65. Awschalom, D.D., Flatté M.E., and Samarth, N., Spintronics. *Sci Am*. 86(6), 66–73, 2002.

66. Heinrich, A.J., Gupta, J.A., Lutz, C.P., and Eigler, D.M., Single-atom spin-flip spectroscopy. *Science*. 306(5695), 466–469, 2004.

67. Clemente-Juan, J.M., Coronado, E., and Gaita-Ariño, A., Magnetic polyoxometalates: From molecular magnetism to molecular spintronics and quantum computing. *Chem Soc Rev*. 41(22), 7464–7478, 2012.

68. Cardona-Serra, S., Clemente-Juan, J.M., Coronado, E., Gaita-Ariño, A., Camón, A., Evangelisti, M., Luis, F., Martínez-Pérez, M.J., and Sesé, J., Lanthanoid single-ion magnets based on polyoxometalates with a 5-fold symmetry: The Series [LnP(5)W(30)O(110)](12−) (Ln(3+) = Tb, Dy, Ho, Er, Tm, and Yb). *J Am Chem Soc*. 134(36), 14982–14990, 2012.

69. Schneider, T.D., Theory of molecular machines. II. Energy dissipation from molecular machines. *J Theor Biol*. 148(1), 125–137, 1991.

70. Shannon, C.E., Communication in the presence of noise. *Proc IRE*. 37, 10–21, 1949.

71. Schneider, T.D., Theory of molecular machines. I. Channel capacity of molecular machines. *J Theor Biol.* 148(1), 83–123, 1991.

72. Schneider, T.D., 70% efficiency of bistate molecular machines explained by information theory, high dimensional geometry and evolutionary convergence. *Nucleic Acids Res.* 38(18), 5995–6006, 2010.

73. Feynman, R.P., Tiny computers obeying quantum mechanical laws, in *New Directions in Physics: The Los Alamos 40th Anniversary Volume*, Metropolis, N., Kerr, D.M., and Rota, G., eds. Academic Press, Boston, MA, pp. 7.25, 1987.

74. Bennett, C.H., Demons, engines and the second law. *Sci Am.* 257(5), 108–116, 1987.

75. Chang, T.M., 50th anniversary of artificial cells: Their role in biotechnology, nanomedicine, regenerative medicine, blood substitutes, bioencapsulation, cell/stem cell therapy and nanorobotics. *Artif Cells Blood Substit Immobil Biotechnol.* 35(6), 545–554, 2007.

76. Dejeu, J., Bechelany, M., Rougeot, P., Philippe, L., and Gauthier, M., Adhesion control for micro- and nanomanipulation. *ACS Nano.* 5(6), 4648–4657, 2011.

77. Song, B., Yang, R., Xi, N., Patterson, K.C., Qu, C., and Lai, K.W., Cellular-level surgery using nano robots. *J Lab Autom.* 17(6), 425–434, 2012.

78. Sharpe, M.A., Marcano, D.C., Berlin, J.M., Widmayer, M.A., Baskin, D.S., and Tour, J.M., Antibody-targeted nanovectors for the treatment of brain cancers. *ACS Nano.* 6(4), 3114–3120, 2012.

79. Poyraz, O., Schmidt, H., Seidel, K., Delissen, F., Ader, C., Tenenboim, H., Goosmann, C., Laube, B., Thünemann, A.F., Zychlinsky, A., Baldus, M., Lange, A., Griesinger, C., and Kolbe, M., Protein refolding is required for assembly of the type three secretion needle. *Nat Struct Mol Biol.* 17(7), 788–792, 2010.

80. Tsutsui, M., He, Y., Furuhashi, M., Rahong, S., Taniguchi, M., and Kawai, T., Transverse electric field dragging of DNA in a nanochannel. *Sci Rep.* 2, 394, 2012.

81. Tsutsui, M., Rahong, S., Iizumi, Y., Okazaki, T., Taniguchi, M., and Kawai, T., Single-molecule sensing electrode embedded in-plane nanopores. *Sci Rep.* 1, 46, 2011.

82. Aksimentiev, A., Heng, J.B., Timp, G., and Schulten, K., Microscopic kinetics of DNA translocation through synthetic nanopores. *Biophys J.* 87(3), 2086–2097, 2004.

83. Smith, L.M., Corn, R.M., Condon, A.E., Lagally, M.G., Frutos, A.G., Liu, Q., and Thiel, A.J., A surface-based approach to DNA computation. *J Comput Biol.* 5(2), 255–267, 1998.

84. Frutos, A.G., Liu, Q., Thiel, A.J., Sanner, A.M., Condon, A.E., Smith, L.M., and Corn, R.M., Demonstration of a word design strategy for DNA computing on surfaces. *Nucleic Acids Res.* 25(23), 4748–4757, 1997.

85. Liu, Q., Wang, L., Frutos, A.G., Condon, A.E., Corn, R.M., and Smith, L.M., DNA computing on surfaces. *Nature.* 403(6766), 175–179, 2000.

86. Seeman, N.C., An overview of structural DNA nanotechnology. *Mol Biotechnol.* 37(3), 246–257, 2007.

87. Mao, C., Sun, W., and Seeman, N.C., Assembly of Borromean rings from DNA. *Nature.* 386(6621), 137–138, 1997.

88. Cantrill, S.J., Chichak, K.S., Peters, A.J., and Stoddart, J.F., Nanoscale Borromean rings. *Acc Chem Res.* 38(1), 1–9, 2005.

89. Adleman, L.M., Molecular computation of solutions to combinatorial problems. *Science.* 266(5187), 1021–1024, 1994.

90. Rogers, H. Jr., *Theory of Recursive Functions and Effective Computability.* McGraw-Hill, New York, 1967.

91. Parker, J., Computing with DNA. *EMBO Rep.* 4(1), 7–10, 2003.

92. Johnston, D.B., NNSA's Sequoia supercomputer ranked as world's fastest. Lawrence Livermore National Laboratory, NR-12-06-07, June 18, 2012. https://www.llnl.gov/news/newsreleases/2012/Jun/NR-12-06-07.html (accessed October 27, 2012).

93. Boehm, F.J., *An Investigation of Nucleic Acid/DNA-Based Manufacturing.* Center for Responsible Nanotechnology, Menlo Park, CA, August 2004. http://wise nano.org/w/Boehm_DNA_Study (accessed October 27, 2012).

94. Wernsdorfer, W., Aliaga-Alcalde, N., Hendrickson, D.N., and Christou, G., Exchange-biased quantum tunnelling in a supramolecular dimer of single-molecule magnets. *Nature*. 416(6879), 406–409, 2002.

95. Giménez-López, M. del C., Moro, F., La Torre, A., Gómez-García, C.J., Brown, P.D., van Slageren, J., and Khlobystov, A.N., Encapsulation of single-molecule magnets in carbon nanotubes. *Nat Commun*. 2, 407, 2011.

96. Kwon, Y.K., Tománek, D., and Iijima, S., "Bucky-shuttle" memory device: Synthetic approach and molecular dynamics simulations. *Phys Rev Lett*. 82(7), 1470–1473, 1999.

97. Cho, S.H., Jung, J.H., Ham, J.H., Lee, D.U., and Kim, T.W., Charge storage variations of organic memory devices fabricated by using C60 molecules embedded in an insulating polymer layer with Au and Al electrodes. *J Nanosci Nanotechnol*. 10(7), 4797–4800, 2010.

98. Ling, Q.D., Lim, S.L., Song, Y., Zhu, C.X., Chan, D.S., Kang, E.T., and Neoh, K.G., Nonvolatile polymer memory device based on bistable electrical switching in a thin film of poly(N-vinyl-carbazole) with covalently bonded C60. *Langmuir*. 23(1), 312–319, 2007.

99. Dresselhaus, P.D., Ji, L., Han, S., Lukens, J.E., and Likharev, K.K., Measurement of single electron lifetimes in a multijunction trap. *Phys Rev Lett*. 72(20), 3226–3229, 1994.

100. Abstreiter, G., Bichler, M., Markmann, M., Schedelbeck, G., Wegscheider, W., and Zrenner, A., Spatially resolved spectroscopy of single and coupled quantum dots. *Jpn J Appl Phys*. 38(1B), 449–454, 1999.

101. Petroff, P.M., Lorke, A., and Imamoglu, A., Epitaxially self-assembled quantum dots. *Phys Today*. 54(5), 46–52, 2001.

102. Nassiopoulou, A.G. and Salonidou, A., Two-silicon-nanocrystal layer memory structure with improved retention characteristics. *J Nanosci Nanotechnol*. 7(1), 368–373, 2007.

103. Gong, W., Han, Y., and Wei, G., Antiresonance and bound states in the continuum in electron transport through parallel-coupled quantum-dot structures. *J Phys Condens Matter*. 21(17), 175801, 2009.

104. Feynman, R.P., Space-time approach to non-relativistic quantum mechanics. *Rev Mod Phys*. 20, 367, 1948.

105. Wineland, D.J., Monroe, C., Itano, W.M., Leibfried, D., King, B.E., and Meekhof, D.M., Experimental issues in coherent quantum-state manipulation of trapped atomic ions. *J Res Natl Inst Stand Technol*. 103(3), 259, 1998.

106. Kielpinski, D., Meyer, V., Rowe, M.A., Sackett, C.A., Itano, W.M., Monroe, C., and Wineland, D.J., A decoherence-free quantum memory using trapped ions. *Science*. 291(5506), 1013–1015, 2001.

107. Monz, T., Kim, K., Villar, A.S., Schindler, P., Chwalla, M., Riebe, M., Roos, C.F., Häffner, H., Hänsel, W., Hennrich, M., and Blatt, R., Realization of universal ion-trap quantum computation with decoherence-free qubits. *Phys Rev Lett*. 103(20), 200503, 2009.

108. Britton, J.W., Sawyer, B.C., Keith, A.C., Wang, C.C., Freericks, J.K., Uys, H., Biercuk, M.J., and Bollinger, J.J., Engineered two-dimensional Ising interactions in a trapped-ion quantum simulator with hundreds of spins. *Nature*. 484(7395), 489–492, 2012.

109. Biercuk, M.J., Uys, H., Vandevender, A., Shiga, N., Itano, W.M., and Bollinger, J.J., High-fidelity quantum control using ion crystals in a Penning trap. *Quantum Inf Comput*. 9, 920–949, 2009.

110. Shiga, N., Itano, W.M., and Bollinger, J.J., Spectroscopy of ground state 9Be+ ions in a 4.5 T Penning trap, in *9th International Workshop on Non-Neutral Plasmas*. Columbia University, New York, 26, June 16–20, 2008.

111. von Neumann, J., *Theory of Self-Reproducing Automata*, Edited and completed by Burks, A.W. University of Illinois Press, Urbana, IL, 1996.

112. Lent, C.S., Isaksen, B., and Lieberman, M., Molecular quantum-dot cellular automata. *J Am Chem Soc*. 125(4), 1056–1063, 2003.

113. Lent, C. and Porod, W., Invention of the "quantum dot cell" and "wireless" electronic computing. University of Notre Dame, Notre Dame, IN, Projects 99, 1999.

114. Amlani, I.I., Orlov, A.O., Toth, G., Bernstein, G.H., Lent, C.S., and Snider, G.L., Digital logic gate using quantum-dot cellular automata. *Science*. 284(5412), 289–291, 1999.

115. Rothemund, P.W., Papadakis, N., and Winfree, E., Algorithmic self-assembly of DNA Sierpinski triangles. *PLoS Biol.* 2(12), e424, 2004.
116. Arima, V., Iurlo, M., Zoli, L., Kumar, S., Piacenza, M., Della Sala, F., Matino, F., Maruccio, G., Rinaldi, R., Paolucci, F., Marcaccio, M., Cozzi, P.G., and Bramanti, A.P., Toward quantum dot cellular automata units: Thiolated-carbazole linked bisferrocenes. *Nanoscale.* 4(3), 813–823, 2012.
117. Wang, X. and Ma, J., Electron switch in the double-cage fluorinated fullerene anions, e(−)@ C20F18(XH)2C20F18 (X = N, B): New contenders for molecular quantum-dot cellular automata. *Phys Chem Chem Phys.* 13(36), 16134–16137, 2011.
118. Wang, Z.F. and Liu, F., Nanopatterned graphene quantum dots as building blocks for quantum cellular automata. *Nanoscale.* 3(10), 4201–4205, 2011.
119. Wang, Z.F., Shi, Q.W., Li, Q., Wang, X., Hou, J.G., Zheng, H., Yao, Y., and Chen, J., Z-shaped graphene nanoribbon quantum dot device. *Appl Phys Lett.* 91, 053109-1-3, 2007.
120. Wang, W.L., Yazyev, O.V., Meng, S., and Kaxiras, E., Topological frustration in graphene nano-flakes: Magnetic order and spin logic devices. *Phys Rev Lett.* 102(15), 157201, 2009.
121. Wang, W.L., Meng, S., and Kaxiras, E., Graphene nanoflakes with large spin. *Nano Lett.* 8(1), 241–245, 2008.
122. Wu, L.A., Lidar, D.A., and Friesen, M., One-spin quantum logic gates from exchange interactions and a global magnetic field. *Phys Rev Lett.* 93(3), 030501, 2004.
123. Orlov, A.O., Amlani, I., Toth, G., Lent, C.S., Berstein, G.H., and Snider, G.L., Experimental demonstration of a binary wire for quantum-dot cellular automata. *Appl Phys Lett.* 74, 2875–2877, 1999.
124. Tougaw, P.D. and Lent, C.S., Dynamic behavior of quantum cellular automata. *J Appl Phys.* 80(8), 4722–4736, 1996.
125. Lent, C.S., Tougaw, P.D., Porod, W., and Berstein, G.H., Quantum cellular automata. *Nanotechnology.* 4, 49–57, 1993.
126. Tulchinsky, D.A., Kelley, M.H., McClelland, J.J., Gupta, R., and Celotta, R.J., Fabrication and domain imaging of iron magnetic nanowire arrays. *J Vac Sci Tech A.* 16(3), 1817–1819, 1998.
127. Vega, V., Böhnert, T., Martens, S., Waleczek, M., Montero-Moreno, J.M., Görlitz, D., Prida, V.M., and Nielsch, K., Tuning the magnetic anisotropy of Co–Ni nanowires: Comparison between single nanowires and nanowire arrays in hard-anodic aluminum oxide membranes. *Nanotechnology.* 23(46), 465709, 2012.
128. Kou, X., Fan, X., Dumas, R.K., Lu, Q., Zhang, Y., Zhu, H., Zhang, X., Liu, K., and Xiao, J.Q., Memory effect in magnetic nanowire arrays. *Adv Mater.* 23(11), 1393–1397, 2011.
129. Mohaddes-Ardabili, L., Zheng, H., Ogale, S.B., Hannoyer, B., Tian, W., Wang, J., Lofland, S.E., Shinde, S.R., Zhao, T., Jia, Y., Salamanca-Riba, L., Schlom, D.G., Wuttig, M., and Ramesh, R., Self-assembled single-crystal ferromagnetic iron nanowires formed by decomposition. *Nat Mater.* 3(8), 533–538, 2004.
130. Vettiger, P., Cross, G., Despont, M., Drechsler, U., Durig, U., Gotsmann, B., Häberle, W., Lantz, M.A., Rothuizen, H.E., Stutz, R., and Binnig, G.K., The "Millipede"—Nanotechnology entering data storage. *IEEE Trans Nanotechnol.* 1(1), 39–55, 2002.
131. Binning, G.K., Rohrer, H., and Vettiger, P., Mass-storage applications of local probe arrays. U.S. Patent 5,835,477, November 10, 1998. http://www.freepatentsonline.com/5835477.html (accessed November 12, 2012).
132. Vettiger, P., Brugger, J., Despont, M., Drechsler, U., Durig, U., Haberle, W., Lutwyche, M., Rothuizen, H., Stutz, R., Widmer, R., and Binnig, G., Ultrahigh density, high-data-rate NEMS-based AFM data storage system. *J Microelectron Eng.* 46(1–4), 11–17, 1999.
133. Lutwyche, M., Andreoli, C., Binnig, G., Brugger, J., Drechsler, U., Haberle, W., Rohrer, H., Rothuizen, H., and Vettiger, P., Microfabrication and parallel operation of 5 × 5 2D AFM cantilever array for data storage and imaging, in Proceedings of the *IEEE 11th International Workshop on Micro Electro Mechanical Systems (MEMS '98)*. Heidelberg, Germany, 8–11, 1998.
134. Armani, D.K., Kippenberg, T.J., Spillane, S.M., and Vahala, K.J., Ultra-high-Q toroid microcavity on a chip. *Nature.* 421(6926), 925–928, 2003.

135. Walters, R.J., Kik, P.G., Casperson, J.D., Atwater, H.A., Lindstedt, R., and Giorgi, M., Silicon optical nanocrystal memory. *Appl Phys Lett*. 85(13), 2622–2625, 2004.
136. Ng, C., Chen, T., Sreeduth, D., Chen, Q., Ding, L., and Du, A., Silicon nanocrystal-based non-volatile memory devices. *Thin Solid Films*. 504(1–2), 25–27, 2006.
137. Inoue, K. and Yoshino, M., Bistability and waveform reshaping in a DFB-LD with side-mode light injection. *IEEE Photon Technol Lett*. 7(2), 164–166, 1995.
138. Chen, C.H., Matsuo, S., Nozaki, K., Shinya, A., Sato, T., Kawaguchi, Y., Sumikura, H., and Notomi, M., All-optical memory based on injection-locking bistability in photonic crystal lasers. *Opt Express*. 19(4), 3387–3395, 2011.
139. Clausen, C., Bussières, F., Afzelius, M., and Gisin, N., Quantum storage of heralded polarization qubits in birefringent and anisotropically absorbing materials. *Phys Rev Lett*. 108(19), 190503, 2012.
140. Gündoğan, M., Ledingham, P.M., Almasi, A., Cristiani, M., and de Riedmatten, H., Quantum storage of a photonic polarization qubit in a solid. *Phys Rev Lett*. 108(19), 190504, 2012.
141. Church, G.M., Gao, Y., and Kosuri, S., Next-generation digital information storage in DNA. *Science*. 337(6102), 1628, 2012.
142. Handt, O., Krings, M., Ward, R.H., and Pääbo, S., The retrieval of ancient human DNA sequences. *Am J Hum Genet*. 59(2), 368–376, 1996.
143. Sennels, L. and Bentin, T., To DNA, all information is equal. *Artif DNA PNA XNA*. 3(3), 2012.
144. dela Torre, R., Larkin, J., Singer, A., and Meller, A., Fabrication and characterization of solid-state nanopore arrays for high-throughput DNA sequencing. *Nanotechnology*. 23(38), 385308, 2012.
145. Schulman, R. and Winfree, E., Synthesis of crystals with a programmable kinetic barrier to nucleation. *Proc Natl Acad Sci USA*. 104(39), 15236–1541, 2007.
146. Cook, M., Rothemund, P.W.K., and Winfree, E., *DNA Computing 9*. Springer, Berlin, 91–107, 2003.
147. Loth, S., Baumann, S., Lutz, C.P., Eigler, D.M., and Heinrich, A.J., Bistability in atomic-scale antiferromagnets. *Science*. 335(6065), 196–199, 2012.
148. Specht, H.P., Nölleke, C., Reiserer, A., Uphoff, M., Figueroa, E., Ritter, S., and Rempe, G., A single-atom quantum memory. *Nature*. 473(7346), 190–193, 2011.
149. Hétet, G., Slodička, L., Hennrich, M., and Blatt, R., Single atom as a mirror of an optical cavity. *Phys Rev Lett*. 107(13), 133002, 2011.
150. Quaade, U.J., Stokbro, K., Lin, R., and Grey, F., Single-atom reversible recording at room temperature. *Nanotechnology*. 12, 265–272, 2001.
151. Pla, J.J., Tan, K.Y., Dehollain, J.P., Lim, W.H., Morton, J.J., Jamieson, D.N., Dzurak, A.S., and Morello, A., A single-atom electron spin qubit in silicon. *Nature*. 489(7417), 541–545, 2012.
152. Morton, J.J.L., Tyryshkin, A.M., Brown, R.M., Shankar, S., Lovett, B.W., Ardavan, A., Schenkel, T., Haller, E.E., Ager, J.W., and Lyon, S.A., Solidstate quantum memory using the 31P nuclear spin. *Nature*. 455, 1085–1088, 2008.
153. Tyryshkin, A.M., Tojo, S., Morton, J.J., Riemann, H., Abrosimov, N.V., Becker, P., Pohl, H.J., Schenkel, T., Thewalt, M.L., Itoh, K.M., and Lyon, S.A., Electron spin coherence exceeding seconds in high-purity silicon. *Nat Mater*. 11(2), 143–147, 2011.
154. Snider, G.S., *Cortical Computing with Memristive Nanodevices*. Hewlett-Packard Laboratories, Bristol, U.K., 2008. http://www.scidacreview.org/0804/pdf/hardware.pdf (accessed October 13, 2012).
155. Kim, S., Jeong, H.Y., Kim, S.K., Choi, S.Y., and Lee, K.J., Flexible Memristive memory array on plastic substrates. *Nano Lett*. 11(12), 5438–5442, 2011.
156. Linn, E., Rosezin, R., Kügeler, C., and Waser, R., Complementary resistive switches for passive nanocrossbar memories. *Nat Mater*. 9(5), 403–406, 2010.
157. Cellan-Jones, R., First human 'infected with computer virus.' BBC News, May 27, 2010. http://www.bbc.co.uk/news/10158517 (accessed October 18, 2012).

Section II

Merging with Reality: Nascent Nanomedical Diagnostics and Therapeutics

8

Nanomaterial-Based Electrochemical Biosensors

Asieh Ahmadalinezhad and Aicheng Chen

CONTENTS

8.1 Introduction

A chemical sensor is a device that transforms chemical information, ranging from the concentration of a specific sample component to total compositional analysis, into an analytically useful signal. Chemical sensors typically contain two basic components that are connected in series: a chemical/molecular recognition system (receptor) and a physicochemical transducer. Biosensors are chemical sensors in which the recognition system functions via a biochemical mechanism (Figure 8.1) [1]. The biological recognition system translates information from the biochemical domain, usually an analyte concentration, into a chemical or physical output signal with a defined sensitivity. The main purpose of the recognition system is to provide the sensor with a high degree of selectivity for the analyte to be measured. While all biosensors are more or less selective (nonspecific) for a particular analyte, some are (by design and construction) only class-specific, since they utilize particular species of enzymes.

For the sensing systems that are present within living organisms, including olfaction, taste, and neurotransmission pathways, actual recognition is performed by cell receptors. Hence, the term receptor or bioreceptor is also often employed to denote the recognition system of a chemical biosensor. These examples are limited to the most common sensing principles, excluding existing laboratory instrumentation systems.

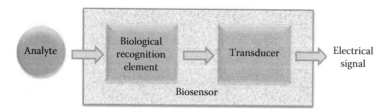

FIGURE 8.1
Basic components of a biosensor.

The transducer component of a sensor serves to transfer the signal from the output domain of the recognition system primarily to the electronic domain. Because of the general significance of the word, a transducer provides bidirectional signal transfer (nonelectrical to electrical and vice versa). A transducer, however, is also called a detector, sensor, or electrode. Hence, the term transducer is preferred in order to avoid confusion.

8.2 Biological Recognition Element

8.2.1 Biocatalytic Recognition Element

In this instance, the biosensor operates via a reaction that is catalyzed by macromolecules, which are either inherently present in biological environments, previously isolated, or manufactured. Thus, the continuous consumption of substrate(s) is achieved by the immobilized biocatalyst that is incorporated into the sensor: transient or steady-state responses are monitored by the integrated detector. Three types of biocatalysts are commonly used:

1. Enzymes (e.g., mono- or multienzymes), which are the most common and well-developed recognition system
2. Whole cells (e.g., microorganisms, such as bacteria, fungi, eukaryotic cells, or yeast), cell organelles, or components thereof (e.g., mitochondria, cell walls)
3. Tissues (e.g., plant or animal tissue layers)

Biocatalytic biosensors are the most well known and studied, and therefore, have been the most frequently applied to biological matrices since the pioneering work of Clark and Lyons [2]. One or more analytes, typically designated as substrates S and S′, react in the presence of enzyme(s), whole cells, or tissue cultures and yield single or multiple products, P and P′, according to the general reaction scheme:

$$S + S' \rightarrow P + P'$$

There are four strategies that utilize adjacent transducers for monitoring the analyte S consumption by this biocatalyzed reaction:

1. Detection of the co-substrate S′ consumption (e.g., oxygen depleted by oxidase), bacteria or yeast reacting layers, and the corresponding signal decrease from its initial value [2,3].
2. Recycling of P, one of the reaction products (e.g., hydrogen peroxide, H^+, CO_2, NH_3). Production by oxidoreductase, hydrolase, lyase, etc. and corresponding signal increase [4–6].

3. Detection of the state of the biocatalyst redox-active center, cofactor, prosthetic group evolution in the presence of substrate S, using an immobilized mediator which reacts sufficiently rapidly with the biocatalyst and is easily detected by the transducer; various ferrocene derivatives, as well as quinones, quinoid dyes, Ru or Os complexes in a polymer matrix, have been used [7–9].

4. Direct electron transfer between the active site of a redox enzyme and the electrochemical transducer [10].

The third strategy attempts to eliminate sensor response dependence on the co-substrate S' concentration and to decrease the influence of possible interfering species. The first goal is attained only when the reaction rates are much higher for immobilized mediators with biocatalysts than those for co-substrates with biocatalysts. An alternative approach to the use of such mediators involves the restriction of the analyte (substrate) concentration within the reaction layer through an appropriate outer membrane, whose permeability strongly favors co-substrate transport. When multiple enzymes are immobilized within the same reaction layer, a number of strategies for improving biosensor performance may be developed [4,11].

8.2.2 Biocomplexing or Bioaffinity Recognition Element

Biosensor operation is based on the interaction of analytes with macromolecules or organized molecular assemblies that have either been isolated from their original biological environment or engineered [5]. Thus, equilibrium is usually attained and there is no further net consumption of the analyte by the immobilized biocomplexing agent. These equilibrium responses are monitored by an integrated detector. In some cases, the biocomplexing reaction itself is monitored using a complementary biocatalytic reaction. Steady-state or transient signals are then monitored by the integrated detector:

1. *Antibody–antigen interaction.* The most developed examples of biosensors that use biocomplexing receptors are based on immunochemical reactions, that is binding of an antigen (Ag) to a specific antibody (Ab). The formation of such Ab–Ag complexes must be detected under conditions where nonspecific interactions are minimized. Each Ag determination requires the production of a particular Ab, its isolation, and typically its purification. Several studies have been described that involved the direct monitoring of the Ab–Ag complex formation on ion-sensitive field-effect transistors (ISFETs) [12]. In order to increase the sensitivity of immunosensors, enzyme labels are frequently coupled to the Ag or Ab, thus requiring additional chemical synthesis steps. Even in the case of the enzyme-labeled Ab, these biosensors will essentially operate at equilibrium, where the sole function of the enzymatic activity is to quantify the amount of complex produced.

2. *Receptor–antagonist–agonist.* Attempts have been made to employ ion channels, membrane receptors, or binding proteins as molecular recognition systems in conductometric, ISFET, or optical sensors. For example, the transport protein, lactose permease (LP), may be incorporated into liposomal bilayers, thus allowing for the coupling of sugar proton transport with a stoichiometric ratio of 1:1, as demonstrated when the fluorescent pH-probe pyranine is entrapped within these liposomes [13]. These LP-containing liposomes have been incorporated within planar lipid bilayer coatings of an ISFET that is gate sensitive to pH. Preliminary results

have shown that these modified ISFETs enable the rapid and reversible detection of lactose in a flow injection analysis (FIA) system. Protein receptor–based biosensors have recently been developed [14]. The result of the binding of the analyte (termed agonist here) to immobilize channel receptor proteins is monitored by changes in ion fluxes through these channels.

8.3 Nanomaterials as Substrates for Biological Recognition Elements

A defining characteristic of nanomaterials is that they have at least one structural dimension on the order of 100 nm or less [15]. Nanomaterials and nanosensors offer several significant advantages owing to their small size. High surface area/volume ratios, allowing for stronger signals, better catalysis, and more rapid movement of analytes through sensors, as well as enhanced optical properties (e.g., quantum dot fluorescence, gold nanoparticle quenching, surface-enhanced Raman scattering [SERS]), represent considerable benefits over macroscale materials [16–18].

Compelling combinations of the dimensional, compositional, and geometric properties of nanomaterials can impart unique functionality and enable diverse applications. With this aim, the synthesis of particular functional nanomaterials with well-defined morphologies that are capable of interacting with specific organic compounds and polymers is a significant and ongoing challenge. The spontaneous adsorption of organic molecules on a variety of nanomaterials can generate films that are only a single molecule in thickness. These nanoscale films have been utilized extensively in the engineering of surfaces with well-defined properties. Figure 8.2 presents the surface morphology and characterization of nanoporous gold, which was used as a substrate for the immobilization of hemoglobin in a hydrogen peroxide biosensor [19].

8.4 Types of Biosensors

8.4.1 Optical Biosensors

Many optical biosensors that are based on the phenomenon of surface plasmon resonance may be considered as evanescent wave techniques. They utilize a property that is inherent to gold and other materials; specifically that a thin layer of gold on a high refractive index glass surface may absorb laser light to produce electron waves (surface plasmons) on the surface of the gold. This occurs only at a specific angle and wavelength of incident light, and is highly dependent on the surface attributes of the gold, such that the binding of a target analyte to a receptor on the gold surface produces a measurable signal [20].

Surface plasmon resonance sensors operate using a sensor chip that consists of a plastic cassette that supports a glass plate, one side of which is coated with a microscopically thin layer of gold. This is the surface that contacts the optical detection apparatus of the instrument. The opposite side is then interfaced with a microfluidic flow system. Contact with the flow system creates channels across which reagents may be passed in solution. This side of the glass sensor chip may be modified in a number of ways to allow for the easy attachment of molecules of interest (Figure 8.3).

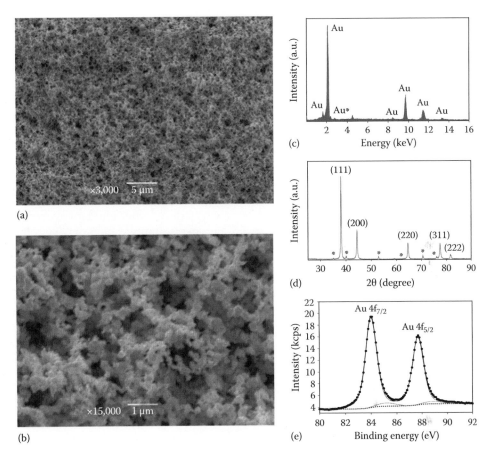

FIGURE 8.2
(a and b) SEM images of nanoporous Au networks recorded at various magnifications. (c) EDS spectrum of the synthesized nanoporous Au networks, peak labeled by an asterisk, is attributed to the Ti substrate. (d) XRD spectrum recorded from the synthesized nanoporous Au network. (e) XPS spectra of the Au 4f region for the as-synthesized nanoporous Au network. (Reprinted from *Biosens. Bioelectron.*, 25(11), Kafi, A.K.M., Ahmadalinezhad, A., Wang, J.P., Thomas, D.F., and Chen, A., Direct growth of nanoporous Au and its application in electrochemical biosensing, 2458–2463, Copyright 2010, with permission from Elsevier.)

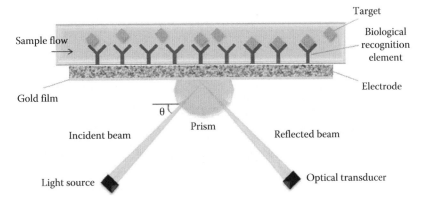

FIGURE 8.3
Schematic diagram of an optical biosensor (surface plasmon resonance biosensor).

Light of a fixed wavelength is reflected from the gold side of the chip at the angle of total internal reflection and is detected inside the instrument. This induces the evanescent wave to penetrate through the glass plate and some distance into the liquid that is flowing over the surface.

The refractive index at the flow region of the chip surface has a direct influence on the behavior of the light that is reflected from the gold region. Binding to the flow region of the chip has an effect on the refractive index, and in this way biological interactions may be measured with a high degree of sensitivity when facilitated by a source of energy.

Other evanescent wave biosensors have been commercialized that utilize waveguides where the propagation constant through the waveguide is altered by the absorption of molecules to the waveguide surface. One such example, dual polarization interferometry employs an embedded waveguide as a reference against which the change in propagation constant is measured. Other configurations such as the Mach–Zehnder have reference arms lithographically defined on a substrate. Higher levels of integration may be achieved using resonator geometries where the resonant frequency of a ring resonator changes when molecules are absorbed.

Other optical biosensors are based primarily on changes in absorbance or fluorescence of an appropriate indicator compound and do not require a total internal reflection geometry. For example, a fully operational prototype device for the detection of casein in milk has been fabricated. This device is based on the detection of changes in absorption of a gold layer [21]. A widely used research tool, the microarray, may also be considered as a biosensor.

Biosensors often incorporate a genetically modified form of a native protein or enzyme. The protein is configured to detect a specific analyte and the ensuing signal is read by a detection instrument such as a fluorometer or luminometer. An example of a recently developed biosensor is one that detects cytosolic concentrations of the analyte, cyclic adenosine monophosphate (cAMP). cAMP is a second messenger that is involved in cellular signaling, which is in turn triggered by ligand–receptor interactions on the cell membrane [22]. Similar systems have been created to study cellular responses to native ligands or xenobiotics (toxins or small molecule inhibitors). Such "assays" are commonly utilized in drug discovery development by pharmaceutical and biotechnology companies. Most cAMP assays in current use require the lysis (decomposition) of the cells prior to the measurement of cAMP. A live-cell biosensor for cAMP may be used in non-lysed cells with the additional advantage of multiple reads for studying receptor response kinetics.

8.4.2 Electrochemical Biosensor

Over the past few decades, a number of reports have highlighted the growing importance of electrochemical biosensing devices in both clinical and environmental analysis. This may not seem as surprising when one considers that electrochemical transduction processes have inherent advantages such as low cost, high sensitivity, independence from solution turbidity, simple miniaturization that is well suited to microfabrication, low power requirements, and relatively straightforward-associated instrumentation. These characteristics make electrochemical sensing methods highly attractive in myriad applications, including the detection of cancer, infectious diseases, glucose and cholesterol, and biological warfare agents, to name but a few.

Electrochemical biosensors are normally based on the enzymatic catalysis of a reaction that produces or consumes electrons (such enzymes are rightly called redox enzymes). The sensor substrate typically contains three electrodes: a reference electrode, an active electrode, and a sink electrode. An auxiliary electrode (also known as a counter electrode) may also be present as an ion source. The target analyte is involved in the reaction that takes place on the active electrode surface, and the ions produced create a potential which is subtracted from that of the reference electrode to provide a signal. The current (flow rate of electrons proportional to the analyte concentration) may either be measured at a fixed potential, or the potential may be measured at zero current (this gives a logarithmic response). Note that the potential of the working or active electrode is space charge–sensitive (space charge domains are formed as the result of heterogeneous phenomena, and hence, are often used). Figure 8.4 illustrates the electron transfer mechanism in a typical biosensor. Further, the label-free and direct electrical detection of small peptides and proteins is made possible via their intrinsic charges using biofunctionalized ISFETs [23,24]. These devices measure a property of the substrate (such as conductance) that is affected by charges near the surface of the sensor or the pH of the solvent. As the concentration of the analyte changes, the charge near the surface or the pH changes, either as the result of enzymatic reactions or competitive binding that causes the sensor to register a change in the measured property. This allows for the indirect quantification of the analyte concentration, although pH changes in the bulk solution may affect the measured response.

Another example, in the form of a potentiometric biosensor, works contrary to the current understanding of its ability. Such biosensors are screen-printed [25], conductive polymer-coated, open circuit potential biosensors that are based on conjugated polymeric immunoassays [26]. They contain only two electrodes and are extremely sensitive and robust, enabling the detection of analyte levels that were previously only achievable using high-performance liquid chromatography (HPLC) and liquid chromatography–mass spectrometry (LC/MS), without rigorous sample preparation. The signal is generated by electrochemical and physical modifications within the conductive polymer layer due to changes that occur at the surface of the sensor. Such alterations may be attributed to ionic strength, pH, hydration, and redox reactions. The latter is due to the enzyme label turning over a substrate.

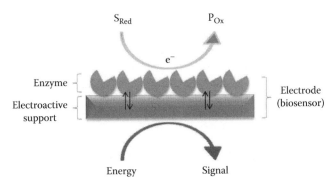

FIGURE 8.4
Schematic diagram of the electron transfer in an enzyme-based electrochemical biosensor.

8.5 Biosensor Construction

8.5.1 Immobilization of Biological Receptors

Since the initial development of enzyme-based biosensors for glucose (first described by Clark in 1962), in which glucose oxidase (GO_x) was entrapped between two membranes [2], an impressive volume of literature that describes immobilization techniques and related biosensor development has appeared. These methods have been extensively reviewed elsewhere [1,27]. Biological receptors, that is enzymes, antibodies, cells, or tissues with high biological activity, may be immobilized within a thin layer at the transducer surface by using different procedures. The following protocols are the most generally employed:

1. Adsorption of enzyme to the surface of electrode to develop a surface-modified biosensor [28]

2. Entrapment behind a membrane: a solution of enzyme, suspension of cells, or a slice of tissue is simply confined by an analyte permeable membrane as a thin film, which covers the electrochemical detector [4]

3. Entrapment of biological receptors within a polymeric matrix such as polyacrylonitrile, agar gel, polyurethane (PU) or poly(vinylalcohol) (PVAL) membranes, sol gels, or redox hydrogels with redox centers [5], or entrapment of biological receptors within self-assembled monolayers (SAMs) or bilayer lipid membranes (BLMs) [6]

4. Covalent bonding of receptors onto membranes or surfaces activated by means of bifunctional groups or spacers such as glutaraldehyde, carbodiimide, SAMs, or multilayers, or avidin–biotin silanization. Several of these activated membranes are commercially available [28]

Figure 8.5 illustrates schematic diagrams of four different approaches for the immobilization of biological receptors. Receptors are either individually immobilized or mixed with additional proteins, such as bovine serum albumin (BSA), directly onto the transducer surface or on a polymeric membrane that coats it. In the latter case, pre-activated membranes may be used directly for enzyme or antibody immobilization without the requirement of further chemical modification of the membrane or macromolecule.

Apart from the final example, reticulation and covalent attachment procedures are more complex than those that involve entrapment, but are especially useful in cases where the

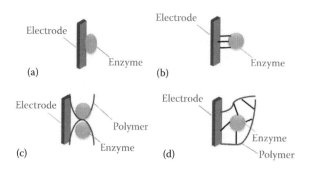

FIGURE 8.5
Scheme of primary types of enzymatically modified electrodes. (a) Modification of the electrode surface through adsorption, (b) covalent bonding, (c) gel/polymer entrapment, and (d) entrapment via cross-linking.

sensor is so diminutive that the appropriate membrane must be fabricated directly onto the transducer. Under such conditions, more stable and reproducible activities may be obtained via covalent attachment.

8.6 Biosensor Applications

There are myriad potential applications of biosensors of various classes. The chief prerequisites for a biosensor approach in terms of its value in research and for commercial applications include the identification of a target molecule, the availability of a suitable biological recognition element, and the potential for disposable portable detection systems as preferable to sensitive laboratory-based techniques in particular situations. A number of examples are given as follows [4–6,12,14,16–19,21,23,25]:

- Glucose monitoring for diabetes patients (historical market driver)
- Other medical/health-related targets
- Environmental applications (e.g., detection of pesticides in ecosystems and water-resident contaminants)
- Remote sensing of airborne bacteria (e.g., in counter-bioterrorist activities)
- Detection of pathogens
- Determination of toxic substance levels prior to and following bioremediation
- Detection and quantification of organophosphates
- Routine analytical measurement of folic acid, biotin, vitamin B12, and pantothenic acid as an alternative to microbiological assay
- Determination of drug residues in food, such as antibiotics and growth promoters, particularly in meat products and honey
- Drug discovery and the evaluation of biological activity of new compounds
- Protein engineering in biosensors
- Detection of toxic metabolites such as mycotoxins

Among the diverse applications of biosensors, we highlight the most important advances in the area of glucose and cholesterol detection due to their critical impacts on human health. Diabetes and cardiovascular diseases are rapidly increasing problems that can effectively be prevented by controlling the glucose and cholesterol levels in human blood. Toward this aim, nanomaterial-based biosensors have been intensely investigated.

8.6.1 Electrochemical Glucose Biosensor

Diabetes is a rapidly growing problem; the number of people with diabetes increased from 153 million in 1980 to 347 million in 2008 [29]. In 2004, an estimated 3.4 million people died as a result of the consequences of high blood sugar. This number is estimated to double by 2030 [30]. Diabetes may lead to serious complications such as lower limb amputations, blindness, as well as cardiovascular and kidney diseases.

There are three types of diabetes:

1. Type 1 diabetes usually affects the young and occurs when the pancreas no longer produces any (or very little) insulin. Approximately 10% of diabetics have Type 1.

2. Type 2 diabetes commonly affects middle-aged or older patients and occurs when the pancreas does not produce enough insulin or when the body does not use the insulin that is produced effectively. Ninety percent of people with diabetes have Type 2.

3. Gestational diabetes is a temporary condition that occurs during pregnancy. It affects 2%–4% of all pregnancies with an increased risk of developing diabetes for both mother and child.

Both glycemia and diabetes are on the rise globally and are driven by population growth, aging, and an increasing age-specific prevalence. Effective preventive interventions are essential, and health systems should prepare to sufficiently detect and manage diabetes and its sequel. To attain optimal control, patients must continually monitor their blood glucose levels. This requires a patient to obtain a small sample of blood, usually via a finger prick. Blood is placed onto a sensor test strip that is then read by a handheld electronic reader, which reports the blood glucose concentration. These sensors are based on electrochemical enzymatic measurements with screen-printed electrodes that provide rapid and accurate measurements of blood glucose without the need for laboratory analysis. However, there are limitations to this approach including painful sampling; analyses cannot be performed if the patient is otherwise occupied (e.g., sleeping); and large fluctuations that occur between sampling intervals can be missed [31]. To facilitate the resolution of inherent problems with discrete blood glucose measurement, new commercial products focus on continuous glucose interrogation. Early-stage nanotechnology and nanomedical research involving nanosensors and nanomaterials is also focused on continuous monitoring.

The incorporation of nanomaterials into these sensors offers a variety of advantages including increased surface area, more efficient electron transfer from enzyme to electrode, and the ability to include additional catalytic steps. Although a detailed discussion of all possible modifications to standard electrodes would be prohibitively long, we highlight recent advances that demonstrate the range of options for integration of nanomaterials for enabling advanced glucose sensors.

The use of carbon nanotubes (CNTs) for the enzymatic detection of glucose is a heavily investigated modification, partly due to the enhanced electron transfer capabilities of CNTs as well as their large surface areas. The electrode can be replaced with a highly porous nanofiber onto which glucose oxidase is immobilized [32]. This structure contains a much higher electronic surface area than do bulk metal electrodes and accordingly may immobilize higher volumes of enzymes to generate stronger signals. Another approach is to modify the nanotubes with an electrochemical mediator such as ferrocene to improve the electron transfer between the enzyme and electrode [33]. Recently, a glucose biosensor was fabricated via the co-immobilization of GO_x and horseradish peroxidase (HRP) on activated buckypaper (physically aggregated buckypaper) [34]. Figure 8.6 shows a photograph (a), along with the microscopic images of the buckypaper surface (b and c), and its elemental surface analysis (d).

The buckypaper-based glucose biosensor exhibited a long lifetime (over 80 days). Figure 8.7 presents the amperometric response of the buckypaper-based biosensor at the beginning (red line) and after 80 days (black line) upon the addition of glucose, revealing that the biosensor retained 94% of its initial current response when it was used in the continuous daily measurement of glucose for a period of 80 days. This property of

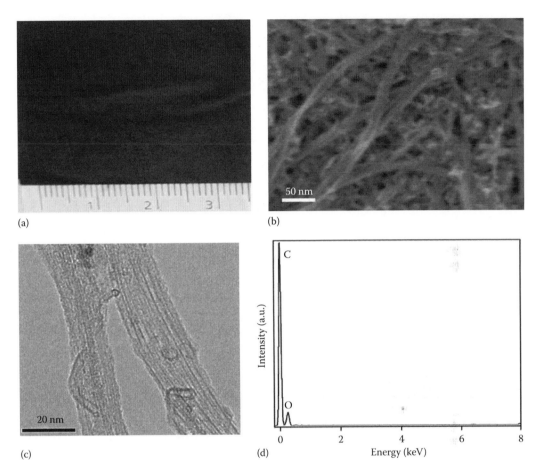

FIGURE 8.6
(a) A photograph, (b) FESEM image, (c) TEM image, and (d) the corresponding EDS spectrum of the buckypaper. (Reprinted from *Biosens. Bioelectron.*, 30(1), Ahmadalinezhad, A., Wu, G., and Chen, A., Mediator-free electrochemical biosensor based on bucky paper with enhanced stability and sensitivity for glucose detection, 287–293, Copyright 2011, with permission from Elsevier.)

the biosensor was attributed to the interconnectivity of physically aggregated CNTs that comprise the internal structure of the buckypaper. On the one hand, its compatibility and strong interaction with chitosan; and on the other, the interaction of chitosan with enzymes significantly enhanced the interfacial adhesion and mechanical strength of the biosensor.

CNTs may be coupled with other nanomaterials or polymers to form nanocomposites for glucose detection. Combining CNTs with additional nanomaterials serves to improve functional aspects such as catalytic activity. Nanocomposite membranes have recently been fabricated via the layer-by-layer assembly of CNTs and gold nanoparticles [35,36]. Similar approaches have also coupled CNTs with silver [37] and platinum nanoparticles [38], in addition to nonmetals such as silica [39].

A variety of nanostructures may serve to improve conventional macrostructured electrodes. Zinc oxide, when configured as nanotube arrays [40], has been used for glucose detection. Nanowire arrays fabricated from ruthenium [41] and gold [42] have an increased surface area and improved electrochemical interrogation compared with conventional electrodes. In addition to creating nanoscale features on the surfaces of electrodes,

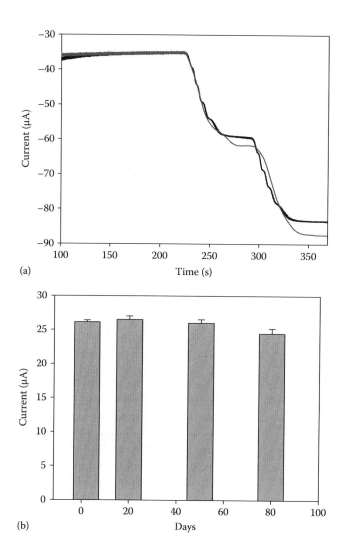

FIGURE 8.7

(a) Amperometric response of the buckypaper-based glucose biosensor initially (red line) and after a period of 80 days (black line) upon addition of 1.2 mM glucose at −0.1 V in PBS of pH 7.4. (b) Comparison of the current response of the biosensor to 1.2 mM glucose during the 80 day stability tests. (Reprinted from *Biosens. Bioelectron.*, 30(1), Ahmadalinezhad, A., Wu, G., and Chen, A., Mediator-free electrochemical biosensor based on bucky paper with enhanced stability and sensitivity for glucose detection, 287–293, Copyright 2011, with permission from Elsevier.)

nanostructures may be generated through the use of nanoparticles. Gold [35], platinum [43], and palladium [44] nanoparticles have been used in membranes to enhance electron transfer and increase the surface area of the sensor.

Magnetic nanoparticles, commonly made from iron oxide, have also been used in the construction of glucose sensors [45,46]. The magnetic nature of these nanoparticles simplifies the assembly of GO_x-labeled nanoparticles onto the electrode [45], as well as enabling the formation of nanoparticle-comprised conductive wires on the electrode surface [46]. In both of these examples, the nanoparticles were attracted to the electrode surface with magnetic fields, which highlights one advantage in using magnetic nanoparticles in the fabrication of nanoparticle-based electrode assemblies.

Nanostructured polymers can improve the development of glucose sensors. Hollow spheres of conductive polymers may be used to transfer electrons from GO_x to the electrode [47]. Conductive polymer electrodes can be utilized in a method similar to other nanostructured surfaces, where GO_x is immobilized directly on the modified electrode. In one example, the electrode surface was covered with highly ordered polyaniline nanotubes, which had GO_x immobilized within lumen of the nanotubes [48]. The use of polymers introduces a range of different electrochemical properties, including options for operation at varying potentials. The use of different potentials helps to minimize electrochemical interference from common electroactive compounds in blood (e.g., acetaminophen, ascorbic acid, and uric acid), which can cause nonspecific signals using standard electrochemical detection approaches.

Nanomaterials-based sensors can also be designed to detect glucose through changes in pH or charge, often through a field-effect transistor (FET). The breakdown of glucose, when catalyzed by GO_x, decreases solution pH by liberating hydrogen ions and generates negative charges by producing gluconate ions. Risveden and colleagues used an ISFET to detect gluconate generation in order to quantify glucose concentrations [49]. The ISFET focuses the gluconate between the sensing electrodes, whereby an increase in current is proportional to the amount of glucose present. The layer-by-layer assembly of CNTs with GO_x allows changes in pH that are generated by glucose degradation to be monitored by measuring the conductance changes in the CNT layer [50]. Modified nanoparticles can also improve the sensitivity of capacitive electrolyte–insulator–semiconductor (EIS) structures. The use of gold nanoparticles modified with both GO_x and ferrocene improved sensitivity nearly twofold over nanoparticles that were modified with only GO_x [51].

8.6.2 Cholesterol Biosensor

Cholesterol is produced by the liver as well as being part of a healthy dietary intake of fats. Cholesterol and triglycerides are important building blocks in the structure of cells and are used in making hormones and vitamin D, and for the production of energy. However, having a high total cholesterol (the sum of free cholesterol and cholesterol esters) level, particularly those of the low-density lipoprotein type, can cause blood vessel damage and result in diseases such as coronary heart disease (CHD) and peripheral vascular disease. The assertion that elevated plasma cholesterol concentrations may lead to an increased chance of developing either atherosclerosis or CHD has now been long established [52] and has become a central tenet of the "lipid hypothesis."

The need to limit dietary fat and cholesterol intake was recognized by the UK government in the 1992 Health of The Nation Report [53], and in the United States from the recommendations of the National Research Council [54]. Nevertheless, the role of cholesterol remains controversial. It is not yet clear whether cholesterol is a causal agent for inducing atherosclerosis, or if it is the primary exacerbating factor in the formation of foam cells after initial artery wall injury, which might be incurred via some other means. The requirement for the accurate determination of serum cholesterol has, as a consequence, stimulated a large amount of work on the development of methods for its assay that are rapid enough for routine assessments, while simple and reproducible. The general analysis of serum cholesterol is currently accomplished by utilizing a three-enzyme assay and indicator method as originally devised by Richmond [55].

Since ≈70% of the cholesterol present in serum samples is esterified, a typical assay for total serum cholesterol usually begins with the incubation of serum with cholesterol esterase in order to isolate free cholesterol, which is amenable to oxidation via cholesterol oxidase. A peroxidase enzyme subsequently reduces the hydrogen peroxide that is produced when one molecule of cholesterol is oxidized. Oxidation of an indicator molecule in turn reactivates the peroxidase and produces a chromogen, which when measured, facilitates the indirect estimation of total serum cholesterol. To develop the electrochemical cholesterol biosensor, Aravamudhan et al. attached the enzymes to the surface of aligned gold nanowires through direct physical adsorption [56]. Their studies demonstrated that the fabricated biosensor had a sensitivity of 0.85 μA/mM. To improve sensitivity, Gopalan et al. recently reported the fabrication of a biosensor for the detection of free cholesterol by combining the advantageous features of MWNT (multiwalled CNTs), Au nanoparticles, chitosan, and an ionic liquid [57].

Ahmadalinezhad and Chen fabricated a cholesterol biosensor by co-immobilizing cholesterol oxidase, cholesterol esterase, and HRP on nanoporous gold networks [58]. The developed biosensor showed a highly selective behavior when tested with common interfering species such as ascorbic acid, uric acid, lactic acid, and glucose. Under physiological conditions (pH 7.4), the designed biosensor exhibited a wide linear range up to 300 mg/dL. Since the desired total plasma cholesterol for an individual is <5.2 mM (200 mg/dL), with a high level being considered as greater than 6.2 mM (240 mg/dL), the fabricated biosensor spans a wide range of cholesterol concentrations, which is promising in clinical diagnostics for total cholesterol. The developed biosensor was also used to measure the total cholesterol in off-the-shelf food samples. The authors claimed that the proposed cholesterol biosensor would be promising for the detection of total cholesterol in both clinical diagnostics and the food industry [58].

Other versions of cholesterol biosensors exist [6,30,59]; however, only a few of these have been successfully commercially launched. One of the reasons for this originates from the optimization of critical parameters, such as enzyme stabilization, quality control, and instrumentation design. Cholesterol biosensors must be easy to use, self-testing, have rapid response, be portable, etc. Further, the proper marketing of the product is essential for attracting the attention of potential users. Increased understanding of immobilized bioreagents, improved immobilization techniques and technological advances in microelectronics are likely to speed up the commercialization of a much-needed cholesterol biosensor.

8.7 Conclusion and Perspectives

Advanced biosensors have the capacity for addressing diverse practical challenges in the medical, industrial, agricultural, and environmental sectors. A variety of methodologies are envisaged to expand the area of biosensors with utility in additional analytical tasks. For example, the development of new biosensors may be seen as essential in solving difficulties that are inherent to a variety of challenging in situ and in vivo analyses. Although other types of biosensors exist; in all cases, an important challenge that remains is their miniaturization, which imparts dual advantages: (i) limits the required amount of immobilized enzyme and (ii) yields tools for direct use and possible implantation within living tissues. The increased integration of biological materials within these patterned geometries may be accomplished through the use of nanostructures. Subsequently, very promising pathways toward the development of "ideal" amperometric biosensors have been opened.

References

1. Turner, A.P.F., Karube, I., and Wilson, G.S., *Biosensors, Fundamentals and Applications*. Oxford, U.K.: Oxford University Press, 1987.
2. Clark, L.C. and Lyons, C., Electrode systems for continuous monitoring in cardiovascular surgery. *Ann. N.Y. Acad. Sci.* 102(1), 29–45, 1962.
3. Tecon, R., van der Meer, and Roelof, J., Bacterial biosensors for measuring availability of environmental pollutants. *Sensors*. 8(7), 4062–4080, 2008.
4. Sternberg, R., Bindra, D.S., Wilson, G.S., and Thevenot, D.R., Covalent enzyme coupling on cellulose acetate membranes for glucose sensor development. *Anal. Chem.* 60(24), 2781–2786, 1988.
5. Shin, J.H., Marxer, S.M., and Schoenfisch, M.H., Nitric oxide-releasing sol–gel particle/polyurethane glucose biosensors. *Anal. Chem.* 76(15), 4543–4549, 2004.
6. Omodeo, S.F., Marchesini, S., Fishman, P.H., and Berra, B., A sensitive enzymatic assay for determination of cholesterol in lipid extracts. *Anal. Biochem.* 142(2), 347–350, 1984.
7. Degani, Y. and Heller, A., Direct electrical communication between chemically modified enzymes and metal electrodes. I. Electron transfer from glucose oxidase to metal electrodes via electron relays, bound covalently to the enzyme. *J. Phys. Chem.* 91(6), 1285–1289, 1987.
8. Qiu, J.-D., Zhou, W.-M., Guo, J., Wang, R., and Liang, R.-P., Amperometric sensor based on ferrocene-modified multiwalled carbon nanotube nanocomposites as electron mediator for the determination of glucose. *Anal. Biochem.* 385(2), 264–269, 2009.
9. Bucur, B., Mallat, E., Gurban, A.M., Gocheva, Y., Velasco, C., Marty, J.L., and Noguer, T., Strategies to develop malic acid biosensors based on malate quinone oxidoreductase (MQO). *Biosens. Bioelectron.* 21(12), 2290–2297, 2006.
10. Ghindilis, A., Direct electron transfer catalysed by enzymes: Application for biosensor development. *Biochem. Soc. Trans.* 28(2), 84–89, 2000.
11. Guilbault, G.G., *Handbook of Immobilized Enzymes*. New York: Marcel Dekker, 1984.
12. Park, H.-J., Kim, S.K., Park, K., Yi, S.Y., Chung, J.W., Chung, B.H., and Kim, M., Monitoring of C-reactive protein using ion sensitive field effect transistor biosensor. *Sens. Lett.* 8(2), 233–237, 2010.
13. Kiefer, H., Klee, B., John, E., Stierhof, Y.-D., and Jähnig, F., Biosensors based on membrane transport proteins. *Biosens. Bioelectron.* 6(3), 233–237, 1991.
14. Sugawara, M., Hirano, A., Rehák, M., Nakanishi, J., Kawai, K., Sato, H., and Umezawa, Y., Electrochemical evaluation of chemical selectivity of glutamate receptor ion channel proteins with a multi-channel sensor. *Biosens. Bioelectron.* 12(5), 425–439, 1997.
15. Chopra, N., Gavalas, V.G., Bachas, L.G., and Hinds, B.J., Functional one dimensional nanomaterials: Applications in nanoscale biosensors. *Anal. Lett.* 40(11), 2067–2096, 2007.
16. Smith, A.M., Dave, S., Nie, S., Tru, L., and Gao, X., Multicolor quantum dots for molecular diagnostics of cancer. *Expert. Rev. Mol. Diag.* 6(2), 231–244, 2006.
17. Wang, W., Chen, C., Qian, M., and Zhao, X.S., Aptamer biosensor for protein detection using gold nanoparticles. *Anal. Biochem.* 373(2), 213–219, 2008.
18. Yuan, W., Ho, H.P., Lee, R.K.Y., and Kong, S.K., Surface-enhanced Raman scattering biosensor for DNA detection on nanoparticle island substrates. *Appl. Opt.* 48(22), 4329–4337, 2009.
19. Kafi, A.K.M., Ahmadalinezhad, A., Wang, J.P., Thomas, D.F., and Chen, A., Direct growth of nanoporous Au and its application in electrochemical biosensing. *Biosens. Bioelectron.* 25(11), 2458–2463, 2010.
20. Rich, R.L. and Myszka, D.G., Advances in surface plasmon resonance biosensor analysis. *Curr. Opin. Biotechnol.* 11(1), 54–61, 2000.
21. Hiep, H.M., Endo, T., Kerman, K., Chikae, M., Kim, D.-K., Yamamura, S., Takamura, Y., and Tamiya, E., A localized surface plasmon resonance based immunosensor for the detection of case in milk. *Sci. Technol. Adv. Mater.* 8(4), 331–338, 2007.

22. Fan, F., Binkowski, B.F., Butler, B.L., Stecha, P.F., Lewis, M.K., and Wood, K.V., Novel genetically encoded biosensors using firefly luciferase. *ACS Chem. Biol.* 3(6), 346–351, 2008.

23. Lud, S.Q., Nikolaides, M.G., Haase, I., Fischer, M., and Bausch, A.R., Field effect of screened charges: Electrical detection of peptides and proteins by a thin-film resistor. *Chemphyschem.* 7(2), 379–384, 2006.

24. Ghindilis, A.L., Atanasov, P., and Wilkins, E., Enzyme-catalyzed direct electron transfer: Fundamentals and analytical applications. *Electroanalysis.* 9(9), 661–674, 1997.

25. Trivedi, U.B., Lakshminarayana, D., Kothari, I.L., Patel, N.G., Kapse, H.N., Makhija, K.K., Patel, P.B., and Panchal, C.J., Potentiometric biosensor for urea determination in milk. *Sens. Actuat. B Chem.* 140(1), 260–266, 2009.

26. Arshak, K., Velusamy, V., Korostynska, O., Oliwa-Stasiak, K., and Adley, C., Conducting polymers and their applications to biosensors: Emphasizing on foodborne pathogen detection. *IEEE Sens. J.* 9(12), 1942–1951, 2009.

27. Wollenberger, U., Schubert, F., Pfeiffer, D., and Scheller, F.W., Enhancing biosensor performance using multienzyme systems. *Trend Biotechnol.* 11(6), 255–262, 1993.

28. Wilson and Wilsons, *Comprehensive Analytical Chemistry Volume XLIV: Biosensors and Modern Biospecific Analytical Techniques*, Gorton, L. ed. Amsterdam: Elsevier, 285–327, 2005.

29. Danaei, G., Finucane, M.M., Lu, Y., Singh, G.M., Cowan, M.J., Paciorek, C.J., Lin, J.K., Farzadfar, F., Khang, Y.-H., Stevens, G.A., Rao, M., Ali, M.K., Riley, L.M., Robinson, C.A., and Ezzati, M., National, regional, and global trends in fasting plasma glucose and diabetes prevalence since 1980: Systematic analysis of health examination surveys and epidemiological studies with 370 country-years and 2.7 million participants. *Lancet.* 378(9785), 31–40, 2011.

30. WHO, Diabetes. updated August 2011, Fact sheet N° 312, http://www.who.int/mediacentre/factsheets/fs312/en/index.html (accessed 06/23/13).

31. Burge, M.R., Mitchell, S., Sawyer, A., and Schade, D.S., Continuous glucose monitoring: The future of diabetes management. *Diabetes Spectrum.* 21(2), 112–119, 2008.

32. Cai, C. and Chen, J., Direct electron transfer of glucose oxidase promoted by carbon nanotubes. *Anal. Biochem.* 332(1), 75–83, 2004.

33. Qiu, J.-D., Zhou, W.-M., Guo, J., Wang, R., and Liang, R.-P., Amperometric sensor based on ferrocene-modified multiwalled carbon nanotube nanocomposites as electron mediator for the determination of glucose. *Anal. Biochem.* 385(2), 264–269, 2009.

34. Ahmadalinezhad, A., Wu, G., and Chen, A., Mediator-free electrochemical biosensor based on bucky paper with enhanced stability and sensitivity for glucose detection. *Biosens. Bioelectron.* 30(1), 287–293, 2011.

35. Ahmadalinezhad, A., Kafi, A.K.M., and Chen, A., Glucose biosensing based on the highly efficient immobilization of glucose oxidase on a Prussian blue modified nanostructured Au surface. *Electrochem. Commun.* 11(10), 2048–2051, 2009.

36. Wang, Y., Wei, W., Liu, X., and Zeng, X., Carbon nanotube/chitosan/gold nanoparticles-based glucose biosensor prepared by a layer-by-layer technique. *Mater. Sci. Eng. C.* 29(1), 50–54, 2009.

37. Lin, J., He, C., Zhao, Y., and Zhang, S., One-step synthesis of silver nanoparticles/carbon nanotubes/chitosan film and its application in glucose biosensor. *Sens. Actuat. B Chem.* 137(2), 768–773, 2009.

38. Wen, Z., Ci, S., and Li, J., Pt nanoparticles inserting in carbon nanotube arrays: Nanocomposites for glucose biosensors. *J. Phys. Chem. C.* 113(31), 13482–13487, 2009.

39. Zhang, Y., Guo, G., Zhao, F., Mo, Z., Xiao, F., and Zeng, B., A novel glucose biosensor based on glucose oxidase immobilized on AuPt nanoparticle–carbon nanotube–ionic liquid hybrid coated electrode. *Electroanalysis.* 22(2), 223–228, 2010.

40. Kong, T., Chen, Y., Ye, Y., Zhang, K., Wang, Z., and Wang, X., An amperometric glucose biosensor based on the immobilization of glucose oxidase on the ZnO nanotubes. *Sens. Actuat. B Chem.* 138(1), 344–350, 2009.

41. Chi, B.-Z., Zeng, Q., Jiang, J.-H., Shen, G.-L., and Yu, R.-Q., Synthesis of ruthenium purple nanowire array for construction of sensitive and selective biosensors for glucose detection. *Sens. Actuat. B Chem.* 140(2), 591–596, 2009.

42. Liu, Y., Zhu, Y., Zeng, Y., and Xu, F., An effective amperometric biosensor based on gold nano-electrode arrays. *Nanoscale Res. Lett.* 4(3), 210–215, 2008.
43. Li, C.-T., *Telecommunications, Information and Multimedia*, Sorell, M. ed. Berlin Heidelberg: Springer, 173–178, 2009.
44. Santhosh, P., Manesh, K.M., Uthayakumar, S., Komathi, S., Gopalan, A.I., and Lee, K.P., Fabrication of enzymatic glucose biosensor based on palladium nanoparticles dispersed onto poly(3,4-ethylenedioxythiophene) nanofibers. *Bioelectrochemistry.* 75(1), 61–66, 2009.
45. Luo, L., Li, Q., Xu, Y., Ding, Y., Wang, X., Deng, D., and Xu, Y., Amperometric glucose biosensor based on $NiFe_2O_4$ nanoparticles and chitosan. *Sens. Actuat. B Chem.* 145(1), 293–298, 2010.
46. Jimenez, J., Sheparovych, R., Pita, M., Narvaez Garcia, A., Dominguez, E., Minko, S., and Katz, E., Magneto-induced self-assembling of conductive nanowires for biosensor applications. *J. Phys. Chem. C.* 112(19), 7337–7344, 2008.
47. Santhosh, P., Manesh, K.M., Uthayakumar, S., Gopalan, A.I., and Lee, K.P., Hollow spherical nanostructured polydiphenylamine for direct electrochemistry and glucose biosensor. *Biosens. Bioelectron.* 24(7), 2008–2014, 2009.
48. Wang, Z., Liu, S., Wu, P., and Cai, C., Detection of glucose based on direct electron transfer reaction of glucose oxidase immobilized on highly ordered polyaniline nanotubes. *Anal. Chem.* 81(4), 1638–1645, 2009.
49. Risveden, K., Ponténa, J.F., Calander, N., Willander, M., Danielsson, B., The region ion sensitive field effect transistor, a novel bioelectronic nanosensor. *Biosens. Bioelectron.* 22(12), 3105–3112, 2007.
50. Dongjin, L. and Tianhong, C., Layer-by-layer self-assembled single-walled carbon nanotubes based ion-sensitive conductometric glucose biosensors. *Sens. J. IEEE.* 9(4), 449–456, 2009.
51. Gun, J., Schöning, M.J., Abouzar, M.H., Poghossian, A., and Katz, E., Field-effect nanoparticle-based glucose sensor on a chip: Amplification effect of coimmobilized redox species. *Electroanalysis.* 20(16), 1748–1753, 2008.
52. Rose, G. and Shipley, M.J., Plasma lipids and mortality: A source of error. *Lancet.* 315(8167), 523–526, 1980.
53. Department of Health. The health of the nation: A strategy for health in England. HMSO, London, 1992.
54. Committee on Diet and Health, Food and Nutrition Board, Commission on Life Sciences, National Research Council, Diet and health implications for reducing chronic disease risk, National Academy Press, Washington, D.C., 1989.
55. Richmond, W., Preparation and properties of a bacterial cholesterol oxidase from *Nocardia* sp. and its application to enzyme assay of total cholesterol in serum. *Clin. Chem.* 19(12), 1350–1356, 1973.
56. Aravamudhan, S., Kumar, A., Mohapatra, S., and Bhansali, S., Sensitive estimation of total cholesterol in blood using Au nanowires based micro-fluidic platform. *Biosens. Bioelectron.* 22(9–10), 2289–2294, 2007.
57. Gopalan, A.I., Lee, K.-P., and Ragupathy, D., Development of a stable cholesterol biosensor based on multi-walled carbon nanotubes-gold nanoparticles composite covered with a layer of chitosan-room-temperature ionic liquid network. *Biosens. Bioelectron.* 24(7), 2211–2217, 2009.
58. Ahmadalinezhad, A. and Chen, A., High-performance electrochemical biosensor for the Detection of total cholesterol. *Biosens. Bioelectron.* 26(11), 4508–4513, 2011.
59. Filippova, N., Rodionov, I., and Ugarova, N.N., The chemiluminescent determination of cholesterol. *Lab Delo.* 9, 20–23, 1991.

9

Gold Nanorods in Sensing and Nanomedical Applications

Gautam Das

CONTENTS

9.1 Introduction

Research in the field of plasmonics has become very promising over a diverse range of areas, including nanoelectronics, energy harvesting, photothermal therapeutics, subwavelength domain optics, as well as in the development of sensing devices for applications in medicine, biotechnology, and environmental monitoring. In order to control the plasmonic characteristics of isolated or aggregated metallic nanostructures, one must have the capacity for specifically "tuning" the dimensions, morphology, and milieu within which they reside [1]. Surface plasmon attributes may be significantly modified when metallic nanostructures are brought into close proximity as a consequence of the robust interplay of localized surface-bound plasmons [2].

The application of noble metal nanoparticles has attracted attention due to their unique optical, chemical, and physical properties. When electromagnetic waves of an optical frequency interact with nanoparticles, which are much smaller than the wavelength of light, the interacting beam of light induces resonant oscillations in the conduction electrons of the metal. These nonpropagating resonant oscillation modes are known as localized surface plasmon resonance (LSPR). This phenomenon enhances the absorption, as well as the linear and nonlinear scattering of light. The amplitude and spectral peak position of the resonance frequency are contingent on the size, shape, and dielectric environment of the nanoparticle. The dielectric environment is formed by an adsorbed biomolecule or the surrounding buffer media with which the nanoparticles may be attached. Localized surface plasmon resonance can give rise to exponential (million-fold) amplification of the domains in the near-field outside the particle, which is the basis of surface-enhanced Raman scattering (SERS)/spectroscopy [3]. The interactions between metals and electromagnetic waves can be described on the basis of Maxwell's equations. Details of the optical properties of materials are available in standard textbooks on electricity and magnetism [4].

In this chapter, we describe the optical properties of a particular class of noble metal nanoparticles—gold (Au) nanorods to further elucidate LSPR and SERS. In addition, we survey a number of recent developments that involve the utilization of gold nanorods for applications in nanomedical diagnostics and therapeutics. A brief description of an application that involves the use of an optical fiber to develop a compact, cost-effective biosensing device, utilizing gold nanorods is also provided.

9.2 Synthesis and Functionalization of Gold Nanorods

There are currently several techniques that are employed for the synthesis of nanorods, which include electrochemistry, seed mediation, and templating. Of these, wet chemistry-based seed-mediated growth serves as one of the most suitable methods due to its simple process, cost effectiveness, and high nanorod yields with straightforward control of size and aspect ratios [5,6]. Subsequent to synthesis, biocompatible compounds such as organothiols may be used to activate the nanorods. Truong et al. demonstrated that when a thiol derivative (OEG_6), employed to avert the random attachment of proteins, was used to functionalize cetyltrimethylammonium bromide (CTAB)-capped single gold nanorod LSPR sensors, a very high sensitivity to low concentrations of biological analytes was possible. The CTAB cationic surfactant serves as a structural guiding agent that induces nanorod growth in aqueous media via binding with the particular facets of nanocrystals. The resultant uniform bilayer of CTAB noncovalently coats the nanorods, and subsequent to synthesis, excess amounts of CTAB (which in its free state is highly toxic) may remain bound to the surface. This excess surfactant may contribute to the disruption of the optical properties of nanorods and thus hinder sensing functionality. The nanorods are therefore typically centrifuged multiple times in order to dispense with the extra volume of CTAB [7–10].

In a new development, Vigderman et al. have demonstrated that CTAB can be completely replaced by cationic thiol ligands (16-mercaptohexadecyl) trimethylammonium bromide (MTAB) that contain pendant thiol groups, which provide robust anchoring to gold substrates [11]. It also has the advantage of exhibiting very low cytotoxicity. In addition, it was estimated that the uptake of MTAB-coated nanorods by cancer cells numbered ~2.17 million, in comparison to similarly dimensioned nanorods at quantities that ranged from several hundred to one hundred and fifty thousand, which have been quantified in the literature [12,13].

Wang et al. developed a stable gold nanorod probe that was functionalized with thiolated polyethylene glycol (SH-PEG) and polyacrylic acid (PAA) and loaded with the anticancer drug doxorubicin (DOX). The resultant hybrid entity illustrated the possibility that gold nanorods could serve both as passive drug delivery devices and therapeutic hyperthermia agents to deliver a simultaneous dual assault on cancer cells [14]. Gold nanorods have also shown the capacity to serve as vehicles for the attachment and delivery of nucleic acids into cells [15,16] and to traverse the blood brain barrier (BBB) to deliver particular siRNAs (small interfering/silencing RNA) to neurons in silencing the expression of DARPP-32 (dopamine, cAMP-regulated phosphoprotein of 32,000 kDa) [17].

Huang et al. noted that nanoparticles tend to form aggregates in aqueous environments, which can seriously impact their viable utility as beneficial agents for medical imaging and in diagnostic and therapeutic applications. Indeed, gold nanorods have shown the tendency for swift aggregation in biofluids. Nanoparticle stability may be facilitated through the use of polyethylene glycol (PEG); however, when PEG is adsorbed on to nanoparticle surfaces, it can have a detrimental effect on the ability of nanoparticles to interact with proteins, or to be taken up by cells [18]. Huang reports that when multiple layers of polyelectrolyte were added to gold nanorods, they remained stable for up to a month. When alternating thin film layers of biocompatible anionic (poly(styrene sulfonate)) and cationic (pEI25 or EGDE-3,3′) polyelectrolytes were used to coat gold nanorod assemblages, they also exhibited multiple capacities in a single platform, including the hyperthermic destruction of prostate cancer cells in vitro, the delivery of plasmid DNA, and serving as an optical imaging agent. These entities revealed decreased cytotoxic effects, in contrast to polyethyleneimine (typically utilized in polymer-based gene conveyance), and improved levels of DNA transfection as well [15].

It is possible to functionalize the surfaces of nanoparticles such that they have an affinity for the adsorption, and thus detection of a particular molecule to be sensed. Functionalization becomes necessary when the analytes of interest have a negligible affinity for gold or other noble metal nanoparticles. Self-assembled monolayers (SAMs) consist of highly uniform layers of amphiphilic molecules (both water- and fat-loving) that contain both "head" and "tail" domains, wherein the heads are equipped to have reversible attractions for substrates, and the tails possess terminal functional groups. Self-assembled monolayers may be employed to coat gold nanoparticles toward preventing their aggregation.

Truong et al. developed individual gold nanorod immunosensors for the highly sensitive detection of ultralow (111 attomolar (aM)— equivalent to a 2.79 nm λ_{max} shift) concentrations of a prostate-specific antigen (PSA) protein biomarker via antibody-endowed surfaces. This achievement represents a significant improvement over the detection limits of commercially available PSA assays (~0.005 ng/mL), alternate surface plasmon resonance techniques (0.15–18.1 ng/mL), surface plasmon fluorescence spectroscopy (3 pg/mL), and real-time Immuno-PCR (0.2 pg/mL) [7,19], and is within the range of detection limits (30 aM down to 3 aM) for PSA achieved by Mirkin et al. utilizing a magnetic micro/nanoparticle oligonucleotide-based biobarcode technology [20,21]. Additional details with regard to nanoparticle functionalization procedures are available in the scientific literature [22].

9.3 Theory and Discussion

9.3.1 Surface Plasmon Resonance Spectroscopy

Localized surface plasmon modes arise because of the interaction of the conduction electrons of metal nanoparticles and incident electromagnetic waves. The oscillation frequency of the electron cloud is identical to the incident electromagnetic wave. In fact, the incident light induces a dipole oscillation, which oscillates in resonance with the incident electromagnetic wave. Thus, the LSPR enhances the absorption and scattering of electromagnetic waves in resonance with the LSPR frequency. This also explains the origin of the colors that emanate from colloidal solutions of noble metals. The origin of LSPR can be explained by the theory of scattering of light by subwavelength metallic particles. The theory of the scattering of light by spherical particles was first introduced by Gustav Mie, which was later modified by several researchers when they included studies of linear and nonlinear optical properties (e.g., extinction = scattering + absorption) of nanoparticles of different sizes, shapes, and complex dielectric environments when they interacted with intense light waves [23]. It is possible to find the LSPR frequency quantitatively for nanoparticles with a radius (R), much smaller than the wavelength (λ) of light, by calculating the expression for absorption and emission cross sections for nanoparticles given by [24,25]:

$$C_{abs} = \frac{2\pi}{3\lambda} \varepsilon_m^{3/2} V \sum_i \frac{\varepsilon'' / \left(n^i\right)^2}{\left(\varepsilon' + \left[\left(1-n^i\right)/n^i\right]\varepsilon_m\right)^2 + \varepsilon''^2}, \tag{9.1a}$$

$$C_{sca} = \frac{8\pi^3}{9\lambda^4} \varepsilon_m^2 V^2 \sum_i \frac{\left(\varepsilon' - \varepsilon_m\right)^2 + \left(\varepsilon''^2 / \left(n^i\right)^2\right)}{\left(\varepsilon' + \left[\left(1-n^i\right)/n^i\right]\varepsilon_m\right)^2 + \varepsilon''^2}, \tag{9.1b}$$

$$C_{ext} = C_{abs} + C_{sca}, \tag{9.1c}$$

$$n^a = \frac{2}{D^2-1}\left(\frac{D}{2\sqrt{D^2-1}} \ln \frac{D+\sqrt{D^2-1}}{D-\sqrt{D^2-1}} - 1\right), $$

$$n^b = n^c = (1-n^a)/2, \tag{9.1d}$$

where
   $\varepsilon = \varepsilon'(\lambda) + i\varepsilon''(\lambda)$ is the complex dielectric constant of the material of the nanoparticles
      (e.g., gold)
   ε_m is the dielectric constant of the surrounding medium
   C_{abs}, C_{sca}, and C_{ext} are absorption, scattering, and extinction cross sections, respectively
   V is the volume of a single nanoparticle
   $n^{i=a,b,c}$ (i represents dimensions along the x, y, and z axes of the nanoparticle)
   n is the depolarization factor
   D is the aspect defined as a/b

The extinction maximum occurs at resonance when the wavelength of the incident wave matches the LSPR peak of the nanoparticles. Thus, from the extinction curve, it is possible to find the LSPR peak, which is very important for the application of nanoparticles in sensing, based on SERS.

   Further, it is also possible to obtain LSPR peaks of nanoparticles by solving Maxwell's equations using FDTD method (e.g., FDTD software from RSOFT). However, the simulations are very lengthy and sometimes require significant computational capacity. Figure 9.1a illustrates the absorption spectra of two different sizes of gold nanoparticles. The LSPR peaks are at the visible region of the electromagnetic spectrum. It is evident from the figure that by changing the dimensions of the nanoparticle and the refractive index of the surrounding medium, one may shift the LSPR peak position (Figure 9.1b).

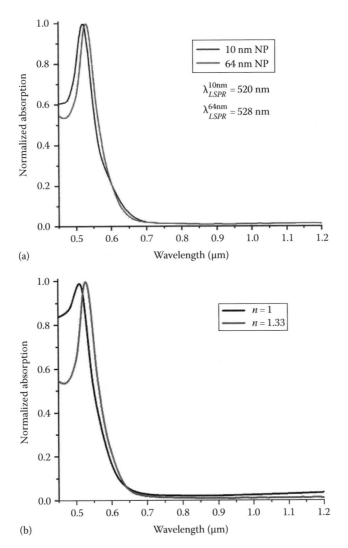

FIGURE 9.1
(a, b) Absorption spectrum of gold nanoparticles.

The LSPR peak may be tuned at any wavelength between the mid-infrared (MID-IR) and UV regions of the electromagnetic spectrum by adjusting the size, shape, and dielectric constant of the metallic nanoparticles and the medium that surrounds them [26]. Gold nanorods are very intriguing and attractive due to their distinct characteristics in comparison to solid gold nanoparticles or gold nanoshells. The structures of the gold nanorods allow LSPR oscillation to occur either along their longitudinal or transverse direction (Figure 9.2). Thus, gold nanorods have two absorption peaks that correspond to the longitudinal and transverse modes, respectively. The transverse surface plasmon resonance peak resides in the visible region, whereas the longitudinal surface plasmon resonance peak is located in the longer wavelength region of the electromagnetic spectrum. These two absorption peaks are also tunable. The LSPR peak corresponding to the longitudinal mode of oscillation is very sensitive to the ratio of length and width, which is known as the aspect ratio

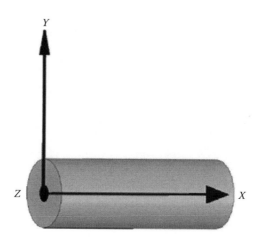

FIGURE 9.2
Single gold nanorod.

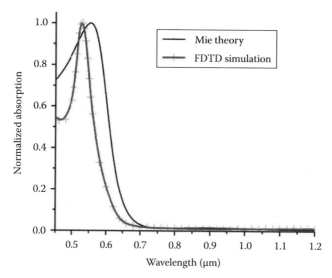

FIGURE 9.3
Absorption spectrum for 64 nm gold nanoparticles.

(D in Equation 9.1). One can obtain a large red-shift in comparison to solid nanoparticles by modifying the aspect ratio. In Equation 9.1, by changing the value of i, one may obtain the cross sections of gold nanorods ($i = a$: for longitudinal surface plasmon resonance and $i = b = c$: for transverse surface resonance oscillations) and spherical solid nanoparticles ($i = 1/3$).

Figure 9.3 depicts the results obtained for a 64 nm gold nanoparticle using the Mie theory and FDTD method. The slight discrepancy in LSPR wavelength is due to the approximation of Maxwell's equations in the Mie theory. Figure 9.4 shows the absorption spectrum of a gold nanorod with a different aspect ratio. The two peaks correspond to the transverse plasmon resonance and the longitudinal plasmon resonance, respectively. By altering the aspect ratio, it is possible to shift the longitudinal surface plasmon resonance peaks at the desired wavelength of interest. It is also clear from Figures 9.1a and 9.4 that in order to

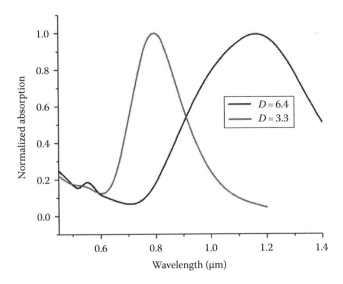

FIGURE 9.4
Absorption spectrum for gold nanorod for different aspect ratios.

obtain a LSPR peak in the MID-IR or IR regions of the electromagnetic spectrum, it is better to utilize gold nanorods rather than nanoparticles. In the latter case, very large particle sizes are required.

The fundamental principle behind the application of nanoparticles in sensing is that the spectral position of the surface plasmon resonance peak shifts with the change of the surrounding dielectric medium. Figure 9.5 shows absorption spectra of the single gold nanorods of aspect ratio 6.4 for two different refractive index media. Higher refractive index corresponds to larger shift in the surface plasmon resonance peak. The refractive indexes of the different protein solutions are not the same, but close to ~1.5. So, by observing the shift in

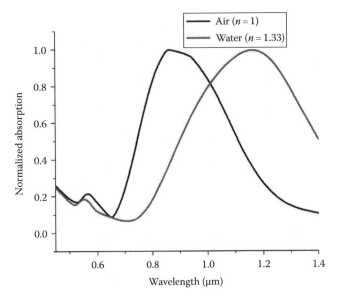

FIGURE 9.5
Absorption spectrum for gold nanorod of aspect ratio 6:4 for two refractive indices.

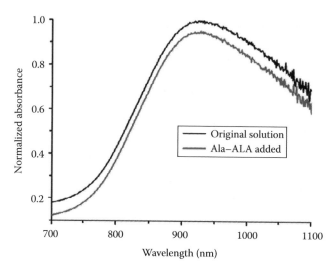

FIGURE 9.6
Absorption spectrum for the solution of gold nanorods and dipeptide.

the resonance peak, one can predict the presence of a particular protein. Figure 9.6 shows the spectrum obtained using the mixture of commercially available gold nanorods solution (Sigma Aldrich, United States) and ALA–ALA dipeptide ($C_6H_{12}N_2O_3$: pH—5, Sigma Aldrich) obtained using a UV–Visible spectrometer. The shift of the resonance peak was only ~2 nm. The addition of the dipeptide changes the refractive index of the solution and thus the shifts in the LSPR peak. As the refractive indices of the protein solutions, are very close, a small shift in LSPR peak is not suitable for practical application, especially for the identification of proteins in biological samples. Further, a biomedical sensing device based on IR radiation (e.g., 0.7–1.1 μm) band is very attractive, because the detrimental effect of fluorescence is absent.

9.3.2 Surface-Enhanced Raman Spectroscopy

Raman spectroscopy is an important analytical tool for the investigation of organic molecules such as proteins in biological samples. It involves detection of inelastic-scattered light from molecules, subsequent to its interaction with a beam of light. The application of Raman spectroscopy for the identification of a single molecule was limited due to a very small scattering cross section (~10^{-30}) of the Raman scattering process. Fleischmann and coworkers found that the Raman spectrum of pyridine was enhanced several fold when adsorbed on the rough surface of a silver electrode, which was verified by other researchers for different molecules and metallic surfaces [27,28]. The discovery of this effect, which is known as SERS has revolutionized the field of Raman spectroscopy [3]. Surface-enhanced Raman scattering applications span biotechnology, biochemistry, environmental monitoring, and homeland security, as it has the ability to detect single molecules. At present, it is possible to obtain field enhancement with a factor of ~10^{10}, via novel noble metal nanostructures and methodologies, which serve to increase the Raman scattering cross section [22]. The mechanisms of SERS enhancement include the augmentation of electromagnetic and chemical properties. The incident electromagnetic waves interact with nanostructures (e.g., gold nanoparticles) and excite localized surface plasmon modes, as described earlier. The LSPR oscillation in nanoparticles enhances the scattering and absorption of the incident wave in resonance with the LSPR frequency. The plasmon energy initiates the Raman process in the molecule that is adsorbed on the nanoparticles [29].

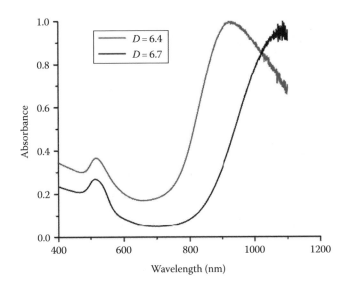

FIGURE 9.7
Absorption spectrum for colloidal gold nanorods.

Gold nanorods are very attractive due to their unique optical properties such as the presence of two resonance peaks and strong SERS [30–32]. The longitudinal surface resonance peak is tunable by virtue of the aspect ratio of the nanorod. Figure 9.7 depicts the absorption spectrum for colloidal gold nanorods (Sigma Aldrich) with an aspect ratio of 6.4 and 6.7, obtained using a UV–Visible spectrometer. It is possible to obtain LSPR peaks at any desired wavelength through the modification of the aspect ratio of the nanorods. In general, biological samples that are excited with a visible laser produce strong fluorescence, which deteriorates the signal-to-noise ratio of the Raman spectra. Very few works have been reported on the sensing of biological samples based on SERS and gold nanorods using near-IR laser radiation, which is free from any detrimental fluorescence effects [30,33].

Fiber lasers are established as robust and reliable photonic conveyance devices. They have wide applications in industry and medicine in that they are compact and cost-effective, with desirable characteristics such as an all-fiber design and lack of the requirements for realignment and external cooling. A tunable laser in the near-IR wavelength band will have strong potential in the development of sensing devices that are based on SERS. It will be possible to excite LSPR oscillation in gold nanorods through the tuning of the laser wavelength, as well as to develop a sensing probe by employing a multimode fiber [34]. Devices that are based on all-fiber technologies will be very attractive for the development of advanced and innovative sensing mechanisms, which may have many applications, potentially including many in the field of nanomedicine.

9.4 Gold Nanorod Mediated Theranostics

Gold nanorods are uniquely suited for theranostic applications, whereby they may be utilized to function simultaneously as diagnostic and therapeutic agents. This is due to their propensity for enabling the controllable manipulation of robust electric fields at their surfaces to either absorb or scatter electromagnetic radiation, resulting in the onset of highly localized heating for nanomedical hyperthermia and the capacity for high-resolution (molecular level) imaging, respectively. When the aspect ratios of these nanoparticles are appropriately configured, they exhibit robust absorption and scattering at near-infrared (650–900 nm) wavelengths.

Huang et al. decorated gold nanorods with monoclonal (anti-EGFR) antibodies that had a high affinity for epidermal growth factor receptors (EGFRs), and cultured them with a noncancerous control epithelial cell line (HaCat) and two species of cancerous oral epithelial cells (HOC 313 clone 8 and HSC 3). It was observed that the targeting enabled nanorods attached selectively to the membrane surfaces of the cancerous cells, as they typically overexpress EGFR. The gold nanorods were shown to scatter intense red light, which clearly differentiated them from the healthy cells. Under sustained irradiation with 800 nm red laser light, the cancerous cells were hyperthermically eliminated, while the healthy cells remained viable. This is because the cancerous cells can be destroyed using only half of the laser power that is necessary to kill healthy cells. This work provided a powerful illustration to the fact that specifically targeted gold nanorods may concurrently diagnose and eradicate cancer cells [35].

In addition to enabling a versatile repertoire of imaging capabilities including two-photon luminescence [36–38], darkfield microscopy [39,40], optical coherence tomography [41,42], and photoacoustic tomography [43–45], gold nanorods have the advantageous concomitant capacity for imparting photothermal therapeutics. The NIR-initiated heating of gold nanorods can impart damage and destruction of diseased cells and tissues that are in close proximity, via the disruption of membranes and cellular equilibrium, which triggers the incursion of Ca^{2+} and subsequent actin network depolymerization [46].

Practically, all (~96%) of the nanorod-absorbed photons are transformed into thermal energy. It was demonstrated by Chou et al. that when polyurethane-encapsulated gold nanorods were irradiated with a 20 mW NIR laser, the temperature increased by more than 100°C within 1 min [47]. The effects of photonically induced hyperthermia in vitro have been investigated by several researchers using cultured tumor cells [48,49], macrophages [50,51], parasites [52], and pathogenic bacteria [46,53–55].

Hypothetically, should nanorods be hollowed and loaded with potent drugs, they may be induced to eject them simultaneously with the onset of hyperthermia, as the nanorods may thermally deform to breach the thin encapsulating walls, enabling the highly localized release of their drug payloads. Further evolution of these capabilities will make possible the noninvasive elimination of in vivo resident diseased entities as an attractive option to surgically imparted physical trauma and may allow the avoidance of accompanying (sometimes extended) surgery recovery times [56].

9.5 Conclusion

Gold nanorods are manifest as advanced and potentially powerful sensing, diagnostic, and therapeutic tools, which may be induced to exhibit single or multiple functionalities, contingent on the particular envisioned application. These capabilities will be made possible via fine control and exploitation of the unique phenomenon of surface plasmon resonance, and by virtue of the properties of the (Au) noble metal itself. The prospective applications of gold nanorods working in conjunction with associated technologies and infrastructures appear indeed to be boundless. A potent example provided in this chapter would consist of a fiber laser that possesses a suitable tuning range, which would serve as an excellent candidate for the application of gold nanorod mediated sensing that is based on SERS. This type of system would be very compact and cost-effective. We are likely to witness the rapidly increased utilization of gold nanorods, encompassing many areas, including potentially dynamic and dramatic illustrations of their benefits in the nascent yet burgeoning disciplines of nanotechnology and nanomedicine.

Acknowledgment

Author acknowledges the financial support of the Natural Sciences and Engineering Research Council of Canada (NSERC) and the Canada Foundation for Innovation (CFI). Also, the contributions of graduate and undergraduate students in the development of Nanophotonics research facilities at Lakehead University.

References

1. Jiang, L., Sun, Y., Huo, F., Zhang, H., Qin, L., Li, S., and Chen, X., Free-standing one-dimensional plasmonic nanostructures. *Nanoscale* 4(1), 66–75, 2012.
2. Halas, N.J., Lal, S., Chang, W.S., Link, S., and Nordlander, P., Plasmons in strongly coupled metallic nanostructures. *Chem. Rev.* 111(6), 3913–3961, 2011.
3. Moskovits, M., Surface-enhanced spectroscopy. *Rev. Mod. Phys.* 57, 783–826, 1985.
4. Jackson J.D., *Classical Electrodynamics*, 3rd edn. Wiley, New York, 1999.
5. Si, S., Leduc, C., Delville, M.H., and Lounis, B., Short gold nanorod growth revisited: The critical role of the bromide counterion. *Chemphyschem* 13(1), 193–202, 2012.
6. Garg, N., Scholl, C., Mohanty, A., and Jin, R., The role of bromide ions in seeding growth of Au nanorods. *Langmuir* 26(12), 10271–10276, 2010.
7. Truong, P.L., Cao, C., Park, S., Kim, M., and Sim, S.J., A new method for non-labeling attomolar detection of diseases based on an individual gold nanorod immunosensor. *Lab. Chip.* 11(15), 2591–2597, 2011.
8. Pérez-Juste, J., Pastoriza-Santos, I., Liz-Marzán, L.M., and Mulvaney, P., Gold nanorods: Synthesis, characterization and applications, *Coord. Chem. Rev.* 249, 1870–1901, 2005.
9. Yu, C., Varghese, L., and Irudayaraj, J., Surface modification of cetyltrimethylammonium bromide-capped gold nanorods to make molecular probes. *Langmuir* 23(17), 9114–9119, 2007.
10. Wang, C., Chen, Y., Wang, T., Ma, Z., and Su, Z., Biorecognition-driven self-assembly of gold nanorods: A rapid and sensitive approach toward antibody sensing. *Chem. Mater.* 19, 5809–5811, 2007.
11. Vigderman, L., Manna, P., and Zubarev, E.R., Quantitative replacement of cetyl trimethylammonium bromide by cationic thiol ligands on the surface of gold nanorods and their extremely large uptake by cancer cells. *Angew Chem. Int. Ed. Engl.* 51(3), 636–641, 2012.
12. Alkilany, A.M., Nagaria, P.K., Hexel, C.R., Shaw, T.J., Murphy, C.J., and Wyatt, M.D., Cellular uptake and cytotoxicity of gold nanorods: Molecular origin of cytotoxicity and surface effects. *Small* 5(6), 701–708, 2009.
13. Hauck, T.S., Ghazani, A.A., and Chan, W.C., Assessing the effect of surface chemistry on gold nanorod uptake, toxicity, and gene expression in mammalian cells. *Small* 4(1), 153–159, 2008.
14. Wang, T., Zhang, X., Pan, Y., Miao, X., Su, Z., Wang, C., and Li, X., Fabrication of doxorubicin functionalized gold nanorod probes for combined cancer imaging and drug delivery. *Dalton Trans.* 40(38), 9789–9794, 2011.

15. Huang, H.C., Barua, S., Kay, D.B., and Rege, K., Simultaneous enhancement of photothermal stability and gene delivery efficacy of gold nanorods using polyelectrolytes. *ACS Nano* 3(10), 2941–2952, 2009.

16. Wijaya, A., Schaffer, S.B., Pallares, I.G., and Hamad-Schifferli, K., Selective release of multiple DNA oligonucleotides from gold nanorods. *ACS Nano* 3(1), 80–86, 2009.

17. Bonoiu, A.C., Mahajan, S.D., Ding, H., Roy, I., Yong, K.T., Kumar, R., Hu, R., Bergey, E.J., Schwartz, S.A., and Prasad, P.N., Nanotechnology approach for drug addiction therapy: Gene silencing using delivery of gold nanorod-siRNA nanoplex in dopaminergic neurons. *Proc. Natl. Acad. Sci. USA* 106(14), 5546–5550, 2009.

18. Huff, T.B., Hansen, M.N., Zhao, Y., Cheng, J.X., and Wei, A., Controlling the cellular uptake of gold nanorods. *Langmuir* 23, 1596–1599, 2007.

19. Healy, D.A., Hayes, C.J., Leonard, P., McKenna, L., and O'Kennedy, R., Biosensor developments: Application to prostate-specific antigen detection. *Trends Biotechnol.* 25(3), 125–131, 2007.

20. Nam, J.M., Thaxton, C.S., and Mirkin, C.A., Nanoparticle-based bio-bar codes for the ultrasensitive detection of proteins. *Science* 301(5641), 1884–1886, 2003.

21. Bao, Y.P., Wei, T.F., Lefebvre, P.A., An, H., He, L., Kunkel, G.T., and Müller, U.R., Detection of protein analytes via nanoparticle-based bio bar code technology. *Anal. Chem.* 78(6), 2055–2059, 2006.

22. Kosuda, K.M., Bingham, J.M., Wustholz, K.L., and Van Duyne, R.P., *Comprehensive Nanoscience and Technology.* Academic Press, New York, 2011, pp. 263–301.

23. Mie, G., Beitrage zur Optik truber Medien, speziell kolloidaler Metallosungen, *Annalen der Physik* 330(3), 377–445, 1908.

24. Jain, P.K., El-Sayed, I.H., and El-Sayed, M.A., Au nanoparticles target cancer, *Nano Today* 2(1), 18–29, 2007.

25. Huang, X.H., Neretina, S., and El-Sayed, M.A., Gold nanorods: From synthesis and properties to biological and biomedical applications. *Adv. Mater.* 21(48), 4880–4910, 2009.

26. Oldenburg, S.J., Jackson, J.B., Westcott, S.L., and Halas, N.J., Infrared extinction properties of gold nanoshells, *Appl. Phys. Lett.* 75(19), 2897–2899, 1999.

27. Fleischmann, M., Hendra, J., and MacQuillan, J., Raman spectra of pyridine adsorbed at a silver electrode, *Chem. Phys. Lett.* 26(2), 163–166, 1974.

28. Kniepp, K., Kneipp, H., Itzkan, I., Dasari, R.R., and Feld, M.S., Surface-enhanced Raman scattering and biophysics. *J. Phys.: Condens. Matter.* 14, 597–624, 2002.

29. McNay, G., Eustace, D., Smith, W.E., Faulds, K., and Graham, D., Surface-enhanced Raman scattering (SERS) and surface-enhanced resonance Raman scattering (SERRS): A review of applications, *Appl. Spectrosc.* 65(8), 825–837, 2011.

30. Nikoobakht, B. and El-Sayed, M.A., Surface-enhanced Raman scattering studies on aggregated gold nanorods, *J. Phys. Chem. A* 107(18), 3372–3378, 2003.

31. Nikoobakht, B., Wang, J., and El-Sayed, M.A., Surface-enhanced Raman scattering of molecules adsorbed on gold nanorods: Off-surface plasmon resonance condition. *Chem. Phys. Lett.* 366(1–2), 17–23, 2002.

32. Wang, Y., Guo, S., Chen, H., and Wang, E., Facile fabrication of large area of aggregated gold nanorods film for efficient surface-enhanced Raman scattering. *J. Colloid Interf. Sci.* 318, 82–87, 2008.

33. Smitha, S.L., Gopchandran, K.G., Ravindran, T.R., and Prasad, V.S., Gold nanorods with finely tunable longitudinal plasmon resonance as SERS substrate. *Nanotechnology* 22, 265705–265712, 2011.

34. Stokes, D.L. and Vo-Dinh, T., Development of an integrated single-fiber SERS sensor, *Sensors Actuators B*, 69, 28–36, 2000.

35. Huang, X., El-Sayed, I.H., Qian, W., and El-Sayed, M.A., Cancer cell imaging and photothermal therapy in the near-infrared region by using gold nanorods. *J. Am. Chem. Soc.* 128(6), 2115–2120, 2006.

36. Ye, E., Win, K.Y., Tan, H.R., Lin, M., Teng, C.P., Mlayah, A., and Han, M.Y., Plasmonic gold nanocrosses with multidirectional excitation and strong photothermal effect. *J. Am. Chem. Soc.* 133(22), 8506–8509, 2011.

37. Wang, D.S., Hsu, F.Y., and Lin, C.W., Surface plasmon effects on two photon luminescence of gold nanorods. *Opt. Express* 17(14), 11350–11359, 2009.

38. Mohamed, M.B., Volkov, V., Link, S., and El-Sayed, M.A., The "lightning" gold nanorods: Fluorescence enhancement of over a million compared to the gold metal. *Chem. Phys. Lett.* 317, 517–723, 2000.

39. Xiao, L., Qiao, Y., He, Y., and Yeung, E.S., Three dimensional orientational imaging of nanoparticles with darkfield microscopy. *Anal. Chem.* 82(12), 5268–5274, 2010.

40. Murphy, C.J., Gole, A.M., Stone, J.W., Sisco, P.N., Alkilany, A.M., Goldsmith, E.C., and Baxter, S.C., Gold nanoparticles in biology: Beyond toxicity to cellular imaging. *Acc. Chem. Res.* 41(12), 1721–1730, 2008.

41. Chhetri, R.K., Kozek, K.A., Johnston-Peck, A.C., Tracy, J.B., and Oldenburg, A.L., Imaging three-dimensional rotational diffusion of plasmon resonant gold nanorods using polarization-sensitive optical coherence tomography. *Phys. Rev. E Stat. Nonlin. Soft Matter Phys.* 83(4 Pt 1), 040903, 2011.

42. Oldenburg, A.L., Hansen, M.N., Ralston, T.S., Wei, A., and Boppart, S.A., Imaging gold nanorods in excised human breast carcinoma by spectroscopic optical coherence tomography. *J. Mater. Chem.* 19, 6407, 2009.

43. Manohar, S., Ungureanu, C., and Van Leeuwen, T.G., Gold nanorods as molecular contrast agents in photoacoustic imaging: The promises and the caveats. *Contrast Media Mol. Imaging* 6(5), 389–400, 2011.

44. Ha, S., Carson, A., Agarwal, A., Kotov, N.A., and Kim, K., Detection and monitoring of the multiple inflammatory responses by photoacoustic molecular imaging using selectively targeted gold nanorods. *Biomed. Opt. Express* 2(3), 645–657, 2011.

45. Chen, Y.S., Frey, W., Kim, S., Kruizinga, P., Homan, K., and Emelianov, S., Silica-coated gold nanorods as photoacoustic signal nanoamplifiers. *Nano Lett.* 11(2), 348–354, 2011.

46. Tong, L., Wei, Q., Wei, A., and Cheng, J.X., Gold nanorods as contrast agents for biological imaging: Optical properties, surface conjugation and photothermal effects. *Photochem. Photobiol.* 85(1), 21–32, 2009.

47. Chou, C.H., Chen, C.D., and Wang, C.R.C., Highly efficient, wavelength-tunable, gold nanoparticle based optothermal nanoconvertors. *J. Phys. Chem. B* 109:11135–11138, 2005.

48. Guo, R., Zhang, L., Qian, H., Li, R., Jiang, X., and Liu, B., Multifunctional nanocarriers for cell imaging, drug delivery, and near-IR photothermal therapy. *Langmuir* 26(8), 5428–5434, 2010.

49. Huff, T.B., Tong, L., Zhao, Y., Hansen, M.N., Cheng, J.X., and Wei, A., Hyperthermic effects of gold nanorods on tumor cells. *Nanomedicine* 2, 125–132, 2007.

50. Pissuwan, D., Valenzuela, S.M., Killingsworth, M.C., Xu, X., and Cortie, M.B., Targeted destruction of murine macrophage cells with bioconjugated gold nanorods. *J. Nanoparticle Res.* 9, 1109–1124, 2007.

51. Choi, R., Yang, J., Choi, J., Lim, E.K., Kim, E., Suh, J.S., Huh, Y.M., and Haam, S., Thiolated dextran-coated gold nanorods for photothermal ablation of inflammatory macrophages. *Langmuir* 26(22), 17520–17527, 2010.

52. Pissuwan, D., Valenzuela, S.M., Miller, C.M., and Cortie, M.B., A golden bullet? Selective targeting of toxoplasma gondii tachyzoites using antibody-functionalized gold nanorods. *Nano Lett.* 7, 3808–3812, 2007.

53. Norman, R.S., Stone, J.W., Gole, A., Murphy, C.J., and Sabo-Attwood, T.L., Targeted photothermal lysis of the pathogenic bacteria, *Pseudomonas aeruginosa*, with gold nanorods. *Nano Lett.* 8, 302–306, 2008.

54. He, W., Henne, W.A., Wei, Q., Zhao, Y., Doorneweerd, D.D., Cheng, J-X., Low, P.S., and Wei, A., Two-photon luminescence imaging of bacillus spores using peptide-functionalized gold nanorods. *Nano Res.* 1, 450–456, 2008.

55. Pissuwan, D., Cortie, C.H., Valenzuela, S.M., and Cortie, M.B., Functionalised gold nanoparticles for controlling pathogenic bacteria. *Trends Biotechnol.* 28(4), 207–213, 2010.

56. Wust, P., Hildebrandt, B., Sreenivasa, G., Rau, B., Gellerman, J., Riess, H., Felix, R., and Schlag, P.M., Hyperthermia in combined treatment of cancer. *Lancet Oncol.* 3, 487–497, 2002.

10

Ophthalmic Glucose Nanosensors for Diabetes Management

Angelika Domschke

CONTENTS

10.1 Introduction: Importance of Diabetes Management

Diabetes represents one of the primary health concerns of the twenty-first century. However, the most common method of glucose level monitoring (e.g., finger-stick method) can be as problematic as the disease itself, as diabetics are required to obtain blood samples up to five times per day. This procedure is painful and inconvenient, and as a result patients tend to test themselves less frequently, which translates to less effective glycemic control. This situation has been described by experts in the field as comparable to a "glycemic" roller coaster ride that diabetes patients must endure on a daily basis, blindfolded. Each finger stick provides only an isolated snapshot of the blood glucose value in real time, devoid of any information in regard to how low or high the level will fall or rise over the next moments (Figure 10.1). This constitutes a frightening situation indeed, albeit one that has bolstered the many research efforts currently underway, in an attempt to assist with remedying this situation. Noninvasive and continuous glucose monitoring (CGM) comprises one of the most highly investigated areas, which may have great potential to increase patient usage. This strategy may significantly improve the lives and health of diabetes patients [1–3].

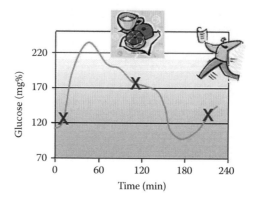

FIGURE 10.1

Exemplary time course of blood glucose levels, depicting high and low glucose values that may go undetected using regular finger-stick glucose measurement.

10.2 Current Continuous Glucose Monitoring Devices

Several CGM devices are currently available: Guardian® REAL-Time (Medtronic), SEVEN® PLUS (DexCom), Paradigm® REAL-Time and insulin pump (Mini-Med), FreeStyle Navigator® (Abbott, discontinued in the United States), GlucoDay® S (Menarini Diagnostics microdialysis system for clinical use, not released in the United States). These monitors consist of a disposable needle sensor wire, a transmitter, and a receiver. The sensor wire is inserted by the patient or is injected clinically under the skin with replacement times from 2 to 7 days. A detailed description of three types of sensor devices has been reported by Brett Ives et al. [4].

The availability of a complete glucose profile, enabled by these methods, was proven to be beneficial for glycemic control [5]. However, for a variety of reasons, large-scale implementation of these monitoring devices in diabetic care still awaits a breakthrough. For example, the method of sensor insertion is painful; frequent replacement increases the risk of inflammation; they are often noticeable, and in some cases have limited water resistance. They are also very expensive (over $5000 per year) [6], and insurance coverage is approved on a case-by-case basis only. Another point of concern is a relatively low accuracy. As evidenced in several studies, the median relative absolute difference (RAD), a measure of sensor accuracy comparing sensor readings to reference glucose levels, ranges from 12% to 20% [6–10]. The newest generation of CGM systems is purported to be within a 20% RAD, yet still does not approach the accuracy of current home glucose monitors. However, it is important to note that sensor accuracy has improved over time and will continue to progress with technological advancements, offering a means to enhance the efficacy of current diabetes care.

10.3 Noninvasive Continuous Glucose Monitoring Devices

In recent years, numerous efforts have been focused on the development of noninvasive or minimally invasive sensors that would allow convenient, pain-free, and CGM for diabetic patients. Noninvasive detection may be achieved by the use of sensing elements that are placed on the skin, combined with a detection device that can sense tissue glucose without piercing the skin. Some examples include iontophoretic extraction of glucose through the epidermis, visible (or near-IR absorption) spectrometry, and polarimetry. A comprehensive evaluation of noninvasive glucose monitoring, spanning 14 technologies and 16 devices has been reported by Tura et al. [11].

10.4 Advantages of Noninvasive and Continuous Ophthalmic/Contact Lens Glucose Sensors

An alternative approach to noninvasive or minimally invasive CGM would be to extract measurements from saliva, urine, or tear fluid. A major disadvantage of this method is that almost all of these fluids have the requirement of being collected prior to measurement and, therefore, truly continuous sensing has not yet been a possibility. Among several available body fluids, tear fluid has a number of distinct advantages insofar as glucose sensing. It is directly assessable in situ from the eye; it possesses a direct correlation to glucose levels in blood [12]; and the fluid is confined to a small area, which is relatively free from interfering compounds that are unrelated to internal metabolism (e.g., saliva may be contaminated with food residues). Contact lenses have been verified as safe for use in diabetic patients [13]. The use of a contact lens that is in direct and continuous contact with ocular tear fluid may provide a unique opportunity for noninvasive and CGM in the eye. Recently, several contact lens sensor designs have emerged that might allow for continuous monitoring and interrogation of the tear fluid. Some of the most advanced designs among those that have succeeded in the exploration of in vivo measurements [14,15] are based on fluorescence and spectrophotometric methods. Other very promising designs make use of micro/nanoelectronic technologies. This chapter will focus on these methods, with a brief excursion to investigate microelectronic contact lens glucose sensors.

10.5 Requirements for Ophthalmic/Contact Lens Glucose Sensors

Ophthalmic glucose sensors, and in particular, contact lens based glucose sensors, operate in a unique physiological environment, which creates a set of equally unique requirements for such sensing devices. One of these is the prerequisite of very high sensitivity to enable the accurate tracking of tear fluid glucose levels, which are substantially lower than those of blood or interstitial fluid. Nondiabetic and diabetic blood glucose values range from ~80 to ~400 mg/dL. Mean values for diabetic and nondiabetic tear glucose, as reported by Morris et al., are 6.3 ± 0.7 mg/dL (0.35 ± 0.04 mmol/L) and 2.9 ± 0.5 mg/dL (0.16 ± 0.03 mmol/L), respectively [16].

Tear fluid glucose concentrations depend strongly on the tear collection methodology. Significantly higher values have been reported for collection methods that mechanically irritate the ocular surface in comparison to nonirritating methods, indicating that disruptive collection methods can trigger the release of glucose from damaged cells and its subsequent diffusion into the tear fluid. A detailed study that relates the historical results of tear glucose levels and tear collection methods for glucose measurement was published by Asher et al. [17]. The mean values reported by Morris et al. were derived from a study that compared the dynamic differences of tear glucose between 121 diabetic and nondiabetic subjects following the administration of a carbohydrate load. A quantitative chromatographic analysis of tear glucose was utilized. These values are representative of the nonirritating values evaluated by Asher, and serve as a good reference point.

A second key requirement is the establishment of a stable, fully reversible, accurate, and sufficiently rapid response over the tear glucose value range. Changes in sensor sensitivity and signal may occur over time due to the degradation of sensing molecules (e.g., conformational changes of protein glucose receptors; photobleaching of organic dye molecules, which may be used for fluorescence sensor devices; or leaching of sensing units from the device). Some of these alterations may be compensated for to a certain degree via recalibration. However, frequent recalibration through the use of blood samples would defeat the purpose and aim of a minimally invasive measurement technique. The response time of the sensor must be on the order of several minutes in order to track accurately and in a timely fashion, increasing and decreasing blood glucose levels. Sensing units as well as the surrounding matrix play a significant role in the response rate.

Many sensing units consist of glucose-binding assays. A key to the success of these sensors resides in optimal binding kinetics under physiological conditions to allow rapid and reversible binding and release. For other enzyme-based tests, the minimal or zero consumption of analytes is important so as to avoid an imbalance in the local levels of glucose, which may impede tracking accuracy.

Some sensor techniques require the encapsulation of sensing molecules prior to embedding the sensor within the contact lens matrix to avoid leaching and/or to stabilize the sensor molecules. In these cases, the morphology of the capsule must be optimized not only to avoid the leaching of the sensor molecules but also to maintain sufficient permeability so as to facilitate the free flow of glucose into and out of the capsule. The leaching of sensing molecules from synthetic sensors may be avoided relatively easily by chemically binding or physically trapping the sensor molecules within the surrounding matrix. Binding or entrapment within protein-based sensors, however, represents a significant hurdle due to the potential loss of sensor activity.

Many reported techniques employ hydrogel contact lens matrices (e.g., polymers and copolymers based on poly(hydroxyethyl methacrylates), poly(vinylalcohols), poly(acrylamides)). The high percentage of water contained within these materials (~50% to 70%) allows for the free flow of glucose through the hydrogel matrix. Over the last decade, hydrogel contact lens materials have been gradually replaced by more advanced silicone hydrogels, which offer superior health benefits due to their high oxygen permeability [18]. These materials have a significantly lower water content (less than ~40%), which greatly reduces or inhibits the glucose flow throughout the matrix. To use these state-of-the art materials, sensor systems must be attached to the surface of the silicone hydrogel contact lenses.

A third requirement is selectivity, which is one of the primary motivations behind the great attention that has been given to the development of enzymatic sensor assays with high specificity for glucose over synthetic glucose-binding ligands, such as boronic acids. Synthetic sensors require optimization in order to obtain higher selectivity for glucose over interfering tear fluid components such as glycosylated proteins and lactate. Synthetic sensors, however, remain attractive due to their high stability and relatively easy immobilization to avoid leaching, which can be a key factor in the production process and shelf-life requirements for contact lens sensors (e.g., today's contact lens production relies on highly efficient sterilization processes such as autoclaving). Heat and pressure ranges applied in this process will degenerate protein-based sensors, but leave boronic acid-based sensors unharmed.

Most contact lens sensors require a handheld readout device that is used in combination with the glucose sensor contact lens to allow for the convenient monitoring of glucose levels by the patient. The development of such a handheld device, however, involves an equivalent level of complexity as the contact lens sensor unit itself.

10.6 Fluorescence-Based Glucose Sensing

One of the most intensely researched glucose-sensing methods is based on fluorescence measurements. Fluorescence is a form of luminescence, whereby an excitable molecule (a fluorophore) absorbs light of a specific wavelength and subsequently releases a lower energy photon. Fluorescence is a rapid (submicrosecond) emission process which accompanies transitions from singlet-excited states to ground states. The emitted light is thereby shifted to a longer wavelength relative to that of the activating light, which enables highly sensitive measurements due to the zero background, as excitation irradiation may be conveniently filtered. Excitation and emission wavelengths, in conjunction with inherent fluorescence kinetics, are dependent on the chemical composition and attributes of the particular fluorophore involved. The chemical environment within which a fluorophore is immersed imparts an influence as well, due to the interactions with the surrounding molecules, once it is raised to an excited state.

These characteristics impart a number of distinct advantages for the utilization of fluorescence measurements in biological environments. An extensive overview is provided by Pickup et al. [19]. The following advantages are of particular interest for tear fluid-based glucose analysis:

- Very high sensitivity, allowing for even single-molecule detection methods [20].

- Versatility of readout options, including not only fluorescence intensity measurements, but also fluorescence decay times: The advantages of time-resolved fluorescence measurements for in vivo sensing [21] are that they may be obtained independent of the effects of tissue resident light scattering and of fluorophore concentration, which become critical in systems that are subject to photobleaching or fluorophore loss via diffusion or degradation.

- Sensitivity to surrounding molecules, as described by Pickup et al. [19] (e.g., the structure and distribution of biomolecules may also be probed by the phenomenon of fluorescence (or Förster) resonance energy transfer (FRET) [22,23]. This involves the nonradiative energy transfer from a fluorescent donor molecule to an acceptor molecule in close proximity (which need not be fluorescent), and is typically brought about by dipole–dipole interactions. In this dynamic, the rate of energy transfer is inversely proportional to R^6 ($1/R^6$ is the long-range van der Waals interaction/attraction that governs the behavior of all atoms and molecules), where R is the distance between the donor and the acceptor. Thus, FRET is an exceptionally sensitive Angstrom-level measure of the subtle changes in molecular distances (e.g., within a molecule, as the tertiary structure undergoes alterations on binding with a ligand, or between molecules, as a ligand displaces a labeled analog from a labeled receptor).

Glucose sensors based on FRET are well known, and numerous devices have been reported and patented worldwide. Detailed reviews of fluorescence-based glucose assays, such as glucose-binding lectins, apoenzymes, and synthetic boronic acid receptors, are conveyed by Cote and McShane and Ballerstadt et al. [24,25].

While fluorescence-based glucose sensing has gained immense academic attention, the implementation of such a technology currently presents significant hurdles, and hence, only a few groups have reported significant advancements that encompass extensive in vitro testing or in vivo proofs of concept. Some of the most promising and advanced technologies toward the realization of ophthalmic fluorescence-based glucose sensors are introduced in the following section.

March et al. ALCON (formerly CIBA VISION) have investigated and developed fluorescence-based contact lens sensors and reported on the initial clinical trials that implemented this technology [14,26]. The team also pioneered the first handheld photofluorometer (Figure 10.2) to track alterations in fluorescence intensity in response to changes in glucose concentration. The sensing units comprise hydrogel-encapsulated nanospheres that contain competitive glucose-binding assay components (tetramethylrhodamine isothiocyanate concanavalin A [TRITC-Con A] and fluorescein isothiocyanate dextran [FITC-dextran]), which operate on the basis of FRET. As glucose levels rise, FITC-labeled dextran molecules are displaced by glucose molecules, which results in decreased FRET and increased fluorescence intensity in alignment with elevated glucose levels. In contrast, as glucose levels fall, higher concentrations of FITC-dextran molecules bind to the TRITC-Con A, and hence, fluorescence intensity is reduced [27] (Figures 10.3 and 10.5). The nanospheres are embedded within a polyvinyl alcohol-based (Nelfilcon A) hydrogel contact lens matrix. The team succeeded in preparing clinical grade contact lenses by UV light polymerization utilizing CIBA VISION's patented Light Stream Technology (Figure 10.4).

The contact lens sensor appeared to track blood glucose concentrations of five diabetic subjects who wore these sensors and one normal (control) nondiabetic subject. Responses had to be individually scaled for each subject in order for the fluorescence signal to fit the blood glucose concentration profile. Nevertheless, these early in situ results clearly demonstrated that there is indeed a correlation between glucose level changes in tears and blood (Figures 10.5 and 10.6). These pioneering results have strongly encouraged further research efforts in the ophthalmic sensor domain.

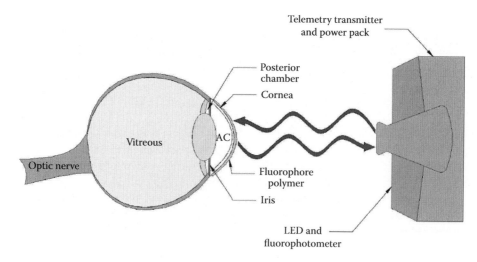

FIGURE 10.2
Depiction of interrogation of a contact lens glucose sensor via a handheld photofluorometer device. (Derived and redrawn from March, W. et al., *Diabetes Technol. Ther.*, 8(3), 312, 2006. With permission.)

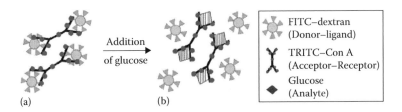

FIGURE 10.3
(a, b) Schematic of hydrogel-encapsulated nanospheres containing competitive glucose-binding FITC-dextran/TRITC-Con A complexes. (Reproduced from Chinnayelka, S., Microcapsule biosensors based on competitive binding and fluorescence resonance energy transfer assays, PhD dissertation, Louisiana Tech University, Ruston, LA, 2005.)

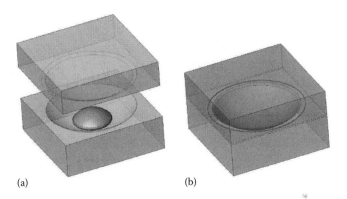

FIGURE 10.4
(a) Nanosphere-infused hydrogel is deposited in a quartz mold having patient-appropriate curvature.
(b) Contact lens is shaped and cured via exposure to UV light. (Derived and redrawn from March, W. et al., *Diabetes Technol. Ther.*, 8(3), 312, 2006. With permission.)

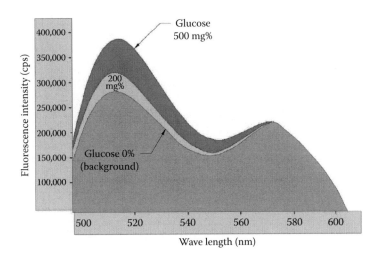

FIGURE 10.5
Fluorescence spectra of contact lens depicting one peak (514 nm) from fluorescein (rises with increases in glucose concentration) and another (574 nm) from rhodamine (remains static with increases in glucose concentration). (Redrawn representation from March, W. et al., *Diabetes Technol. Ther.*, 8(3), 312, 2006. With permission.)

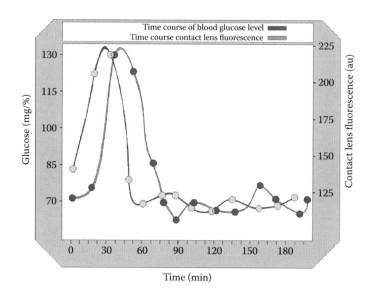

Time (min)

FIGURE 10.6
Depiction of correlation between blood glucose concentration and contact lens fluorescence. (Redrawn representation from March, W. et al., *Diabetes Technol. Ther.*, 8(3), 312, 2006. With permission.)

This sensor technology platform was further technologically advanced by Eyesense (a diagnostic device company spun out from Novartis and CIBA VISION) in the form of an ophthalmic glucose sensor implant. The diminutive ophthalmic implant sensor is inserted beneath the conjunctiva, which is a delicate transparent membrane that lines the inner eyelids and is continuous across the anterior portion of the eye ball, covering the white of the eye (sclera). The implanted subconjunctival sensor may be inserted at the outer zone of the eye in a simple, sutureless, and painless procedure that can be performed by an ophthalmologist within only three minutes. This sensor monitors glucose concentrations in the interstitial fluid, which are in the same range as those of the blood, and therefore far easier to monitor than the much lower tear glucose concentrations.

Eyesense reports via its website [28] that the dimensions, morphology, and composition of its "mini-sensor" are designed and adapted such that no foreign body sensation is elicited. In addition, the sensor is invisible to other individuals and may reside within the eye of the patient for up to 1 year, after which it is replaced by an ophthalmologist. While carrying the insert, the patient requires only an unobtrusive measuring device to quantify blood glucose in a completely noninvasive manner. The device analyzes fluorescence signals, and following a single and simple calibration, displays blood glucose levels in typical units. The biggest advantage of this innovative technology is that the patient may measure glucose levels as often as he or she wishes by simply placing the small photometer in front of the eye. The very rapid (~20 s) and easy measurements incur no extra costs with their frequency of use.

A subconjunctival implant has significant technical advantages over skin-implantable glucose sensors due to the high transparency of the conjunctiva, which contains minimal vascularization and pigmentation. The concept of subconjunctival implants has been reported previously by Abreu as a suitable system for the noninvasive measurement of chemical substances such as glucose [29].

Zhang et al., at the University of Western Ontario, recently developed a fluorescence contact lens sensor based on nanocomposites [30,31]. The sensor units are comprised of fluorescent mesoporous silica nanoparticles (FMSNs) (Ø ~55 nm) (Figure 10.7), which physically

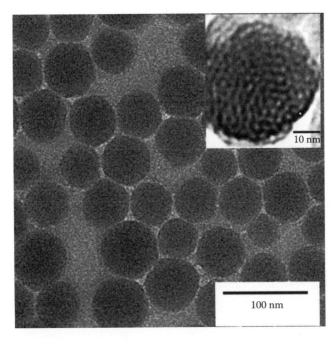

FIGURE 10.7
Transmission electron microscopy (TEM) micrograph of FMSNs. (Reproduced from Zhang, J. et al., *J Diabetes Sci. Technol.*, 5(1), 166, Copyright 2011. With permission.)

entrap and stabilize glucose assay components such as FITC-dextran and TRITC-Con A, via ionic interaction.

The group applied a two-step photopolymerization process in the casting of optical nanoparticles (NPs) into soft hydrogel lens materials. Initially, fluorescent NPs were assembled on a pretreated poly(dimethylsiloxane) slice through spin-coating. Subsequently, the optical probe was embedded within a hydrophilic hydrogel lens material (2-hydroxyethyl methacrylate) through UV polymerization of the monomeric formulation. The device was able to detect glucose concentrations in the range from 0.04 to 4 mM, which is well within tear glucose monitoring parameters. The response times reported for detection in a 0.1 mM glucose solution were less than five minutes, and the sensor response capability remained stable for five days. The stabilizing effect of the porous silica NPs against the photobleaching of FITC (Figure 10.8) (constituting a major concern with this technology) was tested, and significant improvements in the functionality of FMSNs were demonstrated [30,31].

Badugu, Lakowicz, and Geddes (Medical Biotechnology Center, University of Maryland) developed and studied the in vitro response of glucose-sensing contact lenses with fluorescent sensor probes that were based on fluorophore-containing boronic acids. This sensor technique exploits modifications in the electronic properties and geometries of boron atoms, which induce fluorescence spectral changes in the probes when glucose binds to the boronic acid moiety. The boronic acid group is an electron-deficient Lewis acid having a sp2-hybridized boron atom with a trigonal planar conformation. The anionic form of boronic acid, created in the presence of glucose, is characterized by a more electron-rich sp3-hybridized boron atom having a tetrahedral geometry.

Modifications in the electronic properties and geometries at the boron atom induces fluorescence spectral changes in the probes. Upon addition of glucose, the electron density of the boron atom is increased, facilitating partial neutralization of the positively charged

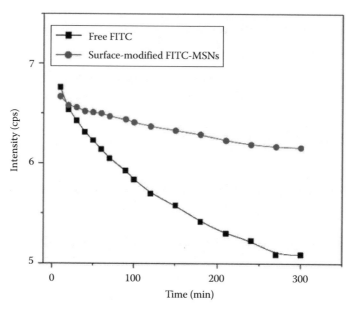

FIGURE 10.8
Photobleaching activity of free and surface-modified FITC. (Reproduced from Zhang, J. et al., *J Diabetes Sci. Technol.*, 5(1), 166, Copyright 2011. With permission.)

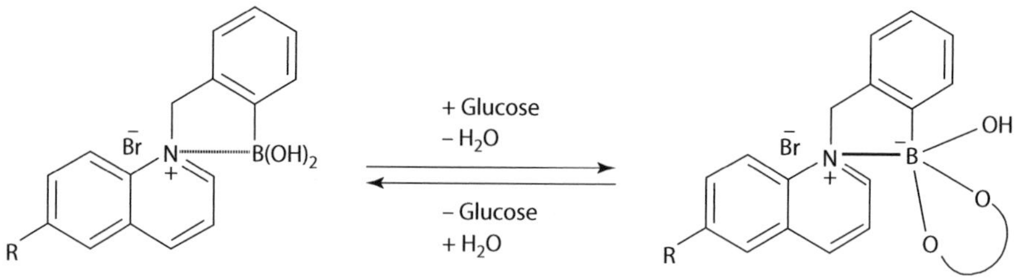

FIGURE 10.9
Schematic representation of the charge neutralization–stabilization mechanism as relates to glucose sensing. The bold line shown between the N+ and boron atom in the structure shown at right indicates an increased interaction between them, and is not intended to show covalent bond formation between the two atoms. (Reproduced from Badugu, R. et al., *Curr. Opin. Biotechnol.*, 16(1), 100, 2005. With permission.)

quaternary nitrogen of the quinolinium moiety. This interaction has been termed a "charge neutralization–stabilization mechanism" [32–34] (Figure 10.9). The lenses detect glucose changes of up to several millimolar in the tear glucose concentration range for diabetics with a 90% response time of ~10 minutes (i.e., time required for the fluorescence signal to deviate by 90% from its original state) [32] (Figure 10.10).

Since the sensor probes of this platform were not chemically bound to the contact lens matrix, the stability of the sensor was investigated by the group, who reported on shelf-life testing over several months, utilizing both wet and dry lens storage. The results revealed identical sugar-sensing capacities, indicating that no lens polymer–fluorophore interactions or probe degradation took place over this time period. While this initial shelf-life testing is encouraging, the leaching of noncovalently bonded molecules from the contact lens matrix may still pose a concern in view of stringent FDA regulations in regard to medical

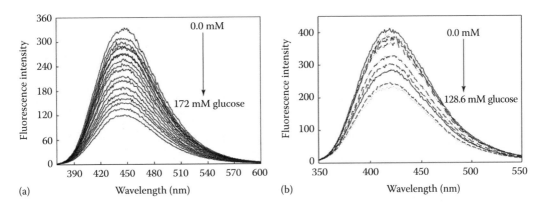

FIGURE 10.10

Illustration of response of contact lens sensors to low concentrations (<2 mM) of glucose. Emission spectra of (a) an *N*-(boronobenzyl)-6-methoxyquinolinium bromide (o-BMOQBA)- and (b) an *N*-(boronobenzyl)-6-ethylquinolinium bromide (o-BMQBA)- doped contact lens under escalating glucose concentrations. (Adapted from Badugu, R. et al., *Curr. Opin. Biotechnol.*, 16(1), 100, 2005; Badugu, R. et al., *J. Fluoresc.*, 14(5), 617, 2004. With permission.)

sensing device safety and efficacy. Other aspects of this technology to be addressed in the future will likely include boronic acid selectivity over interfering tear fluid components such as lactate and glycoproteins, and the design of a robust and highly accurate handheld readout device.

10.7 Colorimetric Sensors Based on Periodic Optical Nanostructures

A unique and different class of glucose sensor incorporates periodic optical nanostructures that are designed to affect the motion of photons. The interaction of light with these nanostructures results in distinct color phenomena that may also be observed in nature, where it is termed "structural" color. A well-known example of structural color operates in the mineral opal. The distinct brilliance of opal colors is caused by a lattice of high-refractive-index material (silica spheres), which are embedded within a low-refractive-index matrix. Other well-researched natural examples are the colors of butterfly wings such as those of the *Lycaenidae* species [36–38] (Figure 10.11). The scales of these butterfly wings contain three-dimensional (3D) photonic structures which are typically composed of a matrix of chitin (high-refractive-index material) containing regularly arranged spherical air spaces (low-refractive-index material) known as an inverse opal structure. Another example is the brilliant coloration found in the feathers of the peacock. Stacked melanin rods, interspersed with air pockets, make up periodic optical nanostructures. Differences in color are achieved by changing the lattice spacing of the rods [39] (Figure 10.12).

Lattices composed of points, spheres, or other structures have found widespread use in the form of thin film optics, with applications ranging from low and high reflective coatings on lenses and mirrors to color-changing inks. Under white light illumination, such lattices diffract light and produce a characteristic spectral peak with a wavelength that is governed in approximation to the Bragg equation: $m\lambda = 2nd\sin\theta$, where m is the diffraction

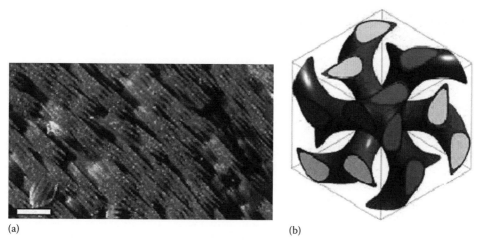

(a)   (b)

FIGURE 10.11
(a) Light micrograph depicting randomly oriented opalescent crystallite domains in the ventral wing cover scales of *Callophrys gryneus (Lycaenidae)*. (Scale bar: 100 μm.) (b) 3D core–shell double gyroid model of a photonic butterfly wing scale cell. (Reproduced from Saranathan, V. et al., *Proc. Natl Acad. Sci. USA*, 107(26), 11676, 2010. Copyright 2003. National Academy of Sciences, U.S.A. With permission.)

order; λ is the wavelength of light; n is the average refractive index; θ is the angle of illumination to the normal; and d is the spacing of the lattice (Figure 10.13). The most subtle variations in the spacing of the nanolattices initiate color shifts that may easily be detected by a spectrophotometer. Ease of fabrication, high sensitivity, and their status as a known technology for integration into readout devices, make optical nanostructures particularly suitable as ophthalmic sensors.

10.8 Holographic Glucose Sensors

A collaborative team led by Domschke ALCON (formerly CIBA VISION) and Lowe (Institute for Biotechnology at the University of Cambridge, United Kingdom) developed a unique holographic platform based on periodic optical nanostructures that are suitable for contact lens applications. The platform combines a simple reflection hologram [40] recorded within a hydrogel matrix with covalently bonded 3-acrylamidophenylboronic acid (3-APB) as the glucose-binding ligand. The construction of such a holographic reflection grating is depicted in Figure 10.14.

When holographic reflection gratings are illuminated by white light, they act as sensitive wavelength filters in the same manner as crystalline colloidal arrays and reflect only a specific narrow wavelength band that is governed by the Bragg equation [42]. Changes in the swelling state of the hydrogel within which the grating is recorded will alter the fringe distance and hence the reflected color that may be detected by a spectrometer. The hydrogels were synthesized using 3-APB, which has the capacity for forming reversible covalent bonds (Figure 10.15) with glucose [43].

The binding of glucose to 3-APB moieties causes the hydrogel to swell, which in turn alters the fringe distances that may be employed to quantify the glucose concentration [43,44].

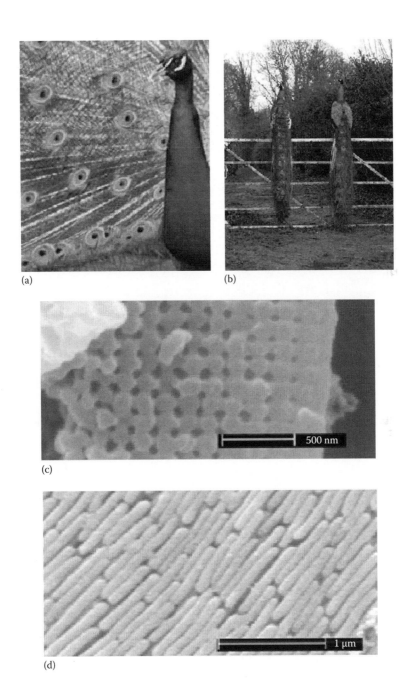

(a)

(b)

(c)

(d)

FIGURE 10.12

(a,b) Examples of iridescent peacock plumage. (Copyright Ian Paterson, and licensed for reuse under Creative Commons License.) (c,d) Scanning electron microscope images of peacock barbule structures. Melanin rods coupled via keratin and interspersed with air pockets comprise periodic optical nanostructures. Differences in color are achieved by alterations in the lattice spacing of the rods. (Reproduced from Zi, J. et al., *Proc. Natl. Acad. Sci. USA*, 100(22), 12576, 2003. Copyright 2003. National Academy of Sciences, U.S.A. With permission.)

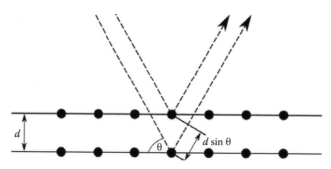

FIGURE 10.13
Schematic of Bragg diffraction. (From Wikimedia Commons.)

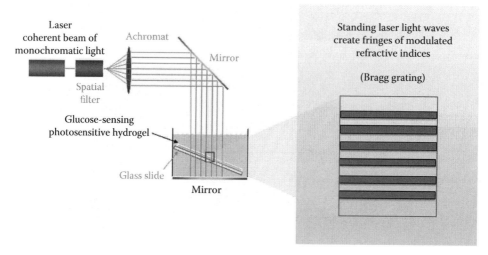

FIGURE 10.14
Schematic drawing of the hologram fabrication process: The hologram is produced by passing a single colli-mated laser beam through the photosensitive hydrogel, backed by a mirror. Interference between the incident and reflected beams creates a permanent modulated refractive index in the form of fringes. (From Domschke, A., Oral presentation at the *International Conference on Nanoscience and Technology (ICN+T)*, Keystone, CO, 2008.)

The team demonstrated the capability of 3-APB (and other derivative)-based holographic glucose sensors to reversibly and continuously function in complex biological media at physiological pH, ionic strength, and glucose levels [43,45]. Boronic acids are known to bind cis-diols, including a variety of sugars [46–48] and hydroxy acids [49]. However, other than glucose, sugars are typically not found in a free state within physiological solutions at high concentrations. Many sugars are present in the form of macromolecular carbohydrate structures and as glycoproteins, but these do not affect the hologram as they cannot dif-fuse into the hydrogel matrix and bind to the pendant phenylboronic acid groups. On the other hand, α-hydroxy acid and lactic acid are present at millimolar concentrations within the blood and other physiological fluids and might therefore interfere with glucose detec-tors that incorporate boronate-based sensing systems. The team also developed various sensor systems with an enhanced selectivity for glucose versus interfering lactic acid [44] (Figure 10.16).

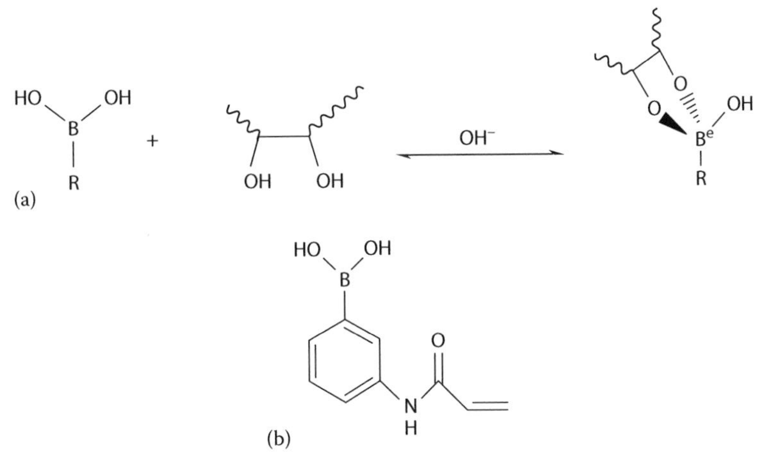

FIGURE 10.15
(a) The reversible binding that occurs between boronic acids and cis-diols in aqueous media. (b) Structure of 3-APB. (Reproduced from Kabilan, S. et al., *Biosens. Bioelectron.*, 20(8), 1602, 2005. Copyright 2005. Elsevier.With permission.)

The holographic sensor units were embedded in a Nelfilcon A, polyvinylalcohol contact lens matrix, and contact lenses were fabricated by UV light polymerization, utilizing CIBA VISION's patented Light Stream Technology. The contact lens glucose sensors were subsequently extracted and autoclaved to render the contact lens sterile and biocompatible. Promising initial clinical studies were performed that indicated the capacity for tracking glucose response for ~30 minutes [45].

Figure 10.17 shows the actual holographic contact lens in a normal patient's eye (subject A), a plot of blood glucose concentration against time after glucose administration in subject A, and the response of the holographic sensor for the same period in the same subject [15]. There appears to be a slight time delay between increased blood glucose and the contact lens sensor response. A polynomial may be derived for each individual patient that can partially correct for this delay, as previously described [50]. While further long-term testing is required to fully develop such a sensor, the method shows considerable promise over the current continuous monitoring systems, as it is less invasive and may be cost-effectively mass-produced.

10.9 Photonic Crystal Glucose Sensors

Photonic crystal contact lens glucose sensors have been investigated by Asher, Department of Chemistry, University of Pittsburgh [51], that consist of a crystalline colloidal array embedded within a polymer network. The network contains pendent phenylboronic acid groups that diffract light in the visible spectral region. The pendent boronic acid groups bind glucose in a "sandwich-like" complex, forming additional cross-links within the hydrogel. As these additional cross-links form, the hydrogel shrinks (Figure 10.18). This alters the lattice spacing of the colloidal array, which results in a blueshift of the diffracted light in proportion to the glucose in solution. Diabetic patients employ a mirror to examine the color of the photonic crystal sensor in the contact lens in comparison to the color

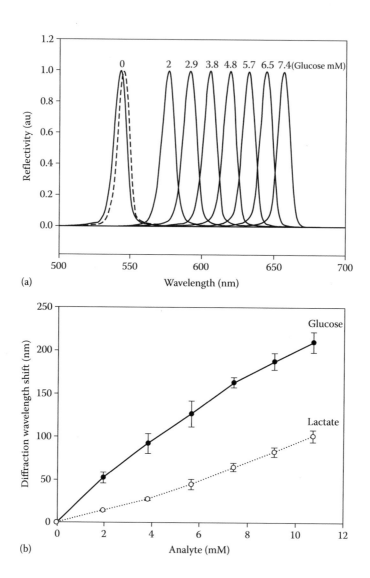

(a)

(b)

FIGURE 10.16

(a) The resulting diffraction spectra of a 25 mol% 3-APB hologram immersed in PBS (pH 7.4) solutions of varying glucose concentrations at 30°C. The dashed line indicates the diffraction peak observed after exposure to
7.4 mM glucose and subsequently rinsing the hologram with PBS. (b) Response of a 20 mol% 3-APB hologram
to variations in glucose and lactate concentrations in PBS (pH 7.4) at 30°C. (From Kabilan, S. et al., *Biosens.
Bioelectron.*, 20(8), 1602, 2005. Copyright 2005. Elsevier. With permission.)

depicted on a calibrated reference color wheel (Figure 10.19). Alternatively, a handheld
spectrophotometer might be developed to discern the color shift.

   Photonic crystals under investigation for their application in prototype contact lens
sensors were fabricated via the self-assembly of highly charged monodispersed polystyrene nanospheres (Ø ~100 nm) within a crystalline colloidal suspension, which
formed photonic crystal templates [51]. The crystal arrays were embedded within a
polyacrylamide-based hydrogel matrix that was functionalized with boronic acid
groups. Sensitivity and response times were optimized, which resulted in changes in
glucose concentrations at rates comparable to the expected rates of glucose concentration

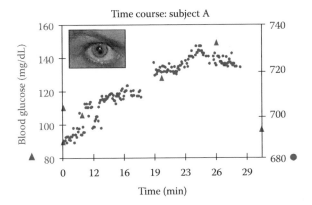

FIGURE 10.17

Photograph of a normal patient (subject A) wearing a holographic contact lens; a plot of response of the holographic sensor for the same period in the same subject. (From Domschke, A.M., *Chimia (Aarau)*, 64(1–2), 43, 2010.)

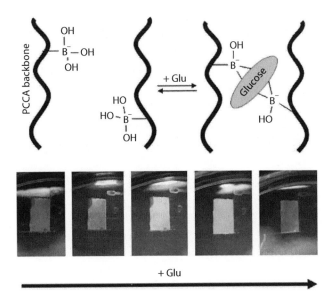

FIGURE 10.18

Schematic of a polymerized crystalline colloidal array (PCCA) with attached glucose binding phenylboronic acid ligands. With increased glucose concentration, the hydrogel shrinks resulting in a blueshift of the diffracted light in proportion to the glucose in solution. (Reproduced from Asher Research Group, Department of Chemistry, University of Pittsburgh, Colloid Group http://www.pitt.edu/~asher/homepage/colgrp.html#pcca, accessed March 12, 2012. With permission.)

changes in blood (~five minute response time in a 0.2 mM D-glucose solution) [53] (Figure 10.20).

Some remaining challenges include the successful demonstration of glucose determination in situ, where factors such as sensor specificity, reproducibility, and robustness will play a significant role. This technology has been licensed for development by Glucose Sensing Technologies, LLC, which is exploring advanced photonic crystal-based platforms such as high-diffraction efficiency two-dimensional (2D) photonic crystals for applications in molecular recognition and chemical sensing [54].

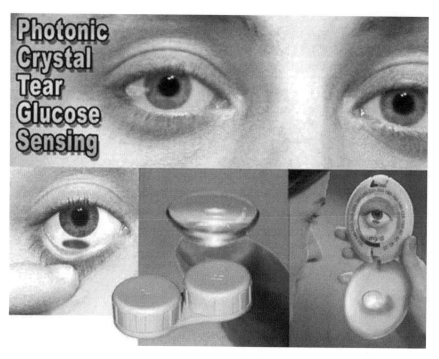

FIGURE 10.19
Conceptual drawing of photonic tear glucose sensing utilizing a mirror to examine the color of the photonic crystal sensor in the contact lens and compare the color to that of a calibrated reference color wheel. (Reproduced from Asher Research Group, Department of Chemistry, University of Pittsburgh, Colloid Group, http://www.pitt.edu/~asher/homepage/colgrp.html#pcca, accessed March 12, 2012. With permission.)

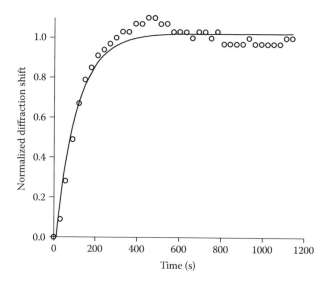

FIGURE 10.20
Response kinetics of n-hexylacrylate PCCA glucose sensors in artificial tear fluid when challenged with freshly prepared 0.15 mM D glucose solutions at pH 7.4 at 37°C. A rapid blueshift of the diffraction (~11 nm) is observed saturating within ~300 s. (Reproduced from Ben-Moshe, M. et al., *Anal. Chem.*, 78(14), 5149, 2006. Copyright 2006. American Chemical Society. With permission.)

10.10 Microelectromechanical-Based Sensors

Techniques for the fabrication of microelectromechanical (MEMS) and nanoelectrome-chanical (NEMS) systems have advanced greatly over the last decade. The implementation of miniaturized sensors interfaced with wireless power delivery systems and sensing readout circuitry is now a reality, which has opened up the new field of small-scale sensor research, including microscale and nanoscale glucose sensors [55]. Microfabrication techniques have been developed to integrate structures into polymeric matrices that are compatible for use in contact lenses. Based on these advancements, MEMS-based contact lens glucose sensors have been developed that bear great promise.

Parviz and his team at the University of Washington have developed a microfabricated (3 μW) wirelessly powered amperometric contact lens glucose sensor. The sensor electrode suite (e.g., working, counter, and reference electrodes) was generated via photoresist and thin metal film deposition techniques, utilizing a poly(ethylene terephthalate) film substrate. The film was then heat-modeled into a lens-like shape and functionalized with a glucose oxidase enzyme/titania sol/gel membrane covered by a layer of Nafion®, a sulfonated tetrafluoroethylene-based fluoropolymer-copolymer. The team also developed an interface chip for contact lens borne electronic circuits for wireless readout, including a wireless power delivery system and sensing readout circuitry (adopting a 2.4 GHz carrier frequency), signal processing and communication subsystems. The sensor system consumes 3 W and may be powered over a distance of 15 cm [56,57].

The sensor exhibited promising sensitivity, repeatability (linear correlation coefficient of 0.9968 over 25 samples), and rapid response times (e.g., response to the subsequent addition of 0.1 mM glucose solution reached 90% of the maximum value in less than 20 s) for low glucose concentrations (0.1–0.6 mM), which are relevant for tear glucose measurements. The sensor can attain a minimum detection of less than 0.01 mM glucose. The team also reported interference rejection for ascorbic acid, urea, and lactate. Future investigations will focus on enhanced stability, the attainment of more efficient interference rejection, and the transfer of the technology into biocompatible contact lens materials [56–58]. This nascent prototype design is intriguing by virtue of its low detection limit, which is of particular interest for diabetes management, as it allows more accurate detection of hypoglycemic glucose levels. Hypoglycemia can ensue following insulin administration and may induce serious complications for patients, including seizures, unconsciousness, and (rarely) permanent brain damage or death.

A very promising soft MEMS contact lens biosensor (SCL-biosensor) for the novel noninvasive biomonitoring of tear fluids was fabricated and tested in an in vivo animal model by Mitsubayashi and coworkers at the Tokyo Medical and Dental University (Figure 10.21). Flexible microelectrode systems with sensor and reference electrodes were fabricated on a 70 μm thin polydimethylsiloxane (PDMS) film. The electrode system was attached to the PDMS lens surface using a PDMS binder. A mixture of glucose oxidase and a copolymer (consisting of 2-methacryloyloxyethyl phosphorcholine and 2-ethylhexylmethacrylate) was applied to the active region of the sensor and cured. Subsequently, an overcoat of the copolymer was applied so as to avoid enzyme leakage. The electrode terminal was connected to a potentiostat to facilitate in vitro and in vivo measurements [59].

The in vitro measurements demonstrated a quick and sensitive response in an appropriate tear glucose concentration range between 0.03 and 5.0 mM. The team successfully conducted an in vivo measurement in a rabbit model, obtaining a stable output current for the basal tear glucose concentration. The estimated basal concentration was 0.11 mM which falls within

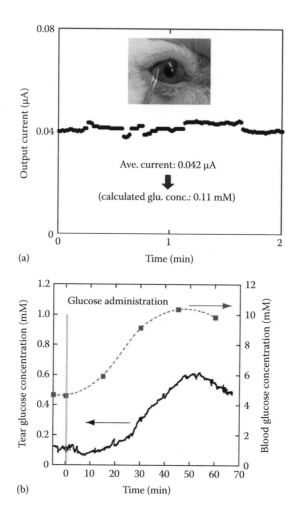

FIGURE 10.21

(a) SCL-biosensor on ocular site of rabbit model generated a stable (0.042 μA) output current, and basal tear glucose concentration was estimated to be 0.11 mM. (b) Plot of chronological alteration in tear and blood glucose concentrations. The registration of changes in tear glucose values lagged ~15 to 20 min behind those of blood glucose values. (Reproduced from Chu, M.X. et al., *Talanta*, 83(3), 960, 2011. With permission.)

the range of human nondiabetic levels. The contact lens sensor was able to track the changes in tear glucose levels induced by changes in blood glucose via the oral administration of glucose. The tear glucose levels followed the blood glucose with a delay of about 10 minutes.

A 3D enzyme-based glucose contact lens sensor was developed by Patel et al. at Simon Fraser University (Burnaby, BC) (Figures 10.22 and 10.23). In this approach, working and reference electrodes with pillar-like geometries were prepared to realize a 3D topography with an enhanced surface area (up to 300% over 2D analogs) contained on a small footprint (1 × 2 mm²). The electrode was fabricated on a flexible PDMS film by employing standard MEMS techniques. Glucose oxidase was immobilized on the gold electrode surface, and glucose responses to selected 3D topographies were tested, which resulted in the achievement of a high sensitivity, utilizing a 200 μm high square pillar pattern. Sensitivities to glucose concentrations as low as 0.04 mM were reported [60].

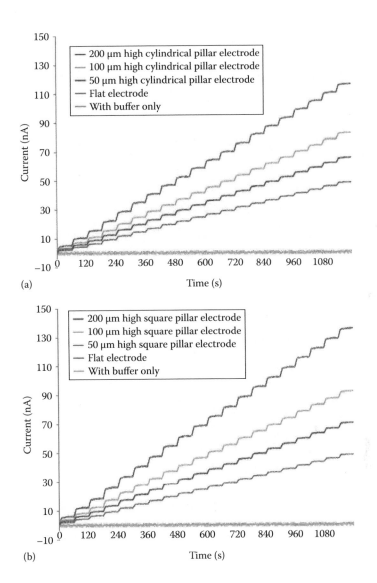

FIGURE 10.22

Measured amperometric responses for different 3D electrode geometries. The response is measured at 0.5 V with respect to the Ag/AgCl (reference) electrode. (a) Amperometric response for different designs with the cylindrical pillars along with the flat electrode response. The amperometric response in phosphate buffer is also shown for comparison of the noise. The amperometric current increases with improvement in the electrode surface area. (b) Amperometric response for different designs with the square pillars along with the flat electrode response. Similar to the cylindrical pillars, the amperometric current increases with improvement in the surface area of the electrode. (Reproduced from Patel, J.N. et al., *J. Diabetes Sci. Technol.*, 5(5), 1036, 2011. Copyright 2011. Journal of Diabetes Science and Technology. With permission.)

Amperometric enzyme-based MEMS systems were further developed and culminated in an interesting alternative ophthalmic sensor. A team led by Wang at Arizona State University and the University of California fabricated a miniaturized flexible film electrochemical biosensor that operated within the lacrimal canaliculus. The lacrimal canaliculi (lacrimal ducts) are the small channels in each eyelid that begin at tiny orifices, termed punta lacrimalia, which are seen on the margins of the lids (Figure 10.24). In vitro testing

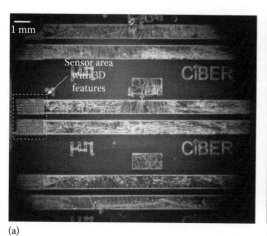

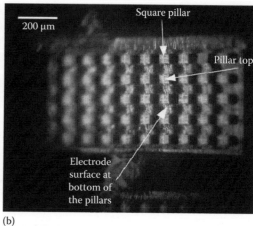

(a)

(b)

FIGURE 10.23
Microscopic image of electrodes immediately following PDMS-based sensor removal from the glass-backing plate. (a) Three consecutive sensors with pillar electrodes are shown along with connecting conductors for testing. The actual sensor area is highlighted in the image. (b) Magnified view of the pillar electrodes with square pillars. Ordered array of square pillars on working electrode are uniformly covered with Cr/Au metal layer. The square pillar feature along with the top and bottom of the metal-covered pillar is indicated in the image. (Reproduced from Patel, J.N. et al., *J. Diabetes Sci. Technol.*, 5(5), 1036, 2011. Copyright 2011. Journal of Diabetes Science and Technology. With permission.)

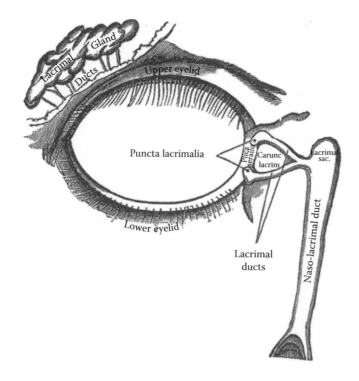

FIGURE 10.24
Schematic depicting the location of lacrimal ducts. (From Gray, H., *Anatomy of the Human Body*, Lea & Febiger, Philadelphia, PA, 1918, Bartleby.com, 2000.)

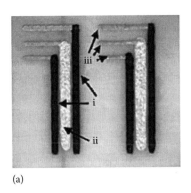 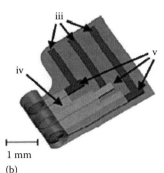 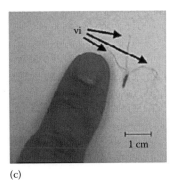

(a) (b) (c)

FIGURE 10.25
(a) Screen-printed tri-electrode microflow electrochemical biosensor: (i) carbon-based working/counter electrodes; (ii) Ag/AgCl reference electrodes; (iii) copper contacts. (b) Rendering of partially rolled sensor: (iii) copper contacts; (iv) insulator; (v) screen-printed inks. (c) Rolled silicone-coated electrode: (vi) electrical contacts. (Reproduced from Kagie, A. et al., *Electroanalysis*, 20(14), 1610, 2008. With permission.)

of the new sensor that employed laterally rolled screen-printed band electrodes and glucose-oxidase containing ink exhibited rapid response when challenged with glucose concentrations in the range between 0.02 and 20 mM (Figure 10.25). The enzyme electrode was covered with electropolymerized polytyramine to minimize contributions from typical electroactive interferant species such as ascorbic and uric acids [61].

10.11 Progress and Remaining Challenges toward the Development of Ophthalmic Glucose Sensors

In recent years, the development of noninvasive and continuous ophthalmic glucose monitoring devices for the progressive management of diabetes has been greatly advanced. Progress toward meeting the challenging requirements for the implementation of such sensing devices has been reported for a large variety of both established and emerging sensor platforms. Very high sensitivity is one example of requisite criteria that has been the centerpiece of enduring efforts over many years. Sensitivity levels have been reported to not only encompass diabetic or normal tear glucose levels, but also hypoglycemic levels. Microelectromechanical-based sensor techniques have been reported with outstanding sensitivities that are up to 10 times lower than normal tear glucose levels. The accurate monitoring of glucose concentrations that may fall to hypoglycemic levels is critical, in that if these levels remain unnoticed, they may culminate in severe health implications, including coma and death.

The development of stable sensing units represents an additional major challenge. A creative solution in this area, however, has been successfully demonstrated via the encapsulation of very sensitive protein-based sensor moieties. Here, one of the most promising advances was realized through the use of a stable fluorescence-based ocular sensing subconjunctival insert that makes possible an annual replacement schedule. A convenient handheld readout device was developed in conjunction with the implanted sensor that enables patients to self-monitor their glucose levels.

Systems based on synthetic sensing units (e.g., boronic acid derivatives) exhibited remarkably short-term stability when subjected to the typical thermal and pressure demands inherent to autoclaving, which is employed as a sterilization method in the process of manufacturing contact lenses. A perceived drawback of boronic acid-based sensors is selectivity for glucose over other interfering tear analytes, specifically lactic acid. Nevertheless, in this area as well, advances have been reported that demonstrate very encouraging selectivity, which significantly increases the importance of boronic acid platforms.

Sufficiently rapid response times, accuracy, and repeatability are the crucial requirements for contact lens integrated sensing devices that have been optimized for many sensors in vitro. A number of well-advanced contact lens sensor platforms have demonstrated the achievement of these requirements in vivo, indicating that measured tear glucose levels can track blood glucose levels well. Variable lag times between tear glucose results and blood glucose levels have been reported that range from ~0 to 20 minutes. Considerable work has been done toward the elucidation and understanding of correlations between blood and tear resident glucose levels. Interestingly, further complex physiological aspects of this relationship have been discovered, such as the variation of lag times and magnitude of response between individuals; single subjects from day to day; and even between the left and right eyes of single subjects. Lag and response times are, to a certain degree, also dependent on the type of sensor and the matrix that surrounds the sensing unit, which adds another layer of complexity. The multifaceted physiological aspects of tear glucose monitoring, and in particular the variations in lag times, remain the most significant challenges.

Accuracy and reliability are absolute necessities for meeting sanctioned safety and efficacy standards, as the long-term well-being of diabetic patients, and in certain cases of hypoglycemia, the lives of the patients are completely dependent on these requirements. Therefore, calibrations of noninvasive glucose sensors are necessary to accurately account for any possible variations in the correlation between the blood and tear glucose levels. Numerous required calibrations, however, greatly reduce the appeal of noninvasive sensors. Consequently, a considerable segment of the overall sensor development must include a very costly clinical evaluation that establishes the need for calibration, which ultimately verifies the value of new noninvasive sensor techniques. This represents a very demanding hurdle for all ophthalmic sensor platforms.

It remains to be seen if the development of contact lens integrated glucose monitoring devices is sufficiently rapid to keep pace with the introduction of alternative approaches such as stem cell treatments [63] and nascent nanomedical therapeutics [64], which may efficiently help fight or even cure diabetes in the future.

10.12 Outlook

Many technologies introduced in this chapter bear the potential for much broader applications, which are yet to be realized. Tear fluid contains a variety of physiological analytes, such as Na^+, K^+, Ca^{2+}, Mg^{2+}, histamine, urea, lactate, and cholesterol, as well as a multitude of biomarkers that could be monitored in the near future through similar contact lens based sensing platforms.

Aside from tear fluid analytes, a different type of contact lens sensor that assists in the management of diabetes-related eye diseases, recently obtained much scientific attention.

A common complication of diabetes is open-angle glaucoma, which is associated with elevated eye pressure in conjunction with typical glaucomatous nerve damage. Most treatments are aimed at lowering the eye pressure to avoid such nerve damage. For efficient glaucoma management, the monitoring of the interocular pressure is very important [65]. To the extent that contact lens sensors which measure interocular pressure have been evolving, some very advanced devices have been developed by companies that anticipate commercial release in the near future. Some of these sophisticated devices include MEMS-based systems that have been developed by companies such as STMicroelectronics to accurately measure very subtle shape changes of the eye [66]. These wireless MEMS sensors act as both a transducer and an antenna within a smart contact lens named "Sensimed Triggerfish" [66], which is an embedded sensor system that incorporates a strain gauge in a smart lens platform, which is designed to monitor the curvature of the eye (Figure 10.26).

Other contact lens based pressure-sensing devices remain in various stages of development [67] with some positive results reported subsequent to comparative studies with a conventional dynamic contour tonometer. Of these, slit-lamp mounted (DCT) and handheld (HH) technologies look promising [68].

Another diabetes-related eye disease is the so-called "dry eye syndrome," also known as keratoconjunctivitis sicca [69]. Dry eye symptoms are conventionally treated with lubricating eye drops. The challenge for an effectual treatment based on eye drops remains a controlled rate of delivery of the eye drop over time, which actually reaches the ocular surface. This is not a trivial matter given the speed at which the administered eye drop drains through the puncta or spills over the lids, and the compliance of the patient with regard to the frequency and dosage. Therefore, the regulated time release of an appropriate lubricant over extended periods by way of a smart contact lens would be advantageous.

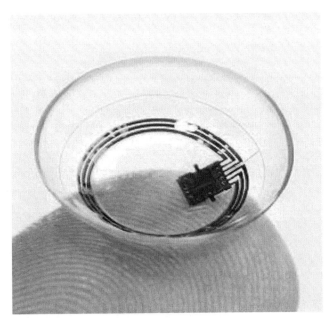

FIGURE 10.26
Sensimed smart lens measures interocular pressure. (Copyright 2012. Sensimed AG, Lausanne, Switzerland. With permission.)

Several institutions are working on strategies for smart drug-releasing contact lenses. One such device developed by a team from the Children's Hospital Boston; the Massachusetts Eye and Ear Infirmary's ophthalmology department; Schepens Eye Research Institute in Boston; and the Massachusetts Institute of Technology's chemical engineering department, sandwiches pharmaceuticals between two layers of polymeric film [70]. In laboratory tests, these multilayered lenses demonstrated the ability to release ciprofloxacin for up to 100 days. Research in the development of drug-releasing contact lenses has been attempted by a number of other research groups, who have reported significant progress [71]. These innovations are raising hopes that such devices might be available in the relatively near future.

Taking into account the many emerging advanced smart contact lens technologies, the future appears to hold great promise for the implementation of state-of-the-art devices for the management of diabetes in the form of multifunctional contact lenses. These lenses might not only monitor multiple diabetes-related analytes and symptoms, but may also be endowed with the capacity for treating ocular discomfort in an all-in-one approach.

References

1. Hirsch, I.B., Clinical review: Realistic expectations and practical use of continuous glucose monitoring for the endocrinologist. *J Clin Endocrinol Metab* 94(7), 2232–2238, 2009.
2. Garg, S.K., Smith, J., Beatson, C., Lopez-Baca, B., Voelmle, M., and Gottlieb, P.A., Comparison of accuracy and safety of the SEVEN and the Navigator continuous glucose monitoring systems. *Diabetes Technol Ther* 11(2), 65–72, 2009.
3. Scaramuzza, A.E., Iafusco, D., Rabbone, I., Bonfanti, R., Lombardo, F., Schiaffini, R., Buono, P., Toni, S., Cherubini, V., and Zuccotti, G.V., Useofintegratedreal-time continuous glucose monitoring/insulin pump system in children and adolescents with type1 diabetes: A 3-year follow-up study. Diabetes Study Group of the Italian Society of Paediatric Endocrinology and Diabetology. *Diabetes Technol Ther* 13(2), 99–103, 2011.
4. Ives, B., Sikes, K., Urban, A., Stephenson, K., and Tamborlane, W.V., Practical aspects of real-time continuous glucose monitors: The experience of the Yale children's diabetes program. *Diabetes Edu* 36(1), 53–62, 2010.
5. Edelman, S.V. and Bailey, T.S., Continuous glucose monitoring health outcomes. *Diabetes Technol Ther* 11(1), S68–74, 2009.
6. Walsh, J. and Roberts, R., Continuous Glucose Monitors, Diabetes Mall, http://www.diabetesnet.com/diabetes-technology/meters-monitors/continuous-monitors/compare-current-monitors (accessed 06/26/13)
7. Diabetes Research in Children Network (DirecNet) Study Group, The accuracy of the guardian RT continuous glucose monitor in children with type 1 diabetes. *Diabetes Technol Ther* 10(4), 266–272, 2008.
8. Wilson, D.M., Beck, R.W., Tamborlane, W.V., Dontchev, M.J., Kollman, C., Chase, P., Fox, L.A., Ruedy, K.J., Tsalikian, E., and Weinzimer, S.A., DirecNet Study Group, The accuracy of the FreeStyle Navigator continuous glucose monitoring system in children with type 1 diabetes. *Diabetes Care* 30(1), 59–64, 2007.
9. Garg, S.K., Schwartz, S., and Edelman, S.V., Improved glucose excursions using an implantable real-time continuous glucose sensor in adults with type 1 diabetes. *Diabetes Care*, 27,734–738, 2004.
10. The Diabetes Research in Children Network (DirecNet) Study Group, Accuracy of the modified continuous glucose monitoring system (CGMS®) sensor in an outpatient setting: Results from a Diabetes Research in Children Network (DirecNet) study. *Diabetes Technol Ther* 7(1), 109–113, 2005.

11. Tura, A., Maran, A., and Pacini, G., Non-invasive glucose monitoring: Assessment of technologies and devices according to quantitative criteria. *Diabetes Res Clin Pract* 77(1), 16–40, 2007.
12. Baca, J.T., Taormina, C.R., Feingold, E., Finegold, D.N., Grabowsk, J.J., and Asher, S.A., Mass spectral determination of fasting tear glucose concentrations in nondiabetic volunteers. *Clin Chem* 53(7), 1370–1372, 2007.
13. March, W., Long, B., Hofmann, W., Keys, D., and McKenney, C., Safety of contact lenses in patients with diabetes. *Diabetes Technol Ther* 6(1), 49–52, 2004.
14. March, W., Lazzaro, D., and Rastogi, S., Fluorescent measurement in the non-invasive contact lens glucose sensor. *Diabetes Technol Ther* 8(3), 312–317, 2006.
15. Domschke, A.M., Continuous non-invasive ophthalmic glucose sensor for diabetics. *Chimia (Aarau)* 64(1–2), 43–44, 2010.
16. Lane, J.D., Krumholz, D.M., Sack, R.A., and Morris, C., Tear glucose dynamics in diabetes mellitus. *Curr Eye Res* 31(11), 895–901, 2006.
17. Alexeev, V.L., Das, S., Finegold, D.N., and Asher, S.A., Photonic crystal glucose-sensing material for non-invasive monitoring of glucose in tear fluid. *Clin Chem* 50(12), 2353–2360, 2004.
18. Sweeney, D., du Toit, R., Keay, L., Jalbert, I., Sankaridurg, P.R., Stern, J., Skotnitsky, C., Stephensen, A., Covey, M., Holden, B.A., and Rao, G.N., Clinical performance of silicone hydrogel lenses. In: Sweeney D, editor. Silicone hydrogels: continuous-wear contact lenses. Edinburgh: Butterworth Heinemann, British Contact Lens Association, 164–216, 2004.
19. Pickup, J.C., Hussain, F., Evans, N.D., Rolinski, O.J., and Birch, D.J., Fluorescence-based glucose sensors. *Biosens Bioelectron* 20(12), 2555–2565, 2005.
20. Yim, S.W., Kim, T., Laurence, T.A., Partono, S., Kim, D., Kim, Y., Weiss, S., Reitmair, A., Four-color alternating-laser excitation single-molecule fluorescence spectroscopy for next-generation biodetection assays. Clin Chem. 58(4), 707–16, 2012.
21. Lakowicz, J.R., Emerging biomedical applications of time-resolved fluorescence spectroscopy. In *Topics in Fluorescence Spectroscopy*, Vol. 4, Lakowicz, J.R., ed. New York: Plenum Press, 1994, pp. 1–19.
22. Selvin, P.R., Fluorescence resonance energy transfer. *Methods Enzymol* 246, 300–334, 1995.
23. Lakowicz, J.R., *Principles of Fluorescence Spectroscopy*, 2nd edn. New York: Kluwer Academic/ Plenum Publishers, 1999.
24. Coté, G.L., McShane, M., and Pishko, M., Chapter 11 Fluorescence-based glucose biosensors, Glucose optical sensing and impact, edited by Valery Tuchin, Taylor & Francis Group, Boca Raton, FL, pp. 319–352, 2009.
25. Ballerstadt, R., Gowda, A., and McNichols, R., Fluorescence resonance energy transfer-based near-infrared fluorescence sensor for glucose monitoring. *Diabetes Technol Ther* 6(2), 191–200, 2004.
26. March, W.F., Mueller, A., and Herbrechtsmeier, P., Clinical trial of a noninvasive contact lens glucose sensor. *Diabetes Technol Ther* 6(6), 782–789, 2004.
27. Chinnayelka, S., Microcapsule biosensors based on competitive binding and fluorescence resonance energy transfer assays, PhD dissertation, Louisiana Tech University, Ruston, LA, 2005.
28. Painless blood glucose measurement for diabetics without blood tests. Eyesense AG. http://www.eyesense.com/ (accessed 06/26/12)
29. Abreu, M.M., U.S. Patent 6,544,193, April 8, 2003.
30. Zhang, J., Hodge, W., Hutnick, C., and Wang, X., Noninvasive diagnostic devices for diabetes through measuring tear glucose. *J Diabetes Sci Technol* 5(1), 166–172, 2011.
31. Zhang, J. and Hodge, W.G., US20100113901, 2010.
32. Badugu, R., Lakowicz, J.R., and Geddes, C.D., A glucose-sensing contact lens: From bench top to patient. *Curr Opin Biotechnol* 16(1), 100–107, 2005.
33. Badugu, R., Lakowicz, J.R., and Geddes, C.D., Fluorescence sensors for monosaccharides based on the 6-methylquinolinium nucleus and boronic acid moiety: Potential application to ophthalmic diagnostics. *Talanta* 65(3), 762–768, 2005.
34. Badugu, R., Lakowicz, J.R., and Geddes, C.D., Boronic acid fluorescent sensors for monosaccharide signaling based on the 6-methoxyquinolinium heterocyclic nucleus: Progress toward noninvasive and continuous glucose monitoring. *Bioorg Med Chem* 13(1), 113–119, 2005.

35. Badugu, R., Lakowicz, J.R., and Geddes, C.D., Ophthalmic glucose monitoring using disposable contact lenses—A review. *J Fluoresc* 14(5), 617–633, 2004.
36. Kumar, C.S.S.R., *Biomimetic and Bioinspired Nanomaterials*. New York: Wiley, 2010.
37. Saranathan, V., Osuji, C.O., Mochrie, S.G., Noh, H., Narayanan, S., Sandy, A., Dufresne, E.R., and Prum, R.O., Structure, function, and self-assembly of single network gyroid (I4132) photonic crystals in butterfly wing scales. *Proc Natl Acad Sci USA* 107(26), 11676–11681, 2010.
38. Vértesy, Z., Bálint, Z., Kertész, K., Vigneron, J.P., Lousse, V., and Biró, L.P., Wing scale microstructures and nanostructures in butterflies—Natural photonic crystals. *J Microsc* 224(Pt 1), 108–110, 2006.
39. Zi, J., Yu, X., Li, Y., Hu, X., Xu, C., Wang, X., Liu, X., and Fu, R., Coloration strategies in peacock feathers. *Proc Natl Acad Sci USA* 100(22), 12576–12578, 2003
40. Denisyuk, Y.N., On the reproduction of the optical properties of an object by the wave field of its scattered radiation. *Opt Spectrosc* 18, 152–157, 1965.
41. Domschke, A., Ophthalmic glucose nano-sensor. Oral presentation at the *International Conference on Nanoscience and Technology (ICN+T)*, Keystone, CO, 2008.
42. Nave, R., Bragg's law. *HyperPhysics*, Section 6.1, Georgia State University. http://hyperphysics.phy-astr.gsu.edu/hbase/quantum/bragg.html. Retrieved September 03, 2011.
43. Kabilan, S., Blyth, J., Lee, M.C., Marshall, A.J., Hussain, A., Yang, X.P., and Lowe, C.R., Glucose-sensitive holographic sensors. *J Mol Recogn* 17(3), 162–166, 2004.
44. Kabilan, S., Marshall, A.J., Sartain, F.K., Lee, M.C., Hussain, A., Yang, X., Blyth, J., Karangu, N., James, K., Zeng, J., Smith, D., Domschke, A., and Lowe, C.R., Holographic glucose sensors. *Biosens Bioelectron* 20(8), 1602–1610, 2005.
45. Domschke, A., March, W.F., Kabilan, S., and Lowe, C., Initial clinical testing of a holographic non-invasive contact lens glucose sensor. *Diabetes Technol Ther* 8(1), 89–93, 2006.
46. Lorand, J.P. and Edwards, J.O., Polyol complexes and structure of the benzeneboronate ion. *J Org Chem* 24, 769–774, 1959.
47. Yang, W.Q., Yan, J., Springsteen, G., Deeter, S., and Wang, B.H., A novel type of fluorescent boronic acid that shows large fluorescence intensity changes upon binding with a carbohydrate in aqueous solution at physiological pH. *Bioorg Med Chem Lett* 13(6), 1019–1022, 2003.
48. Lavigne, J.J. and Anslyn, E.V., Teaching old indicators new tricks: A colorimetric chemosensing ensemble for tartrate/malate in beverages. *Angew Chem Int Ed Engl* 38(24), 3666–3669, 1999.
49. Gray, C.W. Jr. and Houston, T.A., Boronic acid receptors for alpha-hydroxycarboxylates: High affinity of Shinkai's glucose receptor for tartrate. *J Org Chem* 67(15), 5426–5428, 2002.
50. March, W.F., Dealing with the delay. *Diabetes Technol Ther* 4(1), 49–50, 2002.
51. Reese, C.E., Guerrero, C.D., Weissman, J.M., Lee, K., and Asher, S.A., Synthesis of highly charged, monodisperse polystyrene colloidal particles for the fabrication of photonic crystals. *Colloid Interf Sci* 232(1), 76–80, 2000.
52. Asher Research Group, Department of Chemistry, University of Pittsburgh, Colloid Group, http://www.pitt.edu/~asher/homepage/colgrp.html#pcca. Accessed March 12, 2012.
53. Ben-Moshe, M., Alexeev, V.L., and Asher, S.A., Fast responsive crystalline colloidal array photonic crystal glucose sensors. *Anal Chem* 78(14), 5149–5157, 2006.
54. Zhang, J.T., Wang, L., Luo, J., Tikhonov, A., Kornienko, N., and Asher, S.A., 2-D array photonic crystal sensing motif. *J Am Chem Soc* 133(24), 9152–9155, 2011.
55. Deshpande, D.C., Yoon, H., Khaing, A.M., and Varadan, V.K., Development of a nanoscale heterostructured glucose sensor using modified microfabrication processes. *J Micro/Nanolith. MEMS MOEMS* 7, 023005, 2008.
56. Liao, Y.T., Yao, H., and Parviz, B.A., Otis, B., A 3μW wirelessly powered CMOS glucose sensor for an active contact lens, Solid-State Circuits Conference Digest of Technical Papers (ISSCC), 2011 IEEE International, San Francisco, CA., pp. 38–40, 2011.
57. Yao, H., Shum, A.J., Cowan, M., Lähdesmäki, I., and Parviz, B.A., A contact lens with embedded sensor for monitoring tear glucose level. *Biosens Bioelectron* 26(7), 3290–3296, 2011.

58. Yao, H., Afanasiev, A., Lahdesmaki, I., and Parviz, B.A., A dual microscale glucose sensor on a contact lens, tested in conditions mimicking the eye, 5734353 abstract. In *Micro Electro Mechanical Systems (MEMS), 2011 IEEE 24th International Conference*. Cancun, Mexico, pp. 25–28, 2011.

59. Chu, M.X., Miyajima, K., Takahashi, D., Arakawa, T., Sano, K., Sawada, S., Kudo, H., Iwasaki, Y., Akiyoshi, K., Mochizuki, M., and Mitsubayashi, K., Soft contact lens biosensor for in situ monitoring of tear glucose as non-invasive blood sugar assessment. *Talanta* 83(3), 960–965, 2011.

60. Patel, J.N., Gray, B.L., Kaminska, B., and Gates, B.D., Flexible three-dimensional electrochemical glucose sensor with improved sensitivity realized in hybrid polymer microelectromechanical systems technique. *J Diabetes Sci Technol* 5(5), 1036–1043, 2011.

61. Kagie, A., Bishop, D.K., Burdick, J., La Belle, J.T., Dymond, R., Felder, R., and Wang, J., Flexible rolled thick-film miniaturized flow-cell for minimally invasive amperometric sensing. *Electroanalysis* 20(14), 1610–1614, 2008.

62. Gray, H., *Anatomy of the Human Body*. Philadelphia, PA: Lea & Febiger, 1918, Bartleby.com, 2000.

63. Larijani, B., Nasli Esfahani, E., Amini, P., Nikbin, B., Alimoghaddam, K., Amiri, S., Malekzadeh, R., Mojahed Yazdi, N., Ghodsi, M., Dowlati, Y., Sahraian, M.A., and Ghavamzadeh, A., Stem cell therapy in treatment of different diseases. *Acta Med Iran* 50(2), 79–96, 2012.

64. Krol, S., Ellis-Behnke, R., and Marchetti, P., Nanomedicine for treatment of diabetes in an aging population: state-of-the-art and future developments. *Maturitas.* 73(1), 61–7, 2012.

65. Alvarado, J., Diabetes and Your Eyesight, Glaucoma Research Foundation, http://www.glaucoma.org/glaucoma/diabetes-and-youreyesight.php (accessed 06/26/13)

66. Wilson, R., Contact lens has MEMS devise to measure glaucoma. *Electronics Weekly*. 2010. www.electronicsweekly.com/Articles/2010/03/24/48276/contact-lens-has-mems-device-to-measure-glaucoma.htm. Accessed April 2011.

67. Leonardi, M., Pitchon, E.M., Bertsch, A., Renaud, P., and Mermoud, A., Wireless contact lens sensor for intraocular pressure monitoring: Assessment on enucleated pig eyes. *Acta Ophthalmol* 87(4), 433–437, 2009.

68. Twa, M.D., Roberts, C.J., Karol, H.J., Mahmoud, A.M., Weber, P.A., and Small, R.H., Evaluation of a contact lens-embedded sensor for intraocular pressure measurement. *J Glaucoma* 19(6), 382–390, 2010.

69. Chous, P., Dry Eyes and Diabetes Often Go Hand In Hand, High risk of disorder calls for tight control of glucose levels, dLife, LifeMed Media, Inc. 2012. http://www.dlife.com/diabetes/complications/eyecare/chous_sept2006

70. Ciolino, J.B., Hoare, T.R., Iwata, N.G., Behlau, I., Dohlman, C.H., Langer, R., and Kohane, D.S., A drug-eluting contact lens. *Invest Ophthalmol Vis Sci* 50(7), 3346–3352, 2009.

71. Singh, K., Nair, A.B., Kumar, A., and Kumria, R., Novel approaches in formulation and drug delivery using contact lenses, *J Basic Clin Pharm* 2(2), 87–101, 2011.

11

Sensorcyte Artificial Cells for Human Diagnostics and Analytics

Mark J. Schulz, Weifeng Li, Brad Ruff, Rajiv Venkatasubramanian, Yi Song, Bolaji Suberu, Wondong Cho, Pravahan Salunke, Anshuman Sowani, John Yin, David Mast, Vesselin Shanov, Zhongyun Dong, Sarah Pixley, Jianjun Hu, and Chris Muratore

CONTENTS

11.1 Introduction

The diagnosis and treatment of a disease might be significantly enhanced if nanorobotic devices, such as sensors and actuators, could be utilized within the human body [1–53]. Sensors for use in the human patient would have to be minimally invasive and biocompatible for temporary use. Nanorobots, as a general category of novel diminutive devices, are proposed in this chapter for use as sensors and actuators in vivo. Since this is a newly emerging area of research, we must first define what nanorobot devices are. Nanorobotic devices are tiny machines, micron size, that are enabled by nanotechnology for applications in medicine. They are important because they may have greater precision, force, and be easier to control than biological materials. The history of nanorobots or "tiny machine" had its inception in 1959, when Richard Feynman stated that "Development of tiny machines cannot be avoided" [11]. Understandably, some people are skeptical and put forward that nanorobots cannot ever be built or work within the human body. Contrarily, we propose that tiny machines will indeed become the new frontier in medicine and that practically every facet of medicine will benefit from the application of nanorobotic devices.

It has been more than five decades since Richard Feynman gave his talk about tiny machines. Hence, one may rightly inquire in 2013: How many types of nanorobot devices or "Tiny Machines" have been built to date? Unfortunately, the answer is none. Why is this the case? We believe that this is due to cumulative mismatches of appropriate applications with available technologies. Looking at the scale of nanorobotic devices may help to explain how nanorobot devices might come into application. At the nanoscale, particles are being developed for drug delivery and therapy; however, these are not electromechanical devices. At the other size extreme (macroscale), existing technologies such as da Vinci medical robot manipulators, which utilize centimeter-size tools are the current state of the art. However, the domain between the nanoscale and macroscale (microscale) is a little investigated intermediate range where microrobotic electromechanical devices that contain nanoscale components can have unique applications. The Sensorcyte (Figure 11.1) is a conceptual microrobotic device that can be built with nanoscale materials. We believe that the Sensorcyte is feasible to construct using existing technologies and has the potential for meeting a range of critical needs in medicine. The design, methods used, and ongoing efforts to build the Sensorcyte are described in this chapter. The simplest configuration of a Sensorcyte, which is still at the conceptual stage, is a carbon nanotube (CNT) wire coil that is wound around a magnetic nanoparticle (MNP) core which forms the secondary winding of a transformer [44,51]. The primary winding of the transformer is a coil on the skin of the patient that is positioned outside the body. Each time that the Sensorcyte passes the primary coil, it is recharged and responds briefly by transmitting a signal from its antenna. The secondary winding of the Sensorcyte might also be connected to capacitors to store charge. The capacitors will discharge through a timer and circular antenna, embedded within the surface of the Sensorcyte. The Sensorcyte, in its most fundamental form, pings its position as it circulates through the vascular system, and the recording instrumentation worn outside the body determines its position and velocity. The transformer can be moved to any position on the body to transmit and receive signals from the Sensorcyte. The ability of the Sensorcyte to communicate in this manner has not yet been established and is the subject of ongoing research. It is assumed that the Sensorcyte would circulate for a certain period of time and then be cleared from the body, in a manner similar to the operation of biological cells.

Reductions in health-care expenditures will make nanodevices and sensors such as the Sensorcyte cost-effective. Instrumentation is being developed [54–62], and significant research efforts are underway [55–136] toward enabling these advances. Existing technologies and products for diagnosing diseases are mainly in vitro medical devices. These devices are simple, inexpensive, and provide portable and rapid diagnostic tests, but are usually limited to the detection of a single analyte or target. An overarching goal is to develop a generalizable platform for in vivo sensing and actuation that provides continuous monitoring of physiology. Such a platform would provide multimodal monitoring in real time. It is anticipated that there would be broad beneficial impacts through the implementation of this continuous physiologic monitoring technology. Sensorcytes might enable the monitoring of metabolic and infectious diseases of national significance via the precise measurement of analytes such as glucose, urea, lactate, and cytokines. As an example of the commercial potential, the glucometer market alone may reach $6 billion by 2015 in the United States.

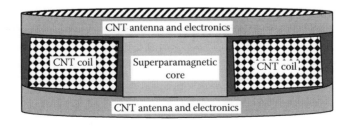

FIGURE 11.1
Sensorcyte concept using lightweight CNT wire, MNP core, and a flexible elastomer matrix material. Dimensions are 8 μm × 2 μm, and the density is ~1.4 g/cc.

11.1.1 Disease Monitoring In Vivo

The monitoring of diseases in vivo has a number of advantages that have motivated the development of biomedical microdevices. In vivo sensing may detect diseases earlier and at lower concentrations using blood-borne sensors, as there is more analyte present in the circulation than in the blood samples used in traditional analysis. Also, circulating sensors may have increased access to be in closer proximity to disease sites where biomarker concentrations may be higher. Many different physical and chemical variables might be detected. Physical variables, including temperature, pressure, strain, force, velocity, waves, light, and vibration may be easier to detect, because they are less affected by sensor biofouling. The detection of biological materials, encompassing proteins, cytokines, bacteria, cells, and viruses is more difficult as the sensor may become biofouled. Linking agents or receptors such as antibodies, aptamers, ligands, and peptides may be used to conjugate analytes to the sensor. Chemical sensors may function by employing enzymes, membranes, or affinity agents. However, the biochemistry and conjugation can be complex, and small nanoparticles (approx. <200 nm) may be cleared from the body by macrophages.

11.1.1.1 Nanoparticles as Sensors

Different strategies are being proposed for in vivo sensing, and the use of nanoparticles as sensors is reviewed here. As an example, an "In vivo Nanoplatforms for Diagnostics" program [DARPA, 114] is developing biocompatible nanosensors employing nontoxic materials for use within the living tissues of animals, plants, and insects. The sensors would provide continuous and noninvasive measurement of a variety of conditions and substances with limited immunogenicity. These sensors would ideally permit the quantitative assessment of small molecules such as glucose, lactate, urea, and large molecules such as proteins, oligonucleotides, infectious agents, and chemical/biological threat agents within organisms and the environment. Optical, electronic, thermal, or magnetic mechanisms might be utilized for sensing.

The chief requirements for in vivo sensors are safety, biocompatibility, and accuracy. Existing implantable sensors, which are comprised mostly of nanoparticles, are limited by toxicity and immunogenic response, and may be rapidly cleared by the reticuloendothelial system or biofouled due to the nonspecific binding of biologic materials onto the surface depending on the size, shape, and coating that exists on the sensor particle. New nanoparticle materials, sizes, shapes, and coatings are needed to limit their toxicity and increase their biocompatibility. Potential approaches might include polymer coatings, surface-modifying additives, and new methods for creating nontoxic nanomaterials of narrow size distribution and tailored shape [114]. Calibration protocols are also required to correct for sensor drift over extended periods, or the nanoparticles must be cleared and replaced. Methods for enhancing the sensitivity and lifetime of in vivo sensors are also needed. New sensing concepts include mixed self-assembled monolayer coatings that include analyte-selective and nonfouling components; self-calibrating multianalyte sensors; fluorescent molecular beacons; oligonucleotide modification enabling tissue targeting and nuclease resistance; and analyte/signal amplification via enzymatic or catalytic mechanisms [114]. A potential problem that might arise with nanometric sensors is that they may become mobile within tissues and thus be difficult to locate. The sensors may also need to be relatively close to the surface of the skin to allow for interrogation when using optical methods.

Adaptable nanoparticle-based sensors could provide distributed and unobtrusive physiologic and environmental sensing and the treatment of physiologic abnormalities, illness, and infectious diseases. In vivo sensing and physiologic monitoring to facilitate diagnostics and subsequent therapeutics should enable a versatile, rapidly adaptable system to provide critical medical information. The multiplexed detection of analytes at clinically relevant concentrations, and the capacity for the external interrogation of the nanoplatform that is free from any implanted communications electronics is desired [114], but may limit the capabilities of the sensing device. Sensor readouts should be considered with respect to parameters such as choice of tissue, analytes, repetitive noncontact signal acquisition, and signal-to-noise ratio. Safe, biocompatible nanoparticles for in vivo multiplexed analyte sensing are needed for defense applications. Imperative to any sensor concept is the overriding requirement to avoid harm to the host. The prudent selection of nanoparticle size, shape, and material to limit clearance by the reticuloendothelial system is an important design consideration, as is the selection of appropriate surface coatings that are nonfouling and biocompatible. One potential approach is to use surface-enhanced Raman spectroscopy nanoparticles within the tissue to detect biologically relevant molecules at low concentration levels, whereby their optical responses would be uniquely altered by analytes of interest. Related to this concept is the design of a selective self-assembled monolayer that has the ability to partition analytes of interest, thereby enhancing sensor specificity. Although a selective self-assembled monolayer has been demonstrated for the detection of glucose, each new analyte of interest will require a unique surface to exploit steric and energetic effects for enhanced selectivity. Mixed self-assembled monolayer coatings that incorporate nonfouling components such as carboxybetaines could also improve sensor sensitivities and lifetimes [114]. Another potential optical approach uses "molecular beacons" that fluoresce upon binding to target analytes. Background subtraction and ratiometric or related techniques were demonstrated to reduce obscurants while maintaining a satisfactory detector response. The choice of wavelength is important for the optimization of tissue penetration and eye safety, while limiting absorption by endogenous chromophores and water. These approaches might increase in vivo sensitivity, specificity, and the lifetime of the nanoparticle sensor components, all of which are critical aspects of sensor development.

11.1.1.2 Microscale Machines as Sensors

An alternate approach to nanoparticle sensors is to build microscale devices that take advantage of advances in electrically conductive nanotube yarn, superparamagnetic nanoparticles, and nanowires. These new nanomaterials are enabling the development of tiny machines that can perform sensing, actuation, and communication functions with unprecedented performance. While inherently more complex, these microdevices have much more extensive functionality than do simple nanoparticles, and are the focus of this chapter.

11.2 Nanoscale Materials for Microscale Devices

Nanoscale materials that may be used to build microscale devices are reviewed here. Processing and characterization of the materials is also discussed.

11.2.1 Carbon Nanotube Materials

Properties of CNT materials are compared to the properties of copper in Table 11.1. The characteristics and performance of nanotubes are being continuously improved. Carbon nanomaterials exhibit unique and extreme properties, because CNT shells are only one atomic layer thick, which implies that they have a low density. The strong triple sp^2 bonding of carbon, combined with the hexagonal tessellated architecture of CNTs, provides high strength.

TABLE 11.1

Approximate Strength and Electrical Conduction of Metals and CNT Materials

Material	Density (10^3 kg/m³)	Strength (MPa)	Specific Strength (MPa/kg/m³)	Electrical Conductivity (1/Ω·m)	Specific Conductivity (1/Ω·m)/(kg/m³)	Current Density in Air (a/m²)	Specific Current Density in Air (A/kg/m)	Resistivity (Ω·cm)	Thermal Conductivity (W/mK)
Copper	8.9	150 Y, 340 U	17 Y, 39 U	59×10^6	6.6×10^6	6×10^6	0.7×10^6	1.7×10^{-6}	400
Aluminum and alloys	2.7	10–600 Y	3.7–222	35×10^6	13×10^6	—	—	2.8×10^{-6}	237
Iron	7.9	140–690 U	17.7–87.3	10×10^6	1.3×10^6	—	—	9.6×10^{-6}	80
CNT	1.8	50,000	27,000	$\sim30 \times 10^6$	$\sim17 \times 10^6$	TBD	TBD	1×10^{-6}	3,000
CNT thread	1.0	2,000	2,000	$\sim10 \times 10^6$	$\sim10 \times 10^6$	1×10^8	1×10^8	1.7×10^{-4}	100

Y, yield strength; U, ultimate strength.

The hexagon structure is the highest order polygon that tessellates, and can be considered as a fundamental platform from which to design novel atomic layer compounds and hybrid inorganic materials with one-, two- or three-dimensionality. Tessellation can be thought of as tiling a floor with abutting shapes that do not overlap or have gaps.

11.2.1.1 Current Status of the Technology to Produce CNT Arrays

CNT technology is advancing to the point where devices can now be made [44,50–72]. Centimeter-long aligned CNT arrays have been synthesized by UC Nanoworld [51]. The method of CNT growth is briefly described in the following paragraph. Vertically aligned centimeter-long CNTs can be grown in a 2 in. diameter quartz tube reactor (Figure 11.2a) or a 3 in. diameter quartz tube reactor (Figure 11.2b), using a water-assisted catalytic chemical vapor deposition (CVD) technique. Substrates are prepared using the following methods. Initially, an Al film buffer layer is deposited on a 4 in. diameter Si (100) wafer with a 500 nm thick SiO_2 layer using an electron beam evaporator. Subsequent to the oxidation of the $Al/SiO_2/Si$ substrate, the catalyst Fe and promoter films are deposited on the $Al_2O_3/SiO_2/Si$ substrates using electron beam deposition. For the synthesis of patterned CNT arrays, different patterned masks may be used to prepare the substrates. The masks covered the $Al_2O_3/SiO_2/Si$ substrates followed by the deposition of catalysts using an e-beam evaporator. Experiments were carried out using the following balanced recipe: 560 mmHg of argon, 60 mmHg of hydrogen, 140 mmHg of ethylene, and 900 ppm of water. The growth temperature varied from 780°C to 820°C.

The characterization of the synthesized nanotube materials is an important step in materials development and quality control. Scanning electron microscopy (SEM) imaging was performed with a Phillips XL30 ESEM. Raman spectroscopy was performed using a Renishaw inVia Reflex Micro-Raman. Figure 11.3a through c show typical SEM images of centimeter-long CNT arrays. Despite the long growth time to produce centimeter-long CNTs, the image reveals well-aligned CNTs at low magnification while individual CNTs show entanglement/adhesion at high magnification. Postprocessing by annealing improves the nanotube quality as shown in Figure 11.3 d,e.

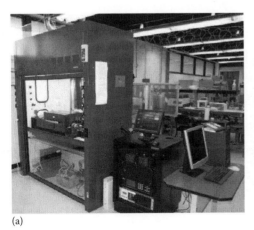
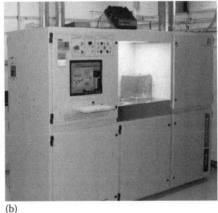

(a)   (b)

FIGURE 11.2
Manufacturing CNT arrays using first nano nanofurnaces. (a) The ET1000 first-generation reactor became operational in 2002, and can produce one 2.5 × 5 cm wafer in each experiment. (b) The ET3000 second-generation reactor became operational in 2007, and can produce one 10 cm wafer in two pieces in each experiment.

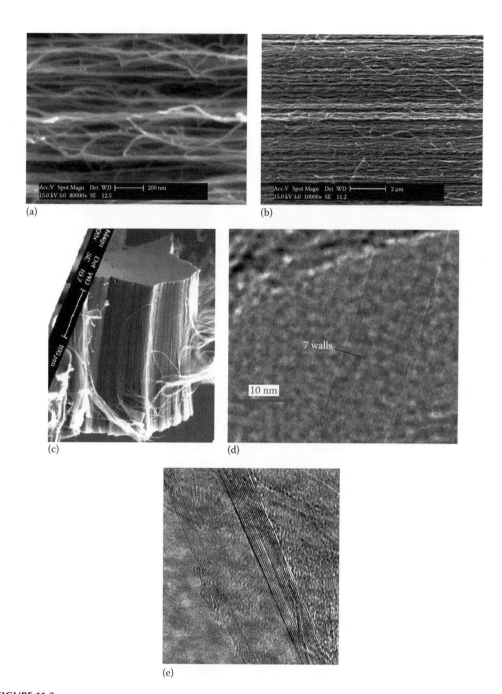

FIGURE 11.3
Characterization of CNT arrays. (a) High-magnification (80,000×) image of CNT array, side view. (b) Low-magnification (10,000×) image of CNT array. (c) A 300 μm tall CNT array. (d, e) CNTs after annealing characterization of CNT arrays.

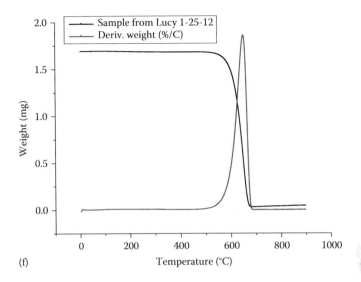

(f)

FIGURE 11.3 (continued)
Characterization of CNT arrays. (f) Thermogravimetric analysis showing the high purity of the CNTs.

Figure 11.4 shows a Raman spectrum of CNTs, which indicates the quality of multiwall CNTs. As can be seen in Figure 11.4a, the D and G peaks are shown at 1350 cm^{-1} and 1590 cm^{-1}. The intensity ratio I_D/I_G which shows the degree of graphitization of CNTs was calculated to be 0.73. For this ratio, the CNTs are well graphitized, but amorphous carbon and other by-products of the reaction reduce the Raman ratio. Annealing may be performed to further graphitize the CNTs. Horizontally grown CNTs show high quality in Figure 11.4b.

There are many applications for CNTs. Each application, however, often requires different types, shapes, or configurations of CNTs, including short length, centimeter-long, bundles, single wall, multiwall, thread, or patterned. Figure 11.5 shows images of different patterned CNT arrays. The images are examples of patterned CNT arrays, tiles of CNT arrays, needle-type CNT posts, and a CNT nanothread that was spun under the microscope. Suitable patterned CNT arrays can be produced for different applications.

11.2.1.2 Producing CNT Yarn

The longest CNT arrays to date have approached the inch-length range. These can be wound into a small diameter coil. However, to form a continuous macroscale material, the spinning of CNT to form yarn is necessary. This CNT yarn can be used for in vivo applications, as the use of electrical wires inside the human body is not new. Conductive wires are currently in use to make connections with pacemakers, and are utilized in veins [99,100]. Table 11.1 lists the properties of CNT, CNT thread/yarn, and traditional materials. Existing CNT yarns are of sufficient quality to build biosensors (strength is ~2 GPa, density is 1 g/cm^3, resistivity may approach 10^{-5} Ω cm, exceeding that of copper on a per-weight basis, max current density is 10^5 A/cm^2). A CNT thread is lighter, more flexible, stronger, chemically inert, and is capable of carrying a large current. The higher resistivity is acceptable, in that an increased voltage or larger diameter thread can be used, and the low duty cycle will allow cooling. Work to improve the electrical conductivity and strength of CNT

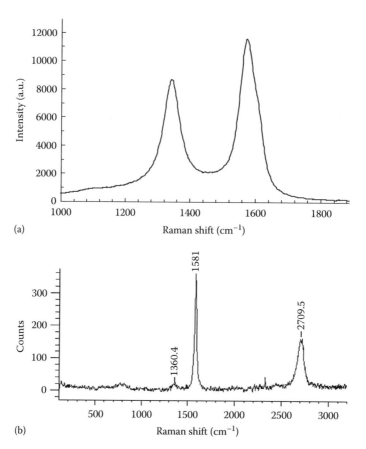

FIGURE 11.4
Raman spectrum of CNTs. (a) Vertically aligned CNT array; typically $I_g/I_d = 1$–2. (b) Horizontally aligned sparse CNTs, $I_g/I_d = 14$–15. The higher the ratio is, the higher will be the CNT quality.

threads using longer CNT elements is ongoing [51,70–72]. The main postprocessing steps in the proper sequence are: (i) functionalization of the array; (ii) doping of the ribbon; (iii) coating (dielectric functionalization) the ribbon; and (iv) twisting into thread. Long CNT will be used to form the coils and antenna of the Sensorcyte. There will be no junctions as with spinning short CNT into thread. The long CNT will have high electrical conductivity, high strength, high thermal conductivity, and be flexible, tough, lightweight, and stronger than steel. However, CNT thread may be required for other applications in vivo. An analysis of the limitations in the strength of the nanotube bundles and thread is shown in the next section.

11.2.1.3 Strength of Bundles of Nanotubes

Since CNTs are small in diameter (e.g., 10 nm) and are not continuous fibers, it is necessary to use bundles of nanotubes to form threads that can be used as an electrical wire. The advantage of using a thread versus a solid metal wire or carbon fiber is that the thread is more flexible and pliable. A disadvantage is that the electrical conductivity may not be as efficient as the metal wire, and the strength may not be as high as carbon fiber. The goal is to create a CNT thread that combines the advantages of both metal wire and carbon fiber, which will also be pliable and flexible. To consider how to produce this type of thread,

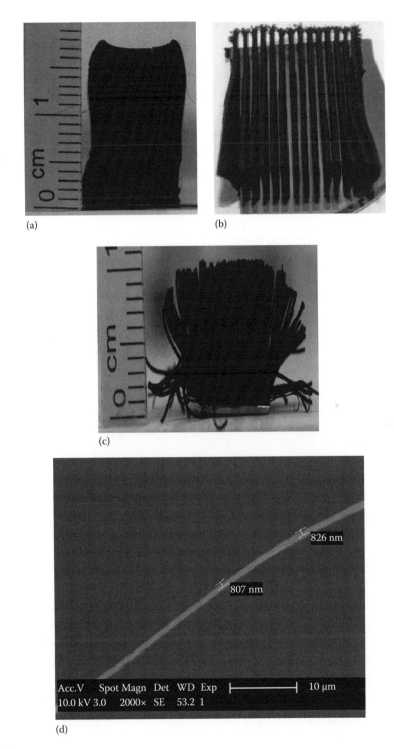

FIGURE 11.5
Forms of nanotube materials. (a) Optical picture of ~18 mm CNT array. (b) 0.5 mm thick CNT tiles. (c) 10 mm needle-type CNT arrays with 0.5 mm diameter. (d) ~816 nm diameter CNT thread.

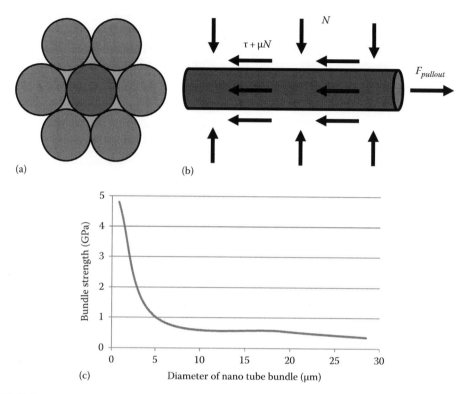

FIGURE 11.6

Modeling the strength of nanotubes. (a) Geometry of a bundle of CNTs; the center tube (red) is coupled to the surrounding tubes (blue) by a polymer (orange) and van der Waals forces and friction forces. (b) Forces acting on an individual nanotube. (c) Measured approximate strength of bundles of nanotubes for different processing conditions and different diameters. (The data is the measured strength from samples that were processed by different methods. Hence, a conclusion cannot be drawn in regard to processing methods; the only qualitative conclusion is that smaller diameter samples may convey enhanced strength.)

we can look at a bundle of CNTs and assess the pullout strength of an individual nanotube from the bundle. The bundle could contain nanotubes that are long, short, straight, or twisted, and the nanotubes could be bonded to each other using a matrix material, or there could be no bonding material. The geometry of the bundle is shown in Figure 11.6a. An individual nanotube is considered in Figure 11.6b, and the forces that act on a single tube are shown.

The strength of the nanotube being pulled out of the bundle will be indicative of the minimum of the strength of the nanotube itself, or the strength of the pullout of the nanotube from the bundle. If the nanotube was very long and spanned the load path of the structure, then the full strength of the nanotube would be achieved, and this would be the ideal case as no twist or matrix material would be necessary. In the following analysis, the nanotube is assumed to not span the loaded length of the material. Also, the strength of the nanotube for engineering design must be based on the full cross-sectional area of the tube (which is mostly space), not only the area of the walls of the tube. The forces that act on the nanotube to resist pullout are the van der Waals force, friction force, and the bonding force of any adhesive that are imparted by adjacent nanotubes. The strength of the nanotube itself depends on its quality, which is contingent on the synthesis process and any posttreatment such as annealing. The strength, stiffness, and straightness of individual nanotubes is a separate area of consideration and is not discussed here, except to say that high-quality multiwall nanotubes are needed to make high-quality thread. The equation for the pullout strength of a single nanotube is

$$S_{pullout} = \frac{F_{pullout}}{A_{cs}} = \frac{\mu N(vdw, F_{radial})}{A_{cs}} + \tau \frac{A_s}{A_{cs}} = \frac{\mu N(vdw, F_{radial})}{(\pi D^2 / 4)} + \tau \frac{(\pi DL)}{(\pi D^2 / 4)} \quad (11.1)$$

where $S_{pullout}$, $F_{pullout}$, A_{cs}, μ, $N(vdw, F_{radial})$, τ, $A_s = (\pi DL)$, $A_{cs} = (\pi D^2/4)$ are the pullout strength of the nanotube in the bundle; pullout force of the nanotube; friction coefficient between adjacent nanotubes; normal force acting on the nanotube where the normal force depends on the van der Waals (*vdw*) force and any radial gripping force if the nanotubes are twisted; the shear strength of any matrix material bonded to the nanotubes that might exist between the nanotubes or the shear strength of any molecular bonding between adjacent nanotubes; the surface area of the nanotube; and the cross-sectional area of the nanotube.

Equation 11.1 can be used to qualitatively explain how to increase the pullout strength of nanotubes from the bundle. If the nanotubes cannot be pulled out of the bundle, then the bundle and the nanotubes will fracture, and the full strength of the thread will be achieved. To maximize Equation 11.1, consider the first term of the right part of the equation. The friction coefficient and normal force should be as large as possible, which is dependant on the *vdw* force, whereas the radial force that depends on the diameter of the thread and the twist angle, as well as the cross-sectional area of the nanotube should be minimized (the diameter of tube should be small). Now, consider the second term in the right part of Equation 11.1. The shear strength of the matrix or any chemical linking should be maximized, and the ratio of surface area to cross-sectional area of the nanotube (A_s/A_{cs}) should be maximized (e.g., length of the nanotube should be maximized, and the diameter of the nanotube should be small). These general guidelines can be utilized in the design of CNT threads.

Figure 11.6c shows the measured approximate strength of bundles of nanotubes for different processing conditions and various diameters. The conditions of the material are all different in the graph, and the only conclusion that can be made is that smaller diameter nanotube bundles have higher strength. Overall conclusions from this analysis, which are very qualitative, include that smaller diameter thread, long nanotubes, and high friction and shear forces between the nanotubes are desired.

Nanotube thread is currently produced using a few different techniques. In one approach, single-wall carbon nanotubes (SWCNTs) are dispersed in an acid and extruded to form a thread. In another approach, multiwall CNTs are dry-spun from a silicon substrate. The most scalable approach might be where single or double wall CNTs are drawn directly from a reactor. In one case of directly drawing nanotubes from the reactor, the nanotube aerogel material is not twisted as it is being drawn, or after being drawn from the reactor. Adding twist acts to reduce the strength of the thread. In a similar approach, the nanotube aerogel is twisted while being drawn from the reactor. These different examples of forming thread indicate that different parameters in Equation 11.1 are more or less important, depending on the process for forming the thread. An overriding consideration is to ensure that the nanotubes are well-aligned for as long as possible. Once this criterion is met, the other parameters become less important. In the limit of continuously long nanotubes, no twisting, no friction, no *vdw*, and no shear forces are needed. We would like to be able to synthesize continuous long nanotube bundles that would be as strong as carbon fiber, but still be flexible, as many nanotubes would make up the bundle.

11.2.1.4 Doping and Coating

The doping of CNTs with iodine [87] and nitrogen is being developed in the Nanoworld Lab and will be used to improve their electrical conductivity. Iodine doping may leach out of the thread; therefore, nitrogen doping may be more reliable. Doping improves DC conductivity but may not improve high-frequency conductivity. Another approach in improving conductivity is to decorate the CNTs with metallic (Au, Ni) nanoparticles. The Air Force Research Laboratory in Dayton, OH is developing this approach. The strength and electrical conductivity of the CNTs are increased by the metal particles, and this augmentation may be greater than expected based on the volume of material used. The best doping/decorating approach will be applied for small-scale use.

The coating of the CNT ribbon is also being developed, and it has shown to improve the mechanical and electrical properties of the thread by ~100%. This improvement is due to the polymer-bonding of the CNTs to each other, as when the solvent in the polymer evaporates, surface tension forces cause the thread to shrink in diameter. The science behind this coating method is based in electrostatics. The fundamental principle is based on the mutual attraction of opposite electrical charges and the mutual repulsion of like charges. Terronics Company has developed a way to safely and effectively charge particles (polymer droplets), so that they are attracted to individual CNT strands in the provision of a thin high-quality coating. Coating individual strands has an advantage in terms of the electrical (tunable R, L, C properties) and mechanical properties (increasing modulus and strength) of the thread. Other techniques coat only the exterior of the thread, and not individual strands; thus, it is important to miniaturize the coating application method so as to coat individual strands of CNT. The electrostatic coating process has been demonstrated with targets that were transiting at line speeds of 20 m/s; hence, it will not slowdown spinning. The full theory of multiple jet electrohydrodynamic coating is described in [54].

11.2.1.5 Densifying Nanotubes

A CNT wire that has a higher current density and smaller diameter will increase the magnetic induction of Sensorcytes. In contrast to superconductors, CNTs conduct electricity more efficiently at high temperatures, and improvements in the conductivity of CNTs are a goal of continuing research. Possible approaches to this end include

1. Improvements in CNT quality
2. Synthesis of all-metallic CNT
3. Synthesis of dense CNT
4. CNT doping

Consider dense CNTs that are operating at high temperature. The resistivity is ρ; the area of the CNT ends to facilitate conduction is A_{cnt}; the cross-sectional area of the CNT is A_{cs}m; which in a MWCNT are $\rho = RA_{cnt}^N / L$, $A_{cs} = \pi D^2/4$, $A_{cnt}^N = nt \sum_{i=1}^{N} D_i$, where $D_i = [D_o-(i-1)2t]$. The area of the CNT walls is shown in Figure 11.7. When the number of walls increases from two to five in a 10 nm diameter nanotube, the properties are enhanced by ~50%.

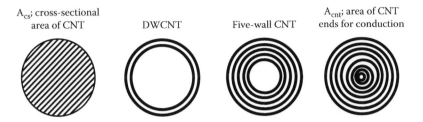

FIGURE 11.7
Increasing the number of walls in a CNT to improve its properties.

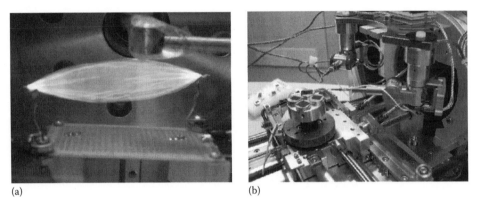

(a)   (b)

FIGURE 11.8
Carbon electromagnetics. (a) Whirling CNT yarn, the first demonstration of the principle of a carbon electric motor. (b) Kleindiek robots used to build microdevices.

11.2.1.6 Electromagnetic Devices Using CNT Yarn

CNTs can be used to form lightweight electromagnetic devices. Figure 11.8a demonstrates the whirling of a CNT yarn, whereas Figure 11.8b depicts the Kleindiek robotic manipulators that are used in the construction of microdevices.

Figure 11.9 illustrates the comparison of a coil that is built using copper wire with that using CNT thread. The equation $B'/B = g'r/gr'$ shows that the magnetic flux density B' of the nanotube-thread-based coil will be larger than the magnetic flux density of the copper coil B, because the maximum current density g' of the nanotube thread is greater than the maximum current density g of the copper wire, and the radius of the nanotube coil r' is smaller than the radius r of the copper coil. The CNT coil is smaller and has a larger flux density. This indicates that microdevices can have better specific performance than macroscale electromagnetic devices, assuming that the duty cycle is low enough to ensure that the cooling of the device is satisfactory. An additional goal is to eliminate copper, iron, and rare earth magnets in electric motors. Using long, high-voltage, high-frequency, parallel CNT windings and a superparamagnetic nanoparticle core, the proposed nanomaterials-based motor will be smaller in radius r, lighter, and will have higher flux density B' for an equivalent current i than conventional motors.

11.2.2 Magnetic Nanotube and Nanowire Materials

The principle of operation of an electric motor is based on Faraday's law of induction which describes the force produced by the interaction between a current-carrying conductor and a magnetic field. The law is immutable, but what can be improved are the

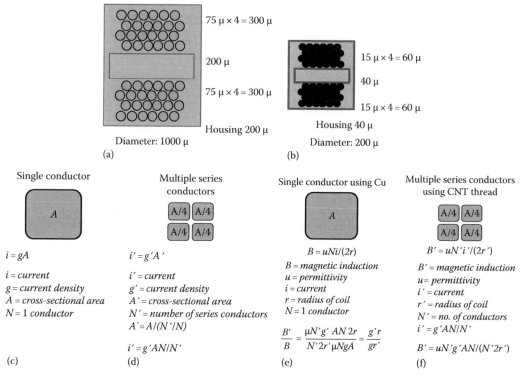

FIGURE 11.9
Design comparison of copper and CNT-based solenoids. (a) Geometry of a copper-wound coil. (b) Geometry of a CNT-wound coil. (c) Current in a single conductor coil. (d) Current in a multiple conductor coil. (e) Magnetic flux in a single conductor coil. (f) Magnetic flux in a multiple conductor coil.

materials that are used to construct the motor, which define its performance characteristics. Materials employed in the fabrication of motors have changed little in the past hundred years. Typically, copper and iron are used, and rare earth magnets are utilized to obtain optimal performance. Herein, nanoscale materials are used to develop next-generation electric motors, transformers, and actuators. The use of nanoscale materials matched to the electromagnetic design of the Sensorcyte will produce a new device that is lightweight with high energy density. New materials used in the Sensorcyte are based on nanometric carbon and iron, which can be readily manufactured. The objective is to reduce the weight of existing electromagnetic devices by 50%, or more, through the integration of nanomaterials. Nanomaterials that will be incorporated are: (1) CNT wire, which is multifunctional, strong, lightweight, electrically and thermally conductive; and (2) superparamagnetic nanoparticles, which are electrical insulators that are exchange-coupled, with little hysteresis. Electromagnetic designs using nanomaterials also provide new concepts that can be used in the development of many types of biomedical microdevices. Different magnetic nanomaterials are being investigated to replace iron for electromagnetic applications. Magnetite nanotubes are shown in Figure 11.10a, and Ni nanowires are shown in Figure 11.10b and c. These materials can be used to build solenoid core materials as well as motor and transformer core materials. Initially, the magnetic nanoparticles (MNPs) described in the next section are used in the design of the Sensorcyte core.

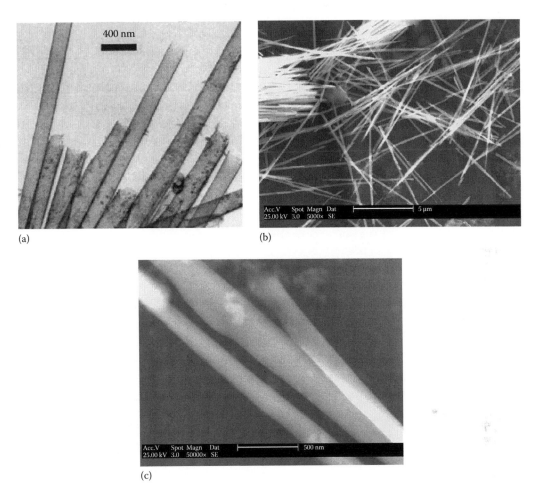

FIGURE 11.10
Magnetic nanoscale materials. (a) Magnetite (Fe$_3$O$_4$) nanotubes. (Vijay K. Varadan, LinFeng Chen, Jining Xie: *Nanomedicine: Design and Applications of Magnetic Nanomaterials, Nanosensors and Nanosystems*. 2008. Copyright Wiley-VCH Verlag GmbH & Co. KGaA.); (b, c) Ni nanowires at different magnifications.

11.2.3 Magnetic Nanoparticle Materials

There are several advantages that make nanoscale materials attractive for electromagnetics design. Superparamagnetic nanoparticles combined with nanotube yarn will be used to enable high-frequency communication and the operation of electromagnetic devices like the Sensorcyte. Carbon nanomaterials reduce the weight and the inertia of components and thus allow higher mechanical rotational velocities. Other advantages of carbon motors are rapid acceleration, high torque, and the ability to operate at higher temperatures and speeds. However, the efficiency of the motor or device must approach that of copper, which is why long CNTs are sought. Small diameter motors will have ultrahigh magnetic field intensities and produce large forces, since the force is proportional to the electrical current/distance between conductors. Eliminating iron cores and losses due to eddy currents within the iron is a significant factor for nanorobots and the Sensorcyte. Carbon materials and electric motor design are discussed next to provide rationale for developing the first nanomaterial transformer to be utilized for nanorobots and the Sensorcyte.

It is envisaged that most of the Sensorcytes might eventually be manufactured from nanoscale materials. The housing could be cast using an elastomer or polymer, and the carbon wire coil will be lighter than metal. The heat conduction of CNTs is very good, and they exhibit a large maximum current density with the capacity for conducting a huge current, in relative terms, to generate strong magnetic fields. Electrical power conduction using lightweight nanotube material is limited only by the temperature range of a given application. Thus, the thermal design and cooling strategies for the Sensorcyte will be critical design considerations. The resistivity of a nanotube yarn decreases with increasing temperature, which is advantageous in comparison to copper. Reducing the electrical resistance of nanotubes and yarn will be an important goal toward increasing the power and improving the efficiency of the Sensorcyte [4]. The long nanotubes that are proposed to be manufactured will exceed the electrical conductivity of copper on a per-weight basis, and potentially match copper on a per-area basis contingent on the doping, functionalization, and postprocess annealing the nanotubes. Improvements are anticipated that will enable the conductivity of CNTs to be equivalent to that of copper (e.g., the electrical conductivity of short perfect armchair nanotubes is indeed better than copper). Currents within the Sensorcyte windings will produce a magnetic field and a significant signal from the antenna to allow the Sensorcyte to communicate via the sensing of a signal through blood and tissue [110–112].

11.2.4 Materials Design for the Sensorcyte

The design of the different materials that are needed to construct the Sensorcyte is discussed in the following section.

11.2.4.1 Magnetic Core Material

Magnetic core materials that are light and carry a similar flux as iron laminations minimize eddy current losses. This core may be possible to fabricate by using MNPs that are coated with an electrical insulator and subsequently distributed within a polymer. When the diameters of MNPs are below ~20 nm, they become superparamagnetic, which means that the nanoparticles consist of a single domain where their magnetization, on average, is equivalent to zero. However, an external magnetic field is able to magnetize the MNPs since their magnetic susceptibility is much larger than that of paramagnets. When an external magnetic field is applied to an assembly of superparamagnetic nanoparticles, their magnetic moments tend to align along the applied field, which leads to a net magnetization. The magnetization curve (magnetization as a function of the applied field) comprises an S shape, which means that the particles behave as paramagnets that possess large magnetic moments. The magnetic field (Figure 11.11) can be switched back and forth at high frequency, which thus opens the possibility for the operation of high-frequency motors and a transformer to power the Sensorcyte. The coating of the nanoparticles will provide electrical insulation and maintain their magnetic properties to serve as a core material.

11.2.4.2 Carbon Wire

A carbon wire that is light and carries a large current with low impedance is possible using long CNTs that are postprocessed and operate at high frequency, where the impedance is low. Annealing, templating, coating, and doping techniques are being developed to lower the resistivity and electrical impedance of CNT yarn. Presently, in the literature,

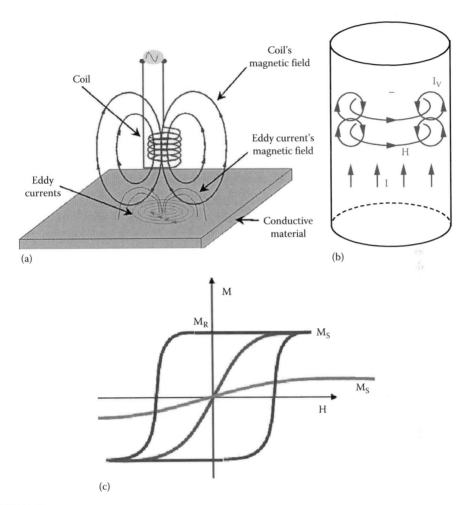

FIGURE 11.11

Eddy currents and magnetic losses are minimized in CNT materials. (a) Eddy currents are circular currents that are formed in a material. When a composite of superparamagnetic nanoparticles and a polymer are used, it does not conduct electrically very well. Thus, eddy currents will be small and eliminate one of the major problems when using soft iron cores in transformers and motors (eddy currents), which cause heating and power loss [138]. (b) Also, the skin effect in CNTs is minimized [138–140] as each CNT shell is so thin that eddy currents are correspondingly small if lateral conduction in the thread is prevented. (c) Superparamagnetic material (red) has high saturation magnetization (M_S), no remanence ($M_R = 0$), and no hysteresis loop, whereas ferromagnetic material (blue) has high remanence, and paramagnetic material (green) has low saturation (From http://en.wikipedia.org/wiki/Electromagnetism; http://en.wikipedia.org/wiki/Superparamagnetism; http://en.wikipedia.org/wiki/Skin_effect.)

the resistivity of CNT thread on a per-weight basis is about equal to that of copper. At high frequencies, the advantage may be greater. Carbon wire is designed by drawing fine CNT strands, coating each strand with a dielectric, and twisting the strands to form threads, and twisting the threads to form yarn. The yarn will essentially be a nano-litz wire that eliminates the skin effect. At high frequency, the impedance of CNT thread is lower than copper due to the capacitance of the thread and absence of the skin effect. As the CNT resistance is reduced, the cross-over frequency is moved to the left. It may be possible to power the Sensorcyte at high frequency, which may reduce the impedance of the CNT.

11.2.4.3 Sensor Structure

A sensor structure that is light and thermally conductive will become possible as the properties of CNT materials improve. CNT thread is much tougher than CNT arrays when subjected to certain postprocessing procedures, and has recently been shown to impart high thermal conductivity. Composite materials reinforced with CNT threads are currently being developed at UC, and will become commercially available as CNT materials production is increased. CNT cast is an elastomer that will be a robust, flexible, and tough material employed for the building of the Sensorcyte structure.

11.2.4.4 Superparamagnetic Particle Core Design and Testing

One approach for the manufacturing of nanomagnetic materials is via powder synthesis using insulator-coated MNPs and the consolidation of the powder into exchange coupled cores [88–97]. When reducing the particle size and the separation between neighboring particles to the nanometer scale, *it was found that Co- or Fe-based nanocomposites can possess permeability that is higher than from bulk Co or Fe metals.* The increased permeability is due to the exchange coupling effect, which leads to magnetic ordering within a grain and extends to the neighboring particles within a characteristic distance called the exchange length L_{ex}. Thus, neighboring grains separated by distances shorter than L_{ex} may be magnetically coupled by exchange interaction. The permeability of an exchange-coupled nanocomposite might be higher than the permeability of its bulk counterpart. Soft nanocomposite magnetic materials possess higher initial permeability and a higher cutoff frequency than iron core materials. This advance opens up greatly the parameter space for motor and transformer design. This nanocomposite material is beginning to be offered commercially [94]. Eddy currents will be minimized in CNT materials as explained in Figure 11.11. We anticipate that nanomagnetics is going to provide a new generation of core materials for the enhancement of electromagnetics design.

Magnetization can be modeled simply for the initial design of the new core material for the Sensorcyte. If all of the MNPs are similar with the same energy barriers and same magnetic moments with their easy axes, all oriented parallel to the applied field, the temperature is low enough, and the particles are closely spaced, then the material behaves like a paramagnet. The magnetization of the assembly of particles is approximated by $M = \mu n \tanh[(\mu \mu_o H)/(k_B T)]$, where n in the density of nanoparticles within the sample, μ_0 is the magnetic permeability of vacuum, μ is the relevant magnetic moment or permeability of a nanoparticle [141], M is the magnetization of the material (the magnetic dipole moment per unit volume measured in amperes per meter), k_B is the Boltzmann constant, T is temperature, and H is the magnetic field strength, also measured in amperes per meter. The magnetic induction B (or flux density in Tesla units) is related to H by the relationship: $B = \mu_o(H + M) = \mu_o(H + \chi_v H) = \mu_o(1 + \chi_v)H = \mu H$, where χ_v is the volume magnetic susceptibility (e.g., degree of magnetization of a volume of material due to an applied magnetic field), and $\mu = (1 + \chi_v)$ is the magnetic permeability of the material. The International System of Units (SI units) should be used for these calculations.

MNPs are shown in Figure 11.12a. A typical sample made in our lab is an MNP composite (Figure 11.12b). The mass of the sample is 0.66 g. The dimensions of the cylindrical sample are: height = 1.28 cm, diameter = 0.64 cm, volume of sample = 0.41 cc, density of sample = 1.62 g/cc, particle type: gamma iron oxide nanoparticles (size: 20 nm), percentage by weight of nanoparticles: 44.7% w/w, binder used: Toolfusion Epoxy (10 parts of Toolfusion

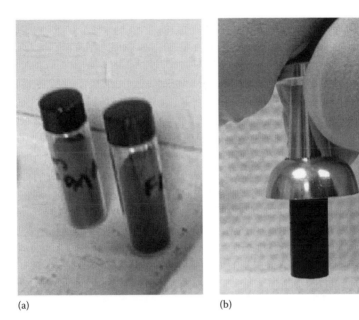

(a)

(b)

FIGURE 11.12
Development of superparamagnetic composites to replace iron. (a) Vial of iron oxide nanoparticles (left) and ferrousoferric oxide powder (right). (b) Hybrid material iron oxide nanoparticles cast in epoxy, picked up by a magnet.

1 A resin + 2 parts of Toolfusion 1 B hardener), percentage by weight of epoxy: 55.3%, density of nanoparticles from MSDS: 5.24 g/cc at 20°C, mass of nanoparticles in sample = 0.30 g, volume of nanoparticles in sample = 0.056 cc, volume fraction of nanoparticles in sample = 0.138.

11.2.4.5 Thermal Analysis and Testing of Components

A key consideration in the design of electromagnetic devices is the dissipation of heat. Metals are good thermal conductors, whereas CNTs are excellent thermal conductors with low thermal mass. When a device is cycled on/off, the temperature of the CNT rises and then drops to ambient temperature almost immediately. In contrast, a copper wire requires several seconds to return to ambient temperature. A CNT thread would allow the heat from the device to be dissipated more rapidly. It could thus allow the motor or solenoid to run at very high loads or for the Sensorcyte to charge quickly for short periods without building up excessive heat in the system. The thermal conductivity of perfect CNTs is greater than copper, and the specific heat of CNT is lower than that of copper. If the resistivity of CNT is reduced to approach the level of copper, then CNT will be a superior conductor for electromagnetic devices in reducing the buildup of heat in the system. High-temperature dielectric materials such as boron nitride, aluminum oxide, and glass may be needed to coat the CNT thread. Heat transfer in the Sensorcyte device must be modeled including the thermal properties of the nanoparticle core material and the CNT thread. Magnetic and eddy current losses are expected to be greatly reduced through the use of superparamagnetic materials, but high-frequency operation will generate more heat. A thermal analysis must be performed in the future to facilitate the production of a prototype Sensorcyte design.

11.3 Characteristics of Blood and Blood Cells

The characteristics of blood and blood cells are described initially in order to provide requirements on how the artificial blood cell or Sensorcyte should operate. Blood is a non-Newtonian fluid (e.g., its viscosity is altered with velocity) containing cells and proteins that are suspended within it. Blood has a higher viscosity than water and is constantly circulating to provide the body with nutrition, oxygen, and waste removal. An average person houses 5 L of blood. A blood cell, also called a hematocyte, is a cell that is produced by hematopoiesis. In mammals, these cells fall into three general categories: red blood cells called erythrocytes, which carry oxygen to the tissues; white blood cells called leukocytes that fight infections; and platelets called thrombocytes, which are smaller cells that help blood to clot. These three types of blood cells comprise 45% of the blood tissue by volume, while the remaining 55% of the volume is composed of plasma, which is the liquid component of whole blood [115–123]. Plasma contains proteins that help the blood to clot and transports substances through the blood. Blood plasma also contains glucose and other dissolved nutrients. Hemoglobin is the main component of red blood cells and is an iron-containing protein which facilitates the transportation of oxygen and other respiratory gases to tissues. Blood flows through blood vessels called arteries and veins, and blood is prevented from clotting within the blood vessels by their smoothness and the finely tuned balance of clotting factors.

Adult humans have roughly 25 trillion red blood cells that comprise about one quarter of the total number of cells within the human body and are much more common than the other blood elements. There are also about 40 billion white blood cells and about 1.4 trillion platelets in human blood. Human blood cells take ~20 to 60 s to complete one cycle of circulation [121–123]. Red blood cells do not contain a nucleus; thus, protein biosynthesis is currently assumed to be absent in these cells. But, all of the necessary biomachinery for protein biosynthesis appears to be within the cells.

The red color of blood is due to the optical properties of the hemic iron ions present in hemoglobin. Each human red blood cell contains approximately 270 million of these hemoglobin biomolecules, each carrying four heme groups. Hemoglobin comprises about a third of the total cell volume. This protein is responsible for the transport of more than 98% of oxygen within the human body. The remaining oxygen is carried dissolved in the blood plasma. The red blood cells of an average adult human male collectively store about 2.5 g of iron, representing about 65% of the total iron contained in the body [115–122].

11.3.1 Sensorcyte Safety in Whole Blood

Ensuring that the Sensorcyte will operate safely in vivo is the most important consideration in its design. There are many diseases of the blood, and under no circumstances should the Sensorcyte initiate problems or exacerbate existing medical conditions. Three potential issues in particular should be guarded against in the design of the Sensorcyte. In sickle cell disease, which is a genetic condition, red blood cells periodically lose their proper shape and appear morphologically as sickles rather than disks. When these deformed blood cells are deposited in tissues, they cause pain and organ damage. The Sensorcyte shape and flexibility will provide biocompatibility and it is important to ensure that the Sensorcytes do not alter their morphology or elasticity. Deep venous thrombosis is the existence of a blood clot in the deep veins, usually in the leg. This clot is dangerous because it may become dislodged and travel to the lungs, causing a pulmonary embolism. Therefore, the Sensorcytes must not agglomerate.

The superparamagnetic material is important in this regard to prevent the magnetic agglomeration of the Sensorcytes. Myocardial infarction, also called a heart attack, occurs when a sudden blood clot develops in one of the coronary arteries, which supply blood to the heart. The Sensorcyte must also not cause clotting; thus, it will be important to track the motion and distribution of the Sensorcytes to ensure that they do not become coated and cause clotting. The number of Sensorcytes in circulation at a given time will constitute a very small percentage of the total number of cells, and the small sizes of the Sensorcytes are important in minimizing the chances of clotting. Figure 11.13 shows a schematic of major blood components.

The circulation of the blood and that of the Sensorcyte are described next. In the vasculature, CO_2-saturated red blood cells from the body enter the superior (upper) and inferior (lower) vena cava into the right atrium of the heart. This blood then flows through the tricuspid valve into the right ventricle, and through the pulmonary valve into the pulmonary artery, from which it flows to the lungs. The carbon dioxide is then exhaled from the lungs and oxygen is taken in via gas exchange that occurs at the extensive network of capillaries within the alveoli. The oxygen-rich blood returns to the heart through the pulmonary veins, into the left atrium and left ventricle through the mitral valve, and then flows through the aortic valve into the aorta and traverses arteries to the rest of the body. Blood then flows to the veins and back to the heart, and the cycle begins again. The red blood cells or erythrocytes keep tissues alive by supplying them with oxygen and removing carbon dioxide.

Normal human red blood cells have the morphology of concave disks with diameters of approximately 8 µm and thicknesses of 2 µm. Red blood cells can also change their shape as they pass through the smallest of capillaries. The membrane of the red blood cell has the capacity for rotating around its cytoplasm, which may help the cell deform and fit through the capillaries. The red blood cell is similar to a bag that can be easily deformed into almost any shape due to its design in which a membrane is filled with a liquid and gel-like material [119]. The Sensorcyte is a solid, albeit soft material that is very flexible and must be deformable to be circulated safely throughout the body.

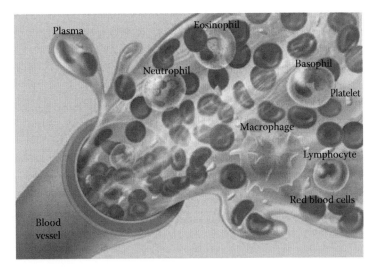

FIGURE 11.13
Schematic of blood composition. Blood plasma is the straw/yellow liquid component of blood, which contains dissolved proteins, glucose, clotting factors, mineral ions, hormones, carbon dioxide, and blood cells. (Source: WebMD, LLC. Copyright 2010. http://www.webmd.com/heart/anatomy-picture-of-blood Accessed August 21, 2013.)

11.3.2 Viscosity and Osmotic Pressure of Plasma

Blood accounts for 8% of the human body weight [115–122] with an average density of approximately 1060 kg/m³, which is 6% greater than the density of pure water. Blood is composed of plasma and several species of cells that are also called corpuscles. The particles in blood are erythrocytes or red blood cells, leukocytes or white blood cells, and thrombocytes or platelets. By volume, red blood cells constitute about 45% of whole blood, the plasma about 54.3%, and white cells about 0.7%. As mentioned earlier, whole blood (plasma and cells) exhibits non-Newtonian fluid dynamics. Blood can flow effectively through tiny capillary blood vessels with low resistance. If all human hemoglobin were free in the plasma rather than being contained within RBCs, the circulatory fluid would be too viscous for the cardiovascular system to function effectively. Normal plasma behaves like a Newtonian fluid at low rates of shear. Typical values for the viscosity of normal human plasma at 37°C, is 1.2 Nsm⁻². The viscosity of normal plasma varies with temperature similar to that of its solvent water. A 5°C increase of temperature in the physiological range reduces plasma viscosity by ~10%.

The osmotic pressure of a solution is determined by the number of particles that are present in a given volume at a specific temperature. A 1 M solution of a substance contains 6.022×10^{23} molecules per liter of that substance and has an osmotic pressure of 2.27 MNm⁻² (22.4 atm) at 0°C. The osmotic pressure of the plasma affects the mechanics of the circulation in several ways. An alteration of the osmotic pressure difference across the membrane of a blood cell will cause a shift of water and alter the cell volume. This change in both shape and flexibility will influence the mechanical properties of whole blood and will alter the hematocrit (volume concentration of red cells within the whole blood), through the redistribution of water between the intravascular and extravascular spaces. This change in RBC concentration will affect the overall mechanics of the whole blood [120–122].

11.3.3 Properties of Red Cells in Blood

Red blood cells are highly flexible concave disks that can deform as the result of shear stress, with cell membranes that have a Young's modulus of 1 MPa. When blood is sheared, the red cells deform and rotate due to the velocity gradient. The rate of deformation and rotation is dependent on the shear-rate and concentration of cells in the blood; hence, such deformation can influence the circulation and blood viscosity. In a steady-state flow of a viscous fluid, the downward gravitational force of the particle is balanced by the viscous drag force. The sedimentation velocity of the particle depends on the square of the radius. In the biomimetic sense, Sensorcytes should optimally match the geometry, density, and flexibility of red cells. The RBC deforms as it enters capillaries and changes color as it alternates in states of oxygenation as it transits the circulatory system. A typical human erythrocyte is smaller than most other human cells, and has an average volume of ~90 fL [122] with a surface area of ~136 µm², and can swell up to a spherical shape of volume 150 fL, without membrane distension. Numerous Sensorcytes may be needed within the blood to transmit signals. The velocities of blood flow are ~20 cm s⁻¹ within the veins that are returning to the heart, and ~100 cm/s within the arteries when being pumped out of the heart [123].

11.3.4 Role in Vascular Disease

Blood vessels are involved in most medical conditions. For example, cancer cannot spread unless tumors initiate the formation of new blood vessels (angiogenesis) to supply malignant cell metabolic demands. The formation of lipid lumps (atheromas) within the blood vessel wall is the most common cardiovascular disease, and constitutes the primary cause of death in the Western world. The circulatory system might possibly be mapped using the Sensorcyte for a person in the healthy condition. If new vessels are formed, then cancer may be indicated if Sensorcytes verify that new vessels exist.

The permeability of blood vessels is increased during episodes of inflammation. Traumatic or spontaneous damage may lead to hemorrhaging due to mechanical damage imparted to the vessel endothelium. In contrast, the occlusion of the blood vessel via atherosclerotic plaque, by an embolized blood clot or a foreign body, may lead to downstream ischemia (insufficient blood supply) and the possibility of necrosis (cell death). Vessel occlusion tends to be a positive feedback system. An occluded vessel creates eddies in the normally laminar flow or plug-flow blood currents. These eddies create abnormal fluid velocity gradients which push blood elements such as cholesterol or chylomicron bodies to the endothelium. These deposit onto the arterial walls which are already partially occluded, and tend to build upon the blockage [135]. The Sensorcytes will be tested in a benchtop flow system that mimics the key characteristics of the human circulatory system.

11.4 Artificial Blood Cells

Natural blood cells transport materials throughout the body; thus, many diseases are related to the cardiovascular system. Artificial blood cells offer the potential opportunity for monitoring overall human health. Recognizing this opportunity, scientists have been attempting for decades to take advantage of the circulation of blood cells through the creation of artificial RBCs. These efforts, for the most part, have failed. Certain concepts have not yet been evaluated due to significant technical barriers or cost.

In general, artificial blood cells are based on the idea that certain functions or structures of biological cells can be replaced or supplemented with synthetic entities. Artificial blood cells are engineered particles that mimic one or more of the functions of biological cells. Often, artificial blood cells comprise biological or polymeric membranes which encapsulate biologically active materials. As such, nanoparticles, liposomes, polymersomes, microcapsules, and various other particles qualify as artificial cells. Microencapsulation allows for metabolism to take place within the membrane and the exchange of small molecules. It also prevents the passage of large substances across it [124–127]. The main advantages of encapsulation include improved mimicry in the body, increased solubility of cargo, and decreased immune response. Notably, artificial cells have undergone successful clinical tests for hemoperfusion. In the area of synthetic biology, a "living" artificial blood cell has been defined as a completely synthetically made cell that can capture energy, maintain ion gradients, contain macromolecules, as well as store information and have the ability to mutate [124]. Although such cells are not technically feasible as yet, a variation of an artificial cell has been created when a completely synthetic genome was introduced into genomically emptied host cells [124–127]. Although not completely artificial, as cytoplasmic components and the membrane of the host cell are retained, the engineered cell is under the control of a man-made genome and is able to replicate. Other efforts described in the following sections elucidate some of the problems encountered in the development of artificial cells.

11.4.1 Artificial Red Blood Cells

Artificial red blood cells were developed to aid drug delivery and imaging [124–127]. The cells look similar to blood cells (Figure 11.14a), but are made of synthetic biodegradable polymers. The artificial RBCs were created by shaping polylactic-co-glycolic acid (PLGA) with rubbing alcohol. The alcohol causes nanospheres of PLGA to deflate into the concave shape of RBCs. PLGA is biodegradable, biocompatible, and is safe for use in the body. Applications for artificial RBCs could potentially include almost any medical procedure that involves circulating a compound or device through the bloodstream. The artificial cells' ability to pass through capillaries makes artificial RBCs ideal for the delivery of drugs or radioactive marking dyes. Conversely, artificial RBCs might circulate throughout the body collecting microbiopsy samples or cleansing the body of contaminants. The chief hurdle for this technology arises from the body's own meticulous upkeep of blood purity. Nanoparticles normally do not reside in the body for longer than 24 h, and indeed some are expelled within 30 s of entering the bloodstream. Hence, if artificial RBCs can be designed and fabricated to emulate the functionality of regular blood cells, a significant milestone will have been achieved.

11.4.2 Designer Cells

NASA-supported researchers have investigated the prospect of designer cells (Figure 11.14b) toward the development of dehydrated blood supplies and advanced space medicine. The artificial RBCs could carry oxygen and medications, and could conceivably be dehydrated and stored for months or years at a time. Hence, it could be carried by medics onto a battlefield or by astronauts into outer space. An additional advantage is that the blood could be transfused with no risk of transmission of AIDS or other diseases. A polymer that forms something akin to a cell membrane was used to form artificial cells, or polymersomes, which are robust and easily handled [124].

11.4.3 Electronic Artificial Cell

An electronic artificial cell (Figure 11.14c) was investigated and sponsored by the European Commission. A Programmable Artificial Cell Evolution program outlined the creation of "microscopic self-organizing, self-replicating, and evolvable autonomous entities built from simple organic and inorganic substances that can be genetically programmed to perform specific functions" [125] for eventual integration into information systems. The project led to the creation of the European Center for Living Technology, which is now continuing similar research. A new research initiative is in the area of electronic chemical cells through a new endowment by the Commission. The Programmable Artificial Cell Evolution program was created by the foundation for a new generation of embedded IT using programmable chemical systems that approach artificial cells in their capacities for self-repair, self-assembly, self-reproduction, and evolvability.

11.4.4 Respirocyte

A respirocyte is a theoretical engineering design for an artificial RBC [126]. Respirocytes are micron-scale spherical robotic RBCs built of nanometer-scale components, which contain an internal pressure of 1000 atm of compressed oxygen and carbon dioxide. The intense pressure would be safely contained within two separate high-pressure vessels, likely made of pure diamondoid materials. At this intense pressure, a respirocyte could

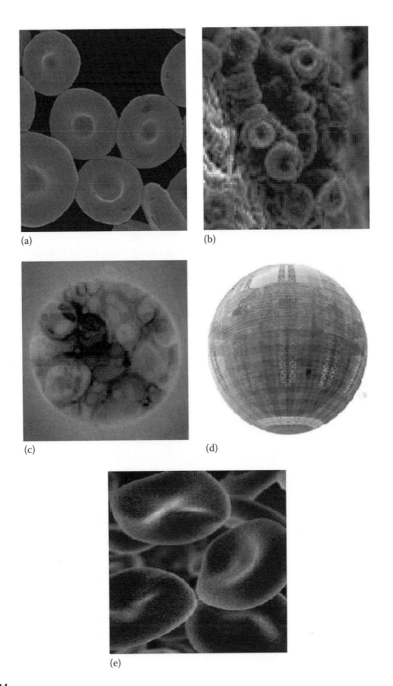

FIGURE 11.14
Different artificial blood cells. (a) Artificial red blood cells. (b) Designer cells. (c) Electronic artificial cell. (d) Respirocyte. (e) Jelly-like synthetic particles. (From http://en.wikipedia.org/wiki/Artificial_cell; http://www.ecltech.org/ecltech_j/index.php; http://www.ruhr-uni-bochum.de/ECCell/; http://www. thenanoage.com/respirocytes.htm; http://zeenews.india.com/news/health/others/artificial-blood-cells-breakthrough_679870.html. Accessed August 21, 2013)

hold 230 times more oxygen and carbon dioxide than natural RBCs. Respirocytes are of an elegantly simplistic design, powered by glucose in the blood and able to manage carbonic acidity via an onboard internal nanocomputer and a multitude of chemical/pressure sensors. Three-dimensional nanoscale fabrication will allow respirocytes to be manufactured in practically unlimited supply very inexpensively, directly from a computer design. This complex tiny machine cannot yet be constructed with current technologies.

Respirocytes would be delivered by injection and would enable a person to run at top speed for 10 min or remain underwater for several hours on a single breath. Because of their smaller form factor (1 μm diameter) compared with the 8 μm diameter of a RBC, respirocytes would have potentially unique medical applications, including the prevention and treatment of ischemia (inadequate oxygen delivery to tissues). Being smaller in diameter, respirocytes could squeeze into much thinner blood vessels, delivering vital oxygen to cells. A respirocyte consists of three major design components: rotors to take in oxygen from the lungs for release into the bloodstream; rotors to gather carbon dioxide from the bloodstream for release in the lungs; and rotors to sequester glucose from the bloodstream for generating energy in a process that is similar to cellular respiration. Preliminary studies have found that extremely smooth diamondoid surfaces would be practically invisible to white blood cells, making the devices biocompatible. Respirocytes were designed and analyzed in detail by Robert Freitas, a nanotechnology researcher at the Institute for Molecular Manufacturing [12,13,22]. The dramatic enhancement of human performance that might be possible via respirocytes could cause the body to overheat. It is also possible that such enhancements in one part of the body will have unforeseen consequences to other bodily systems. Only the actual testing of nanotechnological respirocytes in a living body will determine, for certain, exactly how these devices will behave under real-world conditions.

11.4.5 Synthetic Jell Particles

Jelly-like synthetic particles (Figure 11.14e) that mimic some of the key properties of RBCs have been developed [127]. The jelly-like synthetic particles which mimic tiny cells in size and shape may be the first step toward developing truly artificial blood. The "hydrogel" nanoparticles are 6 μm in size and could also be employed to fight cancer. They have the important property of being highly flexible, as are real RBCs, meaning that they will likely remain longer in the circulation before being filtered out, and can slip through narrow capillaries or microscopic pores in organs. The particles' ability to perform functions such as transporting oxygen or carrying anticancer drugs has not yet been evaluated. But early experiments indicate that they have exciting medical potential. One possible, and welcome, application would be the potential for producing unlimited supplies of man-made blood. To date, the most promising research with the so-called synthetic blood has seen RBCs created from stem cells, which were extracted from umbilical cords. Red blood cells have also been harvested from spare IVF embryos; however, attempts to mimic nature with an artificial method for carrying oxygen throughout the body have not proved successful. Lack of flexibility has been the major stumbling block. Naturally occurring blood cells gradually become stiffer during their lifetime, and as a consequence are eventually filtered out of the circulation when they are no longer pliable enough to pass through the pores within the spleen. It remains difficult to develop particles that can reside for extended periods within the bloodstream. The tailoring of particle deformability and achieving the ability to synthesize artificial cells that can circulate through the body provides a new capability in medicine. Different artificial cells are shown in Figure 11.14. In the long run, we might well expect that many elements of the human body will be replaced incrementally, one component at a time. Artificial white blood cells may be developed subsequently to augment the human immune system, and eventually tissues and organ systems may be considered for replacement with advanced and resilient bioengineered constructs.

11.5 Sensorcyte Design

The Sensorcyte (Figure 11.15) is an electromagnetic device that behaves like an artificial blood cell or fixed cell to screen diseases, including cancer and arteriosclerosis. The Sensorcyte is formed using an elastomer, which is flexible and contains superparamagnetic nanoparticles that exhibit exchange coupling, with an onboard CNT coil and antenna [43] that form a tracking and communication system. The Sensorcyte is designed to be tracked magnetically while in the body, although this capability has not yet been demonstrated. The concept includes that the Sensorcyte will act as the secondary coil of a transformer that is charged by a transformer coil that is located on the skin outside the body, and when charged, the Sensorcyte will transmit a signal through an antenna that will identify its positional coordinates and velocity. When blood vessels are constricted by plaque, blood velocity increases may cause an increase in the induced current in the Sensorcyte, which may be utilized to identify the constricted vessel. Sophisticated, higher level Sensorcytes developed in the future could possibly measure specific charges on the tissues or the membrane potential of biological cells, which indicate the presence of a wound or cancer cells. It is envisaged that many classes of Sensorcytes will be possible. We believe that different Sensorcytes will eventually be able to measure blood velocity, detect cancerous tissues by measuring impedance, pH, or charge using a sensitive galvanometer, as well as temperature, pressure, acceleration, vibration, rotation, and various chemicals.

One might query: Why is such a small particle necessary? Sensorcytes would reside within the blood, which circulates throughout the body and permeates tumors, and might detect tumor tissues by their location in the body, by its electronic potential, or via pH, and send a signal to identify the existence and spatial coordinates of the tumor. Subsequently, other classes of Sensorcytes may provide therapy that involves heating, the puncturing of cells, or the release of drugs. It is not certain what the actual effects of administering Sensorcytes would be, because the presence of electromagnetic nanorobots within the human body is unprecedented.

The mass production of these devices is another vital aspect that must be considered and developed. There might be many Sensorcytes within the body, each having different sensing capabilities. In comparison to existing technologies, such as gold nanoshells, the Sensorcyte is much larger and is active by virtue of having electromagnetic or possibly electromechanical capabilities. No other nanoparticle to date has these capacities. The Sensorcyte can avoid being filtered out of the body before it does its work through the use of biocompatible polymer coatings. Whole body diagnostics and therapies are additional capabilities of the Sensorcyte that no other particle has. The Sensorcyte is envisioned to be recharged while passing a transformer that is positioned outside of the patient, and could also be tracked by a magnetic resonant imaging (MRI) system [146], because it is an electromagnet and will have a larger magnetic signature than superparamagnetic iron oxide or gadolinium nanoparticles that serve as contrast agents. The design of the Sensorcyte is described in the following section.

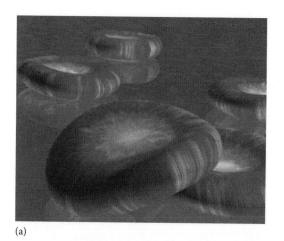

(a)

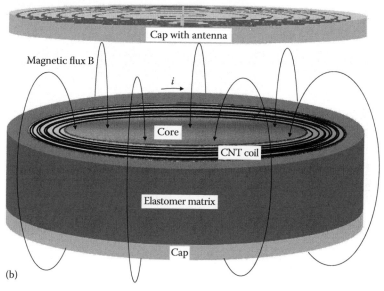

(b)

FIGURE 11.15

(a) The Sensorcyte is a blood-borne 8 μm in diameter nanomedical device designed by the Nanoworld Lab at UC and inspired by the respirocyte, which was envisaged by Robert A. Freitas Jr. [12–13,22,50] (Image reproduced and modified from Forrest Bishop (http://www.foresight.org/Nanomedicine/Gallery/Images/RespCell2c.gif (accessed August 26, 2013))With permission). (b) The Sensorcyte is a tiny and flexible device that may be tracked in the body and might have simple functions to sense electrical charge and flow velocity, which can be remotely triggered by the physician to deliver drugs via externally applied magnetic signals.

11.5.1 Structural Design

The body of the Sensorcyte, depicted in Figure 11.15a, will be composed of an elastomeric material to provide flexibility. The core, Figure 11.15b, will contain superparamagnetic metal nanoparticles dispersed in an elastomer to form the magnetic core material for a transformer. Long CNT thread will be wound into a coil around the core, and the elastomer will be impregnated into the coil. Both the MNPs and the nanotube thread will be encapsulated within the elastomer and thus will not be in contact with the blood, thereby imparting nontoxicity. A biocompatible coating on the exterior of the Sensorcyte will be employed to prevent the Sensorcyte from being removed from the body until a certain period of time. The mass, mass moments of inertia, and flexibility will be analyzed and designed to match those of biological cells as closely as is possible. Biological cells are constructed of a cell membrane that encloses fluid and gel-type biological materials that can easily deform and conform to pass through the circulatory system. The Sensorcyte will, however, not be as deformable as biological cells. There is also the possibility of designing Sensorcytes with different morphologies that might have advantages insofar as passing through small capillaries or to prevent their being removed from the body. The geometry of the Sensorcyte can be designed by considering the complete flow paths of RBCs and the various constraints on their motion.

11.5.2 Powering the Sensorcyte

The Sensorcyte will essentially be the secondary winding of a transformer. A core made of magnetic iron nanoparticles that are cast into an elastomer will be used, as it will be lightweight and paramagnetic. Long CNT will be wound into a coil around the core, and the elastomer will be impregnated into the coil. The number of turns of CNT are computed as: $L = \pi D n$, where L, D, n are the length of the CNT, the diameter of the CNT bundle, and number of turns. Solving, $n = L/(\pi D) = 2 \times 10^{-2}/(\pi 5 \times 10^{-6}) = 1200$. The equation in Figure 11.9 may be used to compute the magnetic flux density of the core. Large flux densities were shown to be possible using small coils. Sensorcytes moving relative to the walls of blood vessels may generate charge, because in actuality, an electrical conductor is moving relative to electrical charges. This constitutes a low-efficiency coulomb drag mechanism. The transformer approach for powering the Sensorcyte is quite straightforward, and multiple Sensorcytes may respond simultaneously to increase the strength of the signal to the receiver antenna. Sensorcytes within a vein being charged by the external magnetic field are shown in Figure 11.16a. Another approach for tracking the Sensorcyte is to move a transformer over the patient to locally map the velocity of the Sensorcyte. The Sensorcyte would charge and discharge underneath the transformer, somewhat like an ultrasound measurement. In this case, however, magnetic fields are used. The Sensorcyte may also perform other functions besides responding with signals that can be tracked to identify its location.

11.5.3 Communication

Different types of miniaturized robots are being developed such as Kilobots and Smart Sand [128–133], which are millimeters in size or larger. Comparatively, the Sensorcyte is ~10 μm in size (100 times smaller). The manufacturing of robots becomes exponentially more difficult at smaller scales. Communication with the Sensorcyte will be wireless, using an antenna. The antennae comprise nanotube bundles that are wound in a spiral configuration in the two caps of the Sensorcyte. The modeling of this antenna has not been completed in detail. Hence, this design is still at the conceptual stage. The directionality of the antenna and the best location for the receivers must still be analyzed. The use of a nanotube supercapacitor and diodes to charge the capacitor for discharge into the antenna is a design concept that is being considered.

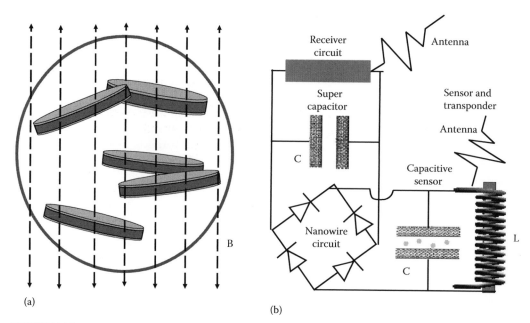

FIGURE 11.16
(a) Cells in blood vessel aligned in magnetic field for charging. A transformer could be moved over the patient to locally map the velocity of the Sensorcyte. The Sensorcyte would charge and discharge underneath the transformer, somewhat like an ultrasound measurement, but in this case magnetics is used. The Sensorcyte may perform other functions besides simply responding with its location. (b) An antenna [43] embedded within the Sensorcyte can also be used to transmit its location.

Larger wireless and battery-free in vivo sensors have been built [144,145]. An initial circuit design for the Sensorcyte is shown in Figure 11.16b. The circuit is formed using nanotube and nanowire electrical components. The resonant frequency of the circuit is $f = 1/2\pi\sqrt{1/LC_{eq}} = 1.2$ GHz.

11.6 Large Size Coil Prototype

11.6.1 Large Size CNT Coil and Composite Core Prototype

MNPs encapsulated within a polymer were used to form a magnetic composite material. The CNT thread was utilized as an electrical wire, which was wound as a coil around the magnetic composite. This coil and core formed the secondary winding of a transformer and provided the means to power the Sensorcyte. The construction and initial bench testing of the large size prototype core and coil are described in the following.

1. *Core material.* The core material is a composite that was prepared by combining nanoparticles and a polymer. The nanoparticles were carefully weighed on a balance and added to an acetone–polymer solution. This mixture was stirred using a Silverson High Shear mixer. The mixture was then poured into a beaker with

a large surface area (exposed to the atmosphere) and held under a fume hood to evaporate the acetone. Subsequent to the evaporation of the acetone, the mixture was transferred to an aluminum mold with a lid. The mold contained multiple small orifices, which were filled with the composite. The block was sealed with the lid to facilitate pressurization and then transferred to a heat press, where it was heated and removed. The composite mass was then carefully extracted from the mold, and the tiny molded cores were separated from the aggregate. These exterior surfaces of the cores were then wound with the insulated CNT wire. This prototype Sensorcyte did not contain any additional electronics beyond the coil and core. The final design might integrate diodes, capacitors, and antennae, and have the capacity for sampling fluids.

2. *Insulated CNT wire.* The "wire" utilized to wrap the flexible magnetic core was a thread that was spun from a vertically aligned CNT array, which was synthesized using water-assisted CVD. A dry spinning method was employed; hence, the thread was comprised of highly aligned, pristine CNT. The thread was subsequently thermally treated and doped so as to increase its conductivity. The CNT thread must be sheathed with an insulated coating in order to be used as a wire and wrapped into a coil in an electromagnetic device. This was accomplished by initially coating the bare thread with a thin layer using an automated coating system. This coating adheres well to the CNT thread, and the coating system provides for a very uniform coating. The thin layer consists of a base coat that is preparatory for a second, thicker polymeric layer, which is highly insulating and flexible. The second coating comprises the primary insulating layer and bonds well to the thin base layer.

3. *Transformer testing.* As Sensorcytes will be circulating throughout the vasculature of the patient, it may be difficult to wirelessly transfer power to them when they are transiently located at random sites within the body. A potentially viable option in addressing this issue might be to power the Sensorcytes at a single location when they pass in close proximity to an external coil, which might be worn as a wrist strap. A Helmholtz Coil configuration may be considered as a strong candidate for powering the Sensorcyte (Figure 11.17a). This might be one possible configuration of the primary coil. By using two identical coils of wire placed at approximately one radius apart, a nearly uniform magnetic field can be generated at the central axis of the two coils. By alternating the current in the Helmholtz Coils, an alternating magnetic field may be generated in the Sensorcyte coil. The integrated flexible core acts to increase the magnetic flux density and provides the electromotive force required to power the Sensorcyte. The polymer core with the CNT wire wound onto it is shown in Figure 11.17b. Using this configuration, an 18 mV peak voltage was generated in the prototype Sensorcyte, as pictured in Figure 11.17c, to demonstrate the concept. An increased number of windings can increase the power that may be transferred to the device. Future work will endeavor to reduce the diameter of the core and coil for use in the circulatory system. The construction of the diminutive coil and core elements will require the development of a miniaturized winding machine. A closed-loop fluidic system that mimics the flow/shear conditions of the human vasculature is available for the testing of the Sensorcyte. Should these benchtop trials be successful when utilizing the devices with simulated blood, smaller Sensorcytes would then be tested in animal models under appropriate animal testing protocols.

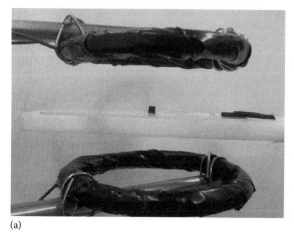
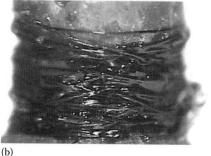

(a)   (b)

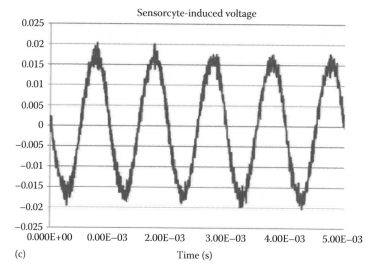

(c)   Time (s)

FIGURE 11.17
Testing of the large-size prototype CNT and magnetic composite coil. (a) The large upper and lower coils are
the primary circular coil windings of a Helmholtz coil transformer (25 windings per coil, 3 in. coil diameter,
1.5 in. coil spacing); no core is used for the primary coils; the small CNT coil and composite core are shown
in the center. (b) Close-up of the hand-wound CNT coil and composite core transformer; diameter is 0.1 in.
and height is ~0.15 in. (c) Voltage generated by the CNT coil and composite core. The peak voltage is 18 mV
at 5 kHz.

11.7 Sensing

First-generation Sensorcytes will simply ping their location in a similar manner to the
black box in an aircraft. The Sensorcyte will be tracked through the circulatory system
based on these pinging signals; hence, its position and velocity in the body will always
be known. Problems within the circulatory system may be identified by the local velocity of the Sensorcyte, that is, the flow velocity of the blood. More sophisticated second
and third generation Sensorcytes will likely be endowed with advanced functions such
as sensing (e.g., impedance, pH, and temperature) a capacity for the collection of biopsy

samples, or the administration of drugs for various therapies. Multiple Sensorcytes may be used simultaneously in the body and could be removed magnetically. The performance of microsurgery and the sensing of physiological variables, chemicals, and biological materials in the body may be some of the future Sensorcyte capabilities.

11.8 Biodegradability

It is highly desirable to include biodegradability as an inherent feature of Sensorcyte design. The materials used to construct the Sensorcyte should be biodegradable and nontoxic, as are the superparamagnetic nanoparticle cores. Biodegradable polymers such as PLGA, or an elastomer are likely available. Contingent on their type and geometry, CNTs can potentially be toxic; hence, there have been investigations into the potential biodegradability of CNTs [142]. Investigations into the biodegradability of each element utilized in the fabrication of Sensorcytes would have to be conducted as future work.

11.9 Manufacturing the Sensorcyte

There are currently no standard tools or commercial instrumentation available for the construction of biomedical microdevices. This section surveys the instrumentation that may be employed in the construction of Sensorcytes and other nanomedical devices described in this volume. A small research facility or "pilot microfactory" will be required to develop prototypes of biomedical micro/nanodevices using nanoscale materials. The pilot microfactory will integrate nanotechnology and medicine, thereby enabling the creation of new collaborations and synergies between scientists, engineers, physicians, and industry. Novel microscale and nanoscale devices produced in these facilities will answer important scientific, engineering, and medical questions. Also, it will take 13 steps of scale reduction, by factors of two, in the factory to go from the precision of producing millimeter-scale features in current devices to the precision of producing submicron scale features in microscale devices.

A fundamental pilot microfactory will be needed to fabricate diminutive mechanical and electrical parts and microdevices. In the scheme of molecular manufacturing, robot tools in the factory will be used to grip, apply force, twist, measure, and build smaller robots, and then these new robots will be utilized to build even smaller robots. Since this work will proceed at the microscale, only a single research instrument is envisioned to be required. This instrument will manipulate nanotube materials that can be used to develop prototype biomedical microdevices and the Sensorcyte. This conceptual instrument consists of several modules and submodules, each of which has specific functionality, and when assembled will comprise a single, albeit large, unified system. The terms "pilot factory" or "pilot microfactory" are used, because "pilot" refers to experimental and "factory" is derived from the analogy of molecular manufacturing to develop new machines as proposed by Robert Freitas Jr. in his book *Nanomedicine* [12]; though, the envisaged pilot microfactory will operate at one level of scale higher. A significant research effort will be necessary to develop this conceptual research instrument or pilot microfactory. In order to be proven successful, as a matter of course, we will need to demonstrate that we can use this instrument or pilot microfactory to manipulate raw nanomaterials into actual functional microdevices.

Toward the development of this microfactory instrument, one can also attempt to answer several key scientific or engineering research questions such as: What practical capabilities might be developed under the purview of micro/nanofabrication? What advances are possible in micro/nanofabrication technology using the synergistic combination of equipment and instrumentation? Since the practical working envelope/distances are very short (e.g., in the submicron range), will micro/nanoscale machinery enable extreme productivity by enabling motion cycles at ultrahigh frequencies? Utilizing microfactory strategies, will the high throughput/low cost manufacturing of high-performance micro/nanoscale products be possible? Finally, after the microfactory is developed, other key scientific and engineering research questions related to the application of devices made by the developed instrument will also be addressed: Can tough biodegradable, nontoxic materials be developed for biomedical implants/devices? What are the most promising areas of nanomedicine to focus these resources on? What advances in medical science can this type of facility most likely enable? Carbon machines? Cancer screening? in vivo biosensing? Artificial blood cells (Sensorcytes) for whole-body diagnostics/therapy?

In view of these questions, the development and construction of the envisaged microfactory system itself is essential for advancing the field of nanomedicine. This type of instrumentation is not available from any manufacturer, anywhere, and addresses several key research areas when investigating applications of nanotechnology. This pilot microfactory will be used, not only to create novel nanomaterials, but also to create new nanodevices. It is our vision that this "instrument" can do for nanotechnology what "molecular foundries" have done for biology. Addressing the issue of toxicity is also important to ensure that tiny devices will be accepted by patients. In these applications, nanomaterials will be confined within polymeric materials, and therefore nanoscale materials should not be released in the body. The development of such a small and complex research instrument to manipulate nanoscale raw materials and to develop intermediate materials and miniaturized electrical/mechanical components, which will be further used to develop prototype biomedical microdevices is unprecedented, and will open many new avenues of research in nanotechnology and nanomedicine that will be of significant benefit to the society.

The pilot microfactory is a new approach for the manufacture of devices that combines the bottom up approach using nanoscale materials and top down approach using conventional materials, depending on the device being constructed. The research microfactory is envisioned to be composed of four modules (Figure 11.18) wherein each module can perform several operations including the assembly of microsystems (bonding, curing, annealing, pressing, high-precision assembly); quality control; inspection; machining and surface patterning; and other operations. The primary advantages of the microfactory include: high-precision manufacturing; frugal energy consumption, small and highly controlled work envelopes, small cost-effective machine components with low power draws; highly precise and reliable production; robustness against environmental perturbations, ultrafast automated operations; modularity—easy configuration and reconfiguration of dynamic modules; and mobility (the entire factory may be easily transferred via compact conventional transport) for strategic or economical reasons.

The microfactory modules are

> Module 1—Doping, coating, spinning, and magnetic nanoparticles
> Module 2—Machining and joining
> Module 3—Characterization and quality control
> Module 4—Assembly and packaging

The research facility uses nanoscale materials such as CNT, iron nanowires (NW), and polymers to build biomedical devices that will function within the human body. The modules (Figure 11.18) have the capacity for interacting in any sequence, which is contingent on the desired product. The new and advanced biomedical devices produced (e.g., Sensorcytes) may improve the detection and treatment of diseases by virtue of working in vivo. This research facility should provide a full contingent of machining and manipulation capabilities at the microscale, including rotational and ion beam machining, bonding, lapping, polishing, and other surface improvement techniques which photolithography-based MEMS does not. CNTs will be used to form electrical fibers and to build microscale devices that are smaller and more precise than existing electromechanical devices. The envisioned microfactory will enable the development of new and advanced devices to improve human health in ways that cannot be accomplished using any other approach, and its myriad applications will impart huge impacts in the medical field, which will drive its extensive use.

The microfactory may also initiate a Research and Education program in the nascent area of implantable biomedical devices. Biosensors, electrodes, capsules, micro/nanoparticles, robots, actuators, and other devices will be built by the microfactory. In the hands of physicians, these devices will produce life-saving advances in medicine. The development of the microfactory will involve the processing of raw materials,

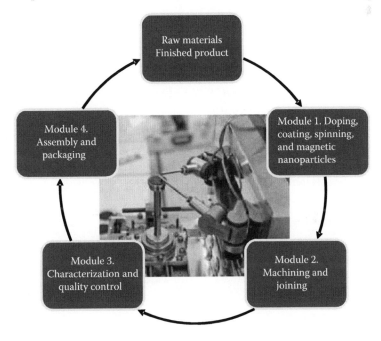

FIGURE 11.18
Four modules in the pilot microfactory.

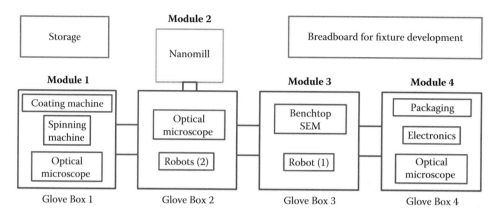

FIGURE 11.19
Plan view layout of the pilot microfactory. All modules are air/load locked together.

development of machines, assembly of devices, inspection, clinical device deployment, and feedback loops to facilitate continual improvements. There are a plethora of envisaged devices that physicians would like to have available in their armamentarium. The microfactory will enable the manipulation and assembly of submicron- and micron-scale components. Nanotube-based electrical fibers will allow for the extreme miniaturization of medical electronic and mechatronic devices. Smaller and increasingly noninvasive devices would allow for enhanced performance in medicine, spanning the areas of in-body sensors, pacemakers, artificial retinas, hearing aids, neural electrodes, tissue scaffolds, surgical robots, haptic devices, and so on. The conceptual layout of the research facility is shown in Figure 11.19. The four microfactory modules are described in the following sections.

11.10 Module 1: Doping, Coating, Spinning, and Magnetic Nanoparticles

Nanoworld Labs at UC has developed CNT arrays and yarns which are strong and electrically conductive for bioengineering applications [44]. Briefly, a spinning machine is used to draw ribbon from a CNT array and twist the ribbon into thread. Multiple threads may be spun to form yarn. This technology must be scaled down for the microfactory. This spinning technology is described in the following sections.

11.10.1 Current Technology to Produce CNT Arrays

CNT technology is advancing to the point where functional devices can now be made [44,51]. Recently, the world's longest (2.2 cm) aligned CNT array was synthesized at UC Nanoworld [51], which represents a new horizon for CNT materials.

11.10.2 Drawing Ribbon and Spinning Yarn

Long CNTs can be used to spin small diameter coils. However, to form a continuous material, and larger diameter coils, the spinning of CNT to form yarn is necessary. The use of electrical wires inside the body is not a new idea. They are employed for pace-makers including within the lumen of veins [99,100]. Existing CNT yarns are of sufficient quality to build biosensors (strength is ~2 GPa, density is 1 g/cm^3, resistivity may approach 10^{-5} Ω cm, maximum current density is 10^5 A/cm^2). A CNT thread is lighter, more flexible, stronger, chemically inert, and accommodates more current than copper. The higher resistivity is acceptable, because a higher voltage or larger diameter thread can be used, and the low duty cycle will allow for cooling. Improvements in the electrical conductivity and strength of CNT threads using long CNTs are ongoing [51]. The purpose of Module 1 of the research facility is to improve the properties of thread by adding postprocessing steps to the spinning process. The main postprocessing steps in the proper sequence are: (i) ribbon doping; (ii) ribbon coating (dielectric functionalization); and (iii) twisting into thread. In Module 1, a small assembly line is envisioned to perform the doping and coating operations (Figure 11.20).

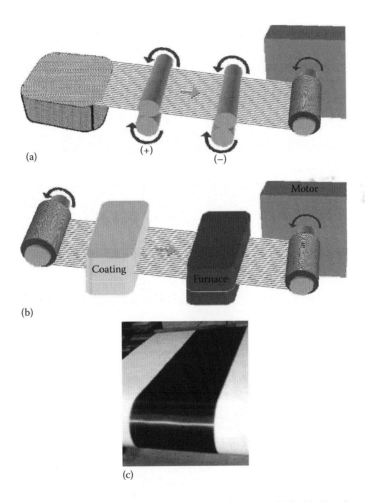

FIGURE 11.20
Assembly line to be built for Module 1 with two stages of manufacturing. (a) Inside the glove box (inert atmosphere), the CNT ribbon will be drawn, doped, and wound onto a roll. (b) In-air processing, where the ribbon is unwound, coated, dried, and rewound onto a roll; the coating will be applied using a custom system developed by collaborators Terronics Development Corporation and Atkins & Pearce. (c) CNT sheet, the sheet manufacturing process will be scaled down in order to fabricate microscale devices.

11.10.3 Doping and Coating

Doping, involving iodine [87] and nitrogen will be used in the research facility to improve the electrical conductivity of the CNT. Since doping with iodine may result in its leaching out of the thread, nitrogen-doping may be more reliable. Although doping improves DC conductivity, it may not have utility in high-frequency conductivity. Another approach for improving conductivity is to decorate the CNT with metal (Au, Ni) nanoparticles. The Air Force Research Laboratory [143] is assisting with the development of this alternative. Strength and electrical conductivity are increased via the presence of the metal particles, and these increases may be greater than expected, based on the volume of material used. The optimal doping/decorating approach will be applied for small-scale use in the research facility.

The coating of the CNT thread improved its mechanical and electrical properties by ~100%. This improvement is due to the polymer bonding of the CNT to each other. Because the solvent in the polymer evaporates, the surface tension forces cause the thread to shrink in diameter. The science behind the coating method involves electrostatics. The fundamental principle is based on the mutual attraction of opposite electrical charges and mutual repulsion of like charges. Terronics [70] has developed a technique for safely and effectively charging particles (polymer droplets), so that they are attracted to individual strands of the CNT to provide a thin high-quality coating. The coating of individual strands has advantages in terms of electrical (tunable resistor/inductor/capacitor (RLC)) properties and mechanical properties (increased modulus and strength) of the thread. Other techniques coat only the outside of the thread and not individual strands. It is important to miniaturize the operation for coating the individual strands of CNT. When optimized, Module 1 will produce a material that will itself have significant commercial potential as an electrical fiber and structural material. The electrostatic coating process has been demonstrated on targets moving at line speeds of 20 m/s. Thus, the coating process will not slowdown spinning. The full theory of multiple jet electrohydrodynamic coating is described elsewhere [54]. A miniaturized coating system will be designed for use in Module 1.

11.10.4 Magnetic Nanoparticles

Superparamagnetic nanoparticles combined with nanotube yarn will be utilized to allow for the high-frequency operation of electromagnetic devices like the Sensorcyte. The MNPs will be integrated within an elastomer using a special approach.

11.11 Module 2: Machining and Joining

Similar to macroscale counterparts, the pilot microfactory also requires the performance of metrological and toolroom activities in addition to production/assembly line activities for sustained operation. Materials, components, and tools will be machined, joined, and inspected in this module [57–59], which is built around an ion beam NanoMill or a focused ion beam (FIB) instrument that will also make use of robotic manipulators. The NanoMill will employ an ultralow energy concentrated ion beam to produce the highest quality specimens. The concentrated ion beam has scanning capabilities and has the capacity for removing material without redeposition. Room temperature to cryogenically cooled NanoMilling is envisioned as possible. The system will be computer-controlled, fully programmable, and easy to use. The variable energy ion source generates ion energies as low as 50 eV. In addition, the beam size is as small as 10 nm–2 µm, enabling the precise removal of material from targeted areas. The 1 µm spot size beam can mill at a rate of 8 nm/min through hard materials like Si, and more rapidly through soft materials such as polymers. The concentrated ion beam can be operated in either point mode, for the milling of a specific area of the specimen, or rastered mode, for the creation of an increased electron transparent area. A secondary electron detector, used to image ion-induced secondary electrons, is ideal for determining the position of the ion beam relative to the specimen.

A liquid-nitrogen-cooled specimen stage eliminates thermally induced specimen damage.

An oil-free vacuum system ensures processing within a clean environment. The user will define all operating parameters through an easy-to-use interface. An air lock enables rapid specimen exchange for high throughput applications and is connected to the glove box. Sensors including the Sensorcyte will be machined using the NanoMill. The NanoMill and robot manipulators will be fully exploited for the nanometric trimming of CNT, stitching of CNT ribbons, nanomachining for patterned CNT growth, machining nanoscale parts for microdevices, and bonding with SEM adhesive. A FIB ion beam machine is ideal for faster milling using a smaller spot size. There is also the possibility of using advanced 3D printing technologies to form Sensorcyte components.

11.11.1 Manipulation and Machining

A considerable challenge in the development of the microfactory is to enable physical manipulation and characterization at the microscale and nanoscale. Kleindiek robots are utilized to work from the nanoscale up to the centimeter scale using fine and coarse modes of operation. This is a powerful system that makes precise, high-end manipulation practical where critical dimensions reside in the nanometer range. The module-based system offers high versatility and flexibility to perform numerous and variable specialized applications by simply swapping tools (Figure 11.21) that are attached to the front of the manipulator, whether it is moving, assembling, preparing, rotating, pushing, probing, sensing,

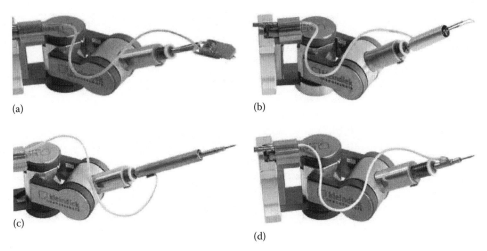

(a) (b)

(c) (d)

FIGURE 11.21

Kleindiek robotic manipulators will be used in the research facility for current and force measurement, rotation, gripping, and other operations (a–d). Concentricity requirements are currently under discussion with Kleindiek. Resolution of $10e^{-7}$ rad per step allows ion milling, tomography, and STEM to be performed. The nanomanipulators will be utilized to machine parts and measure properties. (Reproduced with courtesy of Stephan Kleindiek, Copyright 2013. Kleindiek Nanotechnik GmbH. With Permission) monitoring, gripping, or any other task that is needed in the factory. Kleindiek Inc. also has multiple accessories for drilling, pulling, etc. that will be required for specific operations in the nanofactory. The Kelindiek manipulator system will be spread over several different modules. We have accumulated 4 years of experience using the Kleindiek manipulators in SEM microscope, and they are deemed as the best option for robotic tools to use in a microscope. Important plug-in tools will be used to spin submicron CNT thread, including a micromanipulator with (a) normal probe; (b) force measurement system; (c) rotational tip; (d) low-current measurement kit. The four-armed robotic nanomanipulator produced by Kleindiek is able to manipulate and handle nanoscale objects, including CNTs, and is a critical tool for the characterization of nanotube fibers and the provision of feedback to facilitate synthesis and modeling.

11.12 Module 3: Assembly and Characterization

Module 3 of the research facility will be used to characterize and assemble materials and components. The chief instruments to be used in the module are a benchtop SEM and an electrical characterization equipment. An inherent challenge for component characterization in the research facility is that they will have dimensions that range from the tens of nanometers to the millimeter range. Electron microscopy enables the imaging of morphologies at the nanoscale. However, it requires a significant investment and operation by highly trained personnel. Optical microscopes are affordable and produce quick results, but they can only resolve up to the 500 nm level and have a limited depth of focus and contrast. Imaging tools can make high-end imaging practical and affordable by combining light and electron optical technologies in one integrated, easy-to-use microscope system. An integrated desktop SEM will be an ideal tool for the characterization of materials and components that are built in the research facility. This high-resolution imaging tool is fast and easy to use. It transitions through the world of optical and electron microscopy (from millimeters to the nanoscale) in seconds. Having a magnification range from 20× to 20,000× with an ultimate resolution of 30 nm, it is ideal for the inspection of nanotube thread materials and the detailed imaging of components [55]. Optical microscopes will also be employed in all of the modules of the research facility. The electrical characterization of the CNT thread will be done using an RLC analyzer [56]. A vector network analyzer in the Nanoworld Lab will be used to measure the electrical impedance and antenna properties of the CNT materials and devices. The analyzer and microscopes will be interfaced with a computer network for the research facility, and results will be available to all researchers. Glove boxes will house the instruments in each module and instrumentation will be distributed between modules as needed. For example, robotic tools will be used in the SEM for assembly operations.

11.13 Module 4: Quality Control and Packaging

Module 4 is required to maintain quality and to specially package devices for medical use. Small and large manipulator systems in this module will perform precision testing operations on nanoscale and macroscale materials and devices. The quality control of microcomponents and the Sensorcyte will be critical because of their medical applications and due to the fact that there may be highly stringent dimensional accuracies required in the building of these tiny devices. Quality control protocols will be developed for each manufactured component.

11.13.1 Packaging Products within the Microfactory

Many of the devices produced in the microfactory will operate within the human body. We foresee final manufacturing operations that will be related to the disinfection and packaging of the micro/nanodevices. Thus, we envision that additional interchangeable stages will be developed (e.g., disinfection stage and packaging stage). For both stages, we will apply the existing experience and standards that are practiced in the pharmaceutical sector, albeit scaled down to the footprint of the research facility. The uniqueness of the research facility is in the design of the modules and the combination of tools for processing, diagnostics, and observation at low and high magnification. Finally, the research facility is envisaged to be relatively easily reproduced, which makes it scalable for high throughput production. The overall design is based on modular structures, where selected modules will be dedicated to specific operations needed to manufacture materials such as CNT nanoscale yarn. The four-module configuration of the research facility does not claim universal functionality that allows for the mass production of any of the medical devices described earlier. This preliminary research ensemble has to be considered as a prototyping system rather than a complete manufacturing facility. It will be designed to have an open architecture that may be enriched with more modules to form platforms, which can be multiplied for production scale-up. We expect that through the proposed dissemination of design requirements and initial trial results that the engineering community will continue to contribute to the research facility. This offers unlimited opportunities for the augmentation or customization of the research facility for specific operations, where lasers, microwave modules, plasma disinfection guns, microetchers, drillers, welders, microrobot packaging, and many other tools can be incorporated in order to serve specific goals. This chapter presents the concept of the microfactory for the benefit of the engineering and medical communities.

11.13.2 Risk Assessment

The risks involved with the development of the microfactory are mainly in terms of the performance and timelines associated with the doping and coating of the CNTs, the machining of parts, and assembly operations. The properties of CNT thread are currently satisfactory for many applications, including the building of Sensorcytes. Initial results indicate that the electrostatic coating technology is very promising, though further development will be required. It is envisioned that the microfactory will be continuously under development with new modules added for specific applications. Machining will be achieved using a NanoMill combined with tool-wielding robots. The assembly of components will be accomplished using Kleindiek robot manipulators, and the computer programming of these robots could speed up assembly operations, though it will take some time to optimize the modules. New modules will be added as specific needs arise.

An important point to make in the assessment of risk is that nanometer precision will not be necessary for most microfactory operations, as most work will involve bundles of nanotubes, particles, and nanowires that have dimensions spanning hundreds of nanometers to microns to millimeters. It is possible to work at the nanoscale, but is too high resolution for the fabrication of microdevices. We have also considered the effects of dispersion forces (van der Waals, Casimir) in developing the tools for the microfactory. The Casimir force is more of a concern for flat materials and not for circular tubes. In a vacuum, the Casimir force is two orders of magnitude smaller than the van der Waals force on two parallel nanotubes (based on our calculation for the van der Waals force and the order of magnitude of the Casimir pressure reported in the literature). Thermal fluctuations and surface tension are not deemed significant for the motions that will be utilized. The problems encountered involve fabrication-related vibrations that tend to cause the blurring of SEM images, EMI in the local environment that causes the robot manipulator to tremble, e-beam that initiated charging of nanoparticles, and van der Waals forces that cause the nanotubes to stick together, which are difficult to release. As we have been using two nanomanipulators for years in a SEM with probes, we understand the problems. We have also considered material handling as a potential safety risk. Nanotube arrays, ribbons, threads, and devices will be used in place of powdered nanotubes, and individual nanotubes will not be released into the ambient air. In CNT thread spinning, there is the possibility of particle release; therefore, we have incorporated a glove box for safety. As most work is done with microscale devices, in terms of considerations of biocompatibility and toxicity within the research facility environment, we have concluded that the microdevices themselves are inherently safe.

The facilities described earlier reflect the integrated goal of developing a pilot microfactory in order to fabricate prototype nanomedical devices. Carefully selected modules, components, and instrumentation will serve the objectives of building Sensorcytes and other microdevices. The internal logic of the design of the microfactory follows the major perceived sequential processing steps that will be required for the construction of micronscale medical devices. The first group includes appropriate instrumentation for the coating, doping, and spinning of nanomaterials. The latter are considered as "raw materials" that will be processed by the nanofacility. Next, these materials will be machined and joined, and the related instrumentation to be used is described. Further steps require the characterization and quality control of the processed materials and devices, which will be performed by several high-tech units. Finally, the manufacturing chain will be completed via assembly, testing, and packaging backed up by several dedicated instruments and robots. The nanofacility has been designed with two important considerations in mind: (1) It has to be developed using available components and instrumentation which are functional and affordable, and (2) The facility should be easily replicated, thus providing opportunities to share and disseminate the knowledge and experience gained through this chapter and future work. The nanotechnology devices market (microwires, sensors, actuators, motors, biomedical devices) is nascent at present, and the proposed research facility is necessary in order to expand nanomedical device technologies beyond the confines of university research. The research facility will be continuously improved over time to produce revolutionary biomedical devices, which we will get into the hands of physicians and subsequently to industry as quickly as possible. Components within the microfactory will be used to make even smaller components and fixtures. The pilot microfactory will constitute a long-term investment in research, technology, innovation, and education that will transition nanotechnology and nanomedical discoveries to practical applications. We perceive that physicians are keen to implement the many prospective nanomedical devices and technologies that are described in this volume, most of which may be developed in the microfactory.

11.14 In Situ Diagnostics and Analytics

There are many different diseases that the Sensorcyte might help to diagnose or treat, and several potential applications are described in this section. The detection of plaque in the arteries is an obvious application of the Sensorcyte. Clinicians would like to know if the plaque material is of the dangerous variety that may be dislodged from vascular walls (Figure 11.22). The luminal dimensions of the arteries range from 0.5 to 8.5 mm (500–8500 µm), whereas vein dimensions range from 0.5 to 2 mm (500–2000 µm), and capillaries are 0.0062 mm (~6 µm). Since Sensorcytes can be tracked, changes in velocity and/or trajectories can assist with elucidating the condition of the vasculature.

Another possible Sensorcyte application is the identification of cancer based on the characteristics of the vasculature within tumor tissue. The tumor vasculature is the target for cancer diagnosis and anticancer therapies. It is generally accepted that most tumors remain dormant and fail to develop beyond a few millimeters in size in the absence of angiogenic growth [115,136]. The application of vascular targeting strategies as adjuvants to standard therapeutic modalities may offer unique opportunities to develop more effective cancer therapies. Tumor vasculature is morphologically and functionally abnormal and differs from that which is found in most normal adult tissues. Some of the common features of vessels that comprise tumor microcirculation are dilated and elongated shapes, blind ends, bulges and leaky sprouts, abrupt changes in diameter, extensive tortuosity, and evidence of vascular compression [134–136]. It is this abnormal nature of the tumor vasculature that not only gives rise to the physiologic characteristics associated with treatment failures but also offers the opportunity for novel therapeutic targeting approaches. Sensorcytes may identify a tumor via the flow patterns within the tumor. Moreover, Sensorcytes might be engineered such as to agglomerate within tumor tissues to initiate localized blood-flow blockage, provide hyperthermia, or deliver drugs more effectively due to their larger onboard volume capacity, when compared with nanoparticles, and because they may be remotely actuated on demand.

11.15 Summary and Conclusions

This chapter describes how biomedical devices that are microscale in size might be built using nanoscale materials. The devices may be called nanorobots as they are built using nanomaterials such as long CNTs, nanowires, and MNPs [137]. One such device is a Sensorcyte. The Sensorcyte is an artificial blood cell that circulates within the cardiovascular system and communicates its position and velocity, which may help in identifying certain diseases and may possibly be useful for cancer diagnostics and therapy. Future advanced features of the Sensorcyte, such as impedance measurements, may be valuable in decision making when physicians are considering biopsies and surgery. The communicative abilities, sensitivity, and reproducibility of the Sensorcyte are yet to be established. Sensorcytes with different functionalities, such as the breaking of blood clots, and other tiny machines that are built using the same technology being developed for the production of the Sensorcyte may improve outcomes for patients. Such nanotechnological devices will serve as crucial elements in driving the future of medicine.

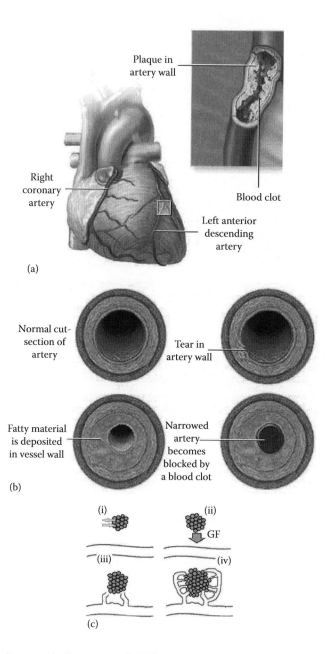

FIGURE 11.22

Diseases that may be diagnosed by Sensorcytes. (a, b) Plaque in arteries. (Figures from the web, Adam Company http://www.adameducation.com/adam_images.aspx.) Stages of tumor-induced angiogenesis: (i) When a tumor reaches 1–2 mm size, its growth cannot be sustained by the diffusion of nutrients from external vessels; (ii) The tumor then produces growth factors (GF); (iii) that induce the external vessels to form new branches; (iv) which extend to reach the tumor and then grow within it. (Derived and redrawn from Van Vliet, M. et al., *Radiographics* 25, 2005, S85–S97.)

Acknowledgments

The authors thank Dr. Sergey Yarmolenko and student Svitlana Fialkova for collaboration on developing carbon nanotube materials; Drs. William Heineman, Frank Witte, William Wagner, Yeoheung Yun, and Sarah Pixley, and students, Xuefei Guo, Julia Kuhlmann, and Amos Doepke for their help in developing sensors for in vivo applications. This research was supported by the National Science Foundation (NSF) ERC for Revolutionizing Metallic Biomaterials (EEC-0812348) and the NSF SNM GOALI: Carbon Nanotube Superfiber to Revolutionize Engineering Designs (1120382). The instrumentation described in the chapter is partly funded by the NSF (MRI award CBET-1239779), the University of Cincinnati, and the state of Ohio. Any opinions, findings, and conclusions or recommendations expressed in this material are those of the authors and do not necessarily reflect the views of the National Science Foundation.

References

1. University Hospital, UC Health, Greater Cincinnati Specialists in Cardiology, Neurology, Cancer, Diabetes and Endocrinology. http://universityhospital.uchealth.com/ (accessed June 6, 2013); Cincinnati VA Medical Center Home. http://www.cincinnati.va.gov/ (accessed June 6, 2013); Cincinnati Children's Hospital Medical Center. http://www.cincinnatichildrens.org/default/ (accessed June 6, 2013).
2. School of Dynamic Systems Research Foci—Mechanical Engineering. http://www.min.uc.edu/me/research (accessed June 6, 2013).
3. Patwardhan, M., Schulz, M., Dong, Z., Yin, J., and Xue, D., Tissue differentiation using electrochemical impedance spectroscopy, A Report, October 2, 2011, http://www.min.uc.edu/nanoworldsmart, under research.
4. Shanov, V., Yun, Y.-H., and Schulz, M.J., Synthesis and characterization of carbon nanotube materials (Review), *J. Univ. Chem. Technol. Metall.* 41(4), 377–390, 2006.
5. Yoon, H., Deshpande, D.C., Ramachandran, V., and Varadan, V.K., Aligned nanowire growth using lithography-assisted bonding of a polycarbonate template for neural probe electrodes, *Nanotechnology*, 19(2), 025304, 2008.
6. Chen, L., Xie, J., Srivatsan, M., and Varadan, V.K., Magnetic nanotubes and their potential use in neuroscience applications, *Proc. SPIE—Int. Soc. Optic. Eng.* 6172, 61720J-1-8, 2006.
7. Varadan, V.K., Hollinger, R.D., Varadan, V.V., Xie, J., and Sharma, P.K., Development and characterization of micro-coil carbon fibers by a microwave CVD system, *Smart Mater. Struct.* 9, 413–420, 2000.
8. NSF press release 07-055: The longest carbon nanotubes you've ever seen, Published May 10, 2007. http://www.nsf.gov/news/news_summ.jsp?cntn_id=108992 (accessed June 6, 2013).
9. Press release: University of Cincinnati researchers grow their longest carbon nanotube ever. Published 11/29/2006. http://www.uc.edu/news/NR.aspx?id=4811 (accessed June 6, 2013).
10. Ball, P., *Made to Measure, New Materials for the 21st Century*, Princeton University Press, Princeton, NJ, 1999.
11. Feynman's Talk. http://www.zyvex.com/nanotech/feynman.html (accessed June 10, 2013).
12. Freitas Jr., R.A., *Nanomedicine, Volume I: Basic Capabilities*, Landes Bioscience, Georgetown, TX, 1999; http://www.nanomedicine.com/NMI.htm
13. Freitas Jr., R.A., Progress in nanomedicine and medical nanorobotics. In *Handbook of Theoretical and Computational Nanotechnology*, Volume 6 (Bioinformatics, Nanomedicine, and Drug Design), Michael Rieth, Wolfram Schommers (eds.), American Scientific Publishers, Stevenson Ranch, CA, 619–672, 2006. http://www.nanomedicine.com/Papers/ProgressNM06.pdf

14. Montemagno, C., Integrative technology engineering emergent behavior into materials and systems, *Int. Conf. MEMS, NANO Smart Sys.(ICMENS'04)*, 2, 2004.
15. Kunzelmann, K., Ion channels and cancer, *J. Memb. Biol.* 205, 159–173, 2005.
16. Wang, Q., Liew, K.M., and Varadan, V.K., Molecular dynamics simulations of the torsional instability of carbon nanotubes filled with hydrogen or silicon atoms, *Appl. Phys. Lett.* 92(4), 043120-1-3, 2008.
17. Xie, J., Chen, L., Varadan, V., Yancey, J., and Srivatsan, M., The effects of functional magnetic nanotubes with incorporated nerve growth factor in neuronal differentiation of PC12 cells, *Nanotechnology* 19, 10, 2008.
18. Hede, S. and Huilgol, N., Nano: The new nemesis of cancer, *J. Cancer Res. Ther.*, 2(4),186–195, 2006. Available from: http://www.cancerjournal.net/text.asp?2006/2/4/186/29829.
19. Halas Nanophotonics Group http://halas.rice.edu/ (accessed June 10, 2013); Nanospectra Biosciences, Inc. http://www.nanospectra.com/ (accessed June 10, 2013).
20. Hogg, T. and Kuekes, P., Mobile microscopic sensors for high-resolution in vivo diagnostics, *Nanomed.: Nanotechnol. Biol. Med.* 2, 239, 2006.
21. NANOROBOTICS CONTROL DESIGN AND 3D SIMULATION http://www.nanorobotdesign.com/ (accessed June 10, 2013).
22. Freitas Jr., R.A., Nanotechnology and radically extended life span, *Life Extension Mag.* January 2009, http://www.lef.org/ (accessed June 21, 2013).
23. NSF ERC revolutionizing metallic biomaterials, http://erc.ncat.edu/ (accessed June 21, 2013).
24. Denkena, B. and Lucas, A., Biocompatible magnesium alloys as absorbable implant materials adjusted surface and subsurface properties by machining processes, *Annals CIRP* (*CIRP Annals—Manufact. Technol.*), 56(1), 113–116, 2007.
25. Radio Interview Features "Engineering In Medicine" Research. http://www.min.uc.edu/nanoworldsmart/news_folder/radio-interview-features-engineering-in-medicine-research (accessed June 21, 2013).
26. Yun, Y.-H., Bange, A., Shanov, V.N., Heineman, W.R., Halsall, H.B., Dong, Z., Jazieh, A., Tu, Y., Wong, D., Pixley, S., Behbehani, M., and Schulz, M.J., A carbon nanotube needle biosensor, *J. Nanosci. Nanotechnol.* 7, 1–8, 2007.
27. Schulz, M.J., Yun, Y.-H., Dong, Z., Shanov, V.N., and Berger, M., Nanowerk Spotlight web article: http://www.nanowerk.com/spotlight/spotid=3115.php, *On Beating Cancer (With Nanotechnology)* (accessed June 21, 2013).
28. Yun, Y.-H., Dong, Z., Shanov, V., Heineman, W., Halsall, H.B., Bhattacharya, A., Conforti, L., Narayan, R.K., Ball, W.S., and Schulz, M.J., NanoToday Article: http://www.nanotoday.com, *Nanotube Electrodes Biosensors*, 2(6), 30–38, 2007.
29. Yun, Y.-H., Dong, Z., Shanov, V.N., and Schulz, M.J., Electrochemical impedance measurement of prostate cancer cells using carbon nanotube array electrodes in a microfluidic channel, *Nanotechnology* 18, 2007.
30. Abraham, J.K., Yoon, H., Chintakuntla, R., Kavdia, M., and Varadan, V.K., Nanoelectronic interface for lab-on-a-chip devices, *IET Nanobiotechnology* 2(3), 55–61, 2008.
31. Yan, X.D., Ji, H.F., and Thundat, T., Microcantilever (MCL) biosensing, *Curr. Anal. Chem.* 2(3), 297, 2006.
32. Dong, Z., YeoHeung, Y., Heineman, W., Halsall, B., Bange, A., Shanov, V., Seth, G., Dadhania, M., Spatholt, A., and Schulz, M.J., Invention disclosure, Active sensor to monitor particles in biology, medicine, and the environment, submitted 12/06, UC 107–066.
33. Yun, Y., Shanov, V., Tu, Y., Schulz, M. J., Yarmolenko, S., Neralla, S., Sankar, J., and Subramaniam, S., A multi-wall carbon nanotube tower electrochemical actuator, *Nanoletters* 6, 689–693, 2006.
34. Yun, Y.-H., Shanov, V., Tu, Y., Subramaniam, S., and Schulz, M.J., Growth mechanism of long aligned multiwall carbon nanotube arrays by water-assisted chemical vapor deposition, *J. Phys. Chem* 110(47), 23920, 2006.

35. Yun, Y.-H., Shanov, V., Schulz, M.J., Narasimhadevara, S., Subramaniam, S., Hurd, D., and Boerio, F.J., Development of novel single-wall carbon nanotube–epoxy composite ply actuators, *Smart Mater. Struct.* 14, 1526–1532, 2005. (Among top twenty downloaded papers of 2005 for SMS journal.)

36. Yeo-Heung, Y., Miskin, A., Kang, P., Jain, S., Narasimhadevara, S., Hurd, D., and Srivinas, S. Carbon nanofiber hybrid actuators, Part I: Liquid electrolyte-based, *J. Intell. Mater. Syst. Struct.* 17(2), 107–116, 2006.

37. Yeo-Heung, Y., Miskin, A., Kang, P., Jain, S., Narasimhadevara, S., Hurd, D., and Srivinas, S., Carbon nanofiber hybrid actuators, Part II: Solid electrolyte-based, *J. Intell. Mater. Syst. Struct.* 17(3), 191–197, 2006.

38. Jung, S., Ji, T., Xie, J., and Varadan, V.K., A novel strain sensor using carbon nanotubes-organic semiconductor matrix composite on polymeric substrates, *Proc. SPIE—The Int. Soc. Opt. Eng.: Smart Struct. Devices Syst. III*, 6414, 641409, 2007.

39. Jung, S., Ji, T., Xie, J., and Varadan, V.K., Flexible strain sensors based on pentacene-carbon nanotube composite thin films, *Proc. 7th IEEE Int. Conf. Nanotechnol.* 375–378, 2008.

40. Mallik, N., Abot, J., Song, Y., Maheshwari, G., Chu, W., Head, E., Dadhania, M., Li, W., Shanov, V., Jayasinghe, C., Salunke, P., Lee, L., Hurd, D., Yun, Y.H., Yarmolenko, S., Sankar, J., Phillips, P., Komoroski, R.A., Chu, W.J., Bhattacharya, A., Watts, N., and Schulz, M.J., Chapter 9: Carbon nanotube array based smart materials. In *Carbon Nanotubes: Multifunctional Materials*, Applied Science Innovations, Prakash R. Somani and M. Umeno, eds. Pvt. Ltd., India, 2009.

41. Ativanichayaphong, T., He, J.W., Hagains, C.E., Peng, Y, B., and Chiao, J-C., A combined wireless neural stimulating and recording system for study of pain processing, *J. Neurosci. Methods* 170, 25–34, 2008.

42. Ativanichayaphong, T., Tang, S.J., Hsu, L.C., Huang, W.D., Seom, Y.S., Tibbals, H.F., Spechler, S., and Chiao, J., An implantable batteryless wireless impedance sensor for gastroesophgeal reflux diagnosis, 2010 IEEE MTT-S International, 608–611, 2010.

43. Press release: Spinning carbon nanotubes spawns new wireless applications. Published March 5, 2009. http://www.uc.edu/news/NR.aspx?id = 9743 (accessed June 6, 2013).

44. Schulz, M.J., Shanov, V.N., and Yun, Y.-H., *Nanomedicine Design of Particles, Sensors, Motors, Implants, Robots, and Devices, with a Supplementary Materials and Solutions Manual*, Artech House Publishers, Boston, MA, 2009.

45. Narayan, R.J., Aggarwal, R., Wei, W., Jin, C., Monteiro-Riviere, N.A., Crombez, R., and Shen, W., Mechanical and biological properties of nanoporous carbon membranes, *Biomed. Mater.* 3(3), 034107, 2008.

46. Tabbara, M.R., O'Hara, P.J., Hertzer, N.R., Krajewski, L.P., and Beven, E.G., Surgical management of infected PTFE hemodialysis grafts: Analysis of a 15-year experience, *Annals Vasc. Surg.* 9(5), 378–384, 1995.

47. Dr. Roy-Chaudhury, P., Professor of medicine/Nephrology & Hypertension, Private communication, July 24, 2009.

48. Park, K., Nanotechnology: What it can do for drug delivery, *J. Controlled Rel.* 120, 1–3, 2007.

49. American Society for Nanomedicine http://www.amsocnanomed.org/ (accessed June 21, 2013).

50. Nanotechnology - Foresight Institute http://www.foresight.org/ (accessed June 21, 2013).

51. Nanoworld Laboratory, University of Cincinnati, http://www.min.uc.edu/nanoworldsmart (accessed June 21, 2013).

52. Nanofactory Instruments AB Home Page http://www.nanofactory.com/ (accessed June 21, 2013).

53. Personal Nanofactories (PNs) http://www.crnano.org/bootstrap.htm (accessed June 21, 2013).

54. Almekinders, J.C., and Jones, C., Multiple jet electrohydrodynamic spraying and applications, Technical note, *J. Aerosol Sci.* 30(7), 969–971, 1999.

55. Products, Hitachi High Technologies America, Inc. http://www.hitachi-hta.com/products/electron–and-focused-ion-beam/tabletop-microscopes/tm-1000-tabletop-microscope (accessed June 21, 2013).

56. http://www.home.agilent.com/agilent/commonlanding.jspx?lc=eng&cc=US

57 Sundaram, M.M., Alkhaleel, A.H., Rajurkar, K.P., and Malshe, A.P., Nontraditional nanostructuring using SPM. In International Conference on Computational & Experimental Engineering and Sciences (ICCES'05); Chennai, 2005.

58. Alkhaleel, A.H., Sundaram, M.M., Rajurkar, K.P., and Malshe, A.P., Study of gap control and electrostatic force in nano electro machining, *Proc. 22nd Ann. Meeting of the American Society for Precision Engineering* 42, 40–43, 2007.

59. Nanomill for TEM and other machining, www.fischione.com (accessed June 21, 2013).

60. Okazaki, Y., Mishima, N., and Ashida, K., Microfactory— Concept, history, and developments, *J. Manuf. Sci. Eng.* 126(4), 837, 2004.

61. Homnatti, M. and Hughes, G., Zyvex application note 9719, Enabling subcellular nanotechnology: An applications overview, Rocky Draper, http://www.zyvex.com.

62. Kleindiek nanomanipulators, Kleindiek Nanotechnik: Home http://www.nanotechnik.com/ (accessed June 21, 2013). Kleindiek Nanotechnik: Home http://www.nanotechnik.com/ nw-em.html (accessed June 21, 2013).

63. Donovan, M.S., Bransford, J.D., and Pellegrino, J.W., *How People Learn: Bridging Research and Practice*, National Academy Press, Washington, DC, 1999.

64. Yun, Y.-H., Li, W., Shanov, V., Sundaramurthy, S., and Schulz, M.J., Revolutionizing biodegradable metals, *Mater. Today*, 12(10), 22–32, 2009.

65. *Small Times Magazine*, Advancements in spinnable CNT arrays, invited article, Summer 2009 Issue, July 2009, http://www.smalltimes.com/

66. Yun, Y.H., Eteshola, E., Bhattacharya, A., Dong, Z., Shim, J.S., Conforti, L., Kim, D., Schulz, M.J., Ahn, C.H., and Watts, N., Tiny medicine: Nanomaterial-based biosensors, *Sensors* 9(11), 9275–9299, 2009.

67. The full FY 2011 S&T Priorities memorandum: http://ostp.gov/galleries/press_release_files/ Final%20Signed%20OMB-OSTP%20Memo%20-%20ST%20Priorities.pdf

68. Mearian, L., FCC mobile network plan could revolutionize health care, Pros say bandage-like monitoring devices could one day cost as little as $5 to $10, March 31, 2010. Development of an Implantable Biodegradable Electrical Stimulator for Bone Repair.

69. Finamore, B., Fedder, G., Khairi, A., Paramesh, J., Schultz, L., Burgess, J., Campbell, P., and Weiss, L., *Development of an Implantable Biodegradable Electrical Stimulator for Bone Repair*, BMES 2009 poster, Department of Electrical and Computer Engineering, The Robotics Institute, Department of Biomedical Engineering, The Institute for Complex Engineered Systems, Carnegie Mellon University, Pittsburgh, PA 15213, and Allegheny General Hospital, Pittsburgh, PA 15212.

70. Terronics Development Corporation http://www.terronics.com/ (accessed June 7, 2013).

71. Atkins and Pearce - Home http://www.atkinsandpearce.com/ (accessed June 7, 2013).

72. Home, General Nano LLC http://generalnanollc.com/ (accessed June 7, 2013).

73. http://news.sciencemag.org/sciencenow/2011/07/magnetic-nanoparticles-fry-tumor.html

74. Microminiature DVRT®, Microstrain Little Sensors. Big Ideas. http://www.microstrain.com/ displacement/dvrt#specs] (accessed June 21, 2013).

75. Carbon (C) - Chemical Properties, Health and Environmental Effects http://www.lenntech. com/periodic/elements/c.htm#ixzz1gFI0wISE (accessed June 21, 2013).

76. Magrez, A., Kasas, S., Salicio, V., Pasquier, N., Seo, J.W., Celio, M., Catsicas, S., Schwaller, B., and Forró, L., Cellular toxicity of carbon-based nanomaterials, *Nano Lett.*, 6(6), 1121–1125, 2006.

77. Biodegradation of Carbon Nanotubes Could Mitigate Potential Toxic Effects http://www. nanowerk.com/spotlight/spotid=8093.php (accessed June 21, 2013).

78. An Alternate Miniature Cotton Spinning System (CSIRO) http://www.cottoncrc.org.au/ industry/Publications/Fibre_Quality/Linking_Farming_Systems/An_alternate_miniature_ cotton_spinning_system (accessed June 21, 2013).

79. Mini Spinning (Miniature spinning machine) http://www.equiptex.com/mini_spinning.htm (accessed June 21, 2013).

80. Hawkins, S., CSIRO, http://www.csiro.au/Organisation-Structure/Divisions/Materials-Science—Engineering/StephenHawkins.aspx

81. Kleindiek Nanotechnik: Nanoindentation. http://www.nanotechnik.com/nanoindentation.html (accessed June 6, 2013).

82. Lu, A-H., Salabas, E.-L., and Schuth, F., Magnetic nanoparticles: Synthesis, protection, functionalization, and application, *Angew. Chem. Int. Ed.*, 46, 1222–1244, 2007.

83. Amanda S. Wu and Tsu-Wei Chou, Carbon nanotube fibers for advanced composites - Review article, Materials Today. 15, 7–8, 302–310, 2012.

84. Yun, Y.-H., Shanov, V.N., Balaji, S., Tu, Y., Yarmolenko, S., Neralla, S., Sankar, J., Mall, S., Lee, J., Burggraf, L.W., Li, G., Sabelkin, V.P., and Schulz, M.J., Developing a sensor, actuator, and nanoskin based on carbon nanotube arrays. In *SPIE Smart Structures and NDE Conference*, San Diego, CA, March 2006.

85. Yun, Y.-H., Kang, I., Gollapudi, R., D.D.S., Lee, J.W., Hurd, D., Shanov, V.N., Schulz, M.J., Kim, J., Shi, D., Boerio, J.F., and Subramaniam, S., Multifunctional carbon nanofiber/nanotube smart materials. In *SPIE Smart Structures Conference*, San Diego, CA, March 6–10, 2005.

86. Schulz, M.J., Li, W., Ruff, B., Mast, D., and Shanov, V.N., UC Invention Disclosure No. 112–016, Carbon Electromagnetic Materials to Replace Copper, Iron and Rare Earth Metals in Electric Motors, August, 2011.

87. Zhao, Y., Wei, J., Vajtai, R., Ajayan, P.M., and Barrera, E.V., Iodine doped carbon nanotube cables exceeding specific electrical conductivity of metals, *Sci. Rep.* 1, 83, 2011, DOI:10.1038/srep00083.

88. http://www.journalamme.org/papers_amme06/192.pdf; Nanocrystalline iron based powder cores for high frequency applications.

89. Magnetic Nanoparticles, Imego AB http://www.imego.com/Expertise/electromagnetic-sensors-and-systems/magnetic-nanoparticles.aspx (accessed June 21, 2013).

90. Hasegawa, D., Yang, H., Ogawad, T., and Takahashia, M., Challenge of ultra high frequency limit of permeability for magnetic nanoparticle assembly with organic polymer—Application of superparamagnetism, *J. Magn. Magn. Mater.* 321(7), 746–749, 2009, *Proc. Fourth Moscow Int. Symp. Magnetism.*

91. Lu, A-H., Salabas, E.-L., and Schuth, F., Magnetic nanoparticles: Synthesis, protection, functionalization, and application, *Angew. Chem. Int. Ed.*, 46, 1222–1244, 2007.

92. Reiss, G., and Hütten, A., Magnetic nanoparticles, applications beyond data storage, *Nature Mater.* 4, 2005, www.nature.com/naturematerials.

93. Raj, P.M., Sharma, H., Reddy, G.P., Reid, D., Altunyurt, N., Swaminathan, M., Tummala, R., and Nair, V., Novel nanomagnetic materials for high-frequency RF applications. In *2011 Electronic Components Technol. Conf.*, Lake Buena Vista, FL, IEEE, 1244–1249, May 31–June 3, 2011.

94. Inframat - Nanomaterials for Your Infrastructure http://www.inframat.com/magnetic.htm (accessed June 21, 2013).

95. Dey, T., Polymer-coated magnetic nanoparticles: Surface modification and end-functionalization, *J. Nanosci. Nanotechnol.* 6(8), 2479–2483, 2006.

96. New Nanocomposite Magnets Could Reduce the Demand for Rare Earth Elements http://www.popsci.com/science/article/2011-01/new-nanocomposite-magnets-could-reduce-demand-rare-earth-elements (accessed June 22, 2013).

97. Park, J.-W., W-S Chang, W.-S., Ju, Chung, H.B., and Kim, B.S., Magnetic moment measurement of magnetic nanoparticles using atomic force microscopy, *Meas. Sci. Technol.* 19, 017005, 2008.

98. Moghimi, S.M., Hunter, A.C., and Murray, J.C., Nanomedicine: Current status and future prospects, *The FASEB J.* 19(3), 311–330, 2005.

99. Artificial Cardiac Pacemaker - Wikipedia, the Free Encyclopedia http://en.wikipedia.org/wiki/Artificial_pacemaker (accessed June 7, 2013).

100. What Is an Implantable Cardioverter Defibrillator? - NHLBI, NIH http://www.nhlbi.nih.gov/health/health-topics/topics/icd/ (accessed June 22, 2013).

101. Kleismit, R.A., Kozlowski, G., Foy, B.D., Hull, B.E., and Kazimierczuk, M., Local complex permittivity measurements of porcine skin tissue in the frequency range from 1 GHz to 15 GHz by evanescent microscopy, *Phys. Med. Biol.* 54, 699–713, 2009.

102. Wang, K., Wang, T., Fu, F., Ji, Z.Y., Liu, R.G., Liao, Q.M., and Dong, X.Z., Electrical impedance scanning in breast tumor imaging: Correlation with the growth pattern of lesion, *Chin. Med. J.* 122, 13, 1501–1506, 2009.

103. Halter, R.J., Schned, A., Heaney, J., Hartov, A., Schutz, S., and Paulsen, K.D., Electrical impedance spectroscopy of benign and malignant prostatic tissues, *J. Urol.* 179, 1580–1586, 2008.

104. Deana, D.A., Ramanathanb, T., Machadoa, D., and Sundararajan, R., Electrical impedance spectroscopy study of biological tissues, *J. Electrostat.* 66, 165–177, 2008.

105. O'Rourke, A.P., Lazebnik, M., Bertram, J.M., Converse, M.C., Hagness, S.C., Webster, J.G., and Mahvi, D.M., Dielectric properties of human normal, malignant and cirrhotic liver tissue: In vivo and ex vivo measurements from 0.5 to 20 GHz using a precision open-ended coaxial probe, *Phys. Med. Biol.* 52, 4707–4719, 2007.

106. Laufer, S., Ivorra, A., Reuter, V.E., Rubinsky, B., and Solomon, S.B., Electrical impedance characterization of normal and cancerous human hepatic tissue, *Physiol. Meas.* 31, 995–1009, 2010.

107. Gersing, E., Impedance spectroscopy on living tissue for determination of the state of organs, *Bioelectrochem. Bioenerg.* 45, 145–149, 1998.

108. Miklavcic, D., Pavselj, N., and Hart, F.X., Electric properties of tissues, In *Wiley Encyclopedia of Biomedical Engineering*, Copyright © 2006 John Wiley & Sons, Inc.

109. Haltiwanger, S., The electrical properties of cancer cells, http://www.royalrife.com/haltiwanger1.pdf (accessed June 21, 2013).

110. McAdamst, E.T., and Jossinett, J., Tissue impedance: A historical overview, *Physiol. Meas.* 16, ALA13, 1995.

111. Casas, O., Bragos, R., Riu, P.J., Rosell, J., Tresanchez, M., Warren, M., Rodriguez-Sinovas, A., Carreno, A., and Cinca, J., *Annals of the New York Academy of Sciences* 873, 51–58, 1999.

112 Toso, S., Piccoli, A., Gusella, M., Menon, D., Bononi, A., Crepaldi, G., and Ferrazzi, E. Altered tissue electric properties in lung cancer patients as detected by bioelectric impedance vector analysis, *Nutrition* 16, 120–124, 2000.

113. 3-d tessellation - Google Image Search http://www.google.co.uk/search?q=3-d+tessellation&hl=en&prmd=imvns&tbm=isch&tbo=u&source=univ&sa=X&ei=UcNGT722NY2XhQeS2oywDg&ved=0CFEQsAQ&biw=1600&bih=882.

114. DARPA Broad Agency Announcement, In vivo Nanoplatforms for Diagnostics (IVN:Dx), Microsystems Technology Office (MTO), DARPA-BAA-12-33, March 15, 2012.

115. Circulatory system - Wikipedia, the free encyclopedia http://en.wikipedia.org/wiki/Cardiovascular_system#Human_cardiovascular_system (accessed June 21, 2013).

116. Blood vessel - Wikipedia, the free encyclopedia http://en.wikipedia.org/wiki/Blood_vessels (accessed June 21, 2013).

117. Blood Cell Pictures http://www.bacteria-world.com/blood-cell-pictures.htm (accessed June 22, 2013).

118. Blood cell Stock Photos and Images. http://www.fotosearch.com/photos-images/blood-cell.html (accessed June 22, 2013).

119. Pictures: Human Anatomy - Blood - Cells, Plasma, Circulation, and More http://www.webmd.com/heart/anatomy-picture-of-blood (accessed June 22, 2013).

120. Complete Blood Count (CBC): Results and Interpretation http://www.webmd.com/a-to-z-guides/complete-blood-count-cbc (accessed June 22, 2013).

121. Blood flow - Wikipedia, the free encyclopedia http://en.wikipedia.org/wiki/Blood_flow (accessed June 21, 2013).

122. Blood - Wikipedia, the free encyclopedia http://en.wikipedia.org/wiki/Blood (accessed June 21, 2013).

123. Zhong, Z., Petrig, B.L., Qi, X., and Burns, S.A., In vivo measurement of erythrocyte velocity and retinal blood flow using adaptive optics scanning laser ophthalmoscopy, *Optics Express* 16(17), 12746–12756, 2008.

124. Artificial cell - Wikipedia, the free encyclopedia http://en.wikipedia.org/wiki/Artificial_cell (accessed June 21, 2013).

125. Università Ca' Foscari Venezia http://www.unive.it/nqcontent.cfm?a_id=144110ecltech_j/index.php (accessed June 22, 2013), Electronic Chemical Cells | Electronic Chemical Cell http://www.ruhr-uni-bochum.de/ECCell/ (accessed June 22, 2013).

126. Respirocytes - Artificial Red Blood Cells http://www.thenanoage.com/respirocytes.htm (accessed June 22, 2013).

127. Artificial blood cells breakthrough http://zeenews.india.com/news/health/others/artificial-blood-cells-breakthrough_679870.html (accessed June 22, 2013).

128. Bite-size Kilobots robots ready to swarm | Cutting Edge - CNET News http://news.cnet.com/8301-11386_3-57334719-76/bite-size-kilobots-robots-ready-to-swarm/?tag=mncol (accessed June 22, 2013).

129. Self-organizing Systems Research Group http://www.eecs.harvard.edu/ssr/projects/progSA/kilobot.html (accessed June 22, 2013).

130. Martin LaMonica - MIT "smart sand" and "robot pebbles" replicate objects | Cutting Edge CNET News http://news.cnet.com/8301-11386_3-57408038-76/mit-smart-sand-and-robot-pebbles-replicate-objects/ (accessed June 22, 2013).

131. Smartdust - Wikipedia, the free encyclopedia http://en.wikipedia.org/wiki/Smartdust (accessed June 21, 2013).

132. http://userweb.elec.gla.ac.uk/j/jbarker/sdd1a.htm

133. SMART DUST http://robotics.eecs.berkeley.edu/~pister/SmartDust/ (accessed June 22, 2013).

134. Siemann, D.W., Tumor vasculature: A target for anticancer therapies. In *Vascular-Targeted Therapies in Oncology*, Siemann, D.W. (ed.), John Wiley & Sons, Ltd., Hoboken, NJ, 2006, Chapter 1.

135. Plaque buildup in arteries, Adam Multimedia Encyclopedia, Maimonides Medical Center http://www.maimonidesmed.org/Main/AdamMultimediaEncyclopedia/Plaque-buildup-in-arteries-219314.aspx (accessed June 22, 2013).

136. van Vliet, M., van Dijke, C.F., Wielopolski, P.A., ten Hagen, T.L., Veenland, J.F., Preda, A., Loeve, A.J., Eggermont, A.M., and Krestin, G.P., MR angiography of tumor-related vasculature: From the clinic to the micro-environment, *Radiographics* 25, S85–S97, 2005.

137. Varadan, V.K., Chen, L., and Xie, J., *Nanomedicine: Design and Applications of Magnetic Nanomaterials, Nanosensors and Nanosystems*, John Wiley & Sons, Chichester, U.K. 2008.

138. Electromagnetism - Wikipedia, the free encyclopedia http://en.wikipedia.org/wiki/Electromagnetism (accessed June 22, 2013).

139. Superparamagnetism - Wikipedia, the free encyclopedia http://en.wikipedia.org/wiki/Superparamagnetism (accessed June 22, 2013).

140. Skin Effect - Wikipedia, the free encyclopedia http://en.wikipedia.org/wiki/Skin_effect (accessed June 22, 2013).

141. Permeability (electromagnetism) - Wikipedia, the free encyclopedia http://en.wikipedia.org/wiki/Permeability_(electromagnetism) (accessed June 22, 2013).

142. Bianco, A., Kostarelos, K., and Prato, M., Making carbon nanotubes biocompatible and biodegradable, *Chem. Commun.* 47, 10182–10188, 2011.

143. Air Force Research Laboratory, Materials and Manufacturing Directorate, Thermal Materials and Sciences Branch, 2941 Hobson Way, Room 136, Wright-Patterson Air Force Base, OH 45433.

144. Farnsworth, B.D., Taylor, D.M., Triolo, R.J., and Young, D.J., Wireless in vivo EMG sensor for intelligent prosthetic control, electrical engineering and computer science department, Department of Biomedical Engineering, Case Western Reserve University, Cleveland, Ohio, 44106.

145. Ketterl, T.P., Arrobo, G.E., Sahin, A., Tillman, T.J., Arslan, H., and Gitlin, R.D., In vivo Wireless Communication Channels, WAMICON 2012.

12

Liposome-Entrapped Antibiotics: Recent Progress and Clinical Applications

Misagh Alipour, Abdelwahab Omri, and Zacharias E. Suntres

CONTENTS

12.1 Introduction

This chapter covers the history of liposomes and their recent applications in nanomedicine. As the field of liposomology has evolved over the past 50 years, it is impossible to comprehensively address every topic here. Readers are thus encouraged to refer to reviews in the literature, henceforth, regarding topics and techniques that are not discussed in detail here. While a general review of liposomes as nanocarriers of antimycotic, antineoplastic, and antimicrobial agents will be discussed throughout the text, the main aim of this chapter is the discussion of liposome-loaded antibiotics, which have been under development and increasingly cited in the literature over the last decade.

12.1.1 History and Description of Lipid Vesicle Carriers (Liposomes)

In 1961, Dr. Alec D. Bangham (1921–2010) at the Babraham Institute in Cambridge discovered spheres under electron microscopy which he called "multilamellar smectic mesophases," later unofficially titled "banghasomes [1]." The discoveries were published in 1964 in the *Journal of Molecular Biology*, and these spheres were later termed "liposomes" by Dr. Weissmann [2]. Liposomes have many applications, and subsequent to 50 years of research, a literature search on PubMed lists more than 39,000 articles. The advances in the field of liposomology have generated many patents over 25 years, including five United States Food and Drug Administration (FDA)-approved liposome-entrapped formulations for fungal infections and cancer therapy, with ongoing clinical trials for other therapies, including those targeting lung infections.

Liposomes are spherical bilayered nanocarriers that have the capacity for entrapping a diverse number of compounds within their inner aqueous cores (e.g., hydrophilic compounds), or for incorporating them into their lipid bilayers (e.g., hydrophobic compounds). Entrapment efficiency may vary depending on: (1) the compound itself (charge, size, solubility, etc.); (2) the lipid variations (a single type or a mixture of lipids, composition, charge, etc.); and (3) the preparation methods. The manipulation and design of liposomes that are endowed with the ability for targeting specific cell sites (or alternately, the temporary avoidance of these sites), result in long circulation times, increased biodistribution, and favorable pharmacodynamics. Lipids utilized as drug nanocarriers offer additional advantages for research due to their relative safety (e.g., the popular neutral lipid called phosphatidylcholine also exists in the lungs where it serves as a natural surfactant); capacity for reducing the toxicity of entrapped compounds; biocompatibility; and safe clearance from the body [3,4]. Despite purported advantages, only a handful of formulations have been approved by the FDA [5]. Some of the setbacks and disadvantages of liposomes include time-consuming preparation techniques, low entrapment volumes, and toxicity concerns due to the presence of residual toxic organic compounds during preparation [6].

12.1.2 Liposomes as Models Mimicking Cell Membranes

As liposomes garnered interest in the mid-1960s, Sessa and Weissmann proposed a new application of liposomes as models for biological membranes [2]. The utilization of liposomes to mimic cellular membranes served as a cost-effective alternative method for experiments involving in vitro cell cultures and in vivo models. Depending on the xenobiotics and cells under study, researchers had the flexibility to select single phospholipids or mixtures thereof (e.g., zwitterionic or charged), with or without cholesterol. Established methods of assessing xenobiotic–cell interaction and toxicity include (1) electron micros-copy of liposomes to elucidate pore formations and morphological changes [7–9]; (2) leak-age of cations (e.g., K^+, Ca^{2+}, Mg^{2+}) and fluorescent dyes (e.g., carboxyfluorescein, calcein, and 1,6-diphenyl-1,3,5-hexatriene) to measure alterations of, and impediments to, cell surface permeability [10–14]; and (3) differential scanning calorimetry (DSC), suggesting changes in lipid bilayer fluidity [15]. A variety of antioxidant, antineoplastic, antimycotic, natural or semisynthetic membrane-active peptides (e.g., bacteriocin, cathelicidins), and antibiot-ics (e.g., aminoglycoside, macrolide, and lipopeptides) have also been examined [10,15–19]. Different interactions of xenobiotics with liposomes have been found (e.g., exchange of lipids, the penetration and incorporation of xenobiotic into the liposomes, leakage of lipo-some content, and pore formations). Liposomes are still utilized as one of the cheapest methods for assessing cellular membrane interactions.

12.1.3 Drug Delivery Systems

Over the last quarter century, the pharmaceutical industry has been developing a num-ber of new products to combat the emergence of resilient cancers and infectious diseases. However, only a fraction of these is clinically relevant today, and researchers continue to struggle to formulate new drugs that have reduced toxicity and increased efficacy [20,21]. Liposomes have been studied for decades as potential nanocarriers for the targeting of healthy or cancerous cells, macrophages, parasites, fungi, and pathogenic bacteria with reduced toxicity to the patient. Years of empirical research in liposomology, along with the development of efficient production methods, have brought forth credited successes from work that was once only seen with in vitro and in vivo models [22].

With liposomal delivery systems aimed at increasing the accumulation of loaded drugs precisely at the sites of action, an enthusiastic interest has flourished that is parallel to the research and development of other novel pharmaceuticals. Particularly, the liposomology of the last decade has focused on rectifying the deficiencies inherent to conventional phar-maceuticals by enhancing pharmacokinetics and pharmacodynamics, encompassing the importance of lipid charges and lipid to drug ratios. The building of these strong founda-tions have led to the development of liposomal doxorubicin (Doxil®, Myocet®), liposomal daunorubicin (DaunoXome®), and liposomal amphotericin B (Ambisome®, Abelcet®). As yet, there is no class of liposomal antibiotic that is approved by the FDA. However, ami-kacin (Arikace™) and ciprofloxacin (ARD-3100™, ARD-3150™) are in phase I/II clinical trials. In the following sections, the general preparation and characterization of liposome-loaded drugs as related to some of the nanomedicines mentioned earlier will be discussed.

12.2 Liposome Preparation Techniques

Various techniques may be employed in the laboratory or in large-scale factory synthe-sis of liposomes, and often, some of these methods are combined (Table 12.1) [23]. The methods described in the following sections are critical for the assembly of multilamel-lar (MLV), dehydrated–rehydrated (DRV), small unilamellar (SUV), large unilamellar (LUV), reverse-phase evaporation (REVs), or heating method (HMV) vesicles (Figure 12.1a). Each method may create empty liposomes that may be loaded with drug com-pounds via other techniques, or loaded liposomes having entrapped drugs within the

TABLE 12.1

Liposomal Preparation Techniques: Advantages and Disadvantages

Preparation Techniques	Advantages	Disadvantages
Dehydration–rehydration	• Simple procedure • Minimal chemicals and equipment required • Various lipids and drugs can be used	• Low entrapment • Low retention • Wide vesicle size distribution • Use of organic chemicals
Extrusion	• Large inner hydrophilic layer • High retention and improved stability in solution • Efficient drug entrapment • Narrow vesicle size distribution	• Time-consuming • High material and equipment costs • Possibility of contamination through handling
Reverse-phase evaporation	• Larger inner hydrophilic layer • Efficient loading of macromolecules	• Use of organic chemicals • Produces a mixture of MLVs and LUVs • Requires extrusion technique for LUV production
Remote-loading	• Very efficient drug loading • FDA-approved for the production of antitumor drugs	• Time-consuming • High material costs
Nontoxic • Heating • ISCRPE • Ethanol injection	• Reduction of organic solvent use • Ease of preparation • Sterility via heating • Narrow vesicle size distribution	• Time-consuming • High equipment costs

liposomal interior encapsulating structure [24]. The loading of the desired compound can be further adjusted with techniques which load at very efficient yields (e.g., remote-loading technique), or can be developed in a large-scale factory setting (e.g., ethanol injection method) [25,26]. Newer techniques, which do not employ volatile organic solvents, are also briefly mentioned [27].

12.2.1 Freeze-Drying Method: Multilamellar Vesicles

The generation of any liposomal formulation proceeds with the composition of its lipid(s). Depending on the characteristics of the drug (e.g., size, solubility, charge), lipids must be selected for their loading efficiency as well as their retention of encapsulated drugs [28]. For example, if the drug to be loaded is positively charged, then anionic lipids are the ideal choice. Conversely, if the drug is water-insoluble, it is desirable to add it directly to the lipid mixture to ensure its incorporation within the hydrophobic lipid bilayer. Precursor mixtures are introduced into an Erlenmeyer flask and are then dissolved in an organic phase (e.g., chloroform, methanol, or diethyl ether). The organic solution is evaporated by heating under vacuum in a rotary evaporator, leaving a thin lipid film. The lipid is hydrated via heating in a buffer (or the drug to be entrapped with the buffer) under agitation above the gel-to-liquid critical transition temperature (T_c), forming a mixture of MLVs, SUVs, and LUVs. For example, if the lipid mixture contains a mixture of

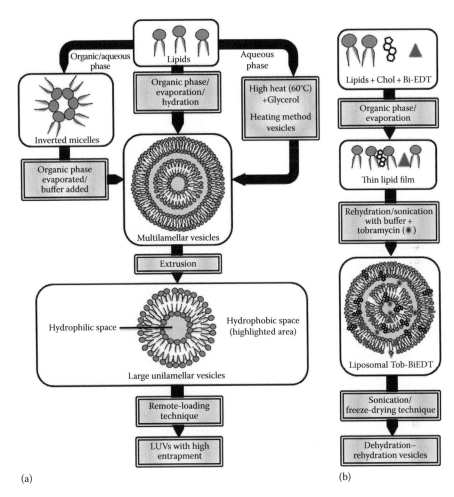

FIGURE 12.1

Classification of liposomes by various techniques. (a) Various techniques could be employed to produce liposomes. Lipids may be dissolved in an organic phase and/or hydrated with an aqueous phase to form liposomes. The multilamellar vesicles can be extruded to form large unilamellar vesicles, and further methods like remote-loading may increase yield of entrapped drug in the liposomes. (b) Dehydrated–rehydrated vesicles loaded with hydrophilic (tobramycin) and lipophilic drugs (bismuth bound to ethanedithiol [Bi–EDT]) can be formed with good loading efficiency using the freeze-drying method. Lipids are dissolved in an organic phase in the presence of bismuth, then dried, and hydrated with buffer. The suspension is sonicated and tobramycin added. The multilamellar vesicles are sonicated again and freeze-dried for higher loading and long-term storage. (Note: The change in lipid sizes are for illustration purposes only.)

dipalmitoylphosphatidylcholine (DPPC) and cholesterol (carbon chain length of 16), the suspension is heated above 41°C. The vesicles are heterogeneous and contain a wide size distribution (50 nm to 5 µm), and typically have low entrapment efficiencies. It is often recommended that the mixture of oligolamellar vesicles be further processed to form smaller and less lamellar vesicles by utilizing sonication.

The sonication technique was one of the first methods employed for the reduction of liposome size by introducing the tip of a probe-type sonicator directly in contact with the liposome suspension, or by placing the suspension in a bath sonicator. After sonication, SUVs (in the supernatant) can be separated from MLVs and LUVs (in the pellet) by centrifugation for 1 h at 100,000*g*. The liposome suspension consisting of MLVs and LUVs having a wide size distribution and fairly low entrapment efficiency are then ready for use or may be freeze-dried to increase entrapment and/or stability for long-term storage.

Freeze-drying, as the name implies, is a procedure where the liposome suspension is frozen and dried under vacuum, using a lyophilizer, which leaves a caky porous solid. As the suspension is slowly cooled down (−80°C) and later dried under vacuum and kept cooled (−10°C), the drugs come into frequent contact with the lipid bilayer as the volume shrinks, allowing diffusion into the inner aqueous layer. Lyoprotectants (e.g., sucrose) with a *w/w* ratio of 1:1 may also be added for the structural stability of the liposomes in freezing temperatures. After drying, the liposomes can be stored at −20°C until needed and rehydrated to form DRVs.

Our laboratory has produced a number of DRVs over the years, and a schematic diagram of this technique for the production of liposome-loaded tobramycin and bismuth–ethanedithiol (Bi–EDT) by the Halwani method is described briefly (Figure 12.1b) [29,30]. A lipid mixture (DSPC: Chol; 2:1 molar ratio) with Bi and EDT (5 mM; 1:1 molar ratio) is dissolved in an organic phase until a clear yellow homogenous solution is formed. The solvents are evaporated from the mixture with a rotary evaporator. The lipid–bismuth film is then rehydrated with a buffered solution (pH 7.4) including 1,2-propanediol (to ensure Bi solubility), and the mixture is sonicated. Tobramycin is then added and sonicated once more. The MLVs are lyophilized and stored at −20°C. When required, the formulation is rehydrated with buffer, and centrifuged twice to remove free bismuth, 1,2-propanediol, and tobramycin. Tobramycin loading and bismuth incorporation can be determined by ELISA and graphite furnace atomic absorption spectroscopy, respectively [31].

12.2.2 Extrusion Technique: Unilamellar Vesicles

The extrusion technique generates LUVs and has many attractive features, including a large inner layer, high retention, and efficient drug loading. If the production of LUVs is desired, MLVs (without freeze-drying) or DRVs are subjected to extrusion. Note that freeze-drying LUVs after extrusion is not recommended due to the fusion of LUVs, which form MLVs, and increase the propensity for leakage of the entrapped drug, even in the presence of lyoprotectants. Although the technique is simple and does not use any volatile organic compounds, it requires an extruder with high-pressured nitrogen gas. The procedure begins with passing the liposome suspension through pores of gradually reduced sizes (e.g., starting from 1 to 0.2 μm) repeatedly up to 10 times under high pressure (100–400 psi). With every pass, the MLVs are forced through smaller pores which reduce the size and lamellarity to form a homogenous suspension with a narrow size distribution that is equal to or lower than the pore size previously used. The suspension is then ready for use or can be stored at 4°C for weeks, or even months, depending on the lipid composition and the inclusion of cholesterol and cryoprotectants.

12.2.3 Reverse-Phase Evaporation Method

Another method for the entrapment of compounds (including macromolecules) is the reverse-phase evaporation method, which yields REVs [32,33]. The REVs are known to have larger inner aqueous layers than LUVs, and are efficient in loading, depending on the lipid mixtures [34,35]. The method begins with introducing a buffered saline solution (containing a hydrophilic compound) to an organic phase (containing the dissolved lipids) at a higher *v/v* ratio for the organic phase. Sonication is applied, which forms an opaque dispersion that contains small inversed micelles, with the head groups oriented to the center and the tails extending outward. The organic phase is removed by heating, forming a viscous gel which then collapses, becoming an aqueous suspension. Excess buffer is added, forcing the phospholipid tails (hydrophobic) to interact with the micelles and form MLVs and LUVs. If only LUVs are desired, the extrusion technique can be followed as described earlier.

12.2.4 Remote-Loading Technique

In order to produce nanomedicines that are superior to conventional pharmaceuticals, the liposomes must first contain high entrapment yields. In addition to the extrusion technique to produce LUVs, the remote-loading technique elevates the yield of drug entrapped via the diffusion of weakly based drugs down a proton gradient. The method has been successful in producing high yields and has been implemented in the production of FDA-approved formulations such as liposomal doxorubicin and liposomal ciprofloxacin [25,36]. Three methods for the production of these LUVs by the remote-loading technique are described herein (Figure 12.2).

In the first method, thin lipid films are hydrated in a citrate buffer (pH 4), and the LUVs are prepared by the extrusion technique as described earlier, forming an acidic interior [25,37]. The external pH is neutralized to 7.5 ($\Delta pH = 3.5$) with HEPES buffer, thereby creating a proton gradient. A weakly basic drug which is neutral at pH 7.5 (e.g., doxorubicin) is introduced which diffuses to the inner acidic membrane. Doxorubicin is protonated and is trapped due to its charge (charged drugs cannot pass through the lipid bilayer). The exchange continues until the drug is loaded, or until the internal/external $\Delta pH = 0$.

A second method involves using an amine gradient [38]. This method is more popular for ciprofloxacin due to the low solubility of the drug in neutral pH and its poor loading. The amine gradient involves forming liposomes in an unbuffered ammonium sulfate solution (LUVs with ammonium [NH_4] in the inner membrane) and using saline as the external buffer. Ammonia (NH_3) leaks from the liposomes, leaving a proton behind, and hence creates an acidic internal pH. Neutral ciprofloxacin is introduced, which diffuses into the inner membrane and becomes charged and trapped. Doxorubicin can also

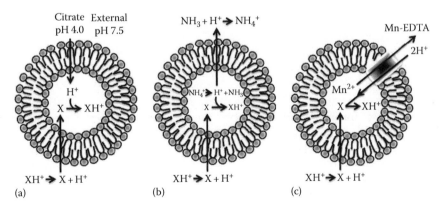

FIGURE 12.2
The remote-loading technique with three methods of drug (X) loading: (a) using citrate buffer and forming a proton gradient; (b) using an ammonium sulfate solution and forming an amine gradient; (c) using an ionophore, cations, and an ion gradient.

be trapped by this method and is known to precipitate in the aqueous layer [37]. Recently, a similar method involving EDTA-disodium or EDTA-diammonium salt for the loading of idarubicin has also been described [39].

The third method requires an ion gradient involving an ionophore and EDTA [36,40]. LUVs by the extrusion method are formed with divalent cations ($MnSO_4$ or $MgSO_4$), thereby creating an ion gradient in an external sucrose buffer. The drug to be entrapped is added (e.g., ciprofloxacin, vincristne, or topotecan) along with an ionophore (e.g., calcymycin) and EDTA. The ionophore transports one divalent cation out of the inner membrane and transports two protons in, thereby acidifying the interior, while EDTA binds to a free cation in the external buffer. The resulting gradient subsequently drives the diffusion of the drug into the inner membrane.

12.2.5 Production of Liposomes without Toxic Solvents

Numerous methods of liposome preparation, including the aforementioned techniques, involve the application of toxic organic solvents for solubilizing lipids and drugs. Despite best efforts to extract and evaporate these chemicals, small residual concentrations either remain in the final product, oxidize, chemically breakdown the lipids, and/or inactivate the drugs during the loading process. There are, however, several methods that do not use organic solvents, namely the Mozafari method and the improved supercritical reverse phase evaporation (ISCRPE) method [41,42]. Another strategy worth mentioning is the ethanol injection method [43]. Although ethanol is used to dissolve the lipids, this method is widely used as it is amenable to industrial scale-up, and it is considered to be safe [26]. The method is currently in practice for the production of Arikace in FDA clinical trials [44,45].

The Mozafari method involves the addition of the lipid ingredients (whether charged or neutral, with or without cholesterol) directly into a preheated mixture of drug to be loaded in buffer with glycerol within a glass vessel [46,47]. After an hour of heating (60°C for noncholesterol liposomes; 120°C for cholesterol liposomes), the lipids dissolve and form HMVs which may be freeze-dried (DRVs) and/or extruded to form LUVs if desired. Mozafari reported that at these high temperatures the phospholipids are not degraded (confirmed by TLC) [41]. The HMVs have advantages due to their benign chemical composition, ease of preparation, sterility via heating, and presence of glycerol as a nonhazardous lyoprotectant for freeze-drying. The ISCRPE method also negates the use of any organic solvent. This method involves the mixing of lipids (with or without cholesterol) with the drug to be loaded under high pressure (200 bar), CO_2, and heating at 60°C. CO_2 pressure is reduced to allow the extraction of LUVs, which have a narrow size distribution, are very stable, and have higher loading efficiencies than is possible using the Bangham method [42,48].

The ethanol injection method can be employed to produce fairly small MLVs, which can incorporate hydrophilic and hydrophobic compounds [26,49,50]. This method involves the dissolution of the desired lipids (and hydrophobic drugs if required) in warm ethanol. An equal volume of heated distilled water (and hydrophilic drug if required) is then injected (with a syringe) into the lipid–ethanol solution or vice versa under constant stirring. The introduction of these two phases spontaneously produces a milky suspension of liposomes. The ethanol is then removed by heating in a rotary evaporator. The pH of the suspension can subsequently be adjusted to within physiological pH parameters. The mechanical filtration of the lipids (dissolved in ethanol) or hydrophilic compounds (in water) using 0.2 μm filters, prior to injection, also assures that the formulations are sterile and free from bacterial contamination.

TABLE 12.2

Lipid Modifications: Advantages and Disadvantages

Surface Modifications	Advantages	Disadvantages
Conventional liposomes	• Lowered toxicity/immunogenicity • Wide variety of natural/synthetic, neutral, or charged lipids can be used	• High MPS clearance • Low stability • Short biodistribution
Targeted liposomes	• Modification of lipid surface elevates delivery to the site of action • Increased binding capacity to target cell	• Possible immunogenic response
pH-sensitive liposomes	• Direct tumor cell or macrophage drug targeting	• Requires uptake and high circulation time to be effective
Long circulating liposomes	• Increased sterical stability • Evasion of MPS uptake • Increased pharmacokinetics and pharmacodynamics	• Slow drug release

12.3 Lipid Modifications and Enhanced Targeting

Despite effective techniques toward the improvement of liposome loading and size, in vivo model experiments pointed to flaws in practical drug delivery. The intravenous administration of neutral liposomes, which are typically comprised of egg phosphatidyl-choline and cholesterol were rapidly cleared from the bloodstream by Kupffer cells (part of the mononuclear phagocyte system [MPS]) of the liver and spleen [51]. Various methods, including alternate routes of delivery and overloading of the MPS by administering empty liposomes, or modifying liposomes with different charges or moieties have been explored (Table 12.2). Herein, we describe a number of methods for the modification of liposomes more popularly used and cited in literature over the last decade, which hold promise for longer circulation times, cellular/tissue interactions, and the controlled release of drugs (Figure 12.3).

12.3.1 Conventional Liposomes

Conventional liposomes consist of natural and/or synthetic lipids, which may be neutral or charged, with no surface modifications. The liposomes are easily prepared by utilizing the techniques described earlier, and have been studied extensively. The selection of surface charge has a major impact on the disposition of the liposomes (and the entrapped drugs) post-administration. Abraham et al. recently explored the distribution of neutral (egg PC: Chol), anionic (egg PC: Dicetylphosphate), and cationic (egg PC: Stearylamine) liposomes that were loaded with an aminoglycoside (gentamicin) after intraperitoneal administration in rodents [52]. Cationic gentamicin-loaded liposomes were shown to accumulate primarily in the brain and liver, while liposomal charge did not influence accumulation in the lungs and kidney. In comparison to the clearance of gentamicin alone over time, cationic liposomes sustained high concentrations of gentamicin in the tissues. The authors concluded that cationic liposomes were superior to anionic and neutral formulations.

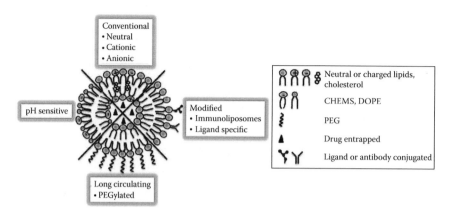

FIGURE 12.3
Lipid composition and modifications. Liposomes can be modified to be (1) neutral (phosphatidylcholines) or charged (anionic phosphatidylinositol and cationic DDAB); (2) conjugated with antibodies or sugar-binding lectins to increase specificity toward the target cells; (3) more sensitive to the physiological environment and release their load by introducing lipids (dioleoylphosphatidylethanolamine, cholesteryl hemisuccinate) which change the liposome shape at different pH; (4) STEALTH by evading clearance and increasing drug levels in the circulation by conjugating PEG to the liposome surface.

Neutral liposomes are considered for certain drug delivery formulations due to their attributes of safety and nontoxicity, owing to minimal interactions between liposomes and cellular membranes [34,53,54]. However, the delivery of their drug payloads is more efficient than that which is possible using conventional formulations. Anderson et al. reported on the blood clearance and organ distribution of neutral (DSPC: Chol) ^{3}H-cholesteryl ether incorporated or ^{14}C-inulin loaded liposomes (~200 nm) administered intravenously [55]. Liposome-loaded formulations were highly distributed (sixfold higher than conventional forms) in the liver and spleen, and lower levels were found in the lung, kidney, and heart. Other routes which have minimal exposure and bypass the circulatory system (e.g., intratracheal instillation) have been proposed. These routes can also target specific organs such as the lungs, where certain infections and diseases can be targeted [56,57]. Omri et al. proposed treatment of *Pseudomonas aeruginosa* (a Gram-negative opportunistic pathogen) lung infection model in rodents [58]. Neutral (DPPC: Chol) polymyxin B-loaded liposomes administered by intratracheal instillation increased drug concentrations in the lungs of the rodents, reduced pro-inflammatory markers, and significantly reduced the *P. aeruginosa* infection in comparison to conventional polymyxin B. Our laboratory has extensively studied neutral liposomes which can also be used to target resistant pathogens like *P. aeruginosa* and *Burkholderia cenocepacia* with interaction and uptake of liposomal antibiotics by these strains, which have low permeability in response to conventional formulations [29–31,59–67].

Charged liposomes, on the other hand, tend to interact with negatively charged cellular membranes (including macrophages), and sometimes these interactions can be unfavorable (potentially toxic) [51]. Cationic liposomes have shown toxicity in both in vitro and in vivo models, while anionic liposomes exhibit minimal toxicity (due to repulsive charges) [53,68,69]. Cationic, anionic, or surface-charged liposomes can also interact with bacterial cells through binding with negatively charged lipopolysaccharides (LPS) and exopolysaccharides (e.g., alginate) in the outer membrane of Gram-negative bacteria, or with zwitterionic lipoteichoic acid and peptidoglycans of Gram-positive bacteria [60,70–73]. Charged liposomal antibiotics have been studied extensively and display greater ability to bind and eradicate bacterial growth compared to conventional antibiotics [74–77]. Catuogno et al. prepared a novel system for delivery of charged liposomes (adsorbed to zinc particles) to oral bacterium *Streptococcus oralis* biofilms [78]. The liposomes successfully delivered bactericidal concentrations of Triclosan and penicillin G in anionic phosphatidylinositol and cationic didecyldimethylammonium bromide (DDAB) carriers. Although the presence of charge did not affect liposomal adsorption to the biofilms, elevated DDAB concentrations increased biofilm binding, suggesting that electrostatic attraction may be playing a part as an integral mechanism.

Other antimicrobial activities of charged liposomes bearing glycopeptides, aminoglycosides, and fluoroquinolones have been reported [77,79,80]. Sachetelli et al. elucidated the activity of fluidosomes (composed of DPPC: DMPG) loaded with tobramycin and having direct fusion of fluidosomes with membranes via flow cytometry, lipid-mixing assay, and transmission electron microscopy [81]. Furneri et al. developed anionic ofloxacin-loaded liposomes against Gram-positive and Gram-negative bacteria [73]. The authors concluded that the anionic liposomes interacted with LPS of Gram-negative, and peptidoglycans of Gram-positive bacteria, hence inhibiting growth. Drulis-Kawa et al. also described the activity of neutral and charged liposomes against Gram-negative bacteria, reporting the superiority of cationic liposomes [71,82,83].

As mentioned earlier, charged liposomes can be toxic to human cells, but the interaction and the engulfment of the liposomes can also be taken as an advantage [84]. Liposome phagocytosis by macrophages has been studied extensively since it was learned that intracellular pathogens residing within cells can be eradicated by liposomal antibiotics (discussed in detail later). Neutral and charged liposomes can be phagocytosed, but charged formulations seem to have a higher activity against intracellular pathogens [51]. Vyas et al. reported the strong bactericidal activity of anionic liposomes (PC: Chol: Dicetylphosphate) loaded with rifampicin [85]. The authors found a significant drop in bacteria residing in alveolar macrophages owing to the uptake of anionic liposomes. El-Ridy et al. prepared neutral and anionic liposomes loaded with pyrazinamide, with the latter formulation being superior in the treatment of mice infected by *M. tuberculosis* [86]. The authors noted that lower doses of liposomes were required for a reduction in bacterial counts toward achieving high therapeutic efficacy.

12.3.2 Targeted Liposomes

Various methods of modifying lipid surfaces with proteins, carbohydrates, and other ligands to increase the interaction between liposomes and their targets have been investigated. Modification of the liposome surface allows for the targeted delivery of the liposomal drug payload to the site of action. These modifications may increase binding capacities to target cells or bacteria, or increase the residency of the carrier, which in turn increases the probability of liposome–cell interaction [87]. Among protein-conjugated liposomes, immunoliposomes (antibody-conjugated) have been considered to target bacteria. The first experiments to examine immunoliposomes, loaded with antibiotics, were conducted by Robinson et al [88–90]. Chlorhexidine or Triclosan-loaded immunoliposomes were prepared using antigens generated by the bacterium *S. oralis*. Immunoliposomes displayed greater affinity than did liposomes without antibodies; yet antibiotic-loaded stearylamine (cationic) liposomes had even greater affinity than did the antibiotic-loaded immunoliposomes.

Saccharide-modified liposomes have also exhibited activity in eradicating bacterial growth. Vyas et al. prepared stearylamine metronidazole-loaded liposomes and surface-coated the liposomes with concanavalin A (con A), a lectin protein. The formulations inhibited *S. mutans* biofilms, and the authors concluded that the binding of conA targeted to the biofilm surface and that the subsequent release and uptake of antibiotics were the mechanisms of liposomal drug delivery [91]. Zaru et al. also investigated polysaccharide chitosan that was coated with neutral and anionic liposomes loaded with rifampicin [92]. The anionic formulations were not only coated more efficiently, but were less toxic to lung cells. Bardonnet et al. explored the affinity of another saccharide (fucose) in glycosylated liposomes loaded with ampicillin against *Helicobacter pylori* [93,94]. The authors concluded that modified liposomes with an inner pH of 4 were stable and would specifically bind to an outer membrane protein of *H. pylori* for targeted delivery. Wijagkanalan et al. explored mannosylated cholesterol liposomes for the targeting of alveolar macrophages in vitro and in vivo after intratracheal administration in rats [95]. The authors noted that the uptake capacity of mannose-modified liposomes was dependent on the mannose density via mannose–receptor-mediated endocytosis.

Other ligand-specific liposomes have also been prepared including vancomycin-loaded anionic liposomes with a folic acid–poly(ethylene oxide)–cholesterol construct for the targeting of folic acid receptors, which exhibited an increased uptake in Caco-2 cell cultures and rat gastrointestinal tract [79]. Vyas et al. reported neutral liposomes (PC: Chol) that were coated with macrophage-specific ligands (maleylated-bovine serum albumin and O-stearoyl amylopectin) and loaded with rifampicin, which resulted in an increased uptake of antibiotic in alveolar macrophages and the maintenance of high entrapment over longer time periods [85]. Liposome formulations with modified lipids have also been investigated for the targeting of cancerous cells, as Huang et al. have reported in regard to a new class of disterol-modified lipids [96]. The authors demonstrated its significance via its ability to form liposomes without the transfer of cholesterol from the bilayer, hence imparting an increase in stability. The cholesterols were covalently linked to the phospholipids which were loaded with doxorubicin (remote-loading technique). The resulting antineoplastic activity was equivalent to Doxil.

12.3.3 pH-Sensitive Liposomes

Sensitive liposomes that respond to low pH environments (PSL) by leaking their encapsulated cargo could be used as potential carriers of drugs to tumor cells or macrophages [97,98]. pH-sensitive liposomes and their opsonization by macrophages have been investigated for over a decade. The key to low pH release resides in the lipid composition. pH-sensitive liposomes are formed from lipids that self-assemble into a spherical shape at neutral pH. In an acidic pH environment, the formation of a fusogenic hexagonal H_{II} phase geometry favors the fusion to, and leaking of entrapped content from, a defective membrane. The most popular lipids used to produce PSLs are a mixture of temperature-sensitive phosphatidylethanolamine (DOPE) with a second lipid that is usually acidic and contains a carboxyl group (CHEMS, fatty acids [oleic acid]) forming anionic liposomes.

Polyethylene glycol (PEG) can also be used for sterical stability (described in the next section) [98]. Although PEG tends to increase the circulation of the liposomes, it reduces the release efficiency of the loaded compound. However, the delivery of the entrapped compound is not jeopardized, which hints at other possible mechanisms of delivery besides a decrease in endosomal pH [99,100]. Research involving PSL-entrapped antibiotics to treat intracellular infections has only scratched the surface. Cordeiro et al. and Lutwyche et al. developed pH-sensitive PEG-coated liposomes loaded with gentamicin that were superior over DPPC (non-PSLs) in lowering intracellular *Salmonella typhimurium* and *Listeria monocytogenes* in an in vitro macrophage and in vivo mouse infection model [101,102].

12.3.4 Long Circulating Liposomes

In order to decrease liposome clearance by the MPS and increase the duration of blood circulation residency, subsequent to intravenous administration, long circulating liposomes (LCLs), which involved the coating of liposome surfaces with PEG (PEGylated or STEALTH liposomes) were introduced in the 1990s [103–106]. The LCLs are hydrophilic negatively charged liposomes, which display excellent pharmacokinetics and biodistribution, and are ideal for long-term therapy. Doxil, a FDA-approved drug, is a PEGylated form of doxorubicin in liposomes, and is one example (discussed in later sections). Previous work with PEG-coated liposomal aminoglycosides for the treatment of pneumonia caused by *Klebsiella pneumoniae* has been described by Bakker-Woudenberg et al., and further modifications of LCL-loaded isoniazid and rifampicin have also been reported by Deol et al. In the past, tagged O-stearoyl amylopectin have been utilized for the targeting of tuberculosis infection in macrophages [107–109]. Bakker-Woudenberg et al. also examined the activity of ciprofloxacin-loaded LCLs in a *P. aeruginosa* infection model [110]. Conventional ciprofloxacin alone (twice daily for 7 days) was not effective in an acute infection model; however, ciprofloxacin-loaded LCLs along with conventional form (one injection on the first day) was 100% effective. In a chronic infection model, ciprofloxacin-loaded LCLs were equally effective when administered once daily in comparison to the conventional form administered twice daily.

The LCLs can also be characterized as having better localization in tissues and in sites of infection with the careful selection of PEG density, size, and lipid charge. Schiffelers et al. investigated the localization of characterized LCLs based on their PEG density, liposomal size, bilayer fluidity, and lipid charge in a *K. pneumoniae* infection model [111,112]. Long circulating liposomes localization increased in phagocytes with decreased PEG density and increased LCL size, reduced biodistribution and lung localization. Negatively charged lipids reduced localization within the lungs. The investigators also noted that inflammation and increased capillary permeability promoted LCL localization in the lung infection site. Schiffelers et al. also examined LCLs loaded with gentamicin compared to the conventional form in a rat *K. pneumoniae* infection model [113–115]. The authors concluded an unsuccessful treatment with no differences between the formulations. However, the combination of the formulations achieved greater survival rates, and the substitution of lipid compositions from a rigid bilayer (containing cholesterol) to a more fluid bilayer (no cholesterol) resulted in the complete survival of rats.

Ellbogen et al. developed LCLs that were loaded with ciprofloxacin and compared their antimicrobial activity against conventional ciprofloxacin and ceftriaxone in a rat model of pneumococcal pneumonia [116]. The LCLs increased ciprofloxacin circulation time and pharmacokinetics, but survival rates were similar between treatments, and ceftriaxone was shown to be even more effective than ciprofloxacin. Recently, Labana et al. reported the synergistic administration of isoniazid and rifampicin in LCLs [117]. At a third of the recommended dose, the LCLs sustained drug release for 1 week, and weekly administrations for 6 weeks eliminated mycobacterium load in mice. de Steenwinkel et al. also demonstrated that LCLs loaded with amikacin resulted in the rapid and complete elimination of M. avium in all infected organs within 12 weeks of treatment, without relapse. On the other hand, the treatment of infected mice with clarithromycin and/or ethambutol, and rifampicin was not as effective, even after 24 weeks of treatment, where a substantial number of mycobacteria within the infected organs were still observed [118].

12.4 Liposome Administration In Vivo

Unlike the poor stability, systemic toxicity, and inactivation of conventional antibiotics, once administered, liposomes provide a protection barrier which entraps hydrophobic and hydrophilic compounds within its compartments. The formulations can be characterized to retain their load and leak slowly; release their payloads only when certain conditions are met (e.g., PSLs); and/or evade detection and uptake by the MPS of the lymph nodes (e.g., STEALTH liposomes). Many modes of liposomal antibiotic delivery have been examined in preclinical and clinical trials. Routes of administration include invasive (e.g., intraperitoneal, intramuscular, intravitreal, intravenous) or noninvasive (e.g., topical, enteral, inhalation) methods.

12.4.1 Invasive Methods

Invasive routes such as intraperitoneal injection are often used in animal models for the slow release of drugs systemically [28,52,119]. Although the method is widely preferred due to its ease of access and large dosage increments, it is not widely used as a method of liposomal drug therapy in humans [120]. Intramuscular injections allow for the sustained release of antibiotics into the circulatory system with elevated tissue levels of antibiotics conveyed by the liposomes. Such routes of administration are used for some conventional antibiotics, yet they are not popular methods for liposomal drug delivery [86,121,122]. Intrathecal injection is an attractive method of administration which avoids the blood–brain barrier. Although antibiotic delivery by this route is unavailable, antineoplastic drugs like the conventional or liposomal cytarabine (Depocyt®; phase II/IV FDA clinical trial) are currently being administered for the treatment of neoplastic meningitis [123,124].

The intravitreal route of administration requires the direct injection of antibiotics (e.g., cephalosporins, aminoglycosides) into the posterior segment of the eye [125]. Although intravitreal injections are successful, adverse effects such as retinal hemorrhage from repeated injections and patient noncompliance have increased the attractiveness of the sustained release properties of liposomes [126]. Liposomal aminoglycosides, delivered by intravitreal injections, have shown sustained therapeutic effects in comparison to conventional forms in rabbit infection models [127,128]. The intravenous route of administration is the most popular method of liposomal drug delivery. It is also the route which requires the application of liposomes with a narrow size distribution (ca. 100–200 nm), which circulate in the blood stream for long periods and slowly release their drug contents and evade destruction (STEALTH liposomes) via natural physiological processes [103]. All liposomal antineoplastic and antimycotic drugs approved by the FDA have been modified to a certain degree to make them more amenable for the intravenous route. Liposomal antibiotics for the treatment of lung infections in clinical trials are not administered by this route, but it is effective for the clearance of intracellular mycobacterial infections due to the superior uptake of the liposomes by the MPS [117,129].

12.4.2 Noninvasive Methods

Noninvasive application methods such as liposomal antibiotic topical treatments have been investigated in soft tissue and burn wound infections, ocular, and facial acne treatment, but the latter has received more attention recently [103,130,131].

Topical administration is an attractive mode of therapy since it is painless, cost-effective, no preparation or devices are required, and patients are more likely to be compliant [125]. There are antibiotic (e.g., clindamycin phosphate, erythromycin) and nonantibiotic (salicylic acid, benzoyl peroxide) treatments available, but topical liposomal antibiotics may be favored because of their sustained release properties. Additionally, the specific attributes of the lipids may facilitate greater adsorption, penetration, and binding to the skin layers and resident pathogens [130,132–134]. Clindamycin-loaded liposomes and conventional forms have been compared in a clinical trial, with the former group being superior in the treatment of acne vulgaris [135]. Other routes like enteral administration are cited in literature, since drugs enter the circulation prior to the first-pass effect by the liver; hence, there is higher bioavailability of lipophilic and hydrophilic drugs in the plasma and lymph nodes [136].

Inhalation (or intratracheal instillation) is the most popular route of administration for liposomal antibiotics as dry powders (using an inhaler), or in aqueous aerosol form (using a nebulizer). Over the past two decades, pulmonary infections in animal models and their subsequent treatment with liposomal antibiotics (aminoglycosides, fluoroquinolones) have promoted the effectiveness of liposomes via their slow targeting and release at the sites of infection [56–58,80,137,138]. Successes in animal models have been beneficial for paving the way for nebulized liposomal amikacin and inhaled liposomal ciprofloxacin in clinical trials for the treatment of cystic fibrosis (CF) and non-CF bronchiectasis [139–143]. The formulations have been characterized, and are tolerable, with prolonged retention in healthy humans [44]. The inhalation route has also been studied as a method to treat tuberculosis infections, and certain formulations like liposomal rifampicin and isoniazid have been reported to retain their drug concentrations in the plasma and remain longer in the lungs and the alveolar macrophages, eliminating the need for multiple dosing regimens [129,144,145].

12.5 Advantages and Successes of Liposomal Antibiotics

It has been more than 40 years since it was suggested that liposomes could become nanocarriers of antibiotics to drug-resistant pathogens, and research and development has produced effective liposomal drug delivery systems with multiple advantages over conventional drug delivery formulations. The goal of any liposome formulation is to improve drug biodistribution and pharmacokinetics while lowering toxicity. Other aims include increasing drug uptake by resistant intracellular and extracellular pathogens. The limitations of conventional antibiotics typically include adverse side effects combined with limited biodistribution or pharmacokinetics in patients. In addition, there are drawbacks such as elevated bacterial resistance, low drug permeability levels, and thus interaction with pathogens. In order to achieve these goals, it is important to characterize the liposomes for their specific activity by the techniques described in the earlier sections. Presently, accomplishments in liposomology have been the production of nanocarriers with reduced toxicity, which not only increase, but also sustain drug levels in the circulation and at the site of infection (lymph nodes, the lungs) [6,34,146]. These achievements overwhelmingly promote the utilization of liposomes as carriers in the treatment of fungal infections, certain cancers, and chronic or resistant lung infections.

12.5.1 Protection from Degradation or Inactivation

At the basic level, liposomes selectively "screen" particular antibiotics for their bacterial targets. In contrast, for example, β-lactams are broad-spectrum antibiotics that are regularly used against Gram-positive and Gram-negative pathogens [147]. Due to their popular clinical use, pathogens like methicillin- or vancomycin-resistant *Staphylococcus aureus* have emerged [148]. Their resistance is usually due to β-lactamases, which have prompted the production of β-lactamase-resistant β-lactams (e.g., meropenem). However, newer forms of semiresistant mutations of penicillin-binding proteins, or proteins with resistance to antibiotic compound diffusion across bacterial membranes have developed [149]. Since liposomes tend to encapsulate compounds which act to mask and protect the internalized antibiotics, many resistance factors like β-lactamase degradation and poor diffusion are assumed to be bypassed [147]. As liposomal β-lactam research is only in the formative stages of in vitro experimentation, in vivo models are lacking [75,82,83]. Schiffelers et al. explored the synergistic activity of liposome co-encapsulated gentamicin and ceftazidime in a rat *K. pneumoniae* infection model [115]. The investigators reported that the co-encapsulation allowed for a shorter treatment course and a lower dose of antibiotics compared to the conventional form, warranting further studies.

Opportunistic pathogens that proliferate in the lungs of CF patients reside within biofilms (an extracellular matrix made up of negatively charged alginate) that are covered with endotoxins generated by pathogens and patient-excreted polyanionic sputum (a mixture of DNA and glycoproteins from host neutrophils) [61,150]. Different classes of cationic antibiotics (e.g., aminoglycosides, polymyxins) with broad-spectrum activity against these pathogens are inactivated in the presence of polyanions. The aggregation of these factors (owing to their charges) with antibiotics retards further diffusion through the biofilm matrix, and hence contact with the pathogens. Liposome entrapment of antibiotics, however, inhibits the antibiotic–polyanion interaction. We have previously shown this to be true for neutral liposomes (which do not favor electrostatic interactions) that were loaded with tobramycin or polymyxin B [60]. While the activity of conventional antibiotics against *P. aeruginosa* was inhibited at low concentrations of the factors, liposomal formulations were superior by 2- to 100-fold, dependant on the inhibiting factors. The liposomal formulations also reduced endogenous bacterial counts in expectorated sputum at a concentration lower than that of the conventional form, but failed to completely eradicate growth. Further investigations have shown that the viscous sputum hampers liposomal diffusion, and that recombinant human DNase and alginate lyase are important components toward the improvement of conventional or liposomal antibiotic diffusion across this barrier [70,151–153].

12.5.2 Reduction of Toxicity

The reduction of cytotoxicity of antimycotics (e.g., amphotericin B, nystatin) and antineoplastic drugs (e.g., doxorubicin, daunorubicin, cytarabine) have popularized liposomal drug delivery. In addition to this, liposomal antibiotics (e.g., amikacin, ciprofloxacin) administered by inhalation reduce systemic toxicity by reducing the circulation time. Popular antibiotics like aminoglycosides, fluoroquinolones, and polymyxins contain broad activity against Gram-negative pathogens, but are restricted due to the risk of adverse systemic events. For example, aminoglycosides like tobramycin are well known for their renal and cochlea toxicity. Only with careful monitoring of serum tobramycin levels and lung-targeting methods like inhalation are the toxicities reduced. The loading of antibiotics in liposomes has also demonstrated reduced toxicity in animal models and in human clinical trials [57,154,155].

Our group has recently developed a neutral liposome formulation of an antibiotic (tobramycin) and a metal (Bi–EDT), which displays synergistic activity against a variety of susceptible or resistant clinical isolates of *P. aeruginosa* (mucoid or nonmucoid). The formulation has shown equal or greater inhibitory and bactericidal activity compared to the conventional form against *P. aeruginosa* [30]. In addition to this, the formulation exhibits a greater ability to attenuate quorum-sensing (bacterial cell-to-cell communication), virulence factors, and biofilms [31]. We have also reported that the liposomal formulation tends to modulate alginate production and increase the penetration of the tobramycin into resistant mucoid *P. aeruginosa* (confirmed by electron microscopy). However, the presence of bismuth was not found inside the bacteria (unpublished data). But perhaps, what brightens the future of this formulation is its lowered toxicity in vitro. The liposomal formulation was bactericidal against *P. aeruginosa* at concentrations which were not toxic to carcinoma A549 lung cells. The conventional form at an equal concentration was not bactericidal to *P. aeruginosa* and was toxic to the lung cells, confirmed by MTT (cell viability) and lactate dehydrogenase (biomarker of cell membrane integrity). Multiple in vivo rodent models are currently being investigated for their efficacy and pharmacokinetics, using liposomal formulations. We have also investigated other potential liposomal therapeutics that co-entraps gentamicin and gallium. The gentamicin–gallium formulation displayed promising results similar to our tobramycin–bismuth formulation, with increased activity against resistant *P. aeruginosa* biofilms, and reduced toxicity in A549 lung cells.

12.5.3 Enhanced Delivery to Intracellular Pathogens

Persistent intracellular pathogens (e.g., *Mycobacterium avium* complex (MAC), *L. monocytogenes*, *S. typhimurium*) may reside in phagocytic cells (an essential component of the immune system) after opsonization, hindering any treatment [51,156,157]. The majority of conventional antibiotics (e.g., aminoglycosides, β-lactams) cannot readily penetrate or diffuse across the phagocyte membrane, while others (e.g., macrolides, fluoroquinolones) are inactivated by acidic pH of lysosomes, or do not reach critical bactericidal concentrations [51]. When antibiotics are loaded within liposomes, these nanocarriers not only show enhanced activity in vitro, but also improve the clearance of bacterial infections in vivo with greater survival capacities [158].

As shown in Figure 12.4, small liposome-loaded antibiotics above 100 nm are normally opsonized by contact with the plasma membrane, which forms a vesicle upon internalization. This is followed by fusion with early endosomes (slightly acidic pH 6.5) and transport to late endosomes (pH 5–6), and then degradation in lysosomes (pH 4–5). It is believed that liposomes release their drug content into the cytosol, where bacteria reside, before lysosome degradation by enzymes. The release of the liposome payload may occur during the process of liposome–endosome fusion, or by passive diffusion through the endosome lipid membrane [51,97]. This concept and the efficient opsonization of liposomes by macrophages have been aggressively exploited to clear the host of an innate immune response with liposomal dichloromethylene diphosphonate (clodronate). The administration can be invasive (e.g., intravenous) or noninvasive (e.g., intratracheal) in experimental animal models, and deplete macrophages completely [159,160].

To date, an array of conventional (e.g., neutral, charged) and modified formulations (e.g., pH-sensitive, protein ligands, PEGylated) have been produced and loaded with aminoglycosides, fluoroquinolones, macrolides, and rifamycins [97,103,118,137,161]. The formulations deliver a higher dose of antibiotics to macrophages and act to clear infections, and reduce toxicity in animal models; however, clinical trials have not yet begun. In 1998, the pharmacokinetics and toxicity of liposomal amikacin (Mikasome™) in a male patient

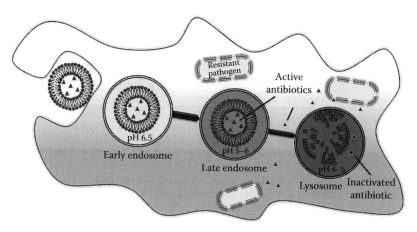

FIGURE 12.4

Opsonization of liposome-loaded antibiotics by macrophages. Liposomes are opsonized after contact with the plasma membrane forming a vesicle upon internalization. This is followed by fusion with early endosome (slightly acidic pH 6.5) and transport to late endosome (pH 5–6), and then degradation in lysosomes (pH 4–5). The liposomes may release their drug content into the cytosol (where pathogens reside) before lysosome degradation in the process of liposome–endosome fusion, or by passive diffusion through the endosome lipid membrane.

suffering from multidrug-resistant tuberculosis concluded that the liposomal formulation was well-tolerated, and that serum levels of amikacin were found to be greater than for conventional forms. Although the patient showed clinical improvement, the liposomal formulation failed to completely eradicate bacterial growth.

12.5.4 Enhanced Delivery to Extracellular Pathogens

Liposomes can also increase the delivery of antibiotics to resistant extracellular pathogens like the opportunistic *S. aureus, K. pneumoniae, P. aeruginosa*, and *B. cenocepacia*, which reside in the lungs of immunocompromised patients. Although liposomes enhance biodistribution and elevate concentrations of the antibiotics at the sites of infection, bacterial resistance owing to low permeability and overexpression of active efflux systems (e.g., mexA-mexB-oprM of *P. aeruginosa* efflux system) retard bactericidal activity [6]. In order to deliver bactericidal concentrations to the resistant pathogens, the direct interaction and uptake (fusion) of the liposomal antibiotics is required. Drulis-Kawa et al. recently described an 18 kDa protein on the outer membrane of *P. aeruginosa*, which may be crucial to the fusion with cationic liposomes [71]. Our laboratory group has focused solely on the uptake of liposomal antibiotics by resistant pathogens [30,31,59,62,66]. The methods used to confirm the fusion included bacterial inhibition assays, and visual techniques like lipid-mixing assay, flow cytometry, and transmission electron microscopy, coupled with immunogold labeling of the antibiotic (immunocytochemistry) [62,66,81].

12.6 Disadvantages and Drawbacks of Liposomal Antibiotics

As mentioned earlier, there are currently a number of drawbacks as per liposome-encapsulated antibiotics, including low entrapment efficiency, short shelf-life, and they may contain lipid peroxides and toxic solvents, owing to their preparation methods [6]. Also, upon intravenous administration, low stability and short circulation in the bloodstream have been reported [51,162]. The primary disadvantages of liposomes, which have not been fully addressed as yet, are the sterility of the lipids, their time-consuming expensive production on a large scale, and the lack of clinical data required to validate liposomal drug delivery as a viable pharmaceutical strategy.

12.6.1 Large-Scale Production and Sterility Issues

Some of the shortcomings mentioned earlier can be remedied by using safer production techniques (e.g., nonvolatile organic solvents, oxygen-free environment), utilizing high-quality lipids, and introducing antioxidant additives (tocopherols) to reduce the formation of lipid radicals [6,47]. Low entrapment and stability issues have been resolved through improvements in loading techniques (remote-loading), increasing shelf-life (freeze-drying), the addition of cholesterol, and longer circulating carriers (STEALTH liposomes) [36,105,138]. Liposome preparation (lipid costs, equipment, etc.) in a laboratory setting is expensive, and the production of liposomes through the techniques mentioned earlier is time-consuming.

In addition, these procedures require mechanisms that may require handling of the lipids for long periods, which can expose the liposomes to bacteria or viruses. Gamma irradiation techniques are available, but are not considered due to the chemical degradation of the lipid components [163]. Although mechanical filtration (with pore sizes smaller than bacteria) may sterilize the samples, it does not separate viruses and spores from the suspension. It is surprising that after decades of animal research, which have consistently validated the efficacy of liposomal antibiotics, clinical trials are slowly starting for only two liposomal formulations in this class. While many liposome formulations have proven to be efficacious against intracellular and extracellular pathogens, the only antibiotic liposomes that have been developed for use against extracellular pathogens involving lung infections are in phase II FDA clinical trials.

12.6.2 Reduced Antibacterial Activity

To favor an antibiotic formulation in liposomes over its conventional form, the liposomes must (1) increase the susceptibility of the resistant pathogen to the antibiotic; (2) be non-toxic to the host; and (3) reduce (or not increase) the toxicity of the loaded antibiotic. Some liposomal antibiotic formulations have shown successes in vitro but have failed to reproduce such results in vivo. Others have been successful in reducing toxicity in the host but have not been able to prevent or eradicate pathogenic growth [164]. Different compositions of lipids have different activities against pathogens, but may not exhibit improvement when compared to conventional formulations. Drulis-Kawa et al. explored different compositions of liposome-loaded meropenem (cationic or anionic lipids with cholesterol) against susceptible and resistant *P. aeruginosa* [83]. The investigators reported that the β-lactam cationic liposomes were more effective against susceptible strains than anionic liposomes (as in agreement with other investigators). However, none of the formulations were effective against resistant strains (due to low permeability) compared to conventional meropenem.

Our laboratory has investigated the activity of neutral liposome-loaded aminoglycosides extensively. We have shown that liposomes tend to reduce the toxicity of antibiotics, and reduce inhibitory concentrations against susceptible or resistant Gram-negative clinical isolates. However, they do not fare better than conventional antibiotics against endogenous bacteria in sputum or against mature biofilms [60]. The polyanionic sputum and biofilms have proven to be perfect barriers against antibiotics and liposomes, owing to their charged polyanionic nature, viscosity, and lowered permeability to molecules. We concluded that in order to completely eradicate the bacteria from sputum and biofilms, "liquefiers" like DNase and alginate lyase must be used for the breakdown, penetration, and subsequent delivery of the liposomal antibiotics [31,61]. The superiority of liposomal antibiotics over conventional forms cannot be achieved without these liquefiers, and further research is warranted. Although the activity of alginate lyase has not been confirmed for in vivo models or clinical trials, DNase (Pulmozyme™) has demonstrated improvements in the lung function of CF patients in clinical settings [165,166].

Delivery of antibiotics by liposomal carriers to attenuate or eradicate intracellular pathogens has been successful in vitro and with some in vivo models, however clinical trials are deficient [158]. The only long-term infection treatment known was conducted using a NeXstar liposomal amikacin formulation in a pharmacokinetics and efficacy study against *M. tuberculosis* infection in a patient more than a decade ago. The drug was well-tolerated, and elevated serum levels of amikacin were verified. However, the infection was not eradicated [164]. The in vivo models have shown a greater superiority of liposome-loaded antibiotics, but some models have failed to eradicate pathogenic growth, which raises questions as to whether liposomal treatment is appropriate for therapeutic applications against intracellular pathogens. Investigators have reported on the excellent retention of conventional (e.g., charged, neutral) or modified (e.g., pH-sensitive, PEGylated) liposome-loaded gentamicin, amikacin, rifabutin, pyrazinamide, or ciprofloxacin in the spleen, liver, and lungs of rodents infected with intracellular pathogens. However, none have reported complete pathogen eradication, even though the liposomal formulations fared better than the conventional therapy in every parameter [86,101,110,167,168]. The failures are multifactorial, and can be explained by lower biodistribution and penetration at the site of infection (due to biofilms and sputum formation), lowered uptake (by the pathogen), or the formation of persister and dormant cells [6,169,170].

12.6.3 Increased Cytotoxicity

Some liposomal formulations require interaction with cells and may be beneficial when opsonized by macrophages or healthy cells to release their payload. However, depending on the composition of the lipids, the carriers can also be harmful to certain cells, and their interaction must be avoided in liposomal drug delivery. It is clear that cationic liposomes (more than anionic liposomes) interact and deliver a higher load of antibiotics to bacterial biofilms. However, these charged liposomes also tend to interact with human cells unfavorably [78]. Stensrud et al. reported that anionic DSPG liposomes promoted the aggregation of red blood cells [163]. Parallel work concluded that liposomes composed of unsaturated lipids were toxic to macrophages, while saturated lipids (except for DMPC) were nontoxic [171].

Smistad et al. have shown that cationic liposomes are toxic to buccal cells, while anionic liposomes were less toxic [53]. The toxicity was dependent on the lipid charges, and not on the liposomal size or concentration. Lipid types also displayed different toxicities, with cationic diacyl-TAP or DPPC lipids being less toxic than stearylamine or DMPC. Filion et al. also examined different cationic lipids and their toxicity toward phagocytes. As opsonization is key for drug release into the cytosol, cationic liposomes (e.g., DOPE: DDAB) were found to be toxic. However, the addition of DPPC or DPPE-PEG$_{2000}$, instead of DOPE, eliminated these toxicities [172]. Berrocal et al. examined the prolonged exposure of skin fibroblasts to elevating doses of soy PC or DMPC. The soy PC liposomes were found to be more toxic than DMPC liposomes [173]. However, when liposomes were loaded with vitamin E, DMPC liposomes were equally toxic to the cells.

12.7 Recent Advances in Clinical Trials

Liposomes have evolved considerably since their discovery as potential drug carriers. As liposomes potentially provide a reduction in cytotoxicity and longer circulation, it is no surprise that the approved formulations to date are medicines that have limited dosing and diffusion across tissues. The first mention of liposomal antibiotics used in humans was by Peyman et al. in a successful treatment (by intravitreal administration) of a patient with chronic intraocular inflammatory disorders [174]. The clinical trials (phase I/II) in the past 20 years have also focused on treating tuberculosis caused by MAC bacteremia with liposomal aminoglycosides [175,176]. Although liposomal aminoglycosides have shown superiority and were well-tolerated, there are no antituberculosis liposomal treatments that are commercially available at this point.

At the present time, two liposomal antimycotics and three liposomal antineoplastic drugs have been developed and are in current use in clinical settings, but liposomal antibiotics have only just entered clinical trials (Table 12.3). Every year, newer formulations are developed, and some progress successfully to enter clinical trials. Recently, the European Medicines Agency (EMEA) and the US FDA granted orphan drug designation to fluidosome-loaded tobramycin by Axentis Pharma [177]. The fluidosomes are to be administered via a nebulizer in the treatment of chronic infections in CF patients caused by *P. aeruginosa* and *B. cenocepacia,* at half the dose of conventional tobramycin. As described earlier, fluidosomes with anionic charge have shown increased efficacy and delivery of antibiotics against Gram-negative pathogens in in vitro experiments through direct fusion with bacterial membranes. The experiments were expected to be completed in 2010; however the results are not publicly available, and since experiments beyond in vitro models have not been performed, the enhanced performance of fluidosomes over conventional forms cannot be speculated.

12.7.1 Nonantibiotic FDA Formulations

Two liposome-loaded amphotericin B formulations have been approved by the FDA. Amphotericin B is a broad-spectrum antimycotic drug which is insoluble in water and is well known for its nephrotoxicity in patients [178]. Its incorporation into the lipid bilayer of anionic liposomes administered intravenously has been approved for the treatment of aspergillosis, candidiasis, and cryptococcal meningitis [179]. The formulations are produced as liquid suspensions (Abelcet) and lyophilized powders (Ambisome). Although higher doses of liposomal amphotericin B (compared to the conventional form) are required, clinical trials have noted a reduction in renal toxicity and improvements in fungal clearance, with no significant difference between the two liposomal formulations [180–182]. Additional clinical trials are also progressing, employing Ambisome in combination with other drugs in the treatment of fungal visceral leishmaniasis [183]. Newer liposomal formulations loaded with nystatin (Nyotran™) have also been developed and compared to conventional amphotericin B in clinical phase III trials. Nyotran was as effective as conventional amphotericin B, with the added benefits of reduced renal toxicity and metabolic disorders [184–186].

Two different formulations of doxorubicin have also been approved for the treatment of some cancers. Doxil (a product of Johnson & Johnson) is a PEGylated liposomal doxorubicin formulation developed for the treatment of ovarian cancer and Kaposi's sarcoma [22]. Doxil's modified structure allows for longer blood circulation, thereby elevating drug

TABLE 12.3

Liposome-Entrapped Medications Approved or in FDA Clinical Trials

Product Name (Manufacturer)	Lipid Composition	Administration Route	Class	Target	Status
Amphotericin B					
• Ambisome (Gilead Sciences)	Hyd. Soy PC: DSPG: Chol	Intravenous	Antimycotic	• Aspergillosis • Candidiasis • Cryptococcal meningitis	FDA-approved
• Abelcet (Enzon Pharm.)	DMPC: DMPG	Intravenous	Antimycotic	• Aspergillosis • Candidiasis • Cryptococcal meningitis	FDA-approved
Doxorubicin					
• Doxil (Johnson & Johnson)	MPEG-DSPE: Chol: Hyd. Soy PC	Intravenous	Antineoplastic	• Ovarian cancer • Kaposi's sarcoma	FDA-approved
• Myocet (Sopherion Therapeutics)	Egg PC: Chol	Intravenous	Antineoplastic	• Metastatic breast cancer	FDA-approved
Daunorubicin • DaunoXome (Gilead Sciences)	DSPC: Chol	Intravenous	Antineoplastic	• Acute myeloid leukemia • Kaposi's sarcoma	FDA-approved
Nystatin • Nyotran (Aronex)	DMPC: DMPG	Intravenous	Antimycotic	• Fever • Neutropenia • Leukemia	Phase III
Cytarabine • Depocyt (Pacira Pharm.)	DOPC: Chol: DMPG	Intrathecal	Antineoplastic	• Neoplastic meningitis	Phase IV
Amikacin • Arikace (Transave)	DPPC: Chol	Inhalation	Antibacterial	• CF • Non-CF bronchiectasis	Phase II
Ciprofloxacin • ARD-3100, ARD-3150 (Aradigm)	Egg PC: Chol	Inhalation	Antibacterial	• CF • Non-CF bronchiectasis	Phase II

accumulation. However, side effects such as palmar plantar erythrodysesthesia (peeling of skin) are prevalent [187,188]. Despite the side effects, Doxil is less cardiotoxic than conventional doxorubicin, and clinical trials that combine Doxil with other antineoplastic and anti-inflammatory drugs are progressing [189–191]. Myocet (a product of Sopherion Therapeutics) is a non-PEGylated liposomal doxorubicin formulation approved for use in combination with cyclophosphamide for the treatment of metastatic breast cancer [192,193]. Unlike Doxil, Myocet has a shorter blood circulation residency since it is not PEGylated, and induces milder side effects. The combination of Myocet with supplementary drugs like trastuzumab and docetaxel to treat metastatic breast cancer are currently in phase II clinical trials [194,195].

Daunorubicin, which is closely related to doxorubicin has also been approved by the FDA in liposomal formulations (DaunoXome), and is produced by Gilead Sciences. The formulation is used in treating Kaposi's sarcoma and acute myeloid leukemia, and has demonstrated reduced toxicity and increased efficacy [196,197]. Moreover, phase III trials have shown that DaunoXome alone is more tolerable and has comparable survival rates to synergistic treatment using doxorubicin, bleomycin, and vincristine [198]. Phase II trials of DaunoXome (in combination with cyclophosphamide, vincristine, and prednisolone), in treating non-Hodgkin's lymphoma, resulted in high survival rates, although one-third of the patients were hospitalized for febrile neutropenia. It was concluded that DaunoXome dosing was too high [199]. Recently, the synergistic activity of DaunoXome with another chemotherapeutic drug (cytarabine) was also compared to the conventional form (phase III clinical trials), and displayed improved overall survival and disease-free survival in the long-term follow-up [200]. The success of cytarabine has also produced liposomal cytarabine (Depocyt) under phase IV clinical trial in the treatment of neoplastic meningitis, imparting elevated dose levels of cytarabine to tumors over a longer time period [124,201,202].

12.7.2 Liposomal Amikacin (Arikace)

The efficacy and superiority of liposomal amikacin has been studied for more than a decade in preclinical models of infection (e.g., CF, tuberculosis) [45,61,118,154,203,204]. The extensive research was conducted mostly by NeXstar Pharmaceuticals and Gilead Sciences. In 2009, Transave initiated preclinical and clinical trials of liposomal amikacin (marketed as Arikace) [140,141,143,154]. The formulation is intended as an inhaled application for the treatment of pulmonary infections (CF, non-CF bronchiectasis). The uncharged, unmodified liposomes (DPPC: Chol) are loaded with amikacin by the ethanol injection method, and are produced with an average size of 300 nm (~170 to 700 nm) [45].

Preclinical studies demonstrated the ability of Arikace to penetrate expectorated CF sputum, and the sustained release of amikacin significantly attenuated bacterial counts in a rat infection model compared to free amikacin [45]. Short-term clinical studies (phase I/II) have been completed [141,143,154]. The studies determined the safety, tolerability, pharmacokinetics, and pharmacodynamics of Arikace (14 or 28 days; 280 or 560 mg daily Arikace inhalation) in CF or non-CF bronchiectasis patients in comparison to a placebo. The trials noted that the administration of Arikace was well-tolerated and was safe. In addition, CF patients receiving Arikace had an increase in amikacin in the lungs and sputum above bacterial inhibitory concentrations; increased forced expiratory volume and weight; reduction in *P. aeruginosa* density, exacerbations, and hospital stays. Long-term FDA clinical trials (phase I/II) are ongoing for the multiple dosing and tolerability of aerosolized Arikace in CF patients (18 months; 28 days on 560 mg daily Arikace inhalation; 56 days off) [140]. These promising results warrant further clinical trials in larger CF populations.

12.7.3 Liposomal Ciprofloxacin (ARD-3100, ARD-3150)

Methods like the remote-loading technique to increase drug loading in LUVs and PEG modifications to increase blood circulation have promoted the use of liposomal ciprofloxacin for the treatment of intracellular, pulmonary, and intraocular infections [36,110,116,137,205,206]. In 2006, Aradigm introduced liposomal ciprofloxacin for the treatment of CF (ARD-3100) and non-CF bronchiectasis (ARD-3150). Aradigm initiated preclinical studies in 2006, and by 2007, an Australian 7-day phase I study to assess the safety and efficacy of the formulation was completed. It was concluded that there were no adverse effects, but for a reduced ciprofloxacin concentration in the blood compared to oral and intravenous administered groups [207]. The phase II trials with administration of liposomal ciprofloxacin for inhalation (450, 350, or 150 mg; 14 or 28 days), studying safety, tolerability, and pharmacokinetics with increasing doses were reported in 2010 [208,209]. The investigators reported an increase in forced expiratory volume, tolerability of the formulations, and a sustained release of ciprofloxacin in plasma. Once-daily treatments in CF and non-CF bronchiectasis patients resulted in elevated ciprofloxacin levels in sputum and reduced *P. aeruginosa* density over 28 days. The liposomal formulations resulted in prolonged activity in the lungs, with lower system levels compared to other administration routes (enteral and intravenous). Further phase II clinical trials to assess the safety and efficacy of liposomal ciprofloxacin in CF and non-CF bronchiectasis patients were completed in the March of 2011. However, no results have as yet been released [139,142].

12.8 Concluding Remarks

The potential for liposomes as dynamic and efficient carriers of drugs, antioxidants, proteins, DNA, and other compounds is growing every year. Some formulations have been produced solely for their lower toxicity profile, and others for their improved pharmacokinetics and pharmacodynamics. Additional formulations have been produced that have the capacity for enhancing the delivery of antibiotics to drug-resistant intracellular or extracellular pathogens. The limitations of low liposomal loading yields, minimal interactions with biological membranes, and clearance from the circulation, which were reported decades ago, are now deemed as marginal. The introduction of more efficient and safer loading techniques, coupled with the capacity for finely "tuning" liposome parameters such as size, charge, lipid composition, and the conjugation of ligands, cumulatively position liposomes favorably to revolutionize drug delivery. The combinations of stable unilamellar vesicles with high drug-loading capacities, modifications to lipid surfaces with the addition of charges, and PEGylation have been the most successful techniques being developed for clinical trials. Cost-effective methods for the large-scale production and sterilization of liposomal formulations will require a thorough review and assessment.

Further enhancements in liposome fluidity have allowed for better targeting and interaction with bacterial biofilms and the delivery of antibiotics to persistent pathogens. Hundreds of in vivo model experiments have been required to finally culminate in trials with patients suffering from cancers and severe infections. Liposomal antineoplastic and antimycotic therapies are becoming more popular, and although there are not, as yet, any liposomal antibiotics approved by the FDA, large multicenter trials are ongoing. The extensive research efforts that have proceeded over the last decade have elevated and transitioned liposomal drug delivery from the small laboratory environment to hospitals. The next decade is certain to witness significant advancements and an influx of several new liposome-based antibiotics for use in clinical settings.

References

1. Bangham, A.D. and Horne, R.W., Negative staining of phospholipids and their structural modification by surface-active agents as observed in the electron microscope, *J Mol Biol* 8, 660–8, 1964.
2. Sessa, G. and Weissmann, G., Phospholipid spherules (liposomes) as a model for biological membranes, *J Lipid Res* 9(3), 310–8, 1968.
3. Kshirsagar, N.A., Pandya, S.K., Kirodian, G.B., and Sanath, S., Liposomal drug delivery system from laboratory to clinic, *J Postgrad Med* 51 Suppl 1, S5–S15, 2005.
4. Goyal, P., Goyal, K., Vijaya Kumar, S.G., Singh, A., Katare, O.P., and Mishra, D.N., Liposomal drug delivery systems—clinical applications, *Acta Pharm* 55(1), 1–25, 2005.
5. Allison, S.D., Liposomal drug delivery, *J Infus Nurs* 30, 89; quiz 120, 2007.
6. Drulis-Kawa, Z. and Dorotkiewicz-Jach, A., Liposomes as delivery systems for antibiotics, *Int J Pharm* 387(1–2), 187–198, 2010.
7. Naghmouchi, K., Drider, D., and Fliss, I., Action of divergicin M35, a class IIa bacteriocin, on liposomes and Listeria, *J Appl Microbiol* 102(6), 1508–17, 2007.
8. Zepik, H.H., Walde, P., Kostoryz, E.L., Code, J., and Yourtee, D.M, Lipid vesicles as membrane models for toxicological assessment of xenobiotics, *Crit Rev Toxicol* 38(1), 1–11, 2008.
9. Park, S.C., Kim, M.H., Hossain, M.A., Shin, S.Y., Kim, Y., Stella, L., Wade, J.D., Park, Y., and Hahm, K.S., Amphipathic alpha-helical peptide, HP (2–20), and its analogues derived from *Helicobacter pylori*: Pore formation mechanism in various lipid compositions, *Biochim Biophys Acta* 1778(1), 229–41, 2008.
10. Katsu, T., Imamura, T., Komagoe, K., Masuda, K., and Mizushima, T., Simultaneous measurements of K⁺ and calcein release from liposomes and the determination of pore size formed in a membrane, *Anal Sci* 23(5), 517–22, 2007.
11. Jelokhani-Niaraki, M., Prenner, E.J., Kay, C.M., McElhaney, R.N., and Hodges, R.S., Conformation and interaction of the cyclic cationic antimicrobial peptides in lipid bilayers, *J Pept Res* 60(1), 23–36, 2002.
12. Pasupuleti, M., Schmidtchen, A., Chalupka, A., Ringstad, L., and Malmsten, M., End-tagging of ultra-short antimicrobial peptides by W/F stretches to facilitate bacterial killing, *PLoS One* 4(4), e5285, 2009.
13. Sung, W.S. and Lee, D.G., The combination effect of Korean red ginseng saponins with kanamycin and cefotaxime against methicillin-resistant *Staphylococcus aureus*, *Biol Pharm Bull* 31(8), 1614–7, 2008.
14. Falck, E., Hautala, J.T., Karttunen, M., Kinnunen, P.K., Patra, M., Saaren-Seppälä, H., Vattulainen, I., Wiedmer, S.K., and Holopainen, J.M., Interaction of fusidic acid with lipid membranes: Implications to the mechanism of antibiotic activity, *Biophys J* 91(5), 1787–99, 2006.
15. Jia, Y., Joly, H., Leek, D.M., Demetzos, C., and Omri A., The effect of aminoglycoside antibiotics on the thermodynamic properties of liposomal vesicles, *J Liposome Res* 20(1), 84–96, 2010.
16. Chauhan, A.S., Negi, P.S., and Ramteke, R.S., Antioxidant and antibacterial activities of aqueous extract of Seabuckthorn (*Hippophae rhamnoides*) seeds, *Fitoterapia* 78(7–8), 590–2, 2007.
17. Strömstedt, A.A., Pasupuleti, M., Schmidtchen, A., and Malmsten, M., Evaluation of strategies for improving proteolytic resistance of antimicrobial peptides by using variants of EFK17, an internal segment of LL-37, *Antimicrob Agents Chemother* 53(2), 593–602, 2009.

18. Yoneyama, F., Shioya, K., Zendo, T., Nakayama, J., and Sonomoto, K., Effect of a negatively charged lipid on membrane-lacticin Q interaction and resulting pore formation, *Biosci Biotechnol Biochem* 74(1), 218–21, 2010.

19. Zhang, L., Rozek, A., and Hancock, R.E., Interaction of cationic antimicrobial peptides with model membranes, *J Biol Chem* 276(38), 35714–22, 2001.

20. Weiss, D., Naik, P., and Weiss, R., The "big pharma" dilemma: Develop new drugs or promote existing ones? *Nat Rev Drug Discov* 8(7), 533–4, 2009.

21. Kraus, C.N., Low hanging fruit in infectious disease drug development, *Curr Opin Microbiol* 11(5), 434–8, 2008.

22. Cattel, L., Ceruti, M., and Dosio, F., From conventional to stealth liposomes: A new frontier in cancer chemotherapy, *J Chemother* 16 Suppl 4, 94–7, 2004.

23. Barenholz, Y., Relevancy of drug loading to liposomal formulation therapeutic efficacy, *J Liposome Res* 13(1), 1–8, 2003.

24. Fenske, D.B. and Maurer, N., Encapsulation of weakly-basic drugs, antisense oligonucleotides, and plasmid DNA within large unilamellar vesicles for drug delivery applications, in *Liposomes: A Practical Approach*, Torchilin, V.P. and Weissig, V., Eds., Oxford University Press, Oxford, U.K., p. 167, 2003.

25. Harrigan, P.R., Wong, K.F., Redelmeier, T.E., Wheeler, J.J., and Cullis, P.R., Accumulation of doxorubicin and other lipophilic amines into large unilamellar vesicles in response to trans-membrane pH gradients, *Biochim Biophys Acta* 1149(2), 329–38, 1993.

26. Wagner, A., Platzgummer, M., Kreismayr, G., Quendler, H., Stiegler, G., Ferko, B., Vecera, G., Vorauer-Uhl, K., and Katinger, H., GMP production of liposomes—a new industrial approach, *J Liposome Res* 16(3), 311–9, 2006.

27. Mozafari, M.R., A new technique for the preparation of non-toxic liposomes and nanolipo-somes: The heating method, in *Nanoliposomes: From Fundamentals to Recent Developments*, Mozafari, M.R. and Mortazavi, S.M., Eds., Trafford Publishing Ltd, Oxford, U.K., p. 91, 2005.

28. Sadzuka, Y., Hirama, R., and Sonobe, T., Effects of intraperitoneal administration of liposomes and methods of preparing liposomes for local therapy, *Toxicol Lett* 126(2), 83–90, 2002.

29. Halwani, M., Hebert, S., Suntres, Z.E., Lafrenie, R.M., Azghani, A.O., and Omri, A., Bismuth-thiol incorporation enhances biological activities of liposomal tobramycin against bacterial bio-film and quorum sensing molecules production by *Pseudomonas aeruginosa*, *Int J Pharm* 373(1–2), 141–6, 2009.

30. Halwani, M., Blomme, S., Suntres, Z.E., Alipour, M., Azghani, A.O., Kumar, A., and Omri, A., Liposomal bismuth-ethanedithiol formulation enhances antimicrobial activity of tobramycin, *Int J Pharm* 358(1–2), 278–84, 2008.

31. Alipour, M., Suntres, Z.E., Lafrenie, R.M., and Omri, A., Attenuation of *Pseudomonas aeruginosa* virulence factors and biofilms by co-encapsulation of bismuth-ethanedithiol with tobramycin in liposomes, *J Antimicrob Chemother* 65(4), 684–93, 2010.

32. Duzgunes, N., Preparation and quantitation of small unilamellar liposomes and large unila-mellar reverse-phase evaporation liposomes, *Methods Enzymol* 367, 23–7, 2003.

33. Szoka, F., Jr. and Papahadjopoulos, D., Procedure for preparation of liposomes with large inter-nal aqueous space and high capture by reverse-phase evaporation, *Proc Natl Acad Sci USA* 75(9), 4194–8, 1978.

34. Wu, P.C., Tsai, Y.H., Liao, C.C., Chang, J.S., and Huang, Y.B., The characterization and biodistri-bution of cefoxitin-loaded liposomes, *Int J Pharm* 271(1–2), 31–9, 2004.

35. Sezer, A.D., Bas, A.L., and Akbuga, J., Encapsulation of enrofloxacin in liposomes I: Preparation and in vitro characterization of LUV, *J Liposome Res* 14(1–2), 77–86, 2004.

36. Fenske, D.B., Wong, K.F., Maurer, E., Maurer, N., Leenhouts, J.M., Boman, N., Amankwa, L., and Cullis, P.R., Ionophore-mediated uptake of ciprofloxacin and vincristine into large unilamellar vesicles exhibiting transmembrane ion gradients, *Biochim Biophys Acta* 1414(1–2), 188–204, 1998.

37. Cullis, P.R., Hope, M.J., Bally, M.B., Madden, T.D., Mayer, L.D., and Fenske, D.B., Influence of pH gradients on the transbilayer transport of drugs, lipids, peptides and metal ions into large unilamellar vesicles, *Biochim Biophys Acta* 1331(2), 187–211, 1997.

38. Lasic, D.D., Ceh, B., Stuart, M.C., Guo, L., Frederik, P.M., and Barenholz, Y., Transmembrane gradient driven phase transitions within vesicles: Lessons for drug delivery, *Biochim Biophys Acta* 1239(2), 145–56, 1995.

39. Gubernator, J., Chwastek, G., Korycińska, M., Stasiuk, M., Grynkiewicz, G., Lewrick, F., Süss, R., and Kozubek, A., The encapsulation of idarubicin within liposomes using the novel EDTA ion gradient method ensures improved drug retention in vitro and *in vivo*, *J Control Release*, 146(1), 68–75, 2010.

40. Tardi, P., Choice, E., Masin, D., Redelmeier, T., Bally, M., and Madden, T.D., Liposomal encapsulation of topotecan enhances anticancer efficacy in murine and human xenograft models, *Cancer Res* 60(13), 3389–93, 2000.

41. Mozafari, M.R., Reed, C.J., Rostron, C., Kocum, C., and Piskin, E., Construction of stable anionic liposome-plasmid particles using the heating method: A preliminary investigation, *Cell Mol Biol Lett* 7(3), 923–7, 2002.

42. Otake, K., Shimomura, T., Goto, T., Imura, T., Furuya, T., Yoda, S., Takebayashi, Y., Sakai, H., and Abe, M., Preparation of liposomes using an improved supercritical reverse phase evaporation method, *Langmuir* 22(6), 2543–50, 2006.

43. Batzri, S. and Korn, E.D., Single bilayer liposomes prepared without sonication, *Biochim Biophys Acta* 298(4), 1015–9, 1973.

44. Weers, J., Metzheiser, B., Taylor, G., Warren, S., Meers, P., and Perkins, W.R., A gamma scintigraphy study to investigate lung deposition and clearance of inhaled amikacin-loaded liposomes in healthy male volunteers, *J Aerosol Med Pulm Drug Deliv* 22(2), 131–8, 2009.

45. Meers, P., Neville, M., Malinin, V., Scotto, A.W., Sardaryan, G., Kurumunda, R., Mackinson, C., James, G., Fisher, S., and Perkins, W.R., Biofilm penetration, triggered release and in vivo activity of inhaled liposomal amikacin in chronic *Pseudomonas aeruginosa* lung infections, *J Antimicrob Chemother* 61(4), 859–68, 2008.

46. Colas, J.C., Shi, W., Rao, V.S., Omri, A., Mozafari, M.R., and Singh, H., Microscopical investigations of nisin-loaded nanoliposomes prepared by Mozafari method and their bacterial targeting, *Micron* 38(8), 841–7, 2007.

47. Mozafari, M.R., Nanoliposomes: Preparation and analysis, *Methods Mol Biol* 605, 29–50, 2010.

48. Otake, K., Shimomura, T., Goto, T., Imura, T., Furuya, T., Yoda, S., Takebayashi, Y., Sakai, H., and Abe, M., One-step preparation of chitosan-coated cationic liposomes by an improved supercritical reverse-phase evaporation method, *Langmuir* 22(9), 4054–9, 2006

49. Wagner, A., Vorauer-Uhl, K., Kreismayr, G., and Katinger, H., The crossflow injection technique: An improvement of the ethanol injection method, *J Liposome Res* 12(3), 259–70, 2002.

50. Maitani, Y., Soeda, H., Junping, W., and Takayama, K., Modified ethanol injection method for liposomes containing beta-Sitosterol beta-D-Glucoside, *J Liposome Res* 11(1), 115–25, 2001.

51. Briones, E., Colino, C.I., and Lanao, J.M., Delivery systems to increase the selectivity of antibiotics in phagocytic cells, *J Control Release* 125(3), 210–27, 2008.

52. Abraham, A.M. and Walubo, A., The effect of surface charge on the disposition of liposome-encapsulated gentamicin to the rat liver, brain, lungs and kidneys after intraperitoneal administration, *Int J Antimicrob Agents* 25(5), 392–7, 2005.

53. Smistad, G., Jacobsen, J., and Sande, S.A., Multivariate toxicity screening of liposomal formulations on a human buccal cell line, *Int J Pharm* 330(1–2), 14–22, 2007.

54. Tikhonov, S.N., Rotov, K.A., Khrapova, N.P., Alekseev, V.V., Snatenkov, E.A., Zamarin, A.A., and Simakova, N.A., Effect of liposomal tetracycline hydrochloride on enzymatic function of the liver, *Bull Exp Biol Med* 145(4), 443–5, 2008.

55. Anderson, M., Paradis, C., and Omri, A., Disposition of ^{3}H-cholesteryl ether labeled liposomes following intravenous administration to mice: Comparison with an encapsulated ^{14}C-inulin as aqueous phase marker, *Drug Deliv* 10(3), 193–200, 2008.

56. Marier, J.F., Brazier, J.L., Lavigne, J., and Ducharme, M.P., Liposomal tobramycin against pulmonary infections of *Pseudomonas aeruginosa*: A pharmacokinetic and efficacy study following single and multiple intratracheal administrations in rats, *J Antimicrob Chemother* 52(2), 247–52, 2003.

57. Marier, J.F., Lavigne, J., and Ducharme, M.P., Pharmacokinetics and efficacies of liposomal and conventional formulations of tobramycin after intratracheal administration in rats with pulmonary *Burkholderia cepacia* infection, *Antimicrob Agents Chemother* 46(12), 3776–81, 2002.
58. Omri, A., Suntres, Z.E., and Shek, P.N., Enhanced activity of liposomal polymyxin B against *Pseudomonas aeruginosa* in a rat model of lung infection, *Biochem Pharmacol* 64(9), 1407–13, 2002.
59. Alipour, M., Halwani, M., Omri, A., and Suntres, Z.E., Antimicrobial effectiveness of liposomal polymyxin B against resistant Gram-negative bacterial strains, *Int J Pharm* 355(1–2), 293–8, 2008.
60. Alipour, M., Suntres, Z.E., Halwani, M., Azghani, A.O., and Omri, A., Activity and interactions of liposomal antibiotics in presence of polyanions and sputum of patients with cystic fibrosis, *PLoS One* 4(5), e5724, 2009.
61. Alipour, M., Suntres, Z.E., and Omri, A., Importance of DNase and alginate lyase for enhancing free and liposome encapsulated aminoglycoside activity against *Pseudomonas aeruginosa*, *J Antimicrob Chemother* 64(2), 317–25, 2009.
62. Halwani, M., Mugabe, C., Azghani, A.O., Lafrenie, R.M., Kumar, A., and Omri, A., Bactericidal efficacy of liposomal aminoglycosides against *Burkholderia cenocepacia*, *J Antimicrob Chemother* 60(4), 760–9, 2007.
63. Halwani, M., Yebio, B., Suntres, Z.E., Alipour, M., Azghani, A.O., and Omri, A., Co-encapsulation of gallium with gentamicin in liposomes enhances antimicrobial activity of gentamicin against *Pseudomonas aeruginosa*, *J Antimicrob Chemother* 62(6), 1291–7, 2008.
64. Jia, Y., Joly, H., and Omri, A., Characterization of the interaction between liposomal formulations and *Pseudomonas aeruginosa*, *J Liposome Res* 20(2), 134–46, 2010.
65. Mugabe, C., Azghani, A.O., and Omri, A., Liposome-mediated gentamicin delivery: Development and activity against resistant strains of *Pseudomonas aeruginosa* isolated from cystic fibrosis patients, *J Antimicrob Chemother* 55(2), 269–71, 2005.
66. Mugabe, C., Halwani, M., Azghani, A.O., Lafrenie, R.M., and Omri, A., Mechanism of enhanced activity of liposome-entrapped aminoglycosides against resistant strains of *Pseudomonas aeruginosa*, *Antimicrob Agents Chemother* 50(6), 2016–22, 2006.
67. Rukholm, G., Mugabe, C., Azghani, A.O., and Omri, A., Antibacterial activity of liposomal gentamicin against *Pseudomonas aeruginosa*: A time-kill study, *Int J Antimicrob Agents* 27(3), 247–52, 2006.
68. Campbell, P.I., Toxicity of some charged lipids used in liposome preparations, *Cytobios* 37(145), 21–6, 1983.
69. Goodman, C.M., McCusker, C.D., Yilmaz, T., and Rotello, V.M., Toxicity of gold nanoparticles functionalized with cationic and anionic side chains, *Bioconjug Chem* 15(4), 897–900, 2004.
70. Sanders, N.N., Van Rompaey, E., De Smedt, S.C., and Demeester, J., On the transport of lipoplexes through cystic fibrosis sputum, *Pharm Res* 19(4), 451–6, 2002.
71. Drulis-Kawa, Z., Dorotkiewicz-Jach, A., Gubernator, J., Gula, G., Bocer, T., and Doroszkiewicz, W., The interaction between *Pseudomonas aeruginosa* cells and cationic PC:Chol:DOTAP liposomal vesicles versus outer-membrane structure and envelope properties of bacterial cell, *Int J Pharm* 367(1–2), 211–9, 2009.
72. Davies, M., Stewart-Tull, D.E., and Jackson, D.M., The binding of lipopolysaccharide from *Escherichia coli* to mammalian cell membranes and its effect on liposomes, *Biochim Biophys Acta* 508(2), 260–76, 1978.
73. Furneri, P.M., Fresta, M., Puglisi, G., and Tempera, G., Ofloxacin-loaded liposomes: In vitro activity and drug accumulation in bacteria, *Antimicrob Agents Chemother* 44(9), 2458–64, 2000.
74. Pasquardini, L., Lunelli, L., Vanzetti, L., Anderle, M., and Pederzolli, C., Immobilization of cationic rifampicin-loaded liposomes on polystyrene for drug-delivery applications, *Colloids Surf B Biointerf* 62(2), 265–72, 2008.
75. Kim, H.J. and Jones, M.N., The delivery of benzyl penicillin to *Staphylococcus aureus* biofilms by use of liposomes, *J Liposome Res* 14(3–4), 123–39, 2004.
76. Hui, T., Yongqing, X., Tiane, Z., Gang, L., Yonggang, Y., Muyao, J., Jun, L., and Jing, D., Treatment of osteomyelitis by liposomal gentamicin-impregnated calcium sulfate, *Arch Orthop Trauma Surg* 129(10), 1301–8, 2009.

77. Kadry, A.A., Al-Suwayeh, S.A., Abd-Allah, A.R., and Bayomi, M.A., Treatment of experimental osteomyelitis by liposomal antibiotics, *J Antimicrob Chemother* 54(6), 1103–8, 2004.
78. Catuogno, C. and Jones, M.N., The antibacterial properties of solid supported liposomes on *Streptococcus oralis* biofilms, *Int J Pharm* 257(1–2), 125–40, 2003.
79. Anderson, K.E., Eliot, L.A., Stevenson, B.R., and Rogers, J.A., Formulation and evaluation of a folic acid receptor-targeted oral vancomycin liposomal dosage form, *Pharm Res* 18(3), 316–22, 2001.
80. Beaulac, C., Sachetelli, S., and Lagace, J., Aerosolization of low phase transition temperature liposomal tobramycin as a dry powder in an animal model of chronic pulmonary infection caused by *Pseudomonas aeruginosa*, *J Drug Target* 7(1), 33–41, 1999.
81. Sachetelli, S., Khalil, H., Chen, T., Beaulac, C., Sénéchal, S., and Lagacé J., Demonstration of a fusion mechanism between a fluid bactericidal liposomal formulation and bacterial cells, *Biochim Biophys Acta* 1463(2), 254–66, 2000.
82. Drulis-Kawa, Z., Gubernator, J., Dorotkiewicz-Jach, A., Doroszkiewicz, W., and Kozubek, A., A comparison of the in vitro antimicrobial activity of liposomes containing meropenem and gentamicin, *Cell Mol Biol Lett* 11(3), 360–75, 2006.
83. Drulis-Kawa, Z., Gubernator, J., Dorotkiewicz-Jach, A., Doroszkiewicz, W., and Kozubek, A., In vitro antimicrobial activity of liposomal meropenem against *Pseudomonas aeruginosa* strains, *Int J Pharm* 315(1–2), 59–66, 2006.
84. Changsan, N., Nilkaeo, A., Pungrassami, P., and Srichana, T., Monitoring safety of liposomes containing rifampicin on respiratory cell lines and in vitro efficacy against *Mycobacterium bovis* in alveolar macrophages, *J Drug Target* 17(10), 751–62, 2009.
85. Vyas, S.P., Kannan, M.E., Jain, S., Mishra, V., and Singh, P., Design of liposomal aerosols for improved delivery of rifampicin to alveolar macrophages, *Int J Pharm* 269(1), 37–49, 2004.
86. El-Ridy, M.S., Mostafa, D.M., Shehab, A., Nasr, E.A., and Abd El-Alim, S., Biological evaluation of pyrazinamide liposomes for treatment of *Mycobacterium tuberculosis*, *Int J Pharm* 330(1–2), 82–8, 2007.
87. Vyas, S.P., Sihorkar, V., and Jain, S., Mannosylated liposomes for bio-film targeting, *Int J Pharm* 330(1–2), 6–13, 2007.
88. Robinson, A.M., Creeth, J.E., and Jones, M.N., The use of immunoliposomes for specific delivery of antimicrobial agents to oral bacteria immobilized on polystyrene, *J Biomater Sci Polym Ed* 11(12), 1381–93, 2000.
89. Robinson, A.M., Creeth, J.E., and Jones, M.N., Adsorption of immunoliposomes to bacterial biofilms, *Biochem Soc Trans* 23(4), 583S, 1995.
90. Robinson, A.M., Creeth, J.E., and Jones, M.N., The specificity and affinity of immunoliposome targeting to oral bacteria, *Biochim Biophys Acta* 1369(2), 278–86, 1998.
91. Vyas, S.P., Sihorkar, V., and Dubey, P.K., Preparation, characterization and in vitro antimicrobial activity of metronidazole bearing lectinized liposomes for intra-periodontal pocket delivery, *Pharmazie* 56(7), 554–60, 2001.
92. Zaru, M., Manca, M.L., Fadda, A.M., and Antimisiaris, S.G., Chitosan-coated liposomes for delivery to lungs by nebulisation, *Colloids Surf B Biointerf* 71(1), 88–95, 2009.
93. Bardonnet, P.L., Faivre, V., Boullanger, P., Ollivon, M., and Falson, F., Glycosylated liposomes against *Helicobacter pylori*: Behavior in acidic conditions, *Biochem Biophys Res Commun* 383(1), 48–53, 2009.
94. Bardonnet, P.L., Faivre, V., Boullanger, P., Piffaretti, J.C., and Falson, F., Pre-formulation of liposomes against *Helicobacter pylori*: Characterization and interaction with the bacteria, *Eur J Pharm Biopharm* 69(3), 908–22, 2008.
95. Wijagkanalan, W., Kawakami, S., Takenaga, M., Igarashi, R., Yamashita, F., and Hashida, M., Efficient targeting to alveolar macrophages by intratracheal administration of mannosylated liposomes in rats, *J Control Release* 125(2), 121–30, 2008.
96. Huang, Z., Jaafari, M.R., and Szoka, F.C., Jr., Disterolphospholipids: Nonexchangeable lipids and their application to liposomal drug delivery, *Angew Chem Int Ed Engl* 48(23), 4146–9, 2009.

97. Simões, S., Moreira, J.N., Fonseca, C., Düzgüneş, N., and de Lima, M.C., On the formulation of pH-sensitive liposomes with long circulation times, *Adv Drug Deliv Rev* 56(7), 947–65, 2004.

98. Simões, S., Slepushkin, V., Düzgüneş, N., and Pedroso de Lima, M.C., On the mechanisms of internalization and intracellular delivery mediated by pH-sensitive liposomes, *Biochim Biophys Acta* 1515(1), 23–37, 2001.

99. Slepushkin, V., Simões, S., de Lima, M.C., and Düzgüneş, N., Sterically stabilized pH-sensitive liposomes, *Methods Enzymol* 387, 134–47, 2004.

100. Slepushkin, V.A., Simões, S., Dazin, P., Newman, M.S., Guo, L.S., Pedroso de Lima, M.C., and Düzgüneş, N., Sterically stabilized pH-sensitive liposomes. Intracellular delivery of aqueous contents and prolonged circulation *in vivo*, *J Biol Chem* 272(4), 2382–8, 1997.

101. Cordeiro, C., Wiseman, D.J., Lutwyche, P., Uh, M., Evans, J.C., Finlay, B.B., and Webb, M.S., Antibacterial efficacy of gentamicin encapsulated in pH-sensitive liposomes against an in vivo *Salmonella enterica* serovar typhimurium intracellular infection model, *Antimicrob Agents Chemother* 44(3), 533–9, 2000.

102. Lutwyche, P., Cordeiro, C., Wiseman, D.J., St-Louis, M., Uh, M., Hope, M.J., Webb, M.S., and Finlay, B.B., Intracellular delivery and antibacterial activity of gentamicin encapsulated in pH-sensitive liposomes, *Antimicrob Agents Chemother* 42(10), 2511–20, 1998.

103. Schiffelers, R., Storm, G., and Bakker-Woudenberg, I., Liposome-encapsulated aminoglycosides in pre-clinical and clinical studies, *J Antimicrob Chemother* 48(3), 333–44, 2001.

104. Awasthi, V.D., Garcia, D., Klipper, R., Goins, B.A., and Phillips, W.T., Neutral and anionic liposome-encapsulated hemoglobin: Effect of postinserted poly(ethylene glycol)-distearoylphosphatidylethanolamine on distribution and circulation kinetics, *J Pharmacol Exp Ther* 309(1), 241–8, 2004.

105. Bakker-Woudenberg, I.A., Schiffelers, R.M., Storm, G., Becker, M.J., and Guo, L., Long-circulating sterically stabilized liposomes in the treatment of infections, *Methods Enzymol* 391, 228–60, 2005.

106. Moribe, K. and Maruyama, K., Pharmaceutical design of the liposomal antimicrobial agents for infectious disease, *Curr Pharm Des* 8(6), 441–54, 2002.

107. Bakker-Woudenberg, I.A., Long-circulating sterically stabilized liposomes as carriers of agents for treatment of infection or for imaging infectious foci, *Int J Antimicrob Agents* 19(4), 299–311, 2002.

108. Bakker-Woudenberg, I.A., ten Kate, M.T., Guo, L., Working, P., and Mouton, J.W., Improved efficacy of ciprofloxacin administered in polyethylene glycol-coated liposomes for treatment of *Klebsiella pneumoniae* pneumonia in rats, *Antimicrob Agents Chemother* 45(5), 1487–92, 2001.

109. Deol, P. and Khuller, G.K., Lung specific stealth liposomes: Stability, biodistribution and toxicity of liposomal antitubercular drugs in mice, *Biochim Biophys Acta* 1334(2–3), 161–72, 1997.

110. Bakker-Woudenberg, I.A., ten Kate, M.T., Guo, L., Working, P., and Mouton, J.W., Ciprofloxacin in polyethylene glycol-coated liposomes: Efficacy in rat models of acute or chronic *Pseudomonas aeruginosa* infection, *Antimicrob Agents Chemother* 46(8), 2575–81, 2002.

111. Schiffelers, R.M., Bakker-Woudenberg, I.A., Snijders, S.V., and Storm, G., Localization of sterically stabilized liposomes in *Klebsiella pneumoniae*-infected rat lung tissue: Influence of liposome characteristics, *Biochim Biophys Acta* 1421(2), 329–39, 1999.

112. Schiffelers, R.M., Bakker-Woudenberg, I.A., and Storm, G., Localization of sterically stabilized liposomes in experimental rat *Klebsiella pneumoniae* pneumonia: Dependence on circulation kinetics and presence of poly(ethylene)glycol coating, *Biochim Biophys Acta* 1468(1–2), 253–61, 2000.

113. Schiffelers, R.M., Storm, G., and Bakker-Woudenberg, I.A., Therapeutic efficacy of liposomal gentamicin in clinically relevant rat models, *Int J Pharm* 214(1–2), 103–5, 2001.

114. Schiffelers, R.M., Storm, G., ten Kate, M.T., and Bakker-Woudenberg, I.A., Therapeutic efficacy of liposome-encapsulated gentamicin in rat *Klebsiella pneumoniae* pneumonia in relation to impaired host defense and low bacterial susceptibility to gentamicin, *Antimicrob Agents Chemother* 45(2), 464–70, 2001.

115. Schiffelers, R.M., Storm, G., ten Kate, M.T., Stearne-Cullen, L.E., den Hollander, J.G., Verbrugh, H.A., and Bakker-Woudenberg, I.A., In vivo synergistic interaction of liposome-coencapsulated gentamicin and ceftazidime, *J Pharmacol Exp Ther* 298(1), 369–75, 2001.

116. Ellbogen, M.H., Olsen, K.M., Gentry-Nielsen, M.J., and Preheim, L.C., Efficacy of liposome-encapsulated ciprofloxacin compared with ciprofloxacin and ceftriaxone in a rat model of pneumococcal pneumonia, *J Antimicrob Chemother* 51(1), 83–91, 2003.

117. Labana, S., Pandey, R., Sharma, S., and Khuller, G.K., Chemotherapeutic activity against murine tuberculosis of once weekly administered drugs (isoniazid and rifampicin) encapsulated in liposomes, *Int J Antimicrob Agents* 20(4), 301–4, 2002.

118. de Steenwinkel, J.E., van Vianen, W., Ten Kate, M.T., Verbrugh, H.A., van Agtmael, M.A., Schiffelers, R.M., and Bakker-Woudenberg, I.A., Targeted drug delivery to enhance efficacy and shorten treatment duration in disseminated *Mycobacterium avium* infection in mice, *J Antimicrob Chemother* 60(5), 1064–73, 2007.

119. Sadzuka, Y., Hirota, S., and Sonobe, T., Intraperitoneal administration of doxorubicin encapsulating liposomes against peritoneal dissemination, *Toxicol Lett* 116(1–2), 51–9, 2000.

120. Cabanes, A., Tzemach, D., Goren, D., Horowitz, A.T., and Gabizon, A., Comparative study of the antitumor activity of free doxorubicin and polyethylene glycol-coated liposomal doxorubicin in a mouse lymphoma model, *Clin Cancer Res* 4(2), 499–505, 1998.

121. Elmas, M., Yazar, E., Baş, A.L., Traş, B., Bayezit, M., and Yapar, K., Comparative pharmacokinetics of enrofloxacin and tissue concentrations of parent drug and ciprofloxacin after intramuscular administrations of free and liposome-encapsulated enrofloxacin in rabbits, *J Vet Med B Infect Dis Vet Public Health* 49(10), 507–12, 2002.

122. Cabanes, A., Reig, F., Garcia-Anton, J.M., and Arboix, M. Evaluation of free and liposome-encapsulated gentamycin for intramuscular sustained release in rabbits, *Res Vet Sci* 64(3), 213–7, 1998.

123. Gaviani, P., Silvani, A., Corsini, E., Erbetta, A., and Salmaggi, A., Neoplastic meningitis from breast carcinoma with complete response to liposomal cytarabine: Case report, *Neurol Sci* 30(3), 251–4, 2009.

124. Pacira Pharmaceuticals Inc, DepoCyt therapy in patients with neoplastic meningitis from lymphoma or a solid tumor. Last accessed November 1, 2011. Available from: http://www.clinicaltrial.gov/ct2/results?term=NCT00029523

125. Gaudana, R., Jwala, J., Boddu, S.H., and Mitra, A.K., Recent perspectives in ocular drug delivery, *Pharm Res* 26(5), 1197–216, 2009.

126. Janoria, K.G., Gunda, S., Boddu, S.H., and Mitra, A.K., Novel approaches to retinal drug delivery, *Expert Opin Drug Deliv* 4(4), 371–88, 2007.

127. Frucht-Perry, J., Assil, K.K., Ziegler, E., Douglas, H., Brown, S.I., Schanzlin, D.J., and Weinreb, R.N., Fibrin-enmeshed tobramycin liposomes: Single application topical therapy of *Pseudomonas keratitis*, *Cornea* 11(5), 393–7, 1992.

128. Zeng, S., Hu, C., Wei, H., Lu, Y., Zhang, Y., Yang, J., Yun, G., Zou, W., and Song, B., Intravitreal pharmacokinetics of liposome-encapsulated amikacin in a rabbit model, *Ophthalmology* 100(11), 1640–4, 1993.

129. Pandey, R., Sharma, S., and Khuller, G.K., Lung specific stealth liposomes as antitubercular drug carriers in guinea pigs, *Ind J Exp Biol* 42(6), 562–6, 2004.

130. Castro, G.A. and Ferreira, L.A., Novel vesicular and particulate drug delivery systems for topical treatment of acne, *Expert Opin Drug Deliv* 5(6), 665–79, 2008.

131. Danion, A., Arsenault, I., and Vermette, P., Antibacterial activity of contact lenses bearing surface-immobilized layers of intact liposomes loaded with levofloxacin, *J Pharm Sci* 96(9), 2350–63, 2007.

132. Jaafari, M.R., Bavarsad, N., Bazzaz, B.S., Samiei, A., Soroush, D., Ghorbani, S., Heravi, M.M., and Khamesipour, A., Effect of topical liposomes containing paromomycin sulfate in the course of *Leishmania major* infection in susceptible BALB/c mice, *Antimicrob Agents Chemother* 53(6), 2259–65, 2009.

133. Shanmugam, S., Song, C.K., Nagayya-Sriraman, S., Baskaran, R., Yong, C.S., Choi, H.G., Kim, D.D., Woo, J.S., and Yoo, B.K., Physicochemical characterization and skin permeation of liposome formulations containing clindamycin phosphate, *Arch Pharm Res* 32(7), 1067–75, 2009.

134. Amin, K., Riddle, C.C., Aires, D.J., and Schweiger, E.S., Common and alternate oral antibiotic therapies for acne vulgaris: A review. *J Drugs Dermatol* 6(9), 873–80, 2007.
135. Honzak, L. and Sentjurc, M., Development of liposome encapsulated clindamycin for treatment of acne vulgaris, *Pflugers Arch* 440(5 Suppl), R44–5, 2000.
136. Ling, S.S., Magosso, E., Khan, N.A., Yuen, K.H., and Barker, S.A., Enhanced oral bioavailability and intestinal lymphatic transport of a hydrophilic drug using liposomes, *Drug Dev Ind Pharm* 32(3), 335–45, 2006.
137. Chono, S., Tanino, T., Seki, T., and Morimoto, K., Efficient drug delivery to alveolar macrophages and lung epithelial lining fluid following pulmonary administration of liposomal ciprofloxacin in rats with pneumonia and estimation of its antibacterial effects, *Drug Dev Ind Pharm* 34(10), 1090–6, 2008.
138. Misra, A., Jinturkar, K., Patel, D., Lalani, J., and Chougule, M., Recent advances in liposomal dry powder formulations: Preparation and evaluation, *Expert Opin Drug Deliv* 6(1), 71–89, 2009.
139. Aradigm Corporation, Evaluation of ciprofloxacin for inhalation to cystic fibrosis patients with *P. aeruginosa*. Available from: http://www.clinicaltrial.gov/ct2/results?term=NCT01090908. (accessed November 1, 2011).
140. Transave, Multidose safety and tolerability study of dose escalation of liposomal amikacin for inhalation (ARIKACE™). Available from: http://www.clinicaltrial.gov/ct2/results?term=NCT00777296 (accessed November 1, 2011).
141. Transave, Multidose safety and tolerability study of (arikace™) for inhalation in cystic fibrosis patients. Available from: http://www.clinicaltrial.gov/ct2/results?term=NCT00558844 (accessed November 1, 2011).
142. Aradigm Corporation, Safety and efficacy study of ciprofloxacin for inhalation in patients with non-cystic fibrosis bronchiectasis "ORBIT-1". Available from: http://www.clinicaltrial.gov/ct2/results?term=NCT00889967 (accessed November 1, 2011).
143. Transave, A study to determine the safety and tolerability of Arikace™ versus placebo in patients who have bronchiectasis. Available from: http://www.clinicaltrial.gov/ct2/results?term=NCT00775138 (accessed November 1, 2011).
144. Chimote, G. and Banerjee, R., Evaluation of antitubercular drug-loaded surfactants as inhalable drug-delivery systems for pulmonary tuberculosis, *J Biomed Mater Res A* 89(2), 281–92, 2009.
145. Justo, O.R. and Moraes, A.M., Incorporation of antibiotics in liposomes designed for tuberculosis therapy by inhalation, *Drug Deliv* 10(3), 201–7, 2003.
146. Fielding, R.M., Moon-McDermott, L., Lewis, R.O., and Horner, M.J., Pharmacokinetics and urinary excretion of amikacin in low-clearance unilamellar liposomes after a single or repeated intravenous administration in the rhesus monkey, *Antimicrob Agents Chemother* 43(3), 503–9, 1999.
147. Abeylath, S.C. and Turos, E., Drug delivery approaches to overcome bacterial resistance to beta-lactam antibiotics, *Expert Opin Drug Deliv* 5(9), 931–49, 2008.
148. Petrosillo, N., Capone, A., Di Bella, S., and Taglietti, F., Management of antibiotic resistance in the intensive care unit setting, *Expert Rev Anti Infect Ther* 8(3), 289–302, 2010.
149. Nitzan, Y., Deutsch, E.B., and Pechatnikov, I., Diffusion of beta-lactam antibiotics through oligomeric or monomeric porin channels of some gram-negative bacteria, *Curr Microbiol* 45(6), 446–55, 2002.
150. Weiner, D.J., Bucki, R., and Janmey, P.A., The antimicrobial activity of the cathelicidin LL37 is inhibited by F-actin bundles and restored by gelsolin, *Am J Resp Cell Mol Biol* 28(6), 738–45, 2003.
151. Sanders, N.N., De Smedt, S.C., Van Rompaey, E., Simoens, P., De Baets, F., and Demeester, J., Cystic fibrosis sputum: A barrier to the transport of nanospheres, *Am J Resp Crit Care Med* 162(5), 1905–11, 2000.
152. Broughton-Head, V.J., Smith, J.R., Shur, J., Shute, J.K., Actin limits enhancement of nanoparticle diffusion through cystic fibrosis sputum by mucolytics, *Pulm Pharmacol Ther* 20(6), 708–17, 2007.
153. Alkawash, M.A., Soothill, J.S., and Schiller, N.L., Alginate lyase enhances antibiotic killing of mucoid *Pseudomonas aeruginosa* in biofilms, *APMIS* 114(2), 131–8, 2006.

154. Okusanya, O.O., Bhavnani, S.M., Hammel, J., Minic, P., Dupont, L.J., Forrest, A., Mulder, G.J., Mackinson, C., Ambrose, P.G., and Gupta R., Pharmacokinetic and pharmacodynamic evaluation of liposomal amikacin for inhalation in cystic fibrosis patients with chronic pseudomonal infection, *Antimicrob Agents Chemother* 53(9), 3847–54, 2009.

155. Wang, D., Kong, L., Wang, J., He, X., Li, X., and Xiao, Y., Polymyxin E sulfate-loaded liposome for intravenous use: Preparation, lyophilization, and toxicity assessment *in vivo*, *PDA J Pharm Sci Technol* 63(2), 159–67, 2009.

156. Gamazo, C., Prior, S., Concepción Lecároz, M., Vitas, A.I., Campanero, M.A., Pérez, G., Gonzalez, D., and Blanco-Prieto, M.J., Biodegradable gentamicin delivery systems for parenteral use for the treatment of intracellular bacterial infections, *Expert Opin Drug Deliv* 4(6), 677–88, 2007.

157. Pandey, R. and Khuller, G.K., Antitubercular inhaled therapy: Opportunities, progress and challenges, *J Antimicrob Chemother* 55(4), 430–5, 2005.

158. Zaru, M., Sinico, C., De Logu, A., Caddeo, C., Lai, F., Manca, M.L., and Fadda, A.M., Rifampicin-loaded liposomes for the passive targeting to alveolar macrophages: In vitro and in vivo evaluation, *J Liposome Res* 19(1), 68–76, 2009.

159. Kurahashi, K., Sawa, T., Ota, M., Kajikawa, O., Hong, K., Martin, T.R., and Wiener-Kronish, J.P., Depletion of phagocytes in the reticuloendothelial system causes increased inflammation and mortality in rabbits with *Pseudomonas aeruginosa* pneumonia, *Am J Physiol Lung Cell Mol Physiol* 296(2), L198–209, 2009.

160. Nakamura, T., Abu-Dahab, R., Menger, M.D., Schäfer, U., Vollmar, B., Wada, H., Lehr, C.M., and Schäfers, H.J., Depletion of alveolar macrophages by clodronate-liposomes aggravates ischemia-reperfusion injury of the lung, *J Heart Lung Transplant* 24(1), 38–45, 2005.

161. Lira, M.C., Siqueira-Moura, M.P., Rolim-Santos, H.M., Galetti, F.C., Simioni, A.R., Santos, N.P., Tabosa Do Egito, E.S., Silva, C.L., Tedesco, A.C., and Santos-Magalhães, N.S., In vitro uptake and antimycobacterial activity of liposomal usnic acid formulation, *J Liposome Res* 19(1), 49–58, 2009.

162. Azarmi, S., Roa, W.H., and Löbenberg, R., Targeted delivery of nanoparticles for the treatment of lung diseases, *Adv Drug Deliv Rev* 60(8), 863–75, 2008.

163. Stensrud, G., Passi, S., Larsen, T., Sandset, P.M., Smistad, G., Mönkkönen, J., and Karlsen, J., Toxicity of gamma irradiated liposomes. 1, in vitro interactions with blood components, *Int J Pharm* 178(1), 33–46, 1999.

164. Whitehead, T.C., Lovering, A.M., Cropley, I.M., Wade, P., and Davidson, R.N., Kinetics and toxicity of liposomal and conventional amikacin in a patient with multidrug-resistant tuberculosis, *Eur J Clin Microbiol Infect Dis* 17(11), 794–7, 1998.

165. Jones, A.P. and Wallis, C., Dornase alfa for cystic fibrosis, *Cochrane Database Sys* 17(3), CD001127, 2010.

166. Bonestroo, H.J., Slieker, M.G., and Arets, H.G., No positive effect of rhdnase on the pulmonary colonization in children with cystic fibrosis, *Monaldi Arch Chest Dis* 73(1), 12–7, 2010.

167. Gaspar, M.M., Cruz, A., Penha, A.F., Reymão, J., Sousa, A.C., Eleutério, C.V., Domingues, S.A., Fraga, A.G., Filho, A.L., Cruz, M.E., and Pedrosa, J., Rifabutin encapsulated in liposomes exhibits increased therapeutic activity in a model of disseminated tuberculosis, *Int J Antimicrob Agents* 31(1), 37–45, 2008.

168. Dhillon, J., Fielding, R., Adler-Moore, J., Goodall, R.L., and Mitchison, D., The activity of low-clearance liposomal amikacin in experimental murine tuberculosis, *J Antimicrob Chemother* 48(6), 869–76, 2001.

169. Lewis, K., Persister cells, *Ann Rev Microbiol* 64, 357–72, 2010.

170. Høiby, N., Bjarnsholt, T., Givskov, M., Molin, S., and Ciofu, O., Antibiotic resistance of bacterial biofilms, *Int J Antimicrob Agents* 35(4), 322–32, 2010.

171. Stensrud, G., Mönkkönen, J., and Karlsen, J., Toxicity of gamma irradiated liposomes. 2, in vitro effects on cells in culture, *Int J Pharm* 178(1), 47–53, 1999.

172. Filion, M.C. and Phillips, N.C., Toxicity and immunomodulatory activity of liposomal vectors formulated with cationic lipids toward immune effector cells, *Biochim Biophys Acta* 1329(2), 345–56, 1997.

173. Berrocal, M.C., Buján, J., García-Honduvilla, N., and Abeger, A., Comparison of the effects of dimyristoyl and soya phosphatidylcholine liposomes on human fibroblasts, _Drug Deliv_ 7(1), 37–44, 2000.

174. Peyman, G.A., Charles, H.C., Liu, K.R., Khoobehi, B., and Niesman, M., Intravitreal liposome-encapsulated drugs: A preliminary human report. _Int Ophthalmol_ 12(3), 175–82, 1988.

175. Nightingale, S.D., Saletan, S.L., Swenson, C.E., Lawrence, A.J., Watson, D.A., Pilkiewicz, F.G., Silverman, E.G., and Cal, S.X., Liposome-encapsulated gentamicin treatment of _Mycobacterium avium-Mycobacterium intracellulare_ complex bacteremia in AIDS patients, _Antimicrob Agents Chemother_ 37(9), 1869–72, 1993.

176. Wiley, E.L., Perry, A., Nightingale, S.D., and Lawrence, J., Detection of _Mycobacterium avium-intracellulare_ complex in bone marrow specimens of patients with acquired immunodeficiency syndrome, _Am J Clin Pathol_ 101(4), 446–51, 1994.

177. Fluidosomes™ (fluid liposomes), Available from: http://www.axentispharma.com/ (accessed November 1, 2011).

178. Blyth, C.C., Hale, K., Palasanthiran, P., O'Brien, T., and Bennett, M.H., Antifungal therapy in infants and children with proven, probable or suspected invasive fungal infections, _Cochrane Database Sys Rev_ 17(2), CD006343, 2010.

179. Moen, M.D., Lyseng-Williamson, K.A., and Scott, L.J., Liposomal amphotericin B: A review of its use as empirical therapy in febrile neutropenia and in the treatment of invasive fungal infections. _Drugs_ 69(3), 361–92, 2009.

180. Cagnoni, P.J., Liposomal amphotericin B versus conventional amphotericin B in the empirical treatment of persistently febrile neutropenic patients, _J Antimicrob Chemother_ 49 Suppl 1, 81–6, 2002.

181. Cagnoni, P.J., Walsh, T.J., Prendergast, M.M., Bodensteiner, D., Hiemenz, S., Greenberg, R.N., Arndt, C.A., Schuster, M., Seibel, N., Yeldandi, V., and Tong, K.B., Pharmacoeconomic analysis of liposomal amphotericin B versus conventional amphotericin B in the empirical treatment of persistently febrile neutropenic patients, _J Clin Oncol_ 18(12), 2476–83, 2000.

182. Subirà, M., Martino, R., Gómez, L., Martí, J.M., Estany, C., and Sierra, J., Low-dose amphotericin B lipid complex vs. conventional amphotericin B for empirical antifungal therapy of neutropenic fever in patients with hematologic malignancies—a randomized, controlled trial, _Eur J Haematol_ 72(5), 342–7, 2004.

183. Shaheed Surhawardy Medical College and Hospital, Drugs for neglected diseases. Phase III, Study of three short course combination regimens (AmBisome®, Miltefosine, Paromomycin) compared with AmBisome® alone for the treatment of visceral leishmaniasis in Bangladesh. Available from: http://www.clinicaltrial.gov/ct2/results?term=NCT01122771 (accessed November 1, 2011).

184. Arikan, S. and Rex, J.H., Nystatin LF (Aronex/Abbott), _Curr Opin Investig Drugs_ 2(4), 488–95, 2001.

185. Groll, A.H., Mickiene, D., Petraitis, V., Petraitiene, R., Alfaro, R.M., King, C., Piscitelli, S.C., and Walsh, T.J., Comparative drug disposition, urinary pharmacokinetics, and renal effects of multilamellar liposomal nystatin and amphotericin B deoxycholate in rabbits, _Antimicrob Agents Chemother_ 47(12), 3917–25, 2003.

186. Aronex Pharmaceuticals, National Cancer Institute. Antifungal therapy for fever and neutropenia in patients receiving treatment for hematologic cancer. Available from: http://www.clinicaltrial.gov/ct2/results?term=NCT00002742 (accessed November 1, 2011).

187. de la Fouchardière, C., Largillier, R., Goubely, Y., Hardy-Bessard, A.C., Slama, B., Cretin, J., Orfeuvre, H., Paraiso, D., Bachelot, T., and Pujade-Lauraine, E., Docetaxel and pegylated liposomal doxorubicin combination as first-line therapy for metastatic breast cancer patients: Results of the phase II GINECO trial CAPYTTOLE, _Ann Oncol_ 20(12), 1959–63, 2009.

188. Miolo, G., Baldo, P., Bidoli, E., Lombardi, D., Scalone, S., Sorio, R., and Veronesi, A., Incidence of palmar-plantar erythrodysesthesia in pretreated and unpretreated patients receiving pegylated liposomal doxorubicin, _Tumori_ 95(6), 687–90, 2009.

189. Bafaloukos, D., Linardou, H., Aravantinos, G., Papadimitriou, C., Bamias, A., Fountzilas, G., Kalofonos, H.P., Kosmidis, P., Timotheadou, E., Makatsoris, T., Samantas, E., Briasoulis, E., Christodoulou, C., Papakostas, P., Pectasides, D., and Dimopoulos, A.M., A randomized phase II study of carboplatin plus pegylated liposomal doxorubicin versus carboplatin plus paclitaxel in platinum sensitive ovarian cancer patients: A Hellenic Cooperative Oncology Group study, *BMC Med* 8, 3, 2010.

190. Trudeau, M.E., Clemons, M.J., Provencher, L., Panasci, L., Yelle, L., Rayson, D., Latreille, J., Vandenberg, T., Goel, R., Zibdawi, L., Rahim, Y., and Pouliot, J.F., Phase II multicenter trial of anthracycline rechallenge with pegylated liposomal doxorubicin plus cyclophosphamide for first-line therapy of metastatic breast cancer previously treated with adjuvant anthracyclines, *J Clin Oncol* 27(35), 5906–10, 2009.

191. Johnson & Johnson and Tibotec Therapeutics, Vincristine, DOXIL (doxorubicin HCl liposome injection) and dexamethasone vs. vincristine, doxorubicin, and dexamethasone in patients with newly diagnosed multiple myeloma. Available from: http://www.clinicaltrial.gov/ct2/results?term=NCT00344422 (accessed November 1, 2011).

192. Del Barco, S., Colomer, R., Calvo, L., Tusquets, I., Adrover, E., Sánchez, P., Rifà, J., De la Haba, J., and Virizuela, J.A., Non-pegylated liposomal doxorubicin combined with gemcitabine as first-line treatment for metastatic or locally advanced breast cancer. Final results of a phase I/II trial, *Breast Cancer Res Treat* 116(2), 351–8, 2009.

193. Batist, G., Ramakrishnan, G., Rao, C.S., Chandrasekharan, A., Gutheil, J., Guthrie, T., Shah, P., Khojasteh, A., Nair, M.K., Hoelzer, K., Tkaczuk, K., Park, Y.C., and Lee, L.W., Reduced cardiotoxicity and preserved antitumor efficacy of liposome-encapsulated doxorubicin and cyclophosphamide compared with conventional doxorubicin and cyclophosphamide in a randomized, multicenter trial of metastatic breast cancer, *J Clin Oncol* 19(5), 1444–54, 2001.

194. Theodoulou, M., Batist, G., Campos, S., Winer, E., Welles, L., and Hudis, C., Phase I study of nonpegylated liposomal doxorubicin plus trastuzumab in patients with HER2-positive breast cancer, *Clin Breast Cancer* 9(2), 101–7, 2009.

195. Catharina Ziekenhuis Eindhoven; Cephalon; Sanofi-Aventis, Liposomal doxorubicin, trastuzumab, and docetaxel in HER2 positive metastatic breast cancer (MYOHERTAX). Available from: http://www.clinicaltrial.gov/ct2/results?term=NCT00377780 (accessed November 1, 2011).

196. Petre, C.E. and Dittmer, D.P., Liposomal daunorubicin as treatment for Kaposi's sarcoma, *Int J Nanomed* 2(3), 277–88, 2007.

197. Latagliata, R., Breccia, M., Fazi, P., Iacobelli, S., Martinelli, G., Di Raimondo, F., Sborgia, M., Fabbiano, F., Pirrotta, M.T., Zaccaria, A., Amadori, S., Caramatti, C., Falzetti, F., Candoni, A., Mattei, D., Morselli, M., Alimena, G., Vignetti, M., Baccarani, M., and Mandelli, F., Liposomal daunorubicin versus standard daunorubicin: Long term follow-up of the GIMEMA GSI 103 AMLE randomized trial in patients older than 60 years with acute myelogenous leukaemia, *Br J Haematol* 143(5), 681–9, 2008.

198. Gill, P.S., Wernz, J., Scadden, D.T., Cohen, P., Mukwaya, G.M., von Roenn, J.H., Jacobs, M., Kempin, S., Silverberg, I., Gonzales, G., Rarick, M.U., Myers, A.M., Shepherd, F., Sawka, C., Pike, M.C., and Ross, M.E., Randomized phase III trial of liposomal daunorubicin versus doxorubicin, bleomycin, and vincristine in AIDS-related Kaposi's sarcoma, *J Clin Oncol* 14(8), 2353–64, 1996.

199. Mitchell, P.L., Marlton, P., Grigg, A., Seymour, J.F., Hertzberg, M., Enno, A., Herrmann, R., Bond, R., and Arthur, C., A phase II study of liposomal daunorubicin, in combination with cyclophosphamide, vincristine and prednisolone, in elderly patients with previously untreated aggressive non-Hodgkin lymphoma, *Leuk Lymphoma* 49(5), 924–31, 2008.

200. Candoni, A., Michelutti, A., Simeone, E., Damiani, D., Baccarani, M., and Fanin, R., Efficacy of liposomal daunorubicin and cytarabine as reinduction chemotherapy in relapsed acute lymphoblastic leukaemia despite expression of multidrug resistance-related proteins, *Eur J Haematol* 77(4), 293–9, 2006.

201. Bomgaars, L., Geyer, J.R., Franklin, J., Dahl, G., Park, J., Winick, N.J., Klenke, R., Berg, S.L., and Blaney, S.M., Phase I trial of intrathecal liposomal cytarabine in children with neoplastic meningitis, *J Clin Oncol* 22(19), 3916–21, 2004.
202. Phuphanich, S., Maria, B., Braeckman, R., and Chamberlain, M., A pharmacokinetic study of intra-CSF administered encapsulated cytarabine (DepoCyt) for the treatment of neoplastic meningitis in patients with leukemia, lymphoma, or solid tumors as part of a phase III study, *J Neurooncol* 81(2), 201–8, 2007.
203. Donald, P.R., Sirgel, F.A., Venter, A., Smit, E., Parkin, D.P., Van de Wal, B.W., and Mitchison, D.A., The early bactericidal activity of a low-clearance liposomal amikacin in pulmonary tuberculosis, *J Antimicrob Chemother* 48(6), 877–80, 2001.
204. Garrison, A.E., Bendele, R., Knauer, S., Wolf, J., Moon-McDermott, L., Gill, S., and Colagiovanni, D.B., Evaluating the efficacy of amikacin in low-clearance unilamellar liposomes in a *S. aureus* local infection model, *J Liposome Res* 11(2–3), 243–54, 2001.
205. Budai, L., Hajdú, M., Budai, M., Gróf, P., Béni, S., Noszál, B., Klebovich, I., and Antal, I., Gels and liposomes in optimized ocular drug delivery: Studies on ciprofloxacin formulations, *Int J Pharm* 343(1–2), 34–40, 2007.
206. Chono, S., Tanino, T., Seki, T., and Morimoto, K., Efficient drug targeting to rat alveolar macrophages by pulmonary administration of ciprofloxacin incorporated into mannosylated liposomes for treatment of respiratory intracellular parasitic infections, *J Control Release* 127(1), 50–8, 2008.
207. Liposomal ciprofloxacin, Available from: http://www.aradigm.com/ (accessed November 1, 2011).
208. Bruinenberg, P., Serisier, D., Cipolla, D., and Blanchard, J., Safety, tolerability and pharmacokinetics of novel liposomal ciprofloxacin formulations for inhalation in healthy volunteers and non-cystic bronchiectasis patients, In *American Thoracic Society International Conference. Am J Respir Crit Care Med* A3192, 2010.
209. Bilton, D., De Soyza, A., Hayward, C., and Bruinenberg, P., Effect of a 28-day course of two different doses of once a day liposomal ciprofloxacin for inhalation on sputum *Pseudomonas aeruginosa* density in non-CF bronchiectasis, *Am J Respir Crit Care Med* A3191, 2010.

13

Progress and Potential of Nanomedicine to Address Infectious Diseases of Poverty

Rose Hayeshi, Boitumelo Semete, Lonji Kalombo,
Yolandy Lemmer, Lebogang Katata, and Hulda Swai

CONTENTS

13.1 Introduction

Nanotechnology is a multidisciplinary field that encompasses the design, manipulation, characterization, production, and application of structures, devices, and systems at the nanometer scale range (~1 to 500 nm), which present unique and/or superior physicochemical properties. This diminutive scale represents the domain of atoms, molecules, and macromolecules [1]. Nanomedicine is the application of nanotechnology to the medical sciences for imaging, diagnosis, drug delivery (e.g., via nanocarriers), and therapeutics that are utilized in the treatment and prevention of diseases.

Nanomedicine has rapidly gained ground over the past several years as may be observed from the increase in the number of nanopharmaceutical patents filed (over 1000 by the year 2008) [2]. Nanomedicine-based drug delivery systems offer an enabling tool for the expansion of current drug markets as they might facilitate the reformulation of classical drugs and failed leads, resulting in improved half-life, precisely controlled release spanning short or long durations, and highly specific site-targeted delivery of therapeutic compounds. Examples of nanocarriers that are utilized in nanomedicine include nanocapsules, liposomes, dendrimers, gold nanoparticles, polymeric micelles, nanogels, and solid lipid nanoparticles, among others. This technology has successfully revolutionized therapies for diseases such as cancer and, indeed, a number of nanomedical products against cancer, such as Doxil® (liposome) and Abraxane® (albumin-bound nanoparticles), are already on the market [3]. The current robust growth in this discipline is due primarily to advances in the nanosciences toward improved approaches for molecular assembly and the design of better controlled and efficient nanomaterials.

The area of drug development experiences very low success rates with regard to drugs that compete to enter the marketplace. These insufficiencies are due to factors such as therapeutic compound toxicity, poor solubility (translating to lowered bioavailability), and thus reduced efficacy. These challenges are even more pronounced in the case of infectious diseases of poverty (IDPs) such as tuberculosis (TB), malaria, and human immunodeficiency virus (HIV). The cumulative annual global death toll from HIV/AIDS, malaria, and TB presently approaches ~6 million people. According to the World Health Organization (WHO) 2010 Global TB report, one-third of the world's population is currently infected with the pathogenic bacteria *Mycobacterium tuberculosis* (*M.tb*) and an estimated 1.7 million individuals died from TB in 2009, with the highest number of deaths occurring in Africa [4]. It has been reported that malaria remains one of the world's most prevalent infectious diseases. Forty percent of the world's population is at risk of infection, and in 2009, there were an estimated 225 million cases of malaria reported worldwide, resulting in approximately 781,000 deaths [5]. Sub-Saharan Africa continues to bear a disproportionately large share of the global HIV burden with the highest number of people living with HIV, new HIV infections, AIDS-related deaths, and the highest prevalence of adult HIV [6]. In addition, due to the weakened state and vulnerability of the immune systems of HIV/AIDS patients, the propensity for co-infection with other diseases such as TB, malaria, and leishmaniasis is beginning to gain serious attention. Apart from HIV, malaria, and TB, neglected tropical diseases (NTDs) such as leishmaniasis further affect more than 1 billion people, primarily low-income populations that reside in tropical and subtropical climates. Visceral leishmaniasis is typically fatal in the absence of treatment [7], and there are an estimated 500,000 new cases that annually affect mostly South East Asia and East Africa.

Although effective therapeutic regimens against these diseases are available, treatment failure due to poor adherence (which in turn leads to the emergence of drug-resistant strains) remains a considerable challenge. Many of these drugs require high doses and high dose frequency due to their poor bioavailability, resulting in protracted treatment times and associated negative side effects. Together, these deficits lead to poorer treatment outcomes and increased treatment costs. In addition to drug-related challenges, drug discovery and developmental research against these IDPs is not at a scale that corresponds with the impact of these diseases in the developing world [8].

The field of drug development for IDPs could benefit greatly from nanomedicine in terms of addressing the aforementioned shortfalls such as poor solubility and limited bioavailability. However, nanomedicine has not been widely applied in the development of transformative therapies for IDPs and other neglected diseases, with only a few groups in Africa [9,10], including the authors of this chapter (CSIR Drug Delivery platform) [11–13], who are exploring the applications of this nascent, yet potentially powerful technology against IDPs. The CSIR group, as well as a group at the University of Witwatersrand, South Africa, are investigating sustained release nanodrug delivery systems that will enable anti-TB drugs to be administered at lower, albeit perhaps more concentrated doses, due to target specificity [10,13]. Another group at the University of KwaZulu-Natal, South Africa, is investigating a similar approach for antiretroviral (ARV) drugs [9].

Although statistics indicate an urgent need for the development of novel and/or improved drugs, the investment allocated for the research and development (R&D) of these drugs is woefully inadequate. Pharmaceutical companies have lagged in the discovery of drugs for the diseases of the developing world due to the cost of R&D, the risk involved, and the time-consuming nature of this field. In the case of NTDs which, unlike HIV, malaria, and TB, do not spread widely to high-income countries, there is even less incentive for the industry to invest in the development of new or better products for a market with low returns. Thus, as relates to the discovery and development of drugs against IDPs, where minimal (if any) returns can be expected, new approaches involving nanotechnology and nanomedicine must be explored.

In addressing the challenges for the treatment of IDPs, investigations into nanomedicine have revealed promising strategies for the improved treatment of TB, HIV, Malaria, and Leishmaniasis, as will be outlined in this chapter.

13.2 Pharmacokinetics in Drug Development and the Benefits of Nanomedicine

Pharmacokinetics (PK) is a facet of science that describes the processes of bodily absorption, distribution, metabolism, and excretion (ADME) of compounds and medicines. In drug development, PK parameters are required in order to determine the optimal route of administration and dose regimen. Absorption describes the movement of molecules from the site of administration to the systemic circulation. Distribution is the molecular transference from the systemic circulation to extravascular sites. Metabolism involves the enzymatic biotransformation of molecules, and excretion is the passive or active transport of molecules for egress (e.g., via bile and urine) [14].

The oral route of drug administration is preferred due to its convenience and cost-effectiveness. However, in order to be absorbed into the systemic circulation and attain its target site, drug molecules must have the capacity for traversing cell membranes. In fact, each of the ADME processes involves passage of compounds across cell membranes. Several routes may be utilized, contingent on the physicochemical properties of the compound. Generally, lipophilic compounds are rapidly absorbed as they distribute into the cell membranes of epithelia via the passive transcellular route. Hydrophilic compounds are absorbed more slowly due to their poor distribution into cell membranes. Such compounds are, therefore, more likely to be transported by carrier-mediated pathways.

Bioavailability refers to the fraction of an administered drug dose that reaches the systemic circulation. When administered intravenously, the bioavailability is 100%. When administered by other routes such as orally, the drug must first be absorbed in the intestine, which may be limited by efflux transporters such as P-glycoprotein (Pgp) within the intestinal epithelium. As drug molecules pass through the liver and intestine, metabolism, mainly by the cytochrome P450 (CYP) family of enzymes (first-pass metabolism), and further excretion may take place, thus reducing bioavailability.

Nanomedicine offers an alternative in addressing PK-related shortfalls in drug development, and the following sections will discuss the properties that make them advantageous as emerging therapies.

13.3 Factors Affecting Drug Development for IDPs

Poor PK is a major cause of IDP treatment failure due to the inability to achieve effective drug concentration levels (poor solubility and intestinal permeability leading to poor bioavailability for orally administered drugs), production of toxic effects (poor elimination or levels above therapeutic values), and drug interactions. For example, the ARV drug, Zalcitabine, was discontinued due to its adverse side effects and drug interactions [15]. The ultimate result is poor patient compliance, which in turn leads to the emergence of resistance. Since the small number of drugs currently available for IDPs is inadequate to address these important treatment challenges, the development of new drugs is high on the agenda.

Drug discovery and development is lengthy and complex; more so for those drugs that are intended as therapeutics against IDPs, which in addition to being pharmacologically active must meet the following criteria: oral administration with good bioavailability, good tolerance with minimal side effects, and short treatment course [16]. A survey of the IDP drug development pipeline reveals that there are too few compounds in clinical development, with 10 for TB [17], 17 for malaria [18], and even fewer for NTDs [19]. It is well-known that the majority of compounds that undergo clinical testing never make it to market due to poor PK, low efficacy, side effects, or toxicity [20]. The clinical success rate for infectious diseases has been estimated at 15% with a failure rate of about 60% at Phase II human clinical trials [20]. Therefore, it is critical that the drug pipeline for IDPs be strengthened considerably to ensure that new products emerge on a timely basis. This goal must be fulfilled through the redoubled efforts of a significantly expanded pool of dedicated researchers and administrators in the generation and implementation of a significant array of innovative solutions.

Strategies to augment the development of new treatments include the reoptimization of currently used drugs; the repurposing of specific drugs to treat other diseases; the exploration of natural/biomimetic resources; and the nanometric modification/enhancement of existing drugs [18]. This chapter will endeavor to demonstrate the advantages of including nanomedicines in the current and future drug development programs. The modification of existing drugs utilizing nanomedicines has revolutionized the treatment of diseases such as cancer. However, nanomedicine has not been extensively applied to addressing IDPs. Doxil® and Abraxane® constitute two of several nanomedicine-based cancer therapies that are already on the market. Doxil® is a liposomal formulation of the anthracycline drug doxorubicin, which is employed in the treatment of cancer in AIDS-related Kaposi's sarcoma and multiple myeloma. Advantages over free doxorubicin include greater efficacy and lower cardiotoxicity due to altered PK [3]. Abraxane® consists of the anticancer drug paclitaxel that is bound to human albumin nanoparticles, which confers it with a longer circulation half-life [3].

13.4 Pharmacokinetics of Nanomedicines

Nanomedicine-based therapies might lead to improved half-life, controlled release over short or long time lines, and highly specific site-targeted delivery of therapeutic compounds. This section will explain how nanomedicine might attain these improvements.

Nanopharmacokinetics [21] is distinct from the PK of small molecules. The latter depends primarily on diffusion and transport (through blood), or metabolism (see Section 13.2). However, nanopharmacokinetics is defined by an array of physiological processes that nanomaterials are involved with, including cellular recognition, opsonization, adhesion, lymphatic transport, and uptake processes such as phagocytosis [21]. A reduction in blood concentrations of nanomaterials might be related to their movement into tissue from which further excretion does not occur. Indeed, the fate of many nanomaterials includes the tendency for accumulation within the liver, sequestration via the reticuloendothelial system (RES), or binding to tissue proteins. In addition, nanomaterials may be transported through lymphatic pathways, which must be taken into account in pharmacokinetic analyses based on blood sampling. However, these altered PK at the nanoscale indicate that nanomedicines have strong potential for presenting pharmaceutic improvements as drug delivery systems in that they can

- Improve drug stability ex vivo (long shelf-life) and in vivo (protection from first-pass metabolism) [22,23]
- Have a high carrying capacity (ability to encapsulate large quantities of drug molecules) [23]
- Incorporate hydrophilic and hydrophobic substances [23]
- Increase drug dissolution rate, leading to enhanced absorption and bioavailability [24]
- Specifically target tissues due to selective uptake by those tissues [3]
- Reduce clearance to increase drug half-life for prolonged pharmacological effects [3]

- Present the capacity to be formulated for the purpose of controlled release [25], therefore posing the possibility to reduce dose frequency and subsequent dose-related side effects [26]
- Be actively targeted to specific sites via the functionalization of nanoparticle surfaces with specific molecules or ligands such as monoclonal antibodies, RNA/DNA aptamers, or peptides to enhance binding and interactions with specific receptors that are expressed by cell populations at the diseased sites [27] thereby reducing toxicity

Protection from first-pass metabolism is an important factor in enhancing systemic bioavailability. However, in terms of intracellular PK, targeting with specific ligands further enhances intracellular bioavailability due to enhanced drug delivery directly into target cells [24].

13.4.1 Physicochemical Factors Influencing PK of Nanocarriers

When materials approach the nanometer size domain, they acquire unique physical and chemical properties. In nanomedicine, their enhanced physicochemical performance may be attributed to nanoscale dimensions, surface properties, and relative hydrophobicity.

13.4.1.1 Advantages of Nanoparticle Size

Submicron-sized particles offer a number of distinct advantages (e.g., the ability to access virtually all tissues within the human body), particularly for nanoparticles of less than 100 nm in diameter [28]. Desai et al. demonstrated that Ø100 nm nanoparticles had a 2.5-fold greater uptake in comparison to those at Ø1 µm, and a sixfold higher uptake when compared to Ø10 µm microparticles in a Caco-2 (human epithelial colorectal adenocarcinoma) cell line [29]. This aspect of intracellular uptake is especially critical for intracellular pathogens such as infectious diseases, where drugs need to act intracellularly. Thus, through nanoencapsulation, one may enable the intracellular delivery of drugs. Furthermore, these nanoparticles have the capacity for crossing biological barriers that in general make it difficult or simply block conventional therapeutic compounds from reaching their targets. Nanoparticles have been reported to traverse the blood brain barrier (BBB), the stomach epithelium, and even to pass through the skin [30]. In addition, orally administered nanoparticles can enter the lymphatic system through intestinal Peyer's patches, followed by M-cell uptake.

13.4.1.2 Nanoparticle Surface Properties

The surface charges of nanoparticles reflect their electrical potential, which is influenced by their chemical composition as well as the medium within which they are dispersed. A positive nanoparticle surface charge, which can be attained by adsorbing positively charged polymers, such as chitosan, onto their surfaces enhances their attachment to negatively charged cellular membranes, thus improving cellular uptake. Chitosan-based or coated nanoparticles have been reported to be efficiently taken up by cells and to pass through cellular barriers such as BBB. A unique function of chitosan is that it can induce the transient opening of the tight junctions between cells, thus facilitating transcellular nanoparticle transport [31]. The surface charge in nanoparticles reflects the electrical potential of particles and is influenced by the chemical composition of the particle and the medium in which it is dispersed. In the case of drug delivery, opsonization (a process that involves the adsorption of proteins, particularly of the complement system, to any foreign material) is also influenced by zeta-potential (electrokinetic potential of colloidal system constituents). These proteins make nanoparticles more susceptible to phagocytosis, thus leading to their clearance from the body.

To circumvent this effect, various groups have coated nanoparticles with hydrophilic polymers, such as polyethylene glycol (PEG), or pluronics, etc., thus affecting both the surface charge and hydrophobicity of the nanoparticles, increasing their circulation time in the blood, and in turn prolonging the release of the drugs from the nanoparticles [32,33]. Therefore, minimizing opsonization through the alteration of the surface charge is important for controlled release formulations. In addition, by coating polymeric nanoparticles with hydrophilic polymers, the half-life and thus efficacy of the drugs may be improved. This approach allows for reductions in dose and dose frequency of many effective, albeit poorly soluble drugs, and thus can dramatically decrease adverse side effects since smaller doses are administered. Furthermore, nanometric particles possess significantly larger surface areas due to the fact that decreased nanoparticle size results in an increase in surface-to-volume ratio, and that size is inversely proportional to specific surface area. This extensive surface area allows for higher loadings of drug molecules, thus enabling the diminution of the required dose to be administered [34].

13.4.1.3 Nanocarrier Hydrophobicity

Aqueous solubility, gastrointestinal permeability, and low first-pass metabolism are critical elements for the achievement of high oral bioavailability. Nanoscale drug delivery systems can increase drug dissolution rates, leading to enhanced absorption and bioavailability [24]. A combination of both nanoparticle surface charge and increased hydrophobicity of the material has been observed to improve gastrointestinal uptake in the case of oral delivery. Hydrophobicity also plays a role in drug release profiles as it impacts the kinetics of the degradation of the polymeric shell. Mittal et al. reported that by changing the hydrophobicity of a nanocarrier, the structure/composition of the polymer/copolymer, or the molecular weight, the polymer degradation and thus the drug release mechanism and/or release duration is impacted [35]. Nanoparticles have the advantage of improving the solubility of drugs, particularly for very hydrophilic or poorly soluble drugs, which in most cases are not easy to formulate and have poor bioavailability. By encapsulating these drugs within polymeric nanocarriers, which are coated with hydrophilic polymers, the solubility of the drugs may be greatly enhanced, which in turn improves the bioavailability of the drug. Kondo et al. documented an increase in bioavailability as a result of a 10-fold reduction in particle size, which was a direct consequence of the increased available surface area and consequently the improvement in the dissolution rate [34].

13.5 Functional Nanocarriers Utilized in Drug Delivery

A drug delivery system is defined as a formulation or a device that enables the introduction of a therapeutic substance within the human body and improves its efficacy and safety by controlling the rate, time, and location of the release of drugs within the body.

TABLE 13.1

Nanotechnology-Based Drug Delivery Systems

Nanocarrier	Characteristics
Liposomes	Self-assembling closed spherical, colloidal structures composed of phospholipid bilayers that surround an aqueous central space [3].
Polymeric micelles	Supramolecular assembly of amphiphilic block copolymers or polymer–lipid-based conjugates [37–39].
Dendrimers	Globular repeatedly bifurcated macromolecules that exhibit controlled patterns of branching with multiple arms extending from a central core [40].
Solid lipid nanoparticles	Particulate systems comprised of melted lipids, which are dispersed within an aqueous surfactant by high-pressure homogenization or emulsification [41].
Polymeric nanoparticles	Solid colloidal particles existing as nanospheres (matrix structure) or nanocapsules (polymeric shell and inner liquid core). Engineered from synthetic or natural polymers. The former are essentially polyesters and polyacids including polylactic acid (PLA), poly(D,L-lactic-co-glycolic acid) (PLGA), polycaprolactone (PCL), and poly(butyl-2-cyanoacrylate) (PBCA). The latter include oligomers that are abundant in nature such as chitosan, alginate, and starch [42,43].

Nanotechnology has increasingly been employed in drug delivery via the nanoencapsulation of medicinal drugs (nanomedicine) [36]. Several nanocarrier devices (Table 13.1 and Figure 13.1) have been used in drug delivery applications. The nanocarriers may be further modified for active disease targeting via the functionalization of their surfaces with ligands such as antibodies, aptamers, peptides, or small molecules that recognize disease-specific antigens (Figure 13.2). In this way, the nanoparticles become "multiple nanocarriers." For example, nanoparticles may be functionalized with aptamers to selectively recognize macrophages that are infected with TB.

Several nanomedical products currently on the market are summarized in Table 13.2, from which it can be noted that very little progress in the area of IDPs has been made. In comparison, Table 13.3 gives an example of some of the research on nanomedicine for IDPs and the stage of development. This table is indicative of the situation in regard to nanomedicine research for IDPs, where little progress has been made beyond basic research and the preclinical development stage, with only a single product on the market against Leishmaniasis and other fungal infections. This is likely because Leishmaniasis is endemic in several European countries [44], affecting both humans and dogs. Thus, a need was identified and incentivized by a market with the potential for high returns. The information in Table 13.3 is further expanded upon in Section 13.4.

13.6 Application of Nanomedicine for IDP Treatment

Due to the advantageous pharmacokinetic properties of nanocarriers, as discussed in Section 13.4, their application in the delivery of drugs for IDPs is being investigated by several research groups, albeit only a few of these groups are African. The following sections will discuss the shortcomings of therapies for Leishmaniasis, malaria, TB, and HIV, and highlight research into the application of nanomedicine for potentially addressing these shortcomings.

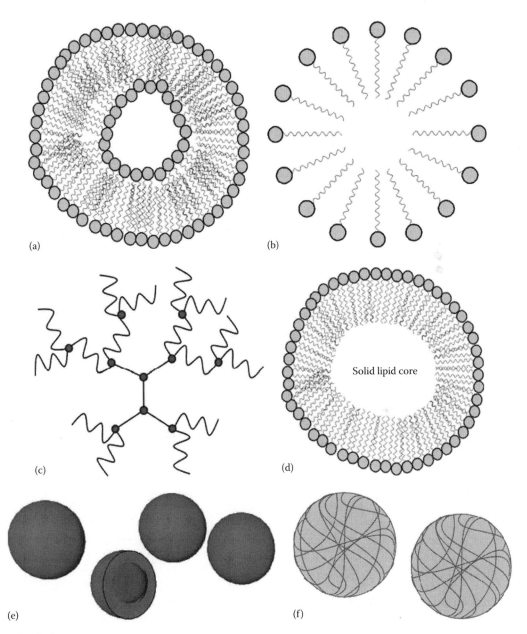

FIGURE 13.1
(a–f) Schematic illustration of nanotechnology-based drug delivery systems.

13.6.1 Current Treatment of IDPs

The challenges inherent to the present therapies against IDPs have been widely attributed to poor pharmacokinetic profiles and toxicity of the chemotherapy, leading to patient non-compliance and ultimately the emergence of drug-resistant strains. On the other hand, drug development for these diseases (as is the case for any other disease) continues to experience very low success rates due to problems with toxicity, solubility, stability, and PK, and thus bioavailability.

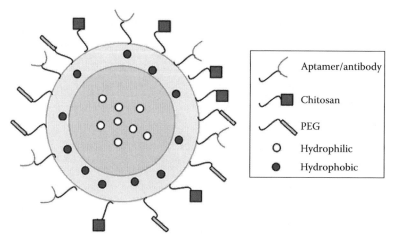

FIGURE 13.2
Schematic illustration of a multifunctional nanocarrier.

13.6.1.1 Treatment of Leishmaniasis

Unfortunately, there is a limited choice for the treatment of leishmaniasis. Four out of the five available first-line drugs must be administered by parenteral routes due to poor oral bioavailability. Pentavalent antimonials, meglumine antimoniate (Glucantime), and sodium stibogluconate (Pentostam) remain the treatments of choice against this disease in Africa, South America, and South East Asia. However, they are no longer effective against visceral leishmaniasis in India, with resistance in 70% of the population in Bihar, which is burdened with 90% of India's cases and 45% of those worldwide [7,52,53]. In addition, the treatment is prolonged, potentially toxic, and painful. The pentavalent antimonials have poor oral absorption and are given intravenously or intramuscularly every 2–3 days, for a period of 28 days. This means that infected individuals must spend every other day for an entire month to travel to a health-service provider, or face hospitalization for the duration of the treatment [7]. The antimonials have a short half-life of 2 h [54,55], and ~50% of antimony is excreted over 24–76 h through the urine [56]. Common side effects include cardiac dysrhythmia, nausea, vomiting, and pancreatitis, which may be fatal.

Amphotericin B is a powerful antileishmanial agent and serves as a first-line drug in India, where resistance to pentavalent antimonials is common. It is effective in advanced mucocutaneous leishmaniasis, against which pentavalent antimonial treatment has a high failure rate [7]. The drug is poorly absorbed from the gastrointestinal tract; hence, it must be administered intravenously. The optimal amphotericin B regimen incudes an intravenous infusion of 1 mg/kg daily, or on alternate days, with a total dosage of 1.5–2 g [56]. Its use requires prolonged hospitalization and close monitoring. Therefore, a strict adherence to the treatment regimen by patients is required. The major limiting factor of amphotericin B is its toxicity. Adverse reactions include fever with rigor and chills, thrombophlebitis, and occasional serious toxicities including myocarditis, severe hypokalemia, renal dysfunction, and even death.

The initial oral drug for visceral leishmaniasis, Miltefosine, was registered in India in 2002 [57]. Miltefosine opened the door to self-administered outpatient therapy; however, it must be taken as a single dose daily for 28 days, thus raising concerns in regard to the development of resistance to this highly effective drug due to poor compliance by

TABLE 13.2

Nanomedicine-Based Products Currently on the Market

Product	Drug	Formulation	Route of Administration	Application	Company
Abraxane	Paclitaxel	Albumin-bound nanoparticles	IV injection	Metastatic breast cancer	American Biosciences (Blauvelt, NY)
Amphocil	Amphotericin B	Lipocomplex	IV infusion	Serious fungal infections	Sequus Pharmaceuticals
Ambisome	Amphotericin B	Liposome	IV infusion	Serious fungal infections	NeXstar Pharmaceutical (Boulder, CO)
Abelcet	Amphotericin B	Lipid complex	IV infusion	Serious fungal infections	The Liposome Company (Princeton, NJ)
Dauno Xome	Daunorubicin citrate	Liposome	IV	Kaposi's sarcoma in AIDS	NeXstar Pharmaceutical (Boulder, CO)
Doxil	Doxorubicin	Liposome	IV injection	Kaposi's sarcoma in AIDS	Sequus Pharmaceuticals
Elestrin	Estradiol	Calcium-phosphate-based nanoparticles	Transdermal	Moderated to severe vasomotors symptoms (hot flashes) in menopausal women	BioSante (Lincolnshire, IL)
Emend	Aprepitant, MK869	Nanocrystal particles	Oral	To delay nausea and vomiting	Merck/Elan (Whitehouse Sation, NJ)
Megace ES	Megestrol acetate	Nanocrystal particles	Oral	Anorexia, cachexia, or unexplained significant weight loss	PAR Pharmaceutical (WoodCliff Lake, NJ)
Rapamune	Sirolimus	Nanocrystal particles	Oral	Immunosuppressant in kidney transplant patients	Wyeth/Elan (Madison, NJ)
Tricor	Fenofibrate	Nanocrystal particles	Oral	Primary hypercholesterolemia, mixed lipidemia, hypertriglyceridemia	Abbott (Abbot Park, IL)

IV, intravenous.

TABLE 13.3

Progress in Nanomedicine-Based Products for IDPs

Application	Drug	Formulation	Development	References
Tubercolosis	RIF, INH, EMB, PZA	PLGA nanoparticles	Preclinical	[11,12,45–47]
Tuberculosis	Moxifloxacin	PBCA nanoparticles	Preclinical	[48]
Malaria	Qunine	PCL nanocapsules	Preclinical	[49]
Malaria	Primaquine	Lipid nanoemulsion	Preclinical	[50]
Leishmaniasis and other fungal infections	Amphotericin B	Liposome	Market	[51]

outpatients [53]. The long half-life of 30 days [58] also increases the risk of development of parasite resistance [59]. Adverse effects of Miltefosine include mild and transient gastrointestinal disturbances and renal toxicity. As Miltefosine is teratogenic, it is contraindicated in pregnancy and women of child-bearing age, not observing contraception.

Paromomycin is an aminoglycoside antibiotic that is effective against visceral leishmaniasis. It is poorly absorbed into systemic circulation subsequent to oral administration, but rapidly absorbed from intramuscular sites of injection. Intramuscular injections must be given daily for 21 days. Peak concentration in plasma occurs within 30–90 min, and its apparent volume of distribution is 25% of body weight. Its half-life varies between 2 and 3 h in patients with normal renal function, and clearance is almost entirely via glomerular filtration [56].

Therefore, the treatment of leishmaniasis has many limitations. With the exception of Miltefosine, all of these drugs have to be given parenterally, and the treatment duration is protracted. Due to the toxicity of these drugs, patients may require hospitalization for close monitoring, which makes the treatments costly and beyond the reach of most patients.

13.6.1.2 Treatment of Malaria

Currently, no effective vaccine against malaria is yet available, although efforts in discovering one are ongoing. Thus, chemotherapy remains the most effective tool to fight this disease along with insecticide (e.g., deltamethrin) treated bed nets. Chloroquine (CQ) has been the mainstay of malaria treatment for many decades, but the development of drug resistance by the parasite has led to therapeutic failure [60]. Chloroquine has several pharmacokinetic and pharmacological advantages over all of the other antimalarial drugs, which account for its excellent performance over eight decades of malaria therapy [61,62]. The primary advantages of CQ therapy include rapid action in blood parasite stages, low toxicity, good bioavailability in oral dosage form, water solubility, and high distribution volume throughout the body [61–63]. Chloroquine is also cost-effective, relatively safe, easy to administer, and was extremely effective until 1989, when CQ resistance emerged. Due to its efficacy, patients felt better soon after taking CQ. However, they ceased taking it prior to completing the required course of treatment.

Where the resistance to CQ appears, Sulphadoxine-Pyrimethamine (SP) typically replaces it, but often resistance to this drug also soon develops [62–64]. Sulphadoxine-Pyrimethamine was one of the first-line treatments for uncomplicated malaria; however, patterns of resistance and frequent adverse side effects to the drug have made it extremely unpopular to both patient and physician [65]. Second- and third-line treatments are Amodiaquine and Quinine (QN) [66]. Quinine is the drug of choice for complicated manifestations of the disease, such as cerebral malaria, but resistance to the drug has been widely reported, and QN also presents high toxicity when administered intravenously. Another drug of choice is Primaquine (PQ), which is characterized by drug-related side effects that can lead to hemolytic anemia, gastrointestinal disturbances, heart failure, and abdominal cramps [67]. The *Plasmodium* strains have developed complex mechanisms of drug resistance [68]; thus, the vast majority of widely used antimalarial therapies have lost their efficacy over time, making drug resistance one of the greatest challenges in malaria treatment.

The artemisinins are the most effective antimalarial drugs known today. They possess a remarkably wide therapeutic index and have the ability to rapidly kill a broad range of asexual parasite stages at safe concentrations that are consistently achievable via standard dosing regimens [68]. In an effort to minimize the risk of developing resistance, WHO has recommended artemisinin to be used to treat uncomplicated malaria in combination with other antimalarials as artemisinin-based combination therapies (ACTs). With the deployment of ACTs in 2005/2006 as a first-line treatment in several endemic countries in Africa, malaria cases and deaths had been reported to be on the decline [69]. However, the reported parasites that have low sensitivity to ACTs in South East Asia have threatened these advances [60,70]. In the past, parasites that were resistant to CQ and antifolates emerged from this region, and spread to the East Coast of Africa, and subsequently to the rest of continent. Should resistance emerge against ACTs, the result will be catastrophic, considering the limited number of antimalarial drugs that are currently available. Furthermore, the artemisinins are known for their very short half-life [60,70]. In view of the earlier findings, there is an urgent need to expedite the development of efficacious intravenous formulations, which are able to reduce the side effects of QN, as well as to improve the solubility and pharmacokinetic profile of artemisinins (particularly in the treatment of cerebral malaria), and also to curtail or ideally negate progressive drug resistance.

13.6.1.3 Treatment of Tuberculosis

The current treatment for drug-susceptible TB involves a combination of four first-line anti-TB drugs administered over a 2 month period. These antibiotics include isoniazid (INH), rifampicin (RIF), pyrazinamide (PZA), and ethambutol (EMB). Thereafter, the patient is placed on INH and RIF treatment for a period of 4 months, which can be extended to 6 months if the culture test remains positive [17]. These drugs are administered in high daily doses essentially as the result of poor bioavailability. This is the case as they have low solubility and undergo premature degradation prior to reaching target sites, in addition to drug–drug interactions. Due to adverse side effects related to the daily administration of high doses, most patients fail to comply with the prescribed treatment. The prevalence of multidrug-resistant TB (MDR-TB) is therefore high due to this lack of adherence to treatment. Addressing MDR-TB is much more expensive than drug-sensitive TB and necessitates the utilization of more toxic second-line drugs that are, for the most part, intravenously injected for a period extending up to 24 months.

In KwaZulu-Natal, South Africa (2005), noncompliance to first- and second-line TB treatment, plus the coinfection of TB-HIV/AIDS led to the emergence of a deadly form of TB strain that has resisted all forms of anti-TB drugs. This is referred to as extensively drug-resistant TB (XDR-TB), and has no cure at present [71].

The first-line drugs described earlier were discovered nearly a half a century ago. Efforts are being expended globally to produce new and effective anti-TB drugs that aim to address the shortfalls of the conventional therapy. Various molecules that exhibit potency against TB in vitro have entered the drug development pipeline, where some are already progressing to very advanced stages of clinical trials. The most promising of these, among others, includes TCM 207, a diarylquinoline-type drug that has shown efficacy against MDR-TB, which is presently in phase IIa clinical trials [72] and PA-824, a nitroimidazopyran compound that demonstrates a lowered minimum inhibitory concentration (MIC) (0.015–0.25 mg/L) against drug-susceptible *M.tb* [31]. It is worth noting that only these two drugs have progressed into advanced phases of clinical trials.

In summary, first-line anti-TB drugs are still effective and are able to eradicate drug-susceptible *M.tb* if proper treatment procedures are strictly complied with, in terms of dose and dose frequency. The course of treatment remains lengthy because most of the drugs involved are characterized by a short half-life and have only slight solubility in biological media, which ultimately translates to reduced bioavailability.

13.6.1.4 Treatment of HIV

Therapeutic regimens currently available for the treatment of HIV are based mainly on ARVs. The aim of these therapeutic compounds is to prolong the life of the patient and to improve the quality of life by maintaining the suppression of viral replication for as long as possible in order to prevent the progression of HIV toward AIDS. Cutting-edge research over the past several years has produced major insights into the pathogenic mechanisms of HIV. This has resulted in the development of more than 20 ARV medications that target HIV, which have been approved by the Food and Drug Administration (FDA), as well as novel prevention strategies and vaccine development. The existing therapy using ARV drugs for HIV/AIDS is available under categories such as nucleoside reverse transcriptase inhibitors (NRTIs), nucleotide reverse transcriptase inhibitors (NtRTIs), nonnucleoside reverse transcriptase inhibitors (NNRTIs), protease inhibitors (PIs), and more recently, fusion and integrase inhibitors [73].

Many ARV drugs pose a hurdle in the fulfillment of HIV chemotherapy, as some undergo extensive first-pass metabolism and gastrointestinal degradation, leading to low bioavailability. Several drugs such as indinavir (800 mg taken three times a day) require frequent administration of large doses owing to their short half-life, culminating in patient noncompliance. Epidemiological studies have revealed that optimal therapeutic results are attained when treatment adherence levels are greater than 95% (no more than two doses missed monthly in a twice-daily regime); adherence levels of below 95% could diminish therapeutic effectiveness by up to 50% [74]. In addition, the major challenge in HIV/AIDS is to develop drugs that can either prevent the transmission of the virus, or at least prevent the progression to AIDS. A compounding factor in the treatment of HIV/AIDS is the chronic intake of highly active antiretroviral therapy (HAART). Furthermore, the rapid mutation rate of the virus initiates multidrug resistance (MDR) against ARV agents. In the case of TB/HIV coinfection, some ARV therapies have shown a reduction in their dose levels and are not compatible with the current TB regimen due to shared toxicities and drug–drug interactions. Therefore, there is an urgent call for superior drugs and more effective drug delivery systems that might address the earlier-mentioned challenges and also improve the efficacy of both the existing and new ARVs [75].

13.6.1.5 Combination Therapies and Drug–Drug Interactions

In an effort to reduce the risk of resistance and improve efficacy, many of the drugs used to treat IDPs are utilized in combination therapies. This strategy brings with it the potential for drug–drug interactions.

Due to their ability to metabolize and transport a large number of compounds, CYPs and Pgp are involved in many drug–drug interactions. When a drug is co-administered with another drug, a pharmacokinetic drug interaction may occur, whereby one drug might proceed to alter the concentration of another within the body fluids and tissues, thereby impacting the efficacy and toxicity of both. Pharmacokinetic drug interactions may be due to an alteration in the content or activity of CYPs or Pgp as a result of induction or inhibition. Clinically significant interactions are more likely to occur for drugs with a narrow therapeutic window. The FDA has removed many drugs from the market due to drug interactions, and several of these drugs are substrates for both CYPs and Pgp [76].

Drug interactions are common in HAART due to the metabolism of protease inhibitors and NNRTIs by CYPs. Protease inhibitors are substrates of CYP3A4. Saquinavir has a low oral bioavailability due to metabolism by CYP3A4 and efflux by Pgp. Ritonavir was found to increase the bioavailability of saquinavir due to the inhibition of CYP3A4. The plasma levels of both indinavir and saquinavir are reduced by nevirapine, which induces CYP3A4. Therefore, doses of indinavir must be increased in the presence of nevirapine [77].

The TB drug RIF is a potent inducer of both CYP3A4 and Pgp. This induction may result in significant drug interactions with many drugs, including ARVs, in the treatment of TB/HIV coinfection. The use of RIF with protease inhibitors and some NNRTIs has been contraindicated due to a significant decrease of the plasma levels of the ARVs via RIF [78].

13.7 Application of Nanomedicine to Overcome Shortfalls of IDP Therapies

Given the discussions in Section 13.6.1, the ideal drug for the treatment of any given IDP would possess the following pharmaceutic properties:

- Allow for oral administration and have high oral bioavailability to permit administration in a nonhospital setting.
- Short duration of therapy and few doses to promote patient compliance to treatment and to reduce the risk of the development of resistance. This translates to rapid and robust therapeutic activity.
- Access to intracellular pathogens in affected tissues (via increased circulation and tissue penetration).
- No potential for drug interactions in combination therapies.
- Safe and efficacious, even toward resistant strains.

The application of nanomedicine to bring about these ideals is discussed in the following sections, which will highlight important advances that have been made in the reformulation of old drugs for the treatment of IDPs, utilizing the nanotechnological approach.

13.7.1 Enhancement of Oral Bioavailability

The oral administration of drugs is the most desirable form of treatment for any disease due to its convenience and cost-effectiveness. However, many of the drugs used to treat IDPs are either not available as oral formulations or have poor oral bioavailability. Aqueous solubility, gastrointestinal permeability, and low first-pass metabolism are important considerations for high oral bioavailability [79]. Nanomedical drug delivery systems have the capacity for increasing drug dissolution rates, leading to enhanced absorption and bioavailability [24].

13.7.1.1 Nanomedicine for Oral Administration of Leishmaniasis Drugs

As mentioned earlier, the treatment choices for leishmaniasis are quite restricted. Only a single drug, miltefosine, is available as an oral formulation. Consequently, there is an urgent requirement for additional oral formulations to improve the chances for treatment success. Further negative factors inherent to conventional treatments include a lengthy course of treatment, potential toxicity, and attendant pain. Current therapeutics are also no longer effective against visceral leishmaniasis in India, with resistance in 70% of the population in Bihar, which is fraught with 90% of India's cases and 45% of global cases [7,52,53].

Only a small number of oral nanomedical drug delivery systems have been explored for leishmaniasis to date. Nanosuspensions comprised of AmB in an aqueous solution of Tween 80, Pluronics F68, and sodium cholate (via a high-pressure homogenization technique) were observed to reduce the liver parasite load by ~28.6% when administered orally [80].

Meglumine antimoniate-β-cyclodextrin complexes administered orally to mice brought about threefold higher antimony plasma levels in comparison to the free drug, which was also administered orally. Mice infected with *L. amazonensis* were given daily oral treatments of the cyclodextrin complex (32 mg/kg), free meglumine antimoniate (120 mg/kg), or a saline solution. Animals treated with the cyclodextrin complex showed significantly smaller skin lesions when compared to those that were treated with the free drug and saline [81]. A single cyclodextrin complex dose exhibited the same efficacy as a double dose of the free drug given intraperitoneally.

13.7.1.2 Polymeric Micelles Improve Bioavailability of Efavirenz

Efavirenz is a NNRTI that has been recommended as one of the first-line treatments against HIV by WHO; however, it has poor oral bioavailability at only 40%–45%. The encapsulation of efavirenz within polymeric micelles has led to a significant dose-independent increase in bioavailability (more than 8400 times at ~34 mg/mL) as was demonstrated by an increase of the area under the curve (AUC) by 1.7-fold [82]. This was likely due to the dramatic increase in aqueous solubility of the drug enabled by the micellar system [83].

13.7.2 Reduction of Therapy Duration and Dose Frequency via Nanomedicine

The longer that a patient must adhere to a treatment and the more side effects that he/she endures, the more likely they are to discontinue treatment midcourse, or as soon as they perceive that they are feeling better. This is exemplified by TB treatments which require at least 6 months of therapy. Therefore, for diseases like TB, a shorter duration of therapy with fewer doses is highly desirable. Sustained release therapeutics and a long elimination half-life will ensure that fewer doses are required. Nanomedical drug delivery systems present the capacity to be formulated for the purpose of controlled release [25], therefore facilitating the possibility for reduced dose frequency, and subsequently, the minimization of dose-related side effects [26].

13.7.2.1 Nanomedicine against TB: Reduction of Dose and Dose Frequency

Pandey and colleagues [45,46] have extensively utilized PLGA for the encapsulation of first-line anti-TB drugs (i.e., RIF, INH, EMB, and PZA). They have shown that when anti-TB drug-loaded PLG nanoparticles were orally administered to mice, the drug was detected in the plasma at concentrations that were well above the MIC for a period of 9 days, whereas free drugs were cleared from the body within 21 h. Additional studies revealed that only five oral doses of drug-loaded PLGA nanoparticles, given over 50 days, were sufficient to completely eliminate the pathogen from various vital organs, such as the lungs, kidneys, and spleen [69]. The researchers went further to investigate a four-drug combination (INH, RIF, PZA, and EMB) co-encapsulated within PLGA nanoparticles [45]. They found that the MICs of all the four drugs were maintained in the blood for more than 5 days, and these drugs continued to be detected in the plasma until day 9. When they administered five doses (once every 10 days), the complete elimination of bacteria in the meninges was observed. Pandey et al. prepared anti-TB drug-loaded PLGA nanoparticles via the multiple emulsion technique. Subsequent to subcutaneous injection in a murine model of TB, they observed that the drug concentration in plasma, lungs, and spleen was maintained above MIC for more than 1 month, and significantly reduced the bacteria counts in most organs [84].

Kisich et al. investigated moxifloxacin-loaded PBCA nanoparticles, which were produced by anionic polymerization of poly(butyl-2-cyanoacrylate) in the presence of the drug [48]. A slow release profile was observed following an early burst release, corresponding to approximately 55% of the formulated drug content. The same study showed that increased cytotoxicity was observed when moxifloxacin-loaded nanoparticles were incubated with macrophages as compared to the free drug [48]. A further study, where similar nanocarriers were administered intravenously in TB-challenged mice, resulted in a significant decrease of mycobacteria counts within the lungs [85].

Wu et al. designed spherical micelles that were comprised of PLA-modified chitosan oligomers with nanoparticle sizes that ranged between Ø154 and Ø181 nm. When they incorporated 10% RIF into the nanocarriers, their dimensions increased to Ø163 and Ø210 nm [86]. This system showed sustained release in vitro for 5 days, following an early burst of 35% of the drug over the initial 10 h.

Another research group synthesized a self-assembled system consisting of INH–poly(ethylene glycol)–poly(aspartic acid) conjugates [87]. This micelle-forming prodrug sustained the release of the drug over time and demonstrated a sixfold increase in anti-TB activity in vitro in comparison to the free drug [87]. In the same way, PZA and RIF were also adsorbed to copolymeric chains and subsequently formed stable micelles with sizes that ranged between Ø70 and Ø100 nm, and a level of drugs conjugated in the range from 65% to 86% [88,89]. These conjugates showed an enhanced activity against TB. Although micelle-like systems are less attractive due to their propensity for leakage, it has been shown that a sustained release of the anti-TB drug, as well as enhanced efficacy were observed for prodrug-like materials.

Ahmad et al. investigated the use of natural polymers in the production of nanocarriers to accommodate anti-TB drugs. The group managed to load anti-TB drugs into alginate nanoparticles via ionotropic gelation [90]. They incorporated first-line anti-TB drugs into alginate nanoparticles at relatively high (>90%) encapsulation efficiency. When orally administered to mice, encapsulated drugs were observed in the plasma up to 7, 9, and 11 days subsequent to administration for EMB, RIF, INH, and PZA, respectively, and in the tissues until day 15. In another study, Ahmad et al. administered nebulized alginate nanoparticles at three doses that were spaced 15 days apart for 45 days, whereas free drugs were orally administered daily for 45 days to *M.tb*-infected guinea pigs. This resulted in undetectable mycobacterial colony-forming units (cfu) in the lungs and the spleen, in contrast to guinea pigs that were administered empty alginate nanoparticles. Untreated controls exhibited elevated cfu counts [91].

13.7.2.2 Nanomedicine against Malaria: Reduction of Dose and Dose Frequency

The primary goal of malaria therapy is to promote a high drug concentration within the intracellular parasitophorous vacuoles where *Plasmodium* is hosted. Antimalarial drugs must traverse barriers (e.g., membranes) in order to access parasite targets within infected red blood cells (RBCs). The ability of a nanocarrier to maintain residency within the bloodstream for a long enough period of time in order to improve interactions with infected RBCs and parasite membranes is critical. This has been confirmed when artemether (AM) was entrapped in a long-circulating and site-specific system prepared with PEG-lysine-type dendrimers and chondroitinsulfate A for sustained and controlled delivery of the drug via the intravenous administration route. It was observed that the mean residence time was increased by fourfold in comparison to free AM [68].

13.7.2.3 Nanomedicine against Leishmaniasis: Reduction of Dose and Dose Frequency

Despite its superior activity, the use of amphotericin B for the treatment of leishmaniasis is limited due to its toxicity. Liposomal amphotericin B (LAB) was consequently developed in an effort to reduce this toxicity, consisting of spherical Ø45 to Ø80 nm liposomes. A number of studies performed in India have shown that the dose of LAB and the treatment duration may be reduced without loss of efficacy [59]. In a recent Phase III study involving 304 patients, a single infusion (10 mg/kg) of LAB was compared to 15 infusions (1 mg/kg) of conventional amphotericin B given on alternate days over 29 days, involving 108 patients in hospital [51]. Cure rates at 6 months were approximately 96% for both groups. The single, lower dose of LAB was not only as effective as the conventional treatment, but was also calculated to be cost-effective, as only 1 day of hospitalization was required.

13.7.3 Nanomedicine for Intracellular Delivery: Passive and Active Targeting

The infectious diseases of poverty are often characterized by the attack of specific cells or tissues by disease-carrying parasites. Drugs must therefore be transported through biological membranes in order to enable the eradication of parasitic targets within infected cells and tissues. The size of nanoparticles and their surface charges play crucial roles in intracellular drug delivery. Nanocarriers may be passively targeted due to their diminutive sizes, as they can permeate the capillaries (the smallest being ~Ø3 µm) throughout the human body. However, this mode of targeting is less efficient due to lack of selectivity. Therefore, in order to increase the localization of nanocarriers at specific sites in vivo, various methods of actively targeting infected cells have been explored. The precise delivery of drugs to specific targets will decrease the risk of drug interactions during combination therapy, as there will be limited exposure of drugs to inhibit or induce CYPs or Pgp.

13.7.3.1 Nanocarrier Targeting of HIV-Infected Cells

Macrophages are well-recognized phagocytic cells of the RES and one of the main cells that are responsible for the uptake and clearance of administered drug-loaded nanoparticles. Schäfer et al. studied the uptake effect of HIV-infected macrophages using polymethylmethacrylate and albumin-based nanoparticles that were loaded with zidovudine [92]. They found that nanoparticle uptake by macrophages was enhanced when these cells were infected with HIV, that is, up to 60% more than that for uninfected macrophages. This higher amount of phagocytosis was attributed to a likely activated state of these infected cells, which might have allowed for the preferential phagocytosis of drug-loaded nanoparticles, thus resulting in the targeted delivery of drugs to these cells [92].

In recent years, poly(ethylene oxide)-modified poly(epsilon-caprolactone) (PEO–PCL) nanoparticles loaded with radiolabeled [3H]-saquinavir were synthesized by Shah and Amiji [93]. The nanoparticles were further evaluated for in vitro uptake by monocytes/macrophages (human THP-1 cell line), and the results showed a higher cellular uptake of [3H]-saquinavir when compared to the free drug. Microscopic observations confirmed qualitatively that a significantly high percentage of nanoparticles was internalized within monocytes/macrophages.

13.7.3.2 Lymphatic System Delivery of ARVs

It has been reported that the presence of a large amount of HIV-susceptible immune cells in the lymphoid organs makes ARV drug targeting to these sites of tremendous interest in HIV chemotherapy. Dembri et al. studied the applicability for the oral administration of azidothymidine (AZT)-loaded poly(iso-hexylcyanoacrylate) nanoparticles (average particle size Ø250 nm) in rats [94]. The concentration of AZT in Peyer's patches was found to be four times higher for AZT-loaded nanoparticles than for the free drug solution. Furthermore, significantly higher tissue concentrations (30–45 µM) were found than those reported for AZT IC50 (0.06–1.36 µM). This work illustrated that it was possible to target important sites related to HIV replication and perpetuation, which improved the concentration of AZT within the gastrointestinal tract and thus gastrointestinal associated lymphoid tissue (GALT). In addition, the release of the drug, which is characterized by a short half-life of 1.1 h, was increased to more than 8 h due to the slow degradation of the polymeric matrix.

The use of liposomes in transdermal delivery for ARV drug administration has also been reported [95,96]. In vitro permeability studies of liposomes using rat skin indicated that they are able to augment skin permeation. Furthermore, when AZT-loaded liposomes were topically administered to rats, the results showed that these systems enhanced plasma concentrations by nearly 12-fold when compared to the drug when it was formulated as a hydrophilic ointment. In the same studies, a preferential distribution to RES organs (e.g., spleen and lymph nodes) was also observed for liposomal formulations, particularly in the case of PEGylated liposomes (up to 2- and 27-fold of the concentrations observed for non-PEGylated liposomes and AZT-hydrophilic ointment, respectively). According to the authors, PEGylation of these systems possibly prevents interaction with the components of the subcutaneous interstitium because of the PEG chains that minimize interactions with membranes, which could cause their partial deposition within this tissue. However, further studies are required in order to assess the significance of these results in terms of the concentrations that are required in order to achieve therapeutic levels using transdermal delivery systems [73,97].

13.7.3.3 Nanocarriers for Targeting Tuberculosis

Deol et al. produced lung-specific Stealth® liposomes, consisting of phosphatidylcholine, cholesterol, dicetyl-phosphate, O-steroyl amylopectin, and monosialogangliosides-distearylphosphatidylethanolamine-poly(ethylene glycol) 2000 for the targeted delivery of anti-TB drugs to the lung [98]. Following intravenous injection of the different liposomes, the findings revealed a significant increase of accumulation of nanoparticles within the lungs (i.e., from 5.1% using conventional liposomes to 31% with PEGylated systems containing O-steroyl amylopectin). These reports have shown that liposomes might also be used as carriers to target tissues that are infected by TB.

In order to target the drug delivery vehicle to macrophages, Kumar et al. incorporated RIF into mannosylated fifth generation (5G) poly (propylene imine) (PPI) dendrimeric nanocarriers [99]. It was established that the modification of the surface with sugar molecules, which are recognizable by lectin receptors located on the surfaces of phagocytic cells, improved the selective uptake of the drug-loaded nanocarriers by macrophages [99]. Moreover, they showed that mannosylation significantly reduced the hemolytic toxicity of the nanocarrier materials from 15.6% to 2.8%. In a further study, Kumar et al. investigated the incorporation of RIF in 4G and 5G PEGylated-PPI dendrimers for sustained release [100]. The findings demonstrated that PEGylation resulted in a 70% increase in the drug entrapment capacity for both 4G and 5G derivatives.

13.7.3.4 Active Targeting Strategies for TB

Most pathological conditions initiate physiological changes within cells and tissues. Specific ligands/molecules may be synthesized that recognize these unique molecular signatures, and when conjugated to nanoparticles, they enable selective delivery of drug molecules to the infected sites. This approach, therefore, has the potential for improving the specificity of the drug action.

   With the aim of enhancing the localization of nanocarriers to specific sites in vivo, various techniques for actively targeting TB-infected cells have been investigated. Irache et al. explored the possibility of utilizing sugars (e.g., mannose) that are recognized by lectin receptors, which are localized on the surfaces of infected macrophages [101]. In another study, Chono et al. demonstrated increased macrophage uptake of mannose-coated liposomes in contrast to unmodified liposomes, whereby an abundant deposition of these mannosylated nanocarriers was found within the lungs, following their administration to rats [102]. Furthermore, the same group evaluated ciprofloxacin-loaded mannosylated liposomes as a lung-targeting delivery system [103]. They observed a substantial increase in uptake by macrophages and more than a twofold increase in AUC and maximum plasma concentration (C_{max}) [103]. Another group evaluated the use of pulmonary surfactant-grafted liposomes to target the respiratory tract [104]. A threefold increase in uptake by epithelial cells as compared to alveolar macrophages, subsequent to intratracheal administration in rats was observed when the pulmonary surfactant was used as a targeting ligand [105].

13.7.3.5 Passive Nanocarrier Targeting for Malaria

Quinine acts on the RBC stage of malaria; however, its use is limited by its narrow therapeutic index and toxicity. Haas et al. investigated the PK and erythrocyte partition coefficient of QN-loaded nanocapsules that were prepared in polycaprolactone (PCL) [49]. The PK were found to be identical to the free drug; however, the partition coefficient into infected erythrocytes was doubled for the QN nanocapsules, indicating an increase in the interaction between QN and erythrocytes. Interestingly, this was also accompanied by an increase in efficacy with a 30% reduction in the QN-effective dose [49].

13.7.4 Safety and Efficacy of Nanomedicines for IDPs

One of the motivations behind poor patient compliance and premature cessation of therapy in the treatment of IDPs has its source in the attendant adverse side effects of the drugs. Therefore, efforts should be invested, when developing any new formulations, to ensure that they convey negligible or no toxicity.

   In the case of malaria, halofantrine was formulated and encased within nanocapsules (having oily cores) that were prepared from PLA, which was surface-modified with PEG chains in order to prolong residency within the circulation [13]. When this formulation was administered to a *Plasmodium*-infected mouse model, the drug concentration in plasma was increased sixfold in comparison with the free drug throughout the experimental period of 70 h. An additional benefit was that no toxic effects, which are typically associated with halofantrine, were observed when the drug was nanoencapsulated, while the same dose of the free drug was toxic.

Primaquine is one of the most widely utilized second-line antimalarials that acts specifically on pre-erythrocytic schizonts, which are concentrated predominantly in the liver. However, PQ is also characterized by dose-dependent toxicities [50]. Following the incorporation of PQ into an oral lipid nanoemulsion with particle sizes in the range of Ø10–Ø200 nm, its efficacy against *Plasmodium bergheii* in infected mice was observed to be satisfactory at a 25% lower dosage level than the unencapsulated form [50]. The lipid nanoemulsion of PQ exhibited improved oral bioavailability and was taken up preferentially by the liver with drug concentrations of at least 45% higher when compared with the unencapsulated drug. It was concluded that lipid nanoemulsion holds a great promise for the delivery of PQ to the liver with strong potential for the treatment of latent stage malaria and toward the minimization of toxicity [49,50,106]. Therapeutic efficacy at reduced doses in these systems might also be explored for the chemoprophylaxis of malaria in high-risk areas [50].

Amphotericin B is a powerful antileishmanial agent whose major limiting factor is its toxicity. Adverse reactions include fever with rigor and chills, thrombophlebitis, and occasional serious toxicities such as myocarditis, severe hypokalemia, renal dysfunction, and even death. Liposomal amphotericin B (see Section 13.7.2.3) was developed to overcome these adverse effects, and has been shown to improve tissue penetration and overall effectiveness at lower doses [59].

13.8 Conclusions

The number of discovery programs for IDPs are far too low to ensure that a steady stream of treatments will make it to market [107]. Unfortunately, only 1.3 products are expected to reach the market out of 100 that enter the screening phase of drug discovery [107]. These bleak figures indicate that there is indeed an urgent necessity for new strategies in the drug discovery and development programs of IDPs. Although nanomedicine has been successfully applied for the treatment of cancer with several products on the market, it has not yet been seriously considered and exploited in the mainstream as a viable, and in many cases superior, option against IDPs, while the technology clearly and increasingly demonstrates enormous potential in effectively addressing them.

Some of the critical properties of nanomedical systems include the protection of unstable drugs, improved cell adhesion properties, the capacity for the intracellular delivery of drugs, and amenability for surface modification, via the conjugation of specific ligands, to enable specifically targeted delivery and controlled release. In effect, nanomedical drug delivery systems can reduce drug dosage frequency, treatment time, and toxicity [13] due to their improved bioavailability and efficacy. Thus, nanoscale drug delivery systems appear to be a promising and feasible strategy for improving the treatment of IDPs and should urgently be considered for drug development programs. Their inclusion will likely decrease patient noncompliance. Therefore, redoubled efforts are required to be focused on increasing the exploitation of nanomedical strategies in drug development as new and potent therapeutics against IDPs.

References

1. Bawa, R., Bawa, S.R., Maebius, S.B., Flynn, T., and Wei, C., Protecting new ideas and inventions in nanomedicine with patents. *Nanomedicine* 1(2), 150–158, 2005.
2. Mishra, B., Patel, B.B., and Tiwari, S., Colloidal nanocarriers: A review on formulation technology, types and applications toward targeted drug delivery. *Nanomedicine* 6(1), 9–24, 2010.
3. Malam, Y., Loizidou, M., and Seifalian, A.M., Liposomes and nanoparticles: Nanosized vehicles for drug delivery in cancer. *Trends Pharmacol Sci* 30(11), 592–599, 2009.
4. WHO, *Global Tuberculosis Control: WHO report 2010.* World Health Organisation, Geneva, Switzerland, 2010.
5. WHO, *World Malaria Report 2010.* World Health Organisation, Geneva, Switzerland, 2010.
6. UNAIDS, UNAIDS report on the global AIDS epidemic, 2010.
7. Davidson, R.N., Leishmaniasis. *Medicine* 33(8), 43–46, 2005.
8. Anwabani, G.M., Drug development: A perspective from Africa. *Paed Perinatal Drug Ther* 5(1), 4–11, 2002.
9. Ojewole, E., Mackraj, I., Naidoo, P., and Govender, T., Exploring the use of novel drug delivery systems for antiretroviral drugs. *Eur J Pharm Biopharm* 70(3), 697–710, 2008.
10. Choonara, Y.E., Pillay, V., Ndesendo, V.M., du Toit, L.C., Kumar, P., Khan, R.A., Murphy, C.S., and Jarvis, D.L., Polymeric emulsion and crosslink-mediated synthesis of super-stable nanoparticles as sustained-release anti-tuberculosis drug carriers. *Colloids Surf B: Biointerf* 87(2), 243–254, 2011.
11. Semete, B., Booysen, L., Lemmer, Y., Kalombo, L., Katata, L., Verschoor, J., and Swai, H.S., In vivo evaluation of the biodistribution and safety of PLGA nanoparticles as drug delivery systems. *Nanomedicine* 6(5), 662–671, 2010.
12. Semete, B., Booysen, L., Lemmer, Y., Kalombo, L., Katata, L., Verschoor, J., and Swai, H.S., In vivo uptake and acute immune response to orally administered chitosan and PEG coated PLGA nanoparticles. *Toxicol Appl Pharmacol* 249(2), 158–165, 2010.
13. Swai, H., Semete, B., Kalombo, L., and Chelule, P., Potential of treating tuberculosis with a polymeric nano-drug delivery system. *J Control Release* 132(3), e48, 2008.
14. Jang, G.R., Harris, R.Z., and Lau, D.T., Pharmacokinetics and its role in small molecule drug discovery research. *Medicinal Res Rev* 21(5), 382–396, 2001.
15. M.D./alert http://www.fda.gov/downloads/Drugs/DrugSafety/DrugShortages/UCM086099.pdf (accessed June, 23, 2011).
16. Nzila, A. and Chilengi, R., Modulators of the efficacy and toxicity of drugs in malaria treatment. *Trends Pharmacol Sci* 31(6), 277–283, 2010.
17. Ma, Z., Lienhardt, C., McIlleron, H., Nunn, A.J., and Wang X., Global tuberculosis drug development pipeline: The need and the reality. *The Lancet* 375(9731), 2100–2109, 2010.
18. Grimberg, B.T. and Mehlotra, R.K., Expanding the antimalarial drug arsenal-now, but how? *Pharmaceuticals (Basel)* 4(5), 681–712, 2011.
19. Chatelain, E. and Ioset, J.R., Drug discovery and development for neglected diseases: The DNDi model. *Drug Des Devel Ther* 5, 175–181, 2011.
20. Kola, I. and Landis, J., Can the pharmaceutical industry reduce attrition rates? *Nat Rev Drug Discov* 3(8), 711–715, 2004.
21. Riviere, J.E., Pharmacokinetics of nanomaterials: An overview of carbon nanotubes, fullerenes and quantum dots. *Wiley Interdiscip Rev Nanomed Nanobiotechnol* 1(1), 26–34, 2009.
22. Couvreur, P. and Vauthier, C., Nanotechnology: Intelligent design to treat complex disease. *Pharm Res* 23(7), 1417–1450, 2006.
23. Gelperina, S., Kisich, K., Iseman, M.D., and Heifets, L., The potential advantages of nanoparticle drug delivery systems in chemotherapy of tuberculosis. *Am J Respir Crit Care Med* 172(12), 1487–1490, 2005.
24. Li, S.D. and Huang, L., Pharmacokinetics and biodistribution of nanoparticles. *Mol Pharm* 5(4), 496–504, 2008.

25. Pandey, R., Ahmad, Z., Sharma, S., and Khuller, G.K., Nano-encapsulation of azole antifungals: Potential applications to improve oral drug delivery. *Int J Pharm* 301(1–2), 268–276, 2005.
26. Medina, C., Santos-Martinez, M.J., Radomski, A., Corrigan, O.I., and Radomski, M.W., Nanoparticles: Pharmacological and toxicological significance. *Br J Pharmacol* 150(5), 552–558, 2007.
27. Kingsley, J.D., Dou, H., Morehead, J., Rabinow, B., Gendelman, H.E., and Destache, C.J., Nanotechnology: A focus on nanoparticles as a drug delivery system. *J Neuroimmune Pharmacol* 1(3), 340–350, 2006.
28. McNeil, S.E., Nanotechnology for the biologist. *J Leukocyte Biol* 78(3), 585–594, 2005.
29. Desai, M.P., Labhasetwar, V., Walter, E., Levy, R.J., and Amidon, G.L., The mechanism of uptake of biodegradable microparticles in Caco-2 cells is size dependent. *Pharm Res* 14(11), 1568–1573, 1997.
30. Koziara, J.M., Lockman, P.R., Allen, D.D., and Mumper, R.J., In situ blood-brain barrier transport of nanoparticles. *Pharm Res* 20(11), 1772–1778, 2003.
31. Park, J.H., Saravanakumar, G., Kim, K., and Kwon, I.C., Targeted delivery of low molecular drugs using chitosan and its derivatives. *Adv Drug Deliv Rev* 62(1), 28–41, 2010.
32. Freiberg, S. and Zhu, X.X., Polymer microspheres for controlled drug release. *Int J Pharm* 282(1–2), 1–18, 2004.
33. Mohanraj, V.J. and Chen, Y., Nanoparticles—A review. *Trop J Pharm Res* 5(1), 561–573, 2006.
34. Kondo, N., Iwao, T., Kikuchi, M., Shu, H., Yamanouchi, K., Yokoyama, K., Ohyama, K., and Ogyu, S., Pharmacokinetics of a micronized, poorly water-soluble drug, HO-221, in experimental animals. *Biol Pharm Bull* 16(8), 796–800, 1993.
35. Mittal, G., Sahana, D.K., Bhardwaj, V., and Ravi Kumar, M.N., Estradiol loaded PLGA nanoparticles for oral administration: Effect of polymer molecular weight and copolymer composition on release behavior in vitro and in vivo. *J Control Release* 119(1), 77–85, 2007.
36. Kumari, A., Yadav, S.K., and Yadav, S.C., Biodegradable polymeric nanoparticles based drug delivery systems. *Colloids Surf B Biointerf* 75(1), 1–18, 2010.
37. Bae, Y. and Kataoka, K., Intelligent polymeric micelles from functional poly(ethylene glycol)-poly(amino acid) block copolymers. *Adv Drug Deliv Rev* 61(10), 768–784, 2009.
38. Gaucher, G., Dufresne, M.H., Sant, V.P., Kang, N., Maysinger, D., and Leroux, J.C. Block copolymer micelles: Preparation, characterization and application in drug delivery. *J Control Release* 109(1–3), 169–188, 2005.
39. Jones, M. and Leroux, J., Polymeric micelles—a new generation of colloidal drug carriers. *Eur J Pharm Biopharm* 48(2), 101–111, 1999.
40. Svenson, S. and Tomalia, D.A., Dendrimers in biomedical applications—Reflections on the field. *Adv Drug Deliv Rev* 57(15), 2106–2129, 2005.
41. Muller, R.H., Mader, K., and Gohla, S., Solid lipid nanoparticles (SLN) for controlled drug delivery—a review of the state of the art. *Eur J Pharm Biopharm* 50(1), 161–177, 2000.
42. Couvreur, P., Barratt, G., Fattal, E., Legrand, P., and Vauthier, C., Nanocapsule technology: A review. *Crit Rev Ther Drug Carrier Sys* 19(2), 99–134, 2002.
43. Sosnik, A., Carcaboso, A.M., Glisoni, R.J., Moretton, M.A., and Chiappetta, D.A., New old challenges in tuberculosis: Potentially effective nanotechnologies in drug delivery. *Adv Drug Deliv Rev* 62(4–5), 547–559, 2010.
44. Ready, P.D., Leishmaniasis emergence in Europe. *Euro Surveill* 15(10), 1–11, 2010.
45. Pandey, R. and Khuller, G.K., Oral nanoparticle-based antituberculosis drug delivery to the brain in an experimental model. *J Antimicrob Chemother* 57(6), 1146–1152, 2006.
46. Pandey, R., Zahoor, A., Sharma, S., and Khuller, G.K., Nanoparticle encapsulated antitubercular drugs as a potential oral drug delivery system against murine tuberculosis. *Tuberculosis (Edinb)* 83(6), 373–378, 2003.
47. Semete, B., Kalombo, L., Katata, L., Chelule, P., Booysen, L., Lemmer, Y., and Swai, H., Potential of improving the treatment of tuberculosis through nanomedicine. *Mol Cryst Liq Cryst* 556(1), 317–330, 2012.

48. Kisich, K.O., Gelperina, S., Higgins, M.P., Wilson, S., Shipulo, E., Oganesyan, E., and Heifets, L., Encapsulation of moxifloxacin within poly(butyl cyanoacrylate) nanoparticles enhances efficacy against intracellular Mycobacterium tuberculosis. *Int J Pharm* 345(1–2), 154–162, 2007.

49. Haas, S.E., Bettoni, C.C., de Oliveira, L.K., Guterres, S.S., and Dalla Costa, T., Nanoencapsulation increases quinine antimalarial efficacy against Plasmodium berghei in vivo. *Int J Antimicrob Agents* 34(2), 156–161, 2009.

50. Singh, K.K. and Vingkar, S.K., Formulation, antimalarial activity and biodistribution of oral lipid nanoemulsion of primaquine. *Int J Pharm* 347(1–2), 136–143, 2008.

51. Sundar, S., Chakravarty, J., Agarwal, D., Rai, M., and Murray, H.W., Single-dose liposomal amphotericin B for visceral leishmaniasis in India. *N Engl J Med* 362(6), 504–512, 2010.

52. Richard, J.V. and Werbovetz, K.A., New antileishmanial candidates and lead compounds. *Curr Opin Chem Biol* 14(4), 447–455, 2010.

53. Murray, H.W., Berman, J.D., Davies, C.R., and Saravia, N.G., Advances in leishmaniasis. *The Lancet* 366(9496), 1561–1577, 2005.

54. Jaser, M.A., el-Yazigi, A., and Croft, S.L., Pharmacokinetics of antimony in patients treated with sodium stibogluconate for cutaneous leishmaniasis. *Pharm Res* 12(1), 113–116, 1995.

55. Cruz, A., Rainey, P.M., Herwaldt, B.L., Stagni, G., Palacios, R., Trujillo, R., and Saravia, N.G., Pharmacokinetics of antimony in children treated for leishmaniasis with meglumine antimoniate. *J Infect Dis* 195(4), 602–608, 2007.

56. Monzote, L., Current treatment of leishmaniasis: A review. *Open Antimicrob Agent J* 1, 9–19, 2009.

57. Desjeux, P., Leishmaniasis: Current situation and new perspectives. *Comp Immunol Microbiol Infect Dis* 27(5), 305–318, 2004.

58. Dorlo, T.P., van Thiel, P.P., Huitema, A.D., Keizer, R.J., de Vries, H.J., Beijnen, H., and de Vries, P.J., Pharmacokinetics of miltefosine in Old World cutaneous leishmaniasis patients. *Antimicrob Agents Chemother* 52(8), 2855–2860, 2008.

59. Moore, E. and Lockwood, D., Treatment of visceral leishmaniasis. *J Glob Infect Dis* 2(2), 151–158, 2010.

60. Thanh, N.V., Cowman, A.F., Hipgrave, D., Kim, T.B., Phuc, B.Q., Cong, L.D., and Biggs, B.A., Assessment of susceptibility of Plasmodium falciparum to chloroquine, quinine, mefloquine, sulfadoxine-pyrimethamine and artemisinin in southern Viet Nam. *Trans R Soc Trop Med Hyg* 95, 513–517, 2009.

61. Crawley, J., Malaria: New challenges, new treatments. *Curr Paediatr* 9, 34–41, 1999.

62. Scholte, E.J., Knols, B.G.J., and Takken, W., Infection of the malaria mosquito Anopheles gambiae with the entomopathogenic fungus Metarhizium anisopliae reduces blood feeding and fecundity. *J Invertebr Pathol* 91, 43–49, 2006.

63. Willcox, M.L., Rakotondrazafy, E., Andriamanalimanana, R., Andrianasolo, D., and Rasoanaivo, P., Decreasing clinical efficacy of chloroquine in Ankazobe, Central Highlands of Madagascar. *Trans R Soc Trop Med Hyg* 98(5), 311–314, 2004.

64. Talisuna, A.O., Langi, P., Mutabingwa, T.K., Van Marck, E., Speybroeck, N., Egwang, T.G., Watkins, W.W., Hastings, I.M., and D'Alessandro, U., Intensity of transmission and spread of gene mutations linked to chloroquine and sulphadoxine-pyrimethamine resistance in falciparum malaria. *Int J Parasitol* 33(10), 1051–1058, 2003.

65. Obonyo, C.O., Juma, E.A., Ogutu, B.R., Vulule, J.M., and Lau, J., Amodiaquine combined with sulfadoxine/pyrimethamine versus artemisinin-based combinations for the treatment of uncomplicated falciparum malaria in Africa: A meta-analysis. *Trans R Soc Trop Med Hyg* 101(2), 117–126, 2007.

66. Smrkovski, L.L., Buck, R.L., Alcantara, A.K., Rodriguez, C.S., and Uylangco, C.V., Studies of resistance to chloroquine, quinine, amodiaquine and mefloquine among Philippine strains of Plasmodium falciparum. *Trans R Soc Trop Med Hyg* 79(1), 37–41, 1985.

67. Murray, M. and Farrell, G.C., Effects of primaquine on hepatic microsomal haemoproteins and drug oxidation. *Toxicology* 42(2–3), 205–217, 1986.

68. Santos-Magalhaes, N.S. and Mosqueira, V.C., Nanotechnology applied to the treatment of malaria. *Adv Drug Deliv Rev* 62(4–5), 560–575, 2010.
69. O'Meara, W.P., Bejon, P., Mwangi, T.W., Okiro, E.A., Peshu, N., Snow, R.W., Newton, C.R., and Marsh, K., Effect of a fall in malaria transmission on morbidity and mortality in Kilifi, Kenya. *The Lancet* 372(9649), 1555–1562, 2008.
70. Lindegardh, N., Hanpithakpong, W., Kamanikom, B., Singhasivanon, P., Socheat, D., Yi, P., Dondorp, A.M., McGready, R., Nosten, F., White, N.J., and Day, N.P., Major pitfalls in the measurement of artemisinin derivatives in plasma in clinical studies. *J Chromatogr B Anal Technol Biomed Life Sci* 876(1), 54–60, 2008.
71. Martin, A. and Portaels, F., Drug resistance and drug resistance detection. Tuberculosis 2007: From basic science to patient care 2007 [cited June 2, 2011], 635–660. Available from: http://www.tuberculosistextbook.com/tb/drugres.htm
72. Lounis, N., Veziris, N., Chauffour, A., Truffot-Pernot, C., Andries, K., and Jarlier, V., Combinations of R207910 with drugs used to treat multidrug-resistant tuberculosis have the potential to shorten treatment duration. *Antimicrob Agents Chemother* 50(11), 3543–3547, 2006.
73. Rathbun, R.C., Lockhart, S.M., and Stephens, J.R., Current HIV treatment guidelines—an overview. *Curr Pharm Des* 12(9), 1045–1063, 2006.
74. Shah, C.A., Adherence to high activity antiretrovial therapy (HAART) in pediatric patients infected with HIV: Issues and interventions. *Indian J Pediatr* 74(1), 55–60, 2007.
75. Amiji, M.M., Vyas, T.K., and Shah, L.K., Role of nanotechnology in HIV/AIDS treatment: Potential to overcome the viral reservoir challenge. *Discov Med* 6(34), 157–162, 2006.
76. Huang, S.M. and Lesko, L.J., Drug-drug, drug-dietary supplement, and drug-citrus fruit and other food interactions: What have we learned? *J Clin Pharmacol* 44(6), 559–569, 2004.
77. Gerber, J.G., Using pharmacokinetics to optimize antiretroviral drug-drug interactions in the treatment of human immunodeficiency virus infection. *Clin Infect Dis* 30 Suppl 2, S123–S129, 2000.
78. Forrest, G.N. and Tamura, K., Rifampin combination therapy for nonmycobacterial infections. *Clin Microbiol Rev* 23(1), 14–34, 2010.
79. Thomas, V.H., Bhattachar, S., Hitchingham, L., Zocharski, P., Naath, M., Surendran, N., Stoner, C.L., and El-Kattan, A., The road map to oral bioavailability: An industrial perspective. *Expert Opin Drug Metab Toxicol* 2(4), 591–608, 2006.
80. Kayser, O., Olbrich, C., Yardley, V., Kiderlen, A.F., and Croft, S.L., Formulation of amphotericin B as nanosuspension for oral administration. *Int J Pharm* 254(1), 73–75, 2003.
81. Demicheli, C., Ochoa, R., da Silva, J.B., Falcão, C.A., Rossi-Bergmann, B., de Melo, A.L., Sinisterra, R.D., and Frézard, F., Oral delivery of Meglumine Antimoniate-{beta}-Cyclodextrin complex for treatment of leishmaniasis. *Antimicrob Agents Chemother* 48(1), 100–103, 2004.
82. Chiappetta, D.A., Hocht, C., Taira, C., and Sosnik, A., Oral pharmacokinetics of the anti-HIV efavirenz encapsulated within polymeric micelles. *Biomaterials* 32(9), 2379–2387, 2011.
83. Chiappetta, D.A. and Sosnik, A., Poly(ethylene oxide)-poly(propylene oxide) block copolymer micelles as drug delivery agents: Improved hydrosolubility, stability and bioavailability of drugs. *Eur J Pharm Biopharm* 66(3), 303–317, 2007.
84. Pandey, R. and Khuller, G.K., Subcutaneous nanoparticle-based antitubercular chemotherapy in an experimental model. *J Antimicrob Chemother* 54(1), 266–268, 2004.
85. Shipulo, E., Lyubimov, I., Maksimenko, O., Vanchugova, L.V., Oganesyan, E.A., Sveshnikov, P.G., Biketov, S.F., Severin, E.S., Heifets, L.B., and Gel'perina, S.E., Development of a nanosomal formulation of moxifloxacin based on poly(butyl-2-cyanoacrylate). *Pharm Chem J* 42(3), 145–149, 2008.
86. Wu, Y., Li, M., and Gao, H., Polymeric micelle composed of PLA and chitosan as a drug carrier. *J Polym Res* 16(1), 11–18, 2009.
87. Silva, M., Lara, A.S., Leite, C.Q.F., and Ferreira, E.I., Potential tuberculostatic agents: Micelle-forming copolymer poly(ethylene glycol)-poly(aspartic acid) prodrug with isoniazid. *Archiv der Pharmazie* 334(6), 189–193, 2001.

88. Silva, M., Ricelli, N.L., El Seoud, O., Valentim, C.S., Ferreira, A.G., Sato, D.N., Leite, C.Q., and Ferreira, E.I., Potential tuberculostatic agent: Micelle-forming pyrazinamide prodrug. *Archiv der Pharmazie* 339(6), 283–290, 2006.

89. Silva, M., Ferreira, E.I., Leiti, C.Q.F., and Sato, D.N., Preparation of polymeric micelles for use as carriers of tuberculostatic drugs. *Trop J Pharm Res* 6(4), 815–824, 2007.

90. Ahmad, Z., Pandey, R., Sharma, S., and Khuller, G.K., Pharmacokinetic and pharmacodynamic behaviour of antitubercular drugs encapsulated in alginate nanoparticles at two doses. *Int J Antimicrob Agents* 27(5), 409–416, 2006.

91. Ahmad, Z., Sharma, S., and Khuller, G.K., Inhalable alginate nanoparticles as antitubercular drug carriers against experimental tuberculosis. *Int J Antimicrob Agents* 26(4), 298–303, 2005.

92. Schäfer, V., von Briesen, H., Andreesen, R., Steffan, A.M., Royer, C., Tröster, S., Kreuter, J., and Rübsamen-Waigmann H., Phagocytosis of nanoparticles by human immunodeficiency virus (HIV)-infected macrophages: A possibility for antiviral drug targeting. *Pharm Res* 9(4), 541–546, 1992.

93. Shah, L.K. and Amiji, M.M., Intracellular delivery of saquinavir in biodegradable polymeric nanoparticles for HIV/AIDS. *Pharm Res* 23(11), 2638–2645, 2006.

94. Dembri, A., Montisci, M.J., Gantier, J.C., Chacun, H., and Ponchel, G., Targeting of 3′-azido 3′-deoxythymidine (AZT)-loaded poly(isohexylcyanoacrylate) nanospheres to the gastrointestinal mucosa and associated lymphoid tissues. *Pharm Res* 18(4), 467–473, 2001.

95. Jain, S., Tiwary, A.K., and Jain, N.K., Sustained and targeted delivery of an anti-HIV agent using elastic liposomal formulation: Mechanism of action. *Curr Drug Deliv* 3(2), 157–166, 2006.

96. Jain, S.K., Gupta, Y., Jain, A., Saxena, A.R., Khare, P., and Jain, A., Mannosylated gelatin nanoparticles bearing an anti-HIV drug didanosine for site-specific delivery. *Nanomedicine* 4(1), 41–48, 2008.

97. McGee, B., Smith, N., and Aweeka, F., HIV pharmacology: Barriers to the eradication of HIV from the CNS. *HIV Clin Trials* 7(3), 142–153, 2006.

98. Deol, P. and Khuller, G.K., Lung specific stealth liposomes: Stability, biodistribution and toxicity of liposomal antitubercular drugs in mice. *Biochim Biophys Acta* 1334(2–3), 161–172, 1997.

99. Kumar, P.V., Asthana, A., Dutta, T., and Jain, N.K., Intracellular macrophage uptake of rifampicin loaded mannosylated dendrimers. *J Drug Target* 14(8), 546–556, 2006.

100. Kumar, P.V., Agashe, H., Dutta, T., and Jain, N.K., PEGylated dendritic architecture for development of a prolonged drug delivery system for an antitubercular drug. *Curr Drug Deliv* 4(1), 11–19, 2007.

101. Irache, J.M., Salman, H.H., Gamazo, C., and Espuelas, S., Mannose-targeted systems for the delivery of therapeutics. *Expert Opin Drug Deliv* 5(6), 703–724, 2008.

102. Chono, S., Tanino, T., Seki, T., and Morimoto, K., Uptake characteristics of liposomes by rat alveolar macrophages: Influence of particle size and surface mannose modification. *J Pharm Pharmacol* 59(1), 75–80, 2007.

103. Chono, S., Tanino, T., Seki, T., and Morimoto, K., Efficient drug targeting to rat alveolar macrophages by pulmonary administration of ciprofloxacin incorporated into mannosylated liposomes for treatment of respiratory intracellular parasitic infections. *J Control Release* 127(1), 50–58, 2008.

104. Vermehren, C., Frokjaer, S., Aurstad, T., and Hansen, J., Lung surfactant as a drug delivery system. *Int J Pharm* 307(1), 89–92, 2006.

105. Poelma, D.L., Zimmermann, L.J., Scholten, H.H., Lachmann, B., and van Iwaarden, J.F., In vivo and in vitro uptake of surfactant lipids by alveolar type II cells and macrophages. *Am J Physiol Lung Cell Mol Physiol* 283(3), L648–L654, 2002.

106. Date, A.A., Joshi, M.D., and Patravale, V.B., Parasitic diseases: Liposomes and polymeric nanoparticles versus lipid nanoparticles. *Adv Drug Deliv Rev* 59(6), 505–521, 2007.

107. Lowell, J.E. and Earl, C.D., Leveraging biotech's drug discovery expertise for neglected diseases. *Nat Biotechnol* 27(4), 323–329, 2009.

14

Nanorobotics for Targeted Medical Interventions

Sylvain Martel

CONTENTS

14.1 Introduction

Nanorobotics often integrates nanotechnology and robotics with the aim of developing new tools and instruments for specific applications. Nanotechnology is attractive in this respect since the physics inherent to nanoscale entities differ significantly from those at the macroscale. Hence, by exploiting the forces and phenomena that operate at both scales, the range of possibilities for generating solutions at the engineering level (where the laws of physics are applied) may be enhanced considerably. When targeted medical interventions are integrated with robotics, which provide techniques for closed-loop control and actuation based on informational feedback, the resulting systems can be envisioned as leading to future nanorobotics applications.

Although many targeted medical interventions could benefit from the techniques being developed in nanorobotics over the longer term, there is one particular medical intervention where nanorobotics might play a huge role in the shorter term, which could translate to an important impact on medical practice. Such an application may be realized as targeted drug delivery in cancer therapy. Indeed, present cancer therapeutics frequently fail because of severe side effects that are related to the fact that drugs accumulate in insufficient concentrations at tumor sites while being distributed to, and negatively impacting, healthy tissues and organs. Due to the lack of an effective means for the direct targeting (DT) of drugs to tumoral areas, systemic chemotherapy often remains the only available drug delivery option, resulting in unnecessary systematic exposure and severe toxicity. Therefore, the use of specifically targeted drug-loaded vehicles that deliver their payloads precisely to areas that are to be treated is pivotal for the creation of improved tumor killing effects, while minimizing the toxic side effects that are initiated by drug activity in nontargeted regions.

It is quite perplexing that the engineering sciences have been ignored as a complementary resource of expertise for assisting in the development of more effective methods for targeted cancer therapies. Certainly, it is well known that engineering has proved to be highly efficient in finding solutions for other targeting applications. Therefore, the integration of these proven techniques, albeit adapted to targeted cancer therapy while taking advantage of the present know-how in drug delivery, may prove to be highly beneficial. One particular engineering domain that may fulfill this role is medical nanorobotics, where robotics is linked with nanotechnology and nanomedicine. However, the introduction of engineering toward the provision of complementary techniques in targeted cancer therapy will most likely influence the way in which future nanoscale drug delivery might be performed and how therapeutic nanocarriers will be synthesized.

Indeed, although chemotherapeutic agents have been widely used in oncology over the past 25 years, they continue to offer poor tumor specificity, and therefore, exhibit dose-limiting toxicity. In recent years, efforts have been undertaken to develop targeted vectors, most often in the form of nanoparticles, for the chemotherapeutic treatment of various types of cancer. A number of systems have demonstrated encouraging results in clinical trials. However, conventional targeted delivery systems are still lacking and have need of considerable improvement. One of the major problems that remain unsolved so far is the low extent of deposition and accumulation of drug carriers and their therapeutic payloads within the tumor tissue. Various approaches that have been explored to date, such as conjugation with targeting molecules including small molecules, peptides, or antibodies, have led to only limited success. As such, there is an urgent requirement for new types of carriers that are capable of delivering most, if not all, of their therapeutic payloads to targeted tumoral sites.

14.2 Recent Targeted Delivery Drug Carriers

Over the last few years, various targeted delivery vehicles have been designed and evaluated in animal model studies as well as in clinical trials. These vehicles include water-soluble polymers to which cytostatic drugs are covalently attached, polymeric nanoparticles, stabilized solid amorphous hydrophobic drug nanoparticles, polymeric micelles loaded in particular with hydrophobic drugs, and liposomes loaded with both hydrophobic and hydrophilic drugs. Doxil, a liposomal formulation that incorporates the cytostatic agent doxorubicin (DOX) is one example of the first systems that have entered the market. Although encouraging results with targeted nanomedicines have been obtained, the extent of their adsorption to and accumulation within tumor tissue remains to be significantly improved through the enhancement of targeting strategies.

14.3 Improved Targeting Strategies

Improved targeting of drug-carrying nanoparticles can be achieved by different means. Initially, the intrinsic properties of tumors were utilized in order to achieve the passive accumulation of nanoparticles by the so-called enhanced penetration and retention (EPR). It is well known that due to the high proliferation rate of cancer cells, which requires high amounts of nutrients, the blood-supplying vessels of the tumor are characterized by the so-called leaky endothelium, with relatively large gaps that are present between endothelial cells, whereas drainage is greatly suppressed by the tight gaps in lymphatic endothelium. If drug nanoparticles are relatively small (e.g., below 200 nm), they may inflow from the blood into the tumor tissue and accumulate there due to the poor outflow of the lymphatic vessels. Since this is a slow process and the goal is to enable continuous inflow into the tumor, the nanoparticles must be characterized by relatively long circulation retention times within the blood vessels.

Toward this end, nanoparticles may be synthesized to achieve "stealth" properties, which can often be done by coating their surfaces with a thin layer of hydrophilic polymer (e.g., PEG). However, the efficiency of this process still remains rather low [1] due to diffusion back into the blood circulation, whereas the stealth properties of the nanoparticles prevent their internalization into the tumor cells. Thus, a certain enrichment of the tumor over surrounding healthy tissues can be observed, and only a small percentage of the applied nanoparticles is able to accumulate within the tumor. The introduction of receptor-specific ligands (e.g., antibodies, folate) onto the surfaces of drug-carrying nanoparticles results in their enhanced internalization within tumor cells and continuous uptake from the extracellular compartments of tumors, with increased rates of intracellular accumulation. However, only a moderate improvement may be achieved. The reasons are that the nanoparticle inflow into the tumor is governed by diffusion from the blood vessel, and also by a relatively low and steadily decreasing concentration of the nanoparticles within the circulation, making their accumulated volumes remain rather low [2].

14.4 Principal Constraints for Controlled Navigation within the Vascular Network

The human adult vascular network provides close to 100,000 km of pathways to access the various regions in the human body. Furthermore, tumors are also accessible by a network of capillaries known as the angiogenesis network, which fuse with normal blood vessels for the purpose of obtaining oxygen and nutrients to facilitate tumor growth. As such, the vascular network appears to be the ideal pathway for many critical targeted medical interventions performed with nanorobotics. However, navigating through the vascular network is highly technologically challenging for several reasons. First, physiological conditions vary considerably from larger blood vessels to the most diminutive of capillaries, and this translates to significant technical complexities. Indeed, the diameters of blood vessels can range from a few millimeters in the arteries, down to a few micrometers in the capillaries, with respective blood flow velocities ranging from approximately one-third of a meter per second down to a millimeter per second. This fact demands relatively robust propulsive forces, with operations being executed in both high and low Reynolds number regimes. This is quite challenging, considering that to reach tumors through the angiogenesis network, the overall diameter of the navigable core or microrobot must ideally not exceed approximately 2 µm.

Second, there is no existing medical imaging modality that is capable of imaging the tiniest blood vessels, including small arterioles and capillaries. For example, medical imaging techniques such as x-ray, computed tomography (CT) and magnetic resonance imaging (MRI) for humans have a spatial resolution of a few hundred micrometers, sufficient to image larger blood vessels such as arteries but far from adequate for the imaging of the ultrafine blood vessels that connect to a tumor. Without the capability of imaging the prospective routes that must be followed to reach targeted tumors, traditional closed-loop navigation control strategies, such as those often encountered in robotics are not possible. The latter is another example of the myriad challenges that call for new innovative approaches that can potentially be fulfilled with the assistance of nanorobotics.

14.5 Overview of Potential Methods of Transport within the Vascular Network

Despite the many challenges and constraints imposed by human physiology, a first step toward in vivo navigation would be to identify potential methods of transport within the vascular network. Each method of transport calls for a propelling or motile force, which in turn requires a source of power. Such an energy source might be embedded within the microcarriers themselves or may be typically located outside the patient. Considering the miniaturized volume of such microcarriers, the generation of sufficient motile force via embedded piezoelectric or electrostatic actuators (to name but two popular strategies) coupled with the provision of a local energy source and frequent voltage conversions are unlikely. This is the case, at least in the short term, as none of these capacities at present may be integrated at such small scales. Microfuel cells are not yet advanced enough; the induction of energy from an external source (as with the use of embedded photovoltaic cells) is problematic as they still occupy a large area which is not suitable for travel within blood vessels, especially through the capillaries, and photonic penetration, even with the use of near infrared (IR), is still depth-limited.

Wireless power induction to activate a small propeller or flagellated propulsion system under low Reynolds' hydrodynamic conditions as encountered in the microvasculature is also difficult to integrate at such a scale, considering the dimensions of the receiving antenna that must be embedded. Thermovoltaic systems, relying on differences in temperature (e.g., Seebeck effect), are also difficult at such a scale, and are limited when operating within the body, considering the relative homogeneity of the body temperature within the vascular system. Microturbines actuated by the blood flow to produce electrical energy that might be transformed as a motile force have been investigated, but it is still improbable that such a technology can be effectively scaled down to provide sufficient energy for moving nanocarriers, taking into account physiological data in terms of blood volume and flow velocities. Chemically mediated catalytic reactions resulting in a propulsive force could potentially be an interesting concept to investigate, but many questions remain unresolved at the present time in regard to its possible utility for therapeutic purposes. One of the most probable methods in the short term that may prove successful, and where substantial efforts and progress in medical nanorobotics have been made in recent years, would be the induction of a motile force for microcarriers from an external source that is capable of generating sufficient magnetic gradients.

14.6 Magnetic Microcarriers

Superparamagnetic iron oxide nanoparticles (SPIONs), in clinical use, for disease detection by MRI have also been considered as targeted drug delivery vectors that are endowed with the capacity for detection. For instance, sustained and elevated tissue concentrations were achieved with intra-articularly administered ultrasmall superparamagnetic iron oxide nanoparticles (USPIONs) when an external magnet was applied to the joint [3]. Nonetheless, although targeting can be enhanced by an external magnetic field, the therapeutic results obtained with these magnetic carriers are still generally far from optimal. This is especially true when attempting targeting operations deeper beneath the skin. There are two primary causes to explain the suboptimal targeting results of this approach. First, these magnetic vectors are still released systematically such that a relatively great proportion accumulates in untargeted regions prior to reaching the tumor. Second, the gradient field from the external magnet decreases exponentially as the distance below the surface of the skin increases—since for a given magnetic material such as iron oxide (which is intensively used in such target interventions), a very high-intensity magnetic field is required to compensate for the very small volume of these magnetic nanoparticles (MNPs), as the force induced is proportional to the overall volume of the magnetic cores. Thus, the efficiency in magnetic targeting is then restricted to the sites that are very close to the surface of the skin, above which the magnet is located. Nonetheless, these preliminary results suggest that magnetism is still a viable noninvasive force to be considered in future research for achieving enhanced targeting efficacy.

14.7 Magnetic Resonance Navigation (MRN)

A recent study, validated with experimental data published in 2007 [4], showed that by immersing a patient (or the region of interest [ROI]) inside a high homogeneous static magnetic field and by superimposing directional magnetic gradients, it was possible to induce a displacement force on a magnetic carrier that, unlike the use of an external magnet, becomes independent of the distance between a potential deeply located target and the skin surface (i.e., the method can be as effective at the core of the torso, for instance, as it is near the surface of the skin). In this experiment, a living swine was placed inside the bore of a 1.5 T clinical MR scanner, and a 1.5 mm magnetic bead was navigated automatically (i.e., without human intervention) back and forth along a preplanned trajectory in the carotid artery of the animal at an average velocity of 10 cm/s. In this experiment, the MR scanner typically used as medical imaging modality, not only tracked the ferromagnetic bead through a special real-time MR-tracking (MRT) technique (capable of gathering 20–30 positions/s), but the high homogeneous static field (the B_0 field of 1.5 T or 3 T in conventional clinical MRI scanners) and the superposed 3D gradients typically used for MR image slice selection (and generated by the MRI scanner's orthogonal imaging coils) provided the required environment for propelling the magnetic object deeply within the body. With this robotically inspired approach, applied corrective actions necessary to propel and maintain the ferromagnetic bead along the planned trajectory were computed and translated onto 3D gradient forces acting on the untethered magnetic core using the MRI gradient coils.

This led to the first experimental demonstration of what would later be referred to as MRN. Not only can MRN perform effectively in deep tissues while avoiding healthy tissues and organs, but it also suggests a new paradigm in targeted cancer therapy, where efforts in increasing the systemic circulation time for drug-loaded carriers is no longer a priority, or a requirement, for specific types of cancer since the influence of the systemic circulation can potentially be eliminated, or at least substantially reduced, using MRN. In other words, MRN brings forth the concept of what is referred to here as DT, rather than the notion of targeting with prior release being conducted systematically, which is typically referred to in oncology. Indeed, unlike all targeting methods proposed thus far, DT based on MRN is most likely the only strategy that has the potential for, and the aim of, avoiding systemic circulation.

14.8 Fundamental Principles of MRN

An MRN agent will contain a quantity of magnetic material that when integrated would correspond to a magnetic entity (ME) (i.e., only typically made of soft magnetic materials, unlike MRN agents that may contain nonmagnetic materials in addition to magnetic material). The ME, behaving similarly to a propulsive and steering entity inside the MRN agent, will experience a force when in the presence of an external magnetic gradient. Such force will depend on the magnetization of the ME (M) and the magnitude of the external magnetic gradient. If the external field is nonuniform (e.g., when applying an external permanent magnet or an active electromagnet on one side of the patient at any particular instant during the intervention), the ME will experience a gradient force that will move the same ME toward the regions of higher magnitude of the field. As the ME moves in the direction of the higher field (toward the magnet), its magnetization level will also increase to the saturation magnetization of the magnetic material that is embedded within the ME ($M \rightarrow M_S$). This increase in magnetization concurrent with motion and combined with an increase of the strength of the magnetic field gradient occurring in a nonlinear fashion would lead to an acceleration of the ME so significant that it might make real-time navigational control extremely difficult, if not impossible, while potentially reducing the effectiveness of feedback control. This would be due to prolonged latencies in the control loop compared to the time required to perform corrective actions on the ME for navigation and/or targeting purposes.

The use of a hard magnetic material within the navigable entity would eliminate the variation in magnetization of the ME while offering the high magnetization level required for inducing a high force for a given gradient intensity. However, the use of hard magnetic materials (e.g., permanent or hard magnets) would restrict the types of targeted interventions that could be supported in comparison to those utilizing ME, which rely, for instance, on soft magnetic materials such as ferromagnetic or superparamagnetic nanoparticles. Another approach employing ME with a soft magnetic material would be to operate them in the linear or quasi-linear region (e.g., in a field below the saturation magnetization of the material embedded within the ME). Although this could potentially simplify the control task, it would limit the area where navigation can be performed, as well as the force induced on the ME, and would impose limitations on its navigability in constrained regions, including smaller diameter blood vessels, since the force induced depends not only on the magnetization of the ME, but also on the effective volume of the magnetic material embedded within the ME. An additional critical issue and limitation of using only external source magnetic gradients is that the decay in the strength of the magnetic gradient at a certain distance from the source is significant, which limits the effective magnetization of the ME, and hence limits effective navigation when positioned at a further distance from the magnets, such as when operating deeper within the patient's body.

To correct the previously mentioned issues, MRN has been proposed. MRN relies on a homogeneous magnetic field (such as the 1.5 T (or more) B_0 field of a clinical MRI scanner, depicted in Figure 14.1) with a magnitude typically and ideally sufficient for the ME to reach (or in a nonideal case, close to reaching) saturation magnetization. In this instance, a proper coil design (referred to here as the steering gradient coil—SGC), shown as a propulsion coil set in Figure 14.1 is mounted in a configuration (such as those found in clinical MRI scanners for image slice selection) that is used to produce

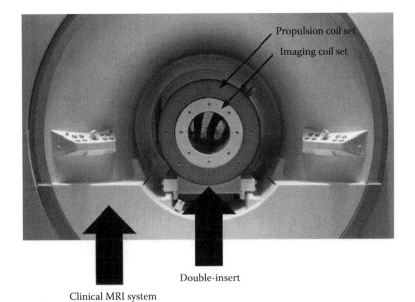

FIGURE 14.1
Photograph of a double-insert used for MRN inside the tunnel of a clinical MRI scanner.

controlled and linear or (quasi-linear) magnetic gradients. This approach makes navigation control easier and more effective while being depth-independent, that is, the motion
behavior of the ME due to the SGC is independent of the depth below the skin surface
where the ME is being navigated.

With an imaging gradient coil (IGC) configuration mounted next to the SGC, the resulting double-insert also provides an imaging modality to potentially assess targeting efficacy by gathering data as to the distribution and quantification of the navigable agents
subsequent to MRN. Additionally, the acquisition of tracking information that might be
necessary for the computation of corrective actions during MRN may be obtained in the
form of 3D gradients, so as to maintain the MRN agents along a planned trajectory and/or
to direct them toward a target.

14.9 Fundamental Theory of MRN

The theory behind the fundamental principle of MRN may be explained mathematically
as follows. The magnetic vectored force F responsible for propelling and/or steering a
single magnetic particle, also referred to here as the "pulling force," is dependent on the
magnetic susceptibility difference $\Delta\chi$ of the particle and its surrounding fluid or environment, the magnetic field strength B, and the gradient of the field, according to the following general equations:

$$\vec{F} = (\vec{m} \cdot \nabla)\,\vec{B}, \tag{14.1a}$$

$$\vec{m} = \frac{V_P \Delta\chi \vec{B}}{\mu_0}. \tag{14.1b}$$

In Equation 14.1b, V_P is the volume of the magnetic particle and μ_0 is the magnetic permeability of free space.

Within the bore (tunnel) of a MRI scanner or a platform such as the MRN system, where
there is a homogeneous static magnetic field with a magnitude sufficient to bring the magnetic particle to full saturation magnetization (referred to here as the B_0 field), the magnetic
moment of the particle will align with B along the z-axis, in our particular case being in
alignment with the longitudinal axis of the tunnel or bore of the MRI scanner, or the MRN
system. In such a condition, we have

$$\vec{m} = m_Z = V_M \cdot M_{SZ}. \tag{14.2}$$

In Equation 14.2, V_M is the total volume of soft magnetic material (typically ferromagnetic
or superparamagnetic) that constitutes the ME within an MRN agent, where $V_M = N\,V_P$ for
N magnetic particles of the same dimensions embedded in an MRN agent with $V_M \leq V_A$,
where V_A is the volume of the same MRN agent, $\tau_M = V_M / V_A$ is the ratio of the total volume
of embedded magnetic material over the total volume of the MRN agent, and M_S is the
corresponding saturation magnetization level of the magnetic material, or ME embedded within the MRN agent. Since the magnetic moment is saturated in the z-direction

(along the bore of the MRI scanner or MRN system having a sufficiently high B_0 field), M_S can be rewritten as M_{SZ}, while Equation 14.1a can be rewritten as

$$\vec{F} = R \cdot V_M \left(M_{SZ} \cdot \nabla \right) B_z, \tag{14.3}$$

where R defined in the interval 0 to 1 represents the duty cycle of the pulling force being applied, that is, the fraction of the time within a cycle where the pulling gradient responsible for inducing a pulling force on the ME is being applied. In Equation 14.3, the gradient operator is expressed as

$$\nabla = \left[\frac{\partial}{\partial x} \quad \frac{\partial}{\partial y} \quad \frac{\partial}{\partial z} \right]^T. \tag{14.4}$$

Hence, in terms of magnetic gradients that are responsible for inducing a directional pulling force along the x-, y-, and z-axes, and denoted G_X, G_Y, and G_Z, respectively, Equation 14.3 may be rewritten as

$$\vec{F} = R \cdot V_M \cdot M_{SZ} \left[\frac{\partial B_Z}{\partial x} \quad \frac{\partial B_Z}{\partial y} \quad \frac{\partial B_Z}{\partial z} \right]^T \tag{14.5}$$

$$= R \cdot V_M \cdot M_{SZ} [G_X \quad G_Y \quad G_Z]^T = R \cdot V_M \cdot M_{SZ} \cdot \vec{G}.$$

The magnitude of the resulting directional force from each of the vectored forces along x, y, and z, as defined in Equation 14.6, and generated by the directional gradient G achieved from the combination of specific values of G_X, G_Y, and G_Z, must be sufficiently high not only to correct various forces or turbulence/perturbations that may cause trajectory errors but also to counteract forces acting against the MRN agents.

$$[F_X \quad F_Y \quad F_Z]^T = R \cdot V_M \cdot M_{SZ} \left[\frac{\partial B_X}{\partial z} \quad \frac{\partial B_Y}{\partial z} \quad \frac{\partial B_Z}{\partial z} \right]^T. \tag{14.6}$$

These forces may include, but are not limited to the blood flow (e.g., if the agent is forced to move in a reciprocal (opposite direction to the flow)), various perturbations such as vortices, sliding friction, drag force, and wall retardation effects, to name but a few potential forces acting upon the MRN agent. As such, in many instances, some of these forces and particularly the blood flow are often exploited to reduce or eliminate the gradient required for effective propulsion. For instance, the blood flow will typically be used for propulsion, while G will be primarily employed to steer, that is, to provide directional forces to navigate the MRN agent into the desired (targeted) branch at vessel bifurcations. Nonetheless, considering the relatively small value of V_A and hence the corresponding V_M, especially in smaller diameter vessels, and the physiological conditions that exist, the trend in the implementation of an MRN system compared to a clinical MRI scanner is to maximize the amplitude of G and to increase its frequency or switching rate within human limits/tolerances. While the trend for the implementation of new MRI scanners is to maximize B_Z, for the MRN system, in terms of inducing a force on the ME for propulsion/steering purposes alone, there is no real advantage to increasing B_Z (also referred to as B_0) being defined as the homogeneous field required to bring ME to M_S.

14.10 MRI as Imaging Modality for MRN

MRN should rely on the fact that single entities as small as a few tens of micrometers (μm) in size should be detectable inside the human body with the aim of collecting information that will guide real-time decisions and navigation control processes to direct them toward specific targets such as those which are accessible through the vascular network. However, the highest spatial resolution of all conventional medical imaging modalities, including x-rays, MRI, PET, and ultrasound, when applied to humans, is far from being sufficient to detect a single object that is as diminutive as a few tens of micrometers.

As such, using MRI techniques as the basis for MRN systems are not only suitable for providing the high homogeneous field required to bring the ME to saturation magnetization, but may also gather tracking information to retrieve the positional information of individual MRN agents, or an aggregate of MRN agents. Even though these entities have overall dimensions of below the spatial resolution of currently available medical imaging modalities, these MRI techniques may facilitate the assessment of targeting effectiveness by quantifying the number of MRN agents within a targeted region and to gather information about the distribution of these agents within a given area. The latter is fundamental to MRN applied to very small agents (i.e., less than the spatial resolution of the imaging/tracking modality), or aggregates of agents, which may often be the case for specific types of interventions.

Indeed, susceptibility-based negative contrast in MRI, for instance, can provide a means to detect these micro-entities. Identical ferromagnetic materials used for propulsion via gradients generated by the SGC may also induce a perturbation in the primary magnetic field homogeneity of the B_0 field of a MRI scanner (or MRN system). The use of a ferromagnetic sphere (to minimize shape anisotropy), for instance, induces a field distortion/perturbation similar to that of a magnetic dipole. Local magnetic field distortions initiated by such a sphere can be estimated at a point P of coordinates r (x, y, z) by that of a magnetic dipole as

$$\vec{B}'(P) = \frac{\mu_0}{4\pi}\left(3\frac{(\vec{m}.\vec{r})\vec{r}}{r^5} - \frac{\vec{m}}{r^3}\right), \tag{14.7}$$

where $\mu_0 = 4\pi \cdot 10^{-7}$ H·m^{-1} is the permeability of free space, with m being generally defined in Equation 14.1b.

This perturbation may attain an overall size that is much larger than the ME itself. When such an artifact reaches the size of a typical MRI voxel (~0.5 × 0.5 × 0.5 mm^3), with a field perturbation that is sufficiently high to be detectable by the MRI scanner (or the MRN system), the ME becomes visible by MRI methods in the form of a susceptibility artifact. More precisely, the intravoxel dephasing in the gradient echo (GE) sequence provides an effective method to amplify the effect of a ME that is physically too small to be visualized in the MR image. Experimental data have demonstrated that a single ME with a diameter as small as 15 μm, which relies on materials with high susceptibility may indeed be detected by the intravoxel dephasing using GE scans. Although this proves to be very advantageous in comparison to other medical imaging modalities, including x-rays, where navigable agents must be at least a few hundred micrometers across to be detectable, MRI-based real-time tracking performance for carriers of this size while operating at full velocity is still a challenging task that requires further investigation. Indeed, although an MRN agent of 1.5 mm might be tracked in real time between 20 and 30 times/s using a special algorithm known as MS-SET, decreasing the size of the magnetic agents results in smaller artifacts, and hence, a weaker signal that requires more time for proper tracking. This may require as long as a few seconds to a few minutes, dependant on the overall dimensions of the agents and the MRI sequence that is being employed for imaging.

14.11 Ideal Closed-Loop MRN Control

Ideally, closed-loop MRN control would be performed as depicted schematically in Figure 14.2, with feedback control performed at a sufficient frequency to guarantee control stability. Initially, images of the blood vessels are gathered. This is typically achieved using x-ray or MRI with contrast agents being injected into the vessels during imaging. After the filtering of gathered images, only the blood vessels of interest remain visible. Subsequently, a reference is indicated in the form of a trajectory or a series of waypoints along the preferred path. This reference is compared with the measured output corresponding to the position of the MRN agent navigating within the vascular network. This comparison leads to a measured error that corresponds to the positional deviation of the MRN agent from the planned trajectory, which is being used as the reference. Based on

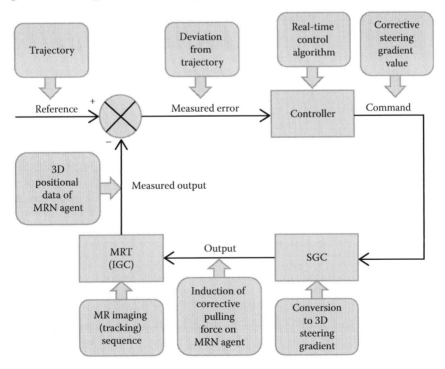

FIGURE 14.2
Schematic of the ideal closed-loop MRN control of an MRN agent.

this measured error, the controller computes a corrective action that needs to be applied in order to maintain such an MRN agent along the planned trajectory. This navigational control action can be based on various algorithms, but real-time performance must be maintained. The result of the control algorithm is translated to a command that indicates the corrective steering gradient that must be applied to the MRN agent. This command is transmitted to the SGC after it is converted to an analog form and is amplified. The output of the SGC then takes the form of a corrective steering gradient with a magnitude that may attain several hundred mT/m. This steering gradient induces a directional pulling force on the magnetic core or MNPs of the MRN agent that influences the displacement of the MRN agent, which ideally returns to the planned trajectory.

Once the corrective steering gradient has been applied, a MRT sequence is performed to gather data in regard to the new position of the MRN agent. To reiterate, many different types of MRI sequences may be developed and used for this purpose, where the most appropriate will depend on various parameters such as acquisition time, or the time necessary to acquire the tracking information, and the requirement in terms of sensibility of the imaging sequence, which would depend on the size of the image artifacts that are generated by the MRN agent, etc. During MRT, the IGC is used to generate a 3D gradient that is employed to select an image slice of the patient. The amplitude of this gradient is typically much less than the maximum amplitude of the steering gradient; however, the transition time (e.g., the rise time) is comparatively much shorter. A radio frequency (RF) pulse generated by an antenna that is located between the patient and the IGC is also used, and the signal that is recovered by the same RF antenna is then either utilized to reconstruct the MR-image, or during MRN, to determine the tracked position of the MRN agent that will be compared against the reference to recompute the next corrective action. Ideally in practice, this execution loop must be repeated at a sufficient rate to guarantee that the MRN agent/s will remain within a given margin of error from referenced pathways in order to reach the targeted site by steering through the appropriate branching vessels along each of the encountered bifurcations.

14.12 Deviations from Ideal Closed-Loop MRN Control

Although an ideal closed-loop MRN control as depicted in Figure 14.2 has been demonstrated experimentally in the carotid artery of a living swine, achieving such optimal real-time MRN control for most targeted medical interventions is unlikely due to several constraints. Without delving into too much detailed information, we mention here the main constraints that would prevent, or at least make such an ideal closed-loop MRN control difficult to achieve in a formal clinical setting.

The first major constraint is the time that is required to track the position of the MRN agent. For the first experimental demonstration of MRN in the carotid artery of a pig, a ferromagnetic bead with a diameter of 1.5 mm was used. At such a dimension, the ME generated a relatively large artifact or distortion of the B_0 homogeneous field where the intensity of such distortion at the edge of the voxel (3D pixel with an edge of ~500 μm in this particular case) was sufficiently large with regard to the sensitivity of the MRI hardware in executing rapid MRT sequences (in this case being between 20 and 30 times/s), which proved to be adequate for real-time MRN operations within the carotid artery. However, 1.5 mm in diameter MRN agents are much too large to be considered for most targeted medical interventions. As such, MRN agents must typically be reduced in size to allow them to be navigated within smaller diameter vessels, ideally well beyond the catheterization limit, which is approximately 1 mm in diameter. However, an MRN agent with a diameter of below 1 mm would already result in a much lower distortion of the homogeneous field, which would make MR detection more difficult and would require a longer acquisition time that might require from a few seconds to a few minutes, contingent on the characteristics of the artifact produced by the MRN agent and the sensitivity level of the MRI hardware. Such delays place a critical constraint on the performance of real-time MRN.

A second major constraint is that such MRT cannot be accomplished when the steering gradient is present, since it would interfere with the imaging gradient. Therefore, the output of the SGC (see Figure 14.2) must be set to zero prior to using the IGC. Because the SGC is typically characterized with a larger inductance compared to IGC in order to achieve larger magnitudes, the corresponding slew rate translates into a relatively longer time to reach the steering gradient magnitude, and similarly, to settle back to the zero level prior to the activation of the IGC. This additional delay prevents adequate real-time performance from being achieved if tracking information must be gathered as is illustrated in Figure 14.2. In turn, setting the steering gradient back to zero so as to gather tracking feedback information would constrain the time during which corrective gradients are applied to the MRN agents, which may lead to an increase in deviations from the planned trajectory. Furthermore, since the acquisition time of MR physiological images is far longer than what is allowable for it to be performed within real-time MRN constraints, such images are typically gathered prior to the procedure.

Since real-time MRT of the MRN agent may be performed much more rapidly, the tracking data are typically superimposed on the pre-acquired images of the blood vessels. Although such an approach results in higher real-time performance, it is also more sensitive to errors that are caused by movements of the patient during MRN. Although registration techniques can compensate in part for the errors that are caused by the movements of the patient during MRN, they have limitations. As the overall diameters of the blood vessels where MRN is performed are reduced, sensitivity to such movements becomes more problematic, and as such, registration techniques must be developed to sufficiently compensate both spatially and timewise to allow for proper MRN to be performed.

These limitations, and particularly the extent of time required to acquire feedback information, could prevent the execution of the scheme of the traditional closed-loop MRN control that is illustrated in Figure 14.2, within the required real-time constraints. Hence, variations on this ideal control scheme must be envisioned that may call for predictive algorithms to be included, based on additional physiological data that are gathered during MRN interventions. Computer modeling may also assist in the potential prediction of MRN agent behaviors and might, therefore, facilitate the determination of the best/optimal MRN control strategy within a known set of physiological and technological constraints.

14.13 Therapeutic Magnetic Microcarriers

The first demonstration of the potential of DT using MRN (also referred to as MRT) of drug-loaded magnetic vectors has recently been reported [5]. These MRN-compatible vectors, depicted in Figure 14.3, referred to as therapeutic magnetic microcarriers (TMMCs),

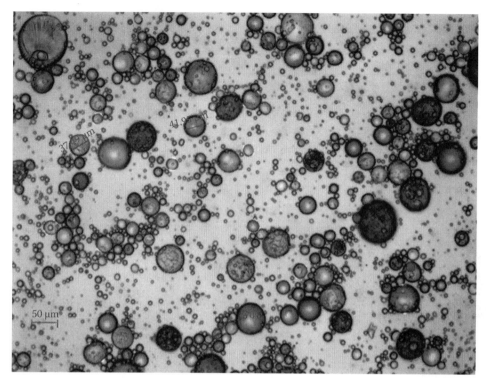

FIGURE 14.3
Photograph of the MRN-compatible therapeutic agents known as TMMCs made of MNPs and the therapeutic agent DOX embedded within biodegradable polymeric spheres and synthesized, in this particular case, for the treatment of liver tumors.

consisted of biodegradable poly(D,L-lactic-co-glycolic) (PLGA) microparticles, which were loaded with 30% iron–cobalt (FeCo) MNP (*w/w*) and DOX, a drug often used in chemotherapy.

FeCo MNPs were preferred over iron oxide MNPs because of their higher saturation magnetization (M_S), allowing for a significantly superior propelling/steering force for MRN purposes, over iron oxide MNPs. To date, TMMCs have been tested in vivo in rabbit models and designed for the treatment of hepatocellular carcinoma (HCC) via transarterial chemoembolization (TACE). TMMC characteristics such as diameter (50 μm in this particular case) and the drug release profile (which was validated experimentally) were similar to drug-eluting beads (DEB), which are recognized as promising chemoembolic systems due to their capacity for inducing tumor anoxia via physical obstruction and the sustained release of cytotoxic agents such as DOX.

The MNPs embedded within the TMMCs are not only used to induce a directional pulling force from the magnetic gradients generated by the MRN system, but also to distort the homogeneous magnetic field to allow for the assessment of targeting efficacy in terms of the quantity and distribution of the TMMCs at targeted regions. Although more highly concentrated populations of MNPs would lead to greater pulling forces being induced, the number of MNPs within each TMMC is also limited by biochemical synthesis constraints, while sufficient space for the embedding of therapeutic cargo must be made available.

The overall diameter of the TMMCs is selected with respect to the width of the vessel at the embolization site where the therapeutic agent would be released. In the case of liver, chemoembolization in the respective lobes of the liver has the potential for relatively positive therapeutic outcomes in comparison to other types of cancers.

Finally, it is likely that the specifications of such therapeutic carriers being used will be influenced by several factors including physiological conditions (e.g., diameter of blood vessels, complexity of the vascular network, blood flow rate) versus the volume of therapeutics that must be delivered. Additional considerations will encompass the specifications of the MRN platform, such as the gradient specifications of the SGC and the control method used, including the type of MRT sequences being employed for MRN purposes.

14.14 Perspective of MRN for Targeted Cancer Therapy

Although in vivo targeting of the right and left lobes of the liver in rabbit models has been achieved by MRN through the hepatic artery located 4 cm beneath the skin using TMMC [5], a number of issues need to be considered for MRN to be recognized as a potential clinical therapeutic method. For instance, although MNP aggregates within each microcarrier (e.g., TMMC) add to the effective magnetic volume, which results in enhanced propelling/ steering force, additional magnetic gradients beyond what are available in clinical MR scanners are still required to induce sufficient force on the MRN-compatible therapeutic vectors, especially those with diameters of a few tens of micrometers that are designed to travel in narrower blood vessels. Depending upon the type of intervention, the physiological environment, and the characteristics of the TMMC, for instance, the required maximum magnitude of the gradient field has been estimated, based on prior calculations (e.g., technological constraints, in vitro tests, and in vivo experiments performed with animal models and extrapolated for human physiological models), to be approximately 400–500 mT/m (about 10-fold larger than what is available in standard clinical MRI systems).

Although the tendency in new models of MR scanners is to enhance imaging by increasing the homogeneous B_0 field (e.g., 1.5–3 T in more recent models), this improvement is of no real help for MRN actuation, since the best magnetic material has already attained saturation magnetization (and hence, maximally induced propelling/steering force) at 1.5 T. But, the fact that manufacturers of clinical MR scanners maintained the amplitude of the imaging gradients, which is approximately equivalent to that of older models, suggests that additional 3D SGCs would need to be added within the bore of clinical MR scanners to allow for effective MRN interventions. This could represent a significant obstacle for the clinical acceptance of MRN in the shorter term.

To illustrate, a 400 mT/m SGC unit intended for small animals (up to the size of a rabbit) has already proved feasible for being fitted inside the bore of a clinical scanner, while it could be removed at will without the requirement of hardware modifications to the MR scanner. Conversely, SGC intended for human applications would require that the imaging coils be replaced by what is referred to as a double-insert, which consists of a SGC with an inner set of imaging coils (since MRI through SGC, although this has never been attempted as yet, is most unlikely), which possess a bore diameter that is large enough to accommodate a human adult. Unless triggered by commercial motivation, it is unlikely that such clinical MRN platforms, which are capable of competitive MR image quality, will be available soon. However, considering that the MNP used for MRT and the provision of a displacement force on the TMMC are fully saturated in a relatively low homogeneous magnetic field, and the fact that such MRN-compatible microcarriers provide strong contrast on T2*-weighted images, suggests that a lower cost MRN system based on MRI technology might be implemented, and hence may potentially shorten the delay for the acceptance of MRN-based targeted cancer interventions in clinical settings.

14.15 Perspective of TMMC for Clinical Interventions

The primary limitation of TMMC is the effective volume of superparamagnetic or ferromagnetic materials that may be embedded within carriers while maintaining the capability of transporting a therapeutic load. The higher propulsive/steering force (also referred to as motive force) achieved by integrating FeCo MNP into the TMMC required the application of a several nanometer thick protective layer made of graphite, not only to prevent the release of toxic cobalt ions (which may not be considered a critical issue for some clinicians compared with the level of toxicity that is involved with relatively large doses of therapeutic agents resident within the systemic circulation during chemotherapy), but also to avoid corrosion which would decrease the magnetization level and hence the MRN performance of the TMMC. Because this graphite shell would prevent biodegradation for a very long period of time, little is known to date in regard to the corresponding immune response and its effects in the body. As such, additional studies are warranted prior to the consideration of the use of FeCo-based TMMC in cancer therapies. On the other hand, the impact of iron oxide MNP in the body are well known (since they are already in use as MRI contrast agents) and have been proven to be relatively safe. Nevertheless, as mentioned earlier, the use of iron oxide MNP would result in lower MRN performance.

Even with the integration of the highest magnetization saturating MNP, such as those based on appropriately synthesized FeCo, some chemoembolization targets may prove to be extremely difficult to reach, if possible at all with TMMC, due to the number of successive changes in the directional motion at vessel bifurcations relative to the distance between them and the surrounding blood flow velocity. Indeed, due to the limited amount of magnetic material embedded within each microcarrier, large gradients from the SGC are required. Any changes in the 3D interventional space would cause fluctuations in the gradient amplitude generated by each of the x–y–z coils, resulting in heat. To limit the heat produced to a manageable level, the amount of electrical current that is circulating in the SGC must be limited to a specific value while having the capacity for generating the required directional gradient amplitude for the effective MRN of TMMC.

Such an engineering challenge will necessitate the addition of extra turns onto the windings of each coil, which would increase their inductance and hence reduce the slew rate, that is, a longer time would be required to change the amplitude level of the magnetic gradient in each axis. Such sluggish response of the SGC would make MRN more complex and potentially less effective when a change in direction of the TMMC is performed between successive vessel bifurcations, especially when separated by a relatively short distance and/or when impacted by a higher blood flow rate. Furthermore, since the propelling/steering gradients prevent the MRT of the TMMC to be performed simultaneously, this additional delay due to the higher inductance of the SGC would put additional constraints on proper MRN operations by limiting the volume of tracking data that could be gathered for servo navigation purposes. Nonetheless, the approach still offers great potential for targeted cancer therapy and may benefit from complementary techniques that rely on the synthesis of other types of MRN-compatible microcarriers. In all cases, for MRN-based technology to be effective within the human body would typically limit the miniaturization of TMMC to a few tens of micrometers in diameter. Although this represents a great advance with major prospects for interventions such as targeted chemoembolization, this limitation in miniaturization would prevent TMMC from reaching specific regions inside tumors.

14.16 Propulsion within the Microvasculature

The microvasculature, which is comprised of small arterioles and capillaries including the angiogenesis network, must be traversed in order to arrive within close proximity of a targeted solid tumor. The major obstacle here is that the tiniest capillaries in humans can be as small as 4 μm in diameter. Therefore, in order to travel effectively without wall retardation effects while providing the largest surface areas for the maximum attachment of therapeutic payloads, the microcarriers must ideally be ~2 μm in diameter. It is therefore obvious that at the present time, the principle of pulling force of MRN cannot be used to effectively navigate a therapeutic agent of this size.

One strategy for the determination of a valuable propulsion method is to consider a biomimetic approach. For instance, nature has already developed systems for effectively propelling micron-sized entities in vivo within aqueous media. Flagellated bacterium serves as a very good example. Indeed, the rotational movement of long filaments referred to as flagella, are well-adapted to low Reynolds' hydrodynamics, as is the case when operating within the microvasculature. Indeed, it is well known that at small scales, the physics of swimming is fundamentally different compared to those at the macroscopic and mesoscopic scales. Indeed, at the microscopic scale, viscous forces dominate while inertial forces become negligible. In such a viscous environment that is characterized by low Reynolds' number hydrodynamics, propeller designs may be replaced by a more effective synthetic "corkscrew" or artificial implementation that is similar to the flagellum that is used to propel bacteria. It is evident that practical technological constraints prevent the implementation of such an approach with an embedded power source, which is capable of powering such synthetic systems in the provision of sufficient thrust to navigate effectively, when considering the physiological conditions that exist within the microvasculature. Such an artificial approach requires an externally mediated translatable power source, and again, magnetism is still the preferred choice. Although a simplified implementation that is based on an elastic flagellum (similar to what is utilized by the spermatozoid) could be investigated, an artificial flagellum, as found in bacteria and based on preliminary studies, is more likely to provide an appropriate thrust in comparison to the elastic flagellum at such small scales under these environmental conditions, but requires a slightly more complex magnetic field generation strategy in the form of directed rotational magnetic fields in order to be functional.

14.17 ABF-Based Microcarriers

In a recent review [6] of propelling methods for microrobots, dedicated to minimally invasive medicine, artificial bacterial flagella (ABF) that are based on helical propulsion have been identified as one feasible propulsion method that could potentially be miniaturized using today's technologies for use in targeted therapeutic delivery through the vasculature under low Reynolds' hydrodynamic conditions, as encountered by microcarriers that are traveling in the narrower vessels such as capillaries. An ABF relies on a torque being applied using a rotating magnetic field and has a distinct advantage with respect to displacement alone, since the induction of torque involves a magnetic field of less magnitude when compared with a pulling force, as is the case with MRN. Nonetheless, the induction of a sufficient directional torque at such small scales for targeted interventions remains nonobvious. In addition, ABF-based microcarriers that are capable of acting as effective drug-targeting delivery vehicles within the vasculature at the systemic level, while being recognized as a therapeutic tool, may also prove very difficult for further reasons.

First, these ABF-based microcarriers, unlike spherical MRN-compatible species, are anisotropic in shape and hence, within the bore of a MRI scanner, they would only travel along the easy axis under the influence of a torque that is generated by the high homogeneous field (the B_0 field) along the z-axis of the MRI scanner or MRN platform. Due to the lack of directional control, targeted delivery using ABF-based microcarriers within the bore of a MRI scanner is dubious, and hence, other medical imaging modalities such as x-ray or CT, for example, might be considered instead. However, the lack of sufficient spatial resolution that is inherent to these medical imaging modalities would prevent the detection of these microcarriers, and hence, they would fail at providing essential tracking information for their navigation along a planned path. This is not necessarily true with MRI, since, as discussed earlier, it was shown through simulation, and has been confirmed via experiments, that the distortions created within the scanner's homogeneous field by a micron-scale magnetic core can be much larger than the physical core itself, such that a single spherical microcarrier with a diameter as small as from 10 to 15 μm (well below the spatial resolution of any current medical imaging modalities), if synthesized appropriately, may be detected and then tracked to conduct MRN that is supported by conventional clinical MRI technology.

Another critical issue is the biocompatibility of the material that is used to implement such ABF-based microcarriers. Indeed, targeting through the microvasculature means that it is most unlikely that all such devices can be recovered, and hence, biodegradation will be required once these entities have located their targets and released their payloads. However, developing such biocompatible ABF-based microcarriers may prove to be a challenging task.

14.18 Steerable Self-Propelled Entities as Therapeutic Carriers

Since in the shorter term, no external source is liable to be able to induce a displacement force on appropriately diminutive therapeutic microcarriers to allow for their utility within clinical system requirements in order to reach a tumor located in deep tissue using the most direct route (using DT), and hence avoiding systemic circulation, a steerable self-propelled therapeutic entity (SSPE) or vector with sufficient propulsive thrust would be highly desirable. Each of these microcarriers would have the prerequisite of suitable dimensions to facilitate effective travel within the narrowest of capillaries in a human patient with a sufficiently robust self-propulsive force (self-propulsive referring to the fact that the propulsive force does not rely on an external source), while being less dependent on external navigational control, due to the lack of spatial resolution in current medical imaging modalities. The approximate ideal diameter of these self-propelled therapeutic microcarriers to travel through the angiogenic network was estimated to be 2 μm, as mentioned earlier. A slightly larger diameter (e.g., 3 μm) would result in wall retardation effects, causing a reduction in motion (decrease in thrust force efficiency) caused by a reciprocal drag force on the microcarrier in the narrowest of vessels, whereas smaller diameters would result in a reduction of the available surface area upon which therapeutic payloads may be attached.

Furthermore, another major obstacle that hinders the achievement of efficient targeting is the lack of autonomy in the form of a path-finding capability (PFC) for artificial or synthetic microcarriers. PFC as defined here enables a microcarrier to travel in a general direction that is indicated by an external source while avoiding obstacles en route, without being controlled by the external source. Since the microvasculature and particularly the sizes of capillary vessels in the vicinity of the tumor are well beyond the spatial resolution of any existing medical imaging techniques, no path information may be gathered, and as such, no trajectory can be computed to achieve DT. Hence, servo-controlled navigation is negated as an option in this case. Therefore, to become more independent of such external controls, a PFC capability that is embedded within the microcarriers would prove to be pivotal for the enhancement of the targeted delivery of cytotoxic agents into tumors.

Although such a steerable self-propelled microcarrier is at present technologically impossible to produce, and will likely remain so for some time, one intriguing strategy has been proposed that would involve the search for a suitable steerable self-propelled microcarrier with PFC from nature, and if available, to harness its potential capability for tumor targeting. Such a natural SSPE was indeed identified in the form of a flagellated magnetotactic bacterium (MTB), known as the MC-1 cell. The MC-1 bacterium has the capacity for emulating a microcarrier that is capable of transporting a therapeutic payload, contains its own propulsion system and is a nonpathogenic spherical cell with an ideal diameter that ranges from 1 to 2 μm. It is propelled by two flagellar bundles (connected to rotary molecular motors) that provide propulsive thrust forces exceeding 4 picoNewtons (pN) (approximately 10 times the thrust force of other known species of flagellated bacteria), allowing each cell to travel between 100 and 150 times its own body length per second. Such thrust would result in a complementary range of propulsive force in regions not covered as yet, and beyond the limits of magnetic resonance propulsion (MRP), that is, induced MRI-based propulsive force during MRN within a human.

Directional control of the MC-1 bacterium is based on magnetotaxis, whereby a low-magnitude directional magnetic field (the cells respond to magnetic fields with magnitudes that are slightly less than the Earth's geomagnetic field of 0.5 Gauss) is utilized to induce a torque on a chain of aligned membrane-based iron oxide MNP called magnetosomes that behave as an embedded magnetic nanocompass, which is synthesized within each cell during cultivation as performed in a laboratory. As shown in Figure 14.4, when one inspects this bacterium more carefully, it becomes evident that indeed, it is very similar in design to a futuristic synthetic or artificial microscale nanorobot (e.g., a microscale robot that relies on nanoscale components to embed new functionalities) that might be conceived by using engineering approaches that are beyond the capabilities of today's technologies.

As depicted in Figure 14.4, the MC-1 MTB (shown in the top figure) provides characteristics similar to a futuristic hypothetical self-propelled microscale robot, illustrated schematically in the bottom figure and designed to navigate within the microvasculature. The flagella-based propulsion system is designed for high performance under low Reynolds' number conditions. To achieve high thrust for overcoming blood flow velocity

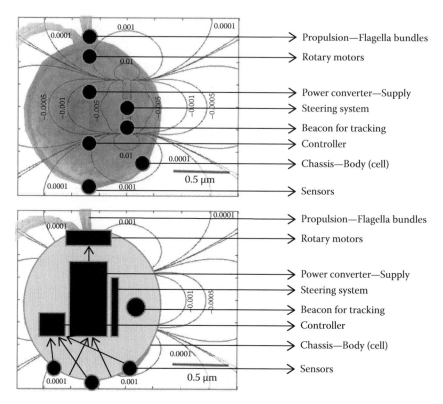

FIGURE 14.4

A natural bacterial microrobot represented by the MC-1 magnetotactic bacterium versus a hypothetical version of an artificial microrobot with the required components suited for targeted medical interventions, requiring such robots to travel within the microvasculature.

in the microvasculature and to allow for deeper penetration into solid tumors, the design is based on not one, but dual flagella bundles that are capable of providing between 4.0 and 4.7 pN of thrusting force. This is sufficient to achieve travel speeds of from 100 to 150 body lengths per second, as stated previously. This propulsion system is tethered to rotary motors which are similar in design to modern electric motors, except for their size and the type of materials employed. As with their macroscale counterparts, they also rely on a rotor that operates inside a stator while being separated by bearings. The flagella are connected to the rotors, providing full 360° rotation. The direction of rotation of the rotors can also be changed. Forward and reverse movements are achieved via counterclockwise and clockwise rotations, respectively. A "fuel line" and the power converter that is used to supply the "fuel or proton flow" necessary for the activation of the motors is connected between them. It also converts nutrients that are gathered from the environment via an intake mechanism, to onboard protons.

To allow for external computer-mediated directional control, a steering system is also available in the form of a single magnetic domain of nanoparticles that are arranged in a chain-like structure. This arrangement allows for external computer-based magnetotactic control, where a directional magnetic torque may be induced with minimal energy, allowing for operations at any depth within the human body. The same nanoparticles may also serve as beacons or MRI contrast agents, allowing a MTB aggregate with a sufficiently large size and density to be visible using MRI sequences. This may prove to be a valuable tool for tracking, or for assessing the distribution and density of the bacteria that have reached the targeted sites. The bacteria have additional onboard sensors that may potentially be used to influence their motion toward a target.

Aerotaxis-based migration, wherein the bacteria move toward lower level oxygen concentrations is but one potential example that might be used in targeted medical interventions. Indeed, tumoral lesions are characterized by a reduced concentration of oxygen, and as such, although more studies are required for its confirmation, aerotaxis may prove useful in this particular case. But, since oxygen gradients are confined to within the vicinity of the tumor, magnetotaxis using an external directional magnetic field would typically be employed to bring the bacteria in closer proximity to the tumor. Finally, it may be observed that all of the components are integrated within what might be described (for an artificial microrobot) as a chassis, which can also be utilized for the attachment of therapeutic payloads. As illustrated, the functionalities that are embedded within such bacterium are very similar to those that would be required for a futuristic artificial microrobot.

The possibility of accurate magnetotactic control of these cells while carrying a payload has been documented [7], and the mass control of an aggregate has been demonstrated using approximately 5000 of these bacteria to build a miniature pyramid in less than 15 min [8]. In vivo experiments using a special platform (distinct from MRI), and referred to as a magnetotaxis system, generated an artificial magnetic pole (to indicate the general direction of the target) that was located inside one of the two xenografts, which were grown in the flanks of mice. This confirmed not only that targeting may be achieved, but also the ability of the bacteria (previously injected intravenously in the tail) to navigate without external control (PFC) through the malformed angiogenesis capillary networks before dying approximately 30–40 min subsequent to injection.

14.19 Applicability of MRN Therapeutic Agents

As mentioned earlier, MRN therapeutic agents such as TMMC are limited by the level of miniaturization that can be achieved, which curtails their usage for interventions in cancer therapies such as chemoembolization. As such, an initial targeted medical intervention that was, and still is, considered against cancer is the liver tumor treatment, which is based on this new magnetic targeting strategy. HCC is the most frequent liver tumor, which rates as the third leading cause of death related to cancer. Its incidence is increasing worldwide and is characterized by a poor prognosis (3–6 months). It should also be mentioned that 70% of the patients may receive only palliative treatments and that chemoembolization remains the most efficient treatment. This particular intervention, when used in conjunction with TMMC, combines two treatment modalities known as chemotherapy with the injection of an antitumor drug being released from the TMMC and embolization caused by the TMMC being blocked in the vessel due to their overall size, which induces an ischemia of the tumor. The efficacy of the treatment can potentially be enhanced with secondary effects, and thus toxicity may be reduced substantially by performing chemoembolization at a targeted location in close proximity to the tumor. This can be significant considering that the targeting is actually limited by the placement of the catheter used for the injection of the cytotoxic agent in the blood vessels at several bifurcations upstream of the tumor. As the distribution of the chemoembolizing agents cannot be adequately controlled, healthy cells are also affected by the treatment.

14.20 Applicability of MTB-Based Therapeutic Agents

Although the MC-1 magnetotactic bacteria proved to be effective in the microvasculature, they are not suitable for traveling within larger blood vessels for two main reasons. First, the blood flow velocity in larger vessels such as the arteries is too high, and as such, systemic circulation of the bacteria would occur resulting, as with chemotherapy, in drug-loaded bacteria accumulations in untargeted organs with significantly less bacteria in the desired targeted regions. Second, even if (hypothetically) the blood velocity would be reduced significantly, or at the extreme, temporarily completely stopped (if the medical protocol would permit such a drastic approach), the swimming distance between the injection site in the artery and the tumor would be too far. Indeed, although this bacterium may reach an average velocity of 200 μm/s, the thrust force responsible for such swimming velocity decreases when it operates at body temperature, and becomes nonmotile after 30–40 min. This constraint is related to the fact that MC-1 is nonpathogenic and will not have the time to reproduce in the body, which would otherwise result in another serious medical issue. As such, it is critical to utilize these bacteria in the microvasculature as early as possible subsequent to injection in order to exploit their motile force, not only for reaching tumor/s, but also to allow them to attain the deeper regions within the patient for the potential enhancement of therapeutic outcomes.

In this respect, there are two primary strategies that may be applied. The first involves the injection of the drug-loaded magnetotactic bacteria, as close as is possible to the tumor, since injecting directly to the tumor mass is not a medical option for various reasons, including the potential risk of metastasis (the spread of cancerous cells throughout the body). Among several types of cancer, colorectal or rectal cancer has been of special interest for MTB-based therapeutic microcarriers, since such sites may be accessed through localized rectal injection, which bypasses the requirement of traveling through the arterial vessels from a more distant injection site. More specifically, an attempt is already underway to inject SN-38-loaded MTB at the periphery of colorectal tumors in animal models and to guide this complex to diffuse within the tumor using an external magnetic field, followed by MRI scans for monitoring and assessment. This work also includes toxicity and biocompatibility studies in primates, with the goal of gathering all of the necessary data toward obtaining the required permission for human trials.

Hence, before these bacteria-based therapeutic agents may be used in humans, several critical questions need to be answered. Among them, one of the fundamental questions (besides biocompatibility) concerns the level of cytotoxicity that might be associated with these MTB-based therapeutic agents. More specifically, the question regards whether an appropriate volume of bacteria may be injected that is below the cytotoxicity level of the patient so as to allow for the delivery of sufficient therapeutics for achieving adequate results in colorectal cancer. This is also an important question when one considers that the therapeutic cargo per bacterium is relatively small and that the time period that is available to perform such interventions with humans is relatively short, as an immune system response could occur within a few days of the initial injection. However, to date, this remains to be confirmed. The second strategy would be to transport, at high speed, MTB-based therapeutic agents closer to the location of the tumor and at the entry of the microvasculature through specialized MRN-compatible carriers. This will be discussed in further detail in the next section.

14.21 Combining MRN with MTB-Based Approaches

As discussed in the preceding sections, each prospective approach has advantages and limitations. For MRN, the minimum size of the magnetic agents is on the order of a few tens of micrometers, which remain too large for reaching solid tumors through the microvasculature. On the other hand, MTB-based agents are very effective in the microvasculature but are ineffective in larger vessels, where MRN becomes much more effectual. MRN also requires some form of external navigation control, and as such, it is more appropriate in larger vessels that can be imaged to provide the pathway information necessary for the development of control algorithms. In tinier vessels, this external control is not possible due to a lack of spatial resolution in clinical imaging modalities. Therefore, the resolution of external control is reduced to an external guidance capability, where only the direction of the target is communicated without the desired fine control to facilitate the avoidance of obstacles, or to maintain a predetermined track en route to tumors. These complementarities suggest that a powerful and logical approach would be to transport MTB-based therapeutic agents to the entry of the microvasculature with specialized MRN-compatible microcarriers.

Such a concept is still under investigation. Although MTB have been successfully encapsulated with sustained viability within MRN microcarriers in the form of micelles containing MNP (which were used to propel the microcarriers), additional work is warranted before such a concept may be initially applied for in vivo experiments. Other aspects such as the optimization of release strategies are also under investigation. Nonetheless, the concept is progressing relatively quickly toward near-term implementation, which might be suitable for the targeting of tumors that are only attainable via more complex vascular networks.

14.22 Conclusion

For some types of cancers, enhanced therapeutic efficacy can be obtained by DT, where a minimal dose of drug-loaded microcarriers can be navigated through the shortest route while avoiding systemic circulation. Such an approach would require the assistance of more sophisticated interventional platforms and engineering techniques that will most likely impact the synthesis of such navigable therapeutic vectors and the development of medical interventional protocols. Computer-assisted interventions that are capable of managing such complexity may become an additional and possibly indispensable tools for achieving enhanced tumor targeting. Cancer therapies will likely become increasingly interdisciplinary, providing additional tools and methods that might be combined in order to achieve improved therapeutic efficacy. Using magnetism to enhance such targeting, these microcarriers, in the form of synthetic TMMC or biological MTB, to name but only two recent types, would have the advantage of being visible under MRI such that one may assess the targeting efficacy and distribution of administered drugs in specific regions. Although further research is needed, preliminary experimental results clearly indicate that the new and innovative paradigms offered by nanorobotics may likely influence and guide the manner by which nanoscale delivery systems for cancer will be achieved.

14.23 To Probe Further

The preceding sections provide only a brief glimpse of the field of nanorobotics as applied to targeted medical interventions. Additional studies and elucidations may be found in the literature. For instance, more detailed information on the modeling of forces on soft magnetic materials can be found [9], while the fundamentals of robotic actuation at small scales are also provided [10,11]. A good introduction to magnetotactic bacteria is available [12], as well as more detailed descriptions of magnetotaxis [13,14]. An overall assessment of the fundamentals of using magnetotactic bacteria for targeted medical interventions is conveyed [15] in addition to an overview of MRN with magnetotactic bacteria [16–18]. The aggregation of MRN agents required to deliver a higher therapeutic dose, which poses additional challenges is also discussed [19]. For readers more interested in the fundamental medical protocols required for MRN, an overview is available [20]. The difficulties of MRN control shown through a simple PID controller is explained [21], and good reading is offered to those more interested in understanding the fundamental constraints of MRI as a platform for MRN [22]. Details on the MRT MS-SET mentioned in the text may be found [23], as well as an example of other MRN agents with enhanced functionality that might be implemented [24]. The previously mentioned publications constitute but a short list of references that describe just some of the techniques and methods currently being utilized, or that are under consideration for medical nanorobotics dedicated exclusively to targeted interventions in cancer therapies. This is to say that the discipline of medical nanorobotics offers tremendous and broad potential for further research and development, toward beneficial pragmatic and enhanced clinical applications.

References

1. Jain, R.K., Delivery of molecular and cellular medicine to solid tumors. *Adv. Drug Deliv. Rev.* 46, 149–168, 2001.
2. Dreher, M.R., Liu, W., Michelich, C.R., Dewhirst, M.W., Yuan, F., and Chilkoti, A., Tumor vascular permeability, accumulation, and penetration of macromolecular drug carriers. *J. Nat. Cancer Inst.* 98, 335–344, 2006.
3. Galuppo, L.D., Kamau, S.W., Steitz, B., Hassa, P.O., Hilbe, M., Vaughan, L., Koch, L., Fink-Petri, A., Hofman, M., Hofman, H., Hottiger, M.O., and von Rechenberg, B., Gene Expression in Synovial Membrane Cells After Intraarticular Delivery of Plasmid-Linked Superparamagnetic Iron Oxide Particles—A Preliminary Study in Sheep. *J. Nanosci. Nanotechnol.* 6, 2841–2852, 2006.
4. Martel, S., Mathieu, J.-B., Felfoul, O., Chanu, A., Aboussouan, É., Tamaz, S., Pouponneau, P., Beaudoin, G., Soulez, G., Yahia, L.H., and Mankiewicz, M., Automatic navigation of an unte-thered device in the artery of a living animal using a conventional clinical magnetic resonance imaging system. *Appl. Phys. Lett.* 90, 114105, 2007.
5. Pouponneau, P., Leroux, J.-C., Soulez, G., Gaboury, L., and Martel, S., Co-encapsulation of magnetic nanoparticles and doxorubicin into biodegradable microcarriers for deep tissue targeting by vascular MRI navigation. *Biomaterials* 32(13), 3481–3486, 2011.
6. Nelson, B.J., Kaliakatsos, I.K., and Abbott, J.J., Microrobots for minimally invasive medicine. *Annu. Rev. Biomed. Eng.* 12, 55–85, 2010.
7. Martel, S., Tremblay, C., Ngakeng, S., and Langlois, G., Controlled manipulation and actuation of micro-objects with magnetotactic bacteria. *Appl. Phys. Lett.* 89, 233804–233806, 2006.
8. Martel S. and Mohammadi M, video presented at IROS, 2009. http://www.youtube.com/watch?v=fCSOdQK5PIY

9. Abbott, J.J., Ergeneman, O., Kummer, M.P., Hirt, A.M., and Nelson, B.J., Modeling magnetic torque and force for controlled manipulation of soft-magnetic bodies. *IEEE Trans. Robotics* 23(6), 1247–1252, 2007.

10. Abbott, J.J., Nagy, Z., Beyeler, F., and Nelson, B., Robotics in the small: Part 1 microrobotics. *IEEE Robotics Automat. Mag.* 14(2), 92–103, 2007.

11. Abbott, J.J., Peyer, K.E., Lagomarsino, M.C., Zhang, L., Dong, L.X., Kaliakatsos, I.K., and Nelson, B., How should microrobots swim? *Int. J. Robotics Res.* 28, 1434–1447, 2009.

12. Blakemore, R.P., Magnetotactic bacteria. *Science*, 190, 377–379, 1975.

13. Frankel, R.B., and Blakemore, R.P., Navigational compass in magnetic bacteria. *J. Magn. Magn. Mater.* 15–18(3), 1562–1564, 1980.

14. Debarros, H., Esquivel, D.M.S., and Farina, M., Magnetotaxis. *Sci. Progr.* 74, 347–359, 1990.

15. Martel, S., Mohammadi, M., Felfoul, O., Lu, Z., and Pouponneau, P., Flagellated magnetotactic bacteria as controlled MRI-trackable propulsion and steering systems for medical nanorobots operating in the human microvasculature. *Int. J. Robotics Res.* 28(4), 571–582, 2009.

16. Martel, S., Collective methods of propulsion and steering for untethered microscale nanorobots navigating in the human vascular network. *J. Mech. Eng. Sci.* 224(C), 1505–1513, 2010.

17. Martel, S., Combining aggregates of synthetic microscale nanorobots with swarms of computer-controlled flagellated bacterial robots to enhance target therapies through the human vascular network. *Int. J. Adv. Sys. Meas.* 3(3–4), 92–98, 2010.

18. Martel, S., Felfoul, O., Mathieu, J.-B., Chanu, A., Tamaz, S., Mohammadi, M., Mankiewicz, M., and Tabatabaei, N., MRI-based nanorobotic platform for the control of magnetic nanoparticles and flagellated bacteria for target interventions in human capillaries. *Int. J. Robotics Res.* 28(9), 1169–1182, 2009.

19. Mathieu, J.-B. and Martel, S., Aggregation of magnetic microparticles in the context of targeted therapies actuated by a magnetic resonance imaging system. *J. Appl. Phys.* 106, 044904-1-7, 2009.

20. Martel, S., Mathieu, J.-B., Felfoul, O., Chanu, A., Aboussouan, E., Tamaz, S., Pouponneau, P., Yahia, L., Beaudoin, G., Soulez, G., and Mankiewicz, M., A computer-assisted protocol for endovascular target interventions using a clinical MRI system for controlling untethered micro-devices and future nanorobots. *Comp. Aided Surg.* 13(06), 340e–352, 2008.

21. Tamaz, S., Chanu, A., Mathieu, J.-B., Gourdeau, R., and Martel, S., Real-time MRI-based control of a ferromagnetic core for endovascular navigation. *IEEE Trans. Biomed. Eng.* 55(7), 1854–1863, 2008.

22. Mathieu, J.-B. and Martel, S., Magnetic microparticle steering within the constraints of an MRI system: Proof of concept of a novel targeting approach. *Biomed. Microdev.* 9(6), 801–808, 2007.

23. Felfoul, O., Mathieu, J.-B., Beaudoin, G., and Martel, S., In vivo MR-tracking based on magnetic signature selective excitation. *IEEE Trans. Med. Imag.* 27(1), 28–35, 2008.

24. Tabatabaei, S.N., Lapointe, J., and Martel, S., Shrinkable hydrogel-based magnetic microrobots for interventions in the vascular network. *Adv. Robotics* 25(6), 1049–1067, 2011.

Section III

Beyond the Event Horizon: Nanomedical Visions

15

Nanomedical Device and Systems Design in Remote Regions and the Developing World

Hayat Sindi and Frank J. Boehm

CONTENTS

15.1 Current Status of Remote Medicine

The developing world comprises approximately 82% of the current overall population on Earth (approx. >7.16 billion—July/2013) and constitutes the greatest challenge insofar as the provision of at least rudimentary and sustainable medical technologies and expertise [1–3]. The chronic lack of medical adequacy in these regions (e.g., sub-Saharan Africa, Asia, South America) pervades smaller towns and villages that are relatively easily accessed. One might rightly surmise that the situation for the inhabitants of locales that are scarcely accessible at the best of times is likely to be abysmal and overwhelming. Individuals in these regions often have no option but to travel hundreds of miles to access the closest doctor or health facility. What we take for granted and consider as elemental infrastructural components (e.g., drivable roads, clean water, basic sanitation) are nonexistent; hence, there are significant, or indeed severe, logistical restrictions.

Bagchi revealed in 2006 that "In a developing country such as India, there is huge inequality in health-care distribution. Although nearly 75% of Indians live in rural villages, more than 75% of Indian doctors are based in cities [4]. Most of the 620 million rural Indians lack access to basic health-care facilities [5]. The Indian government spends just 0.9% of the country's annual gross domestic product on health, and little of this spending reaches remote rural areas [6]." [7]. It would appear that in 2011, this situation has improved only slightly, as Prathiba indicates: "While 72% of India's 1.2 billion people live in rural areas, over 70% of the doctors practice in urban areas" [8].

Health care in Ghana faces a particularly dire situation, as its citizens must travel by foot (average of 16 km) to the nearest health-care facility. In 2006, WHO estimated that the 20 million population of Ghana (at that time) had 0.15 physicians for every 1000 patients [9]. Health facilities, of which there were only ~1500 in 2008, are not evenly distributed and are typically accessible to only one-third of Ghana's population of ~25 million. In addition, most hospitals lack basic and proper supplies, and core equipments such as CT scanners are frequently in need of repair or obsolete. Rural populations face acute poverty and poor sanitation, and lack even the most basic of health services [10]. Thus, it seems obvious that the establishment of a telemedicine infrastructure might be of immense benefit, not only for the people of Ghana but for the whole of the African continent. To bring home this point, in 2009 there was but a single dermatologist for every 3–4 million people in Africa [11].

In assessing the efficacy of telemedicine in Ghana, Darkwa found that most physicians were computer-literate but less so when it came to the utilization of telemedicine technologies. The primary factors that limited the implementation of telemedicine in health facilities were financial, technological, and organizational. Urban practitioners were more familiar with, and had easier access to information technology, than their rural counterparts [11].

This chapter will briefly survey the development of remote medicine; how it has evolved and is being practiced today. A review of the state-of-the-art technologies in this domain will be followed by a prospective exploration of how nanomedical technologies might facilitate the provision of access to important medical technologies in some of the most geographically challenging and remote regions on the globe.

It is prudent to note/suggest that concurrent with humanitarian development and the provision of medical technologies in remote regions, no matter how advanced, the conveyance and promotion of sound health practices via simultaneous educational activities, and the supply of basic tools to facilitate/implement them, whenever and wherever possible in the developing world, and particularly for populations in remote regions, will hold an equivalent weight of importance.

15.1.1 Telemedicine

Telemedicine involves the rapid electronic exchange of medical data and imagery between local and distant sites, increasingly separated by thousands of miles, to facilitate improvements in the health status of patients [12]. Advanced telecommunications technologies now enable the capacity for patients in underserved and remote rural areas to gain access to specialized expertise. In the United States alone, there are currently ~200 telemedicine networks that connect 2000 medical facilities. Various sources have estimated the value of the telemedicine market to range from $6 billion to $17.8 billion in 2012, and Schooley Mitchell Consultants have predicted that home-based telemedicine will be worth $4.4 billion in 2013 [13]. One of the most significant users of telemedicine is the U.S. military, as its personnel are widely dispersed across the globe. It has implemented the MERMAID (medical emergency aid through telematics) system to provide 24-h tertiary care in the field, which is enabled via multiple telecommunications capabilities. The efficacy of medical support for sailors at sea is facilitated via the transfer of live two-way imagery [14,15].

The current state-of-the-art *modus operandi* for medical technologies in remote regions of the world involves various manifestations of telemedicine, including teleconsultation and teleradiology, telepathology, teledermatology, telecardiology, telepsychiatry, and so on. Medical data that are typically conveyed encompass computed tomography (CT) and ultrasound scans, mammograms, echocardiograms, and frozen sections [16]. The perspective in ~2005 was that these technologies were futuristic and quite advanced. However, soon afterward, to the surprise of the researchers and technicians who were working to implement these "innovative" technologies, they were already being generally regarded and accepted as commonplace. It is reasonable to assume that there have been, and continue to be, human factor problems that are inherent with the adoption of any new technologies, as is evidenced by a more or less initial fundamental resistance to change. This tendency has been observed by some medical practitioners who favor the modification of preexisting technologies rather than the adoption of completely new ones.

Telemedicine has advantages in the provision of cost-effective health care and access to medical specialists to those in distant and remote areas in countries where there exist considerable monetary, geographic, and social obstacles to conventional health care. However, the prerequisite is that it must involve coordinated efforts between the medical communities and governments of developing countries and developed nations. In 2009, it was concluded by Rao and Lombardi, in regard to its use in developing countries that, "Although current efforts using telemedicine have demonstrated positive effects in countries in need, they have not substantially reduced or compensated for a fundamental lack of healthcare. Countries with inadequate healthcare must incorporate telemedicine into their healthcare system through volunteer efforts of doctors in countries worldwide" [10].

Recent developments in telemedicine have seen the emergence of wireless sensor networks (WSNs) and specific derivative applications such as body area sensor networks (BASN) in enabling the remote monitoring of patients' vital signs. A BASN system is comprised of an array of interconnected nodes (Figure 15.1) that have integrated capacities for sensing and data processing, as well as the conveyance of data via wireless communications. Individual nodes may be positioned in close proximity, on the skin or within the patient. Although the prospective applications of BASNs are promising, there remain a number of obstacles to overcome prior to their extensive implementation [17]. These challenges include the following criteria:

1. Optimally noninvasive and inconspicuous, and when utilized for in vivo applications, they must be biocompatible [18].

2. Must adhere to established safety and security protocols. High-level encryption must be employed to protect sensitive/confidential data [19–22].

3. User-friendly operation and intuitive controls for user/device interface.

Body area sensor network nodes, which might incorporate multiple external units (distributed motes) (to monitor close patient proximity environmental factors such as "ambient temperature, background light, atmospheric pressure, or the patient's exact position"

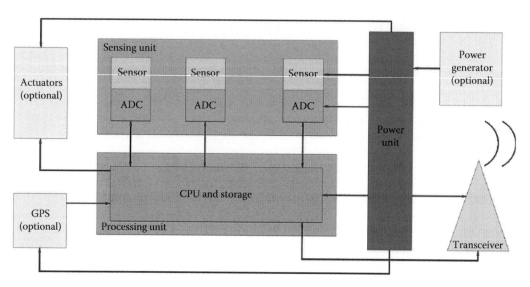

FIGURE 15.1
BASN architecture. (Redrawn from Grgić, K. et al., *Med. Glas. Ljek. Komore. Zenicko-doboj kantona.* 9(1), 23–31, 2012. With permission.)

through GPS) and implants, which could be endowed with various sensing capabilities may cumulatively enable them to monitor and analyze a patient's overall physiological status [23–27]. The most critical of these parameters might include continual observations of the heart (electrocardiography—ECG), muscles (electromyography—EMG), and the brain (electroencephalography—EEG) [28,29]. Other sensors may be dedicated to tracking temperature (thermistors), glucose levels, blood pressure, respiration, and arterial blood oxygen saturation (SpO$_2$) levels via photoplethysmography—(PPG) [23–25]. In order to detect patient falls, integrated microelectromechanical systems (MEMS)-based accelerometers may also be included in the system [30,31] (Refs. [17–31] from [32]).

The extent of applications for these types of systems is virtually limitless and has been made possible via the advent of MEMS that operate seamlessly in conjunction with wireless communications. Smart, configurable, and economical sensing devices endowed with onboard power supplies, data processing, storage, and transceivers may be individually tuned to allow for a range of medical monitoring applications, as listed earlier, and wireless interdevice and networked systems communications. The large-scale implementation of these sensors and systems will, however, be contingent on the acceptance and use of standardized low power system architectures (e.g., ZigBee) in order to assure ease of use and compatibility, as well as broad interconnectivity and interoperability.

With the advent of sophisticated nanosensors/nanodevices, the long-term implantation of nanomedical "sentinel" class micro- or nanomotes may be feasible. These multiple nanodevices in effect would function as 24/7/365 physiological monitors and cumulative would serve as a potent immune system augmentation (Chapter 17) with the capacity for administering an array of nanomedical diagnostics and therapeutics (via dynamic nanodevices that are imperceptibly tethered within the tissues of host patients) to neutralize practically any detected threat to the host "system."

The nascent field of telepathology involves the long-distance electronic transfer of images, typically generated via a microscope, for the transfer of various pathological conditions to query/convey expert opinion, provide emergency data when there is no resident pathologist available, and for educational purposes. A pilot project is being implemented by the Laval University Integrated Health Network in the provision of an "intraoperative frozen section service to small hospitals (17 in this study) in sparsely populated areas which are experiencing a severe shortage of on-site pathologists." [33]. Puppa et al. assessed the efficacy of a multicenter/multinational interobserver virtual microscope in the reproducible early diagnosis of gastrointestinal (GI) tumor budding (TB) among experienced pathologists. The researchers found an "overall fair level of diagnostic agreement for TB in CRC [colorectal cancer], which was improved significantly among experienced GI pathology observers and, above all, in early cancer" [34].

Costa and Oliveira explore the establishment of a telecardiology system to facilitate diagnoses via the secure exchange of ECG and echocardiography examinations through ubiquitous Internet services rather than a server-based infrastructure, which would necessitate IT resources. The three primary elements of such as system were identified as including "central storage capacity, normalized communication channel, and universal access." Protected communications were ensured by utilizing a secure SMTP connection with a secure sockets layer (SSL) to enable contact with service requesters as well as a secure IMAP protocol (via SSL) linking the reviewing software and a central mailbox. The data (exam files), destined for transmission, were also encrypted using the "Advanced Encryption Standard (AES) algorithm is used to encrypt each exam file inside the ZIP archive with a 256-bit key encryption key" [35].

One may surmise that when advanced nanomedical devices are in common use and wirelessly transmit their data to local computers (which in turn may be transmitted online to virtually any destination of the globe to communicate with physicians and other medical personnel), technologies with an aim to infiltrate wireless data streams and online exchanges will also have evolved. Therefore, to ensure the robustly secure global transmission of medical data that are generated by nanomedical devices (such as the vascular cartographic scanning nanodevice (VCSN)), the development of multitiered quantum encryption architectures will be required [36].

15.1.2 Digital Medical Informatics

Medical informatics is a very useful tool for the assessment of patients in remote areas. In the military, it has taken the form of the Battlefield Medical Information System-Tactical (BMIS-T), which consists of a handheld personal digital assistant (PDA) that is utilized to convey and retrieve critical patient-in-the-field data and to access databases that contain patient medical histories [37]. This technology was superseded by the "electronic dogtag," which was first introduced in 2005 by the company Irvine Sensors. Modern electronic dog tag personal information carriers (PICs) are designed to interface with a field medic's handheld device. They are endowed with 8 Gbs of data capacity, are USB-compatible, and are powered by long-lived rechargeable batteries [38]. They can be connected via secure wireless transmission to the Army's central medical information system. In the near future, it is envisioned that they will be enabled with GPS tracking and the capacity for monitoring the vital signs of any soldier in the field. Hence, the Army will be aware of the exact location of each of their soldiers in conjunction with their health status. By differentiating the physiological parameters of individual soldiers, a treatment prioritization strategy can be formulated. The DARPA Virtual Soldier Project includes what it calls the personalized "Holomer structure," which would be a "compilation of all imaging and medical data, for each soldier…." The segmentation of an individual's previous CT scan would be utilized to personalize certain anatomical regions. As stated on the project website: "The ultimate goal is the construction of a complete, functioning, accessible simulation of the human thorax-from the physiology of individual cells to the operation of entire organ-tissue systems. This virtual representation of the human thorax will provide capabilities to diagnose battlefield injuries, specifically ballistic wounds to the heart" [39].

When extrapolated to the micron scale, one can envision that nanomedical informatics platforms will likely be internalized in the form of tissue-embedded implants. Multiple copies of these archival/sentinel class of nanodevices would contain the entire medical history of an individual and might be employed as the primary reference against which any physiological deviations that transgress pre-established thresholds would be spontaneously transmitted to the appropriate medical practitioner. They would also function as ultrasensitive physiological nanosensors that might continually monitor perhaps hundreds of physiological parameters. When any of these established parameters are deemed to have significantly deviated from established norms for a particular individual, medical personnel would be notified, who would then prescribe the appropriate nanomedical therapeutics. In effect, one's doctor would "always" know how one is. Further into the future, multiple classes of interacting nanodevices, encompassing archival, sentinel, diagnostic, and therapeutic might all be "patient resident," meaning that they would cumulatively serve as a highly dynamic and robust extension of the patient's natural immune system to thwart practically any perceived assault on the host.

15.1.3 Digital Communications

It has been estimated that there are ~6 billion mobile device users globally, with ~500 million cell phone subscribers centered in Africa alone. Greater than half of all users worldwide reside in low- and middle-income countries where access to medical care is limited at best. In rural Africa, where there is widespread malaria, poor health-care systems, inadequate infrastructures, and poverty have typically prevented basic communications between patients, health workers, and health-service managers that might lead to more efficient health care. However, a cost-effective and user-friendly mobile phone function called short message service (SMS) may effectively bridge this communication gap and lead to potential improvements in both health-service delivery and patient outcomes [40–43].

Zurovac et al. investigated the potential impacts of text messaging and real-time reporting on malaria control and found that there were six primary deficient areas where they would likely accrue benefits, including

1. Disease and treatment effectiveness surveillance
2. Monitoring of the availability of health commodities
3. Pharmacovigilance and postmarketing surveillance of the safety and quality of antimalarial drugs
4. Health worker adherence to guidelines
5. Patient adherence to medication regimens
6. Posttreatment

Although several pilot projects involving SMS-based text messaging (primarily relating to surveillance and commodity monitoring) in regard to malaria have been undertaken in Zambia [44], Madagascar [45], Tanzania, and Uganda [46], there remain potential challenges to its widespread implementation for individual patients. The benefits remain uncertain for the use of text messaging toward the control of malaria in Africa in the areas of routine adoption and malarial drug adherence, posttreatment review, and overall/ actual cost effectiveness. Additional interventional hurdles, from the individual patient care perspective, may also include "high facility workload or illiteracy" [40].

Recently (2010), an open source software platform called Sana ("healthy" in Spanish) was developed by students and researchers at MIT's Computer Science and Artificial Intelligence Laboratory (CSAIL). This app was designed to run on Google's Android platform and enabled remote health practitioners to transmit pictures, x-ray, ultrasound imagery, and videos to a database. These images were then uploaded and analyzed by a physician who responded with a preliminary diagnosis via texting. Since the software is an open source, it can be adapted to suit the requirements of specific regions and customized for particular disease states. In a pilot project based in Bangalore, 400 high-risk oral cancer patients had their mouths photographed. The images were transferred to an oncologist at Bangalore's Narayana Hrudayalaya Hospital to be assessed for evidence of precancerous lesions. As a consequence, two patients were referred for treatment of these lesions [47].

Inspired by the prevalence of mobile phones in the developing world, Breslauer et al. have developed an effective, yet straightforward and economical technique to screen and diagnose hematologic and infectious diseases. They have devised a light microscope that can be mounted to a mobile phone to facilitate diagnostic imaging and telemedicine and demonstrated its value by imaging *Plasmodium falciparum* infected cells and sickle red blood cells in brightfield, as well as sputum samples that were infected with *Mycobacterium tuberculosis* using fluorescence microscopy with LED excitation. The resolution surpassed that which is required for the detection of the morphologies of microorganisms and blood cells. To augment this capability further, the digitized tuberculosis sample images were exploited, using image analysis software, in conducting automated bacillus counting. "An additional advantage to using a phone-based microscope is that mobile phones are essentially computers that can be used for digital image processing as well as electronic medical record keeping and communication." The researchers suggest that this technology will serve as a critical boon for the screening and diagnoses of diseases, especially in the developing world, where access to laboratory facilities are very limited, yet mobile phone use is ubiquitous [48].

Anderson et al. endeavored to learn if the breath sounds recorded by a mobile phone might enable remote heath practitioners to differentiate between normal and asthmatic patients. Tracheal breath sounds were recorded from 20 subjects ranging in age from 12 to 61 years; half of the subjects were women and 7 of the 20 subjects were asthma patients on treatment. The standard computer used in the laboratory to process the recordings was objective in that it received no indication of any history of asthma. The breath sounds were recorded using a free Internet-based voice mail service, and each was received as a date-stamped audio file (GSM 6.10 format, 16 bit resolution, 8 kHz sampling frequency). As the investigators explain, "Normal lung function was assessed by measurement of peak flow, forced expiratory volume in 1 s (FEV1), and forced vital capacity using a handheld portable spirometer (Vitalograph 2120, Vitalograph, Ireland). We could detect a significant difference in lung function between patients with healthy lungs and those with asthma (median FEV1 3·55 L [IQR 3·07–4·16] vs 1·43 L [1·3–1·7]; $p = .0004$, Mann–Whitney U test)." It was found that the sound quality, when the wave file was replayed in the laboratory, approached that of "direct auscultation with a stethoscope." Lung sound analysis and spectrograms could be calculated and viewed rapidly (>5 min) from the onset of the initial breath recording. Thus, it was demonstrated that the efficacy of remotely recorded breath sounds might be accurately reproduced for rapid spectral analysis to reveal the presence of asthma. This may facilitate the remote diagnosis of asthma by health practitioners, or assist in the adjustment of drug dosages [49].

15.1.4 Magnetic Resonance Imaging in Remote Regions and the Developing World

MRI constitutes one of the greatest medical inventions of the twentieth century, and has the capacity to identify arthritis, osteoarthritis, cancer, arteriosclerosis, epilepsy, and physical damage due to trauma, with objective measurements that are clear markers of clinical issues [50]. Yet, over 60 years since its inception, MRI has not yet reached the hands of clinicians in remote regions and the developing world in sufficient numbers.

15.1.4.1 Overlap between MRI Products and the Developing World

The explanation may be derived from the poor fit that exists between conventional MRI products and the developing world: MRI products that are sold for millions of dollars in the developed world are in obvious misalignment with the socioeconomic conditions of the developing world [51]. Clinicians in these countries have insufficient resources to maintain these products with their huge cryogenic magnets, software and hardware servicing requirements, let alone for their initial purchase. As a result, countless patients are deprived of the best possible health care. Clearly, a MRI product that is more portable and less of a burden to operate for users is required to recover picture-perfect images, in helping to recognize broken hands, arms, and legs; problems with the brain, spine, and vertebrae; heart and organ failure; epilepsy, arthritis, cancer, arteriosclerosis, and more.

The potential diversity of images that might be available to clinicians is illustrated in Figure 15.2. As radio waves, rather than x-rays, are utilized to capture imagery, this

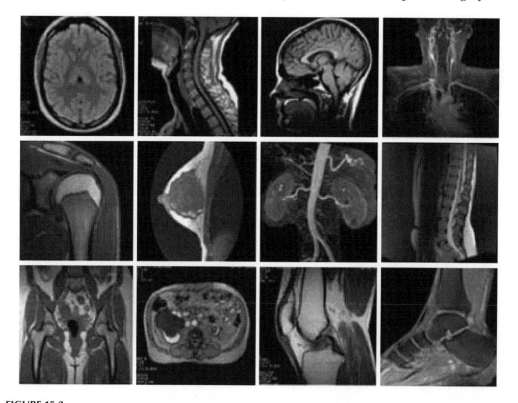

FIGURE 15.2
The diversity of MRI images available for detecting human pathologies. (Adapted with courtesy from Timothy Nagel, Copyright 2013. Advanced MRI, accessed August 12, 2013. With permission.)

method is regarded as intrinsically safe. However, MRI technologies are quite challenging to master; they require state-of-the-art knowledge and procedures, spanning engineering, physics, biology, biochemistry, and medicine. Thus, the cost burden is extensive, placing it out of reach of the developing world.

This was the scenario in the developing world approximately 5 years ago. Today, however, the situation has evolved, and GE Healthcare is targeting the developing world [52]. As a multinational company with offices in Waukesha, WI, it is selling some of the first MRI products that are designed to fit the needs of patients in the developing world. In contrast to what the prevailing perspective in the developed world might be, developing countries have growing economies, with health-care budgets that are on the increase. In China, there is but a single MRI scanner per 1 million people in comparison to 50 MRI scanners per million individuals in the United States. Hence, GE anticipates significant growth potential, and potential for profit, on the proviso that it can manufacture these systems at significantly lower cost in China and India. GE will initially target top-tier hospitals with the notion that they do not wish to compromise quality. Rather, they are striving to simplify products and to provide enhanced value [53].

15.1.4.2 Budget MRI Systems for the Developing World

Since cost is the primary barrier to the acquisition of MRI systems for the developing world, a prudent first step must involve the modification of current systems to facilitate cost reductions. Let us survey the characteristics of these systems to assess how far they might go to satisfy users in the developing world. GE has re-engineered a full MRI system to cut the purchase price by half, that is, to $700 k (Figure 15.3). The specific product, contingent on the market, is named either the 1.5 T Brivo MR355 or the Optima 360, which utilizes a short tunnel for more patient freedom [54]. This system is also less complex and has a smaller footprint, making it attractive for clinicians insofar as they are being portable enough to move to different locations within a hospital, and perhaps to other medical facilities if necessary.

GE has endeavored to cover almost any clinical scenario, spanning routine orthopedic exams, to breast, organ, or neurological cases. Of further attraction is that the power consumption of the system has been lowered by 34% to better align with the usage in the developing world; it comprises one of their most energy-efficient systems.

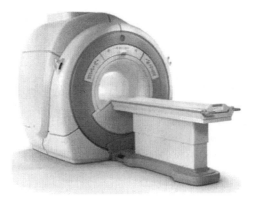

FIGURE 15.3
GE Optima 360 1.5 T for Indian and Chinese health-care markets. (Reproduced from General Electric Company, Optima MR360 1.5T (available in 2012). http://www.gehealthcare.com/euen/mri/products/optima_mr360/index.html (accessed November 4, 2012). With permission.)

The majority of this character is derived from the short bore magnet design, which offers strong magnetic fields and a 48 × 48 cm^2 field of view. Conventional power is used, but importantly, the equipment room and software have been integrated into the instrument. With the negation of the equipment room and only a single separate box of electronics, the system footprint of this unit has been reduced to 25 m^2. Antennas are integrated into the patient table, which further simplifies the setup. Contrast is of high quality as the signals from patient adipose tissues may be suppressed via software. As a result, the appropriate levels of detail and quality have been recognized and met, which considerably augment the human value. Software enhancements have also been integrated in order to provide, for example, detailed breast or spine scans that are contrasted with VIBRANT software. The main compromise is associated with the short bore design, which fits well with the highly variable conditions present in the developing world, albeit at the cost of slightly lower patient throughput. With respect to the unit's smaller overall dimensions translating to only a minimal loss of functionality, it is an excellent compromise in trade for significant expenditure savings. This scanner is currently being produced in China and sold in India. The Achilles' heel of this system, however, remains the cryogenic magnets. Nevertheless, as much as they increase cost and inconvenience, they do improve performance with images that are 5–10 times clearer, which is a critical factor in diagnostic accuracy.

Bruker managed to decouple cryogenic magnets from MRI, as they are unpopular and costly to maintain, and as a result created the Bruker Icon 1.0 T [55], while still managing to retain image quality. Bruker BioSpin is a major global company that has its U.S. headquarters in Billerica, MA, with multiple distribution points in China and India. It is clear that this company has the developing world in its sights. Its technical innovation involves an aspect magnet that utilizes a patented method to increase image resolution via a type of electronic magnet stabilizer for a Halbach magnet array. It is evident that this design constitutes an improved fit for all markets.

From a technical perspective, there are a number of advances that make this system special. First, it provides an exceptional resolution of 100 μm without the use of cryogenic magnets. Of particular appeal for portable use in remote and developing countries is a low fringe field, which constitutes a key selling point. This means that the magnetic field does not leak out of the system, which can indeed pose a dangerous hazard. (Unfortunately, some deaths have occurred from ballistic metal objects, which were sucked into a patient-occupied MRI). Therefore, this feature enhances patient and operator safety and likely enables the unit to be compatible for all outdoor environments. Further, the system employs a 1 T permanent magnet; hence, it does not have the requirement for being maintained, which makes running costs very low indeed [55].

Clearly, there is great potential for portability, which will allow for its use in isolated environments with integrated software packages such as ParaVision that control radio pulses and alter signal processing. This capability expands the range of tissues that may be analyzed; for example, the use of rapid acquisition software packages enables the visualization of tissues and structures that possess a short radio emission character, such as lung and cartilage, respectively, the latter being frequently damaged by arthritis. Other examples of software include arterial scanning that employs the pulsed arterial spin tagging package, or diffusion tensor analysis (DT-MRI), which elucidates the structures of nerve fibers and the brain by monitoring the trajectories of water molecules. This software is inclusive of rapid image readouts [55]. What prevents the Bruker Icon 1.0 T from being a true success for human use is its size. The operating volume is far too small for patients; hence, it may only be used to image rodents, rats, and mice. Regrettably, this technology is not yet being utilized in the developing world and is currently more likely to be found in research laboratories, where it is used for preclinical analyses such as the tracking of responses to drugs. Nevertheless, considering its attractive virtues, this type of scanner might eventually expand into the clinical domain and take the developing world by storm (see M2 which is related).

15.1.4.3 Mobile MRI Systems: Serving the Wider Community

The renting of MRI units as an on-the-road mobile solution constitutes an additional strategy that might dramatically increase accessibility and lower the costs for their use in the developing world. GE has developed a rentable mobile solution, which consists of a self-contained MRI that is housed within a trailer (GE mobile LX) [56]. The upfront rate may be as low as 10% of the normal cost, should a refurbished MRI system be used. Another important advantage is the option for its transport to myriad locations that require MRI services (e.g., towns, villages, cities, or any rural area where services are limited, or small-sized hospitals that have no budget to purchase a MRI system outright). Service companies normally own these vehicles and maintain them. In the developed world, their role is to assist, to a large measure, parent metropolitan area hospitals in dealing with overcapacity and backlog issues. The MRI is typically custom-installed into the interior of the trailer, where the vehicle is divided into a room for the scanner and a room for the instrument console/control center. Telemetry systems transfer the resulting images to the clinicians who have requested them. Price and flexibility make these MRI units attractive for the developing world, in that low- to mid-budget rural centers can begin to offer MRI services. As a developed world example, a complete mobile MRI system is available in California for only US$65,000. Clearly, there is strong potential for MRI solutions of this type in the developing world, albeit the path to their extensive implementation will likely initially require teams of motivated entrepreneurs, more so than any further improvements in the technology itself.

A mobile Ingenia 3.0 T system produced by Philips offers high patient throughput with the fastest scan times available with high image quality. Philips Healthcare (headquartered in Andover, MA) has found that per-patient costs can be lowered through the use of superfast scans. This system does not use antennas that are built into patient tables, but rather utilizes a number of flexible multitransmitting coils (e.g., via a shoulder coil or Flex coverage spinal coil). This strategy provides a remarkable 300 μm resolution, or better, and results in very smooth images, as well as the suppression of signal distorting adipose tissues. Due to radio adaptation to the unique anatomies of every individual, scans are only 2–4 min in duration, which is more rapid and more detailed than many 3D x-ray solutions, without the risk. For example, a 32-year-old male patient with back pain was examined via a CT scan. The image quality, however, was insufficient for a diagnosis, whereas the Ingenia system provided excellent images that enabled the identification of a small protrusion of disk L5/S1. System accessory technologies also make cardiac measurements possible, using Vascular Explorer and Cardiac Explorer, giving quantitative analyses of vascular pathologies (e.g., hemorrhaging and plaque deposits within the body). Achieva is a very similar system that is offered by Philips, with the most frequent uses involving children's abdominal areas, breast, spine, and pediatric issues within 2 min [57].

Inland imaging offers mobile MRI systems in the eastern Washington area that integrates smart single-click protocols for reproducible MRI exams, and an "exam card" which neatly categorizes scans, dependant on the pathology. Magnetic resonance images

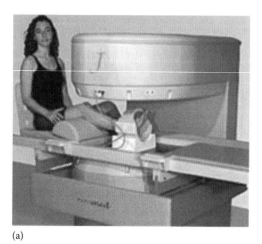
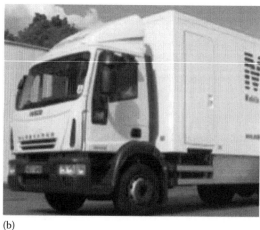

(a)   (b)

FIGURE 15.4
(a, b) MRJ mobile deployed in the Indian subcontinent to investigate hip, shoulder, and spine. (Reproduced from Shiva Medicare, Mobile MRI Unit (MrJ 0.22T), 2012. www.shivamed.com (accessed November 4, 2012). With permission.)

are transmitted over a wireless network to a radiologist with a referring physician to read them, typically within 24 h of an exam. Although overall the upfront purchase prices of these systems do not align well with the economic realities of the developing world, rental packages with a lower price point, coupled with the emphasis on the speed of the scans and exceptional image quality suggest that these types of systems might be taken up in developing regions by higher tier hospitals and private health-care groups.

With its 2200 0.22 T mobile MRI system, MRJ produces a low-cost rentable mobile system that Shiva Medicare, Mobile Diagnostics, Berlin offers for one-third of the cost of comparable systems to the Indian subcontinent. This technology utilizes a low-field, maintenance-free permanent magnet MRI system (produced by Paramed Medical Systems—head office at Genova, Italy) (Figure 15.4) to address orthopedic issues, which is mounted within an 18 ton truck. Patients are scanned in a comfortable open magnet system, where children can hold their parents' hands. The entire system is ultracompact and supports telehealth and telemedicine, including videoconference teleradiology for remote access to medical consultants. This system is intended to serve rural areas within India and has the capacity for being powered by solar energy, making available for the first time, access to MRI in remote locations [58].

15.1.4.4 Portable MRI Systems on Wheels: New Hope for Patients

Technical innovations have led to MRI systems that are mounted on wheels for portability within hospitals. Without the constraint of heavy and cumbersome cryogenic magnets, they can be moved to wherever they are needed, whether for the prescreening of patients or in the operating theater. These systems produce clear images of joint-related injuries/conditions, particularly in the extremities, and can support surgical use as well. The Magnevu scanner 0.20 T, introduced in ~2000, was the first wheeled system of this type with an innovative design that exploited nonuniform fields [59].

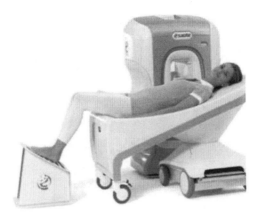

FIGURE 15.5
Esaote O-Scan for knee, hand, foot, ankle, and elbow. (Reproduced from Esaote, O-Scan dedicated MRI system, 2012. http://www.esaote.co.uk/modules/core/page.asp?p=MRI (accessed November 4, 2012). With permission.)

Esaote (Genova, Italy) is also a producer of medical diagnostic systems that has developed a suite of 0.2–0.31 T MRI systems based on this low field technology, which offers high-resolution imagery despite very low field strengths (fractions of a Tesla) to accommodate hip, shoulder, spine, and extremity joints. The Esaote O-Scan system, shown in Figure 15.5, is one of the company's latest unit offerings, which is ultraportable and redefines the classical look of a MRI unit. At present, Esaote has set its focus on musculoskeletal imaging only, not claiming to offer the contrast of other tissues outside of this domain. The various types of systems are listed in the following paragraphs and appear to retain the core system but with different antennas, and form adapted to particular extremities. Performance may be classified in three tiers: 0.2 T, 0.25 T, and 0.31 T, where the 0.2 T machines include the Magnevu (also called Orthovu), C-scan, E-scan (Opera), and Artoscan-m. The 0.25 T machines are called the G-scan and S-scan, which preceded the wheeled 0.31 T O-scan [60].

Recently, the PoleStar N-30 (Figure 15.6) went a step further in introducing a portable real-time imaging MRI system to hospitals for guiding surgical procedures. Medtronic (world headquarters, MN) manufactures the latest version of this remarkably compact

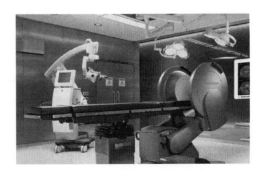

FIGURE 15.6
Ultracompact PoleStar N-30 for brain tumor removal. (Reproduced from Medtronic ST Neurosurgery (launched 2010). http://www.medgadget.com/2010/04/polestar_n30_surgical_mri_system_launched_1.html (Accessed August 24, 2013) (With permission)

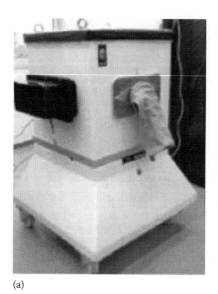 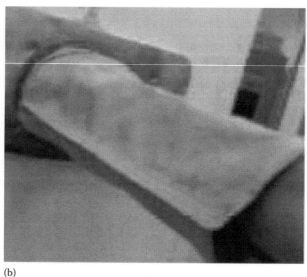

(a)   (b)

FIGURE 15.7
(a, b) Aspect's M2 wrist scanner for a doctor's office, clinic, or hospital. (Reproduced from Aspect Imaging, Aspect Imaging's M2™ compact high-performance MRI imaging system selected as a "Top 10 Innovation" in life science by *The Scientist*, 2012. http://www.aspectimaging.com/press-releases/m2-selected-as-a-top-10-innovation-in-life-science/(accessed November 4, 2012). With permission.)

portable MRI system for operating theater use, which makes available a close-to-real-time imaging solution. In conjunction with a "stealthstation," it provides a facile working environment for the surgeon who wishes to conduct in-theater scanning for thoracic and brain surgeries [61].

The Aspect M2 MRI wrist scanner 1.0 T [62] may hold the record for the smallest medical MRI scanner, which is a small box-shaped scanner, on wheels (Figure 15.7). This first generation system can scan wrists in any environment. It was pioneered by Uri Rapoport, Aspect's Founder and CEO, with his headquarters, research, development, and manufacturing all based in Shoam, Israel, with worldwide commercial operations in Toronto, Canada. His Aspect M2 has won awards for its design, which furnish the high-resolution, high-clarity images that are needed for accurate medical diagnoses. A resolution of less than 100 μm is exemplary without the use of cryogenic magnets. Further, the containment of the magnetic field and an operating size of just over a cubic foot suggest that similar systems might be available in the future for scanning larger body segments and extremities. At the other end of the scale, in the more distant future, we may also see this system working as a 3D microscope for living cells to confirm malaria, leukemia, and other afflictions associated with blood. One might also envision its use with functionalized nanoparticles, and in the longer term, potentially operating in conjunction with autonomous nanomedical devices (Chapter 1).

Although the company Magritek [63] does not manufacture medical MRI systems, they are included in this list as they offer MRI systems that can operate in remote regions. Their Terranova product contains no magnet and is a part of range of equipment that is produced in New Zealand, which offers MRI portability for the developing world. This system is the only MRI device that has operated in the harsh conditions of Antarctica [64], where it was employed to measure ice structures.

15.1.4.5 Developing Trends in MRI

Definite technical trends are under development and progressing, which are evident via a survey of existing commercial systems. Table 15.1 lists a surprising number of portable MRI systems with costs that should be affordable to medical facilities in the developing world. It spans the very fast and expensive mobile Ingenia systems that have full body imaging capabilities, to the lower cost and more portable (on wheels) Esaote systems that measure only the musculoskeletal system. It also covers the open magnet designs and the closed "polo"-like designs used for body segment analysis. Apart from the Terranova system, all of the previously mentioned systems have sufficient performance to construct 3D images from within the human body and can be transported to different locations. Those units with permanent magnets are truly portable; thus, with an appropriately dedicated business plan, these units may begin to have positive impacts on the developing world.

The magnetic field is a good indicator of performance, resulting in better quality images and faster scans. However, it can sometimes overshadow other patented technologies that are utilized to reduce noise and to make use of lower field levels for certain purposes. For example, surgical applications are only possible at 0.15 T, suggesting that a unique technology is at work here, which is not always recognized or advertised. Also, what Table 15.1 does not reveal is exactly how efficient a portable system might be in the detection of different tissue types and subsequently alerting the clinician of any problems. MRI performance numbers alone are obviously not sufficient criteria with which to recommend a system. Clinicians will have to judge the recognition and contrast for various tissue types, which is a more subtle performance parameter that is disseminated by medical opinion leaders. For the moment, the ultracompact Aspect M2 system appears to be distinct from the other systems; it exceeds the performance of Bruker, a market leader for several decades, who has moved to incorporate the M2 technology into their Icon system. Hence, this decade may indeed flag the start of a trend in high-resolution portable MRI that will be of benefit to those in remote regions and the developing world.

TABLE 15.1

Comparison of Mobile and Portable MRI Systems

MRI System	Field (T)	Medical Use	Scan (min)	Cost ($)	Cryogenic (Y/N)	Type
GE mobile LX	1.5	All body	20	200 k	Y	Mobile
Magnevu 1000	0.2	Musculoskeletal	25	200 k	N	Portable
MRJ 2200	0.25	Musculoskeletal	20	500 k	N	Portable
Esaote G-Scan	0.25	Musculoskeletal	20	300 k	N	Portable
Esaote O-Scan	0.32	Musculoskeletal	15	300 k	N	Portable
Magritek Kea2		N/A	—	10 k	N	Portable
MRI Achieva	3.0	All body		3 M	Y	Mobile
Magritek Terranova	0.001	N/A	400	5 k	N	Portable
MRI Ingenia	3.0	All body	2–4	3 M	Y	Mobile
Aspect M2	1.0	Wrist	2	100 k	N	Portable
Bruker Icon	1.0	Mice	2	200 k	N	Portable
PoleStar N-30	0.15	Head	<0.01	1 M	N	Portable
GE Optima	1.5	All body	8	700 k	Y	Mobile

15.1.4.6 Innovations Poised to Shift the MRI Paradigm

Several new concepts that may allow for the shrinkage of MRI are listed as follows. These ideas relate to significant changes to the component parts that alter the clarity of the MRI image. The key components encompass

1. The magnet, which induces hydrogen nuclei to resonate and precess
2. The antenna, which sends and receives radio waves from body segments
3. The radio transceiver, which sends and receives radio signals to/from patients

1. *A "mouse" magnet scanner*: Blümich [65] at the University of Aachan has altered the magnet and its geometry in a fundamental way, which has shown promise in other application areas. The result is a "mouse" and a box of electronics that is connected to it (Figure 15.8). The scanner typically utilizes two magnets, with the North Pole and the South Pole residing just beneath the surface. It has the capacity for scanning concrete to reveal its structural composition or to verify the history of famous artworks by elucidating the attributes of its underlying paint layers. The output of the system is normally a graph that shows the concentration of water beneath the surface of a sample.

2. Sensitive gas-based MRI antennas, where the conventional wire coil is replaced by gas atoms. These structures are also known as magnetometers and have the ability to detect very small MRI signals. The best known of these devices is the SQUID (superconducting quantum interference device). However, it requires cryogenic cooling. As an alternative, Savukov and Romalis at Princeton University [66] have suggested the use of a small glass container that is filled with vaporized potassium. In this way, a laser can then quantify the magnetic field through the movement of potassium atoms. This technology is not practical as yet, however, due to the shielding that is needed to block out noise. A more practical solution has come from the National Institute of Standards and Technology in Boulder, CO, where physicist John Kitching [67] has exploited vaporized cesium atoms that are contained within what are called atomic magnetometers. These sensors are equivalent in size to a grain of rice and are comprised of an infrared laser and photodetector in a stacked

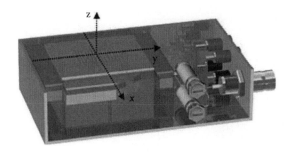

FIGURE 15.8
First-generation hand-based MRI scanning. (Reproduced from Casanova and Blümich J. Magn. Reson. 163(1), 38–45, 2003. With permission.)

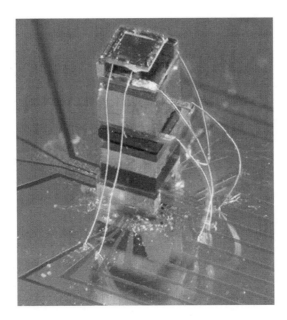

FIGURE 15.9
MRI detector based on cesium gas. Source: http://www2.technologyreview.com/article/409590/tr10-atomic-magnetometers/ (accessed August 26, 2013). (Reproduced from John Kitching. With permission.)

sandwich configuration on silicon. Normally, light passes easily through the cesium gas. However, under exposure to a magnetic field (even a very weak one), the cesium atoms align and absorb light in proportion to the magnetic field strength. Atomic magnetometers are of low power, extremely sensitive, and can operate at room temperature. They may also be reconfigured as arrays to further boost performance. A stack of these devices is shown in Figure 15.9.

3. *Miniature MRI transceiver "phone"*: As mobile phone technologies are based on transceivers, the know-how necessary to develop miniature MRI transceivers is also available. With the correct engineering improvements, sufficient funding, and cooperation of larger multinationals, a smart MRI handset similar to a mobile phone might appear in the next decade.

15.1.4.7 Bold Future: Advent of the Incredible Shrinking MRI

To speculate on the evolution of MRI technologies and the resulting products that might appear in the future is indeed challenging. The prime driver—human health—is a potent one, leading to numerous pioneers who are strongly motivated to innovate. These pioneers work tirelessly toward the "incredible shrinking MRI," as coined by *Scientific American* [68]: These unique individuals include Bernhard Blümich, a professor of macromolecular chemistry at RWTH Aachen University in Germany, Aachen. Blümich created the "mouse" magnet scanner described earlier, wherein the sample does not have to be positioned inside or between the poles of a magnet. Rather, the face of the magnet presents a field gradient in order to obtain composition with depth. In many ways, this format may evolve as the equivalent of an ultrasound scanner, where the MRI mouse is moved manually over an anatomical site of interest to build up an image.

Alexander Pines, a professor at the Pine laboratory at the University of California, Berkeley, has come up with novel ways of compensating for the variations in magnetic fields [69], such that uniform fields do not have to be constructed. This work addresses the bulky magnet problem in that it allows magnets to be used more in their native state. More recently, Pines has begun working on the chemical analysis of fluidic channels [70], which are now commonplace in the analysis of blood and urine. The addition of MRI to these systems might enable reagentless tests for the detection of diseases, which are far more reliable.

Paul Callaghan (Victoria University, Wellington, New Zealand) is behind the Magritek company mentioned previously. His focus is to turn innovative ideas into portable working systems that may beneficially impact medical applications in the future. Systems that support remote MRI are one of Paul Callaghan's interests. To date, two of his portable MRI systems designed for remote diagnostic applications have been deployed in Antarctic studies, conducted by research groups at the University of Wellington [71]. A remote setup using the Magritek Kea mole is depicted in Figure 15.10, which is a forerunner of the Kea2 tomography system. These systems facilitate structural ice studies by providing a deeper understanding of how the mechanical properties of the sea ice are changing. Magritek's Terranova earth field imaging has been used in Antarctica as well, although its performance through the utilization of the Earth's magnetic field has not sufficiently resolved structures. Although medical applications have not yet been reported, these exceptionally portable systems may well inspire equally portable medical systems that serve as the seeds of advanced MRI technologies for remote regions and the developing world.

Mobile support vehicles for these and the other types of portable MRI systems described earlier for remote regions are attractive. These vehicles may conceivably provide mobile infrastructure support for MRI systems in terms of electrical power, stability, automation

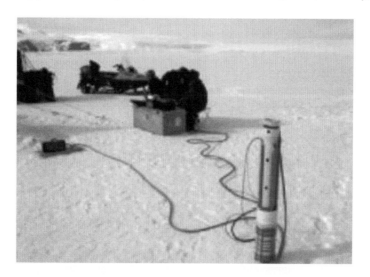

FIGURE 15.10
Kea mole assessing water ice in Antarctica. (Reproduced from Antarctic NMR, University of Victoria, 1994–2009. http://www.victoria.ac.nz/scps/research/research-groups/magnetic-resonance/antarctic-nmr (accessed November 4, 2012). With permission.)

of measurement protocols, and wireless data transmission facilities. Currently, trailer to truck-sized vehicles are available, which can support areas that can be accessed by road. Other less accessible locations will require alternate transport platforms. A four-wheel drive jeep, for example, might be equipped with some of the smaller portable MRIs mentioned, to extend service for remote regions. Two other unusual transportation platforms may help to move these heavy "portable" systems of today. If access to sites can only be achieved by foot, robotic upright vehicles produced by Segway Robotics [72] could follow medics on foot and carry significant payloads, such as a portable MRI that supports musculoskeletal scanning, with batteries and data transmission capabilities. Access by air to carry MRI support might also be a possibility for injured climbers or car crash. For terrestrially inaccessible regions, the soon-to-be manufactured Martin jetpack [73] may provide an option: This personalized hoverable aircraft might potentially fly a medic to a crash scene in conjunction with a robotized version, which would carry a portable MRI system. On arrival at the incident, telemetry systems may access a control center to obtain advice on the scanning protocol.

The targeting of accident cases with portable MRI systems may contribute to and expedite their implementation in remote regions and developing countries. Installed at casualty sites or within ambulances, open magnet designs from MRJ or Esaote could allow a patient to be placed on a table where the system would assist in the recognition of damage to bones and soft tissues, to quickly acquire (and transmit if necessary) critical medical data. The same strategy would apply in remote regions where teams in the field and at hospitals could be much better coordinated if the nature of the damage is known early on.

Transitioning to the future in contemplating what might be possible insofar as advances in MRI, we may expect that the functionality of wheeled portable permanent magnet systems will increase, along with new software plug-ins and incremental, albeit steady, improvements in engineering. In parallel, portable systems such as the Aspect M2 are likely to accommodate additional scannable body segments, whereby image quality and tissue types rendered will increase. Overall, increasing numbers of MRI machines will become available with further cost reductions, making it probable that access to MRI will improve for the developing world. Advancements in systems miniaturization, renewable energy sources, and battery technologies in a decade hence will undoubtedly lower costs even further and virtually guarantee MRI access for these current underserved regions.

Technically, MRI magnets, antennae, and transceivers will shrink in size. Antennae may be replaced by more sensitive cesium gas probes, which will allow smaller magnets and magnetic fields to be utilized. This in turn could lead to the following innovations:

1. MRI jackets to be clipped to the front or back of the patient, with dedicated "hot zones" that will scan critical organs, liver, heart, and lungs.

2. Helmet-integrated MRI scanner that paramedics may fit onto suspected stroke victims to quickly elucidate blood clots, and if appropriate, apply initial treatment while an ambulance is in transit.

3. Handheld "MRI stethoscope" that doctors can directly apply to probe the location of pain such as the stomach, thorax, or head, to expose a high fidelity image of the underlying tissue with accurate dimensions, such that an enlarged heart or a swollen brain may be rapidly recognized.

4. MRI spectacles that might quickly scan the blood vessels and nerves of the retina.

5. In the more distant future, a desktop MRI scanner that would produce microscopic 3D images of blood cells in order to spot pathologies such as leukemia or malaria. Scan data could then be transmitted to the hospital prior to the arrival of the patient, saving significant time. Injected, inhaled, or orally administered magnetic nanoparticles (e.g., superparamagnetic iron oxide nanoparticles—SPIONs) might also, in many cases, dramatically enhance MRI imagery through their use as fine contrast agents [74].

Before MRI coverage can occur in remote regions and the developing world, portable and mobile MRI systems will need to be considered by major hospitals in these areas (e.g., those systems with very high performance, such as the mobile Philips Ingenia that spans the full range of disease pathologies, versus the portable Esaote O-Scan, which is limited to musculoskeletal analysis). When presented with these various products, a clinician must endeavor to balance purchase costs with prospective fees charged. At the Apollo hospital in Bangalore, India (Figure 15.11), for example, the fee for a brain scan is $180 in comparison to $2500 in the United States. Maximum functionality must also be balanced against expenditure; hence, an older refurbished unit may be preferred, at a fraction of the cost of a new system. This suggests that portable MRI systems might be purchased to supplement complete systems that are already installed in hospitals. They will not, however, replace established systems in the near term, as the limited functionality of today's portable systems will leave the clinician with unknowns.

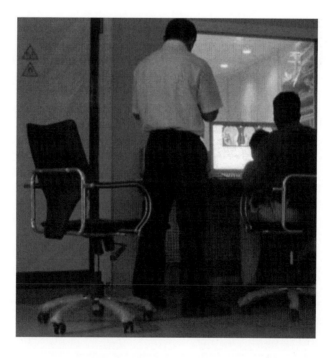

FIGURE 15.11
The MRI exam room in the Apollo Hospital in Bangalore. (Reproduced from TimWit blog, A little review, March 19, 2008, http://timwit.wordpress.com/2008/03/19/a-little-review (accessed November 8, 2012). With permission.)

15.1.5 Remote Robotic Telesurgery

Remote robotic surgery enables the capacity for doctors to conduct surgical procedures on patients who may be at different locations within the same operating theater (as is in most instances practiced today), or in contrast, hundreds or many thousands of kilometers distant, thus essentially anywhere on the globe. The world's two primary robotic surgical systems (ZEUS and Da Vinci) have been reduced to one (Da Vinci), as in 2003, Da Vinci's manufacturer (Intuitive Surgical) acquired ZEUS producer, Computer Motion.

15.1.5.1 ZEUS Remote Intercontinental Surgery

An initial unprecedented long distance robot assisted laparoscopic cholecystectomy (gall bladder removal) in a porcine model was performed in 2001 by surgeon Dr. Jacques Marescaux, who was situated in Strasbourg, France, with joystick in hand. The porcine "patient" was located in Paris; hence, the signals from the surgeon's console were transmitted over a cumulative distance of ~1000 km. One of the purposes of this initial operation was to quantify "variable time delays on surgical manipulations." "The time lag was artificially increased from 20 ms (standard time delay) up to 551.5 ms. The limit of the acceptable time delay in terms of a surgeon's perception of safety was roughly 330 ms." Subsequently, transoceanic "latencies" (signal time delays) were measured during a porcine gall bladder removal procedure in order to determine the viability of intercontinental surgery between New York (surgeon site) and Strasbourg (porcine patient site), with a total two-way distance of >14,000 km.

The actual surgery was executed by the ZEUS surgical system (Computer Motion, California, which in 1999 made medical history by assisting with the world's first beating-heart bypass surgery—Dr. Douglas Boyd), comprised of two distinct subsystems (surgeon side and patient side). These dual sites were linked via a high-speed terrestrial fiber-optic network that transferred data through dedicated connections utilizing "asynchronous transfer mode (ATM) technology" with a reserved bandwidth capacity of 10 Mb/s. A network termination unit (NTU) enabled the provision of a multiservice conduit to different applications. Postprocedure analysis revealed that no ATM packets were lost; two-way delay via ATM transfer was 78–80 ms; 70 ms was allotted to video coding/decoding as well as several ms for "rate adaptation and Ethernet-to-ATM packet conversion." This resulted in nearly seamless functionality, whereby any movement performed by the surgeon in New York made the round trip and was registered on his video screen within 155 ms.

Finally, the team performed a remote human laparoscopic cholecystectomy in a 68-year-old female on securing appropriate ethical committee approval and informed patient consent. Using an identical setup, this procedure was conducted by a surgeon, who was in New York, while the patient was in Strasbourg. The average time delay was 155 ms; robotic system setup time was 16 min, and "the gallbladder was dissected in 54 min, without any intraoperative complication." There were no postoperative issues, and the patient was released within 48 h. These successes facilitated the inception of an entirely new surgical field [76].

15.1.5.2 ZEUS Remote Undersea/Space Surgery

Another notable study in remote robotic surgery involving the ZEUS system included testing for wireless remote surgery in the NASA undersea (67 ft subsurface) research facility Aquarius (Key Largo, Florida) where a simulated performance of a gall bladder removal surgery on a dummy was telementored by Canadian surgeon (Mehran Anvari) located 1300 miles away at the Centre for Minimal Access Surgery, St. Joseph's Hospital (Hamilton, ON). The surgically untrained NASA Extreme Environment Mission Operations (NEEMO) 7 crew was successfully guided through the surgery and suturing process, which verified that minimally trained astronauts might conduct intricate medical procedures. This exercise served as a precursor to potential future use in remote emergency medical situations on the International Space Station (ISS) or during future explorations of the Moon or Mars [77,78]. Since signal latencies of beyond 0.7 s will begin to impair the surgeon's ability to control the robot, signal delays and hence telesurgical procedures in deep space, well beyond the distance of the ISS (330–410 km), would be significant. Two-way signal transmissions from Earth–Moon–Earth at 384,000 km would clock in at 2.5 s, whereas from Earth–Mars–Earth at 55–378 million km would range from 8.7 to 42 min [79]. Hence, one might correctly surmise that future medical robotic and nanomedical device autonomy will play a considerable role in extraterrestrial surgical procedures nearer term, and an exclusive role in the future.

15.1.5.3 Da Vinci Remote 3D Display with Haptic Tactile Feedback

Bornhoft et al. explored the efficacy of integrating a stereoscopic monitor visualization system to potentially enhance remote robotic surgery. The Da Vinci system typically incorporates stereoscopic vision in conjunction with haptic tactile feedback in the provision of an "intuitive environment for remote surgical applications." The researchers compared the performance of surgeons who used a stereoscopic interfacing system with those who used 2D monitors. The illusion of the depth of imagery provided by cameras mounted (at a specific distance/angle) to a miniature multifunctional in vivo robot was conveyed by displaying live video streams on dual (left/right) monitors and four-angled mirrors to imitate human eye depth perception. The haptic interface was comprised of "two PHANTOM Omni® (SensAble, Woburn, MA) controllers." These devices calculate the three degrees of freedom orientation and position of pointed end effectors. These interfaces allowed the surgeons to see a 3D image and to sense force feedback "for collision and workspace limits." Subsequent to the completion of two types of surgical training tasks using 2D monitors and 3D interface, the participants noted that the 3D system was easier to utilize and reduced the time to completion of the given tasks due to the perceived virtual environment. This capacity showed the potential for facilitating the performance of higher complexity surgeries with greater precision. This will likely translate to improved outcomes for remote surgical procedures [80].

15.1.5.4 Trauma Pod

Dr. Richard Satava, a former DARPA Project Manager, and current professor of surgery at the University of Washington, is a pioneer in the discipline of long-distance robotic surgery or "telesurgery." As Satava described it from the perspective of the surgeon: "I never see my patient," …. "I never touch him. But the images I see by going through computer systems allow me to do things that I can't do with my own eyes. The systems are more precise. They allow me to scale up and scale down. They magnify an image so I can see much more than if I was standing and looking right at the patient" [81].

Satava et al. envisage a Trauma Pod (TP) system (Figures 15.12 and 15.13), which would consist of a "rapidly deployable robotic platform, capable of performing critical diagnostics and acute life-saving interventions in the field for an injured person who might otherwise die from

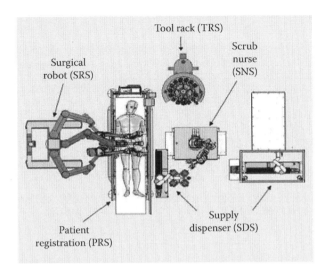

FIGURE 15.12
Primary TP elements. (Reproduced from Garcia, P. et al., *Int. J. Med. Robot.* 5(2), 136, 2009. With permission.)

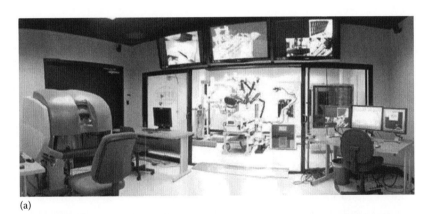

(a)

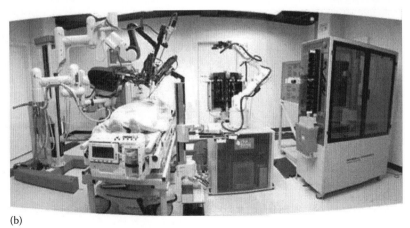

(b)

FIGURE 15.13
Trauma Pod. (a) Control cell; (b) surgical cell. (Reproduced from Garcia, P. et al., *Int. J. Med. Robot.* 5(2), 136, 2009. With permission.)

TABLE 15.2

List of TP Subsystems

Acronym	Subsystem	Developer
SRS	Surgical Robot Subsystem	Intuitive Surgical, Inc.
AMS	Administrator and Monitoring Subsystem	SRI International
SNS	Scrub Nurse Subsystem	Oak Ridge National Laboratory
TAS	Tool Autoloader Subsystem	Oak Ridge National Laboratory
SDS	Supply Dispenser Subsystem	General Dynamics Robotics
TRS	Tool Rack Subsystem	University of Washington
SCS	Supervisory Controller Subsystem	University of Texas
PRS	Patient Registration Subsystem	Integrated Medical Systems
PIS	Patient Imaging Subsystem	GE Research
MVS	Machine Vision Subsystem	Robotic Surgical Tech., Inc.
RMS	Resource Monitoring Subsystem	University of Maryland
SIM	Simulator Subsystem	University of Texas
UIS	User Interface Subsystem	SRI International

Source: Adapted with permission from Garcia, P. et al., *Int. J. Med. Robot.* 5(2), 136, 2009.

loss of airway, hemorrhage, or other acute injuries, such as tension pneumothorax." These necessarily invasive damage control interventions would come into play only as life-saving measures, when it is determined that the patient will not survive without them, in the absence of the appropriate medical personnel, and when the patient is unable to be transported quickly enough. Hence, the TP surgical robot would serve as a first responder in a remote or precarious location until further treatment can be obtained at a conventional medical facility. In addition to the opening of an airway, TP interventional measures might encompass the insertion of an intravenous or intraosseous line, the performance of hemostasis, performance of a bowel anastomosis, manipulation of damaged tissues, and the placement of monitoring devices. A prototype of the TP was developed by researchers, which was comprised of 13 subsystems (Table 15.2), which would be teleoperated by a remote surgeon via voice commands.

Using a patient phantom in a controlled environment, it was demonstrated that a shunt could be positioned on a major abdominal vessel and that a bowel anastomosis could be performed (SRS). Additionally, a full body CT scan was achieved during operations. Further demonstrated capabilities included automatic surgical tool dispensing/storing (TRS); automatic storing, depacking, dispensing, and supply counting (SDS); automatic surgical tool swapping/delivery and removal of supplies (SNS); speech-based teleoperating surgeon/TP system interface (UIS); automatic synchronization and interaction between SRS and SNS. Future work will include the integration of semi- and fully autonomous functionality, including anesthesia and sterilization protocols, operation during transport, and overall miniaturization of the system [82].

15.1.5.5 Mobile Robotic Telesurgery

Most contemporary telesurgical procedures are configured such that the surgeon console and patient/surgical robot are in close proximity to each other in the operating room. Lum et al. sought to investigate the challenges that are involved with the deployment and operation of a surgical robot system, utilizing a mobile control linkage, in remote or extreme environments, such as the battlefield or the sites of natural disasters. The researchers at the University of Washington, as collaborators in the HAPs/MRT (High Altitude Platform/Mobile Robotic

Telesurgery) project, proposed to use an unmanned aerial vehicle (UAV) (AeroVironment PUMA) as an alternative data link, in contrast to employing standard telecommunications to enable the teleoperation of a surgical robot in the field. A surgical robot was deployed in a desert near Simi Valley, CA, in order to conduct telesurgical trials with a simulated model. It was found that telerobotic surgical tasks could be conducted with a maximum signal latency of 20 ms between the surgeon's console and surgical robot (robotic control signals) and 200 ms (video stream) (still well below the threshold of 330 ms as described earlier).

An initial consideration was the safe packing and transport of the 700 kg surgical robot system. Hard shell foamed lined cases were designed and built to protect the surgical manipulators, surgical tools, and surgeon console components. To protect the operating mechanical elements (e.g., surgical manipulator motor packs and brakes) of the surgical robot system, as well as computer hardware and electronics, from wind-borne dust particles and extreme heat, several customized covers were designed and fabricated. Vents were incorporated into the covers that allowed the mounting of a PC fan to protect the actuators from the heat. An additional concern involved the supply of clean power. Hence, in order to protect the system from generator spikes, dual 1200 W line regulators were employed. Most of the electronic components were housed within two SKB Industrial Roto-Shock Rack cases.

For these trials, the distance between two surgeons in one tent and the surgical manipulators in another was 100 m, to expedite debugging and testing. However, the distance could extend to 2 km, within the range of the AUV. Most of the kinematic control signals for the robot were transmitted at 100 Hz, and the video bandwidth was 800 kB/s, as at higher rates (1 kHz and 2 MB/s) at full bandwidth, there was major (80%) packet loss. Following 3 days of field trials, the results revealed that the surgeons could indeed conduct gross telemanipulation tasks through a mobile wireless communication link in a remote environment [83].

15.1.5.6 Portable Intensive Care Unit

Integrated Medical Systems, Inc. (Signal Hill, CA) has developed a 40 pound (18 kg) suitcase-sized (22 in. × 21 in. × 7 in. – 56 cm × 53 cm × 18 cm) portable intensive care unit (ICU), which it calls the LS-1 (Figure 15.14, Table 15.3) for the treatment of both pediatric and adult patients in the field. The LS-1 integrates a number of important medical device capabilities within a single platform, utilizing a central control interface, and is designed to mount to the support poles of a standard NATO litter (stretcher) or strap to the floor of a terrestrial or airborne vehicle. The unit may operate by battery or via an external power source, and its capabilities encompass "electrocardiogram, invasive pressure monitoring, noninvasive blood pressure monitoring, temperature, pulse rate, blood oxygen saturation, and heart rate; low-rate and high-rate infusion pumps; a fluid warmer; a ventilator with carbon dioxide and oxygen monitoring capabilities; and the ability to deliver oxygen to a patient (using an external oxygen cylinder or oxygen concentrator)" [84].

Future advanced field-deployable nanomedical systems might be packaged similarly, albeit in more compact lightweight, ruggedized, and self-sterilizing cases for use in remote regions and across the developing world. The physician/systems interface might incorporate voice commands, and individual diagnostic and therapeutic components may be semi- or fully autonomous. A multifaceted power-harvesting/generating infrastructure could include integrated piezoelectric zinc oxide nanowire arrays; nanomaterials-based supercapacitors for power storage; and compact, yet high-performance, solar and wind energy harvesting elements. Additional capabilities would encompass conventional and stand-alone GPS systems, as well as a secure broadband wireless telecommunication link to enable rapid data transfer and real-time access to global medical expertise.

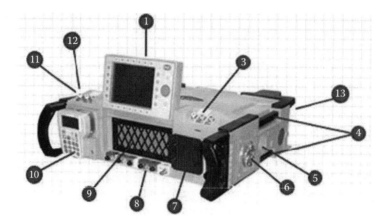

FIGURE 15.14
LS-1 portable ICU. See Table 15.3 for list of components. (Reproduced from LS-1, Integrated Medical Systems, Inc. http://www.lstat.com/showcase/overview.html (accessed July 23, 2012). With permission.)

TABLE 15.3

List of Integrated LS-1 Portable
Intensive Care Unit Components

Item	Description
1	Control and display unit
2	Secondary control and display unit
3	Alarm indicators
4	Auxiliary equipment rails
5	Oxygen inlet
6	Ventilator inlet
7	Ventilator connection
8	Patient connections
9	Cooling filter
10	Infusion pump
11	Auxiliary infusion pump connections
12	Auxiliary connections
13	Battery bays

Source: Reproduced from LS-1, Integrated Medical Systems, Inc. http://www.lstat.com/showcase/overview.html (accessed July, 23, 2012). With permission.

15.2 Nanomedical Devices in Remote Regions and the Developing World

Once the armamentarium of advanced nanomedical diagnostic and therapeutic technologies begins to filter into commercial availability, there will be a number of positive advantages for their utility in the developing world. Important benefits from the perspective of patients and health-care providers will include extreme compactness, high user compatibility, improved efficacy, minimal or noninvasiveness, as well as dramatically reduced side effects. Attractive aspects from the supply and operations perspective will include relatively low cost, high portability, frugal energy consumption, ease of setup and operation (e.g., nanomedical devices and systems will be semi- or fully automated, and most nanodevices intended for in vivo applications will be autonomous, albeit ultimately under external computer control). They will also be amenable to interfacing with a host of electronic devices such as mobile phones for the almost instantaneous conveyance and retrieval of robustly encrypted critical medical data, to and from medical experts globally.

Due to their compactness, it is conceivable that dedicated nanomedical devices and systems might be delivered by unmanned aircraft (subsequent to coordination with regional/local health administrators) to specific sites at remote locations in rough terrain, such as Ethiopia, where 85% of its population resides in remote areas with no available modern health care [85], or India and Pakistan, where ~72% [86] and 70% [87] of its people, respectively, live in rural regions. In addition, their deployment may assist in natural disaster situations where geographic or physical accessibility by first responders and medical personnel may be restricted or completely cut off.

15.2.1 VCSN and GMSD Imaging

A critical issue that might potentially be addressed via the development of the conceptual VCSN and gastrointestinal micro scanning device (GMSD) (Chapter 1) is the potential alleviation of the very limited or nonavailability of advanced medical imaging technologies in remote and impoverished regions of the world. Through the envisaged advancement and extreme miniaturization inherent to these innovative medical imaging technologies, virtually any individual on the globe might have access to important medical diagnostic tools.

As an autonomous device, the VCSN would harvest its power from the in vivo environment, thereby having the advantageous attribute of self-sustainability when in operation. Most of the conventional power required to operate the system would be consumed by "outbody" computers that house the Pixel Matrix image reconstruction software, along with additional hardware associated with the navigational guidance beacons, and communications infrastructure. These power requirements might conceivably be met via photovoltaic cells, wind generation, fuel cells, manual wind-up generators, or other locally appropriate power harvesting/generating sources. Thus, the complete infrastructure required for the scanning procedure might conceivably achieve fully functional status in remote and (if necessary) physically confined areas. The VCSN is envisaged as having the capability for rendering complete systems (vascular, lymphatic, or gastrointestinal) in ultrafine detail, displaying all interior and exterior surfaces with, for instance, the possibility of discerning plaque deposits in arterial lumen and their chemical compositions as well.

Although the GMSD would not be endowed with autonomy or the capacity for energy harvesting or generation, it may have significant utility in remote regions, particularly in the developing world, for the accurate imaging of the GI tract (GIT) toward the diagnosis of various disease states. The infrastructure required for the GMSD would be minimal, as the easily ingestible Bright Ball (BB) (Ø ~3 mm) would be highly portable as well as its external skin adherent activation/monitoring/tracking device, the Pulse Generator/Data Transfer (PGDT) unit. Subsequent to the ~2 to 3 day scanning procedure, the unobtrusive PGDT would simply be removed from the patient and interfaced via an onboard connector with either a laptop computer, mobile phone, or PDA for 3D Pixel Matrix rendering and transmission to the appropriate medical personnel for review/analysis/diagnosis.

Hypothetically, compact nanomedical devices/systems such as the VCSN and GMSD might be deployed (subsequent to coordination with regional and local health-care administrators) via small fixed wing UAVs or Rotorcraft Unmanned Aerial Vehicles (RUAVs) to specific sites in remote areas in rugged terrain to enable vascular, lymphatic, or GIT imaging for those who are deemed by local medical personnel to require it. Aggregates comprised of individual VSCN or GMSD/PGDT "kits" might be packaged and sealed within biodegradable starch-based or bioplastic polymeric foam (e.g., polylactic acid [PLA] or poly-ε-caprolactone [PCL] reinforced with bioplastic flax fiber) [88] encasements to protect them from initial impact damage and the elements. They would also serve as sterile storage containers until utilized. Specific GPS coordinates transmitted by health providers on site would guide the drop at a predetermined demarcated site. This strategy may serve as a viable option in the future toward securing critical advanced imaging capabilities in the absence of the capacity for patients to obtain MRI/CT scan or endoscopic procedures at any location where these imaging technologies are not practicable.

15.2.2 Prospective Nanomedical Contrast Imaging Agents

There are a growing number of nanomaterials-based contrast agents that are increasingly being utilized for cancer diagnostics and the imaging of cancerous tumors. These include fluorescent quantum dots (e.g., CdSe/CdS/ZnS), SPIONs (Fe_3O_4), gold, silica, and carbon nanoparticles. Pöselt et al. synthesized a novel ligand (micelle-forming) system that imparted bioinertness to quantum dots (55 nm hydrodynamic diameter) and SPIONs (60 nm hydrodynamic diameter). The team combined "aminofunctionalized poly(isoprene) preligand (PI-N3) and a polyisoprene-block-poly(ethylene oxide) diblock copolymer (PI-b-PEO), which results in excellent water solubility and bioinertness of the nanocrystals." The conversion of the terminating PEO hydroxyl into carboxylate facilitated the binding with monoclonal antibodies (in this case, T84.1) which target and bind with HT29 cells (human colon adenocarcinoma grade II cell line). This strategy for the biofunctionalization of quantum dots and SPIONs may enable important molecular imaging capabilities in remote areas. As these agents are typically used in conjunction with and enabled by MRI, their utilization in remote areas may be contingent on the ability to reduce the physical footprint and power consumption of these systems, or alternately to develop innately portable field-deployable or handheld devices with the capacity for generating magnetic fields of adequate strength and frequency to enable T_2-weighted scans [89].

Highly fluorescent carbon "quantum" dots (< Ø10 nm), surface-doped with an inorganic salt (zinc sulfide—ZnS), were developed by Cao et al. and functionalized with diamine-terminated oligomeric poly(ethylene glycol) PEG_{1500N} (enabling the decoration of the dots with targeting agents), resulting in a nontoxic bioimaging probe. When tested in mouse models, the carbon dots performed comparably to semiconducting quantum dots, and demonstrated more intense fluorescence than CdSe/ZnS quantum dots in confocal fluorescence images under 458 nm excitation [90]. Since carbon is not a semiconductor, it will not fluoresce on its own. The attribute of fluorescence, therefore, is thought to be facilitated by the nanopores that reside on the carbon surface that serve as "energy traps" when the nanoparticles are doped or coated with PEG to "become emissive upon stabilization as a result of the surface passivation" [91]. These contrast agents may typically be resolved through fluorodeoxyglucose positron emission tomography/computed tomography (F-FDG PET/CT). Ideally, fluorescing contrast agents might be utilized that are activated by lasers in the near-infrared (NIR) range (0.76–1.5 μm), which can harmlessly penetrate several centimeters into human tissues.

15.2.3 Prospective Nanomedical Hyperthermic and Photothermal Therapeutics

In terms of nanomedical therapeutics, hyperthermia is a state at which the temperature of human cells and tissues is artificially induced to be raised above median levels with the aim of eradicating diseased cells and/or tissues. The cooling capacity (via blood flow) of malignant tissues is only 10%–15% of that in normal tissues; thus, heat dissipation within tumors is significantly lacking. This situation results in higher temperatures when compared with surrounding healthy tissues. The maximum survival threshold temperature of cancer cells is ~42°C (therapeutic temperature), whereas healthy cells can withstand 48°C or higher [92,93]. When SPIONs are exposed to oscillating AC or DC magnetic fields, thermal activation ensues via the reorientation of magnetic moments (Néel relaxation) when anisotropic barriers are surpassed. Additionally, Brown relaxation can produce heat as a result of the rotational friction at the interfaces of nanoparticles and their aqueous carrier media [94]. Both phenomena may occur simultaneously or independently [95].

In hyperthermic therapeutics, magnetic nanoparticles have the advantage of treating diseased cells and tissues at anatomically deep sites in contrast to optically activated nanoparticles, whose efficacy is limited by the depth range of NIR photons. Beyond this depth threshold, there is likely to be pronounced photonic dissipation and scattering; hence, the light intensity required for effective treatments will be negated. On the other hand, certain types of magnetic nanoparticle materials that exhibit the strongest magnetic responses are toxic to the human body (e.g., cobalt and nickel). Therefore, they must be shielded from the biological milieu via encapsulation within biocompatible polymers or other materials, which gives rise to additional complexities [92].

Challa et al. synthesized (Ø6.3 nm) SPIONs with ultrathin Au coatings (0.4–0.5 nm thick) (Figure 15.15), and on exposure to low-frequency (44–430 Hz) oscillating magnetic fields it was observed that the amount of heat released was up to five times greater than uncoated control SPIONs (5.4 nm size). When both samples were exposed to 44 Hz magnetic fields at 465 Oe, the increase to the therapeutic temperature of 42°C was more rapid for the gold-coated SPIONs than the controls. Interestingly, thermal release was augmented via control

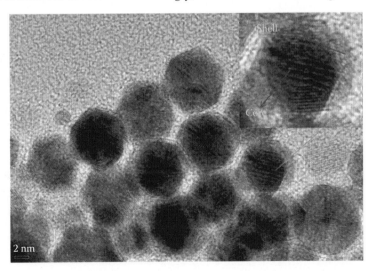

FIGURE 15.15
HRTEM image of Au/SPION nanoparticles with the inset depicting core and shell structure. (Reproduced from Mohammad, F. et al., *J. Phys. Chem. C Nanomater. Interf.* 1(20), 3141–3146. Copyright 2010. American Chemical Society. With permission.)

SPION concentration, whereas the reverse was true for Au/SPIONs. This was surmised to be attributed to heat-quenching due to the higher conductivity of gold. Thermal diffusion was also contingent on a "Brownian-rotation loss mechanism in addition to the Neel relaxation." The researchers also hypothesized that the "higher heat capacity of the gold shell to shield the heat generated within the SPIONs could be responsible for enhancing the temperature rise on application of oscillating magnetic field." They conclude that the outstanding hyperthermic activity imparted by the Au/SPIONs in conjunction with their biocompatibility make them excellent contenders for the "thermolysis of cancer cells" [96].

Biocompatible, multifunctional gold nanoshells were initially conceived and developed by Naomi Halas and Jennifer West (Rice University, Texas) [97]. These dielectric entities (silica core coated with ultrathin gold layer) may be induced, on exposure to NIR laser light (at "water window" wavelengths (690–900 nm) where biological tissues are optimally transparent), to undergo localized surface plasmon resonance, which is a cumulative oscillation of conduction band electrons. Nanoshells may be tuned, via the control of their geometries and core dimension–skin thickness ratios, to either strongly scatter NIR radiation or absorb it. In the case of scattering, the nanoshells can be utilized as imaging agents, whereas when they absorb NIR radiation they radiate heat and thus can be employed as hyperthermic agents for tumor ablation. Additionally, hollow nanoshells may be synthesized, loaded with drugs, and decorated with specific chemical groups or biomolecules for the potential precision targeting and delivery of concentrated drugs directly to diseased cells and tissues without inflicting collateral damage on neighboring healthy cells/tissues.

Gold nanoshells can also be used in theranostic applications where they serve simultaneously as dynamic diagnostic and therapeutic entities. When the nanoshell core is Ø129 nm with a shell thickness of 10–12 nm, they exhibit the capacity for both scattering and absorbing NIR photons at 800 nm. Halas et al. note that "In combining these two functions, it is important to note that the light intensities typically used for imaging are far below those used to induce photothermal effects" [98]. An array of further multifunctional nanoformulations, encompassing polymeric and metallic nanoparticles, liposomes, dendrimers, carbon nanotubes, C_{60} (buckyballs), and quantum dots may enable synergistic theranostics against cancer and myriad other diseases. However, although these approaches have great potential they must be properly vetted to ensure their safety in humans and to elucidate any indirect effects and long-term risks [99].

An alternative technique for inducing hyperthermia involves the use of pulsed ultrasound in combination with metallic nanoparticles or the initiation of microbubble cavitation events. Unfocused ultrasound may be utilized to eradicate tumors at superficial sites and can enhance the uptake of chemotherapeutic drugs with temperatures that range from 43°C to 50°C, and are capable of deep penetration at frequencies from 1 to 3 MHz [100–102]. Kislev described a hyperthermic tissue ablation method that utilized metallic nanoparticle clusters, which were initially heated by a NIR light source (λ 800–1300 nm). Each of the clustered aggregates (Ø20–Ø200 nm) were comprised of from 5–500 nanoparticles. When these entities were photonically induced to a state of surface plasmon resonance, microbubbles were created that further enhanced "the absorption of ultrasound radiation (0.5 and 7.5 MHz) to generate and propagate localized heat to inhibit the viability and propagation of cancer cells…" [92,102].

15.2.4 Prospective Nanomedical Precision Drug Delivery

Many techniques may be utilized for the hyperthermic release of drugs from, for instance, nanoparticle-infused polymeric matrices. Magnetic nanoparticles can be combined with biocompatible thermosensitive polymeric encasements (e.g., polyethylene glycol [PEG], poly (glycolide co-lactide) [PLGA], polylactic acid [PLA], PLA-PEG, poly(glycolic acid) [PGA], poly(ε-caprolactone) [PCL], and poly(methyl methacrylate) [PMMA]), where the melting temperature of the encasement is slightly below or equivalent to the maximum nanoparticle temperature (40°C–45°C), with the subsequent release of a drug payload. When heating is continued postrelease, the effect of the drug against diseased tissue is enhanced [103].

Nanoparticles can be endowed with stealth properties to enhance long circulation and evade macrophage uptake when they are coated with PEG or high-molecular-weight dextran, which act to reduce surface charge [104]. Other types of hydrophilic ligand carrier systems that are employed to functionalize the surfaces of nanoparticles so that they will specifically aggregate at tumor sites include certain polysaccharides, heparin and chitosan [105,106]. Specific polymer compositions can have a considerable impact on the performance and final fate of nanoparticle delivery systems in regard to the variable biological environments within a patient. The molecular weight, hydrophobicity, and hydrophilicity of the parent polymer/s, along with morphology and surface charge, are also important factors to consider. These characteristics play critical roles in the release of drug payloads at specific target sites, which are enabled by one of the following three methods:

1. Drug diffusion from hydrated particles
2. Degradation of polymer network through enzymatic action
3. Cleavage of the drug, subsequent to nanoparticle hydration

An extensive assortment of natural polymers (e.g., albumin, gelatin, chitosan, heparin) and synthetic polymers (e.g., poly(amino acids), poly(alkyl-cyano acrylates) [107], poly(esters), poly(orthoesters), poly(urethanes), and poly(acrylamides)) may be incorporated for enabling novel nanoparticle drug delivery strategies, as well as the targeted transport of DNA segments, oligonucleotides, proteins, and inorganic materials to address myriad disease states [108]. Extensive investigations of poly(lactic acid) (PLA), poly(lactic-glycolic acid) (PLGA), and chitosan have been prompted by their attributes of biocompatibility and biodegradability [109,110] (Refs. [104–109] from [110]).

Hollow nanoporous metallic nanoshells with various morphologies having tunable internal and external diameters (Figure 15.16) may be utilized to encapsulate and deliver drug molecules. When these structures are thermally activated by NIR laser, the thin boundary walls deform/contract and thereby squeeze out encapsulated drug payloads. This functionality may be facilitated by surface-resident nanopores, or should the walls be solid they may be randomly breached due to deformative heating effects.

Schwartzberg et al. synthesized hollow gold nanospheres using cobalt nanoparticles as seed materials that underwent sacrificial galvanic replacement reactions. Finely tuned surface plasmon band absorption of between 550 and 820 nm was obtained through precise control of cobalt nanoparticle dimensions (via the simultaneous modification of sodium borohydride and sodium citrate concentrations, reduction, and capping agents, respectively) and nanosphere wall thickness (through careful control of the addition of gold salts) [111]. Xia et al. synthesized gold nanocages (and nanocubes) through the sacrificial galvanic replacement of Ag with Au. Since the electrochemical potentials of Ag and Au are dissimilar, Ag surrenders its electrons as ions, which diffuse into the solution, whereas Au is deposited onto the exterior of the nanocage. The volume of chloroauric acid was carefully monitored during the reaction to produce Au nanocages that responded to wavelengths of 600–1200 nm [112].

Gene therapies involve the insertion of specific DNA or RNA fragments to downregulate or potentially negate the expression of particular disease-causing/perpetuating proteins.

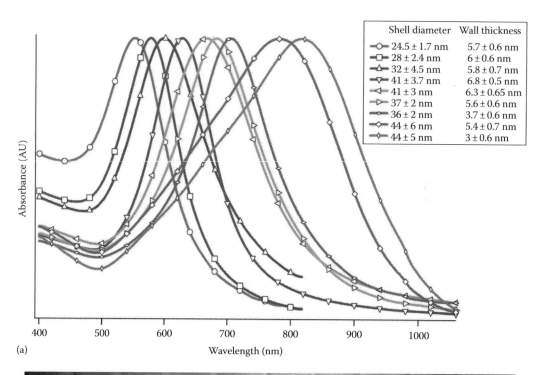

	Shell diameter	Wall thickness
○	24.5 ± 1.7 nm	5.7 ± 0.6 nm
□	28 ± 2.4 nm	6 ± 0.6 nm
△	32 ± 4.5 nm	5.8 ± 0.7 nm
▽	41 ± 3.7 nm	6.8 ± 0.5 nm
◁	41 ± 3 nm	6.3 ± 0.65 nm
▷	37 ± 2 nm	5.6 ± 0.6 nm
⬡	36 ± 2 nm	3.7 ± 0.6 nm
◇	44 ± 6 nm	5.4 ± 0.7 nm
◇	44 ± 5 nm	3 ± 0.6 nm

(a)

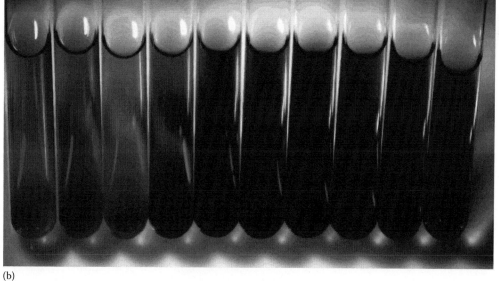

(b)

FIGURE 15.16

(a) Absorption spectra (via UV–Vis–NIR) of nine hollow gold nanoparticle samples with different diameters and wall thicknesses. (b) Color range of hollow gold nanoparticle samples with different diameters and wall thicknesses (vial on far left contains solid gold nanoparticles. (Reproduced from Schwartzberg, A.M. et al., *J. Phys. Chem. B* 110(40), 19935–19944. Copyright 2006. American Chemical Society. With permission.)

Halas et al. have proposed that gene therapies involving antisense ss-DNA and short interfering RNA (si-RNA) may be enabled through the use of gold nanoshells as efficient delivery vehicles. Short (15–30 bases) ss-DNA or si-RNA (19–21 bases) strands that are tethered to the surfaces of gold nanoshells have the capacity for being released at specific sites in vivo through plasmonic light triggering [98,113].

The precise delivery of small molecules into cell nuclei might be possible through the use of DNA duplex-decorated gold nanoshells, where the molecular cargo is intercalated within the minor helical grooves of the duplex [114]. This capacity was demonstrated when DAPI molecules (water-soluble fluorescent blue dye that binds reversibly with the minor groove of the DNA duplex) were initially incubated with Au nanoshell complexes, which were subsequently incubated with H1299 lung cancer cells to facilitate their uptake. When irradiated with an 800 nm continuous wave laser (equivalent to the peak resonant wavelength of the Au nanoshell complexes) at $1 W/cm^2$ for 5 min, the DNA duplex "dehybridizes and the ss-DNA and the DAPI molecules are released within the cells. Subsequent to release, the DAPI diffuses through the cytoplasm and into the cell nucleus, where it preferentially binds to and stains the nuclear DNA." Numerous species of molecules that may be additionally intercalated into the DNA duplex include steroids, antibiotics, and chemotherapeutic molecules, which impart great potential for this controlled intracellular delivery strategy [115].

The hydrophobic nature of the cell membrane typically prevents the entry of the majority of hydrophilic macromolecules, peptides, and proteins. Thus, only a small number of molecules that meet specific criteria as related to dimension, charge, and polarity have the capacity for directly traversing the membrane. Sawant and Torchilin described the use of cell-penetrating peptides (CPPs), specifically TATp ("derived from the transcriptional activator protein encoded by human immunodeficiency virus Type-I HIV-1"), to facilitate the delivery of drug molecules or drug-laden nanocarriers directly into the cell cytoplasm. Interestingly, a variety of therapeutic entities may be delivered that possess molecular weights considerably larger than the CPP itself.

CPPs have demonstrated the ability to traverse the cell membrane to deliver proteins, antibodies and SiRNA, liposomes, micelles, and nanoparticles. They state that "Both in vitro and in vivo studies have shown that by covalently linking TATp to nearly any drug class, including hydrophilic compounds and large protein molecules (MW >150 kDa) it was able to transduce the attached cargoes into cells of all organ types including the brain." When TATp was affixed to dextran-coated SPIONs (Ø41 nm), their uptake into cells was shown to be 100 times higher than nonmodified SPIONs [116,117].

Early investigations showed that when TATp was bound with β-galactosidase (hydrolase enzyme—120 kDa), it was capable of penetrating all tissues including the blood–brain barrier in mice [118]. The protein PTD-HA-Bcl-xL (Bcl-xL is a molecule that acts to prevent neuronal apoptosis) was also induced to cross the blood–brain barrier [119]. In another study, when TATp was conjugated with FITC (fluorescein isothiocyanate)-doped silica nanoparticle (FSNP) bioimaging agents, they were transported to the brain without disrupting the blood–brain barrier [116,120].

The representative nanomedical agents briefly surveyed earlier might likely be amenable for use in remote locations and in developing countries due to their diminutive physical footprint, high portability, presumed cost effectiveness and potent capacity for imaging, hyperthermia, and the precise delivery of therapeutics. What will be required in conjunction with these nanomedical capabilities nearer-term is the practical miniaturization and ruggedization of associated conventional imaging and hyperthermic activation technologies. In the future, as described for VCSN and GMSD, imaging capabilities will be integrated into nanomedical systems.

References

1. United Nations, Department of Economic and Social Affairs, Population Division (2013). http://www.geohive.com/earth/population_now.aspx (accessed July 01, 2013).
2. DeLong, J.P., Burger, O., and Hamilton, M.J., Current demographics suggest future energy supplies will be inadequate to slow human population growth. *PloS ONE* 5(10), e13206, 2010.
3. United Nations (2012) World Population Prospects, the 2012 Revision. http://esa.un.org/wpp/(accessed July 01, 2013).
4. Nair, G.M., Chairman of the Indian Space Research Organisation. India to launch satellite exclusively for telemedicine. Quoted in: *Agence-France Presse.* March 17, 2005 Available: http://servesrilanka.blogspot.com/2005/03/india-to-launch-satellite-exclusively.html. (accessed July 17, 2012).
5. Krishnakumar, A., Healing by wire. 2003 January 18–31 *Frontline.* Available: http://www.hinduonnet.com/thehindu/thscrip/print.pl?file=20030117007309400.htm&date=fl2001/&prd=fline& (accessed July 17, 2012).
6. Rajalakshmi, T.K., India confronts AIDS. 2004 December Multinational Monitor. Available: http://multinationalmonitor.org/mm2004/122004/front.html (accessed July 17, 2012).
7. Bagchi, S., Telemedicine in rural India. *PLoS Med* 3(3), e82, 2006.
8. Prathiba, V. and Rema, M., Teleophthalmology: A model for eye care delivery in rural and underserved areas of India. *Int J Family Med* 683267, 2011.
9. Baidoo, R., Toward a comprehensive healthcare system in Ghana. Master of Arts thesis, Center for International Studies of Ohio University, March 2009.
10. Rao, B. and Lombardi, A., 2nd. Telemedicine: Current status in developed and developing countries. *J Drugs Dermatol* 8(4), 371–375, 2009.
11. Darkwa, O., An exploratory survey of the applications of telemedicine in Ghana. *J Telemed Telecare* 6(3), 177–183, 2000.
12. American Telemedicine Association, 2013. http://www.americantelemed.org/ (accessed July, 01, 2013).
13. Burby, M.J., Global trends in telemedicine Cisco healthcare, *Asia Pacific*, 19 October, 2011. http://www.slideshare.net/ciscoanz/global-telemedicine-trends-final
14. Zajchuk, J.T. and Zajchuk, R., Strategy for medical readiness: Transition to the digital age. *Telemed J* 2(3), 179–186, 1996.
15. Anogianakis, G. and Maglavera, S., Medical emergency aid through telematics (MERMAID). *Stud Health Technol Inform* 29, 255–264, 1996.
16. Hannah, K.J., Ball, M.J., and Edwards, M.J.A., *Introduction to Nursing Informatics,* Springer Science + Business Media, Inc., New York, 2006.
17. Lorincz, K., Malan, D.J., Fulford-Jones, T.R.F., Nawoj, A., Clavel, A., Shnayder, V., Mainland, G., and Welsh, M., Sensor networks for emergency response: Challenges and opportunities. *IEEE Pervasive Comput* 4, 16–23, 2004.
18. Almudevar, A., Leibovici, A., and Tentler, A., Home monitoring using wearable radio frequency transmitters. *Artif Intell Med* 42, 109–120, 2008.
19. Li, M., Lou, W., and Ren, K., Data security and privacy in wireless body area networks. *IEEE Wireless Commun* 1, 51–58, 2010.
20. Malasri, K. and Wang, L., Design and implementation of a secure wireless mote-based medical sensor network. In *Proc 10th Int Conf Ubiquitous Computing,* Seoul, Korea, 21–24 September, 2008. http://netlab.cs.memphis.edu/papers/ubicomp08.pdf (accessed June 1, 2010).
21. Misic, J. and Misic, V.B., Implementation of security policy for clinical information systems over wireless sensor networks. *Ad Hoc Networks* 5, 134–144, 2007.
22. Malasri, K. and Wang, L., Securing wireless implantable devices for healthcare: Ideas and challenges. *IEEE Commun Mag* 7, 74–80, 2009.
23. Benini, L., Farella, E., and Guiducci, C., Wireless sensor networks: Enabling technology for ambient intelligence. *Microelectron J* 37, 1639–1649, 2006.

24. Jones, V.M., Mei, H., Broens, T., Widya, I., and Peuscher, J., Context aware body area networks for telemedicine. In *Proc 8th Pacific Rim Conf Advances in Multimedia Information Processing*, Hong Kong, China, 11–14 December, 2007. http://eprints.eemcs.utwente.nl/11640/01/1569055303.pdf (accessed June 1, 2010).

25. Lee, H.J., Lee, S.H., Ha, K.S., Jang, H.C., Chung, W.Y., Kim, J.Y., Chang, Y.S., and Yoo, D.H., Ubiquitous healthcare service using Zigbee and mobile phone for elderly patients. *Int J Med Inform* 78, 193–198, 2009.

26. Engin, M., Demirel, A., Engin, E.Z., and Fedakar, M., Recent developments and trends in biomedical sensors. *Measurement* 37, 173–188, 2005.

27. Valdastri, P., Rossi, S., Menciassi, A., Lionetti, V., Bernini, F., Recchia, F.A., and Dario, P., An implantable ZigBee ready telemetric platform for in vivo monitoring of physiological parameters. *Sensors Actuators A* 142, 369–378, 2008.

28. Gyselinckx, B., Penders, J., and Vullers, R., Potential and challenges of body area networks for cardiac monitoring. *J Electrocardiol* 40, 165–168, 2007.

29. Lai, C.C., Lee, R.G., Hsiao, C.C., Liu, H.S., and Chen, C.C., A HQoS-demand personalized home physiological monitoring system over a wireless multi-hop relay network for mobile home healthcare applications. *J Network Comp Appl* 6, 1229–1241, 2009.

30. Sneha, S. and Varshney, U., Enabling ubiquitous patient monitoring: Model, decision protocols, opportunities and challenges. *Decision Support Syst* 46, 606–619, 2009.

31. Bang, M. and Timpka, T., Ubiquitous computing to support co-located clinical teams: Using the semiotics of physical objects in system design. *Int J Med Inform* 765, 558–564, 2007.

32. Grgić, K., Zagar, D., and Križanović, V., Medical applications of wireless sensor networks—Current status and future directions. *Med Glas Ljek komore Zenicko-doboj kantona* 9(1), 23–31, 2012.

33. Trudel, M.C., Paré, G., Têtu, B., and Sicotte, C., The effects of a regional telepathology project: A study protocol. *BMC Health Serv Res* 12, 64, 2012.

34. Puppa, G., Senore, C., Sheahan, K., Vieth, M., Lugli, A., Zlobec, I., Pecori, S., Wang, L.M., Langner, C., Mitomi, H., Nakamura, T., Watanabe, M., Ueno, H., Chasle, J., Conley, S.A., Herlin, P., Lauwers, G.Y., and Risio, M., Diagnostic reproducibility of tumour budding in colorectal cancer: A multicentre, multinational study using virtual microscopy. *Histopathology*. 61(4), 562–575, 2012.

35. Costa, C. and Oliveira, J.L., Telecardiology through ubiquitous Internet services. *Int J Med Inform* 81(9), 612–21, 2012.

36. Cincotti, G., Spiekman, L., Wada, N., and Kitayama, K., Spectral coherent-state quantum cryptography. *Opt Lett* 33(21), 2461–2463, 2008.

37. Morris, T.J., Pajak, J., Havlik, F., Kenyon, J., and Calcagni, D., Battlefield Medical Information System-Tactical (BMIST): The application of mobile computing technologies to support health surveillance in the Department of Defense. *Telemed J E Health* 12(4), 409–416, 2006.

38. Irvine Sensors to Show Electronic "Dog Tag" at ATA Conference; Operational Demonstrations Set for April 17–20, 2005 in Denver http://www.thefreelibrary.com/Irvine+Sensors+to+Show+Electronic+'Dog+Tag'+at+ATA+Conference%3B...-a0131058871

39. The DARPA Virtual Soldier Project http://www.virtualsoldier.us/index.htm (accessed July 01, 2013).

40. Zurovac, D., Talisuna, A.O., and Snow, R.W., Mobile phone text messaging: Tool for malaria control in Africa. *PLoS Med* 9(2), e1001176, 2012.

41. International Telecommunication Union (2008), African telecommunication/ICT indicators 2008: At a crossroads. http://www.itu.int/ITU-D/ict/publications/africa/2008/index.html (accessed July 21, 2012).

42. International Telecommunication Union (2010), The world in 2010: ICT facts and figures. Available: http://www.itu.int/ITU-D/ict/material/FactsFigures2010.pdf (accessed July 21, 2012).

43. Rao, M., Mobile Africa Report 2011. Regional hubs of excellence and innovation. http://www.scribd.com/doc/53028350/Mobile-Africa-Report-2011-Regional-Hubs-of-Excellence-and-Innovation (accessed July 21, 2012).

44. Davis, R.G., Kamanga, A., Castillo-Salgado, C., Chime, N., Mharakurwa, S., and Shiff, C., Early detection of malaria foci for targeted interventions in endemic southern Zambia. *Malaria J* 10, 260, 2011.

45. Randrianasol, L., Raoelina, Y., Ratsitorahina, M., Ravolomanana, L., Andriamandimby, S., Heraud, J.M., Rakotomanana, F., Ramanjato, R., Randrianarivo-Solofoniaina, A.E., and Richard, V., Sentinel surveillance system for early outbreak detection in Madagascar. *BMC Public Health* 10, 31, 2010.

46. Barrington, J., Wereko-Brobby, O., Ward, P., Mwafongo, W., and Kungulwe, S., SMS for life: A pilot project to improve anti-malarial drug supply management in rural Tanzania using standard technology. *Malar J* 9, 298, 2010.

47. Bettex, M., In the World: Health care in the palm of a hand MIT-led student team develops mobile-device software to help improve health-care accessibility in remote regions. *MIT News Office*. September 27, 2010. http://web.mit.edu/newsoffice/2010/itw-sana-0927.html

48. Breslauer, D.N., Maamari, R.N., Switz, N.A., Lam, W.A., and Fletcher, D.A., Mobile phone based clinical microscopy for global health applications. *PLoS One* 4(7), e6320, 2009.

49. Anderson, K., Qiu, Y., Whittaker, A.R., and Lucas, M., Breath sounds, asthma, and the mobile phone. *Lancet* 358(9290), 1343–1344, 2001.

50. History of MRI innovations from 1969–1999, FONAR. http://fonar.com/innovations.htm (accessed November 4, 2012).

51. Dai, J., Opportunities and challenges of MRI in the developing world. *Proc. Int. Soc. Mag. Reson. Med.* 14, 2006. http://cds.ismrm.org/ismrm-2006/files/00002.pdf (accessed November 4, 2012).

52. Manufacturing in a two-speed world, Knowledge@Wharton, 2011. http://knowledge.wharton. upenn.edu/article.cfm?articleid=2682 (accessed November 4, 2012).

53. General Electric Company, A $6 billion commitment to healthcare. Better health for more people everywhere, 2012. http://www.gehealthcare.com/euen/healthymagination/healthymagination.html (accessed November 4, 2012).

54. General Electric Company, Optima MR360 1.5T (available in 2012). http://www.gehealthcare. com/euen/mri/products/optima_mr360/index.html (accessed November 4, 2012).

55. Bruker, Icon 1 Tesla desktop MRI scanner (available in 2012). http://www.bruker-biospin. com/icon-overview.html (accessed November 4, 2012).

56. Sound Imaging, Mobile MRI Units: GE Mobile LX units (available since 1995). http://www. soundimaging.com/mobile-mri-unit.asp (accessed November 4, 2012).

57. Monee, I.L., Advanced mobility delivers first mobile Philips Ingenia MRI to Vancouver Island health authority. PRWEB, October 10, 2012 (1.5 and 3T units) http://www.prweb.com/ releases/2012/10/prweb9991772.htm (accessed November 4, 2012).

58. Shiva Medicare, Mobile MRI Unit (MrJ 0.22T), 2012. www.shivamed.com (accessed November 4, 2012).

59. Magnevu 1000 scanner 0.20T (FDA approval 1998). http://www.mr-tip.com/serv1. php?type=db1&gid=1345 (accessed November 4, 2012); Needell, S.D., Value of 3D T1W & STIR MRI sequences in diagnosing erosions in rheumatoid arthritis. http://www.bocaradiology. com/ra/3D/ (accessed November 4, 2012).

60. Esaote, O-Scan dedicated MRI system, 2012. http://www.esaote.co.uk/modules/core/page. asp?p=MRI (accessed November 4, 2012).

61. PoleStar Surgical MRI System (launched 2010). http://www.medtronic.com/for-healthcare-professionals/products-therapies/spinal-orthopedics/surgical-navigation-imaging/polestar-surgical-mri-system/systems-software-instruments/index.htm#tab4 (accessed November 4, 2012).

62. Aspect Imaging, Aspect Imaging's M2™ compact high-performance MRI imaging system selected as a "Top 10 Innovation" in life science by *The Scientist*, 2012. http://www. aspectimaging.com/press-releases/m2-selected-as-a-top-10-innovation-in-life-science/ (accessed November 4, 2012).

63. Magritek, Portable NMR systems (available since 2004). http://magritek.com/products (accessed November 4, 2012).

64. Callaghan, P.T., Eccles C.D., and Seymour. J.D., An Earth's field NMR apparatus suitable for pulsed gradient spin echo measurements of self-diffusion under Antarctic conditions. *Rev Sci Instr* 68(11), 4263–4270, 1997.
65. Eidmann, G., Savelsberg, R., Blümler, P., and Blümich, B., The NMR MOUSE: A mobile universal surface explorer. *J Magn Reson A* 122(1), 104–109, 1996.
66. Savukov, I.M., Seltzer, S.J., Romalis, M.V., and Sauer, K.L., Tunable atomic magnetometer for detection of radio-frequency magnetic fields. *Phys Rev Lett* 95(6), 063004, 2005.
67. Shah, V., Knappe, S., Schwindt, P.D.D., and Kitching, J., Subpicotesla atomic magnetometry with a microfabricated vapour cell. *Nat Photonics* 1(11), 649–652, 2007.
68. Blümich, B., The incredible shrinking scanner: MRI-like machine becomes portable. *Scientific American* 68, 2008.
69. Meriles, C.A., Sakellariou, D., Trabesinger, A.H., Demas, V., and Pines, A., Zero-to low-field MRI with averaging of concomitant gradient fields. *Proc Natl Acad Sci USA* 102(6), 1840–1842, 2005.
70. Pines Lab, Flow Imaging MRI technology, 2012. http://waugh.cchem.berkeley.edu/research/flow_imaging.php (accessed November 4, 2012).
71. Antarctic NMR, University of Victoria, 1994–2009. http://www.victoria.ac.nz/scps/research/research-groups/magnetic-resonance/antarctic-nmr (accessed November 4, 2012).
72. Segway Robotics (robotic vehicles with potential to carry MRI over difficult terrain). http://rmp.segway.com/tag/segway-robotics/ (accessed November 4, 2012).
73. Martin Jetpack (potential to carry future lightweight MRI systems: see commercial applications). http://martinjetpack.com/video-gallery.aspx (accessed November 4, 2012).
74. Shi, Y., Superparamagnetic nanoparticles for magnetic resonance imaging (MRI) diagnosis. Master of Engineering Science Thesis, 2006. http://digital.library.adelaide.edu.au/dspace/bitstream/2440/37879/1/02whole.pdf
75. TimWit blog, A little review, March 19, 2008 http://timwit.wordpress.com/2008/03/19/a-little-review (accessed November 8, 2012).
76. Marescaux, J., Leroy, J., Gagner, M., Rubino, F., Mutter, D., Vix, M., Butner, S.E., Smith, M.K., Transatlantic robot-assisted telesurgery. *Nature* 413(6854), 379–380, 2001.
77. Graham-Rowe, D., Scrubbing up for robotic surgery in space. *New Scientist* October 11, 2004. http://www.newscientist.com/article/dn6512-scrubbing-up-for-robotic-surgery-in-space.html (accessed July 22, 2012).
78. Anvari, M., Telesurgery: Remote knowledge translation in clinical surgery. *World J Surg* 31(8), 1545–1550, 2007.
79. Olson, P., Pfeffer, L., and Fuhrman, L., Boskone 43, Going to a higher domain: Expanding Internet connectivity beyond Earth. http://people.delphiforums.com/peabo/interplanetary.html (accessed July 22, 2012).
80. Bornhoft, J.M., Strabala, K.W., Wortman, T.D., Lehman, A.C., Oleynikov, D., and Farritor, S.M., Stereoscopic visualization and haptic technology used to create a virtual environment for remote surgery—biomed 2011. *Biomed Sci Instrum* 47, 76–81, 2011.
81. Satava, R., Looking for the game changer. http://www.businessinnovationfactory.com/bif-6/storytellers/richard-satava (accessed July 23, 2012).
82. Garcia, P., Rosen, J., Kapoor, C., Noakes, M., Elbert, G., Treat, M., Ganous, T., Hanson, M., Manak, J., Hasser, C., Rohler, D., and Satava, R., Trauma Pod: A semi-automated telerobotic surgical system. *Int J Med Robot* 5(2), 136–146, 2009.
83. Lum, M.J., Rosen, J., King, H., Friedman, D.C., Donlin, G., and Sankaranarayanan, G. et al., Telesurgery via unmanned aerial vehicle (UAV) with a field deployable surgical robot. *Stud Health Technol Inform* 125, 313–315, 2007.
84. LS-1, Integrated Medical Systems, Inc. http://www.lstat.com/showcase/overview.html (accessed July, 23, 2012).
85. Shiferaw, F. and Zolfo, M., The role of information communication technology (ICT) towards universal health coverage: The first steps of a telemedicine project in Ethiopia. *Glob Health Action* 5, 1–8, 2012.

86. Prathiba, V. and Rema, M., Teleophthalmology: A model for eye care delivery in rural and underserved areas of India. *Int J Family Med* 2011, 683267, 2011.

87. Sattar, K., A sustainable model for use of ICTs in rural Pakistan. *Int J Edu Devel Inform Commun Technol (IJEDICT)* 3(2), 116–124, 2007.

88. Wróbel-Kwiatkowska, M., Czemplik, M., Kulma, A., Zuk, M., Kaczmar, J., Dymińska, L., Hanuza, J., Ptak, M., and Szopa, J., New biocomposites based on bioplastic flax fibres and biodegradable polymers. *Biotechnol Prog* 28(5), 1336–46, 2012.

89. Pöselt, E., Schmidtke, C., Fischer, S., Peldschus, K., Salamon, J., Kloust, H., Tran, H., Pietsch, A., Heine, M., Adam, G., Schumacher, U., Wagener, C., Förster, S., and Weller, H., Tailor-made quantum dot and iron oxide based contrast agents for in vitro and in vivo tumor imaging. *ACS Nano* 6(4), 3346–3355, 2012.

90. Cao, L., Yang, S.T., Wang, X., Luo, P.G., Liu, J.H., Sahu, S., Liu, Y., and Sun, Y.P., Competitive performance of carbon "quantum" dots in optical bioimaging. *Theranostics* 2(3), 295–301, 2012.

91. Sun, Y.P., Zhou, B., Lin, Y., Wang, W., Fernando, K.A., and Pathak, P. et al., Quantum-sized carbon dots for bright and colorful photoluminescence. *J Am Chem Soc* 128(24), 7756–7757, 2006.

92. Boehm, F. and Chen, A., Medical applications of hyperthermia based on magnetic nanoparticles, *Recent Patents on Biomed Eng* 2, 110–120, 2009.

93. Hong, Z., Nanometer targeted drug for magneto-thermotherapy of malignant tumors—EPO Patent- EP1952825, 2006.

94. Rovers, S.A., Hoogenboom, R., Kemmere, M.F., and Keurentjes, J.T.F., Relaxation processes of superparamagnetic iron oxide nanoparticles in liquid and incorporated in poly(methyl methacrylate). *J Phys Chem C* 112(40), 15643–15646, 2008.

95. Zahn, M. and Adalsteinsson, E., Systems and methods for tuning properties of nanoparticles, WO2007035871, 2007.

96. Mohammad, F., Balaji, G., Weber, A., Uppu, R.M., and Kumar, C.S., Influence of gold nanoshell on hyperthermia of super paramagnetic iron oxide nanoparticles (SPIONs). *J Phys Chem C Nanomater Interf* 1(20), 3141–3146, 2010.

97. Loo, C., Lin, A., Hirsch, L.R., Lee, M.H., Barton, J., Halas, N.J., West, J.L., and Drezek, R., Nanoshell-enabled photonics-based imaging and therapy of cancer. *Technol Cancer Res Treat* 3, 33–40, 2004.

98. Bardhan, R., Lal, S., Joshi, A., and Halas, N.J., Theranostic nanoshells: From probe design to imaging and treatment of cancer. *Acc Chem Res* 44(10), 936–946, 2011.

99. Fernandez-Fernandez, A., Manchanda, R., and McGoron, A.J., Theranostic applications of nanomaterials in cancer: Drug delivery, image-guided therapy, and multifunctional platforms. *Appl Biochem Biotechnol* 165(7–8), 1628–1651, 2011.

100. Corry, P.M., Barlogie, B., Tilchen, E.J., and Armour, E.P., Ultrasound induced hyperthermia for the treatment of human superficial tumors. *Int J Radiat Oncol Biol Phys* 8(7), 1225–1229, 1982.

101. Liu, Y., Cho, C.W., Yan, X., Henthorn, T.K., Lillehei, K.O., Cobb, W.N., and Ng, K.Y., Ultrasound induced hyperthermia increases cellular uptake and cytotoxicity of P-glycoprotein substrates in multi-drug resistant cells. *Pharm Res* 18(9), 1255–1261, 2001.

102. Kislev, H., Nanoparticle mediated ultrasound therapy and diagnostic imaging. US20080045865, 2008.

103. Chang, W.H., Chao-hung, K., Lin, C., and Wang, S., Thermosensitive nanostructure for hyperthermia treatment. US20070154397, 2007.

104. Avgoustakis, K., Pegylated poly(lactide) and poly(lactide-co-glycolide) nanoparticles: Preparation, properties and possible applications in drug delivery. *Curr Drug Deliv* 1(4), 321–333, 2004.

105. Fahmy, T.M. and Fong, P.M., Goyal, A., Saltzman, W.M., Targeted nanoparticles for drug delivery, *Mater Today (Nano Today)* 8, 18–26, 2005.

106. Chung, Y.I., Kim, J.C., Kim, Y.H., Tae, G., Lee, S.Y., Kim, K., and Kwon, I.C., The effect of surface functionalization of PLGA nanoparticles by heparin- or chitosan-conjugated Pluronic on tumor targeting. *J Control Release* 143(3), 374–382, 2010.

107. Nicolas, J. and Couvreur, P., Synthesis of poly(alkyl cyanoacrylate)-based colloidal nanomedicines. *Wiley Interdiscip Rev Nanomed Nanobiotechnol* 1(1), 111–127, 2009.

108. Kumari, A., Yadav, S.K., and Yadav, S.C., Biodegradable polymeric nanoparticles based drug delivery systems. *Colloids Surf B Biointerf* 75(1), 1–18, 2010.
109. Nagpal, K., Singh, S.K., and Mishra, D.N., Chitosan nanoparticles: a promising system in novel drug delivery. *Chem Pharm Bull (Tokyo)* 58(11), 1423–1430, 2010.
110. Young, J.K., Figueroa, E.R., and Drezek, R.A., Tunable nanostructures as photothermal theranostic agents. *Ann Biomed Eng* 40(2), 438–459, 2012.
111. Schwartzberg, A.M., Olson, T.Y., Talley, C.E., and Zhang, J.Z., Synthesis, characterization, and tunable optical properties of hollow gold nanospheres. *J Phys Chem B* 110(40), 19935–19944, 2006.
112. Sun, Y. and Xia. Y., Mechanistic study on the replacement reaction between silver nanostructures and chloroauric acid in aqueous medium. *J Am Chem Soc* 126, 3892–3901, 2004.
113. Barhoumi, A., Huschka, R., Bardhan, R., Knight, M.W., and Halas, N.J., Light-induced release of DNA from plasmon-resonant nanoparticles: Towards light-controlled gene therapy. *Chem Phys Lett* 482, 171–179, 2009.
114. Neto, B.A.D. and Lapis, A.A.M., Recent developments in the chemistry of deoxyribonucleic acid (DNA) intercalators: Principles, design, synthesis, applications and trends. *Molecules* 14, 1725–1746, 2009.
115. Huschka, R., Neumann, O., Barhoumi, A., and Halas, N.J., Visualizing light-triggered release of molecules inside living cells. *Nano Lett* 10(10), 4117–4122, 2010.
116. Sawant, R. and Torchilin, V., Intracellular delivery of nanoparticles with CPPs. *Methods Mol Biol* 683, 431–451, 2011.
117. Josephson, L., Tung, C.H., Moore, A., and Weissleder, R., High-efficiency intracellular magnetic labeling with novel superparamagnetic-Tat peptide conjugates. *Bioconjug Chem* 10(2), 186–191, 1999.
118. Schwarze, S.R., Ho, A., Vocero-Akbani, A., and Dowdy, S.F., In vivo protein transduction: Delivery of a biologically active protein into the mouse. *Science* 285(5433), 1569–1572, 1999.
119. Cao, G., Pei, W., Ge, H., Liang, Q., Luo, Y., Sharp, F.R., Lu, A., Ran, R., Graham, S.H., and Chen, J., In vivo delivery of a Bcl-xL fusion protein containing the TAT protein transduction domain protects against ischemic brain injury and neuronal apoptosis. *J Neurosci* 22(13), 5423–5431, 2002.
120. Stroh, M., Zimmer, J.P., Duda, D.G., Levchenko, T.S., Cohen, K.S., Brown, E.B., Scadden, D.T., Torchilin, V.P., Bawendi, M.G., Fukumura, D., and Jain, R.K., Quantum dots spectrally distinguish multiple species within the tumor milieu in vivo. *Nat Med* 11(6), 678–682, 2005.

16

Nanomedical Device and Systems Design in Space Applications

Frank J. Boehm

CONTENTS

16.1 Nanomedicine in Space Applications

This chapter will explore how conceptual future nanomedicine might be practiced in a range of space applications, constituting what we might consider to be the ultimate in remoteness from the perspective of our primarily Earth-bound human experience. Within the realms of aerospace and space travel, conjunctive with the further physical size reductions and yet increased capabilities of nanoelectronics blended with artificial intelligence (AI), nanomedicine may be envisaged as enabling a wide variety of advanced diagnostic and therapeutic capabilities. Such medical innovations may be manifest as core components of advanced extravehicular space suits. Space-suit-integrated nanomedical capabilities may impart a number of advantages insofar as the continuous real-time monitoring of astronaut health, and if required, the capacity for virtually instantaneous in situ diagnostics, administration of therapeutics, or in cases of serious or accidental circumstances, and emergency interventions. These capacities would serve to ensure optimal astronaut health and provide for the rapid resolution of practically any health-related issue that may arise at any time when astronauts don their space suits, during space walks, or further into the future, to support potentially extended exploratory terrestrial missions on the Moon and Mars.

Integrated nanomedical suites onboard spacecraft will also impart benefits in that envisioned nanomedical devices, systems, and associated infrastructures will represent the ultimate in extreme compactness and lightness (definite boons for space travel), yet be highly sophisticated, dynamic, and medically powerful with practical utility to rapidly and effectively address virtually any conceivable medical issue or emergency. Indeed, nanomedical technologies may serve as a perfect fit for space travel as they will possess many of the attributes that align well with this noble and adventurous enterprise, albeit, one that is sometimes fraught with extreme risk. The utilization of nanomedical technologies in the support of future Moon and Mars colonies will have positives as well, posing a minimal burden on the tight spatial constraints that will most likely accompany early colonies, while offering an extensive range of highly specific diagnostics and therapeutics (coupled with powerful evolutionary and deductive AI in instances where unknown Lunar or Martian elements are suspected as causative agents in a particular sickness or disease).

Although the nanomedical capabilities of extravehicular space suits will initially operate from strategically positioned nodes via dermal interfacing membranes, or from within the "second skins" wherein they reside, ultimately they might be designed to imperceptibly meld within the physical bodies of the astronauts themselves. An elegant array of circulating nanodevices and/or static subdermally self-implanting nanomedical reservoirs that are resident at the periphery of astronauts' bodies will for the most part sustain a "standby" status. However, they will instantaneously implement appropriate countermeasures in response to any detected form of insult to their accommodating "host." In essence, they would cumulatively operate to serve as an enhanced, highly sensitive "damage immunity" system "on steroids."

16.2 Current Challenges of Space Medicine

Space medicine aims to address specific health risks that are associated with space travel, ranging from brief Earth orbital flight (several days) to long-duration space residency on the International Space Station (ISS) (~6 months), and eventually deep space exploration (a two-way mission to Mars would have a duration of 3 years). In 1992, NASA initiated a protocol (Longitudinal Study of Astronaut Health, LSAH) to establish whether, and what particular astronaut medical conditions and health risks might be associated with the "unique occupational exposures encountered by astronauts." The database is inclusive of the Russian cosmonaut experience, as well as analogous data from other harsh-to-human environments, encompassing submarine fleet crew members, Antarctic and mountaineering expeditions [1]. The medical conditions observed in astronauts during spaceflight have and will inevitably be variable, ranging from nonemergency superficial conditions to those that are increasingly complex and severe, to critical emergencies (Tables 16.1 and 16.2) [2].

A NASA-sponsored Virtual Collaborative Clinic was held in 1999 to demonstrate the viability of utilizing broad bandwidth ground fiber networks, as well as satellite communications and multicasting to link five different sites (some remote and others located in urban centers) for clinical discussion, diagnosis, and the transfer of patient-specific data to experts [3]. This exercise constituted an initial step toward the aim of establishing "telecommunication linkages and virtual reality technology for space applications." A small "immersive workbench" was also demonstrated, which would facilitate a virtual environment that included haptic feedback. It was surmised that in conjunction

TABLE 16.1

List of U.S. Astronaut Medical Issues during the Space Shuttle Program, STS-1–STS-89, April 1981 to January 1998

Medical Event or System by (ICD-9) Category	Number	Percentage of Total
Space adaptation syndrome	788	42.2
Nervous system and sense organs	318	17.0
Digestive system	163	8.7
Skin and subcutaneous tissue	151	8.1
Injuries or trauma	141	7.6
Musculoskeletal system and connective tissue	132	7.1
Respiratory system	83	4.4
Behavioral signs and symptoms	34	1.8
Infectious diseases	26	1.4
Genitourinary system	23	1.2
Circulatory system	6	0.3
Endocrine, nutritional, metabolic, and immunity disorders	2	0.1

Source: ICD-9, *International Classification of Diseases*, 9th edn. Adapted from Risin, D., *Human Health and Performance Risks of Space Exploration Missions: Evidence Reviewed by the NASA Human Research Program.* Chapter 8, pp. 242, 2009. http://humanresearchroadmap.nasa.gov/evidence/reports/ExMC.pdf (accessed July 28, 2012).

TABLE 16.2

Medical Conditions and Recurrences among
International Astronauts on MIR between
March 14, 1995 and June 12, 1998

Medical Condition	Instances
Superficial injury	43
Arrhythmia	32
Musculoskeletal	29
Headache	17
Sleeplessness	13
Fatigue	17
Contact dermatitis	5
Surface burn	5
Conjunctivitis	4
Acute respiratory infection	3
Asthenia	3
Ocular foreign body	3
Globe contusion	2
Dental	2
Constipation	1

Source: Adapted from Risin, D., *Human Health and Performance Risks of Space Exploration Missions: Evidence Reviewed by the NASA Human Research Program.* Chapter 8, pp. 242, 2009. http://humanresearchroadmap.nasa.gov/evidence/reports/ExMC.pdf (accessed July 28, 2012).

with 3D ultrasound imaging, these technologies might "provide nearly instantaneous stereo images of an astronaut's heart daily on the spacecraft, to keep track of changes in heart muscle during flight." Additional microsensors (embedded within clothing or integrated into handheld devices) might be utilized to monitor heart functionality and to quantify parameters such as blood flow, oxygen levels, and electrolytes. In the event of serious medical conditions that are beyond the scope of experience of the astronauts, "telecommunications and a virtual environment can augment astronaut responses to the emergency" and "advice can be sought from Earth even though lag-time in communications would be considerable." The long-range goal of NASA's efforts in CyberMedicine would be to "fulfill humankind's destiny to reach and populate distant sites in the universe, and to do so safely" [4].

Ball and Evans [5] revealed that some of the primary space travel related hazards, which had been identified to date included radiation exposure, loss of bone calcium/density/mass and muscle mass, issues associated with changes in the neurovestibular system as relates to space adaptation syndrome (space motion sickness) and behavioral adaptation to prolonged confined living quarters. The committee on creating a vision for space medicine during travel beyond Earth orbit was formed by the Institute of Medicine in 2001 to make "recommendations regarding the infrastructure for a health system in space, defining the principles that should guide such a system to provide an appropriate standard of care for astronauts, and identifying the nature of clinical and health services research that will be required."

The core findings of the committee were as follows:

1. "Not enough is yet known about the risks to humans of long-duration missions, such as to Mars, or about what can effectively mitigate those risks to enable humans to travel and work safely in the environment of deep space."

2. "Everything reasonable should be done to gain the necessary information before humans are sent on missions of space exploration" [5].

16.2.1 Ophthalmic and Cellular Anomalies

Additional areas of concern as relates to the health of astronauts in long-duration space-flight have recently (2011–2012) been brought to light, which may impact and limit prospective human space exploration. Mader et al. undertook the study of seven astronauts who noted ophthalmic anomalies subsequent to long-duration (6-month) space missions to the ISS, and asked an additional 300 astronauts to complete a questionnaire as related to perceived in-flight vision changes. Ophthalmic findings for the seven ISS astronauts included: disk edema (in five), globe flattening (in five), choroidal folds (in five), cotton wool spots (in three), nerve fiber layer thickening (in six), decreased near-vision (in six). Five of the seven who noted near-vision problems showed a hyperopic shift and globe flattening. Also noted were optic nerve sheath distension and tortuous optic nerves. As to the postflight questionnaires, ~29% and 60% of the 300 astronauts who were engaged on short- and long-duration missions, respectively, reported degradation in both near and distant vision; with some respondents, these conditions persisted for years postflight. The researchers summarized that "although a definitive etiology is unknown, we hypothesize that venous congestion in the brain and/or eye, brought about by cephalad fluid shifts and perhaps exacerbated by choroidal volume changes, may be a unifying pathologic mechanism to explain our findings." They concluded by noting: "the optic nerve and ocular changes we describe may result from cephalad fluid shifts brought about by prolonged microgravity exposure. The findings we report may represent parts of a spectrum of ocular and cerebral responses to extended microgravity exposure" [6].

Further, Kramer et al. reported abnormalities in the pituitary gland and its connection to the brain in 3 out of 27 astronauts who were previously exposed to microgravity. As they explain it, there was "moderate concavity of the pituitary dome with posterior stalk deviation in three (11%) without additional intracranial abnormalities." Also observed in 26 of the 27 astronauts was an increase in the diameter of the optic nerve in conjunction with optic nerve sheath kinking, posterior globe flattening (in seven), and optic nerve protrusion (in four). The conclusion reached here was: "Exposure to microgravity can result in a spectrum of intraorbital and intracranial findings similar to those in idiopathic intracranial hypertension" [7].

Microgravity also has effects on the structures and motility of human mechanosensitive cells such as osteocytes, chondrocytes, and fibroblasts. Clinorotation (induced/simulated weightlessness) has been shown to initiate the remodeling of the cytoskeleton in cultured endothelial cells (ECs), whereas longer-term gravity modification can alter surface adhesion molecule (e.g., ICAM-1, E-selectin, VCAM-1) expression in cultured ECs. In experiments conducted via the Russian onboard facilities of the ISS, it was found that immune (natural killer) cells retained their capacity to distinguish, contact, and eliminate oncogenic cells in vitro. Overall, the data obtained from simulated and actual microgravity showed that "cell-cell interactions are not compromised, thus preserving critical physiological functions of immune and endothelial cells" in spite of effects on the cytoskeleton,

TABLE 16.3

Summation of Systemic Effects of Microgravity

System	Microgravity Impact
Musculoskeletal system	Decreased bone formation
	Increased bone resorption
	Decreased bone mass
	Decreased muscle mass
	Decreased functional capacity
	Increased muscle fatigue
	Postflight muscle necrosis
Cardiovascular system	Reduced heart rate
	Reduced diastolic pressure
	Cardiac dysrhythmias
	Headward fluid redistribution
	Decreased plasma volume
	Postflight hypovolemia
	Postflight postural hypotension
Sensory motor system	Deconditioning of posture and gait control
	Deconditioning of motion sensors
	Deconditioning of somatosensory system
	Altered perception of orientation
	Loss of balance
Immune system	Decreased number of T lymphocytes
	Decreased response of T lymphocytes to potent activator
	Reduced cytotoxic activity of natural killer cells
	Alterations in cytokine/chemokine activity
Would healing	Impaired matrix formation
	Impaired proliferation and migration of cells into wound
	Reduced wound collagen content
	Impaired revascularization
	Impaired keratinocyte migration

Source: Reconfigured from Blaber, E. et al., *Astrobiology* 10(5), 463, 2010. With permission.

cell motility, and expression of adhesion molecules [8]. The systemic effects of microgravity (known to date) are summarized in Table 16.3 [9].

16.2.2 Radiation Exposure: Galactic Cosmic Rays

Cosmic ray energy is typically determined in units of either mega-electron volts (MeV) or giga-electron volts (GeV). A single electron volt refers to the energy that is acquired via the acceleration of an electron through a potential difference of 1 V. Galactic cosmic rays possess energies of from 100 MeV (at proton velocity at 43% of the speed of light) to 10 GeV (at proton velocity at 99.6% of the speed of light). The most extreme cosmic ray energy that has been quantified to date was 10^{20} eV. The composition of cosmic rays spans practically all elements of the periodic table, consisting of 89% hydrogen (proton) nuclei and 10% helium, with ~1% heavier elements (e.g., oxygen, carbon, silicon, iron, and magnesium) in equivalent proportions to the solar system, and ~1% free electrons [10].

Since the initial discovery of galactic cosmic rays by Victor Hess in 1912 [11], there has been concern as to the risks that might be posed to critical biophysical entities, such as the constituents of the central nervous system (CNS) (e.g., neurons, neurotransmitters) when they are traversed by ionizing cosmic ray (HZE) nuclei [12]. The light flash phenomenon of single HZE nuclei traversals of the retina, as foreseen by Tobias in 1952 [13], was later confirmed by Apollo astronauts in 1970 and 1973 [14]. Single high-energy HZE nuclei were found to have the ability to generate a column of seriously damaged or inactivated cells, "microlesions," in the path of their trajectories through biological tissues, as well as possible impacts on neurogenesis. Both of these factors have increased concerns of potentially significant consequences for the CNS of astronauts engaged in space travel [15]. Microlesions in individual cells and hair follicles have also been reported, and there is some proof for isolated secondary electron activity. Damage to the entire organism due to the subtle, albeit cumulative, effects of several hundred microlesions may be contingent on the specific character of the insult to critical cells and tissues. It is conceivable that cancer may be initiated in instances where several cells are destroyed in a linear trajectory and adjacent cells along the path are mutated, presumably via direct hits on/damage to nuclear DNA, as a consequence [16]. Todd has calculated that if "a microlesion is taken as due to a HZE particle track 10 cell diameters long with LET (linear energy transfer) >200 KeV/μm in its core and >25 rad dose in its penumbra at a distance of 10 μm, then the microlesion dose rate in geostationary orbit, for example, is about 9000 microlesions per cm^3 of tissue per month" [17].

Curtis et al. endeavored to calculate HZE particle hit frequencies on vital elements of the CNS, including the macula, and an interior brain point (typical of the genu, thalamus, hippocampus, and nucleus basalis of Meynert) that would be encountered on a mission to Mars at full cosmic ray intensity (during solar minimum). Among other conclusions relating to the spatial distribution and orientation of critical CNS cells (based on the 1977 spectrum of cosmic rays), the investigators calculate that

1. "for a three year mission to Mars at solar minimum... 2% or 13% of the 'critical sites' of cells in the CNS would be directly hit at least once by iron ions, depending on whether 60 μm^2 or 471 μm^2 is assumed as the critical cross sectional area..."
2. "...roughly 6 million out of some 43 million hippocampal cells and 55 thousand out of 1.8 million thalamus cell nuclei would be directly hit by iron ions at least once on such a mission for space travelers inside a simple pressure vessel."
3. "...roughly 20 million out of 43 million hippocampal cells and 230 thousand out of 1.8 million thalamus cell nuclei would be directly hit by one or more particles with z > or = 15 on such a mission" [18].

These calculations do not take into account the peripheral cell impacts, initiated by delta rays (energetic electrons), which are generated through the trajectory of HZE nuclei [19] or "correlated cell damage." Together, these tangential factors can elevate the possible number of damaged cells —approximately two- to threefold from those calculated for single HZE tracks, giving rise to the "possibility of heterogeneously damaged regions," and it is stressed that the "importance of such additional damage is poorly understood" [20–22] (Refs. [15,19–21] from [22]).

Although incremental progress is being made in this area, there is a considerable deficit in data, as well as a means to accurately extrapolate the conditions of deep space and the random manner by which cosmic rays may impact the physiology of astronauts. It is safe to say that the extent of detrimental, microlesion-initiated (reversible or irreversible) biological effects on the overall health and performance, and psychological and cognitive functions of astronauts are not yet close to being quantified and established. It is quite clear that fundamentally robust cosmic ray shielding strategies must be developed for the protection of astronauts who are engaged in both Earth orbital and deep space missions. Once such absorbent or reflective shielding becomes available, at this juncture most likely through advances in nanotechnology and nanomaterials, it will likely be generously integrated into space suits, spacecraft, and within the dwellings of Moon and Mars habitats.

16.2.3 Loss of Bone Density and Mass

Other significant areas of concern to be addressed if astronauts are to safely engage in long-haul space missions in optimally healthy condition include the negation of loss of bone density and mass and muscle atrophy. In the terrestrial environment of Earth, the bones of humans and other vertebrates are in a continuous state of flux as they are constantly being replenished and remodeled as a result of dynamic synergies between osteoblasts (bone-forming cells) and osteoclasts (bone-resorbing cells). In healthy human adults at 1 g, this bone mineral balance (BMB) is ~0, as there is equilibrium between bone formation and resorption. This balance however may be disrupted by the onset of diseases such as osteoporosis, multiple myeloma, and metastatic cancers, which can lead to serious debilitation or fatality. The capacity for precisely quantifying BMB would be of significant benefit for astronauts on space missions [23].

Morgan et al. postulate that any alterations in BMB are likely to be sensitively represented by changes in the concentrations (in blood, urine, and soft tissues) of a number of naturally occurring calcium (Ca) isotopes (^{40}Ca, ^{42}Ca, ^{43}Ca, ^{44}Ca, ^{46}Ca, and ^{48}Ca) [23–26]. Further, variations in the concentrations of Ca isotopes should align directly with bone metabolism and indirectly by way of Ca excretion via the kidneys [23]. The researchers deducted that the average human skeleton contains ~1000 ± 100 g Ca, based on an assumed average skeletal mineral mass of 3000 g and bone mineral Ca content of 32.2% [23,27,28]. A skeletal remodeling rate of 500 ± 100 mg Ca/d was determined from one study by Smith et al., as was an estimated rate of new bone formation, for both men and women volunteers, of 190–635 mg Ca/d [29]. A later study by Smith et al. approximated the bone formation rate of 16 astronauts on the MIR space station at 490 ± 153 mg Ca/d prior to spaceflight and 434 ± 194 mg Ca/d during spaceflight [30].

Since it is known that bone loss is induced by bed rest due to skeletal unloading, it is utilized as an analog to model the impacts of spaceflight on the metabolism of human bone. A study conducted by Morgan et al. was undertaken to assess Ca isotope variations in 12 individuals during and following a 30-day bed rest trial. The results indicated that the median bone mass loss from day 7 to day 30 of bed rest was 0.25% ± 0.07%, which correlated to ~109 mg Ca/d. This value was extrapolated to a bone loss of 1.0% ±0.3% of total skeletal mass over a 90 day period. The researchers conclude that "In the future, the Ca isotope technique may be useful in clinical settings to allow close monitoring of subjects at risk for bone loss and safe, rapid assessment of individual subjects' response to treatment" [23].

It was observed by Bloomfield that the rate of bone loss associated with extended exposure to microgravity is almost double that seen during bed rest at 1 g, which indicates that factors unique to the space environment intensify the effects of a nonweight bearing condition [31]. It was verified by Lang et al. that astronauts resident in low Earth orbit for 4–6 months had cancellous bone loss of the proximal femur at a rate of 2.7% [32]. In a follow-up study, it was revealed by Lang et al. that when weight-bearing activity was resumed for 12 months, a complete recovery of bone mineral content was observed. However, this was due to an increase in the cross-sectional bone dimensions. There was incomplete recovery in "volumetric cancellous and cortical BMD, as well as estimated bone strength" [33].

Sibonga et al. collected postflight data on 45 U.S. and Russian astronauts that had served onboard MIR and the ISS, which was fitted to "an exponential mathematical function, allowing prediction of rate of BMD recovery." It was estimated that 94% of the bone lost during 6 months of spaceflight was recovered over a 3 year period, when normal weight-bearing activity in 1 *g* resumed [34]. Keyak et al. disclosed that regardless of intense exercise schedules, which were intended to mechanically load the skeletons of astronauts aboard the ISS and MIR, they lost areal bone mineral density (aBMD) at a rate of "1.06% per month from the spine and 1.0% to 1.6% per month from the hip," and that in a number of instances the degree of decrease was comparable to "estimated mean lifetime losses associated with aging in Caucasian females, the population most strongly affected by osteoporosis" [35].

It was found by Smith et al. that a reduction in bone loss may be realized through the combination of resistance exercise and careful nutritional intake. With the aim of pro-spectively counteracting bone loss, the early crews of the ISS utilized an "interim resis-tive exercise device" (IRED) (~135 kg resistance load), which had virtually no effect. The advanced resistive exercise device (ARED) (~270 kg resistance load) was transported to the ISS in 2008. The dietary intake, bone densitometry, and biochemical markers were studied for 13 ISS crew members (spanning 2006–2009). While the IRED was used by eight subjects, the remaining five exercised with the ARED. Elevated alkaline phosphatase (bone-specific) was found in both groups near the completion of their mission and for a subsequent 30 days after their return to Earth, as were the majority of markers for bone resorption. A number of mineral density/content parameters quantified by bone densitometry remained unaltered (from preflight) only for those individuals who used the ARED, who also exhibited increased lean mass and lower adipose mass. All subjects dem-onstrated unaltered total body mass and typical vitamin D (75 ± 17 nmol/L) concentrations prior to and during spaceflight. This constituted the first evidence that resistance exercise, in conjunction with adequate energy intake (to maintain body mass) and vitamin D, might counteract the loss of bone mineral density that is associated with long-term (4–6 months) exposure to microgravity [36].

16.2.4 Cardiac Functionality and Muscle Atrophy

A field called bioastronautics, defined as "the study of the biological and medical effects of spaceflight on biological organisms" was established by NASA in 2004, with the release of its bioastronautics critical path roadmap (BCPR) [37]. In addition to prioritizing research and technologies against the hazards of human spaceflight, the aim of the BCPR was to "establish tolerance limits to the space environment and develop countermeasures to over-come these problems." Among a BCPR list of no less than 50 space-travel-associated medi-cal/health risk factors are those related to the potential for serious cardiac dysrhythmias, with cause unknown, which may also initiate hypotension (low blood pressure) and syn-cope (fainting). Significant cardiac rhythm issues such as ventricular tachycardia (rapid heartbeat) were observed in a number of instances during a MIR mission, which is indica-tive of altered cardiac electrical activity and stability [37]. Also, spaceflight (both long and short duration) is linked with reduced cardiac and vascular functionality and a decrease in cardiac mass, which may exacerbate "underlying cardiovascular disease (e.g., arterial atherosclerosis) leading to myocardial infarction, stroke or heart rhythm disturbances that could be irreversible" [9,37]. One reason surmised for the occurrence of cardiac dysrhyth-mias in some astronauts is the reduction in aerobic capacity. Blaber et al. present a number of additional cardiovascular issues including reduced heart rate and diastolic pressure, headward fluid distribution, and decreased plasma volume. Blood and plasma volumes undergo significant changes during spaceflight, and studies have shown plasma volume reductions of from 10% to 17%, and this was thought to be the result of reduced fluid intake and urinary output, a reduction in red blood cell mass, and fluid reallocation from "intravascular to interstitial space due to reduced compression of tissue by gravitational forces" [38–40]. Additionally, when gravity is removed from the human body in space-flight, facial edema occurs, as well as thinning of the legs, due to the headward flow of fluid [9,41] (Refs. [38–41] from [9]).

Rapid cell mass loss and skeletal muscle atrophying that accompany prolonged space-flight result in the reduction of strength and endurance via insufficiencies in the regulation of sensory-motor and muscle force capacities. These deficits leave one at risk for damage to and soreness at muscle/connective tissue interfaces (e.g., muscle fiber/tendon/bone), which will likely lead to further incapacitation. Fitts et al. observed that in microgravity, the muscle mass of rats was reduced by ~37% over the span of 1 week. Studies with human subjects under microgravity indicated that the soleus muscle (component of calf) underwent greater atrophy than the fast-twitch gastrocnemius muscle (component of calf). Both slow type I fibers and fast type II fibers had equivalent susceptibility to atrophy. Muscle peak force was also negatively affected and verified in two instances where "the maximal voluntary contraction of the human plantar flexor muscles declined by 20%–48% following 6 months in space, while a 21% decline in the peak force of the soleus type I fibers was observed after a 17-day shuttle flight." This is ascribed to atrophy of the muscle in conjunction with the "selective loss of contractile protein" [42]. Additional factors that have been determined to play a role in muscle atrophy include a decline in the expression of mRNA muscle genes, a decrease in microRNAs and the translation of proteins, a decrease in neural drive to muscles, and systemic issues relating to hormone modification and changes in metabolism. It was also found that muscle atrophy worsens on return to the 1 g gravity of Earth [43].

16.3 Nanomedical Space Radiation and Microgravity Countermeasures

Incremental progress has been made on several fronts to potentially counteract the degradative effects of galactic cosmic rays and microgravity on human physiology. The implementation of these strategies and the enhancement of their preventative, diagnostic, or therapeutic effects for future orbital, planetary, and deep space missions might be enabled via diverse and potent synergies between unique nanomaterials, nanotechnologies, and nanomedicine.

16.3.1 Potential Nanomedical Antioxidant-Based Space Radiation Mitigation

Rabin et al. investigated the impact of antioxidant diets in rats as a potential approach to mitigate the effects of heavy-particle exposure, which leads to increased oxidative stress. A number of rats were fed an antioxidant diet for 8 weeks (2% blueberry or strawberry extract), while others were given a control diet over the same time period. All rats were subsequently exposed to 1.5 or 2.0 Gy (Gray (Gy) relates to the absorption of 1 J of radiative energy by 1 kg of tissue) of accelerated iron particles. Following several types of response, learning, and memory tests, it was found that the rats sustained with the antioxidant diet faired much better than their control diet counterparts. The antioxidant-fed rats also showed a decrease in radiation-induced tumorigenesis, 1 year after exposure. These findings may culminate in the development of a specialized antioxidant diet/supplementation as a constituent of a multifaceted system, which may enhance the protection of astronauts from cosmic ray-induced physiological and neurological damage [44].

The encapsulation of concentrated antioxidants within nanoscale delivery vehicles (e.g., liposomes, hollow gold nanoshells, polymeric micelles with wall-embedded magnetic nanoparticles, organic and inorganic nanotubes, and in the future, autonomous implanted molecular dispensers) (Figure 16.1) might facilitate their controlled release over extended time periods enabled via protracted (stealth mode) residency within the circulation to cumulatively offer a significant measure of protection for astronauts from heavy-particle exposure during space travel. Ideally, these nanocarriers could be stored within replenishable, strategically implanted reservoirs and incrementally released to provide a (prescribed) sustained concentration of antioxidants within the bloodstream. When nanocarrier payloads approach depletion levels within single or multiple reservoirs, onboard medical personnel would be automatically notified via a unique signal that emanates from the reservoir/s. Subsequently, a new dose of nanocarriers would be administered, which might be introduced via needleless injection, inhalation, or topical gel. The nanocarriers would be decorated with specialized "homing" molecules that are engineered to have an exclusive affinity for the input ports that populate the external surfaces of the reservoirs. Once adhered to a reservoir input port "gate," the nanocarriers would be transferred to an appropriately pressurized (to maximize storage capacity) internal storage compartment via reversible molecular sortation rotors (Figure 16.2) until they are electronically, chemically, or mechanically induced to be released via output ports into the circulation [45].

Schoenfeld et al. have advanced a systemic strategy against the effects of radiation exposure that would conjunctively utilize a mixture of therapeutic medical gases such as nitric oxide (NO), carbon monoxide (CO), hydrogen sulfide (H_2S), hydrogen, which might serve as radical-scavenging antioxidant "chemical radioprotectors." In addition, it is proposed that certain gas molecules may be utilized as "biological signalling molecules to disrupt

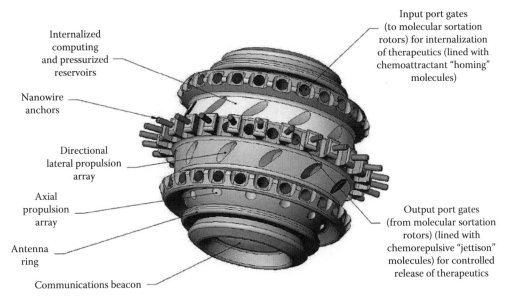

FIGURE 16.1
Conceptual autonomous implantable molecular dispenser.

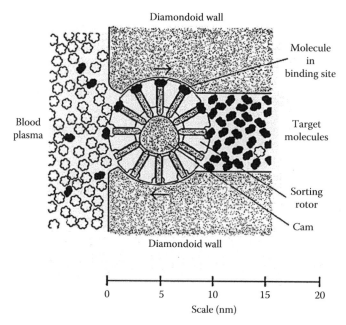

FIGURE 16.2

Reversible molecular sortation rotor. (Reproduced from Freitas Jr., R.A., *Nanomedicine, Volume I: Basic Capabilities*, Landes Bioscience, Georgetown, TX, 1999. With permission.)

the chain of events initiated by radiation exposure and interfere with pathogenesis of disease." It has recently come to light that particular medical gas molecules (e.g., NO, CO, H_2S) play significant roles as biological messengers and radical scavengers. Additionally, the antioxidant medical gases, Xenon (Xe) and Ozone (O_3) have been shown to impart therapeutic vasodilation, anti-apoptotic, and anti-inflammatory effects [46–49].

Free radical and reactive oxygen species (ROS) (e.g., O_2^-, $^1O_2$, $\cdot OH$, $\cdot OOH$, $NO\cdot$, and H_2O_2) that are generated by radiolysis (chemical bond cleavage via nuclear radiation) may impair or destroy healthy cells via oxidative stress via lipid peroxidation or DNA damage. In contrast to the occurrence of single DNA strand (oligonucleotide) breaks (~10 min repair), both strands of the DNA duplex can be cleaved by ballistic heavy HZE particles, which are significantly more difficult for cellular machinery to rectify (several hours) [48]. Human cells are hosts to a number of naturally occurring free radical scavengers, and as Chopping et al. note "As long as they are in excess of the radiolysis products, the DNA may be protected. When the products exceed the amount of scavengers, radiation damage and cancer induction may occur. In principle, there could thus be a threshold dose for radiation damage, at which the free radicals formed exceed the capacity of scavenging. The scavenging capacity may differ from individual to individual depending on his/her physical condition" [50].

16.3.1.1 Fullerene-Based Antioxidants

16.3.1.1.1 C_{60}-Derivative Antioxidants

Pristine C_{60} (~Ø7.0 Å) (Figure 16.3) and several classes of C_{60}-derived fullerenes have demonstrated potent antioxidant properties that may be incorporated into nanomedical formulations toward the potential mitigation of the degradative effects of exposure to space-resident heavy-particle ionizing radiation (Table 16.4). This intriguing molecule has

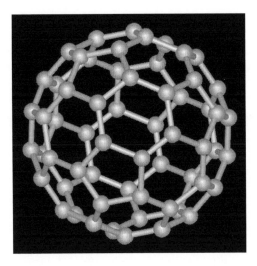

FIGURE 16.3
C_{60} (Buckminsterfullerene) molecule. (From Wikimedia Commons, 2005.)

TABLE 16.4

Examples of C_{60} and Derivative Aantioxidants

C_{60} Species	Antioxidant Effect	References
Polyhyrdoxylated fullerenol ($C_{60}(OH)_{24}$)	Scavenges intermediate free radicals.	[58]
	Eliminates superoxide radicals ($O_2\cdot^-$), radicals (OH and H), and oxidants (H_2O_2 and HO_2).	[59–61]
	Mitochondrial protective antioxidant.	[62]
Hydrated C_{60} fullerene ($C_{60}HyFn$)	Suppresses formation of OH^- radicals in water.	[63]
	Significantly reduces diabetes-induced oxidative stress.	[64]
Carboxyfullerene ($C_{63}(COOH)_6$)	Neuroprotective capacity against superoxide.	[65,66]
	Protects the nigrostriatal dopaminergic system (dopamine transit pathway) from iron-induced oxidative injury.	[67]
	Protects human peripheral blood mononuclear cells from apoptosis via radical oxygen species.	[68]
C_{60}-monomalonic acid (MMA C_{60})	Induces inhibitory effect on nitric-oxide dependant relaxation of aortic smooth muscle.	[60,69]
C60-dimalonic acid ($C_{62}(COOH)_4$)	Decreased toxicity of paraquat and heteropentaline ($O_2\cdot^-$) generators in *E. coli*.	[70,71]
Hexasulfobutylated C_{60} FC(4)S	Vasorelaxation effects due to release of NO or derivatives from vascular endothelium.	[72]
Polyalkylsulfonated C_{60}	Free radical scavenger.	[73]
Pristine C_{60}	Potent liver-protecting agent.	[74]
Colloidal C_{60}	Prevented in vivo protein synthesis disturbances, neurodegeneration, and amyloid-beta 25–35 deposit formation in neurons.	[75]

been dubbed a "radical sponge" as each of its 30 carbon–carbon double bonds provides a binding site for a variety of radicals [51]. Thakral and Mehta revealed that up to 34 methyl radicals were able to be attached to a single C_{60} sphere. The capacity for enhanced solubility of C_{60} derivatives in water and lipid solutions greatly expands their potential for applications in the treatment of myriad disease states [52].

Tabata et al. showed that in vivo tumor necrosis could be robustly initiated by polyethylene glycol-conjugated fullerenes, while healthy tissues in close proximity were left unscathed [53]. It was also found that the antioxidant potency of the carboxylic acid fullerene was hundreds of times that of vitamin E. The Institute of Physiological Active Compounds (Karkov, Ukraine) indicate that hydrated fullerenes may have up to 1000 times the potency of vitamin E. Yin et al. revealed that endohedral metallofullerenols ($[Gd@C_{82}(OH)_{22}]n$) were effective scavengers of superoxide radical anions, hydroxyl radicals, and singlet oxygen ($^1O_2$). They were observed to protect cells from oxidative damage and were potent lipid peroxidation inhibitors. Additionally, they demonstrated efficacy in inhibiting the growth of malignant tumors in vivo; decreased ROS formation from H_2O_2 in human adenocarcinoma cells and rat brain capillary ECs; and acted to protect against mitochondrial damage [54].

The possibility that C_3 carboxyfullerene isomers may provide protection from free radical initiated neurodegenerative conditions such as Alzheimer's and Parkinson's disease has been explored by Dugan et al. They found that C_3 has the capacity for eliminating both superoxide and H_2O_2 free radicals, and "reduce basal mitochondrial production of superoxide in cortical astrocytes" [55]. It has also been shown to obstruct the iron-mediated peroxidation of lipids in vitro [56] and in vivo [57]. This group also showed that two species of polyhydroxylated C_{60} derivatives ($C_{60}(OH)n$ and $C_{60}(OH)nOm$) exhibited remarkable antioxidant properties for the protection of neurons. They were observed to reduce the destruction of neurons from induced excitotoxic (overactivation of neuronal glutamic acid receptor) insults from N-methyl-ᴅ-aspartic acid (NMDA) (by 80%), from 2-amino-3-(5-methyl-3-oxo-1,2-oxazol-4-yl)propanoic acid (AMPA) (by 65%), and from kainite (by 50%). Further, they reduced apoptosis in cortical neurons that were deprived of serum for 24 and 48 h [76].

Lai et al. describe the antioxidant action of fullerene derivative $C_{60}(ONO_2)_{7\pm2}$ to ease ischemia reperfusion (IR) (tissue damage via the return of blood flow to sites that had a previous lack of blood) to induced lung injury, which is characterized by physiological dysfunctions including edema, inflammation, and vascular malfunction. ROS play a significant role in these pulmonary IR injuries. Nitric oxide was also released by $C_{60}(ONO_2)_{7\pm2}$, with activity akin to trinitroglycerol, in the reduction of pulmonary arterial pressure and pulmonary arterial resistance [77].

16.3.1.1.2 Dendritic Fullerene (DF-1) Antioxidants

Daroczi et al. investigated the toxicity and radioprotective effects of dendritic (C_{60}) fullerene (DF-1) nanoparticles in zebrafish embryo models, which were exposed to ionizing radiation in the range of from 20 to 80 Gy, both with and without DF-1. As to the toxicity of DF-1, there were no deleterious effects observed under concentrations that spanned (1–1000 Amol/L). It was shown that an optimized dose of 100 Amol/L imparted "markedly attenuated overall and organ-specific radiation-induced toxicity when given within 3 h before or up to 15 min after radiation exposure." When DF-1 was administered beyond 30 min postexposure, no protection was observed. The activity of DF-1 was comparable to that of the FDA-approved radioprotector amifostine (4 mmol/L), which can, however, impart side effects such as hypotension and vasodilation.

As pristine C_{60} has been shown to impart toxic effects in largemouth bass, presumably through lipid peroxidation [78], the DF-1 derivative, which contains a single branched dendrimer geometry, can be modified through the addition of 18 carboxylic groups to facilitate water solubility and reduce toxicity. When the control (devoid of DF-1) zebrafish embryos were exposed to 10–40 Gy of ionizing radiation, they were subject to morphological and physiological disturbances, including dorsal curvature of the body, neurotoxicity, damaged excretory function, and overall higher fatality. A dose of 100 Amol/L DF-1 was observed to ameliorate these degradative effects when administered 3 h prior to radiation exposure or up to 15 min, following exposure. It was also seen to protect neuromasts (formative nerve cells) from the effects of radiation when exposed to intensities of up to 80 Gy [79].

In humans, specific types of cells are particularly susceptible to radiation. These include erythrocytes, granulocytes, lymphocytes in the blood, and basal epidermal and crypt cells of the intestinal tract [80]. Theriot et al. revealed that DF-1 may serve as a DNA protectant against gamma radiation in human lymphocytes and rat intestinal crypt cells. As fullerenes exhibit strong interactions with species that possess high electron populations, DF-1 had the capacity to reduce crypt cell ROS levels and was shown, in this study, to have greater radioprotective potency than amifostine. This indicated that DF-1 likely had an increased absorptive capacity for electrons per molecule than did amifostine. To elucidate the cytogenetic properties of DF-1 in both lymphocytes and crypt cells, the researchers sought indicators of radiation-induced DNA damage, namely the formation of micronuclei (compacted DNA fragments) external to the cell nucleus [81]. When lymphocytes were pretreated with PBS (phosphate-buffered saline) (controls) and DF-1 (100 µM) and exposed to radiation doses of from 1 to 4 Gy, DF-1 showed lower micronuclei formation. Similarly, crypt cells that were pretreated with PBS, amifostine (0.1 mM and 100 µM), and DF-1 (100 µM), and exposed to 1–4 Gy radiation revealed the least amount of micronuclei formation in the DF-1 pretreated samples [82].

16.3.1.1.3 Single- and Multiwalled Carbon Nanotube Antioxidants

It was revealed by Lucente-Schultz et al. that both pristine and phenolic-functionalized water-soluble single-walled carbon nanotubes (SWCNTs) are potent antioxidants. When the SWCNTs (Ø ~1 nm × 60 nm long) were decorated with a butylated hydroxytoluene (BHT) antioxidant derivative, their radical-scavenging abilities were shown to be 40-fold higher than the DF-1 fullerenes described earlier. However, it was found that the radical-scavenging activity could be decreased contingent on the method of BHT functionalization employed. "When functionalized with the radical scavenger BHT-derivatives through existing functionalities on the sidewall, the antioxidant activity of the system is increased. If, however, the BHT-derivative functionalization occurs through covalent addition to the sidewall, the antioxidant activity of the system is decreased." Hence, the researchers suggested that pristine SWCNTs might themselves be superior radical scavengers. An additional advantage afforded by the SWCNTs was that concentrations of up to 330 nM or 83 mg/L had negligible cytotoxicity on the studied human renal epithelial (HRE) and HepG2 liver cells [83].

As evidenced by Cirillo et al., multiwalled carbon nanotubes (MWCNTs) (in this study 20–30 nested graphene walls with inner diameters 5–25 nm, outer diameters 10–70 nm × 10–30 µm long) also exhibited antioxidant activity when they were covalently functionalized with gallic acid. Gallic acid is a powerful naturally occurring antioxidant that is found in a number of vegetable sources [84]. The functionalization of the MWCNTs served to facilitate their biocompatibility, and the bioactivity of the gallic acid was maintained in the final hybrid system. The specific activity of the gallic acid functionalized MWCNTs included the inhibition of 2,2′-diphenyl-1-picrylhydrazyl (DPPH) radicals by 92% ± 2%, hydroxyl radicals by 63% ± 1%, peroxyl radicals 98% ± 1%, and acetylcholinesterase by 57% ± 2% [85].

16.3.1.2 Halloysite Clay Nanotubes for Delivery of Antioxidants

Halloysite is a naturally abundant biocompatible aluminosilicate clay that is comprised of hollow nanotubes (15 nm outer diameter × 15 nm inner diameter × 500–1500 nm in length; Figure 16.4), which may be employed for the delivery of antioxidants to potentially negate space radiation effects. Vergaro et al. demonstrated that halloysite nanotube lumens can be loaded with the poorly soluble polyphenol antioxidant resveratrol (3,5,40-trihydroxy-trans-stilbene), with a consistent release profile of over 48 h. Halloysite nanotubes have a negative electrical ζ potential of −50 mV that facilitates their colloidal stability and makes them well dispersible in water under variable pH. They are also nontoxic to humans up to concentrations of 75 mg/mL. A layer-by-layer coating technique was utilized to coat and cap the lumen ends of the halloysite nanotubes with six polyelectrolyte layers in order to gain further control of the resveratrol release kinetics against MCF-7 cells (a breast cancer cell line) [86].

16.3.1.3 Nanoparticle-Based Antioxidants

Biological cells typically generate and operate under a basal free radical population, which is essential in facilitating signal transduction (e.g., calcium signaling, phosphatase activity, and for the activation of transcription factors). A certain threshold of excess free radicals and the associated damage that is wrought by oxidative stress may be tolerated and remediated by cells through the utilization of naturally occurring enzymes (e.g., superoxide

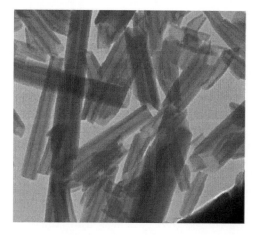

FIGURE 16.4
TEM of halloysite clay nanotubes. (Reproduced from Vergaro, V. et al., *Macromol. Biosci.* August 8, 2012. With permission.) (Since halloysite nanotubes have the potential for hosting a wide range of drug molecules, it is conceivable that they may serve as important nanocarrier elements in antiradiation strategies for, ideally, the full protection of astronauts and future space travellers. For critical neuroprotective applications, they might be exploited to deliver powerful antioxidants such as mitoquinone, which targets coenzyme Q in the mitochondria. This compound has the capacity for obstructing neurodegenerative oxidation reactions at a 1000-fold level over conventional therapeutics.) (*The Handbook of Neuroprotection*, 2011, Jain, K.K., Springer Science+Business Media, LLVC.)

dismutase, glutathione peroxidase, and catalase) and reductants, including vitamins E, C, carotene, melatonin, and n-acetyl cysteine [87]. However, it is not difficult to imagine that in the radiation-permeated space environment, these cellular resources are likely to soon be overwhelmed.

Certain nanoparticles are also endowed with the unique capacity to alleviate oxidative stress in biological systems, and thus may have utility for the mitigation of radiation-induced oxidative stress to benefit spacefaring humans. These include ceria (CeO_2) nanoparticles (Ø20 nm), that when administered as a 10 nM dose have demonstrated the ability to extend the in vitro lifetimes of a mixture of brain cells by up to six times the nominal (decreasing cell death by ~60%), while sustaining "normal neuronal calcium signaling during this extended lifespan." In vitro studies showed that the 10 nM of ceria nanoparticles exhibited sustained neuroprotection for ~3 months without repeating the dose. It was also found that they have the ability to shield neurons from the damage imparted by UV light, H_2O_2, and excitotoxicity [88]. Interestingly, ceria nanoparticles that were larger than Ø30 nm showed no noteworthy impacts.

A comparative study was undertaken by Schubert et al. who demonstrated that yttrium oxide (Y_2O_3) nanoparticles (Ø6 and Ø12 nm) conveyed an even greater radical-scavenging activity than ceria oxide nanoparticles in the protection of both neuronal (HT22) and macrophage (RAW164) cell lines. Each of these species of nanoparticles directly reduced the generation of free radicals and negated the effects of oxidative stress in the studied cells. As the group notes:

> cerium and yttrium oxide nanoparticles are able to rescue cells from oxidative stress-induced cell death in a manner that appears to be dependent upon the structure of the particle but independent of its size within the 6–1000 nm range [89].

A unique class of self-assembling amphiphilic block copolymer nanoparticles (Ø40 nm) has recently been developed by Nagasaki, which has the ability to encapsulate nitroxide radical compounds (2,2,6,6-tetramethylpyperidine-1-oxyl [TEMPO]) within their cores as a potential therapeutic candidate against oxidative stress through the catalyzation of ROS such as superoxides. When administered on its own, nitroxide radicals have a number of disadvantages including a broad dispersion profile within healthy tissues, rapid renal clearance and chemical reduction to hydroxylamine (a pulmonary irritant and potential mutagen), as well as the possible initiation of tachycardia (accelerated heart rate), increased temperature of the skin, and seizures. Nitroxide radical compounds can be encased within the polymeric nanoparticles by virtue of their serving as side chains of the hydrophobic portion of the amphiphilic polymer elements. They demonstrate enhanced circulatory residence and safety for possible therapeutic applications against "cerebral and renal ischemia reperfusions, ulcerative colitis and Alzheimer's disease models." The nitroxide radicals are released into the circulation via a pH-determined phase transition [90]. For instance, a "poly(ethylene glycol)-b-PEAMA block copolymer forms core–shell type polymer micelle above pH 7.5, while it disintegrates under pH 7.4" [91,92].

Aside from their antibacterial and anti-inflammatory properties [93], silver nanoparticles (~Ø4 nm) were shown to be radioprotective when complexed with 6-palmitoyl ascorbic acid-2-glucoside (PAsAG), a vitamin C derivative. On exposure to ionizing radiation, PAsAG was observed to protect against DNA strand cleavage in spleen and bone marrow cells, as well as blood leucocytes (in animal models), against radiation damage from ROS (e.g., hydroxyl radicals, superoxide anions, hydrated electrons, hydroperoxy radical, hydrogen peroxide, and hydronium ions). As ascorbic acid undergoes oxidative and thermal degradation in vivo, derivatives such as PAsAG are more stable and bioavailable with higher radical-scavenging activity in vivo. When administered directly following exposure to radiation, the PAsAG derivative was also shown to improve DNA repair in bone marrow cells and leucocytes [94–99].

When silver nanoparticles (<Ø50 nm) were combined with glyzyrrhizic acid, they exhibited a synergistic free radical-scavenging activity for protection against cellular DNA strand breaks and the formation of micronuclei and chromosomal abnormalities in bone marrow, spleen, and leucocytes as well. Glyzyrrhizic acid is a primary bioactive licorice root (Glyzyrrhiza) triterpene glycoside extract, and among a host of additional beneficial pharmacological properties, it is radioprotective [100]. The hybrid silver nanoparticle/glyzyrrhizic acid complex was thought to have enhanced potency due to cumulative scavenging contributions from both components, as individually, the silver and glyzyrrhizic acid had reduced abilities [101].

16.3.1.4 Naturally Occurring Antioxidants: Potential Integration with Nanocarriers

Nanomedical applications for space radiation protection for astronauts might also be enabled through the integration of naturally occurring systems that possess inherent antioxidant properties, as encapsulant cargoes within biocompatible nanocarriers or as external surface adsorbents. Alternately, it is conceivable that synthetic biomimetic analogs of these systems may be employed to enhance their shelf life, efficacy, and stability for the negation of the degradative physiological effects of space radiation exposure.

The algicolous marine fungus, *Acremonium* sp. was found to contain hydroquinone derivatives with significant antioxidant properties. Their radical-scavenging abilities were determined utilizing free radical 1,1-diphenyl-2-picrylhydrazil (DPPH) and thiobarbituric acid reactive substances (TBARS) assays. At a concentration of 25.0 μg/mL, the radical-scavenging effects of two novel hydroquinone derivatives (acremonin A and acremonin A glucoside) showed DPPH radical-scavenging levels of 85.5% and 17.5%, respectively, whereas known hydroquinone derivatives 2-(1-hydroxy-1-methyl)-2,3-dihydrobenzofuran-5-ol, 2,2 Dimethylchroman-3, 6-diol, and 2-(3-dihydroxy-3-methylbutyl)benzene-1,4-diol exhibited radical-scavenging levels of 85.8%, 72.9%, and 90.2%, respectively [102]. Additional naturally occurring antioxidants have been found in the fungal species *Penicillium roquefortii* [103], *Aspergillus candidus* [104,105], *Mortierella* sp. [106], and *Emericella falconensis* [107], *Acremonium* [108], and 10 natural p-terphenyl derivatives in three species of edible mushrooms (e.g., *Thelephora ganbajun*, *Thelephora aurantiotincta*, and *Boletopsis grisea*) [109]. When administered in high concentrations, albeit in a highly localized manner, or combined in composite doses, these compounds may facilitate enhanced prevention, and ideally, full protection for astronauts from oxidative stress, the provision of biological protection, and efficient repair mechanisms.

Interestingly, the survival, and indeed even growth, of the bacteria *Deinococcus radiodurans* under intense radiation exposure (50 Gy/h), and its recovery from extreme radiation doses (10 kGy) have been correlated to the ability of antioxidants to minimize the degree of oxidative insult. It was discovered by Daly et al. that the inherent capacity of *D. radiodurans* to survive (10 kGy) radiation levels, which can initiate ~100 DNA double-strand breaks (DSB) per genome, is likely associated with a ~300-fold increase of Mn(II) ions and threefold decrease of Fe(II) within its cells, than radiation-sensitive cells such as those of *Shewanella oneidensis*. When *D. radiodurans* was deprived of Mn and exposed to 10 kGy of radiation, they exhibited 1000 times lower survival rates than when their Mn levels were nominal. Although *D. radiodurans* is endowed with a fairly standard compliment of DNA repair mechanisms, they are significantly more efficient than those of bacteria that are sensitive to ionizing radiation. The explanation for this enhanced DNA repair activity following irradiation, however, remains elusive. It appears that proteins, more so than DNA itself, are the entities that are most protected in *D. radiodurans* via the antioxidant activity of well-distributed Mn(II), which reacts robustly with superoxide radicals [110,111].

Beblo et al. investigated the survival rates of 14 species of thermophilic and hyperthermophilic microorganisms following high-dose ionizing radiation exposure, whereupon nine were observed to have high IR tolerance, and only two (*A. pyrophilus* and *I. hospitalis*) were seen to survive even a 20 kGy exposure. The genome of *I. hospitalis* was heavily segmented (~1000 fragments with 1600 bp typical length); yet, it was somehow able to repair the damage even though it contains only several DNA repair genes. The basis and kinetics of this repair mechanism so far remain unknown [112].

16.3.1.5 *Tardigrades and Rotifers*

Tardigrades, also known as waterbears, are intriguing microscopic (~250 to 700 μm) herbivorous invertebrate species, of which there are ~1500 members, in that they can withstand and survive desiccation, extreme (−273°C to 151°C) thermal environments, high pressure (<600 MPa), radiation, and even the ambient vacuum of space. These remarkable creatures also exhibit the capacity for undergoing hibernation for decades and emerging unscathed upon subsequent reanimation (see Section 7.6.6). In terms of radiation exposure, species such as *Milnesium tardigradum* were observed as being capable of surviving levels of up to 5000 Gy (gamma-rays) and 6200 Gy (heavy ions) when hydrated, and 4400 Gy (gamma-rays) and 5200 Gy (heavy ions) when in an anhydrobiotic (desiccated) state, subsequent to 48 h of exposure. Tardigrades in both states, however, became sterile at 1000 Gy and did not attain their natural life spans.

Horikawa et al. surmise that the presence of various concentrations of trehalose (2.3%, <0.2% wt/dry wt, respectively, in *M. tardigradum and R. coronifer* to 15% and 20% wt/dry wt, respectively, in *A. salina* cysts and *P. vanderplanki* larvae) found in anhydrobiotic tardigrades might facilitate their ability to tolerate high radiation exposures [113]. Trehalose (a nonreducing disaccharide that stabilizes cells in their desiccated state), along with maltose and sucrose, is seen to confer radiation protection to DNA [114,115]. Since hydroxyl radical lifetimes are extremely brief (8.7 × 10^{-9} s) with an average diffusion distance in the range of ~60 Å, only those radicals that are generated at a sufficiently intimate proximity can react with and impart damage to DNA [115,116]. Thus, it would seem to follow that sugars such as trehalose might have an enhanced protective impact against radiation, should they be positioned more closely to DNA duplexes.

In 2007, a project entitled Tardigrade Resistance to Space Effects (TARSE) was flown on FOTON-M3 for 12 days to assess the effects of the space environment on both active and anhydrobiotic tardigrades (*Macrobiotus richtersi*). It was found that radiation and microgravity had no effect on the stability of tardigrade DNA, or normal moulting and reproductive cycles (Figure 16.5). Noted were increased glutathione and associated enzyme action, decreased catalase and superoxide dismutase, and no change in TBARS [117]. Interestingly, Rizzo et al. studied a number of antioxidant enzymes in hydrated and anhydrobiotic tardigrades (*Paramacrobiotus richtersi*) and found that superoxide dismutase was increased in desiccated specimens with the generation of glutathione and glutathione peroxidase. Polyunsaturated fatty acid composition and TBARS were also increased in the desiccated animals [118,119]. When a terrestrial tardigrade undergoes desiccation due to lack of available water in its environment, it will contract its body anteriorly-posteriorly

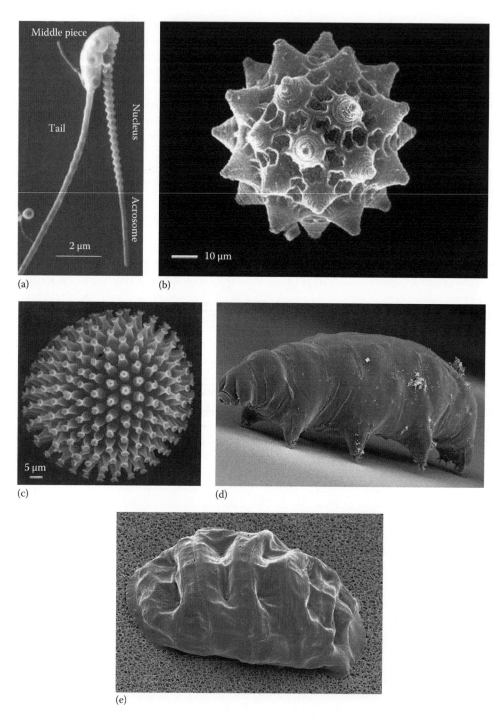

FIGURE 16.5
(a) SEM of tardigrade spermatozoon (*Macrobiotus macrocalix*). (b) In toto tardigrade egg (*Paramacrobiotus richtersi*).
(c) In toto tardigrade egg (*Macrobiotus* cf. *persimilis*). (d) Mature hydrated tardigrade. (e) Tardigrade in desiccated tun state. ((a–c) Reproduced from Lorena Rebecchi, Department of Life Sciences, University of Modena
and Reggio Emilia, Italy. With permission. (d–e) Reproduced from Ralph Schill, Biological Institute, Zoology,
University of Stuttgart, Germany. With permission.)

and retract four pairs of lobopodous legs while transmuting into what is referred to as a "tun." When the conversion is complete, it will have shed 95% of the water content of its body [120].

In the study of an alternate hypothesis as to the resilience of tardigrades (eutardigrade *Richtersius Coronifer*) against ionizing radiation, Jönsson et al. undertook the investigation of 30–50 tardigrades, which were irradiated with gamma-ray doses of between 1.0 and 9.0 kGy (anhydrobiotic specimens) and 0.5–5.0 kGy (hydrated specimens). It was deduced that rather than an exclusive radiation tolerance mechanism involving bioprotectant enzymes and increased concentrations of antioxidants/sugars when tardigrades are in the shrunken tun state, the actual strategy may employ a complementary highly efficacious DNA repair system. The specific kinetics of such a proposed system remains to be fully investigated [121]. However, toward elucidation, it has been learnt that *Ramazzottius varieornatus* has the capacity for the efficient repair of detrimental radiation-induced thymine dimers in its DNA following massive radiation exposure [122]. Likely, it may be a combination of, and synergy between, biochemical protectants and robust DNA repair that enable a high degree of radiation resistance in tardigrades.

Additional model candidates that may assist in the investigation, design, and development of potential nanomedical protectant strategies to negate the degradative effects of space radiation are the rotifers (Figure 16.6) [123]: pervasive invertebrate animals that possess novel characteristics of a similar nature to those of the tardigrades.

The robust ionizing radiation resiliency of bdelloid rotifers has been probed by Gladyshev and Meselson [124]. This species can also undergo desiccation, and any DNA damage that occurs while they are in this state is spontaneously repaired upon rehydration. They can also survive the process of desiccation without the generation of trehalose, which is commonly seen in tardigrades [125,126]. It is thought that the mechanism of protection of

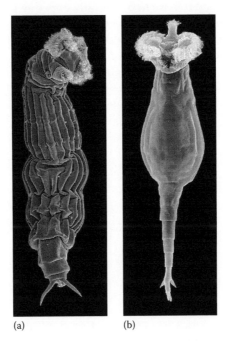

(a)   (b)

FIGURE 16.6
Examples of bdelloid rotifer body plans. (Reproduced from Fontaneto, D. et al., *PLoS Biol* 5(4), e87, 2007. With permission.)

bdelloids from ionizing radiation, despite high rates of DNA duplex breakage and other damage may involve system components (e.g., enhanced radical scavengers) that serve to protect essential proteins and other elements of core repair systems. The multiplicity of DNA DSB may be the result of the close proximity and clustering of hydroxyl radicals or other ROS that are simply out of reach, temporally and spatially (as discussed earlier), of radical scavengers [124,127,128].

A variety of nematode species have also demonstrated radiation resistance up to levels of 4.0 kGy (root-knot nematode *Meloidogyne javanica*) without apparent effect [129], while the pine wood nematode *Bursaphelenchus xylophilus* was observed to withstand up to 6–8 kGy of gamma (cesium-137) radiation [130]. Ye et al. found that resveratrol had protective effects against ionizing radiation and oxidative stress in the radiation-sensitive nematode model *Caenorhabditis elegans*, due to its potent radical-scavenging abilities and capacity for controlling the expression of superoxide dismutase. It also prevented the decrease of superoxide dismutase expression in the mitochondria. When *C. elegans* were pretreated with 100 μM resveratrol and exposed to 100 Gy of gamma-radiation, both the maximum and average life spans of the nematodes were prolonged by 8 days and 3.89 days, respectively [131].

The recognized survival factor, fibroblast growth factor 2 (FGF2), was investigated by Marie et al. to elucidate its DNA repair abilities in epidermoid carcinoma stem cells, subsequent to gamma-radiation exposure (4 Gy). It was learned that the cells demonstrated rapid DNA repair (50% repaired damage within 5 min) concomitant with high levels of nuclear FGF2, in comparison to human A431 squamous carcinoma cells (20% repaired damage within 5 min)[132]. The initiation of FGF2-mediated DNA repair has also been observed in HeLa cells [133] and healthy human epidermal cells [134]. It may be theoretically possible that concentrated FGF2 could be loaded into nanocarriers for delivery to cell nuclei to facilitate its sustained release to potentially expedite DNA repair in all cell types.

As seems apparent from the work surveyed briefly earlier, the primary theme for the protection of cells, tissues, and DNA from the deleterious effects of ionizing radiation appears to be a synergistic combination of highly efficacious antioxidants that work in conjunction with enhanced DNA repair mechanisms. Hence, nanomedical strategies that further augment and sustain these protective mechanisms might be useful in the prevention and repair of ionizing radiation initiated physiological damage in astronauts over extended space missions.

16.3.2 Potential Nanomedical Mitigation of the Effects of Microgravity

Advanced nanomedicine might assist in preventing and/or counteracting the effects of microgravity, such as bone mass loss, neurological damage, the degradation of tissues, and the onset of detrimental ocular issues in enabling humans to endure prolonged spaceflight to Mars and beyond.

16.3.2.1 Nanomedical Countermeasures for Preservation of Bone Mass in Microgravity

16.3.2.1.1 Fullerene-Facilitated Bone Repair and Growth

The composition of bone includes 60%–65% hydroxyapatite (HAP; $Ca_{10}(PO_4)_6(OH)_2$) (calcium phosphate in its most stable form), along with the components chondroitin sulfate, keratin sulfate lipids, and collagen [135]. Bisphosphonate compounds are well-known drugs that have an affinity for, and are active with, the bone matrix. Hence, they are utilized in therapeutics to address osteoporosis and other bone diseases. To date, fluoride (F−) remains one of the only identified substances that can "generate new bone matrix and new mineral from previously inactive areas." It also aids in therapeutics to improve the prognosis of osteoporosis by enhancing bone strength and thus preventing fractures. However, when bisphosphonates are administered via the conventional oral route, they are not properly taken up in the gastrointestinal tract, whereas F− which is given orally as sodium fluoride (NaF) results in toxicity [136]. To boost the maintenance and repair of bones for humans involved in space travel, micron-scale delivery reservoirs might be engineered to enhance the bioavailability, safety, and efficacy of existing therapeutics. Initial novel nanoparticles, giving way in the future to dedicated nanomedical devices, may be employed in the prevention and mitigation of bone loss, and if necessary, for periodic rebuilding of bone mass.

Fullerene derivatives, a number of species of which are described earlier as potent antioxidants (Section 16.3.1.1), could also be utilized in the treatment of bone diseases and to alleviate microgravity-induced skeletal degradation. Bone tissues provide an extensive range of target binding sites for therapeutic entities that are functionalized with phosphonic and carboxylic acids and hydroxyl groups that readily adhere to bone minerals via hydrogen and ionic bonds [137,138]. A bisphosphonate fullerene $C_{60}(OH)_{16}AMBP$ that specifically targeted bone tissue (Figure 16.7) was synthesized by Gonzalez et al. A robust affinity for bone-resident calcium phosphate mineral HAP ($Ca_{10}(PO_4)_6(OH)_2$) was accomplished through the combination of an amide bisphosphonate addend and numerous hydroxyl groups. The fullerenol $C_{60}OH_{30}$ also demonstrated an affinity for HAP, albeit at reduced intensity.

In the targeting of bone tissues, the inhibition of crystal growth is critical, as vectored substances with an affinity to bone characteristically gravitate to sites that are metabolically engaged in bone formation or resorption [139]. Metabolism in diseased bone tissues is highly active, which fortunately serves to attract appropriately functionalized compounds with high specificity directly to sites that require therapeutic treatment [140]. It was found that at a concentration of 1 mM, $C_{60}(OH)_{16}AMBP$ initiated a 50% reduction in the rate of HAP crystal growth, whereas $C_{60}OH_{30}$ achieved a 28% reduction [136].

Carbon nanotubes have been employed as mechanical reinforcing materials in bioactive composite scaffolding material for the repair of bone tissue, comprised of chitosan (a natural chitin-derived polymer from crustacean exoskeletons) and HAP. These bone-rebuilding composites are biocompatible, biodegradable, antibacterial, and amenable to being molded into multiple geometries as porous structures, which make them appropriate for

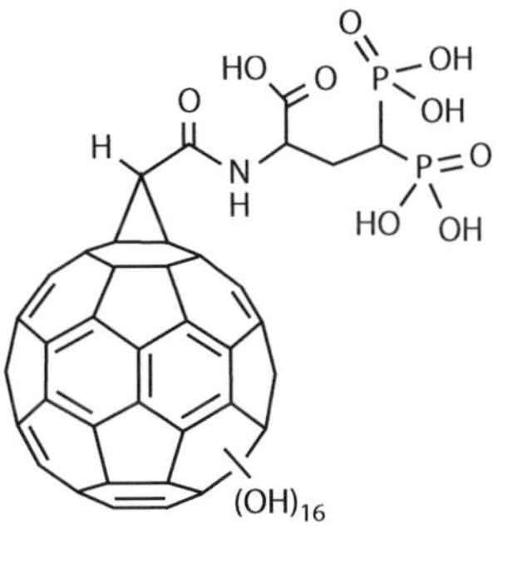

FIGURE 16.7
Tissue-vectored bisphosphonate fullerene $C_{60}(OH)_{16}AMBP$. (Reproduced from Bosi, S. et al., *Eur. J. Med. Chem.* 38(11–12), 913, 2003. Copyright 2003. Editions scientifiques et médicales Elsevier SAS. All rights reserved. With permission.)

the ingrowth of cells and what is known as osteoconduction (a process that mediates the restorative propagation of natural bone) [135,141]. Advantages of such biodegradable materials when applied to bone repair, or the potential therapeutic addition of bone mass for astronauts, include the concurrent distribution of drugs or growth factors to expedite the generation of bone tissue [142].

When MWNTs were functionalized with increased carboxylic and hydroxyl groups, and combined with the chitosan matrix, a marked increase in mechanical strength was observed in the composite. Small loadings of MWNTs with neat chitosan resulted in significant increases of tensile modulus and strength, which were measured to be 78% and 94% (at 0.4 wt% MWNT loading) and 93% and 99% (at 0.8 wt% MWNT loading), respectively, in comparison with unaltered chitosan. Interestingly, the elongation at break (%) decreased in step with higher MWNT loadings (49.5% ± 5.6% for neat chitosan and 13.4% ± 4.5% for MWNT loading at 2.0 wt%) (Table 16.5). This might be a cumulative effect of the presence of MWNT aggregates within the chitosan matrix [143].

Usui et al. discovered that MWNTs exhibited superior compatibility with bone and tissue, showed low levels of inflammation, "and are capable of permitting bone repair and becoming closely integrated with bone tissue and accelerate bone formation stimulated by recombinant human bone morphogenetic protein-2" (rhBMP-2) [144]. The capacity of MWNTs for the repair of bone fractures may encompass their dimensions, structural attributes, and surface properties. The functionalized surfaces of both SWNTs [145] and MWNTs [144] have demonstrated the capacity to serve as core nucleation sites for the crystallization of HAP, which is the initial and critical event in the formation of bone matrices. Further, when MWNTs were blended with type I collagen, which is a prime delivery agent for bone morphogenetic protein, bone formation was expedited in reaction with rhBMP-2, where it was evident that the nascent bone matrix quickly began to encapsulate the MWNT [146].

Recently, Gonçalves et al. conducted a comparative study between functionalized MWNTs (~Ø30 to Ø50 nm × 1.5 μm long) and graphene oxide plates (GOs) (200 nm–3 μm × 1.2 nm thick = ~3 graphene sheets) to learn which bone cement reinforcing agent might be most effective. It was revealed that the considerably higher oxidation level (48.57%) of the graphene surface than the MWNTs (13.96%) and its high surface area, combined with its wrinkled and convoluted morphology contributed to its robust adhesion and interlocking with a poly(methyl methacrylate) (PMMA)/HAP bone cement. In addition, the GO was functionalized with epoxy groups, while the MWNTs were functionalized with a higher population of carboxylic groups. The improved integration with the polymer displayed by GO was hypothesized to be the result of its particular carbon structure, which scavenges

TABLE 16.5

Mechanical Attributes of Neat Chitosan and Chitosan/MWNT Composites

Samples	Tensile Modulus (GPa)	Tensile Strength (MPa)	Elongation at Break (%)
Neat chitosan	1.08 ± 0.04	37.7 ± 4.5	49.5 ± 5.6
Chitosan/0.2% MWNTs	1.33 ± 0.06	56.0 ± 6.8	36.1 ± 3.0
Chitosan/0.4% MWNTs	1.92 ± 0.07	73.1 ± 6.3	20.8 ± 4.3
Chitosan/0.8% MWNTs	2.08 ± 0.05	74.9 ± 4.8	19.5 ± 3.3
Chitosan/2.0% MWNTs	2.15 ± 0.09	74.3 ± 4.6	13.4 ± 4.5

Source: Reconfigured from Wang, S.F. et al., *Biomacromolecules* 6(6), 3067, 2005. With permission.

radicals (generated via the polymerization process) to a lesser degree than do the high-density p-bonds of the MWNTs [147].

Zanello et al. found that osteoblastic cell proliferation was enhanced, and that "plate-shaped crystals" were formed when they were cultured on, as-prepared, and chemically modified SWNTs (Ø1.5 nm × ~300 nm – ~2 to 3 μm long) that possessed a neutral electrical charge. Following 5 days, the as-prepared SWNTs achieved 59% ± 4% growth, whereas polyethylene glycol functionalized SWNTs attained 57% ± 4% growth on glass coverslips, as percentages of the maximal growth achieved by controls over the same timeline [148].

The layer-by-layer application of a SWNT (Ø1–2 nm in × 50 μm long) composite on osteoblasts in vitro and in vivo was investigated by Bhattacharya et al. to learn of its capacity as a substrate for bone formation and as a bone implant material in comparison to pure titanium. The composite was fabricated using a layer-by-layer self-assembly dipping process and consisted of two bilayers of polydimethyldiallylammonium (PDDA) (positively charged) and polystyrene sulfonate (PSS) (negatively charged) to which alternating layers of polyethyleneimine (PEI) and SWNTs were added, giving [(PDDA/PSS)$_2$(PEI/SWCNT)$_6$]$_{10}$PEI, which were assembled on polycaprolactone (PCL) sheets. This composite exhibited physical characteristics of cortical and trabecular bone. It was found that although cell proliferation profiles were alike between the composite and the titanium, the differentiation of cells was enhanced on the surface of the composite, which also stimulated the mineralization of the bone-forming matrix. There were no indications of inflammation or rejection when the composite was implanted in the calvarial (upper cranium) defect of a rat [149].

Stem cells have been transplanted in regenerative medicine to repair human tissues. With the advent of nanomedicine, they might be incorporated into dedicated scaffolds that are comprised of a number of novel nanomaterials, including functionalized graphene, for the regeneration of bone tissues. As Nayak et al. point out, "One of the key objectives for bone regeneration therapy to be successful is to direct stem cells' proliferation and to accelerate their differentiation in a controlled manner through the use of growth factors and osteogenic inducers." These workers demonstrated that graphene does not impede the propagation of human mesenchymal stem cells and serves to hasten their differentiation into bone cells, the rate at which is comparable to that of typically employed growth factors (e.g., BMP-2) [150]. Graphene has many attractive features that make it amenable as a dynamic scaffold material for bone regeneration to counteract the effects of microgravity. As this nanomaterial is essentially a pure carbon mesh of only a single atom in thickness, it is extremely flexible to facilitate intimate form-fitting with any complex bone structure geometries [151]. It can also robustly accelerate bone cell differentiation by virtue of the presence of morphological ripples, which emulate the nanoscale disorder that has been shown to stimulate the differentiation of human mesenchymal stem cells to osteoblasts "in the absence of osteogenic supplements" [152].

The integration of stem cells with nanomaterials-based scaffolds may enable nanomedical layer-by-layer growth of bone tissues in vivo for human space travellers to counteract the degradative effects of microgravity on skeletal structures (see Section 16.3.2.1.3) These treatments might be administered when onboard physicians deem them as necessary supplemental adjuncts to exercise regimens and, when practicably implemented, artificial gravity. These conceptual orthopedic therapeutics might be administered via painless jet injection or taken orally, whereupon targeted elements would adhere to and self-assemble on the surfaces of deficient bones body-wide, if necessary, to add uniform layers of bone tissue at prescribed thicknesses.

As certain bone tissues (e.g., trabecular bone tissue in particular, as well as proximal femur, hip, and spine) are more vulnerable to the effects of microgravity than others, dedicated "inducer" class nanoparticles might be first deployed to locate and bind exclusively with degraded bone sites. This capacity may be facilitated by computer-mediated comparative imaging, whereby full-body skeletal images that have been captured of individuals preflight would be compared with subsequent full-body scans onboard spacecraft, either by ex vivo or in vivo means. The resulting data would specifically demarcate all sites that suffer from reductions in bone mass. The inducer nanoparticles could be specifically functionalized to adhere to these sites while also being endowed with guidance receptors that have specific and robust molecular affinities with subsequently administered stem cell/scaffolding nanocarriers.

Sufficiently sophisticated autonomous nanodevices will, in the future, negate many of these preliminary/preparatory steps as they will be programmed to seek out and proceed directly to impacted bone sites to commence with repairs via the dispensing of self-assembling bone-rebuilding elements, including stem cells or biomimetic analogs thereof. The primary aim here will be to sustain the original 1 g Earth level bone mass of astronauts as required during prolonged space missions, and/or while they are resident in gravity-deficient (in terms of human physiology) Lunar or Martian habitats.

16.3.2.1.2 Nanofiber-Mediated Bone Repair and Growth

Electrospinning involves the application of a voltage to a syringe needle that dispenses a polymer melt onto a plate-like or rotating drum electrode in the production of nanofibers. Shao et al. undertook to investigate randomly arranged and aligned electrically conductive nanofibers that were generated via electrospinning processes. Biodegradable poly-DL-lactide (PDLLA) was infused with MWNTs (Ø10–20 nm × 10–20 µm long) to form nanofiber matrices that served as substrates for the study of the effects of electrical current and nanoscale topological features on the propagation of osteoblasts. It was learned that when no current was applied, the aligned nanofibers augmented the directionality and elongation of osteoblasts over their randomly arranged counterparts [153].

When a direct current of 100 µA was applied to the substrates, osteoblast proliferation was enhanced with growth that was guided by the direction of the current, regardless of their alignment, whereas in this case, the topologies of substrates had little impact. It is known that inherent bioelectrical signaling is vital in the mediation of cellular adhesion and differentiation [154] and that electrical stimulation can influence the migration of cells, the secretion of proteins, and the synthesis of DNA [155–157]. A further elucidation was that the diameters of the electrospun nanofibers had a significant bearing on the growth of osteoblasts. Hu et al. found that electrospun poly(L-lactic acid) (PLLA) nanofibers with diameters in the same range of that of natural collagen (Ø100 and 200 nm) had a direct effect on the enhanced differentiation of mouse osteoblastic cell line (MC3T3-E1), with "dramatically higher bone sialoprotein (BSP) gene expression (two orders of magnitude higher) and significantly higher alkaline phosphatase (ALP) activities" [158]. Badami et al. demonstrated that "topographical factors designed into biomaterial scaffolds can regulate spreading, orientation, and proliferation of osteoblastic cells" through the use of electrospun poly(lactic acid) and poly(ethylene glycol)-poly(lactic acid) diblock copolymers with diameters that ranged from 140 nm to 2.1 µm and MC3T3-E1 cells [159]. Other researchers have explored various synthetic micron-scale materials with nanometric surface topologies (e.g., pits, grooves, pillars, ridges) to further elucidate their effects on cell behaviors [160,161].

16.3.2.1.3 *Osteolaminals: Conceptual Bone Mass Replenishment Strategy*

Enabling the capacity for the maintenance of bone mass, density, and strength will be critical for astronauts who can lose bone mass at the average rates of 1%–1.6% per month from the "spine, femur neck, tibia, trochanter, calcaneus, and pelvis" and 0.3%–0.4% per month from the legs and median whole body [162]. An added level of complexity is that in conjunction with the degradative effects of microgravity on skeletal integrity, ionizing radiation has been observed to exacerbate bone loss in the space environment [163]. Bone rebuilding/maintaining therapeutics (e.g., parathyroid hormone (PTH 1-84), human recombinant PTH peptide 1–34 (Teriparatide) [164,165], oligodeoxynucleotides (ODNs) [166]), nanomaterial/cellular composites [167,168] or nanoscale biomimetic analogs, for instance, of collagen type I fibers, and HAP [169] crystals (~0.74 nm × 11.0 nm × 14.0 nm) for the rebuilding of bone tissues might be encapsulated within liposomes or polymeric nanocarriers, or adsorbed to the external surfaces of targeted nanoparticles. The ingress of these nanocarriers may be achieved by ingestion in pill form, via transdermal infusion, through the use of an adhered patch, or applied as a topical gel (Chapter 2).

Alternately, contingent on the arrival of nanomanufacturing, advanced "osteolaminal" (OSTL) nanodevices might autonomously transit to specific bone sites. Subsequent to these areas being elucidated via imaging and determined to have deficiencies/damage and in need of repair, OSTL's might be deployed as a supplemental bone-rebuilding platform to methodically "topdress" the thinning bones of astronauts with multiple layered laminations as prescribed by medical personnel, in order to maintain and prospectively enhance bone mass, density, and strength. Osteolaminal nanodevices could be administered in doses comprised of millions of distinct nanoscale entities in a colloidal suspension, or as a solidified/dissolvable aggregate in pill form.

Each nanodevice would contain an onboard complement of specific molecules that have robust binding affinities for bone-resident minerals, which can be externally displayed for affinity-based targeting purposes. Their slender/streamlined morphologies may allow them to traverse bone/tissue interfaces at an intimate proximity to bone surfaces (hypothetically) beneath the periosteum (a resilient osteoprogenitor cell-resident membrane that encases all skeletal elements) in an organized fashion as semiparallel arrays that might form travelling segmented "rings" to circumscribe bones that are in need of repair or reinforcement. Although the OSTLs would have the capacity for laterally connecting with each other via docking "keys" located on their sides to form an unbroken ring around a bone of interest, this capacity is likely to be only partially utilized. This is due to certain anatomical features at the cortical bone/subperiosteal interface that contain obstructing tethers that proceed directly from subperiosteal surfaces onto/into bone matrices, as well as vascular elements that traverse and run along the space between the two elements. Sharpey's "perforating" fibers (SF) (5–25 μm thick) comprised of elements such as collagen type VI, elastin, and tenascin, which are utilized to anchor the teeth to their sockets, also securely tether ligaments and tendons to the tough outer surfaces of the periosteum [170]. These strain-absorbing microfibers possess irregular profiles (in cross section) ranging from randomly invaginated to horseshoe-shaped to hollow core. Interestingly, when the periosteum is put under load via connections to muscles, enzymatic activity ensues, thus initiating and facilitating bone remodeling [171,172].

Specific external stimuli would induce the OSTLs to form thin film matrices/scaffolds via the release of their onboard payloads of bone-rebuilding biomaterials. For the sake of higher efficacy, the OSTLs might carry short nanofibers that are interspersed with newly laid bone materials to impart additional mechanical and torsional strength to formed matrices.

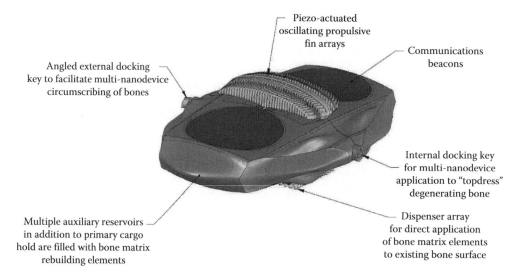

Piezo-actuated
oscillating propulsive
fin arrays

Communications
beacons

Angled external docking
key to facilitate multi-nanodevice
circumscribing of bones

Internal docking key
for multi-nanodevice
application to "topdress"
degenerating bone

Multiple auxiliary reservoirs
in addition to primary cargo
hold are filled with bone matrix
rebuilding elements

Dispenser array
for direct application
of bone matrix elements
to existing bone surface

FIGURE 16.8
Artistic depiction of conceptual autonomous nanomedical osteolaminal bone matrix dispensing device.

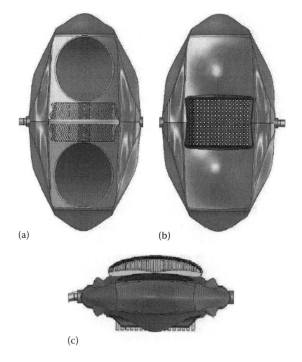

(a)   (b)

(c)

FIGURE 16.9
(a–c) Artistic depiction of top, bottom, and front views of conceptual nanomedical osteolaminal bone matrix dispenser.

In effect, these legions/swarms of autonomous "bone matrix dispensers" [173,174] might methodically transit along the subperiosteal spaces of the entire lengths of bones (under external computer control) to deposit their cargoes as optimally patterned [175] ultrathin layers in a manner analogous to parallel arrays of asphalt "paving" machines (Figures 16.8 through 16.10) Advanced nanomedical bone matrix formulations might rapidly crystallize

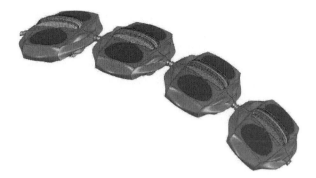

FIGURE 16.10
Artistic depiction of linked conceptual osteolaminals for semicircumscribing segments of microgravity-degraded bones for parallel "topdressing" with bone-rebuilding elements in a nanomedical orthopedic therapeutic procedure.

on contact with existing bone tissues, or contingent on the composition of the formulation, may be simultaneously photonically "cured" via onboard nanoscale UV lasers [176].

Replacement OSTLs would proceed to molecularly tagged sites to take over where initial "first wave" OSTLs have depleted their payloads, to ensure the uniform and complete coverage of affected skeletal elements to compensate for prequantified levels of degradation. OSTLs might refill their internal reservoirs by docking with dedicated microneedles that painlessly protrude through the skin of the patient from the underside of a dermally adhered reservoir patch. This top dressing procedure could conceivably be repeatable as prescribed by medical personnel to ameliorate microgravity-induced bone loss.

Hypothetically, diamondoid or diamond-like carbon nanoparticles may be incorporated within OSTL formulations to cumulatively enhance bone resilience against the deleterious effects of microgravity. Ultrathin films of uniformly thick nanoporous diamondoid for the coating of human bone may facilitate their solid embedment within the existing bone matrix to impart a considerable measure of sustained protection from bone mass loss. Insofar as the amenability of diamond with biological tissues in vivo, diamond-coated zirconium (Zr) has been found to be biocompatible, and demonstrated no inflammation when implanted in Wilster rats for 30 days [177]. A diamond-coated steel implant exhibited a similar benign response when implanted within a human subject for 7 months [178].

Under the assumption that articulating joints might also be coated with nanostructured diamond materials, studies are warranted to elucidate and quantify the volume of diamond nanoparticulates that may be generated over time from diamond-on-diamond wear. In wear simulations of a diamond-coated hip joint conducted by Lappalainen et al., the cumulative debris volume was extrapolated to be $<10^{-4}$ mm^3 year^{-1} [179]. Thomas et al. studied the effect of "nanodiamond wear debris" particulate sizes on the response of RAW 264.7 (mouse leukemic monocyte) macrophages through their incubation with nanodiamonds of variable sizes ranging from Ø6 to 500 nm at concentrations of 0, 10, 50, 100, and 200 µg mL^{-1}. The results verified that the nanodiamonds were indeed phagocytized. However, when observing their effects on the responses of macrophages via cell proliferation, cell morphology, and viability, the genetic expression of pro-inflammatory cytokines and chemokines and other parameters, it was revealed that no inflammation was induced by any size of nanodiamond used in the study at low concentrations ($\leq$50 µg mL^{-1}) [180]. Although, in microgravity environments within spacecraft, on the Moon and on Mars, there will be an obvious reduction in the mechanical forces at joint interfaces, which remains an important issue to be addressed.

Wissner-Gross and Kaxiras reveal an intriguing strategy, based on molecular dynamics simulations, as relates to the wear resistance of diamond, whereby a thin layer of ice may be formed on diamond surfaces in vivo that are treated by a monolayer of sodium Na^+. Their simulations illustrate that this "interfacial ice bilayer" will melt at 130 K above the melting temperature of free ice (265 ± 37 K) at ambient pressure. They stipulate further that "relatively thick ice films (2.6 nm at 298 K and 2.2 nm at 310 K) are stabilized by dipole interactions with the substrate. This unique physical effect may enable biocompatibility-enhancing ice overcoatings for diamond at human body temperature." These pliable diamond ice multilayers (each ~3.7 Å thick) would be hydrophilic, could facilitate abrasion reduction, and prevent the adsorption of clotting proteins such as fibrinogen, thereby increasing biocompatibility. An estimated six ice bilayers (cumulatively 2.2 nm thick) would be required to sustainably remain frozen solid at body temperature (310 K) [181].

16.4 Nanomedical Microgravity Countermeasures: Soft Tissues and DNA

16.4.1 Nanomedical Countermeasures for Microgravity-Induced Muscle Atrophy

Several countermeasures against muscle atrophy as the result of exposure to microgravity have been explored, and include resistance and endurance exercise, as well as nutritional growth factor manipulation [182]. Combined exercise regimens have shown to resist modifications that occur subsequent to long-term bed rest, specifically protein synthesis and degradation, oxidative phosphorylation, and glycolysis [183]. For instance, protein synthesis may be reduced to levels up to 45% in the course of prolonged spaceflight [184], and the mechanical properties of slow-twitch (e.g., soleus) muscle fibers that are utilized in sustained muscle contractions are converted to fast-type muscle fibers, which generate rapid bursts of energy but are rapidly fatigued [185]. Insofar as the identification of potential candidates for nutritional support in the prevention of muscle atrophy, it appears that the anabolic effects of essential amino acids (e.g., branched-chain leucine) have in some, but not all, cases [186,187] demonstrated the capacity for stimulating protein synthesis within skeletal muscle by, for instance, hastening the initiation of peptide chains. Leucine has also been shown to diminish the rate of proteolytic events and "suppress the ubiquitin-proteasome proteolytic pathway and degradation of myofibrillar proteins" [180,188,189].

Muscle gene expression, motility, differentiation, and satellite cell proliferation have been shown to be deeply influenced by certain growth factors such as insulin-like growth factor 1 (IGF-1), a polypeptide protein hormone, fibroblast growth factor (FGF), the cytokine transforming growth factor-beta (TGF-β), and clenbuterol (CB), which stimulates the growth of muscle mass [190,191]. Antioxidants, such as vitamin E [192] and Bowman–Birk inhibitor concentrate (BBIC) [193] have shown to impart some positive effects in counteracting muscle atrophy. Appropriately designed nanocarriers may enable the precise targeting and protracted delivery, as well as optimal distribution of such entities, which may be translatable and reconfigured such that they may function synergistically with nanomedical devices to sustain muscle mass.

Myogenesis is the core process in the development of muscle cells during embryogenesis. The inclusion of heparan sulfate (HS) in the extracellular matrix facilitates the appropriate interplay between FGF-2 and muscle cells to enable their differentiation, proliferation, migration, and adhesion. Due to the large surface areas of gold nanoparticles (AuNPs), a large fraction of their atoms are exposed on their surfaces, thereby making them highly reactive. Gold nanoparticles demonstrate a potent affinity for thiol groups, which enables them to bind preferentially with high efficacy to intracellular substances [194,195]. They also have the capability of entering cells via endocytosis and may be endowed with targeting agents to deliver therapeutic drugs [196], bioactive compounds [197], and nucleic acids [198].

It has been hypothesized by Zielinska and coworkers that when AuNPs are combined with HS that muscle cell formation can be augmented. When chicken embryos were injected with a HS/AuNP complex (50 mg/L concentration, 500 µL dose), the number of breast muscle nuclei was increased considerably from that of controls. An increase in "myocytes and nuclei, and enlarged area of muscle fibers" was observed in the embryos that were treated with HS/AuNP, in contrast to untreated controls or those embryos that were treated with only HP or AuNP [194].

The delivery of small interfering RNAs (siRNAs) (with the capacity for specifically and efficaciously silencing target genes) to the skeletal muscles of healthy and diseased mice via their combination with atelocollagen (ATCOL) as a nanoparticle complex initiated a significant increase in muscle mass over several weeks. Atelocollagen is a highly biocompatible and biodegradable biomaterial that is derived from bovine type I collagen [199], which has been observed to have the capacity for the formation of nanoparticle complexes as small as approx. <$\emptyset$200 nm, with unmodified siRNAs, and enabling effective delivery to metastatic tumors in vivo [200,201]. Kinouchi et al. utilized the siRNA sequence (GDF8 siRNA26, 50 AAGATGACGATTA TCACGCTA-30, position 426–446), which targets myostatin mRNA in humans [202] to downregulate myostatin in the mouse models, and found that the median size of muscle myofibrils of the mice treated with the Mst-siRNA/ATCOL nanoparticle complex was ~1.3 times larger than that of the untreated controls [203].

The delivery of siRNAs to cardiomyocytes, which are typically difficult to transfect, with efficiencies of greater than 95% was accomplished by Ladeira et al. who employed carboxyl-functionalized SWNTs (50–500 nm long) as nanocarriers. The cardiomyocyte beating frequency and overall cell viability were not affected by the introduction of SWNTs within their interiors, at doses of 0.05 mg mL^{-1}. This mode of nanomedical delivery may facilitate the transport of specific cardiac therapeutics to cardiomyocytes in ensuring that the heart muscle maintains optimal physiological integrity in microgravity environments [204]. Martinelli et al. sought to learn if carbon nanotubes might augment the functionality and electrical attributes of cardiac myocytes. A defunctionalized MWNT scaffold (162.75 ± 11.4 nm thick) was synthesized, onto which neonatal rat ventricular myocytes (NRVMs) were cultured. It was found that intimate contacts were formed between the MWNT scaffolding and NRVM membranes, and that the NRVMs modified their "viability, proliferation, growth, maturation, and electrophysiological properties when interacting with carbon nanotube scaffolds." Interestingly, it emerged that the MWNTs both extended cardiac myocyte proliferation, which maintained a portion of the cells in an undifferentiated condition, and hastened the maturation of already differentiated cells. The electrophysiological influence of the MWNT scaffold was that it conveyed a NRVM resting potential, which was more negative in comparison to the controls [205].

The investigators observed that "the resting potential becomes progressively negative as the cells become more adult-like, suggesting that the interaction with carbon nanotubes may promote cell maturation." Other indirect factors involved in the enhancement of myocyte function and proliferation may include influences due to the similarity of the MWNT scaffold to a natural extracellular matrix (ECM) and changes in cell cytoskeletal dynamics [205]. One can envisage that such carbon nanotube based scaffolds might be employed to grow heart muscle cells as part of an advanced tissue engineering capability onboard future spacecraft for the potential replacement of degraded heart muscles of astronauts, due to prolonged exposure to microgravity.

16.4.2 Nanomedical Strategies for the Repair of Microgravity-Induced Brain Damage

The nanomedical transplantation of cells to restore degraded or destroyed cell populations and neuronic circuitry may involve the precisely targeted transport of stem cells via programmable biomaterials or nanocarriers to the brain [206], spinal cord, or any site in the human body that has sustained nerve damage due to microgravity. The growth and repair of brain-resident (neuron and glial) cells and nerve cells might make use of multilayered electrospun polymeric nanowire scaffolds. These scaffolds could be employed in ex vivo tissue engineering or conceivably administered to the patient as targeted nanoscale entities, which would self-assemble at treatment sites. Alhosseini et al. utilized electrospun polyvinyl alcohol (PVA)/chitosan nanofiber (Ø221 nm with a range of 94–410 nm) scaffolds that formed micron-sized pores at their interstices. The inclusion of pores within scaffold matrices is critical in that they enable cell migration, the propagation of blood vessels, and facilitate nutrient and waste product exchange between cells and their immediate surroundings. PC12 nerve cells derived from rat adrenal medulla were cultured in vitro on the PVA/chitosan nanofiber scaffold and were found to react favorably to this substrate, as they remained viable, attached, proliferated, and migrated at higher rates in comparison to a solely PVA nanofiber scaffold. The researchers concluded that this may be attributed to a number of physicochemical and biological properties that are amenable to nerve cells provided by the addition of chitosan, encompassing a smaller nanofiber diameter, an increased amount of amine present at surfaces, and lower water content [207].

Jang et al. showed that E18 rat hippocampal neurite growth followed the biomimetic extracellular matrix-like micropatterns provided by successive "bars" of octadecyltrichlorosilane (OTS) and pristine carbon nanotubes (Figure 16.11), which were subsequently coated with poly-L-lysine (PLL) (a cell adhesion protein), giving substrates of ~20 to 30 nm thickness. It was observed that prolonged E18 cultures were strikingly similar to "in vivo neural circuit structures." It was postulated that the neurite guidance and elongation mechanisms along the carbon nanotube tracks might derive from the higher affinity of the PLL to the carbon nanotubes. It appeared that the application of the PLL was critical for the attachment of neurites, as there was none seen on the carbon nanotube or OTS substrates, which were devoid of the PLL coating [208].

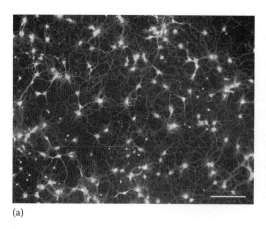
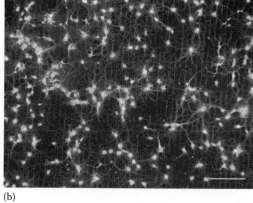

(a) (b)

FIGURE 16.11
Networks of neurons (at seven divisions) cultured on (a) carbon nanotube-only substrate and (b) carbon nanotube/OTS patterned substrate. Cell plating density for (a) was 200 cells/mm^{-2}. Scale bar = 100 μm. (Reproduced from Jang, M.J. et al., *Nanotechnology* 21(23), 235102, 2010. With permission.)

Contingent on the severity of damage to the brain, due to the combination of prolonged exposures to ionizing radiation and microgravity, more intensive (quite radical or indeed impossible from our perspective today—2012) nanomedical procedures might come into play. One of these, as described by Merkle [209], would involve the cryogenic suspension (see Section 16.6.3) of the patient and molecular repair of the brain in its frozen state. An insightful and intriguing observation put forward by Merkle stipulates that as ultra-highly organized assemblages of atoms of which human beings are entirely comprised, the fundamental difference between healthy and diseased states has its source in the specific spatial arrangements of the various species of atoms. As Merkle explains:

> The brain, like all the familiar matter in the world around us, is made of atoms. It is the spatial arrangement of these atoms that distinguishes an arm from a leg, the head from the heart, and sickness from health. This view of the brain is the framework for our problem, and it is within this framework that we must work. Our problem, broadly stated, is that the atoms in a frozen brain are in the wrong places. We must put them back where they belong (with perhaps some minor additions and removals, as well as just rearrangements) if we expect to restore the natural functions of this most wonderful organ.

Hence, it would seem plausible that when we eventually evolve the capacity to image/map the human body (e.g., vital organs and tissues in particular) in situ in their optimal healthy condition at atomic level resolution for utilization as a reference 3D atomic coordinate template, it seems plausible that any misalignment within these elegant atomic puzzles may translate to the ability of being able to identify and conceivably correct molecular level damage or disease anywhere within the human "aggregate" system. Merkle calculates that insofar as the data required in ascertaining where each atom is positioned in 3D space: "If we could record the position of each atom to within 0.01 nm, we would know its position accurately enough to know what chemicals it was a part of, what bonds it had formed, and so on," and further that the positions of individual atoms in the brain could be fully described when allocated to ~100 bits of data, which might be reduced to ~24.5 bits via improved encoding [209,210]. If it is deemed that the brain damage inflicted by ionizing radiation and microgravity can be satisfactorily repaired at molecular resolution, spatial data requirements would likely be significantly reduced. If malconfigurations in the brain can be rectified by sufficiently sophisticated dedicated nanomedical assemblers at atomic or molecular resolution in accordance with original reference spatial data maps, the restoration of optimal health for the patient should be possible. The repair of neurons and their processes, as well as glial cells, astrocytes, oligodendrocytes, and other brain-resident constituents might be repaired by the earlier method without the requirement of cryogenic suspension, which may be reserved for only the most extreme cases of injury or cellular degradation.

As relates to the current status of nanomedical research in brain repair, Santos et al. describe the potential use of multipotent neural stem cells (NSCs) that reside within particular zones of the brain to refresh neurons, astrocytes, and oligodendrocytes. It is surmised that the activation of NCS differentiation might be triggered through the delivery of neurogenesis-inducing biomolecules via targeted nanoparticles, with minimal side effects [211]. In contrast to the earlier perspective that brain physiology is set static and incapable of generating new neurons, recent research provides compelling evidence to the contrary. Two specific regions of the brain (germinal subventricular and hippocampal subgranular zones located "between the lateral ventricles and the parenchyma of the striatum") contain renewable NSCs that may indeed replenish damaged neurons and other brain cells [212–216].

In addition to the specific targeting and delivery of NSCs, the nanocarriers may themselves provide rudimentary structural support matrices to nurture newly transplanted neural cells.

It was demonstrated by Bible et al. that when NSCs were combined with "plasma polymer-ised allylamine (ppAAm)-treated poly(D,L-lactic acid-co-glycolic acid) (PLGA) scaffold parti-cles" (Ø50 and 200 mm) and injected into mice, they facilitated their integration with existing tissues via the generation of an elementary "neural tissue" [217]. A number of nanocarriers have been developed that can enable the transport of NSCs to the brain, including liposomes (Chapter 12), micelles, nanoparticles comprised of solid lipids, various polymeric formula-tions in the Ø10–1000 nm range, encompassing "poly(lactic acid) (PLA), poly(glycolic acid) (PGA), poly[lactide-co-glycolide] (PLGA), poly(alkylcyanoacrylate), polyanhydride, poly[bis-(p-carboxyphenoxy) propane-sebacic acid] (PCCP-SA), [and] polyethyleneimine (PEI)," silica nanoparticles, and dendrimers [211]. These nanocarriers may circumvent the blood–brain barrier (BBB) through intranasal pathways, where they may traverse to the brain within olfactory neuron cells (Chapter 2), or through more direct, albeit invasive means, including the intracerebroventricular route, where pharmaceuticals are administered into the ventri-cles of the brain [218], or via convection-enhanced delivery that employs a small gauge cath-eter that is stereotactically guided into the bulk brain tissue [219]. As relates to this chapter, however, it is probable that in the era of advanced spaceflight and mature nanomedicine that most, if not all, invasive medical procedures will have long been superseded.

The differentiation of NSCs via the intracellular delivery of retinoic acid (RA) to (RXR/RAR) receptors that are present on the surfaces of NSC nuclei was reported by Duester [220], and Maia et al. demonstrated that Ø200 nm polyelectrolyte nanoparticles loaded with RA (86 ± 28 μg of RA per mg of nanoparticle) were quickly internalized by subventricular stem cell cytoplasms and enabled neurogenesis. Due to its combination with PEI, the RA was released at the rate of >63 ng/mL at physiological pH [221]. Although RA is inherently hydrophobic, its water solubility may be electrostatically enhanced when attended by poly-cations such as PEI and chitosan [211].

As microgravity-induced oxidative stress [222], alterations in numerous brain pro-teins (e.g., in the hippocampus and hypothalamus), and distorted cell signaling events are known to negatively impact the brain [223], a prudent therapeutic approach onboard spacecraft may combine the use of potent nanomedical antioxidants, as well as NSC acti-vators, which could be delivered by the appropriate nanocarriers to the affected regions of the brain. Further out, one can envision that dedicated autonomous nanomedical cell repair devices might be tasked with triple duty to monitor, diagnose, and treat the brain, on an as-required basis during extended space exploration missions, and for the protec-tion of those individuals who undertake eventual Lunar and Martian exploration and the establishment of planetary habitats.

16.4.3 Nanomedical Strategies to Attenuate Microgravity-Induced Ocular Anomalies

Though it is well-established that ocular damage to the eye (e.g., cataracts and retinal degeneration) is a consequence of exposure to ionizing radiation, the impacts of micro-gravity alone on ocular cells and tissues require further elucidation. Roberts et al. utilized a NASA-designed rotating wall vessel (RWV) bioreactor that simulates microgravity to study its effects on human retinal pigment epithelial (hRPE) cells in comparison to con-trols in nonrotating wall vessels at ambient gravity. On exposure to 24 h of simulated microgravity, the hRPE cells sustained a considerable degree of single-strand DNA breaks in comparison to the controls, and this damage was not rectified within 48 h postexpo-sure. The number of oligonucleotide breaks was reduced by half, however, when the cells were pretreated with 1 μM cysteine, followed by a 48 h recovery period. Additionally, there was a considerable secretion of prostaglandin E_2 (PGE_2), which indicated an acute inflammatory response to microgravity [224]. Retinal inflammation poses a severe concern for astronauts, as typically, the blood/retinal barrier thwarts access to the retina from the majority of immune cells that generate ROS [225]. Hence, if this barrier is breached and an immune response proceeds, the ensuing damage may result in retinal deterioration and/or retinal detachment. Retinal inflammation and the discharge of PGE_2 can also jeopardize the integrity of the retina by inducing macular degeneration and proliferative vitreoretinopathy [226–229].

A nanomedical strategy for addressing retinal inflammation may involve the delivery of lutein and zeaxanthin-loaded nanocarriers that have the capacity for traversing the blood–retina barrier (BRB), without imparting cytotoxicity, to directly convey their payloads to the retina to preserve its functionality. Lutein, zeaxanthin, and meso-zeaxanthin are xanthophyll carotenoids (cumulatively known as the macular pigment) that provide protection for retinal neurons through beneficial attributes as antioxidants, anti-apoptotics, and anti-inflammatory agents [226,230].

Kim et al. observed that injected AuNPs (~Ø20 nm) could transit through the BRB, where within 24 h, they were found to be distributed throughout all retinal layers (in neurons 75% ± 5%, in ECs 17% ± 6%, and bound to membrane surfaces of peri-endothelial glial cells 8% ± 3%), whereas no Ø100 nm AuNPs were able to traverse the BRB [231]. These macular pigments might be reformulated as a colloidal suspension, as nanocrystals or nanoparticles, and encapsulated within hollow gold nanoshells, or adhered to the outer surfaces of AuNPs for delivery to the retina. This strategy may allow for the delivery of higher concentrations of these constituents to the retina with enhanced bioavailability as their maximum concentrations through dietary intake are likely to be far too low to offset the far greater stresses that must be endured by the retina in the radiation/microgravity-permeated space environment. As a matter of course, a rigorous protocol toward the potential implementation of any nanomedicines should be established, whereby stringent testing would be undertaken to elucidate the maximum allowable concentrations for each of the macular pigments that may be safely employed to optimize their use as retinal therapeutics. In ensuring successful passage across the BRB, the nanocarrier formulation criteria should include that the maximum nanocarrier/lutein, zeaxanthin, or meso-zeaxanthin BRB transit diameter of ~Ø20 nm is maintained.

Thomson and Lotery review a number of nanocarriers that might be tailored specifically for ocular applications. In addition to liposomes and dendrimers, albumin is identified as potentially serving as a viable ocular nanocarrier as it is nontoxic, nonantigenic, and biodegradable. Additionally, albumin contains a significant complement of amino acids that endows it with the ability to bind with either positively or negatively charged oligonucleotides or therapeutic chemical groups [232]. The synthetic polymers PLA and poly(lactide-co-glycolide) (PLGA) may be good candidates as well, in that post-delivery, they degrade to natural metabolites. Kim et al. investigated the release profile of the anti-inflammatory and immunosuppressive glucocorticoid agent dexamethasone (DEX), which was combined with PLGA nanoparticles (~400 to 600 nm) that were embedded within the alginate hydrogel matrices. The nanoparticle DEX loading capacity was found to be 13 wt%, and over 2 weeks ~90% of the drug was released [233]. The advantage of these entities is that they may be fine-tuned to degrade and release their drug payloads over days or up to several years [234,235]. This capability alone would vastly simplify the requirement for sustained drug release over long timelines in ensuring the continual protection of astronaut vision in microgravity.

Cerium oxide nanoparticles can serve as regenerating catalytic antioxidants to protect retinal neurons due to their redox capabilities, whereby their valence may be actively toggled between trivalent and quadrivalent states [236,237]. It was revealed by Deshpande et al. that as the dimensions of ceria nanoparticles shrink (~Ø3–5 nm), the number of resident oxygen vacancies within its crystalline structure is increased [238–240].

Microgravity-induced cerebrospinal fluid flow disturbances within the optic nerve sheath, in conjunction with venous congestion either in the brain or eye or both, due to cephalad fluid shifts and alterations in choroidal volume are ascribed by Mader et al. to explain the globe flattening, choroidal folds, optic disc edema, and hyperopic shifts that are experienced by astronauts [6]. Papilledema, which can also be brought on by microgravity, is correlated with increased intracranial pressure conveyed to the subarachnoid space (surrounding the brain) and the optic nerve [241]. It is thought that all of these conditions stem from a venous obstructive process known as space obstructive syndrome, which involves the proximal internal jugular veins at four susceptible "compression zones," leading to increased intraocular pressure, intracranial hypertension, and swelling [242].

A range of nanocarriers might deliver encapsulated or impregnated formulations of fixed prostaglandin analog–timolol (beta-blocker) combinations, carbonic anhydrase inhibitors, or muscarinic receptor agonists for the reduction of intraocular pressure [243]. Nanospheres comprised of PLGA–PLLA have demonstrated the prolonged delivery (>3 months) of timolol and neurotrophic proteins to boost the viability, regeneration, and differentiation of neural cells [244]. The renewal of axons may also be facilitated through the utilization of self-assembled peptide scaffolds or protein-decorated nanotubes/fibers. The potential regeneration of the optic nerve itself might be enabled through the use of a "glial-derived neurotrophic factor (GDNF)–nanofiber composite scaffold," which was shown by Chen et al., to augment the regeneration of a rat sciatic nerve with "increased myelinated axons, and improved electrophysiologic function" [245,246]. The prevention and treatment of this complex of interrelated ocular conditions in the microgravity environment will likely consist of a multifaceted program that includes an advanced means of applying artificial gravity onboard spacecraft, tailored exercise regimens, as well as dietary and antioxidant supplementation. A dedicated suite of nanomedical therapeutics might be employed to directly target the compression zones mentioned previously, as well as swelling prone sites, and enable the precise delivery of stems cells, anti-inflammatory, and nerve-regenerating compounds.

16.4.4 Nanomedical Strategies for the Repair of Microgravity-Induced DNA Damage

A robust means for the preservation of the integrity and viability of DNA molecules and the proteins that they encode will be absolutely essential for long-haul human space travel and the eventual human habitation of the Moon, Mars, and beyond. Nanomedical interventions will likely play key roles in the development of these capacities.

16.4.4.1 Magnesium Nanoparticles for the Restoration of DNA

There exist within human cell nuclei (~Ø5–10 μm) 12 species of naturally occurring proteinaceous DNA repair mechanisms, which are encoded by ~150 genes. Each of these self-assembling "nanomachines" is dedicated to repairing a particular type of insult that is inflicted on the DNA duplex. Although DNA DSB in humans are quite uncommon in the terrestrial setting, ionizing radiation is their principal cause in the space environment [247]. When both strands of the duplex are cleaved and left repaired, extraordinarily deleterious effects may ensue [248] resulting in genomic instability via the "large-scale loss of information during cell division and consequently, cell death" [249]. The mending of a

DSB is undertaken by two repair mechanisms and occurs nearly instantaneously once the breach has been discovered. One strategy utilizes homologous recombination, whereby an unaffected sequence from a sister chromatid is employed as a repair template [250], while the other makes use of DNA ligase to directly fuse cleaved duplex ends by exploiting nonhomologous end joining (NHEJ), which can result in inaccuracies and thus a distorted sequence segment being left at the repair site [251] (Refs. [248–251] from [247]). The speed of DSB repair in humans has a typical half time of ~15 to 30 min, where NHEJ is initiated by the Ku molecule, a protein that numbers about 300,000 per cell, with a robust affinity for the cleaved DSB sites [252,253].

In addition to ionizing radiation, microgravity has also been observed to have deleterious effects on DNA and its repair mechanisms [254]. It has been elucidated by Rowe that a significant decrease ($p < 0.0001$) in serum magnesium (Mg) (an antioxidant and calcium blocker) is concomitant with human exposure to microgravity, as was revealed by extensive studies of astronauts and cosmonauts [255,256]. Magnesium is critical for the binding of telomerase to DNA, which enables the elongation of telomeres, and hence, the stabilization of chromosomes, as well as the promotion of DNA replication and transcription. Deficient Mg levels are associated with oxidative stress, hastened cell senescence, DNA instability, diminished protein synthesis, and reduced mitochondrial function [257,258]. Human ECs that were deprived of Mg for only 2 h exhibited increased levels of 8-hydroxy-deoxyguanine (primary DNA repair product generated as a consequence of DNA damage due to oxidative stress) in comparison to controls [259].

A potential nanomedical strategy for the maintenance of healthy human Mg concentrations in microgravity may involve the utilization of appropriately formulated Mg nanoparticles for the prolonged release of Mg ions, not only to sustain healthy plasma levels but also Mg levels within intracellular compartments, which decrease with age and may not necessarily be reflected in plasma concentrations [255]. Shafiee et al. demonstrated the use of magnetic, magnesium ($^{25}Mg^{2+}$)-loaded nanoparticles (Porphylleren-MC16 or PMC16) for the transport of Mg to cardiac cells in the hearts of rats to reduce malathion-induced toxicity. The PMC16 was an "iron containing porphyrin monoadduct of a classical buckminster fullerene," and Mg that it delivered acted to boost mitochondrial energy production via the initiation of increased ATP levels [260]. It has been shown that only when Mg is in its magnetic isotopic form of $^{25}Mg^{2+}$ does it serve a critical role in the Mg-associated generation of ATP [261–263].

16.4.4.2 Chromosome Replacement Therapy

In an era of mature nanotechnology and nanomedicine, the complete changeover of defective chromosomes, with replacements synthesized from the patients' own DNA, may be achievable. This capability may be especially useful, if not vital, for the survival of humans on long-duration space missions, where personnel might be required to undergo numerous such replacements to maintain optimal health. Freitas has suggested this possibility, and describes how the procedure might proceed:

> Medical nanorobots will also be able to intervene at the cellular level, performing in vivo cytosurgery. The most likely site of pathological function in the cell is the nucleus – more specifically, the chromosomes. In one simple cytosurgical procedure, a nanorobot controlled by a physician would extract existing chromosomes from a diseased cell and insert new ones in their place. This is called chromosome replacement therapy. The replacement chromosomes will be manufactured to order, outside of the

patient's body in a laboratory benchtop production device that includes a molecular assembly line, using the patient's individual genome as the blueprint. The replacement chromosomes are appropriately demethylated, thus expressing only the appropriate exons that are active in the cell type to which the nanorobot has been targeted. If the patient chooses, inherited defective genes could be replaced with nondefective base-pair sequences, permanently curing a genetic disease. Given the speed with which nanorobots can be administered and their potential rapidity of action, it is possible that an entire whole-body procedure could be completed in one hour or less [264].

Issues to be explored and resolved in order for this prospectively powerful nanomedical procedure to be successful in space and heavily irradiated extraterrestrial environments will include the establishment of stringent protocols for the extraction and expedited replication of the entire genomes of each individual onboard spacecraft, or those individuals who are residents of Lunar and Mars habitats. It may indeed be the case, toward the negation of the otherwise high likelihood that immediate damage may be inflicted on DNA (via ionizing radiation) within the intended replacement chromosomes, that appropriately shielded (radiation-free) laboratories and storage facilities be developed to enable the synthesis and long-term storage of perhaps many multiple copies per patient, of pristine replacement chromosomes.

16.4.4.3 Vasculoid Medical Robotic System

In a radical departure from any biologically based nanomedical therapeutic strategy in dealing with the degradative effects of space radiation and microgravity, Freitas and Phoenix have conducted an intriguing preliminary hypothetical analysis (assuming mature nanomanufacturing) pertaining to the complete replacement of the human vasculature, and blood, with a highly sophisticated aggregate of hundreds of trillions of individual nanorobots. This system would also be cardioplegic (devoid of a heartbeat). As they explain the concept:

> The vasculoid is a single, complex, multisegmented nanotechnological medical robotic system capable of duplicating all essential thermal and biochemical transport functions of the blood, including circulation of respiratory gases, glucose, hormones, cytokines, waste products, and cellular components. This nanorobotic system, a very aggressive and physiologically intrusive macroscale nanomedical device comprised of ~500 trillion stored or active individual nanorobots, weighs ~2 kg and consumes from 30 to 200 watts of power in the basic human model, depending on activity level. The vasculoid system conforms to the shape of existing blood vessels and serves as a complete replacement for natural blood [265].

In addition to the perceived extreme complexity that would be involved with actually developing such a system, a plethora of moral and ethical aversions (understandably from our current biological perspective) to such an invasive procedure, including of the prospect of transgressing the human line to cyborgism (Chapter 17) are highly likely. However, in the event (despite our best efforts) that no plausible or sustainable solutions can be found to ensure the safe traversal of space for humans via complete protection from the harmful effects of ionizing radiation and microgravity, serious future astronaut/space exploration candidates may indeed consider such a transformative procedure if it can, in the distant future, be successfully accomplished. Should this type of drastic nanomedical intervention allow them to explore the stars, and to witness what no other human being has ever seen, they may be willing to boldly attempt to extend their reach.

16.5 Precursors to Nanomedically Enhanced Space Suits

In view of the expansive array of degradative processes, as briefly surveyed earlier, that pose significant health risks (physiological/cognitive/psychological) to astronauts in spaceflight, it is evident that isolating and remedying only several of these maladies, although cumulatively beneficial, will not be adequate. It is clear that if humankind ever hopes to endure long-duration spaceflight and the exploration of deep space while maintaining the vigorous health of its best and brightest astronauts, cosmic explorers, and in the more distant future, human settlers, it is necessary to establish that nothing less than the implementation of a robust holistic strategy for the complete protection of humans in space and planetary environments will suffice. This strategy will likely involve integrated multipronged solutions for protection from the effects of ionizing radiation and weightlessness. In conjunction with tangible macroscale technologies (e.g., sustained 1 g artificial gravity onboard spacecraft, via centrifuge, to directly counteract all microgravity effects, and perhaps in future, localized within human habitats on the Moon and Mars) and solid behavioral and space adaptive countermeasures, nanotechnological and nanomedical approaches might be anticipated to facilitate the negation of myriad radiation and microgravity-induced health issues.

Materials that have conventionally been employed in the composition of shielding against gamma-radiation include lead, steel, tungsten, boron, gold, silver, platinum, palladium, hafnium, tantalum, gadolinium, osmium, or combinations thereof [266]. Investigations of gamma-ray shielding glasses have also been undertaken that include bismuth–borate [267], ZnO-PbO-B_2O_3 [268], CaO-SrO-B_2O_3, Bi_2O_3-PbO-B_2O_3, PbO-B_2O_3 [269], PbO-$BaOB_2O_3$ [270,271], PbO-SiO_2 [272] systems. The attenuation of gamma-ray and thermal neutron beams through the use of open-cell aluminum foams, which were infused with either water or a boric acid solution, was investigated by and showed that the liquid-containing foams had improved performance in blocking gamma-rays than did bulk aluminum. It was surmised that the water-filled metallic foam attenuation could be attributed to the high hydrogen content. By increasing the boric acid solution concentration (2% w/v to 3% w/v), an improvement in a neutron beam attenuation was achieved and was totally negated using a 1-1/2″ thick foam. This was thought to be due to the presence of 10 B isotopes that have a "high cross-section for absorption of low energy (thermal) neutrons" [271].

In terms of the complete individual protection of astronauts from ionizing radiation while they undertake myriad extravehicular/extraterrestrial tasks, ultra-lightweight yet highly effective shielding in-suit technologies will be required. Zhang et al. developed a mechanically resilient microcellular PMMA/graphene (1.8% vol.) nanocomposite foams using subcritical CO_2 as the foaming agent. This nanocomposite material, permeated with semispherical cells in the size range of from 1 to 10 μm, was highly conductive (3.11 S/m) with an enhanced capacity for shielding against electromagnetic interference (EMI) (13–19 dB at 8–12 GHz). The shielding ability of this nanocomposite was ascribed to its absorption of electromagnetic radiation through multicell internal reflective and scattering events; hence, its energy dissipation might also be exploited in energy harvesting [273]. Huang et al. studied the EMI shielding effects of SWNT epoxy composites and found that they had a shielding capacity of 20 dB at 10 MHz–1.5 GHz, with an optimal performance (with SWNT content at 15 wt%) of 15–20 dB from 500 to 1.5 GHz and 49 dB at 10 MHz [274].

It may be prudent toward ensuring such protection that dedicated preventative/reparative nanomedical therapeutics be utilized in vivo to serve as supplemental protective layers in addition to advanced space suit-integrated shielding. Nanomedically enhanced, personalized space suits might be comprised of advanced nanomaterials, as well as numerous sophisticated interlinked components that are electronically intertethered and enabled with pervasive levels of functional redundancy, which are in constant real-time communication. The ultimate purpose of such an advanced space suit would be for the provision of optimal protection and safety of its occupant, inclusive of a rapid and highly competent array of initial medical responses.

An important array of medical capabilities might be driven by dedicated space suit-integrated software that is utilized as a highly detailed physiological database/template to assist in maintaining the best of health for astronauts. A NASA-supported effort by the National Space Biomedical Research Institute has been implemented as an integrative physiology program under the moniker "digital human," with the aim of developing "a quantitative description of a healthy human being that contains state-of-the-art information on each component of the body and on how these components relate to each other." In essence, this program would enable access to the complete knowledge of human biomolecular, organellar, cellular, organ systems, and their interactions [275]. When integrated into a nanomedically enabled space suit, this capacity might allow for exponential advances in the provision of a wide array of real-time medical interventions for astronauts.

Fei et al. investigated and developed a "Space Sock" that contained a series of embedded modular biomedical sensors intended for the real-time monitoring of the physiological parameters of astronauts during extravehicular activities (EVAs) in free space, and when engaged in Lunar or Martian expeditions. The primary elements of this system encompassed a sensing sock, a sensor processor module, and a computer that was enabled with communications, avionics, and informatics capabilities. The sensing sock was fabric-based and housed multiple noninvasive sensors, which interfaced with the skin of the occupant. This system had its focus on peripheral blood flow, and the physiological data acquisition compliment included

1. *Plethysmograph sensor*—employed infrared photoelectric sensing to quantify alterations in tissue/blood perfusion. Blood volume changes could be correlated via respiration.

2. *Galvanic skin resistance sensor*—indicated stress by utilizing two electrodes adhered to the skin surface to measure impaired sweat response.

3. *Skin temperature sensor*—used a low applied voltage to discern skin conductively in the calculation of skin temperature.

4. *Pulse oximetry sensor*—utilized an infrared photoelectric probe that was interfaced with the skin of the astronaut's toe to determine the percentage of hemoglobin oxygen saturation and heart rate.

One of the drawbacks of the Space Sock pertained to the elevated oxygen content of the pressurized space suit, which poses difficulties for the safe in-suit integration of electronic circuitry and batteries. Hence, the cables from each sensor were fed through ports in the space suit to batteries, sensor-processing module (containing stabilization, amplifier, and band-pass filter circuits), and the computer [276]. Extrapolations of this type of integrated sensor system within space suits will likely evolve to increasingly diminutive and sophisticated capabilities for the monitoring of myriad physiological parameters and the development of nanomedical strategies that aim to rapidly respond to almost any medical emergency in situ.

The integration of nanomaterials into a wearable radiation-protective covering has been described in a patent by Chen and Mckay. A wearable radiation-protective strategy utilizing nanomaterials has been devised by NASA (U.S. patent 7,923,709) [277], whereby ionizing radiation is harvested, discharged/dissipated, and converted to electrical energy via multiple substrates of SWNT or MWNT (Ø10–50 nm × 50–100 nm long) arrays with a density of 0.05–0.5 gm/cm^2 and tip-to-tip spacing of ~50–1000 nm. The nanotubes are coated with conductive polymers such as polyethylene or polypyrrole at a thickness of 100–1000 nm. The patent states that an alternate system employs metallic "fingers" (e.g., Ti, Mo, W, Os, Co, Rh, Ir, Ni, Cu, Ag, Au, Zn, or Cd) in place of the carbon nanotubes. The inventors stipulate, "a fabric, body covering or other layered or laminated body protection system that can be used to greatly reduce the effects of radiation incident on a person." Such protective layers, if they function as portrayed, might be integrated into space suits to work in conjunction with potent antioxidant therapeutics (see Section 16.3.1) for the enhanced protection of their occupants.

When humans come to inhabit the Moon and Mars, an important issue to address will involve the exclusion of omnipresent silicon dioxide (SiO_2) dust particulates (Ø10 nm to ~>Ø1 mm) that permeate these environments. Fine powdery regolith particulates may be the source of many potentially serious problems including the coating of essential solar panels and the penetration of seals that are meant to isolate and maintain optimal/pristine conditions within the internal environments of space suits, vehicles, and habitats. The inhalation of these particulates would definitely not be conducive to human health. Thus, a robust dust mitigation capacity embedded into space suits, vehicles, and habitats will have critical implications for the safety and health of future extraterrestrial explorers and settlers. A potential strategy proposed by Chen and Wu would utilize the repellent force of 13.8 kHz 128 dB acoustic standing waves to surmount van der Waals adhesive forces at the surfaces to essentially induce the particles to levitate and dislodge. This capacity is described as potentially being used in conjunction with some type of airflow capacity. It seems, however, that this would indeed be a superfluous use of precious oxygen and other gases in these environments. The efficiency of such a system is also shown to drop for particles that are smaller than Ø2 μm [278]. A potential investigation in this area might involve the use of dense piezoelectric nanowire arrays (e.g., zinc oxide) that are invisible to the naked eye to generate a thin, albeit solid and continuously active ultrasonic dust repellent barrier at surfaces.

At present, space suits are pressurized with 100% oxygen at ~222 mmHg [279]. This condition significantly impedes astronaut freedom of movement and flexibility. A number of researchers have investigated the advantages of elastic mechanical counterpressure (MCP) space suits over conventional designs. This strategy involves the application of negative ambient pressure via the use of a form-fitting elastic suit (in future perhaps utilizing integrated weaves of electrically activated conductive polymeric nanofibers or shape memory alloys acting as a dynamic and resilient morphing membrane of artificial muscle) that would act to uniformly compress the body (except the head) of the occupant as an alternative to pressurizing it. Various segments of such a flexible suit might have the capacity to rapidly relax and tighten in deft response to the slightest movements of its inhabitant. The replacement of stiff and cumbersome joints with tough yet soft and pliable elastic materials will allow for considerable improvements in comfort, limb extension, dexterity, and fine digit articulation [280,281]. Other considerations involve the development of an automated in-suit thermoregulatory capability as well as a self-contained, compact, and light personal life support system (PLSS) with the capacity to sustain and protect astronauts for up to hundreds of hours. A suit-dubbed "Chameleon" utilizes electroactive polymers, in addition to wearable electronics and thermal infrared electrochromic materials, to detect the internal and external environments of the suit to automatically adjust heat conduction between suit layers [282].

16.6 Conceptual Nanomedically Enhanced "Interskin"

Nanotechnology and nanomedicine enhanced extravehicular space suits will allow for a dynamic and intimate interface between astronaut occupants with advanced medical nanodevices, embedded nanomaterials, and AI, which would cumulatively serve to elegantly orchestrate sophisticated nanomedical diagnostic and rapid response therapeutic capabilities. Ideally, light and flexible, yet extremely resilient, "Interskin" (IS) class space suits will be sufficiently advanced such that when donned, they will auto-activate, resize to fit snugly (negative pressure) to the physical contours of the occupant, and proceed immediately with a total body scan and biochemical diagnostic examination and assessment toward the rapid generation of a highly personalized, real-time onboard medical profile. To facilitate this procedure, the astronaut would insert an electronic "medic tab" key into an IS-provided data connection port, which contains his/her complete medical physiological and psychological parameters and history.

The vital signs of the occupant, down to the most subtle physiological and biochemical functions, would be constantly monitored. Any deviation from the occupant's optimal (reference) physiological profile (predetermined and programmed into the IS) would be rapidly assessed by AI and compensated for if required, via an onboard "molecular pharmacy" that is stocked with a full compliment of nanomedical devices, with the ability to quickly addressing almost any conceivable physiological aberration or injury. The IS would henceforth transition to a state of semi-engaged medical readiness and prompt the astronaut to don his or her helmet. The donning of a conceptual "Envisor" helmet would initiate full engagement, full power up, AI integration, sealing, and safety checklist protocols. This helmet would serve as a highly dynamic and advanced multifunctional nanotechnology-enabled system in its own right, and further, would provide a virtually seamless and instantaneous communicative interface between the indwelling astronaut and all configurable aspects of the IS space suit. A thorough Envisor-initiated brain scan would complete the initial in situ health status check. At this stage, the astronaut and the AI-controlled IS would essentially function as a single fully integrated synergistic entity.

The conceptual IS would be light and pliable enough so as to be completely comfortable for indwelling astronauts, to accommodate and sustain them for long periods if necessary (e.g., several months). It would allow for safe, secure, and potentially extended duration "off ship" (e.g., maintenance or repair tasks) or "off base" (e.g., terrestrial exploratory or scientific investigative) expeditions.

16.6.1 Interskin Power

A unique, if not vital, feature of the IS would be its capacity for generating its own power to complement and continually recharge embedded banks of lightweight laminated thin film batteries. Beyond the provision of basic life support, this capability will be critical in terms of powering onboard nanomedical infrastructures. While some classes of in vivo autonomous nanodevices will be self-powered via in vivo energy-harvesting (Chapter 4), others will be activated by external sources that are embedded within the layered IS.

Interskin-generated power might be accomplished by lining the entire suit with a durable thin film layer that is comprised of aligned arrays of billions of piezoelectric nanowires or nanotubes (e.g., zinc oxide, barium titanate, cadmium selenide) [283–285] that will produce voltage in response to being flexed by the slightest movement that is imparted by the occupant. The infinitesimal voltages produced by individual nanowires or nanotubes might cumulatively provide sufficient power to sustainably operate the suit. Lightweight and comfortable, yet ruggedized, footwear would be fitted with similar piezoelectric pressure pads that would generate voltage via bipedal (heel strike) foot pressures [286,287].

Accessory power modalities might also include the generation of electricity via the exploitation of the potentially significant temperature differentials (Seebeck effect) that will exist between the warm interior surfaces of the IS in contrast to frigid or scalding exterior surfaces (e.g., vacuum of free space/planets that are devoid of atmosphere, or on close proximity exposure to the heat of planetary volcanic regions, respectively). In addition, the entire outer surface of the IS might be endowed with high-performance ultrathin film photovoltaic collectors. As described in Section 16.5, electrical energy from cosmic ionizing radiation could also be harvested through the use of unique combinations of conductive nanomaterials.

In the deeper hypothetical realm, it would be interesting to learn if supplemental electrical energy might be generated from "atomic outgassing," whereby atomic elements (e.g., carbon atoms that are stripped from the CO_2 generated by the respiration of the occupant) are induced to slowly seep from the IS. A number of specialized venting "patches" that are perforated with arrays of tortuous ~2 Å piezofiber-lined pores would lead from the warm gaseous interior to the frigid ambient vacuum. The tortuous angstrom-sized pores might be formed through the offsetting of laminated stacks of atomic layer thick graphene layers [288,289].

Carbon atoms with diameters of ~1.8 Å may be simultaneously "pushed" from sequestered reservoirs of C atoms (which have been stripped from CO_2, releasing oxygen atoms for recycling) from the interior of the IS through tortuous arrays of "Åpores" and "pulled" via external vacuum at a certain velocity that would be determined by the internal IS pressure, as well as the diameters and extent of the tortuosity of the pores. The cumulative friction caused by multiple streams of outbound C atoms through these tortuous Åpores may induce the piezo nanofibers to generate voltage. As a potential option, the graphene sheets themselves could be nanoengineered to exhibit piezoelectric properties. Ong and Reed have demonstrated that inherently nonpiezoelectric graphene sheets can be transformed into piezoelectric materials through the patterned atomic (e.g., F, K, and Li) doping of only one side of the structure, which acts to break its inversion symmetry. It was discovered that graphene doped with both Li and F produced the largest d_{31} piezoelectric (length strain) coefficient, while K or Li doping generated the highest e_{31} piezoelectric (transverse) coefficient [290].

16.6.2 Additional Interskin Capabilities

The AI-driven IS may be comprised of a lamination of sophisticated ultrathin, yet highly robust/resilient layers that are electronically integrated. The individual layers that constitute this fused ruggedized composite will be nanoengineered for, and dedicated to specific functionalities. In essence, it will comprise a very powerful wearable computer that is intimately merged within a flexible and form-fitting custom-personalized space suit. In contrast to having AI modules evenly dispersed throughout the IS, this intelligence would be strategically located, with a high level of redundancy, at specific sites for optimal utility and benefit to the occupant.

In an envisaged cross section, proceeding from the inside out, the layers and associated functions of the IS might encompass (a) diagnostic and physiological parameter monitoring nanosensors, nanotherapeutic interface, moisture wicking, and waste transport system (collection and recycling); (b) power harvesting/generation and insulation (e.g., aerogel) [291,292]; (c) integrated AI and extensively distributed nanoelectronic infrastructure; (d) woven, highly durable artificial muscle/exoskeleton infrastructure encased within an ultrastrong, yet pliable shell. It would also have superhydrophobic properties that would act to vigorously repel any liquid and prevent regolith particulates from sticking to the exterior surfaces. It will likely be the case that each of these primary layers would be further subdivided into finer dedicated strata.

The intelligent inner layer of an IS space suit will serve as an interface with all exposed skin surfaces wherein embedded mini-reservoirs that contain the full compliment of primary emergency nanomedicines are stored in readiness for administration should they be required. An extensive network of ultrasensitive diagnostic nanosensors would monitor the health status of the occupant on a continuous basis throughout their residency. Any instance of negative deviation from the occupant's health profile would be rapidly detected by nanosensors and immediately relayed and responded to by the IS, subsequent to practically instantaneous algorithmic analyses via multiple onboard quantum computers.

Nanodevice ingress nodes, strategically placed throughout the IS as transdermal interfaces, or atomizers that are oriented to the nose and mouth within the helmet, would administer appropriate medical countermeasures. The expansive arsenal of IS nanomedical therapeutics would include the capacity for in situ DNA sequencing, the generation and inoculation of artificial blood, and the ability to perform hyperthermic therapeutics to rapidly eradicate any internalized foreign bacteria, viruses, or parasites, be they naturally occurring or extraterrestrial.

In addition to the provision of intrinsic protective security and the potential for extended life support for the indwelling astronaut, the innermost IS layer that interfaces with the skin might be populated with a series of modules that take the form of "patch zones." These specialized zones may be comprised of dense nanoneedle arrays [293] that are in intimate, albeit unnoticeable (to the inhabitant) contact with the skin, which could, if warranted, release nanomedical therapeutics to compensate for practically any physiological imbalance to address most encountered injuries or infections. The IS might also be equipped with onboard reservoirs of functionalized nanobiomaterials that could be quickly deployed to initiate the cessation of rapid blood loss in combination with sequential disinfectant and wound sealant capabilities.

Significant advances wrought by mature nanotechnologies and nanomedicine might allow for the increased mobility of the occupant while resident within the IS via dramatic reductions in the size and weight of conventional pressurized cylinders that typically carry oxygen and water, as well as other containers that are utilized for the disposal and storage of human waste. Breathable oxygen may be continually supplied to the interior of the IS through the use of millions of embedded, AI-controlled micron-sized diamondoid vessels that are equally distributed within dedicated layers of the IS. These highly pressurized entities might accommodate ~1000 atm or more of pressure, containing extremely dense concentrations of gas molecules, and hence, may have the ability to dispense breathable oxygen to the astronaut and recycle exhaled breath for extended periods. In the extremely unlikely event that the onboard IS oxygen-generating capacity is damaged or disabled, additional millions of oxygen-carrying "respirocytes" highly pressurized Ø1 μm nanomedical artificial red blood cells that can "deliver 236 times more oxygen to the tissues per unit volume than natural red cells and to manage carbonic acidity" via reversible molecular sortation rotor pumps [294], may be administered via the nanotherapeutic interfaces described earlier to enable the indwelling individual to obtain his or her requirement of oxygen in vivo.

Most of the primary nanomedical functions of the IS will be autonomous and self-initiated, triggered by any deviation beyond established parameters, in the status of any of myriad physiological parameters. Once any of these personalized and finely calibrated biochemical thresholds are exceeded as either a surplus or deficit, the IS will immediately administer the appropriate nanomedical therapeutic countermeasures to reinstitute homeostasis.

On an equivalent level of vigilant monitoring (as the life of the inhabitant is at stake), any unexpected change within the internal sustaining environment, or mechanical breach/insult to the IS itself, will be addressed with speed and precision. Should astronauts encounter situations in which the IS becomes mechanically punctured, ripped, or somehow breached by thermal, electrical, or chemical means, an immediate self-sealing protocol would be implemented whereby the space suit would instantaneously "heal" itself. This capacity might be inspired by natural systems, albeit radically augmented through the use of novel nanomaterials and nanotechnological processes. Ionov and Synytska have reviewed a number of self-healing strategies that involve polymeric systems [295], which include the rebonding of two segments of the same polymer via molecular interdiffusion at above glass transition temperatures [296], the recombination of polymer chain free ends through photoinduced cross-linking [297], and ambient temperature reversible bond formation [298]. Subsurface nanocapsules might contain healing agents (e.g., dicyclopentadiene with Grubbs catalyst) that can mend a puncture, microcrack, or tear in a material as they will rupture via the impacting mechanical force and release their payloads to fill the resulting voids in enabling repair [299].

16.7 Integrated Nanomedical Suites for Spacecraft and Lunar/Mars-Based Habitats

Future spacecraft might be endowed with an onboard nanomedical suite to ensure the sustained well-being and robust protection of the crew during protracted space voyages. Due to the significant constraints in real estate on space vessels, which seem inevitable for the foreseeable future, it may make sense to endow astronaut attire (e.g., perhaps configured as form-fitting flight suits) with an extensive array of nanomedical competencies, rather than to incorporate space-consuming medical bays. This tenet may also hold true for habitats located on the Moon and Mars, as physically large medical equipments will have long been deemed as obsolete artifacts in the wake of increasingly compact and powerful nanomedical technologies, which are directly adhered to, or operate autonomously within the patient. That said, there will still likely exist room-sized medical facilities within planetary habitats, as space limitations will not be as severe and the number of potential patients may be significantly larger, who present with a diverse array of afflictions or injuries, as is the case with hospitals on Earth. There may be instances where patients require extensive or multiple nanomedical surgeries followed by close monitoring during recovery, treatment for trauma or shock, or psychological conditions. In addition, large-scale decontamination or quarantine facilities may be required in order to contain known transmissible diseases, or unknown conditions of suspected extraterrestrial origin.

Within spacecraft, primary nanomedical capabilities may include continuous real-time health monitoring with extensive periodic checkups, health maintenance via the administration of antioxidant and nutritional supplementation and other nanomedical countermeasures to compensate for the particular degradative effects inherent to space travel, and potent contingencies to effectively deal with a wide range of unforeseen emergencies. Onboard spacecraft and within planetary colonies alike, specialized nanomedical diagnostic, therapeutic and nanosurgical procedures may necessitate that patients be variably interfaced with distinct, albeit compact and powerful accessory nanosystems.

A transfigured version of the IS might be utilized as a lightweight and comfortable form-fitting flight suit of sorts that incorporates a highly sensitive integrated network of nanosensors to acquire comprehensive seamless streams of real-time physiological data from astronauts to be compared with individuated physiological reference data. A series of unobtrusive nanomedical interfaces of the skin could automatically provide personalized highly efficient supplementation or therapeutics via administration using arrays of nanoneedles, supersonic microjet injection [300], or other noninvasive means. While this nanomedically enabled flight suit may serve as a day-to-day accruement, crew sleeping garments/quarters could be similarly outfitted and enabled. Scheduled ocular, auditory, nasal, and oral checkups, as well as brain scans might be accomplished through the use of a specialized modular (or stationary) Envisor-type helmet, as describe earlier. An additional functionality of such a helmet would facilitate the rapid detection of breath-resident, disease-indicating biomarkers via integrated self-refreshing nanosensor assays. For prospective long-haul space travel, it seems logical that, when made available, these nanomedical capabilities may well be considered as indispensable.

In the more distant future, one can envisage that most, if not all, of these capabilities will be enabled by, and manifest as, autonomous long-term patient-resident nanomedical sentinels that serve as extremely robust enhancements to the innate immune system in warding off or quickly neutralizing any physiological threat to its host (again, utilizing the patient's own previously determined optimal physiological profile as a reference template). Further, they will have the ability to deliver antioxidants, drugs, bone-rebuilding (see Section 16.3.2.1.3), and other therapeutic nanomaterials, or to perform myriad nanosurgical procedures. Additionally, the VCSN might provide high-resolution 3D imagery of the entire vasculature and lymphatic system, whereas the GMSD could provide similar high-quality images of the GIT. These measures might be utilized in potent combination with subsequently advanced IS capabilities, such as enhanced radiation protection, an integrated artificial muscle-based exoskeleton, and the faculty for onboard physicians to "visuate" through the surfaces of the IS itself (subsequent to initiating a sequence of confidential security protocols) to scrutinize, as though the skin were transparent, high-resolution 3D imagery of internal organs, tissue sections, cells, etc. of the patient, at any selected depth, to ~organelle level magnification via dynamic zoom. These sophisticated synergistic nanomedical and nanotechnological technologies may provide future space travellers with bolstered defenses against the potential deleterious effects of space and extraterrestrial environments.

16.8 Nanomedical Strategies in Suspended Animation for Space Travel

When humans endeavor to explore beyond Mars (8–9 months—one way), and indeed beyond the furthest reaches of our (classical) solar system (e.g., Pluto, ~9 years—one way), serious consideration must be given to the long-term viable preservation (suspended animation or cryostasis) and reanimation of astronauts, once arrived a target destination. Otherwise, the obvious constraint of human life spans, which will have long expired prior to arriving at even the closest destination from Earth (e.g., the star α Centauri A, at 4.27 light-years from the Sun) will render the prospect of human exploration of interstellar space impracticable. The distance to α Centauri A is equivalent to ~24.8 trillion miles (1 light-year = ~5.8 trillion miles). At the current velocity of Voyager I (~38,000 mph/~61 155 km/h, now (2012) approaching interstellar space), it is estimated that a one-way trip to α Centauri A might require ~70,000 years [301]. Needless to say, even with an extremely radical improvement in propulsive technologies that allow for velocities of from ~10% to 20% of the speed of light (186,000 mps or 299,337 km/s), the length of the trip to α Centauri A would total ~42.7 years and 21.3 years, respectively. Hence, human explorers of deep space would still be in for a quite prolonged sleep.

16.8.1 Cryopreservation

Cryopreservation involves the preservation of deceased "patients" in liquid nitrogen to induce sustained freezing at approx. <–130°C. Options include either full body inversion (inverted contingency against loss of power or other unforeseen event to ensure at least that the head of the patient is thawed last) or heads only. It is anticipated that whatever lead to a patient's demise might be cured when they are prospectively revived, perhaps ~100 years henceforth. In the case of preserved heads, it is hypothesized that these patients might be uploaded to a newly nanobioengineered replicate body using the patient's own DNA as a template [302]. There remain issues with this strategy insofar as cryoprotectant toxicity, osmotic stress, and ultrastructural damage [303]. In addition, even if full revival is successful, there are no guarantees, stemming from damaged neurons' dendrites within the brain, that an individual's original memories or even personalities will remain intact. In a nutshell, will me still be me? Compounding this, as will be the case for all individuals who undergo suspended animation, are associated psychological factors, as suspended individuals who wake up many tens or even hundreds of years from their initial "sleep dates" will be the same physical age, though they will have to come to terms with the knowledge that they are in reality, far older, and their loved ones, barring radical life extension advances (Chapter 17) may all have passed.

In order to minimize the damage to molecular structures, cells, and tissues induced by sharp ice crystals formed during freezing and thawing processes (especially within the brain), recent cryonics techniques employ vitrification, which involves the perfusion of high concentrations of cryoprotectants as a replacement for intercellular H_2O. A vitrification solution dubbed M22 (Table 16.6) has been developed by cryobiologists and is under study by the Alcor Life Extension Foundation [302,304]. It was revealed by Fahy et al. that M22 enabled the recovery and transplantation of whole kidneys subsequent to cooling to –45°C [304].

Potential nanomedical cryopreservation revival operations have been explored by Merkle and Freitas, who propose the use of diamondoid-based molecular machines that can operate at liquid nitrogen temperatures, and a dedicated cryonics version of the vasculoid (see Section 16.4.4.3) to conduct repairs to the vasculature. Fractures that are a consequence of current cryopreservation methods might be stabilized via the use of ~1 nm thick nanosheets to serve as temporary structural supports within the gaps formed as a preventive measure against potentially serious cumulative damage. The vasculoid would also function to reestablish appropriate concentrations of tissue-resident chemicals such as ions, ATP, oxygen, and glucose, as these may likely be disrupted in cryopreservation. Concentrations of cryoprotectants would be diminished over time as well, and completely removed in step with warming procedures. As the patient warms further, "fracture faces

TABLE 16.6

Composition of M22 Vitrification Solution

Chemical	Weight/Volume%
Dimethyl sulfoxide	22.305
Formamide	12.858
Ethylene glycol	16.837
N-methylformamide	3
3-methoxy-1,2-propanediol	4
Polyvinyl pyrrolidone K12	2.8
X-1000 ice blocker	1
Z-1000 ice blocker	2

Source: Fahy, G.M. et al., *Cryobiology* 48(2), 157, 2004.

can be brought together and the support sheets removed and exported from the body." Other classes of nanodevices might subsequently be introduced to conduct cell repair procedures, the replacement of damaged DNA and mitochondria, and to facilitate the removal of various forms of both cellular and intercellular detritus, prior to waking the patient [305].

Fahy proposes a set of feasible and realistic considerations and guidelines for the sequential repair of the frozen human brain, which encompasses an initial replacement of brain-resident ice with "repair networks"; the commencement of "gross structural repairs at temperatures in the range of about −100°C to −30°C," and conducting repairs at the intracellular level under higher temperatures, in part by facilitating biological self-assembly and repair mechanisms [306].

Cryopreservation may evolve to be viable for applications in space travel at some juncture, with further technical refinements, advancements in vitrification, and the establishment of tried, true, and efficient cooling/warming, repair protocols, and revival processes. The reduction of the physical footprint, energy, and chemical requirements of this technology will also constitute major concerns when being considered for use in long-haul spacecraft.

16.8.2 Human Hibernation

For space missions of intermediate duration, nanomedically induced torpor (temporary hibernation) characterized by a marked reduction in metabolism with subsequent decreases in body temperature, oxygen consumption, heart rate, and breathing rate, may serve as a viable solution for astronaut stasis. Blackstone et al. investigated the use of H_2S, which induced a state similar to suspended animation in mice. The functions of H_2S include its role as a reversible inhibitor of complex IV (cytochrome c oxidase), a terminal enzyme complex that is involved in the electron transport chain. It was discovered that within 5 min of the mice being exposed to 80 ppm of H_2S, there was a 50% and 60% drop in oxygen (O_2) consumption and carbon dioxide (CO_2) output, respectively. Subsequent to 6 h of exposure, the metabolic rate fell by 90% followed by a decrease in core body temperature to 15°C at an ambient temperature of 13°C. At this stage, O_2 consumption and CO_2 output were 10% of normal values, concurrent with 10 breaths per minute, in comparison to the normal breath rate of 120. When the mice were returned to ambient air and temperature, all physiological parameters returned to normal. Analysis revealed a correlation between the H_2S concentrations and the intensity of these effects. Though H_2S is toxic at elevated doses, there were no deleterious effects identified in the mice at the 80 ppm exposure [307].

Jinka et al. conducted an investigation of torpor in the seasonal hibernating arctic ground squirrel under the premise that the CNS plays a critical regulatory role in its onset. The initiation of torpor has been hypothesized to occur via a cascade of processes, including alteration in CNS-mediated thermoregulation, sleep extension, metabolic inhibition (e.g., muted mitochondrial oxidative phosphorylation), and metabolic effects induced by temperature changes. It was shown in this study that torpor was induced by the CNS-mediated activation of A_1 adenosine receptors (A_1AR) (sleep promoters) by endogenous adenosine (an inhibitory neurotransmitter), which was also shown to lower the body temperature in hamsters [308,309].

With respect to humans and space travel, highly pressurized (circulating or tissue self-implanting) respirocyte-like (see Section 16.5.3) nanocarriers may be utilized for the precisely calibrated release of H_2S in vivo. Targeted nanoparticles or (when evolved) autonomous nanodevices might be used in conjunction to trigger A_1AR to induce human hibernation and to sustain it over prescribed timelines.

16.8.3 Conceptual Nanomedical "Sustun" Strategy for Suspended Animation

A conceptual nanomedical model for inducing and sustaining long-term human stasis at ambient temperatures may negate the use of cryogenics and associate infrastructures altogether through the use of billions of autonomous tendril-wielding nanodevices that have the capacity for interconnecting via the establishment of trillions of angstrom and nanoscale cross-links with the potential to spatially constrain and, in a sense, induce a state of hibernation in every cell in situ within the bodies of astronauts [310]. The aim would be to radically slow the body's metabolic requirements, as well as oxidation, and hence, biodegradation. Further, a highly resilient encasement comprised of tough, ionizing radiation resistant/diffusing nanomaterials would be self-assembled to encapsulate occupants to complete this "sustun" procedure. In effect, this strategy would enable the completely reversible immobilization and "sealing-off" of the occupant from the local environment (analogous to prehistoric insects being encased and wholly preserved in a dollop of amber) in a condition that might be equivalent to, or even more robust than, that of the desiccated tardigrade tun state. The distinction here would be that H_2O molecules would remain in place within the system, allowing for simplified reanimation procedures without concern, as is the case with cryogenics, for ice crystal damage.

Once the course of the preprogrammed stasis timeline (likely many years) has been run, this intercommunicative population of "preservicytes" would reactivate and operate in a massively parallel fashion to incrementally reverse the sealing and cross-linking procedure, with the concomitant initiation of resuscitation protocols, commencing with revitalization at the molecular level, up to the "unlocking" and activation of neural pathways within the brain, as well as cardiac, pulmonary, and all-organ revival.

16.9 Nanomedicine in Interstellar Space

A recent (May 2012) Defence Advanced Research Projects Agency (DARPA)-seeded initiative named 100 Year Starship™ (100YSS) has been launched to "make the capability of human travel beyond our solar system to another star a reality over the next 100 years." Overseen by former astronaut, engineer, and physician, Mae Jemison, the mission of

100YSS statement includes that it "will pursue national and global initiatives, and galvanize public and private leadership and grassroots support, to assure that human travel beyond our solar system and to another star can be a reality within the next century" [311].

Concomitant with the inevitable human achievement of attaining the level of technological sophistication as the prerequisite to traversing and surviving in deep space, it is likely that nanomedical strategies for the maintenance of health for future astronauts, explorers, and the pioneers who colonize the Moon, Mars, and beyond will be pervasive. As mentioned earlier, nanomedicine has a number of inherently attractive advantages as relates to space travel, encompassing the capacity for the integration of autonomous, highly advanced, and powerful nanomedical technologies in what might be considered as the ultimate in non-invasive compact medical devices. It seems probable, as alluded to earlier, that the onboard medical facilities of dedicated deep-space spacecraft will be devoid of a conventional operating theater and surgical instrumentation, as most physically invasive surgical procedures, including catheter-based and keyhole surgeries, will have long been regarded as obsolete. The majority of cellular, tissue, and organ repairs will likely be accomplished by rapid action, highly coordinated legions of subtly administered (e.g., inhaled, swallowed as pill, applied as topical gel, or needleless/painless injection) nanomedical devices (Chapter 2).

Although one can envision instances where macroscale physical interventions might be necessitated, such as organ transplantation, to address serious hemorrhaging or the setting of broken bones, there may be (hypothetical) nanomedical solutions for these traumas as well.

In the case of a patient that is in need of an organ transplant, "homeostat" class nanodevices (tasked with orchestrating the maintenance of optimal human homeostasis) would contain complete (frequently refreshed) ultrahigh resolution 3D positional molecular and cellular maps of the patient, making it theoretically possible for rows of sufficiently sophisticated nanomedical devices (e.g., "organogrow knitters") to incrementally "disassemble" damaged portions of a particular organ (cell layer, by cell layer) and replace them and their supportive extracellular matrices with identical viable cells and stabilizing structures in situ. In effect, this would enable the seamless "printing" [312–314] of new organ segments or perhaps even an entire organ in vivo (in a manner similar to today's 3D printers). This would be accomplished without ever requiring an invasive incision.

In cases of serious hemorrhaging due to complications in childbirth, injurious or disease-caused internal bleeding, lacerations or the accidental loss of a limb, patient indwelling homeostat and analgesic nanodevices would instantaneously transit to the site/s of injury via the appropriate vascular pathways to quickly seal any severed arteries, veins, and capillaries, while negating nerve impulse traffic [315] for as long as required, and sanitizing the injury site to prevent infection. These first-response nanodevices would maintain a sterile sealed "cap" over the injury while a new identical organ or limb is replaced or regrown by specialized organogrow knitter class nanodevices.

It is anticipated that the likelihood of breaking a bone in the space environment is between 20% and 30% [316]. When considering the case of a patient that is presenting with a broken limb, it is conceivable that multitudes of the appropriate classes of advanced in vivo and ex vivo nanodevices working in a highly coordinated (massively parallel) fashion may set and completely repair broken bone/s, and even compound fractures, within a ~30 min or less time frame.

> Note: Should the patient have broken his/her leg, for instance, at some distance from an established medical facility while on an exploratory mission on the regolith of the Moon or Mars, the following procedure might be administered via the integrated capabilities of the nanomedically enabled IS of his/her extravehicular space suit. As the IS

would be endowed with robust artificial muscles having the capacity for imparting sufficient deformative physical forces (subsequent to anesthetizing the injured limb), its programming could include the capability for logically and sequentially manipulating and setting a broken bone that occurs at almost any site of the body. Should the injury be of such a serious nature as to be beyond the treatment scope of the IS, it might serve (e.g., in cases of serious spinal or neck injuries) to physically immobilize areas that are directly and indirectly related to the injured site/s of the patient to enable their safe transportation to the appropriate medical facilities where their injuries may be properly and fully treated.

A particular class of surface-ambling nanodevices may be administered externally as a viscous gel that is applied in close proximity to the injured site. Prior to their externally mediated activation through portable photonic or ultrasonic sources, which emanate a pulse-coded "start" sequence, internally resident nanodevices will rapidly anesthetize the entire injury site employing a strategy similar to that suggested by Freitas for the prospective administration of anesthesia in nanodentistry [315]. This procedure might involve a contingent of "analgesic" class nanodevices that would autonomously travel to nerve junctions in appropriate proximity to the injury site in order to temporarily secure the control of the flow of localized nerve impulses, with the subsequent effect of almost instantaneously numbing the entire injury site. This "flash freeze" operation would be completely reversible, hence, normal sensation to the injured site upon the completion of repairs will return to normal just as quickly. This condition would be activated, possibly by a handheld remote, and sustained by the attending physician until deemed that the repairs are complete and that default nerve activity may commence.

At this juncture, the previously dermally applied "expander" class nanodevices would be activated. These entities would initially self-organize into solid appearing ultrafine multilayered cross-hatched/mesh-like "cuffs" positioned strategically on opposing sides of the break, which would entirely circumscribe the leg. Subspecies segments of the expander populations located on either side of the break would painlessly traverse through the skin and tissue to self-form perhaps thousands of robust, albeit temporary, ~>micron in diameter filamentous tethers that circumscribe the leg as well, which anchor at inclined angles away from the injury site and directly into unaffected solid bone tissues. When the opposing sides of the break are properly secured, the primary expander cuffs on either side of the injury would proceed to migrate toward and overlap each other. Subsequently, these multitudes of expanders could conceivably cumulatively operate as microscopic sliding and interlocking "expansion/contraction jacks" with the capacity for the fine macroscale manipulation of the leg in any orientation, and being able to push against and away from the opposing anchors, resulting in the potentially (computationally guided) perfect alignment of the broken bone. In many respects, these expander nanodevices would have a functionality that is akin to the "foglet" elements of the polymorphic "utility fog," which is envisioned by Storrs Hall [317].

In all of the earlier-mentioned scenarios, it is assumed that either long indwelling homeostat class nanodevices will convey complete and detailed data on every relevant aspect of the patient physiology to the appropriate nanodevices, or that these data will be transferred to the nanodevices from an external medical database. Indeed, it may be the case, as the timeline for the development of interstellar travel may be ~50 to 100 years out, that advanced autonomous nanomedical devices will be permanent residents within those individuals who select to be imbued with such enhancements.

References

1. Longitudinal Study of Astronaut Health (LSAH), http://lsda.jsc.nasa.gov/docs/research/research_detail.aspx?experiment_type_code=23&researchtype=(accessed July 01, 2013)

2. Risin, D., Risk of inability to adequately treat an ill or injured crew member. *Human Health and Performance Risks of Space Exploration Missions: Evidence Reviewed by the NASA Human Research Program*, pp. 241–244, 2009. http://humanresearchroadmap.nasa.gov/evidence/reports/ExMC.pdf (accessed July 28, 2012).

3. Ross, M.D., Twombly, I.A., Bruyns, C., Cheng, R., and Senger, S., Telecommunications for health care over distance: The virtual collaborative clinic. In: *Medicine Meets Virtual Reality 2000, 13th Humans in Space Symposium*, Westwood, J.D., Hoffman, H.H., Mogel, G., Robb, R., Stredney, D. (eds). IOS Press, Washington, DC, pp. 286–291, 2000.

4. Ross, M.D., Medicine in long duration space exploration: The role of virtual reality and broad bandwidth telecommunications networks. *Acta Astronaut* 49(3–10), 441–445, 2001.

5. Ball, J.R. and Evans, C.H., *Safe Passage: Astronaut Care for Exploration Missions*, National Academy Press, Washington, DC, 2001.

6. Mader, T.H., Gibson, C.R., Pass, A.F., Kramer, L.A., Lee, A.G., Fogarty, J., Tarver, W.J., Dervay, J.P., Hamilton, D.R., Sargsyan, A., Phillips, J.L., Tran, D., Lipsky, W., Choi, J., Stern, C., Kuyumjian, R., and Polk, J.D., Optic disc edema, globe flattening, choroidal folds, and hyperopic shifts observed in astronauts after long-duration space flight. *Ophthalmology* 118(10), 2058–2069, 2011.

7. Kramer, L.A., Sargsyan, A.E., Hasan, K.M., Polk, J.D., and Hamilton, D.R., Orbital and intracranial effects of microgravity: Findings at 3-T MR imaging. *Radiology* 263(3), 819–827, 2012.

8. Buravkova, L., Romanov, Y., Rykova, M., Grigorieva, O., and Merzlikina, N., Cell-to-cell interactions in changed gravity: Ground-based and flight experiments. *Acta Astronaut* 57(2–8), 67–74, 2005.

9. Blaber, E., Marçal, H., and Burns, B.P., Bioastronautics: The influence of microgravity on astronaut health. *Astrobiology* 10(5), 463–473, 2010.

10. Mewaldt, R.A., Cosmic Rays, *Macmillan Encyclopedia of Physics*, 1996. http://www.srl.caltech.edu/personnel/dick/cos_encyc.html (accessed July 28, 2012).

11. Hess, V.F., Über Beobachtungen der durchdringenden Strahlung bei sieben Freiballonfahrten. *Physikalische Zeitschrift* 13, 1084–1091, 1912. (Observations about the penetrating radiation in seven free balloon rides. *Physical Journal*)

12. Newberg, A.B., Changes in the central nervous system and their clinical correlates during long-term spaceflight. *Aviat Space Environ Med* 65(6), 562–572, 1994.

13. Tobias, C.A., Radiation hazards in high altitude aviation. *J Aviat Med* 23(4), 345–372, 1952.

14. Pinsky, L.S., Osborne, W.Z., Bailey, J.V., Benson, R.E., and Thompson, L.F., Light flashes observed by astronauts on Apollo 11 through Apollo 17. *Science* 183(4128), 957–959, 1974.

15. Todd, P., Stochastics of HZE-induced microlesions. *Adv Space Res* 9(10), 31–34, 1989.

16. Todd, P. and Walker, J.T., The microlesion concept in HZE particle dosimetry. *Adv Space Res* 4(10), 187–197, 1984.

17. Todd, P., Unique biological aspects of radiation hazards—an overview. *Adv Space Res* 3(8), 187–194, 1983.

18. Curtis, S.B., Vazquez, M.E., Wilson, J.W., Atwell, W., Kim, M., and Capala, J., Cosmic ray hit frequencies in critical sites in the central nervous system. *Adv Space Res* 22(2), 197–207, 1998.

19. Cucinotta, F.A., Nikjoo, H., Goodhead, D.T., and Wilson, J.W., Comment on the effects of delta-rays on the number of particle-track transversals per cell in laboratory and space exposures. *Radiat Res* 150(1), 115–119, 1998.

20. Cucinotta, F.A., Nikjoo, H., Goodhead, D.T., and Wilson, J.W., Applications of amorphous track models in radiobiology. *Radiat Environ Biophys* 38(2), 81–92, 1999.

21. Ponomarev, A. and Cucinotta, F.A., Nuclear fragmentation and the number of particle tracks in tissue. *Radiat Protect Dosim* 122(104), 354–361, 2006.
22. Cucinotta, F.A., Wang, H., and Huff, J.L., Chapter 6—Risk of acute or late central nervous system effects from radiation exposure. In McPhee, J.C., Charles, J.B. (eds.), *Human Health and Performance Risks of Space Exploration Missions*, NASA Washington, DC, SP-2009-3405, 191–212, 2009.
23. Morgan, J.L., Skulan, J.L., Gordon, G.W., Romaniello, S.J., Smith, S.M., and Anbar, A.D., Rapidly assessing changes in bone mineral balance using natural stable calcium isotopes. *Proc Natl Acad Sci USA* 109(25), 9989–9994, 2012.
24. DePaolo, D.J., Calcium isotopic variation produced by biological, kinetic, radiogenic and nucleosynthetic processes. In Johnson, C.M., Beard, B.L., and Albarede, F. (eds.), *Geochemistry of Non-Traditional Stable Isotopes, Reviews in Mineralogy and Geochemistry*, The Mineralogical Society of America, Washington, DC, Vol. 55, 2004, pp. 255–288.
25. Nielson, L.C., Druhan, J.L., Yang, W., Brown, S.T., and DePaolo, D.J., Calcium isotopes as tracers of biogeochemical processes. In Baskaran, M. (ed.), *Handbook of Environmental Isotope Geochemistry*, Springer, Berlin, Vol. 1, 2011, pp. 105–124.
26. Russell, W.A., Papanastassiou, D.A., and Tombrello, T.A., Ca isotope fractionation on the Earth and other solar system materials. *Geochim Cosmochim Acta* 42, 1075–1090, 1978.
27. Mazess, R.B., Peppler, W.W., and Gibbons, M., Total body composition by dual-photon (153Gd) absorptiometry. *Am J Clin Nutr* 40(4), 834–839, 1984.
28. Martin, A.D., Bailey, D.A., and McKay, H.A., Whiting, S., Bone mineral and calcium accretion during puberty. *Am J Clin Nutr* 66(3), 611–615, 1997.
29. Smith, S.M., Wastney, M.E., Nyquist, L.E., Shih, C.Y., Wiesmann, H., Nillen, J.L., and Lane H.W., Calcium kinetics with microgram stable isotope doses and saliva sampling. *J Mass Spectr.* 31(11), 1265–1270, 1996.
30. Smith, S.M., Wastney, M.E., O'Brien, K.O., Morukov, B.V., Larina, I.M., and Abrams, S.A. et al., Bone markers, calcium metabolism, and calcium kinetics during extended-duration space flight on the mir space station. *J Bone Miner Res* 20(2), 208–218, 2005.
31. Bloomfield, S.A., Disuse osteopenia. *Curr Osteoporos Rep* 8(2), 91–97, 2010.
32. Lang, T., LeBlanc, A., and Evans, H. et al., Cortical and trabecular bone mineral loss from the spine and hip in long-duration spaceflight. *J Bone Miner Res* 19(6), 1006–1012, 2004.
33. Lang, T.F., LeBlanc, A.D., and Evans, J.H. et al., Adaptation of the proximal femur to skeletal reloading after long-duration spaceflight. *J Bone Miner Res* 21(8), 1224–1230, 2006.
34. Sibonga, J.D., Evans, H.J., Sung, H.G., Spector, E.R., Lang, T.F., Oganov, V.S., Bakulin, A.V., Shackelford, L.C., and LeBlanc, A.D., Recovery of spaceflight-induced bone loss: Bone mineral density after long-duration missions as fitted with an exponential function. *Bone* 41(6), 973–978, 2007.
35. Keyak, J.H., Koyama, A.K., LeBlanc, A., Lu, Y., and Lang, T.F., Reduction in proximal femoral strength due to long-duration spaceflight. *Bone* 44(3), 449–453, 2009.
36. Smith, S.M., Heer, M.A., Shackelford, L., Sibonga, J.D., Ploutz-Snyder, L., and Zwart, S.R., Benefits for bone from resistance exercise and nutrition in long-duration spaceflight: Evidence from biochemistry and densitometry. *J Bone Miner Res* 27(9), 1896–906, 2012.
37. Lockheed Martin Space Operations, Bioastronautics Critical Path Roadmap. An Approach to Risk Reduction and Management for Human Space Flight: Extending the Boundaries, NASA JSC 62577, April 2, 2004 http://surc.isas.jaxa.jp/Space_Agriculture/SpaceAgri_Ref/jsc62577_bcpr_040204-1.pdf
38. Bao, J.X., Zhang, L.F., and Ma, J., Angiotensinogen and AT1R expression in cerebral and femoral arteries during hindlimb unloading in rats. *Aviat Space Environ Med* 78(9), 852–858, 2007.
39. Diedrich, A., Paranjape, S.Y., Roberston, D., Plasma and blood volume in space. *Am J Med Sci* 334(1), 80–85, 2007.
40. Blomqvist, C.G., Buckey, J.C., Gaffney, F.A, Lane, L.D., Levine, B.D., and Watenpaugh, D.E., Mechanisms of post-flight orthostatic intolerance, *J Gravit Physiol* 1(1), 122–124, 1994.

41. Norsk, P., Cardiovascular and fluid volume control in humans in space. *Curr Pharm Biotechnol* 6(4), 325–300, 2005.
42. Fitts, R.H., Riley, D.R., and Widrick, J.J., Functional and structural adaptations of skeletal muscle to microgravity. *J Exp Biol* 204(Pt 18), 3201–3208, 2001.
43. Allen, D.L., Bandstra, E.R., Harrison, B.C., Thorng, S., Stodieck, L.S., and Kostenuik, P.J., Effects of spaceflight on murine skeletal muscle gene expression. *J Appl Physiol* 106(2), 582–595, 2009.
44. Rabin, B.M., Shukitt-Hale, B., Joseph, J., and Todd, P., Diet as a factor in behavioral radiation protection following exposure to heavy particles. *Gravit Space Biol Bull* 18(2), 71–77, 2005.
45. Freitas Jr., R.A., *Nanomedicine, Volume I: Basic Capabilities,* Landes Bioscience, Georgetown, TX, 1999.
46. Schoenfeld, M.P., Ansari, R.R., Nakao, A., and Wink, D., A hypothesis on biological protection from space radiation through the use of new therapeutic gases as medical counter measures. *Med Gas Res* 2, 8, 2012.
47. Nakao, A., Sugimoto, R., Billiar, T.R., and McCurry, K.R., Therapeutic antioxidant medical gas. *J Clin Biochem Nutr* 44, 1–13, 2009.
48. Huang, C., Kawamura, T., Toyoda, Y., and Nakao, A., Recent advances in hydrogen research as a therapeutic medical gas. *Free Radical Res* 44(9), 971–982, 2010.
49. Szabo, C., Hydrogen sulphide and its therapeutic potential. *Nat Rev Drug Discov* 6(11), 917–935, 2007.
50. Chopping, G., Liljenzin, J., and Rydberg, J., *Radiation Biology and Radiation Protection. Radiochemistry and Nuclear Chemistry*, 3rd edn., Butterworth-Heinemann, 2002, pp. 474–513.
51. Krusic, P.J., Wasserman, E., Keizer, P.N., Morton, J.R., and Preston, K.F., Radical reactions of c60. *Science* 254(5035), 1183–1185, 1991.
52. Thakral, S. and Mehta, R.M., Fullerenes: An introduction and overview of their biological properties. *Ind J Pharm Sci* 68(1), 13–16, 2006.
53. Tabata, Y., Murakami, Y., and Ikada, Y., Photodynamic effect of polyethylene glycol-modified fullerene on tumor. *Jpn J Cancer Res* 88, 1108–1116, 1997.
54. Yin, J.J., Lao, F., Meng, J., Fu, P.P., Zhao, Y., Xing, G., Gao, X., Sun, B., Wang, P.C., Chen, C., and Liang, X.J., Inhibition of tumor growth by endohedral metallofullerenol nanoparticles optimized as reactive oxygen species scavenger. *Mol Pharmacol* 74(4), 1132–1140, 2008.
55. Dugan, L.L., Lovett, E.G., Quick, K.L., Lotharius, J., Lin, T.T., and O'Malley, K.L., Fullerene-based antioxidants and neurodegenerative disorders. *Parkinsonism Relat Disord* 7(3), 243–246, 2001.
56. Dugan, L.L., Lovett, E., Cuddihy, S., Almli, C.R., Lin, T.S., and Choi, D.W., Carboxyfullerenes as neuroprotective antioxidants. In Kreiglstein, J. (ed.), *Pharmacology of Cerebral Ischernia*, Academic Press, New York, 1987.
57. Lin, A.M., Chyi, B.Y., Wang, S.D., Yu, H.H., Kanakamma, P.P., Luh, T.Y., Chou, C.K., and Ho, L.T., Carboxyfullerene prevents iron-induced oxidative stress in rat brain. *J Neurochem* 72, 1634–1640, 1999.
58. Chaing, L.Y., Wang, L.Y., Swirczewski, J.W., Soled, S., and Cameron, S., Efficient synthesis of polyhydroxylated fullerene derivatives via hydrolysis of polycyclosulfated precursors. *J Org Chem* 59(14), 3960–3968, 1994.
59. Chiang, L.Y., Lu, F.J., and Lin, J.T., Free radical scavenging activity of water-soluble fullerenols. *J Chem Soc Commun I* 1283–1284, 1995.
60. Kadish, K.M. and Ruoff, R.S., *Fullerenes, Chemistry, Physics and Technology,* John Wiley & Sons, Inc., New York, 2000.
61. Zemanova, A., Klouda, K., and Zeman, K., C_{60} Fullerene derivative: Influence of nanoparticle size on toxicity and radioprotectivity of water soluble fullerene derivative. *NANOCON 2011* 1–10, 2011.
62. Cai, X., Jia, H., Liu, Z., Hou, B., Luo, C., Feng, Z., Li, W., and Liu, J., Polyhydroxylated fullerene derivative C(60)(OH)(24) prevents mitochondrial dysfunction and oxidative damage in an MPP(+) -induced cellular model of Parkinson's disease. *J Neurosci Res* 86(16), 3622–3634, 2008.

63. Andrievsky, G.V., Bruskov, V.I., Tykhomyrov, A.A., and Gudkov, S.V., Peculiarities of the anti-oxidant and radioprotective effects of hydrated C60 fullerene nanostuctures in vitro and in vivo. *Free Radic Biol Med* 47(6), 786–793, 2009.

64. Bal, R., Türk, G., Tuzcu, M., Yilmaz, O., Ozercan, I., Kuloglu, T., Gür, S., Nedzvetsky, V.S., Tykhomyrov, A.A., Andrievsky, G.V., Baydas, G., and Naziroglu, M., Protective effects of nanostructures of hydrated C(60) fullerene on reproductive function in streptozotocin-diabetic male rats. *Toxicology* 282(3), 69–81, 2011.

65. Ali, S.S., Hardt, J.I., and Dugan, L.L., SOD activity of carboxyfullerenes predicts their neuroprotective efficacy: A structure-activity study. *Nanomedicine* 4(4), 283–294, 2008.

66. Tsao, N., Luh, T.Y., Chou, C.K., Chang, T.Y., Wu, J.J., Liu, C.C., and Lei, H.Y., In vitro action of carboxyfullerene. *J Antimicrob Chemother* 49(4),641–649, 2002.

67. Lin, A.M., Chyi, B.Y., Wang, S.D., Yu, H.H., Kanakamma, P.P., Luh, T.Y., Chou, C.K., Ho, L.T., Carboxyfullerene prevents iron-induced oxidative stress in rat brain. *J Neurochem* 72(4), 1634–1640, 1999.

68. Monti, D., Moretti, L., Salvioli, S., Straface, E., Malorni, W., Pellicciari, R. Schettini, G., Bisaglia, M., Pincelli, C., Fumelli, C., Bonafè, M., and Franceschi, C., C_{60} carboxyfullerene exerts a protective activity against oxidative stress-induced apoptosis in human peripheral blood mononuclear cells. *Biochem Biophys Res Commun* 277(3), 711–717, 2000.

69. Satoh, M., Matsuo, K., Kiriya, H., Mashino, T., Hirobe, M., and Takayanagi, I., Inhibitory effect of a fullerene derivative, monomalonic acid C_{60}, on nitric oxide-dependent relaxation of aortic smooth muscle. *Gen Pharmacol* 29(3), 345–351, 1997.

70. Okuda, K., Hirobe, M., Mochizuki, M., and Mashino, T., *Proc Electrochem Soc* 97(42), 337, 1997.

71. Okuda, K., Mashino, T., and Hirobe, M., Superoxide radical quenching and cytochrome C peroxidase-like activity of C_{60}-dimalonic acid, $C_{62}(COOH)_4$. *Bioorg Med Chem Lett* 6, 539542, 1996.

72. Huang, S.S., Mashino, T., Mochizuki, M., Chiang, L.Y., Chih, L.H., Hsieh, H.M., Teng, C.M., Okuda, K., Hirota, T., and Tsai, M.C., Effect of hexasulfobutylated C(60) on the isolated aortic ring of guinea pig. *Pharmacology* 64(2), 91–97, 2002.

73. Chen, H.H., Yu, C., Ueng, T.H., Chen, S., Chen, B.J., Huang, K.J., Chiang, L.Y., Acute and subacute toxicity study of water-soluble polyalkylsulfonated C_{60} in rats. *Toxicol Pathol* 26(1), 143–151, 1998.

74. Gharbi, N., Pressac, M., Hadchouel, M., Szwarc, H., Wilson, S.R., and Moussa, F., [60]fullerene is a powerful antioxidant in vivo with no acute or subacute toxicity. *Nano Lett* 5(12), 2578–2585, 2005.

75. Makarova, E.G., Gordon, R.Y., and Podolski, I.Y., Fullerene C60 prevents neurotoxicity induced by intrahippocampal microinjection of amyloid-beta peptide. *J Nanosci Nanotechnol* 12(1), 119–126, 2012.

76. Dugan, L.L., Gabrielsen, J.K., Yu, S.P., Lin, T.S., and Choi, D.W., Buckminsterfullerenol free radical scavengers reduce excitotoxic and apoptotic death of cultured cortical neurons. *Neurobiol Dis* 3(2), 129–135, 1996.

77. Lai, Y.L., Murugan, P., and Hwang, K.C., Fullerene derivative attenuates ischemia-reperfusion-induced lung injury. *Life Sci* 72(11), 1271–1278, 2003.

78. Oberdorster, E., Manufactured nanomaterials (fullerenes,C60) induce oxidative stress in the brain of juvenile largemouth bass. *Environ Health Perspect* 112(10), 1058–1062, 2004.

79. Daroczi, B., Kari, G., McAleer, M.F., Wolf, J.C., Rodeck, U., and Dicker, A.P., In vivo radioprotection by the fullerene nanoparticle DF-1 as assessed in a zebrafish model. *Clin Cancer Res* 12(23), 7086–7091, 2006.

80. Rubin, P. and Casarett, G.W., Clinical radiation pathology as applied to curative radiotherapy. *Cancer* 22(4), 767–778, 1968.

81. Cornforth, M.N., Perspectives on the formation of radiation induced exchange aberrations. *DNA Repair (Amst)* 5(9–10), 1182–1191, 2006.

82. Theriot, C.A., Casey, R.C., Moore, V.C., Mitchell, L., Reynolds, J.O., and Burgoyne, M., Dendro [C(60)] fullerene DF-1 provides radioprotection to radiosensitive mammalian cells. *Radiat Environ Biophys* 49(3), 437–445, 2010.

83. Lucente-Schultz, R.M., Moore, V.C., Leonard, A.D., Price, B.K., Kosynkin, D.V., and Lu, M. et al., Antioxidant single-walled carbon nanotubes. *J Am Chem Soc* 131(11), 3934–3941, 2009.

84. Umadevi, S., Gopi, V., Simna, S.P., Parthasarathy, A., Yousuf, S.M., and Elangovan, V., Studies on the cardio protective role of gallic acid against AGE-induced cell proliferation and oxidative stress in H9C2 (2–1) cells. *Cardiovasc Toxicol* 12(4), 304–11, 2012.

85. Cirillo, G., Hampel, S., Klingeler, R., Puoci, F., Iemma, F., Curcio, M., Parisi, O.I., Spizzirri, U.G., Picci, N., Leonhardt, A., Ritschel, M., and Büchner, B., Antioxidant multi-walled carbon nanotubes by free radical grafting of gallic acid: New materials for biomedical applications. *J Pharm Pharmacol* 63(2), 179–188, 2011.

86. Vergaro, V., Lvov, Y.M., and Leporatti, S., Halloysite clay nanotubes for resveratrol delivery to cancer cells. *Macromol Biosci* August 8, 2012.

87. Jain, K.K., *The Handbook of Neuroprotection*, Springer Science+Business Media, LLVC, New York, 2011.

88. Rzigalinski, B.A., Meehan, K., Davis, R.M., Xu, Y., Miles, W.C., and Cohen, C.A., Radical nanomedicine. *Nanomedicine (Lond)* 1(4), 399–412, 2006.

89. Schubert, D., Dargusch, R., Raitano, J., and Chan, S., Cerium and yttrium oxide nanoparticles are neuroprotective. *Biochem Biophys Res Commun* 342(1), 86–91, 2006.

90. Nagasaki, Y., Nitroxide radicals and nanoparticles: A partnership for nanomedicine radical delivery. *Ther Deliv* 3(2), 165–179, 2012.

91. Xu, P., Van Kirk, E.A., Murdoch, W.J., Zhan, Y., Isaak, D.D., Radosz, M., and Shen, Y., Anticancer efficacies of cisplatin-releasing pH-responsive nanoparticles. *Biomacromolecules* 7(3), 829–835, 2006.

92. Jiang, X., Luo, S., Armes, S.P., Shi, W., and Liu, S., UV irradiation-induced shell cross-linked micelles with pH-responsive cores using ABC triblock copolymers. *Macromolecules* 39(18), 5987–5994, 2006.

93. Wong, K.K., Cheung, S.O., Huang, L., Niu, J., Tao, C., Ho, C.M., Che, C.M., and Tam, P.K., Further evidence of the anti-inflammatory effects of silver nanoparticles. *ChemMedChem* 4(7), 1129–1135, 2009.

94. Takebayashi, J., Tai, A., and Yamamoto, I., Long-term radical scavenging activity of AA-2G and 6-acyl-AA-2G against 1,1-diphenyl-2-picrylhydrazyl. *Biol Pharm Bull* 25(11), 1503–1505, 2002.

95. Mathew, D., Nair, C.K., Jacob, J.A., Biswas, N., Mukherjee, T., Kapoor, S., Kagiya, T.V., Ascorbic acid monoglucoside as antioxidant and radioprotector. *J Radiat Res* 48(5), 369–376, 2007.

96. Fujinami, Y., Tai, A., Yamamoto, I., Radical scavenging activity against 1,1-diphenyl-2-picrylhydrazyl of ascorbic acid 2-glucoside (AA-2G) and 6-acyl-AA-2G. *Chem Pharm Bull (Tokyo)* 49(5), 642–644, 2001.

97. Chandrasekharan, D.K., Kagiya, T.V., Nair, C.K., Radiation protection by 6-palmitoyl ascorbic acid-2-glucoside: Studies on DNA damage in vitro, ex vivo, in vivo and oxidative stress in vivo. *J Radiat Res* 50(3), 203–212, 2009.

98. Chandrasekharan, D.K., Khanna, P.K., Kagiya, T.V., Nair, C.K.K., Studies on radiation protection by silver nanoparticle complexes of palmitoyl ascorbic acid 2-glucoside. *Proc Int Conf Nanosci Technol Chem Health, Environ Energy* 75–79, 2010.

99. Chandrasekharan, D.K., Khanna, P.K., Kagiya, T.V., and Nair, C.K.K., Synthesis of nanosilver using a vitamin C derivative and studies on radiation protection. *Cancer Biother Radiopharm* 26(2), 249–257, 2011.

100. Gandhi, N.M., Maurya, D.K., Salvi, V., Kapoor, S., Mukherjee, T., Nair, C.K.K., Radioprotection of DNA by glycyrrhizic acid through scavenging free radicals. *J Radiat Res* 45(3), 461–468, 2004.

101. Chandrasekharan, D.K., Khanna, P.K., Nair, C.K., Cellular radioprotecting potential of glyzyrrhizic acid, silver nanoparticle and their complex. *Mutat Res* 723(1), 51–57, 2011.

102. Abdel-Lateff, A., König, G.M., Fisch, K.M., Höller, U., Jones, P.G., and Wright, A.D., New antioxidant hydroquinone derivatives from the algicolous marine fungus *Acremonium sp. J Nat Prod* 65(11), 1605–1611, 2002.

103. Hayashi, K., Suzuki, K., Kawaguchi, M., Nakajima, T., Suzuki, T., Numata, M., and Nakamura, T., Isolation of an antioxidant from *Penicillium roquefortii* IFO 5956. *Biosci Biotechnol Biochem* 59(2), 319–320, 1995.

104. Yen, G.C. and Lee, C.E., Antioxidative properties of extracts from *Aspergillus candidus* broth filtrate. *J Sci Food Agric* 75, 326–332, 1997.

105. Yen, G.C., Chang, Y.C., Sheu, F., and Chiang, H.C., Isolation and characterization of antioxidant compounds from *Aspergillus candidus* broth filtrate. *J Agric Food Chem* 49(3), 1426–1431, 2001.

106. Hirota, A., Morimitsu, Y., and Hojo, H., New antioxidative indophenol-reducing phenol compounds isolated from the *Mortierella sp.* fungus. *Biosci Biotech Biochem* 61, 647–650, 1997.

107. Takahashi, N., Tamagawa, K., Kawai, K., and Fukui, T., Antioxidant properties of a new type of polyene, *falconensone A* and its derivatives. *Biol Pharm Bull* 23(8), 989–994, 2000.

108. Teshima, Y., Shin-Ya, K., Shimazu, A., Furihata, K., Chul, H.S., Furihata, K., Hayakawa, Y., Nagai, K., and Seto, H.J., Isolation and structural elucidation of pyridoxatin, a free radical scavenger of microbial origin. *J Antibiot (Tokyo)* 44(6), 685–687, 1991.

109. Liu, J.K., Hu, L., Dong, Z.J., and Hu, Q., DPPH radical scavenging activity of ten natural p-terphenyl derivatives obtained from three edible mushrooms indigenous to China. *Chem Biodivers* 1(4), 601–605, 2004.

110. Daly, M.J., Gaidamakova, E.K., Matrosova, V.Y., Vasilenko, A., Zhai, M., Leapman, R.D., Lai, B., Ravel, B., Li, S.M., Kemner, K.M., and Fredrickson, J.K., Protein oxidation implicated as the primary determinant of bacterial radioresistance. *PLoS Biol* 5(4), 0769–0779, 2007.

111. Daly, M.J., Gaidamakova, E.K., Matrosova, V.Y., Vasilenko, A., Zhai, M., Venkateswaran. A., Hess, M., Omelchenko, M.V., Kostandarithes, H.M., Makarova, K.S., Wackett, L.P., Fredrickson, J.K., and Ghosal, D., Accumulation of Mn(II) in *Deinococcus radiodurans* facilitates gamma radiation resistance. *Science* 306, 1025–1028, 2004.

112. Beblo, K., Douki, T., Schmalz, G., Rachel, R., Wirth, R., Huber, H., Reitz, G., Rettberg, P., Survival of thermophilic and hyperthermophilic microorganisms after exposure to UV-C, ionizing radiation and desiccation. *Arch Microbiol* 193(11), 797–809, 2011.

113. Horikawa, D.D., Sakashita, T., Katagiri, C., Watanabe, M., Kikawada, T., Nakahara, Y., Hamada, N., Wada, S., Funayama, T., Higashi, S., Kobayashi, Y., Okuda, T., and Kuwabara, M., Radiation tolerance in the tardigrade *Milnesium tardigradum. Int J Radiat Biol* 82(12), 843–848, 2006.

114. Wełnicz, W., Grohme, M.A., Kaczmarek, L., Schill, R.O., Frohme, M., Anhydrobiosis in tardigrades—the last decade. *J Insect Physiol* 57(5), 577–583, 2011.

115. Yoshinaga, K., Yoshioka, H., Kurosaki, H., Hirasawa, M., Uritani, M., Hasegawa, K., Protection by trehalose of DNA from radiation damage. *Biosci Biotechnol Biochem* 61(1), 160–161, 1997.

116. Roots, R. and Okada, S., Estimation of life times and diffusion distances of radicals involved in x-ray-induced DNA strand breaks of killing of mammalian cells. *Radiat Res* 64(2), 306–320, 1975.

117. Rebecchi, L., Altiero, T., Guidetti, R., Cesari, M., Bertolani, R., Negroni, M., and Rizzo, A.M., Tardigrade resistance to space effects: First results of experiments on the LIFE-TARSE mission on FOTON-M3 (September 2007). *Astrobiology* 9(6), 581–591, 2009.

118. Rizzo, A.M., Negroni, M., Altiero, T., Montorfano, G., Corsetto, P., Berselli, P., Berra, B., Guidetti, R., Rebecchi, L., Antioxidant defences in the hydrated and desiccated states of the tardigrade *Paramacrobiotus richtersi. Comp Biochem Physiol B Biochem Mol Biol* 156(2), 115–121, 2010.

119. Rebecchi, L., Cesari, M., Altiero, T., Frigieri, A., and Guidetti, R., Survival and DNA degradation in anhydrobiotic tardigrades. *J Exp Biol* 212(Pt 24), 4033–4039, 2009.

120. Rebecchi, L., Altiero, T., and Guidetti, R., Anhydrobiosis: The extreme limit of desiccation tolerance. *Invertebr Survival J* 4, 65–81, 2007.

121. Jönsson, K.I., Harms-Ringdhal, M., and Torudd, J., Radiation tolerance in the eutardigrade *Richtersius coronifer. Int J Radiat Biol* 81(9), 649–656, 2005.

122. Horikawa, D.D., Cumbers, J., Rogoff1, D., Leuko1, S., Harnoto, R., Arakawa, K., Katayama, T., Toyoda, A., Kunieda, T., and Rothschild, L.J., UVC radiation tolerance in the Tardigrade *Ramazzottius varieornatus.* In *12th Int Symp on Tardigrada*, Portugal, June 2012. http://www.tardigrada.net/newsletter/images/symposia/12_Booklet.pdf (accessed July, 01, 2013).

123. Fontaneto, D., Herniou, E.A., Boschetti, C., Caprioli, M., Melone, G., Ricci, C., and Barraclough, T.G., Independently evolving species in asexual bdelloid rotifers. *PLoS Biol* 5(4), e87, 2007.

124. Gladyshev, E. and Meselson, M., Extreme resistance of bdelloid rotifers to ionizing radiation. *PNAS* 105, 5139–5144, 2008.

125. Shannon, A.J., Browne, J.A., Boyd, J., Fitzpatrick, D.A., and Burnell, A.M., The anhydrobiotic potential and molecular pohylogenetics of species and strains of *Panagrolaimus* (*Nematoda, Panagrolaimidae*). *J Exp Biol* 208, 2433–2445, 2005.

126. Tunnacliffe, A., Lapinski, J., and McGee, B., A putative LEA protein, but no trehalose, is present in anhydrobiotic bdelloid rotifers. *Hydrobiologia* 546, 315–321, 2005.

127. Milligan, J.R., Aguilera, J.A., Wu, C.C., Paglinawan, R.A., Nguyen, T.T., Wu, D., and Ward, J.F., Effect of hydroxyl radical scavenging capacity on clustering of DNA damage. *Rad Res* 148(4), 325–329, 1997.

128. Ayene, I.S., Koch, C.J., and Krisch, R.E., DNA strand breakage by bivalent metal ions and ionizing radiation. *Int J Rad Biol* 83, 195–210, 2007.

129. Chinnasri, B., Moy, J.H., Sipes, B.S., and Schmitt, D.P., Effect of gamma-irradiation and heat on root-knot Nematode, *Meloidogyne javanica*. *J Nematol* 29(1), 30–34, 1997.

130. Eichholz, G.G., Bogdanov, A.A., and Dwinell, L.D., Radiation sensitivity of pine wood nematodes in wood chips. *Int J Rad Appl Instrum Part A, Appl Rad Isotopes* 42(2), 177–179, 1991.

131. Ye, K., Ji, C.B., Lu, X.W., Ni, Y.H., Gao, C.L., Chen, X.H., Zhao, Y.P., Gu, G.X., and Guo, X.R., Resveratrol attenuates radiation damage in *Caenorhabditis elegans* by preventing oxidative stress. *J Radiat Res* 51(4), 473–479, 2010.

132. Marie, M., Hafner, S., Moratille, S., Vaigot, P., Mine, S., Rigaud, O., and Martin, M.T., FGF2 mediates DNA repair in epidermoid carcinoma cells exposed to ionizing radiation. *Int J Radiat Biol* 88(10), 688–93, 2012.

133. Ader, I., Muller, C., Bonnet, J., Favre, G., Cohen-Jonathan, E., Salles, B., and Toulas, C., The radioprotective effect of the 24 kDa FGF-2 isoform in HeLa cells is related to an increased expression and activity of the DNA dependent protein kinase (DNA-PK) catalytic subunit. *Oncogene* 21, 6471–6479, 2002.

134. Harfouche, G., Vaigot, P., Rachidi, W., Rigaud, O., Moratille, S., Marie, M., Lemaitre, G., Fortunel, N.O., and Martin, M.T., Fibroblast growth factor type 2 signaling is critical for DNA repair in human keratinocyte stem cells. *Stem Cells* 28, 1639–1648, 2010.

135. Venkatesan, J., Kim, and S.K., Chitosan composites for bone tissue engineering—an overview. *Mar Drugs* 8(8), 2252–2266, 2010.

136. Bosi, S., Da Ros, T., Spalluto, G., and Prato, M., Fullerene derivatives: An attractive tool for biological applications. *Eur J Med Chem* 38(11–12), 913–923, 2003.

137. Orme, M.W. and Labroo, V.M., Synthesis of β-estradiol-3-benzoate-17-(succinyl-12a-tetracycline): A potential bone-seeking estrogen. *Bioorg Med Chem Lett* 4, 1375–1380, 1994.

138. Willson, T.M., Charifson, P., Baxter, A., and Geddie, N., Bone targeted drugs.1. Identification of heterocycles with hydroxyapatite affinity. *Bioorg Med Chem Lett* 6(9) 1043–1046, 1996.

139. Rodan, G.A. and Fleisch, H.A., Bisphosphonates: Mechanisms of action. *J Clin Invest* 97(12), 2692–2696, 1996.

140. Gonzalez, K.A., Wilson, L.J., Wu, W., and Nancollas, G.H., Synthesis and in vitro characterization of a tissue-selective fullerene: Vectoring C(60)(OH)(16)AMBP to mineralized bone. *Bioorg Med Chem* 10(6), 1991–1997, 2002.

141. Di Martino, A., Sittinger, M., Risbud, and M.V., Chitosan: A versatile biopolymer for orthopaedic tissue-engineering. *Biomaterials* 26(30), 5983–5990, 2005.

142. Hu, Q., Li, B., Wang, M., and Shen, J., Preparation and characterization of biodegradable chitosan/hydroxyapatite nanocomposite rods via in situ hybridization: A potential material as internal fixation of bone fracture. *Biomaterials* 25(5), 779–785, 2004.

143. Wang, S.F., Shen, L., Zhang, W.D., and Tong, Y.J., Preparation and mechanical properties of chitosan/carbon nanotubes composites. *Biomacromolecules* 6(6), 3067–3072, 2005.

144. Usui, Y., Aoki, K., Narita, N., Murakami, N., Nakamura, I., Nakamura, K., Ishigaki, N., Yamazaki, H., Horiuchi, H., Kato, H., Taruta, S., Kim, Y.A., Endo, M., and Saito, N., Carbon nanotubes with high bone-tissue compatibility and bone-formation acceleration effects. *Small* 4(2), 240–246, 2008.

145. Zhao, B., Hu, H., Mandal, S.K., and Haddon, R.C., A bone mimic based on the self assembly of hydroxyapatite on chemically functionalized single-walled carbon nanotubes. *Chem Mater* 17(12), 3235–3241, 2005.

146. Geiger, M., Li, R.H., and Friess, W., Collagen sponges for bone regeneration with rhBMP-2. *Adv Drug Deliv Rev* 55(12), 1613–1629, 2003.

147. Gonçalves, G., Cruz, S.M., Ramalho, A., Grácio, J., and Marques, P.A., Graphene oxide versus functionalized carbon nanotubes as a reinforcing agent in a PMMA/HA bone cement. *Nanoscale* 4(9), 2937–2945, 2012.

148. Zanello, L.P., Zhao, B., Hu, H., Haddon, and R.C., Bone cell proliferation on carbon nanotubes. *Nano Lett* 6, 562–567, 2006.

149. Bhattacharya, M., Wutticharoenmongkol-Thitiwongsawet, P., Hamamoto, D.T., Lee, D., Cui, T., Prasad, H.S., and Ahmad, M., Bone formation on carbon nanotube composite. *J Biomed Mater Res A* 96(1), 75–82, 2011.

150. Nayak, T.R., Andersen, H., Makam, V.S., Khaw, C., Bae, S., Xu, X., Ee, P.L., Ahn, J.H., Hong, B.H., Pastorin, G., and Özyilmaz, B., Graphene for controlled and accelerated osteogenic differentiation of human mesenchymal stem cells. *ACS Nano* 5(6), 4670–4678, 2011.

151. Lee, Y., Bae, S., Jang, H., Jang, S., Zhu, S.E., Sim, S.H., Song, Y.I., Hong, B.H., and Ahn, J.H., Wafer-scale synthesis and transfer of graphene films. *Nano Lett* 10(2), 490–493, 2010.

152. Dalby, M.J., Gadegaard, N., Tare, R., Andar, A., Riehle, M.O., Herzyk, P., Wilkinson, C.D.W., and Oreffo, R.O.C., The control of human mesenchymal cell differentiation using nanoscale symmetry and disorder. *Nat Mater* 6(12), 997–1003, 2007.

153. Shao, S., Zhou, S., Li, L., Li, J., Luo, C., Wang, J., Li, X., and Weng, J., Osteoblast function on electrically conductive electrospun PLA/MWCNTs nanofibers. *Biomaterials* 32(11), 2821–2833, 2011.

154. Rivers, T.J., Hudson, T.W., and Schmidt, C.E., Synthesis of a novel, biodegradable electrically conducting polymer for biomedical applications. *Adv Funct Mater* 12(1), 33–37, 2002.

155. Li, X., and Kolega, J., Effects of direct current electric fields on cell migration and actin filament distribution in bovine vascular endothelial cells. *J Vasc Res* 39(5), 391–404, 2002.

156. Kotwal, A. and Schmidt, C.E., Electrical stimulation alters protein adsorption and nerve cell interactions with electrically conducting biomaterials. *Biomaterials* 22(10), 1055–1064, 2001.

157. Ozawa, H., Abe, E., Shibasaki, Y., Fukuhara, T., and Suda, T., Electric fields stimulate DNA synthesis of mouse osteoblast-like cells (MC3T3-E1) by a mechanism involving calcium ions. *J Cell Physiol* 138(3), 477–483, 1989.

158. Hu, J., Liu, X., and Ma, P.X., Induction of osteoblast differentiation phenotype on poly(l-lactic acid) nanofibrous matrix. *Biomaterials* 29(28), 3815–3821, 2008.

159. Badami, A.S., Kreke, M.R., Thompson, M.S., Riffle, J.S., and Goldstein, A.S., Effect of fiber diameter on spreading, proliferation, and differentiation of osteoblastic cells on electrospun poly(lactic acid) substrates. *Biomaterials* 27(4), 596–606, 2006.

160. Flemming, R.G., Murphy, C.J., Abrams, G.A., Goodman, S.L., and Nealey, P.F., Effects of synthetic micro- and nano-structured surfaces on cell behavior. *Biomaterials* 20, 573–588, 1999.

161. Curtis, A. and Wilkinson, C., Topographical control of cells. *Biomaterials* 18, 1573–1583, 1997.

162. LeBlanc, A., Shackelford, L., and Schneider, V., Future human bone research in space. *Bone* 22, 113S–116S, 1998.

163. Willey, J.S., Lloyd, S.A., Nelson, G.A., and Bateman, T.A., Ionizing radiation and bone loss: Space exploration and clinical therapy applications. *Clin Rev Bone Miner Metab* 9(1), 54–62, 2011.

164. Whitfield, J., Morley, P., and Willick, G., The parathyroid hormone, its fragments and analogues— potent bone-builders for treating osteoporosis. *Expert Opin Investig Drugs* 9(6), 1293–1315, 2000.

165. Vescini, F. and Grimaldi, F., PTH 1–84: Bone rebuilding as a target for the therapy of severe osteoporosis. *Clin Cases Miner Bone Metab* 9(1), 31–36, 2012.

166. Feng, Z., Shen, Y., Wang, L., Cheng, L., Wang, J., Li, Q., Shi, W., and Sun, X., An oligodeoxynucleotide with promising modulation activity for the proliferation and activation of osteoblast. *Int J Mol Sci* 12(4), 2543–2555, 2011.

167. Chatterjea, A., Yuan, H., Fennema, E., Chatterjea, S., Garritsen, H., Renard, A., van Blitterswijk, C.A., and de Boer, J., Engineering new bone via a minimally invasive route using human bone marrow derived stromal cell aggregates, micro ceramic particles and human platelet rich plasma gel. *Tissue Eng Part A* 19(3–4), 340–9, 2013.

168. Anyango, J.O., Duneas, N., Taylor, J.R., and Taylor, J., Physicochemical modification of kafirin microparticles and their ability to bind bone morphogenetic protein-2 (BMP-2), for application as a biomaterial. *J Agric Food Chem* 60(34), 8419–8426, 2012.

169. Egli, R.J. and Luginbuehl, R., Tissue engineering—nanomaterials in the musculoskeletal system. *Swiss Med Wkly* 142, w13647, 2012.

170. Aaron, J.E., Periosteal Sharpey's fibers: A novel bone matrix regulatory system? *Front Endocrinol (Lausanne)* 3, 98, 2012.

171. Feik, S.A., Storey, E., and Ellender, G., Stress induced periosteal changes. *Br J Exp Pathol* 68(6), 803–813, 1987.

172. Skerry, T.M., Bitensky, L., Chayen, J., and Lanyon, L.E., Early strain-related changes in enzyme activity in osyeocytes following bone loading in vivo. *J Bone Miner Res* 4, 783–786, 1989.

173. Meister, A., Polesel-Maris, J., Niedermann, P., Przybylska, J., Studer, P., Gabi, M. Behrb, P., Zambellib, T., Lileya, M., Vörösb, J., and Heinzelmanna, H., Nanoscale dispensing in liquid environment of streptavidin on a biotin-functionalized surface using hollow atomic force microscopy probes. *Microelectron Eng* 86, 1481, 2009.

174. Meister, M., Gabi, J., Polesel-Maris, P., Behr, P., Studer, J., Vörös, P., Niedermann, P., Bitterli, J., Polesel-Maris, J., Liley, M., Heinzelmann, H., and Zambelli, T., FluidFM: Combining atomic force microscopy and nanofluidics in a universal liquid delivery system for single cell applications and beyond. *Nano Lett* 9(6), 2501–7, 2009.

175. Tarawnehm, A.M., Wettergreen, M., and Liebschner, M.A., Computer-aided tissue engineering: Benefiting from the control over scaffold micro-architecture. *Methods Mol Biol* 868, 1–25, 2012.

176. Vanmaekelbergh, D. and van Vugt, L.K., ZnO nanowire lasers. *Nanoscale* 3(7), 2783–2800, 2011.

177. Guglielmotti, M.B., Renou, S., and Cabrini, R.L., A histomorphometric study of tissue interface by laminar implant test in rats. *Int J Oral Maxillofac Implants* 14, 565–570, 1999.

178. Zolynski, K., Witkowski, P., Kaluzny, A., Has, Z., Niedzielski, P., and Mitura, S., Implants with hard carbon layers for application in pseudoarthrosis femoris sin. Ostitis post fracturam apertam olim factam. *J Chem Vapor Depos* 4, 232–239, 1996.

179. Lappalainen, R., Selenius, M., Anttila, A., Konttinen, Y.T., and Santavirta, S.S., Reduction of wear in total hip replacement prostheses by amorphous diamond coatings. *J Biomed Mater Res: Appl Biomater* 66B, 410–413, 2003.

180. Thomas, V., Halloran, B.A., Ambalavanan, N., Catledge, S.A., and Vohra, Y.K., In vitro studies on the effect of particle size on macrophage responses to nanodiamond wear debris. *Acta Biomater* 8(5), 1939–1947, 2012.

181. Wissner-Gross, A.D. and Kaxiras, E., Diamond stabilization of ice multilayers at human body temperature. *Phys Rev E Stat Nonlin Soft Matter Phys* 76(2 Pt 1), 020501, 2007.

182. Chopard, A., Hillock, S., and Jasmin, B.J., Molecular events and signalling pathways involved in skeletal muscle disuse-induced atrophy and the impact of countermeasures. *J Cell Mol Med* 13(9B), 3032–3050, 2009.

183. Chopard, A., Lecunff, M., Danger, R., Lamirault, G., Bihouee, A., Teusan, R. Jasmin, B.J., Marini, J.F., and Leger, J.J., Large-scale mRNA analysis of female skeletal muscles during 60 days of bed rest with and without exercise or dietary protein supplementation as countermeasures. *Physiol Genomics* 38(3), 291–302, 2009.

184. Stein, T.P., Leskiw, M.J., Schluter, M.D., Donaldson, M.R., and Larina, I., Protein kinetics during and after long-duration spaceflight on MIR. *Am J Physiol* 276(6 Pt 1), E1014–21, 1999.

185. Basco, D., Nicchia, G.P., Desaphy, J.F., Camerino, D.C., Frigeri, A., and Svelto, M., Analysis by two-dimensional Blue Native/SDS-PAGE of membrane protein alterations in rat soleus muscle after hindlimb unloading. *Eur J Appl Physiol* 110(6), 1215–1224, 2010.

186. Trappe, T.A., Burd, N.A., Louis, E.S., Lee, G.A., and Trappe, S.W., Influence of concurrent exercise or nutrition countermeasures on thigh and calf muscle size and function during 60 days of bed rest in women. *Acta Physiol* 191(2), 147–159, 2007.

187. Trappe, S., Creer, A., Slivka, D., Minchev, K., and Trappe, T., Single muscle fiber function with concurrent exercise or nutrition countermeasures during 60 days of bed rest in women. *J Appl Physiol* 103(4), 1242–1250, 2007.

188. Norton, L.E., Wilson, G.J., Layman, D.K., Moulton, C.J., and Garlick, P.J., Leucine content of dietary proteins is a determinant of postprandial skeletal muscle protein synthesis in adult rats. *Nutr Metab (Lond)* 9(1), 67, 2012.

189. Chen, Y., Sood, S., McIntire, K., Roth, R., and Rabkin, R., Leucine-stimulated mTOR signaling is partly attenuated in skeletal muscle of chronically uremic rats. *Am J Physiol Endocrinol Metab* 301(5), E873–E881, 2011.

190. Allen, R.E. and Boxhorn, L.K., Regulation of skeletal muscle satellite cell proliferation and differentiation by transforming growth factor-beta, insulin-like growth factor I, and fibroblast growth factor. *J Cell Physiol* 138, 311–315, 1989.

191. Yang, Y.T. and McElligott, M.A., Multiple actions of beta-adrenergic agonists on skeletal muscle and adipose tissue. *Biochem J* 261(1), 1–10, 1989.

192. Servais, S., Letexier, D., Favier, R., Duchamp, C., and Desplanches, D., Prevention of unloading-induced atrophy by vitamin E supplementation: Links between oxidative stress and soleus muscle proteolysis? *Free Radic Biol Med* 42(5), 627–635, 2007.

193. Arbogast, S., Smith, J., Matuszczak, Y., Hardin, B.J., Moylan, J.S., Smith, J.D., Ware, J., Kennedy, A.R., and Reid, M.B., Bowman-Birk inhibitor concentrate prevents atrophy, weakness, and oxidative stress in soleus muscle of hindlimb unloaded mice. *J Appl Physiol* 102, 956–964, 2007.

194. Zielinska, M., Sawosz, E., Grodzik, M., Wierzbicki, M., Gromadka, M., Hotowy, A., Sawosz, F., Lozicki, A., and Chwalibog, A. Effect of heparan sulfate and gold nanoparticles on muscle development during embryogenesis. *Int J Nanomed* 6, 3163–3172, 2011.

195. Ghosh, P., Han, G., De, M., Kima, C.K., and Rotello, V.M., Gold nanoparticles in delivery applications. *Adv Drug Deliv Rev* 60(11), 1307–1315, 2008.

196. Gonçalves, A.S., Macedo, A.S., and Souto, E.B., Therapeutic nanosystems for oncology nanomedicine. *Clin Transl Oncol* 14(12), 883–90, 2012.

197. Alkilany, A.M., Lohse, S.E., and Murphy, C.J., The gold standard: Gold nanoparticle libraries to understand the nano-bio interface. *Acc Chem Res* 46(3), 650–661, 2013.

198. Kim, J.H., Yeom, J.H., Ko, J.J., Han, M.S., Lee, K., Na, S.Y., and Bae, J., Effective delivery of anti-miRNA DNA oligonucleotides by functionalized gold nanoparticles. *J Biotechnol* 155(3), 287–292, 2011.

199. Miyata, T., Taira, T., and Noishiki, Y., Collagen engineering for biomaterial use. *Clin Mater* 9(3–4), 139–148, 1992.

200. Takeshita, F., Minakuchi, Y., Nagahara, S., Honma, K., Sasaki, H., Hirai, K., Teratani, T., Namatame, N., Yamamoto, Y., Hanai, K., Kato, T., Sano, A., and Ochiya, T., Efficient delivery of small interfering RNA to bone-metastatic tumors by using atelocollagen in vivo. *Proc Natl Acad Sci USA* 102(34), 12177–12182, 2005.

201. Hanai, K., Takeshita, F., Honma, K., Nagahara, S., Maeda, M., Minakuchi, Y., Sano, A., and Ochiya, T., Atelocollagen-mediated systemic DDS for nucleic acid medicines. *Ann N Y Acad Sci* 1082, 9–17, 2006.

202. Magee, T.R., Artaza, J.N., Ferrini, M.G., Vernet, D., Zuniga, F.I., Cantini, L., Reisz-Porszasz, S., Rajfer, J., and Gonzalez-Cadavid, N.F., Myostatin short interfering hairpin RNA gene transfer increases skeletal muscle mass. *J Gene Med* 8: 1171–1181, 2006.

203. Kinouchi, N., Ohsawa, Y., Ishimaru, N., Ohuchi, H., Sunada, Y., Hayashi, Y., Tanimoto, Y., Moriyama, K., and Noji. S., Atelocollagen-mediated local and systemic applications of myostatin-targeting siRNA increase skeletal muscle mass. *Gene Ther* 15(15), 1126–1130, 2008.

204. Ladeira, M.S., Andrade, V.A., Gomes, E.R., Aguiar, C.J., Moraes, E.R., Soares, J.S., Silva, E.E., Lacerda, R.G., Ladeira, L.O., Jorio, A., Lima, P., Leite, M.F., Resende, R.R., and Guatimosim, S., Highly efficient siRNA delivery system into human and murine cells using single-wall carbon nanotubes. *Nanotechnology* 21(38), 385101, 2010.
205. Martinelli, V., Cellot, G., Toma, F.M., Long, C.S., Caldwell, J.H., Zentilin, L., Giacca, M., Turco, A., Prato, M., Ballerini, L., and Mestroni, L., Carbon nanotubes promote growth and spontaneous electrical activity in cultured cardiac myocytes. *Nano Lett* 12(4), 1831–1838, 2012.
206. Emerich, D.F., Orive, G., and Borlongan, C., Tales of biomaterials, molecules, and cells for repairing and treating brain dysfunction. *Curr Stem Cell Res Ther* 6(3), 171–189, 2011.
207. Alhosseini, S.N., Moztarzadeh, F., Mozafari, M., Asgari, S., and Dodel, M., Samadikuchaksaraei, A. et al. Synthesis and characterization of electrospun polyvinyl alcohol nanofibrous scaffolds modified by blending with chitosan for neural tissue engineering. *Int J Nanomed* 7, 25–34, 2012.
208. Jang, M.J., Namgung, S., Hong, S., and Nam, Y., Directional neurite growth using carbon nanotube patterned substrates as a biomimetic cue. *Nanotechnology* 21(23), 235102, 2010.
209. Merkle, R.C., The molecular repair of the brain. *Cryonics Mag* 15(1, 2), January and April 1994.
210. Dancoff, S.M. and Quastler, H., The information content and error rate of living things. In Quastler, H. (ed.), *Essays on the Use of Information Theory in Biology,* University of Illinois Press, Urbana, 1953, pp. 263–273, 1953.
211. Santos, T., Maia, J., Agasse, F., Xapelli, S., Ferreira, L., and Bernardino, L., Nanomedicine boosts neurogenesis: New strategies for brain repair. *Integr Biol (Camb)* 4(9), 973–981, 2012.
212. Reynolds, B.A. and Weiss, S., Generation of neurons and astrocytes from isolated cells of the adult mammalian central nervous system. *Science* 255(5052), 1707–1710, 1992.
213. Gage, F.H., Coates, P.W., Palmer, T.D., Kuhn, H.G., Fisher, L.J., Suhonen, J.O., Peterson, D.A., Suhr, S.T., and Ray, J., Survival and differentiation of adult neuronal progenitor cells transplanted to the adult brain. *Proc Natl Acad Sci USA* 92(25), 11879–11883, 1995.
214. Quadrato, G. and Di Giovanni, S., Waking up the sleepers: Shared transcriptional pathways in axonal regeneration and neurogenesis. *Cell Mol Life Sci* 70(6), 993–1007, 2013.
215. Kazanis, I., Neurogenesis in the adult mammalian brain: How much do we need, how much do we have? *Curr Top Behav Neurosci* 15, 3–29, 2013.
216. Gage, F.H., Neurogenesis in the adult brain. *J Neurosci* 22(3), 612–613, 2002.
217. Bible, E., Chau, D.Y., Alexander, M.R., Price, J., Shakesheff, K.M., and Modo, M., The support of neural stem cells transplanted into stroke-induced brain cavities by PLGA particles. *Biomaterials* 30(16), 2985–2994, 2009.
218. Cook, A.M., Mieure, K.D., Owen, R.D., Pesaturo, A.B., and Hatton, J., Intracerebroventricular administration of drugs. *Pharmacotherapy* 29(7), 32–45, 2009.
219. Gabathuler, R., Approaches to transport therapeutic drugs across the blood-brain barrier to treat brain diseases. *Neurobiol Dis* 37(1), 48–57, 2010.
220. Duester, G., Retinoic acid synthesis and signaling during early organogenesis. *Cell* 134(6), 921–931, 2008.
221. Maia, J., Santos, T., Aday, S., Agasse, F., Cortes, L., Malva, J.O., Bernardino, L., and Ferreira, L., Controlling the neuronal differentiation of stem cells by the intracellular delivery of retinoic acid-loaded nanoparticles. *ACS Nano* 5(1), 97–106, 2011.
222. Chen, H.L., Qu, L.N., Li, Q.D., Bi, L., Huang, Z.M., and Li, Y.H., Simulated microgravity-induced oxidative stress in different areas of rat brain. *Sheng Li Xue Bao* 61(2), 108–114, 2009.
223. Sarkar, P., Sarkar, S., Ramesh, V., Kim, H., Barnes, S., Kulkarni, A., Hall, J.C., Wilson, B.L., Thomas, R.L., Pellis, N.R., and Ramesh, G.T., Proteomic analysis of mouse hypothalamus under simulated microgravity. *Neurochem Res* 33(11), 2335–2341, 2008.
224. Roberts, J.E., Kukielczak, B.M., Chignell, C.F., Sik, B.H., Hu, D.N., and Principato, M.A., Simulated microgravity induced damage in human retinal pigment epithelial cells. *Mol Vis* 30(12), 633–638, 2006.

225. Xu, H., Manivannan, A., Liversidge, J., Sharp, P.F., Forrester, J.V., and Crane, I.J., Requirements for passage of T lymphocytes across non-inflamed retinal microvessels. *J Neuroimmunol* 142(1–2), 47–57, 2003.

226. Li, S.Y., Fung, F.K., Fu, Z.J., Wong, D., Chan, H.H., and Lo, A.C., Anti-inflammatory effects of lutein in retinal ischemic/hypoxic injury: In vivo and in vitro studies. *Invest Ophthalmol Vis Sci* 53(10), 5976–5984, 2012.

227. Delyfer, M.N., Raffelsberger, W., Mercier, D., Korobelnik, J.F., Gaudric, A., Charteris, D.G., Tadayoni, R., Metge, F., Caputo, G., Barale, P.O., Ripp, R., Muller, J.D., Poch, O., Sahel, J.A., and Léveillard, T., Transcriptomic analysis of human retinal detachment reveals both inflammatory response and photoreceptor death. *PLoS One* 6(12), e28791, 2011.

228. Campochiaro, P.A., Pathogenic mechanisms in proliferative vitreoretinopathy. *Arch Ophthalmol* 115(2), 237–241, 1997.

229. Vingerling, J.R., Dielemans, I., Bots, M.L., Hofman, A., Grobbee, D.E., and de Jong, P.T., Age-related macular degeneration is associated with atherosclerosis. The Rotterdam study. *Am J Epidemiol* 142, 404–409, 1995.

230. Sabour-Pickett, S., Nolan, J.M., Loughman, J., and Beatty, S., A review of the evidence germane to the putative protective role of the macular carotenoids for age-related macular degeneration. *Mol Nutr Food Res* 56(2), 270–286, 2012.

231. Kim, J.H., Kim, J.H., Kim, K.W., Kim, M.H., and Yu, Y.S., Intravenously administered gold nanoparticles pass through the blood-retinal barrier depending on the particle size, and induce no retinal toxicity. *Nanotechnology* 20(50), 505101, 2009.

232. Sahoo, S.K., Dilnawaz, F., and Krishnakumar, S., Nanotechnology in ocular drug delivery. *Drug Discov Today* 13, 144–151, 2008.

233. Kranz, H., Ubrich, N., Maincent, P., and Bodmeier, R., Physicomechanical properties of biodegradable poly(D,L-lactide) and poly(D,L-lactide-co-glycolide) films in the dry and wet states. *J Pharm Sci* 89(12), 1558–1566, 2000.

234. Thomson, H. and Lotery, A., The promise of nanomedicine for ocular disease. *Nanomedicine* 4(6), 599–604, 2009.

235. Chen, J., Patil, S., Seal, S., and McGinnis, J.F., Rare earth nanoparticles prevent retinal degeneration induced by intracellular peroxides. *Nat Nanotechnol* 1(2), 142–150, 2006.

236. Kim, D.H. and Martin, D.C., Sustained release of dexamethasone from hydrophilic matrices using PLGA nanoparticles for neural drug delivery. *Biomaterials* 27(15), 3031–3037, 2006.

237. Zarbin, M.A., Montemagno, C., Leary, J.F., and Ritch, R., Regenerative nanomedicine and the treatment of degenerative retinal diseases. *Wiley Interdiscip Rev Nanomed Nanobiotechnol* 4(1), 113–137, 2012.

238. Deshpande, S., Patil, S., Kuchibhatla, S.V., and Seal, S., Size dependency variation in lattice parameter and valency states in nanocrystalline cerium oxide. *Appl Phys Lett* 87(13), 133113, 2005.

239. Tsunekawa, S., Sahara, R., Kawazoe, Y., and Ishikawa, K., Lattice relaxation of monosize CeO2-x nanocrystalline particles. *Appl Surf Sci* 152, 53–56, 1999.

240. Celardo, I., Pedersen, J.Z., Traversa, E., and Ghibelli, L., Pharmacological potential of cerium oxide nanoparticles. *Nanoscale* 3(4), 1411–1420, 2011.

241. Killer, H.E., Jaggi, G.P., and Miller, N.R., Papilledema revisited: Is its pathophysiology really understood? *Clin Exp Ophthalmol* 37(5), 444–447, 2009.

242. Wiener, T.C., Space obstructive syndrome: Intracranial hypertension, intraocular pressure, and papilledema in space. *Aviat Space Environ Med* 83(1), 64–66, 2012.

243. Aptel, F., Chiquet, C., and Romanet, J.P., Intraocular pressure-lowering combination therapies with prostaglandin analogues. *Drugs* 72(10), 1355–1371, 2012.

244. Bertram, J.P., Saluja, S.S., McKain, J., and Lavik, E.B., Sustained delivery of timolol maleate from poly(lactic-co-glycolic acid)/poly(lactic acid) microspheres for over 3 months, *J Microencapsul* 26(1), 26, 2009.

245. Chew, S.Y., Mi, R., Hoke, A., and Leong, K.W., Aligned protein–polymer composite fibers enhance nerve regeneration: A potential tissue-engineering platform, *Adv Funct Mater* 17(8), 1288–1296, 2007.

246. Chen, D.F. and Rao, R.C., Nanomedicine and optic nerve regeneration—Implications for ophthalmology. *US Ophthal Rev* 4(1), 108–111, 2011.
247. Dynan, W.S., Takeda, Y., and Li, S., Modifying the function of DNA repair nanomachines for therapeutic benefit. *Nanomedicine* 2(2), 74–81, 2006.
248. Ward, J.F., Nature of lesions formed by ionizing radiation. In Nickoloff, J.A., and Hoekstra, M.F. (eds.), *DNA Damage and Repair*, Humana Press, Totowa, NJ, Vol. II, 1998, pp. 65–84.
249. Di Leonardo, A., Linke, S.P., Clarkin, K., and Wahl, G.M., DNA damage triggers a prolonged p53-dependent G1 arrest and long-term induction of Cip1 in normal human fibroblasts. *Genes Dev* 8(21), 2540–2451, 1994.
250. Sonoda, E., Takata, M., Yamashita, Y.M., Morrison, C., and Takeda, S., Homologous DNA recombination in vertebrate cells. *Proc Natl Acad Sci USA* 98(15), 8388–8394, 2001.
251. Featherstone, C. and Jackson, S.P., DNA double-strand break repair. *Curr Biol* 9(20), R759–R761, 1999.
252. Mladenov, E. and Iliakis, G., Induction and repair of DNA double strand breaks: The increasing spectrum of non-homologous end joining pathways. *Mutat Res* 711(1–2), 61–72, 2011.
253. Lieber, M.R., The mechanism of double-strand DNA break repair by the nonhomologous DNA end-joining pathway, *Annu Rev Biochem* 79, 181–211, 2010.
254. Mognato, M., Girardi, C., Fabris, S., and Celotti, L., DNA repair in modeled microgravity: Double strand break rejoining activity in human lymphocytes irradiated with gamma-rays. *Mutat Res* 663(1–2), 32–39, 2009.
255. Rowe, W.J., Correcting magnesium deficiencies may prolong life. *Clin Interv Aging* 7, 51–54, 2012.
256. Leach Huntoon, C.S., Grigoriev, A.L., and Natochin, Y.V., *Fluid and Electrolyte Regulation in Spaceflight 94*, Science and Technology Series, San Diego, CA, pp. 11–13, 1998.
257. Killilea, D.W. and Maier, J.A., A connection between magnesium deficiency and aging: New insights from cellular studies. *Magnes Res* 21(2), 77–82, 2008.
258. Lue, N.F., Sequence-specific and conformation-dependent binding of yeast telomerase RNA to single-stranded telomeric DNA. *Nucl Acids Res* 27(12), 2560–2567, 1999.
259. Wolf, F.I., Trapani, V., Simonacci, M., Ferré, S., and Maier, J.A., Magnesium deficiency and endothelial dysfunction: Is oxidative stress involved? *Magnes Res* 21(1), 58–64, 2008.
260. Shafiee, H., Mohammadi, H., Rezayat, S.M., Hosseini, A., Baeeri, M., Hassani, S., Mohammadirad, A., Bayrami, Z., and Abdollahi, M., Prevention of malathion-induced depletion of cardiac cells mitochondrial energy and free radical damage by a magnetic magnesium-carrying nanoparticle. *Toxicol Mech Methods* 20(9), 538–543, 2010.
261. Buchachenko, A.L., Kouznetsov, D.A., Arkhangelsky, S.E., Orlova, M.A., and Markarian, A.A., Spin biochemistry: Magnetic 24Mg-25Mg-26Mg isotope effect in mitochondrial ADP phosphorylation. *Cell Biochem Biophys* 43(2), 243–251, 2005.
262. Buchachenko, A.L. and Kuznetsov, D.A., Magnetic field affects enzymatic ATP synthesis. *J Am Chem Soc* 130(39), 12868–12869, 2008.
263. Rezayat, S.M., Boushehri, S.V., Salmanian, B., Omidvari, A.H., Tarighat, S., and Esmaeili, S. et al., The porphyrin-fullerene nanoparticles to promote the ATP overproduction in myocardium: $^{25}Mg^{2+}$-magnetic isotope effect. *Eur J Med Chem* 44(4), 1554–1569, 2009.
264. Freitas Jr., R.A., The future of nanofabrication and molecular scale devices in nanomedicine. In Renata, G.B. (ed.), *Future of Health Technology*, IOS Press, Amsterdam, The Netherlands, pp. 45–59, 2002.
265. Freitas Jr., R.A. and Phoenix, C.J., Vasculoid: A personal nanomedical appliance to replace human blood. *J Evol Technol* 111–139, 2002.
266. Tong, X.C., Chapter 11—Special shielding materials in aerospace and nuclear industries. In *Advanced Materials and Design for Electromagnetic Interference Shielding*, CRC Press, Taylor & Francis, Boca Raton, FL, pp. 275–292, 2008.
267. Singh, K., Singh, H., Sharma, V., Nathuram, R., Khanna, A., and Kumar, R. et al., Gamma-ray attenuation coefficients in bismuth borate glasses. *Nucl Instr Meth Phys Res B: Beam Interactions with Materials and Atoms* 194(1), 1–6, 2002.

268. Singh, H., Singh, K., Gerward, L., Singh, K., Sahota, H.S., and Nathuram, R., ZnO–PbO–B_2O_3 glasses as gamma-ray shielding materials. *Nucl Instr Meth Phys Res B: Beam Interactions with Materials and Atoms* 207(3), 257–262, 2003.

269. Singh, N., Singh, K.J., Singh, K., and Singh, H., Comparative study of lead borate and bismuth lead borate glass systems as gamma-radiation shielding materials. *Nucl Instr Meth Phys Res B: Beam Interactions with Materials and Atoms* 225(3), 305–309, 2004.

270. Singh, N., Singh, K.J., Singh, K., and Singh, H., Gamma-ray attenuation studies of PbO-BaOB_2O_3 glass system. *Radiat Meas* 4(1), 84–88, 2006.

271. Xu, S., A novel ultra-light structure for radiation shielding. Master of Science Thesis, North Carolina State University, 2008.

272. Singh, K.J., Singh, N., Kaundal, R.S., and Singh, K., Gamma-ray shielding and structural properties of PbO–SiO_2 glasses. *Nucl Instr Meth Phys Res B: Beam Interactions with Materials and Atoms* 266(6), 944–948, 2008.

273. Zhang, H.B., Yan, Q., Zheng, W.G., He, Z., and Yu, Z.Z., Tough graphene-polymer microcellular foams for electromagnetic interference shielding. *ACS Appl Mater Interfaces* 3(3), 918–924, 2011.

274. Li, N., Huang, Y., Du, F., He, X., Lin, X., Gao, H., Ma, Y., Li, F., Chen, Y., and Eklund, P.C., Electromagnetic interference (EMI) shielding of single-walled carbon nanotube epoxy composites. *Nano Lett* 6(6), 1141–1145, 2006.

275. White, R.J., Averner, M., Humans in space. *Nature* 409(6823), 1115–1118, 2001.

276. Fei, D.Y., Zhao, X., Boanca, C., Hughes, E., Bai, O., Merrell, R., and Rafiq, A., A biomedical sensor system for real-time monitoring of astronauts' physiological parameters during extravehicular activities. *Comput Biol Med* 40(7), 635–642, 2010.

277. Chen, B. and Mckay, C.P., Radiation shielding systems using nanotechnology, United States Patent, 7923709, 04/12/2011.

278. Chen, D. and Wu, J., Dislodgement and removal of dust-particles from a surface by a technique combining acoustic standing wave and airflow. *J Acoust Soc Am* 127(1), 45–50, 2010.

279. Tanaka, K., Gotoh, T.M., Morita, H., and Hargens, A.R., Skin blood flow with elastic compressive extravehicular activity space suit. *Biol Sci Space* 17(3), 227, 2003.

280. Webb, P. and Annis, J., Development of a Space Activity Suit, NASA CR-1892, December 1971.

281. Waldie, J.M.A., *Mechanical Counter Pressure Space Suits: Advantages Limitations and Concepts for Martian Exploration*, The Mars Society, 2005. http://quest.nasa.gov/projects/spacewardbound/australia2009/docs/Waldie%202005%20MCP-Paper.pdf (accessed July, 02, 2013)

282. Hodgson, E., The chameleon suit—a liberated future for space explorers. *Gravitat Space Biol Bull* 16(2), 107–120, 2003.

283. Lee, M., Chen, C.Y., Wang, S., Cha, S.N., Park, Y.J., Kim, J.M., Chou, L.J., and Wang, Z.L., A hybrid piezoelectric structure for wearable nanogenerators. *Adv Mater* 24(13), 1759–1764, 2012.

284. Wang, Z., Hu, J., Suryavanshi, A.P., Yum, K., and Yu, M.F., Voltage generation from individual BaTiO(3) nanowires under periodic tensile mechanical load. *Nano Lett* 7(10), 2966–2969, 2007.

285. Zhou, Y.S., Wang, K., Han, W., Rai, S.C., Zhang, Y., Ding, Y., Pan, C., Zhang, F., Zhou, W., and Wang, Z.L., Vertically aligned CdSe nanowire arrays for energy harvesting and piezotronic devices. *ACS Nano* 6(7), 6478–6482, 2012.

286. Riemer, R. and Shapiro, A., Biomechanical energy harvesting from human motion: Theory, state of the art, design guidelines, and future directions. *J Neuroeng Rehabil* 8, 22, 2011.

287. Donelan, J.M., Li, Q., Naing, V., Hoffer, J.A., Weber, D.J., and Kuo, A.D., Biomechanical energy harvesting: Generating electricity during walking with minimal user effort. *Science* 319(5864), 807–810, 2008.

288. Koenig, S.P., Wang, L., Pellegrino, J., and Bunch, J.S., Selective molecular sieving through porous graphene Nat Nanotechnol. 7(11), 728–32, 2012.

289. Jiang, D.E., Cooper, V.R., and Dai, S., Porous graphene as the ultimate membrane for gas separation. *Nano Lett* 9(12), 4019–4024, 2009.

290. Ong, M.T. and Reed, E.J., Engineered piezoelectricity in graphene. *ACS Nano* 6(2), 1387–1394, 2012.
291. Guo, H., Meador, M.A., McCorkle, L., Quade, D.J., Guo, J., Hamilton, B., Cakmak, M., and Sprowl, G., Polyimide aerogels cross-linked through amine functionalized polyoligomeric silsesquioxane. *ACS Appl Mater Interfaces* 3(2), 546–552, 2011.
292. Paul, H.L. and Diller, K.R., Comparison of thermal insulation performance of fibrous materials for the advanced space suit. *J Biomech Eng* 125(5), 639–647, 2003.
293. Peer, E., Artzy-Schnirman, A., Gepstein, L., and Sivan, U., Hollow nanoneedle array and its utilization for repeated administration of biomolecules to the same cells. *ACS Nano* 6(6), 4940–4946, 2012.
294. Freitas, R.A.Jr., Exploratory design in medical nanotechnology: A mechanical artificial red cell. *Artif Cells Blood Substit Immobil Biotechnol* 26(4), 411–430, 1998.
295. Ionov, L. and Synytska, A., Self-healing superhydrophobic materials. *Phys Chem Chem Phys* 14(30), 10497–10502, 2012.
296. Shi, Q., Wong, S.C., Ye, W., Hou, J., Zhao, J., and Yin, J., Mechanism of adhesion between polymer fibers at nanoscale contacts. *Langmuir* 28(10), 4663–4671, 2012.
297. Chung, C-M., Roh, Y-S., Cho, S-Y., and Kim, J-G., Crack healing in polymeric materials via photochemical [2+2] cycloaddition. *Chem Mater* 16, 3982–3984, 2004.
298. Amamoto, Y., Kamada, J., Otsuka, H., Takahara, A., and Matyjaszewski, K., Repeatable photoinduced self-healing of covalently cross-linked polymers through reshuffling of trithiocarbonate units. *Angew Chem Int Ed Eng* 50(7), 1660–1663, 2011.
299. Jackson, A.C., Bartelt, J.A., Marczewski, K., Sottos, N.R., and Braun, P.V., Silica-protected micron and sub-micron capsules and particles for self-healing at the microscale. *Macromol Rapid Commun* 32(1), 82–87, 2011.
300. Tagawa, Y., Oudalov, N., El Ghalbzouri, A., Sun, C., and Lohse, D., Needle-free injection into skin and soft matter with highly focused microjets. Lab Chip. 13(7), 1357–63, 2013.
301. Overbye, D., Offering funds, U.S. Agency dreams of sending humans to stars. *The New York Times*, August 17, 2011. http://www.nytimes.com/2011/08/18/science/space/18starship.html?pagewanted=all (accessed October 13, 2012).
302. Alcor Life Extension Foundation, 2012. http://www.alcor.org/ (accessed July, 14, 2013)
303. Khalili, M.A., Maione, M., Palmerini, M.G., Bianchi, S., Macchiarelli, G., and Nottola, S.A., Ultrastructure of human mature oocytes after vitrification. *Eur J Histochem* 56(3), 2012.
304. Fahy, G.M., Wowk, B., Wu, J., Phan, J., Rasch, C., Chang, A., and Zendejas, E., Cryopreservation of organs by vitrification: Perspectives and recent advances. *Cryobiology* 48(2), 157–178, 2004.
305. Merkle, R.C. and Freitas Jr., R.A., A cryopreservation revival scenario using molecular nanotechnology. *Cryonics* 4th Quarter, 29(4), 7–8, 2008.
306. Fahy, G., "Realistic" scenario for nanotechnological repair of the frozen human brain. In Wowk, B., Darwin, M. (eds.), *Cryonics: Reaching for Tommorow* , Alcor Life Extension Foundation, Scottsdale, AZ, 1991.
307. Blackstone, E., Morrison, M., and Roth, M.B., H_2S induces a suspended animation-like state in mice. *Science* 308(5721), 518, 2005.
308. Jinka, T.R., Tøien, Ø., and Drew, K.L., Season primes the brain in an arctic hibernator to facilitate entrance into torpor mediated by adenosine A(1) receptors. *J Neurosci* 31(30), 10752–10758, 2011.
309. Tamura, Y., Shintani, M., Nakamura, A., Monden, M., and Shiomi, H., Phase-specific central regulatory systems of hibernation in Syrian hamsters. *Brain Res*1045, 88–96, 2005.
310. Lastapis, M., Martin, M., Riedel, D., Hellner, L., Comtet, G., and Dujardin, G., Picometer-scale electronic control of molecular dynamics inside a single molecule. *Science* 308(5724), 1000–1003, 2005.
311. 100 Year Starship http://100yss.org/initiative
312. Mironov, V., Kasyanov, V., and Markwald, R.R., Organ printing: From bioprinter to organ biofabrication line. *Curr Opin Biotechnol* 22(5), 667–673, 2011.

313. Marga, F., Jakab, K., Khatiwala, C., Shepherd, B., Dorfman, S., Hubbard, B., Colbert, S., and Gabor, F., Toward engineering functional organ modules by additive manufacturing. *Biofabrication* 4(2), 022001, 2012.
314. Koch, L., Deiwick, A., Schlie, S., Michael, S., Gruene, M., Coger, V., Zychlinski, D., Schambach, A., Reimers, K., Vogt, P.M., and Chichkov, B., Skin tissue generation by laser cell printing. *Biotechnol Bioeng* 109(7), 1855–1863, 2012.
315. Freitas, R.A. Jr., Nanodentistry. *J Am Dent Assoc* 131(11), 1559–1565, 2000.
316. Groopman, J., Medicine on Mars, Astronaut Bio-Suit for Exploration Class Missions: NIAC Phase I Report, 2001.
317. Hall, J.S., Utility fog: The stuff that dreams are made of. In Crandall, B.C. (ed.), *Nanotechnology: Molecular Speculations on Global Abundance*, MIT Press, Cambridge, MA, pp. 161–184, 1996.

17

Nanomedicine in Regenerative Biosystems, Human Augmentation, and Longevity

Frank J. Boehm

CONTENTS

17.1 Nanomedicine in Regenerative Biosystems

It seems reasonable to infer, based on the accelerating pace of advances in the field, that fundamental strategies will evolve for the nanomedical repair and subsequent regeneration of myriad cell types (i.e., those damaged or diseased cells that have not crossed the nonrecoverable threshold) in the human body, which will allow for sufficient operational latitude to accommodate the inherent variabilities of distinct cell species. A standardized set of instrumentation onboard nanomedical devices might enable nanometric biopsies and cellular/organellar imaging in situ, facilitate peptide or drug delivery to individual cells, and conduct multiple modes of repair, which can be reconfigured as appropriate to suit different cell types. Distinct classes of nanomedical devices could be implemented to perform dedicated diagnostic (Chapters 1, 8–11) and therapeutic (Chapters 12–17) procedures.

Protocols may stipulate that nanodevices conduct initial diagnostic interrogations of each cell of the group that they are assigned to treat within a predetermined spatial domain. Subsequent to the verification and quantification of the extent of damage within individual cells caused by injury or disease, appropriate sequential repair operations would ensue until it can be verified, via incremental checks, that the prescribed remedial procedures have been completed. A final "outcome" diagnostic assessment would then be performed to ensure the success of the treatment, and that the health of the cell has been recovered.

These restorative "cell-centric" repairs could be performed (if deemed necessary by physicians and/or surgeons) in a massively parallel manner to rapidly accrue cumulative benefits for entire organs (e.g., brain, heart, lung, liver, kidney) and systems (e.g., circulatory, lymphatic, nervous, various sensory, gastrointestinal). When the vital constituents (cells) that comprise these organs and systems are restored to vibrant health, it is likely to follow that the organs and systems themselves, within which they reside, will undergo positive transformations that reflect this condition, and in turn translate to robust overall health for the patient. An exploration (by no means comprehensive) of how nanomedicine may beneficially impact human cellular "patients" is conducted in the following.

17.1.1 Nanomedical Cell Repair

One can envisage that in conjunction with the advent of sophisticated autonomous nanomedical devices and systems, conventional surgical procedures, which entail invasive incision-based access to anatomical sites for the bulk removal, repair, or replacement of damaged or diseased tissues and organs, will become obsolete. Adept, mass orchestrations of micron-sized nanodevices (Figure 17.1) will have the capacity, under the direction of the human surgeons who program them, to perform elegant nanosurgical procedures (under exceptionally stringent safety and efficiency protocols) at the cellular, molecular, and inevitably atomic levels, to swiftly address virtually any conceivable injury or disease state, including aging (Section 17.3).

The manipulation of molecules within cell structures in order to bring them into alignment with those of healthy cells of the same species might be accomplished through guided physiochemical reconstruction, derived from and driven by onboard databases that house templates of healthy cells of specific genera. In highly advanced nanomedical devices, onboard three-dimensional (3D) "atomic maps" (though perhaps considerably excessive in detail) may contain useful data reflected in the identity and spatial positions

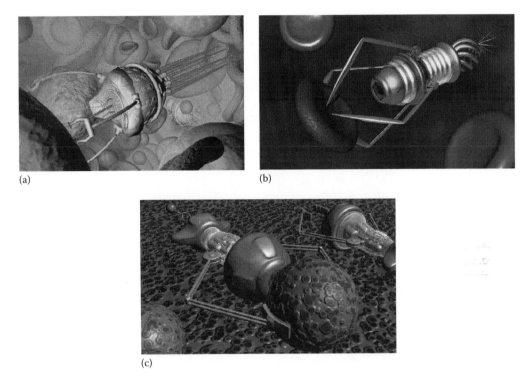

(a)

(b)

(c)

FIGURE 17.1
Conceptual depictions of nanomedical devices: (a) diamondoid cell repair nanodevice, (b) performing RBC inspection, and (c) transporting a drug molecule. (Image (a): created by Yuriy Svidinenko, Nanobotmodels Company; Images (b) and (c): produced by and copyright Christopher Barnatt, ExplainingTheFuture.com. With permission.)

of all atomic species (in relation to a precisely determined central reference datum) of all human cell types. These atomic resolution cell maps might serve as comparative reference templates to guide cell repair nanodevices in the manipulation and reconstruction of aberrant cellular constituents. Aging cells could likely be rebuilt and upgraded to a (user-selected) youthful state, derived from onboard molecular templates of young cells of the same type (Section 17.3). These procedures would also entail the disassembly and removal of accumulated intracellular lipofuscin deposits (Section 17.3.1) (the recalcitrant waxy metabolic end product of lysosome hydrolase enzymatic degradation).

The premise here would not be to have the template replicated exactly in the production of a cloned cell, but rather to make available to cell repair devices the most comprehensive data possible, from which to work. It is virtually guaranteed that individual cells, even if they are of the same type, will not be identical in every way. There are bound to be nuanced variabilities, for instance, insofar as the exact sizes and shapes of the cell exterior; the location, orientation, and geometries of the nucleus and cell-resident organelles (e.g., Golgi complex, endoplasmic reticulum); size and morphologies of membrane-embedded surface proteins, nuclear pores It is likely that there will evolve established standardized parameters (tolerances/margins of error) within which cell repair nanodevices must deftly operate in the repair of individual cell components. Important investigations in this regard might aim to define and quantify thresholds that can be tolerated between differently sized and shaped organelles and variances in their atomic composition, as relates to their optimal functionality.

Drexler suggests that, as relates to cryonics applications, "... to repair a damaged cell, you do have to recognize a complex pattern of molecules and decide what to do about it. Therefore, if you want to have a general, powerful cell repair capability ... you're going to need on-site computers. Fortunately, as we have seen, these turn out to be possible." He supports the notion that all of the mechanistic functionalities that may be required for efficient repair of cells may be analogously extrapolated from biological entities (e.g., white blood cells and viruses [tissue and cell entry strategies], organelles [intracellular mobility], antibodies [protein identification], enzymes, ribosomes, and cytoskeleton [actin, tubulin] proteins [molecular detection, disassembly, and self-assembly]) [1]. Wowk concurs with this idea and brings attention to the fact that all of the capabilities necessary to enable cell repair are regularly evidenced through the process of cell division, which continually replicates new cells within our bodies, utilizing readily available molecules. Nanomedical conceptualists, designers, and engineers will be significantly challenged with the development of biomimetic analogs for each of the functionalities involved in cell replication, which will work in conjunction to make sophisticated cell repair nanodevices possible [2].

As relates to the comprehensive functionality and design of cell repair nanodevices, an optimal logistical strategy may include that multiple species, constituting a cell repair "suite," might be dedicated to specific tasks, for the sake of (relative) simplicity, and to expedite their development and implementation. Nanomedical cell repair devices will likely operate in a massively parallel fashion to facilitate rapid repairs, and hence the swift restoration of the patient to optimal health. When pondering optimized advanced and autonomous cell repair nanodevices (time line ~2020 to 2030), it may be presumed that they will likely not possess universal functionality, and attempts with this aim may well become mired in undue complexities. Hence, a clearly articulated scope of operations will be useful. A potential best case scenario, in terms of strategy and efficiencies, may involve multiple, task-dedicated cell repair nanodevices that are deployed sequentially to address particular conditions that have specific requirements, toward enabling highly streamlined repair procedures for the benefit of the patient. These nanodevices could be assigned to dedicated tasks such as initial interrogative scanning, the supply of modular prefabricated replacement organelles and other cell components, the removal of cellular detritus and plaque materials (e.g., lipofuscin) (Section 17.3), and follow-on repair verification scanning (Section 17.1.2.11).

Some of the fundamental capabilities of cell repair nanodevices may encompass many of those that are required to functionalize the exemplar VCSN (Chapter 1):

1. *Functional autonomy*—driven by an onboard solid-state quantum computer, albeit ultimately under external computer control, administered by attending physicians or surgeons.

2. *Energy-harvesting/generation*—to ensure continuous autonomous operation in vivo and to power all onboard instrumentation.

3. *Propulsion and navigation*—via integrated piezo-fin/piezo-ribbon elements, biomimetic flagella, rotating screws, or nanojets. Alternately, externally assisted systems utilizing embedded magnetic, plasmon resonance generating, or piezo elements that operate in conjunction with external magnetic fields, near-infrared (NIR) laser, or ultrasound, respectively.

4. *Communications*—real-time interdevice and external communications to enable the organization of mass cell repair procedures and to digitally broadcast (real time) the spatial coordinates of all cells that have been repaired, to negate the replication of cell visits and associated tasks.

5. *Cell entry capacity*—minimally invasive traversal of cell membrane bilayers in order to conduct direct cytoplasmic repairs and indirect (using extendable arms) nucleus repairs.

6. *Cell grasping and tethering*—to stabilize the movement of individual cells with the use of extendable, pliable probes, and multiple "end of arm" repair mechanisms (e.g., atomic and molecular "grippers" and "pick and place") to rapidly conduct less complex repairs within the cytoplasm, while the body of the nanodevice remains outside the cell.

7. *Nanobiopsy and nanospectrometry*—entails the probing of cells to expeditiously assess damage toward facilitating the formulation of repair strategies.

8. *Nanoinjection*—to, in some cases, administer powerful reparative drug molecules that have beneficial synergistic effects with the repairs.

17.1.1.1 Nanomedical DNA Repair and Replacement

In nanomedicine, the natural inclination and initial focus will be on the enhancement of various DNA repair mechanisms toward restoring individual damaged cells to robust health. The DNA within every cell in the human body is subject to ~50,000 lesions (primarily base modifications and DNA adducts) and ~10 double-strand breaks (DSBs) per day [3–5]. Hence, highly efficient repair pathways are required to maintain the integrity of the genome. There are no less than five primary mammalian DNA repair pathways (Table 17.1) that function to maintain the integrity of the human genome [6–8]. In swiftly replicating cancer cells, however, a reverse strategy might hold true in that nanomedical interventions could throw a wrench into the gears of cancer cell DNA repair mechanisms, thereby slowing and ideally halting their replication.

The potential modification of innate cancer cell DNA repair "nanomachines" has been investigated by Dynan et al., with a particular focus on the "nonhomologous end-joining (NHEJ) reaction for DNA double-strand break (DSB) repair." Repair foci (a.k.a. ionizing radiation-induced foci) appear at DNA damage sites to perform NHEJ, which are comprised of altered chromatin that is augmented with γ-H2AX (a phosphorylated histone variant). These foci emerge almost immediately following radiation exposure and vanish upon the completion of DSB repairs (~60 to 90 min). Interestingly, the prevalence of DNA-PKcs (a protein involved in NEHJ) was shown to have a direct correlation to the radioresistance of several human lung cancer cell lines [9,10]. The researchers proposed that a single-chain antibody (scFv 18–2) could be utilized to inhibit the DNA repair activity of DNA-PKcs as it binds specifically with a 25-residue peptide located close to its core, thereby thwarting conformation changes that DNA-PKcs typically employs when binding with DNA [11]. Nanocarriers such as liposomes (Chapter 13), cell-penetrating peptides [12], or in the future, autonomous nanodevices might be employed in this strategy to deliver scFv 18–2 antibodies to cancer cell nuclei to prevent their proliferation.

Svidinenko has conceptualized an advanced DNA repair nanorobot (Figure 17.2) that would run along the duplex (analogous to a bead on a chain) with an input port on one end of the mechanism and an output port oriented perpendicular to the central axis and positioned close to the opposite end. DNA damage would be detected soon after entering through the input port. When approaching the output port, the damaged DNA fragment would be held in place, where the deficient base pairs would be excised and rapidly replaced via a dedicated "sequenator"; loosely analogous in operation to a film-editing apparatus. The extricated DNA fragment would be jettisoned from an axial discharge port to be naturally degraded [13].

TABLE 17.1

Primary Mammalian DNA Repair Pathways

DNA Repair Pathway	Active Elements	Result
Direct repair	O6-alkylguanine-DNA alkyltransferase (MGMT, OGAT, ATase)	Altered base is restored without disturbing phosphodiester backbone
Mismatch repair (MMR)	Detection (Msh2–Msh6 complex)	Repairs replication errors (mutated in cancer cells)
	Repairs (Mlh1–Pms1 complex)	
Base excision repair (BER)	XRCC1, glycosylases, endonuclease (APE1), DNA polymerase (Polβ), ligase (LigIII), and poly(ADP ribose) polymerases (PARP1 and PARP2)	Repair of single-strand breaks (protects against ionizing radiation and alkylating agents)
Nucleotide excision repair (NER)	Xeroderma pigmentosum G (XPG) protein	Repair of UV damage and removal of cross-linked DNA
	Replication protein A (RPA)	
DSB	NHEJ Homologous recombinational repair (HR)	Re-establishes the integrity of DNA duplex
Recombinational repair (i) NHEJ (ii) HR	(i) DNA polymerases—Polμ and Polλ (ii) RAD51 paralog proteins (RAD51B, RAD51C, RAD51D, XRCC2, and XRCC3)	Repairs most damage induced by radiotherapy and chemotherapeutic agents such as cisplatin and mitomycin C
Cross-link repair (FANC)		Protects against acetaldehyde damage
Single-strand annealing (SSA)		

Sources: Plummer, R., *Clin. Cancer Res.*, 16(18), 4527, 2010; Hansen, W.K. and Kelly, M., *J. Pharmacol. Exp. Ther.*, 295, 1, 2000; Hombauer, H. et al., *Cell*, 147(5), 1040, 2011; Natarajan, A.T. and Palitti, F., *Mutat. Res.*, 657(1), 3, 2008; Lindahl, T. and Wood, R.D., *Science*, 1286(5446), 1897, 1999; Cloud, K.G. et al., *Mutat. Res.*, 347(2), 55, 1995; Martin, M.J. et al., *Nucl. Acids Res.*, 2012; Suwaki, N. et al., *Semin. Cell Dev. Biol.*, 22(8), 898, 2011.

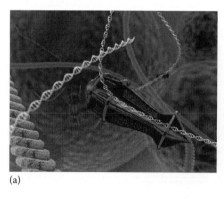

(a)

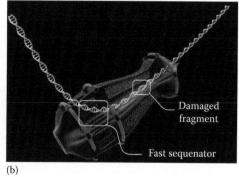

(b)

FIGURE 17.2

(a, b) Conceptual DNA repair nanorobot. (Reproduced from Svidinenko, Y., DNA-repair nanorobot, Nanobotmodels Company, http://www.nanobotmodels.com/node/48?size=preview, accessed November 22, 2012. With permission.)

Looking ahead to prospective nanomedical cell repair capabilities that might potentially be available several decades hence (2020–2030), the damage imparted to human DNA may be remediated considerably beyond the capacity of inherent cellular DNA repair mechanisms. In instances where human DNA damage is determined to be too extensive due to ionizing radiation exposure [21], micronutrient deficiencies that can mimic radiation damage (e.g., single- and double-strand breaks and oxidative lesions) [22], particular types of mutagenic chemicals (e.g., polycyclic aromatic hydrocarbons), heavy metals such as cadmium (Cd) [23], and certain viruses (e.g., Hepatitis B) [24], the most prudent course of action in an era of mature nanomedicine may be the complete replacement of the chromosomes. By today's standards, this may appear quite inconceivable and drastic. However, such a procedure might be made possible by Freitas' conceptual chromallocyte, which would have the capacity to perform what he terms, "full chromosome replacement therapy (CRT)," where "entire chromatin content of the nucleus in a living cell is extracted and promptly replaced with a new set of prefabricated chromosomes which have been artificially manufactured as defect-free copies of the originals."

A theoretical chromallocyte has a rectangular box-like morphology (3.28 μm high × 4.18 μm wide × 5.05 μm long) with a volume of 69 μm^3 and would typically consume 50–200 pW of power in operation. It is estimated, for example, that complete chromosome replacement in each of the 250 billion hepatic cells that make up the liver might require ~1 trillion chromallocytes. This translates to a ~69 cm^3 overall chromallocyte dose dispersed as a 7% colloidal suspension within a 1 L saline solution, which would be administered over a 7 h course of therapy. Freitas articulates a 5-phase, 26-step nanosurgical procedure that involves complete replacement of chromatin-utilizing chromallocytes [25].

It is suggested that whole chromatin replacement is preferred over protracted incremental DNA repair in terms of far reduced complexity (e.g., otherwise, it would be necessary to completely spool through each chromosome to detect and mend specific faulty nucleotides or genes), increased time consumption, and an elevated risk for multiple critical errors. As Freitas puts it, "The whole-genome strategy also permits all defects on multiple chromosomes to be efficiently corrected at once, avoiding subsequent repeat visits to the same cell to correct other deficiencies" [25].

17.1.1.2 Nanomedical Intracellular Interrogation and Therapeutics

Prior to the commencement of any cell repair activities within tissues and organs, it is likely that "reconnaissance" class nanodevices will initially interrogate cells for indicators of organellar and molecular level structural damage and irregularities, create detailed inventories of such damage, and record the exact spatial coordinates of the probed cells. These data would subsequently be uploaded by various species of cell repair nanodevices to guide tasking allocation and the trajectories of their therapeutic missions.

A single cell interrogation strategy, investigated by Schrlau et al., involved the use of tapered carbon nanopipettes (outer diameters of from several 10s to 100s nm) which can be synthesized by the hundreds via chemical vapor deposition of a carbon film on the inner surfaces of quartz pipettes. A short carbon tip was then exposed via wet etching. These carbon nanopipettes were shown to work in conjunction with conventional cell physiology instrumentation and had the capacity to serve as an electrode for the acquisition of electrical measurements (with resistivity 1070 μΩ cm along its length, and ohmic resistance of ~15 kΩ) concurrently with the delivery of fluids. The short hollow carbon nanopipette tip, while flexible, was rigid enough to penetrate into smooth muscle cells (Figure 17.3), oral squamous carcinoma cells, and neurons, without causing damage to the cell membranes,

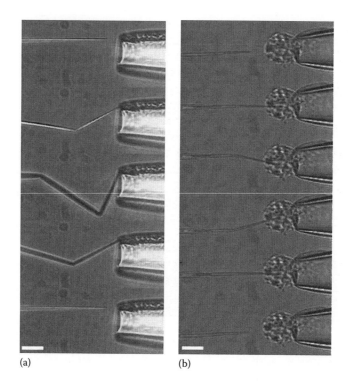

(a)   (b)

FIGURE 17.3
(a) Flexible nanopipette shape memory when pushed against solid surface. (b) Injection of smooth muscle cell. The cell was secured via glass micropipette aspiration (scale bar—15 μm). (Reproduced from Schrlau, M.G. et al., *Nanotechnology*, 19(1), 015101, 2008. With permission.)

and did not hinder cell proliferation. A fluorescent dye (Rhodamine 123) was pressure injected (10–100 hPa over 2 s) into oral squamous carcinoma cells. Following the injection, the fluorescence of the cells was seen to increase, verifying that the fluid had entered the cell [26].

A further study explored the use of Ohmic carbon nanopipe electrodes, which were employed to conduct cell electrophysiology with mouse hippocampal cells (HT-22). It was possible to measure the resting cell membrane potential and transitory potential changes thereof in reaction to extracellular drug compounds [27]. Conventional techniques employed for the measurement of the electronic attributes of cells include the patch-clamp method, which utilizes glass micropipettes (Ø 2–3 μm) that are loaded with intracellular solution, and the sharp (>1 μm) microelectrode method where glass pipettes are loaded with a concentrated sodium electrolyte (Refs. [28,29], from [27]). Both of these techniques, however, suffer from serious disadvantages. The patch-clamp method irreparably damages the cell membrane and disrupts the cytoplasm, negating the possibility of sustained or repeated measurements. Although the microelectrode method is less invasive, injury to cells may still occur during protracted measurements as the electrolyte can seep into and disturb the cytoplasm. In both cases, the pipette tips may become damaged or clogged with detritus during the penetration process [27].

Conversely, robust hollow ohmic nanoelectrodes have the capacity to penetrate cell membranes to both deliver substances and monitor cell physiology-related electrical signals without imparting cellular damage and a decreased propensity for clogging. The resting membrane potential of mammalian cells typically ranges from −30 to −75 mV and is driven by the ion concentration gradients that exist between internal and external environments of cells. The resting membrane potential of the HT-22 cells used in these experiments, subsequent to the insertion of the carbon nanoelectrode through the cell membrane, was found to have a value of -61.5 ± 2.97 mV, in contrast to the value of the extracellular milieu (Hank's balanced salt solution [HBSS]) of 0 mV. When varied amounts of potassium chloride (KCl) (generating K^+ ions) were added to the HBSS cell bath, the membrane potential of the HT-22 cells underwent linear depolarization, where the addition of each 5 mM K^+ to the solution translated to a 10 mV depolarization of the cell membrane potential. The HT-22 resting membrane potential would return to nominal values within 90 s when the solution was perfused with normal HBSS, thereby illustrating the efficacy of the carbon nanoelectrodes in measuring cellular level electrical signals [27].

Singhal et al. investigated the use of a carbon nanotube based endoscope mounted on a glass micropipette to enable nondisruptive cellular interrogation, Raman spectroscopy, fluid transport, and to conduct optical and electrochemical diagnostics in the domain of individual organelles with a spatial resolution of ~100 nm. The multiwalled carbon nanotube (MWNT) endoscope ($\varnothing$ 10–200 nm × 50–60 μm long) could also be filled with magnetic nanoparticles to facilitate remote movement in the acquisition or delivery of attoliter volumes of fluids and nanoparticles from and to specific sites [30]. Further work probed the effects of carbon nanoendoscopes on cell structural, metabolic, and functional integrity and found that there was no significant mechanical or biochemical stress induced, even at penetration depths of several microns. The plasma membranes of HeLa cells were observed to dimple at initial penetration, followed by its disappearance and relaxation around the hydrophobic probe, and neither nanoendoscopic insertion nor retraction incited changes in cell morphology. The plasma membrane and cytoskeletal network remained stable, and organelles were not rearranged under prolonged (>1 h) probing. Cellular metabolic systems involving energy generation, and inositol 1,4,5-trisphosphate-dependent calcium signaling were similarly undisturbed. The researchers propose that these capabilities may portend the possibility of noninvasive single cell diagnostics, drug delivery, and surgery [31].

17.1.2 Nanomedical Cell, Tissue, and Organ Regeneration

Although significant, and indeed welcome, advances are continually being realized as relates to the noninvasiveness of medical procedures, conventional medicine employs comparatively, very crude (no derogation intended) bulk surgery, from the nanomedical perspective, and the administration of drugs in the attempt to induce cells and the tissues that they comprise, to conduct self-repair. The prospective nanomedical repair and regeneration of cells, tissues, and organs holds great promise in taking a more direct, high-resolution individualistic (cellular) approach, where disease or injury-initiated "misalignments" in the molecular composition of myriad structures within individual cells might be rectified to reestablish the robust health of cells, and by extension, tissues, organs, and the patients within which they reside.

Since, by extrapolation, it can be deduced that if all diseased or damaged organellar and cellular constituents of various tissue and organ types are brought back to optimal functional status, associated tissues and organs themselves will have been as well. Hence, it will be useful to investigate how nanomedical interventions may repair/regenerate particular cell species as they are inexorably linked to the regeneration-specific tissues and organs.

It has been proposed by Gupta et al. that low-level laser therapy (LLLT) and photodynamic therapy (PDT) may facilitate the repair and regeneration of tissues via the acceleration of repairs and stimulation of the propagation, promotion, and differentiation of viable stem cells. Nanometric materials may also be recruited for this purpose as their structural attributes and surfaces may biomimetically provide cellular-like microenvironments to encourage their migration, adhesion, proliferation, and segregation. It is further suggested that the synergistic coupling of these two technologies may have strong prospects for the eradication of cancers, infectious and other diseases toward facilitating tissue repair and regeneration. These capabilities might derive from the creation of reactive oxygen species (ROS) (e.g., hydroxyl radicals, superoxide, hydroperoxides, and excited state singlet oxygen) that are generated as the result of the combination of photosensitive (PS) molecules, nanoparticles, or hybrids of the two, with near-infrared (NIR) or visible light at appropriate frequencies. Their interaction can elevate them to excited states such that they will react with ambient oxygen to generate various ROS. As Gupta et al. state, "Suitable PS [photosensitizer] has a high extinction coefficient in the far-red or near infrared (NIR) spectral region and a high yield of the long lived triplet electronic state (formed from the excited singlet state by intersystem crossing). The triplet PS is able to react with surrounding molecular oxygen ..." [32–34].

The majority of efficacious PS are superhydrophobic and have the greatest photoactive effect in a monomeric state. Since they will form relatively nonfunctional aggregates in aqueous media, they should be encapsulated within nanocarriers (Ø 1–100 nm) for optimal operation, to enable the selective targeting and release of ROS in close proximity to diseased cells, while leaving healthy cells untouched. A diverse range of nanoparticles and nanocarriers that may facilitate photodynamic therapies is reviewed in Table 17.2. With the development of advanced nanomedical lasing technologies, it may be envisioned that external ex vivo sources of laser light may transition to nanodevice-integrated lasers to significantly enhance the specificity and efficacy of photodynamic therapies at the individual cell level.

Cells, tissues, and organs may be successfully regenerated through various beneficial synergies that exist at the interface of tissue-engineering technologies and integrated organic and inorganic nanomaterials. These enhancements include the augmentation of interactions between biomaterials and biological entities in vivo. The criteria for nanomedically assisted tissue-engineered regeneration encompass increasing the volume of cells that comprise tissues and the fabrication of a viable extracellular matrix, the physical structures of which cells rely upon for physical support. These matrices also supply specific mechanochemical prompts that activate cellular adhesion, migration, differentiation, and propagation. The nanometric surface features of biomaterials may also be manipulated via nanomaterials that emulate inherent substrates to guide surface binding, interactions between cells, and the reinforcement of mechanical robustness of scaffolds to the degree necessary for the integrity of cartilage and bone tissue. Additionally, a (by no means comprehensive) selection of nanobiomaterials, reviewed in Table 17.3, may facilitate the delivery of DNA fragments and genes, drug molecules, growth factors, and the assembly of various tissue scaffolds using appropriate types of nanofibers, to enable efficient cell, tissue, and potentially organ repair and regeneration.

17.1.2.1 Nanocytotherapeutics

Nanomedicine may have strong prospects for the specific delivery, tracking, and differentiation of stem cells, toward the efficient repair and regeneration of damaged or degraded

TABLE 17.2

Potential Nanoparticles and Nanocarriers that may Facilitate Photodynamic and Low-Level Laser Therapies

Nanoparticle/Nanocarrier Type	Species	Basic Functionality
Lipid-based	Liposomes, lipoplexes, micelles, nanoemulsions.	PS delivery for cancers and microbial infections.
Lipoprotein nanoparticles	Naturally occurring nanoparticles with surface comprised of apoprotein, phospholipid, and cholesterol encapsulating a hydrophobic cholesterol ester and triglyceride core.	Low-density lipoprotein (LDL) exhibits inherent potential for cancer-targeting, facilitated by the overexpression of LDL receptors on malignant cells.
Polymeric nanocomposites	*Natural polymers*: chitosan, alginate, albumin, xanthum, collagen. *Synthetic polymers*: polyacrylamide (PAA), polylactidepolyglycolide co-polymers (PGLA) (PLGA), N-(2-hydroxypropyl) methacrylamide (HPMA). *Dendrimers*: dendrimeric porphyrins, Phthalocyanines, and tetrapyrroles.	Capacity for delivering large volumes of PS to targeted sites; flexibility for surface modification for higher efficacy; prevents degradation in vivo; ability for the attachment of multiple elements (e.g., targeting ligands and diagnostic contrast agents; enhanced permeability retention effects; minimization of immunogenicity and side effects of drugs.
Carbon nanomaterials	SWNTs, MWNTs, Graphene oxide (GO), Fullerenes.	(SWNT/MWNT) amenable to supramolecular modification, enabling multifunctionality; graphene oxide/polymer composites enable cancer targeting; fullerenes facilitate photodynamic inactivation of pathogenic microbial and malignant cancer cells.
Silica-based nanoparticles	Pure silica, organically modified silica (ORMOSIL), porous hollow silica nanospheres.	Amenable to diverse polymerization as well as stabilization of, and functionalization with various PS. Flexible hydrophobic and hydrophilic properties.
Metallic nanoparticles	Gold (Au) nanostructures, gold–silver nanocages.	Biocompatible, high stability, good size control, and facile surface functionality. Dimension-dependent enhancement of intracellular ROS generation. Localized surface plasmon resonance effects enable plasmonic imaging and therapeutic hyperthermia.

(continued)

TABLE 17.2 (continued)

Potential Nanoparticles and Nanocarriers that may Facilitate Photodynamic and Low-Level Laser Therapies

Nanoparticle/Nanocarrier Type	Species	Basic Functionality
Semiconductor nanoparticles	Titanium dioxide (TiO_2), zinc oxide (ZnO), TiO_2/polyethylene glycol (PEG) nanoparticles, quantum dots (QD).	TiO_2 nanoparticles generate hydroxyl radicals and good photocatalytic response; smaller ZnO nanoparticle size increases cytotoxicity for cancer cells; quantum dots can be made water-soluble and target specific sites of pathology, long stability in vivo; CdSe/ZnS QD generate $^1O_2$ and other ROS, with photodynamic, photocatalytic, or antioxidant effects.
Upconversion nanoparticles	Sodium yttrium fluoride (NaYF4) nanocrystals co-doped with Yb^{3+} and Er^{3+} with polymeric coat of poly(ethylenimine) (PEI).	Absorbs light in the NIR and emits higher energy visible light, significant efficacy in the destruction of colon cancer cell subsequent to exposure by NIR laser.
Self-illuminating nanoparticles	BaFBr/Eu2+.	Exhibits three emission bands (400, 500, 640 nm); upon exposure to X-rays emits sustained luminescence and activates PS to produce $^1O_2$; can penetrate deep into tumor tissue.
Magnetic nanoparticles (MNP)	Magnetic Iron(II,III) oxide (Fe_3O_4) core coated with biocompatible layer with covalently tethered PS, Superparamagnetic iron oxide nanoparticles (SPIONs).	Precision delivery of drugs, diagnostic contrast agents, and therapeutic hyperthermia via the application of an external magnetic field.

Source: Derived from Gupta, A. et al., *Biotechnol. Adv.*, 31(5), 607–31, 2013.

human tissues and organs. The use of embryonic stems cells remains fraught with controversy and immunorejection issues, while the relative scarcity of adult stem cells limits their extensive clinical use [62,63]. The timely advent, however, of biotechnologies that enable practically any of a patient's cell species to be reprogrammed into pluripotent stem cells, and further, to be voluminously differentiated into any desired cell type (including germ cells), might bring with them the potential for the establishment of advanced nanocytotherapeutics. As Janowski et al. observe, "The possibility to derive, repair, propagate, and transplant cells specifically for each individual patient takes personalized medicine to an entirely new dimension" [64–66].

Although investigations of stem cell transplantation hold myriad potential benefits for patients, reliable methods for monitoring the in vivo fate of transplanted stem cells, along with quantifying their viability and distribution to facilitate accurate outcome analyses, remain lacking [64]. Indeed, established procedures with which to gauge the efficacy of stem cell treatments are nonexistent. This capability will be absolutely critical, though currently (2013) there is no reliable and reproducible method to guarantee that stems cells will differentiate

TABLE 17.3

Nanobiomaterials with Potential for the Repair and Regeneration of Cells, Tissues, and Organs

Cell or Tissue	Nanobiomaterial and Adjunct	Repair/Regenerative Strategy Functional Mechanism	Outcome
Axons (ocular) Brain Tissue	Self-assembling peptide nanofiber scaffold (SAPNS); includes arginine, alanine, aspartate, and alanine (RADA)16-I.	Initiated the migration of cells into the lesion area, enabling axons to pervade through lesion site. May facilitate closure of lesions via binding with ECM on either side of the lesion and bring them in closer proximity though a "contractile process."	Promoted the closure of neural tissue lesions and enabled the regrowth of axons. Functional recovery demonstrated via the re-establishment of lost vision [35,36].
Bone Osteoblast	Chitosan nanofibers with bone morphogenetic protein-2 (BMP 2)	Directed regenerative bone membrane surface through provision of sustained bioactive substrate, BMP-2 remained on site and stable for longer duration at chitosan membrane surface.	Augmented attachment of osteoblastic cells and increased cell propagation; deposition of calcium and alkaline phosphatase interaction [37].
Bone Osteoblast	Hydroxyapatite (Ø 67 nm)	Nanometric alumina, titania, ceramic, and hydroxyapatite discriminately absorbed vitronectin protein, improves osteoblast bonding.	Improved adhesion of osteoblast; negated competitive fibroblast bonding in contrast to typical (Ø 179 nm) hydroxyapatite [38].
Bone Osteoblast	Calcium phosphate ceramic infused with apatite, calcium, and magnesium ions with Ti.	Nanoapatite coating emulates composition, structure, and formation kinetics of natural bone apatite.	Influenced osteoblast activities; improved bone growth and cell layering [39].
Bone Osteoblast	Biomimetic mineral phase hydroxyapatite precipitate via poly (amino acids), with Ti mesh.	Formation of low-density nanocrystalline organoapatite, which is more disposed to natural remodeling.	Hastened migration and elevated propagation of osteogenic cells [40].
Bone Osteoblast	MWNT in conjunction with electrical stimulation (10 µA at 10 Hz) 6 h/day over variable time periods.	MWNT added to polylactic acid and chloroform emulsions provides conductive composite substrate to facilitate osteoblast exposure to electrical stimulation.	Osteoblast propagation increased by 46% over 2 days; extracellular calcium increased 307% over 21 days; mRNA expression for collagen type-I upregulated at 1 and 21 days [41].

(continued)

TABLE 17.3 (continued)

Nanobiomaterials with Potential for the Repair and Regeneration of Cells, Tissues, and Organs

Cell or Tissue	Nanobiomaterial and Adjunct	Repair/Regenerative Strategy Functional Mechanism	Outcome
Bone tissue	Silk fibroin, poly(ethylene oxide) (PEO) nanohydroxyapatite BMP -2, and mesenchymal stem cells (hMSCs), extracted from bone marrow.	BMP-2 and hydroxyapatite nanoparticle infused silk fibroin fiber scaffolds fabricated by electrospinning. Flexible fiber matrix provided highly porous 3D substrate with high surface area, enabling nutrient and gas exchange and cell interactivity. Effective substrate for delivering nanohydroxyapatite and BMP-2.	Elevated deposition of calcium; augmented bone-specific marker levels for osteogenesis [42].
Cardiac myocytes	Semicrystalline poly(L-lactic acid) (PLLA) in conjunction with primary cardiomyocytes from heart ventricle.	Electrospun poly(lactide) PLLA derived substrates enable design of nanomaterials with adjustable geometries and architectures to facilitate cell and tissue growth. Hydrophobic PLLA provides optimal substrate for the growth cardiomyocytes as they prefer such surfaces.	Substrates comprised of PLLA improved cell adhesion and mature cytoskeletal structure with distinct periodic units within contractile sarcomeres; intercell contact and intercalated disks re-established (inherent in mature cardiac tissue) [43].
Cartilage	Heparin/poly L-lysine with TGF-β3 rabbit bone mesenchymal stem cells (MSC) from bone marrow.	PGL nanosphere-encapsulated heparin/poly (L-lysine) nanoparticles with growth factor payloads coated onto PLGA nanosphere exteriors provided substrates that were highly amenable to ordered growth and binding of cells.	Cartilage formation via mesenchymal stem cells within PLGA nanosphere assembly generated well-ordered circular lacunae geometries, mimicking natural cartilage. Cells aggregated and interacted in nanosphere assembly with uniform movement [44].
Cartilage	Nanofibrous porous scaffold comprised of poly-caprolactone nanofibers (Ø 700 nm) combined with TGF-β1 MSC.	Nanofibrous substrate structure has similarities to collagen fibrillar matrix substrate and enhances MSC chondrogenesis (cartilage development); extensive substrate surface for the accretion of ECM in highly porous substrates enhanced the generation of sulfated glycosaminoglycan (a critical component of ECM).	Production of thick, cartilage-resembling layers, indicative of efficacious segregation into chondrocyte-resembling cells and generation of cartilaginous ECM [45].

TABLE 17.3 (continued)

Nanobiomaterials with Potential for the Repair and Regeneration of Cells, Tissues, and Organs

Cell or Tissue	Nanobiomaterial and Adjunct	Repair/Regenerative Strategy Functional Mechanism	Outcome
Cartilage and bone	Self-assembling peptide KLD-12 hydrogel scaffold.	Peptide hydrogel-cultured chondrocytes sustained round morphology; showed active propagation and clustered aggregation.	Subsequent to 3 weeks in vitro peptide hydrogel culture, chondrocytes sustained capacity for secretion of aggrecan and expression of type II collagen [46,47].
Corneal tissue	Covalently immobilized laminin peptide Tyr-Ile-Gly-Ser-Arg (YIGSR) (a cell adhesion peptide) grafted to collagen – acrylic copolymer scaffold, combined with immortalized human corneal epithelial cells.	Residual dendrimer amine group modified with COOH group, containing YIGSR, into collagen scaffolds. YIGSR-bound dendrimers serve as collagen cross-links to incorporate peptide into collagen gel bulk structure. Modification via cell adhesion peptides instead of immobilizing the complete protein minimizes possible immune response/protein denaturation, maximizes surface density and homogeny—molecular peptides are more accessible to integrin receptors on cell surface.	Integration of YIGSR into the bulk/YIGSR surface modification promoted bonding and propagation of human corneal epithelial cells. Density of nerve cells and extension of neurite from DRG were improved [48].
Extracellular matrix (ECM) (Human) embryonic kidney, epidermal keratinocytes, hepatocytes, osteosarcoma, neuroblastoma, foreskin fibroblast, NSCs, embryonic stem cells	Self-assembling peptides, forming nanotubes, nanofibers, nanovesicles, nanorods, nanoribbons. Lego peptides RADA16-I (PuraMatrix)	Peptide nanofiber scaffolds exhibit remarkable water retention (= >99%), and closely emulate ECMs' porosity and structure.	Provides analogous substrate for a wide variety of tissue cells to grow and migrate; allows slow diffusion of molecular nutrients and growth factors [46,49].

(continued)

TABLE 17.3 (continued)

Nanobiomaterials with Potential for the Repair and Regeneration of Cells, Tissues, and Organs

Cell or Tissue	Nanobiomaterial and Adjunct	Repair/Regenerative Strategy Functional Mechanism	Outcome
Muscle	Electrospun (Ø 237 nm) poly(ε-caprolactone) (PCL) nonwovens.	Deposition of nanometer-thick "oxygen functional hydrocarbon coating" was deposited on PCL onto which C2C12 muscle cells were grown to observe viability, propagation, "spatial orientation, differentiation and contractility."	Oxygen functional hydrocarbons identified as potent activators for myotube differentiation, with high-density sarcomeric striation and contractility were exhibited on plasma-coated substrates. Synergistic structural and chemical attributes induced high levels of myotube formation and alignment of cells [50].
Nerve	MWNT PLCL scaffolds.	Surface properties of electrospun poly (L-lactic acid-co-caprolactone) (PLCL) nanofibers are modified when coated onto MWNTs (hydrophobic to hydrophilic) with increased conductivity.	Enhanced neurite outgrowth of ganglia neurons and focal adhesion kinase expression of PC-12 cells; up-regulated focal adhesion kinase (FAK) (critical in molecular signaling for neurite outgrowth) [51].
Neurons	Carbon nanotubes and polycarbonate urethane with mouse embryo cortical NSCs and bone marrow.	Conductive carbon nanotubes aligned in polycarbonate urethane, displayed nanostructures that emulated proteins of ECM and interacted with stem cells. Discriminately improved survival of mesenchymal cells (MSCs), which favor propagation on carbon nanotubes.	Nanospheres cultivated on carbon nanotube–polycarbonate urethane array promoted astrocyte and neuron segregation. Neuron-like structures adhered to carbon nanotubes, verifying biocompatibility [52].
Neurons	Self-assembling peptide amphiphile molecules combined with neural progenitor cells.	3D nanofiber matrix served as mechanical substrate for migration of cells and diffusion of soluble elements. Nanofibers form highly dense 3D structures around cells in comparison to natural ECM.	Expedited cell differentiation into neurons and inhibited the generation of astrocytes [53].

TABLE 17.3 (continued)

Nanobiomaterials with Potential for the Repair and Regeneration of Cells, Tissues, and Organs

Cell or Tissue	Nanobiomaterial and Adjunct	Repair/Regenerative Strategy Functional Mechanism	Outcome
Neurons	Carbon nanotubes (Ø 20 nm × 20–100 µm long) with 4-hydroxynonenal molecules (impacts neurite growth), and binding promoter for neuronal growth—polyethyleneimine.	4-Hydroxynonenal-coated carbon nanotubes with diameters similar to neuritis promote local molecular interactions necessary for the development of functional neuronal circuitry.	Neurons tend to adhere to and grow on carbon nanotube surfaces promoting growth cone motility and branching of neuritis [54].
Skin tissue wound healing	Chitosan-poly(vinyl alcohol) (C-PVA) nanofiber 2D chitosan-poly(vinyl alcohol) film in conjunction with growth factor - RSpondin1Mouse 3T3 fibroblast cells.	Electrospun chitosan-poly(vinyl alcohol) (C-PVA) nanofiber substrate and 2D chitosan-poly(vinyl alcohol) film generated a PVA nanofiber network saturated with 3T3 fibroblast scaffold.	C-PVA exhibited considerably enhanced catalase and superoxide dismutase activity. Wound closure was 98.6% at 2 weeks post-injury [55].
Skin tissue burn healing	Self-assembling RADA16 peptide nanofiber hydrogel dressing.	Absorbed bodily fluids and toxic exudates, allowed gas exchange, served as nanometric membrane barrier for blood and bacteria, provided humid microenvironment.	This dressing induced fibroblast growth factor and epidermis growth factor [46,56].
Soft connective tissue	Electrospun zein (corn-derived protein) nanofibers (Ø 310 nm) containing curcumin (free radical scavenger).	Zein nanofibers were utilized to fabricate mats for tissue engineering.	Zein/curcumin nanofiber scaffolds had a high surface area-to-volume ratio and well-dispersed nanopores (Ø 3.8–4.5 nm) promoted favorable parameters for cell proliferation of mouse (L929), fibroblast attachment, growth, and proliferation [57].
Spinal cord tissue	Self-assembling peptide nanofiber scaffold (SAPNS), (RADA)16-I spontaneously generates nanofibers (Ø 10 nm), and further, a hydrogel.	Demonstrated the robust migration of neural progenitor cells and Schwann cells, growth of blood vessels and axons into SAPNS scaffolds, verifying that they provide a "true 3D environment for the migration of living cells."	SAPNS have potential for the repair of damaged spinal tissue via the spanning of lesions with the appropriate cells and vasculature subsequent to spinal cord injury [58].

(continued)

TABLE 17.3 (continued)

Nanobiomaterials with Potential for the Repair and Regeneration of Cells, Tissues, and Organs

Cell or Tissue	Nanobiomaterial and Adjunct	Repair/Regenerative Strategy Functional Mechanism	Outcome
Urinary bladder/ urothelial cells	Peptide-amphiphile (PA) on PA/PGA gel substrate.	Poly(glycolic acid) (PGA) fiber scaffold partly immersed in a PA suspension facilitated the restoration of urinary bladder ECM.	Nanotextured film utilized in cultured stem cells enhanced tissue regeneration [59].
Vascular tissue	Poly(caprolactone) gelatin molecules with human coronary artery endothelial cells.	Electrospinning of aligned PCL nanofiber substrate generated by grafted gelatin molecules. Cell culture generation and compatibility were enhanced with guided orientation, while negating the necessity of fluid system. Grafting of gelatin enhanced endothelial cell growth and proliferation on PCL nanofibers.	Appearance of three distinctive markers, encompassing platelet endothelial cell adhesion molecule (PCAM-1), intracellular adhesion molecule 1 (ICAM-1), and vascular cell adhesion molecule 1 (VCAM 1). Orientation of ECs aligns with gelatin-grafted PCL nanofibers to provide orientational control of EC without a fluidic field [60].
Vascular tissue	PLGA	Nanostructured polymeric surface increased adsorption of proteins (e.g., albumin, laminin, collagen, fibronectin, and vitronectin) due to greater surface reactivity in contrast to conventional materials.	Enhanced nanometric surface roughness; increased populations of aortic smooth muscle cells and endothelial cells on nanostructured surface in comparison to traditional PLGA [61].
	Rat aortic endothelial cells		

Source: Derived from Gupta, A. et al., *Biotechnol Adv.*, 31(5), 607–31, 2013.

to specific functional cells in vivo. The absence of directive controls for stem cell differentiation has the potential to be devastating and even deadly for patients (e.g., the unanticipated differentiation of brain implanted stem cells into other than neural tissues) [67].

In the realm of stem cell imaging for personalized medicine, nanomedicine may employ various biocompatible and biodegradable nanomaterials-based cellular labels (e.g., nanoparticles, nanofibers/wires, nanocoatings) to facilitate stem cell trajectory tracking, tissue integration, and functionality to elucidate the ultimate efficacy of treatments. Advanced autonomous nanodevices may be imbued with the capacity for reprogramming any human cell species to a pluripotent state in vivo, as a first response and initial step to assist with tissue repairs and/or the regeneration of organs in situ. They may operate in unison with other classes of nanodevices that are tasked with the precisely targeted delivery of (physician- or surgeon-prescribed) cloned populations of cells (derived from the patients themselves) that have been reprogrammed as pluripotent stem cells.

Kaji et al. demonstrated that both mouse and human fibroblasts could be reprogrammed into pluripotent stem cells through the use of a transfection vector comprised of four cell-reprogramming master control genes (c-Myc, Klf4, Oct4, and Sox2) that were coupled with a self-processing 2A peptide of the foot-and-mouth disease virus. Additionally, once the reprogramming had been completed, the activating vector could be removed. This is important, as any remaining exogenous factors may incite unpredictable genetic dysfunction or ectopic gene expression [68]. Hence, it may be possible that these particular genes, as well as yet still undiscovered factors, might be packaged within future nanodevices and delivered to cells as elements of their reprogramming arsenals, and subsequently recovered once their tasks have been completed. Interestingly, Nizzardo et al. describe a new stem cell research paradigm (transdifferentiation/lineage reprogramming) that proposes the direct reprogramming of somatic cells while circumventing the otherwise requisite process of undifferentiated pluripotency. In adult cells, the overexpression of a sole factor (Oct4) has been observed to initiate complete cell reprogramming (e.g., in the expression of neural stem cells [NSCs]) [69–71]. This strategy, it seems, would take the guesswork out of the determination of cell fates, thereby increasing the accuracy and safety of regenerative procedures.

Murtuza et al. have reviewed the prospective use of implantable micro- and nanopatterned biomaterials (e.g., biopolymers—PLLA, PLGA, PCL, and hydrogels—PEG and methacrylated hyaluronic acid [HA]) based substrates to influence the behaviors (propagation, differentiation, cell fate, and apoptosis) of cardiac stem cells. These 3D "smart" grafted constructs offer a number of advantages, including the provision of a supportive interface between cardiac stem cells and biomaterial substrates, and to provide shelter for nascent cells from potentially destructive biochemical and mechanical factors at the sites of cardiac muscle damage. In addition, they may facilitate the co-integration of host cardiac cells/capillaries and implanted stem cells/capillaries that are prefabricated into the substrate. Further, controlled release elements and specific molecules could be embedded within the substrates toward the enhancement of angiogenesis, promotion of cell adhesion (e.g., via arginine–glycine–aspartic acid) and growth, reduction of apoptosis, and other spatiotemporal modulations as relates to interactions between host cardiac cells and implanted cardiac cells [72].

Santos et al. describe the utilization of nanoparticles for the targeted transport of molecules with the aim of inducing neurogenesis within the brain toward its repair and regeneration. The two primary domains in the human brain that generate self-replenishing multipotent NSCs (giving rise to neurons, astrocytes, and oligodendrocytes) are the subventricular zone (SVZ) and the hippocampal subgranular zone (HSZ). An assortment of nanoparticles (Ø ~10 to 1000 nm) may be employed for the delivery of molecules to aid in the generation of NSCs at specific sites of injury or disease-wrought damage within the brain. These may encompass liposomes (Chapter 13), synthetic (poly(lactic acid), poly(glycolic acid), poly(alkylcyanoacrylate), polyanhydride, poly[bis-(p-carboxyphenoxy) propane-sebacic acid], and polyethyleneimine), and naturally derived (alginate, chitosan, dextran sulfate, and gelatin) polymeric nanoparticles. Inorganic nanoparticles such as nanoporous silica might also be employed [73].

Specific nanoparticle/nanocarrier-transported biomolecules that may assist with NSC generation and differentiation include histamine, which was shown to enhance the differentiation of SVZ cells into mature neurons [74]; nerve-growth factor, which is a neurotrophin that supports the renewal of axons into damaged sites of the CNS and also impacts NSC activity [75]; and retinoic acid (vitamin A derivative), which induces NSC differentiation via coupling with retinoic acid receptors (RXR/RAR) situated on cell nuclei [76].

Silica nanoparticles (Ø ~15 nm) were employed to initiate the self-replenishment of NSCs via the intracellular delivery of an agent that obstructs the active binding site of the protein glycogen synthase kinase-3b. When taken up by NSC cells, this conjugate activated genes that promoted active NSC proliferation while they remained undifferentiated [73,77].

17.1.2.2 Nanomedical Tissue and Organ Printing

A further intriguing modality for human regenerative nanomedicine might involve the layer-by-layer 3D printing of nanostructured biomaterials, specific biomolecules, chemical groups, and whole cells to build up myriad types of implantable tissues and even complete, fully functionalized living organs. One of the principal technological obstacles to overcome, however, relates to the capacity for the establishment of appropriate vascularization within the bulk of layered printed cells to ensure the sustained viability of fabricated organs, as well as to prevent mass apoptosis and necrosis [78–81]. Should these capabilities become a practical reality, they may initially alleviate and subsequently negate the potentially long waiting times that are currently endured by patients for available donor allografts and organs. Physicians and surgeons might have the option of requisitioning the print-fabrication of any of a patient's primary tissue types or major organs, which are derived from the patient's own cells, for rejection-free implantation or transplantation, virtually on demand. If tissues and organs are printed in a manner analogous to today's (2013) 3D printers, fully functional hearts, kidneys, or livers (for example) might be available within 1 or 2 days. Prospectively, patients and healthy individuals (Section 17.2) could be presented with the option of having "auxiliary" tissues and organs printed and stored via cryogenics, freeze-drying, or desiccation [82,83], which would serve as a personalized "biocache" to address the possibilities of future serious injuries or diseases.

Atala et al. have investigated the fabrication of various implantable tissues and organs utilizing an experimental ink-jet printer-like platform. This bioprinting strategy involves the initial volumetric scanning of the patient to obtain layer-by-layer compositional, spatial, and morphological data of the tissue or organ of interest. This information is then transferred to a bioprinting system that draws on reservoirs of hydrogels and stem cells derived from the patient to bioprint heterogeneous tissues or complex organs (e.g., kidney). These constructs are subsequently transferred to a bioreactor, which emulates in vivo physiological conditions to enhance their mechanical properties toward facilitating transplantation [84–86]. The researchers have also investigated the possibility of bioprinting multilayered cross-linking hydrogels (e.g., Extracel UV), directly into deep wounds and full thickness burns of patients to support cell regeneration and healing while decreasing inflammatory responses and scarring [87].

It is likely that bioprinting technologies will continually evolve to the point, where conceivably, print-fabricated tissues and organs will be indistinguishable from their original counterparts. The blending of bionanomaterials and self-assembling nanostructured elements within bioprinting formulations may enable higher resolution constructs with increased complexity. This advance may lead to the development of replacement tissues and organs that are practically identical functional replicas of the originals, and might perhaps even allow for their enhancement in function and resilience.

17.1.2.3 Conceptual Nanomedical Repair of Acute Achilles Tendon Rupture

Acute Achilles tendon rupture is typically sustained in athletes as a consequence of rapid accelerations or jumping when engaged in running sports (e.g., baseball, basketball, soccer) or when involved in racquetball or tennis. The Achilles constitutes the largest and most robust tendon within the human body; is commonly subject to injury [88]; and typically ruptures about 2 in. above the heel bone. Anatomically, the Achilles tendon connects the base of the *calcaneus* bone to the *gastrocnemius* and the *soleus* calf muscles in enabling toes-down (plantar flexion) movements across the ankle. It may be imagined as a rope-like band that the muscles pull on to initiate foot movement, facilitating walking and running. In addition to injuries that are acquired during sports activities, the Achilles tendon may become weak and thin with age, and thus more vulnerable to injury.

The initial nanomedical concept (1) proposed next might be accomplished near-term as it would not involve advanced autonomous nanodevices, but has the requirement of surgical access to the tendon. However, it may enable the highly effective repair of an acute Achilles tendon rupture (Figure 17.4). Alternatively, a preemptive augmentative implant intervention (2) fitted under conventional surgery, might dramatically increase the strength and resilience of the Achilles tendon, which may be accomplished through the combined use of tissue-engineered biomaterials and a novel biomimetic nanoadhesive. Finally, a hypothetical repair scenario (3) is envisioned that would involve autonomous nanodevices, which may achieve restorative Achilles repair in situ without the requirement of invasive surgery. This strategy has similarities to the nanomedical procedure described for the potential mending of broken bones in the space environment (Chapter 16):

1. Subsequent to the surgical exposure of the Achilles tendon, its two free ends would be mechanically brought together by conventional means and held in place. An electrospun ultrathin flexible and highly durable sheet-like allograft comprised of bioengineered nanofibrous and cross-linked collagen scaffolding would then be wrapped around the interface of the two ends of the tendon and affixed in place using a powerful bionanoadhesive [89,90]. Successive layers of allograft would be wrapped and cemented in place to form a very strong and resilient lamination over the injured site and facilitate healing.

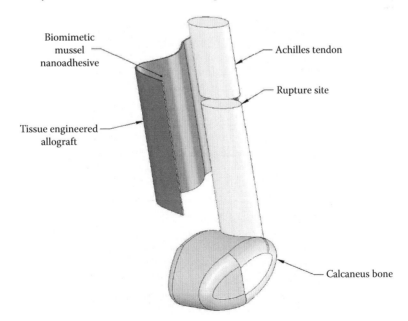

FIGURE 17.4
Conceptual nanomedical rapid repair of Achilles tendon rupture.

2. An augmentative intervention might follow a similar procedural path as the repair. After surgical exposure, several layers of the nanomaterials-based allograft would be wrapped around the Achilles tendon. To ensure the biocompatibility of the allograft, the collagen scaffolding would be generically grown via tissue engineering so as to be biologically inert and would be designed to "breathe" to allow free access to the injured site by nutrients, tenocytes, stem cells, and growth factors [91–93]. The nanoadhesive utilized to powerfully, yet flexibly adhere the allograft layers to the exterior of Achilles tendon could be comprised of a bio-mimetic analog of the adhesive proteins that marine mussels secrete to securely tether themselves to any type of organic or inorganic substrate in aqueous media. These adhesive proteins contain an altered form of the amino acid tyrosine (amino acid 3,4-dihydroxyphenyl-L-alanine—DOPA) [90]. The 25–30 adhesive proteins in the byssus (fine threads) generated by the blue mussel (*Mytilus edulis*) might be produced via contemporary recombinant DNA techniques [94].

3. The repair of Achilles tendon ruptures via autonomous nanomedical devices might ensue through the initial administration of three nanodevice species that would function collectively under external computer control to anchor, incrementally pull together, and fuse the two free ends of the tendon in situ. They would consist of "grappler," "tensor," and "fuser" type nanodevices. The goal of this strategy would be the establishment of several or tens of thousands nanoscale diameter tethers that would anchor to and span the distance between the free ends of the tendons. When the self-assembled (prefusion) construct is complete, for all intents and purposes (to the causal observer), the spanned gap would be completely filled in and appear as a continuous segment of tendon.

Prior to the onset of the procedure, dedicated nanodevices would rapidly migrate to and "turn off" the relevant nerve pathways that surround and terminate at the injury site, to instantly numb the entire area [95]. This function would also be overseen by the attending surgeon and operate under external computer control. Following "nanoesthesia," multiple linearly linked grapplers would "hook" into and along a certain length of individual collagen fibers (Ø 50 nm), which are comprised of structurally fundamental trihelical collagen molecules (Ø 1.5 nm × 200 nm long) [96] on each of the free tendon ends. This process would continue through the full cross-sectional volume of the tendon segments, commencing at their cores and fanning out toward their external perimeters.

Tensor-type nanodevices would then connect with docking clips that are present on each of the grapplers that comprise the multigrappler segments (buckles) at both sides of the gap, and proceed to rapidly self-assemble as linked linear chains that extend across its distance, ultimately meeting at the halfway point. In order to physically draw the two free tendon ends together once the "tensor bridge" has been completed, individual tensor units would follow preprogrammed instructions to sequentially extricate themselves from the centers of each chain, making them incrementally shorter (one to several microns per extrication) over time.

As this process continues, the two free ends of the tendon would slowly be drawn together with friction acting to keep the individual tethers taut, while increasing numbers of tensors depart from their respective chains. A loose analogy here may be to imagine the interleaving of the pages of two telephone books that are held together solely by the friction over the cumulative overlapping surface area. The hosts of the *Mythbusters* television program conducted an experiment and demonstrated (using two military vehicles) that it required ~8,000 lb (3628 kg) of force to finally separate them.

Although detailed experimental investigations will, of course, be critical in quantifying and verifying that a sufficient magnitude of pulling force capacity can be met for this application, it seems plausible that these many thousands of nanometric tethers may cumulatively impart enough pulling strength to successfully abut the free tendon ends to the point where they may be fused. The Young modulus for a single collagen fibril (Ø 40 nm) has been shown to be 32 Mpa (4641 psi) for a fibril, which was stretched far beyond its elastic state [97]. This value, however, is likely much higher than those that would be encountered by the tensor nanomedical tethers given that individual collagen fibrils will remain elasticized and thus impart elastic-relative loads even when the two free tendon ends are abutted.

Once the two free ends of the tendon are aligned and confirmed to be in a proper orientation to be joined, the fuser-type nanodevices would proceed to join individual collagen fibers together. This task might be achieved through the use of bionanoadhesives [98] that are dispensed from internal fuser reservoirs, induced molecular interactions [99], by photochemical cross-linking [100], or in sufficiently advanced nanodevices, via the hierarchical biomimetic synthesis of collagen in situ [101].

When a successful Achilles tendon union has been verified via fuser nanodevice consensus, contingent on the mode of tendon fusion engaged, the few remaining tensors and all of the grapplers would release themselves almost immediately upon completion of the fusion process, or be left in place for an appropriate duration to allow time for fusion "curing." As directed by the surgeon, the nanodevices would vacate the site to egress the patient. The Achilles tendon of the patient would thus be restored to a fully functional state, and the fusion site may be in fact be stronger than the natural tendon, just as a formerly broken, mended bone site might be tougher and more dense than the surrounding original bone.

17.1.2.4 Conceptual Sequential Quadraplanar Whole-Organ Regeneration In Situ

The hypothetical nanomedical concept (sequential quadraplanar whole-organ regeneration in situ) described in this section might serve as an organized whole-organ regeneration strategy, which may be reconfigured and adapted to any tissue or organ in the human body. If such a concept might someday be realized, it would offer a completely new paradigm under which to perform surgical procedures. Advantages of these regenerative procedures might include the following:

1. Rapid regeneration time line (an hour to several hours contingent on the organ involved, extent of damage, and complexity). This would be an outpatient procedure.

2. Painlessness (specialized nanodevices would ensure temporary highly localized anesthesia prior to procedures and rapid return of nerve function as directed by medical personnel) [95].

3. Complete organ restoration (all constituent cells of the organs under treatment would be repaired and restored to robust health, translating to robust health for the entire organ).

4. Repeatability (if it is determined, subsequent to follow-on scans/imaging that there are repair deficits, the procedure can be repeated to effect corrections).

This concept utilizes the human liver as an example (Figure 17.5), and assumes mature mass nanomanufacturing, nanomedicine, and quantum computers (estimated time line ~2020 to 2030).

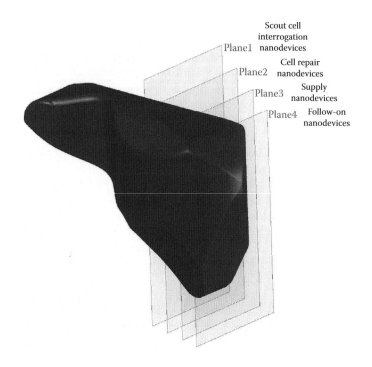

FIGURE 17.5
Artistic representation of conceptual nanomedical sequential quadraplanar whole-organ regeneration in situ, with dedicated nanodevice "planes" progressing through the volume of an exemplar liver.

The cellular complement of human liver encompasses ~250 billion cells that are arranged within ~1 million hepatic lobules. Liver cell species primarily (65%–80%) include parenchymal hepatocytes, sinusoidal endothelial cells, Kupffer cells, hepatic stellate cells, intrahepatic lymphocytes, and nonparenchymal liver connective tissue cells, with a median diameter of ~10 to 20 μm [102,103]. Within individual patients, there will be a certain proportion of each of these cell groups that will be diseased or damaged, versus those that remain in a healthy state.

The hypothetical nanomedical whole-organ regeneration strategy presented here would incorporate four species of sophisticated autonomous nanodevices (each with a specific range of functionality), which could be injected or otherwise administered to the patient. They would remain under the control of external computers for the duration of procedure, which would orchestrate all operations while they transit as steady slowly progressing planar "waves," through the entire liver volume. Once in vivo, these nanodevices would transit to the periphery of the liver and self-organize into four distinct/segregated parallel "planes" (sheets), each of which may be from one to several nanodevices thick, assuming average nanodevice diameters of ~1 to 3 μm. Each of these four planes would be equally spaced relative to one another (~50 to 100 μm or several cell widths). Individual planes might consist of from hundreds of millions to billions of identical nanodevices that are equidistant at a spacing of ~20 μm, spanning an area that extends to the outermost dimensions of the liver.

Under the direction of the human surgeon, this quadraplanar assemblage would proceed in unison to sequentially traverse the liver with one plane following behind the other, similar to the movement of, but much slower than, a 3D laser scan. The strategy being that nanodevices within distinct planes will collect and convey critical data for ensuing planes, or provide operational support for leading planes to facilitate the efficient repair of all defective cells in their path, as the planes progress through the entire liver over a

~1 to 2 h time line. Following the procedure, nanodevice programming would spontane-ously direct all entities to transit to predetermined egress sites, where they would be either excreted or extracted from the patient. Subsequently, they would be collected, sterilized, and pulverized (or disassembled) for recycling. (Note: with mature nanomanufacturing, the disassembly of used nanodevices for reconstitution into atomic feedstock for future nanodevices will likely be commonplace. This might be construed as analogous to the operation of lysosomes, which break down all manner of cellular waste and release the resulting compounds back into the cytoplasm for reuse.)

The sequential order of nanodevices and functionality within their respective planes is described in the following:

1. *Scout Cell Interrogation* nanodevice (leading plane):
   Penetrates cell encasing phospholipid bilayers to conduct interrogative scans of the contents of the cytoplasm and subsequently the nuclei of cells in order to deter-mine the specific cell type, and concurrently, the status of its health to quickly ascertain whether repairs will be required. If affirmative, data will be generated to specify exactly what repairs are necessary and the spatial coordinates of all dam-aged sites. This data will be transmitted in real time to cell repair nanodevices, resident in plane two.

2. *Cell Repair* nanodevice (plane two):
   Would repair cellular damage based on onboard (quantum computer) atomic refer-ence maps of specific cell types in their healthy state, in accordance with the data specified by leading plane nanodevices. Multiple nanodevices may be assigned to work in unison (per cell) to enable expeditious repairs encompassing the disas-sembly and reassembly of cellular structures at the molecular level as required, to reflect those of healthy cells of a particular type. The repair process is also likely to proceed more rapidly if certain modular cell components (e.g., organelles) may be prefabricated beforehand and provided ready-made, rather than burdening the cell repair units with the task of assembling them from scratch on the spot. These cel-lular "supplies" might be provided by third plane nanodevices and could include

   1. Mitochondria: Ø ~0.5 to 1.0 μm (1000–2000 per cell) [104]
   2. Ribosomes: Ø ~20 to 30 nm (4×10^6 per cell) [105,106]
   3. Lysosomes: Ø ~0.05 to 0.5 μm (several hundred per cell) [96,106]

3. *Supply* nanodevice (plane three):
   Upon being summoned to assist, the supply nanodevices would enter the same cells that, by cell repair nanodevices, are "operating" on to provide necessary cellular com-ponents, much like today's surgical assistants, who hand scalpels, sponges, sutures, etc., to surgeons. For the sake of efficiency, when their internalized payloads have been delivered, they would collect any residual detritus (waste elements) that are deemed not necessary for cell functionality or that might impede optimal cell functionality.

4. *Follow-On* nanodevice (plane four):
   This final plane of nanodevices would perform detailed follow-on scans of all liver cells that have been computationally "data tagged" as having been treated, to ensure that repairs have been done correctly. The spatial coordinates of cells that may require further repairs would be registered. Based on this data, if deemed necessary, the quadraplanar procedure could be repeated at an appropriate junc-ture that is determined by the attending surgeon who is overseeing the procedure.

Notes:

1. Any cells in organs that are determined to be beyond remediation will be left alone, as they will naturally undergo apoptosis.

2. An additional plane of chromallocyte-like nanodevices (Section 17.1.1.1) could be added as a second plane, if it is predetermined (via an initial exploratory scan) that the DNA of many-organ resident cells is defective. As described earlier, these nanodevices would replace the entire chromatin of the cell, with an exact copy of the patient's own DNA complement, which is presynthesized, packaged, and stored ahead of the procedure.

3. Precise organ shape and volume is determined ahead of time via high-resolution imaging. These spatial parameters are programmed into all nanodevices to guide optimal orientation and trajectory.

One can envisage that similar nanomedical sequential multiplanar strategies might be employed to facilitate the regeneration of virtually any human organ and tissue. Conceivably, even the human brain might be regenerated to a certain extent utilizing high-resolution imaging as a reference template for the reestablishment of neural pathways. Disease-specific applications may also be hypothesized, such as the comprehensive detection and methodical dissolution or nanomechanical disassembly of pathological physiological elements (e.g., amyloid-β protein and neurofibrillary tangles) that are involved in Alzheimer's. The rectification of mitochondrial dysfunction and aggregation, which are implicated in Parkinson's disease, might also be possible.

17.2 Nanomedicine in Human Augmentation

Concurrent with advances in nanomedicine will likely be the morally/ethically charged potential for its inevitable use, perhaps driven by the intrinsically competitive and survivalist elements of human nature, or unabashed vanity, beyond the purely medicinal therapeutic realms into the uncharted territories of human physical and cognitive augmentation. These possibilities may be especially alluring to some, due to the potentially broad scope of applicability and potency of nanomedicine to enable rapid and highly efficacious treatments. Indeed, there may be those individuals who endeavor to radically enhance specific functional or aesthetic aspects of their physiologies and/or mental capacities to attain some aspect of fulfilment or to gain a form of perceived advantage. An obvious contemporary (2013) example is the diversion from the intended use of anabolic steroids, as agents for assisting patients with recovery from serious injuries, to the enhancement of performance in sports [107,108].

Ethicists, sociologists, politicians, lawmakers, etc. will be especially challenged in arriving at logical and sound determinations as to what degree of nanomedically induced human enhancement will be deemed as acceptable public policy in human society. Will particular facets of nanomedical augmentation be considered as intolerable and subsequently banned, such as reproductive human cloning is today [109]? What parameters should be established insofar as cosmetic, physical, and intelligence augmentation? When such procedures become possible, where and how might these limits impinge on an individual's freedom of expression? Will these types of augmentative nanomedical technologies further exacerbate the divides between socioeconomic classes and among developed and developing worlds, where the disadvantaged and poor are unlikely to have access [110]?

Future nanomedical practitioners will walk a fine line indeed in the assessment of multiple strata of augmentory procedures that constitute beneficial therapies, distinguished from those that edge into pure augmentation. While reconstructive surgeries (e.g., dealing with the regeneration/reconfiguration/restoration of tissues subsequent to injuries or burns) and cosmetic procedures (e.g., those currently sanctioned for aesthetic enhancements such as wrinkle removal, lip and breast augmentation, liposuction) may be somewhat well demarcated, many distinctions may well be blurred, or dissolve altogether, with the availability of myriad nanomedical capabilities. For instance, a nanomedical neurological procedure to address memory degradation might be "overcompensated," at the request of a patient, to enable the capacity for a photographic memory, constituting a significant improvement over the patient's original cognitive abilities. A similar scenario could ensue when a neurological procedure, intended to address a learning impediment, is "over-remediated" and imparts superintelligence [107].

Will moral and ethical compulsions or dilemmas come into play for physicians and surgeons to not only restore patients to their former nominal healthy condition and functionality, but impart a "little extra" (only, of course, if requested/consented to by the patient), to potentially improve their quality of life, simply because it is possible to do so? As transformative nanomedical technologies become commonly available, infused with the ability to positively augment an individual's quality of life (as perceived by physicians/surgeons and their patients), might the Hippocratic dictum "do no harm" integrate the exponent "offer the optimal"? The questions posed here are, of course, complex and profound, and as such are beyond the purview of this chapter. However, they will warrant serious consideration, discussion, and debate on myriad fronts, having, it is hoped, the aim of prudent consensus.

17.2.1 Nanomedical Immune System Augmentation

In terms of nanomedical interventions that may enhance the functionality of the human immune system, Metcalfe and Fahmy have investigated dual nanotherapeutic strategies that may serve to boost immune system functionality. They first studied the possible utility of "smart modular nanoconstructs" (∅ ~100 nm) as immunogenic vaccines. These vaccine nanoparticles were comprised of a core antigen-encapsulating matrix that was infused with ligands for the targeting of dendritic cells (DC), immunopotentiators, agents to assist with transepithelial cell uptake/improved endothelium adhesion, and a protective shell to sustain nanoparticle integrity while en route to targets. Following DC uptake, the nanoparticles can initiate the priming of major histocompatability complex (MHC) class II molecules to activate CD4+ T cells, and thus the "helper-mediated antibody response." Antigen may also be transported to the cytosol, where it primes MHC class I molecules, with the subsequent activation of the "cytotoxic CD8+ T cell response" [111].

The second strategy involved loading the cytokine, leukemia inhibitory factor (LIF) (supports regulatory T cell (Treg) maturation), within PLGA nanoparticles (∅ ~100 nm), to target CD4+ T cells. An immune system master switch, dubbed "Foxp3" is a transcription factor that is critical for the differentiation of Treg T lymphocytes and governs the fine distinction between autoimmune self-tolerance opposed to autoimmune self-destruction. Treg functions to protect the immune system "self" and vigorously suppresses autoimmune attack. The CD4+ T-targeted LIF-loaded nanoparticles were shown to invigorate the generation of Foxp3+ CD4+ T cell numbers in vitro using a nonhuman primate model.

The researchers concluded that "this targeted nanoparticle approach is able to harness endogenous immune-regulatory pathways, providing a powerful new method to modulating T cell developmental plasticity in immune-mediated disease indications" [111,112].

Demento et al. describe advances in the delivery of antigens via nanometric biomaterials (e.g., liposomes [Chapter 13] and biodegradable polymers) to enable nanoparticle-based vaccines for immunostimulatory modulation. Contingent on the invasive species (e.g., bacterium, virus, or protozoa), pattern recognition receptors (PRRs) embedded within DC membranes will respond in different ways. These PRRs can detect what are known as pathogen-associated molecular patterns (PAMPs), which are displayed on the surfaces of microbes. The information gleaned from the microbial PAMPs is subsequently transferred to T cells in the lymph nodes concurrent with antigen presentation, through cytokine release, the expression of CD40 and CD80 co-stimulatory molecules, and an increase in adhesion integrins. The researchers propose that biomaterials-based nanoparticulate vaccines would function by targeting the PRRs on DCs to increase the transfer of antigen and thereby enhance the control and character of the immune response [113]. Another work in this area includes that of Perche et al. who utilized liposomal nanoparticles that were loaded with tumor antigen mRNA in splenic DCs with the aim of inducing an anticancer (B16F10 melanoma) immune response in mice [114].

Broos et al. endeavored to increase the immunostimulatory robustness of agonistic anti-CD40 monoclonal antibodies (anti-CD40 mAb), which hold considerable promise in cancer immunotherapies. Immune-activating amphiphilic poly(g-glutamic acid) nanoparticles (g-PGA NPs) were combined with anti-CD40 mAbs as anti-CD40-NPs, to induce Interleukin 12 (IL-12) secretion as well as the enhancement of CD40 stimulatory abilities, which in turn bolstered the response of CD80 and CD86 molecules present on antigen-displaying cells. The synergistic proliferation of B cells (antibody-secreting lymphocytes) was also activated, presumably via the increased population of CD40 mAbs on the nanoparticle surfaces. Further, in a bladder cancer (MB49 cell) mouse model, localized anti-CD40-NP exposure incited a considerable diminution in IL-6, IL-10, IL-12, and TNF-a cytokines in serum levels. This prospective nanoparticle-based therapy may enable CD40-mediated immunostimulation, while diminishing undesirable side effects such as cytokine release syndrome and liver damage that can occur when anti-CD40 mAbs are administered systemically [115].

17.2.1.1 Conceptual Nanomedical Immune System Sentinels

One can envisage that with the advent of mature nanomedicine, the human immune system might be augmented with the capacity to rapidly identify and eradicate virtually any perceived "nonself" chemical toxin or pathogenic micoorganism that the human body might be exposed to. Conceptual autonomous micron-scale "sentinel" class nanodevices, imbued with comprehensive data on all known toxins and pathogens, might continually "patrol" the human vasculature and lymphatic system for the presence of invasive species (Figure 17.6). They would also be enabled with the capacity for penetrating into tissues via diapedesis (Chapter 2). As relates to instances where the identity of an intrusive agent is unknown, a default protocol would be spontaneously instituted to ensure their complete destruction via chemical, oxidative, hyperthermic, or highly localized nanomechanical disassembly.

These sentinels (at their nascent level of sophistication) could operate in conjunction with the innate human immune system, serving as exceptionally sensitive "first responders" to rapidly identify, engage, disable, and degrade all manner of foreign entities for subsequent

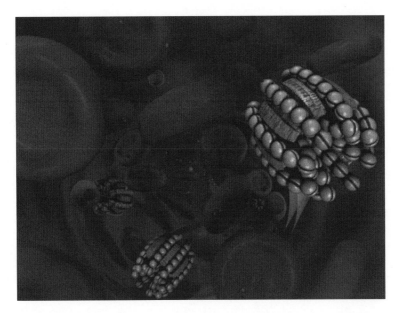

FIGURE 17.6
Artistic representation of Sentinel class nanomedical device. (Reproduced from Svidinenko, Y., DNA-repair nanorobot, Nanobotmodels Company, http://www.nanobotmodels.com/node/48?size=preview, accessed November 22, 2012. With permission.)

molecular tagging, to facilitate recognition, and further degradative processing by the innate immune system. Significant advantages imparted by sentinel-augmented immunity may encompass that it can negate the requirement of vaccines as, in addition to having the ability to quickly detect and eliminate virtually any foreign entities that enter the human system, sentinels could be programmed to scan, distinguish, and rapidly destroy any normal cells that have been commandeered by viruses for stealth infective/replicative purposes. Additionally, paradigm shifts would likely emerge in interventions against malaria (*Plasmodium falciparum*), HIV/AIDS, influenza, so-called superbugs, etc., which can evolve drug resistance (2013) [116–119]. These new paradigms might be enabled by "drugless" sentinel strategies that employ plasma membrane lancing, highly localized hyperthermia, nanomechanical disablement, or disassembly to eliminate any infectious agents and/or cellular aberrations in the human body (including metastatic cancer cells). In essence, this nanomedical armamentarium may serve as an insurmountable obstacle (from the perspective of infectious agents) to their propagation, as any attempted adaptation by these agents to circumvent sentinel capacities would be rendered futile. They would also be eradicated via multiple irreversible mechanical insults to their structural integrity, with the subsequent obliteration of their internal components.

A sentinel nanodevice may be envisioned as having Swiss Army knife-like multifunctionality that makes use of a diverse contingent of tools, such as a retractable cellular lance to puncture and irreversibly disrupt pathogenic microorganism cell membranes, and gold-tipped cell-insertable electrodes for the induction of highly localized hyperthermia via surface plasmon resonance (Chapter 9). These electrodes might work in conjunction with externally (or internally) applied NIR laser light. Sentinels might optimize operational efficiency by recharging themselves during this procedure by harvesting residual electron flow. A chemistry inducing free radical generator might produce highly localized "clouds" of hydroxyl radicals and/or other potent oxidizing agents to destroy intruding pathogens. An onboard "disassembly array" might be manifest as some form of functional grid populated by thousands of manipulator tooltips, to enable the sentinel to immobilize and progressively proceed "through" (only designated external computer/physician/surgeon consensus verified) pathogenic entities, while rapidly nanomechanically disassembling them, molecular layer by molecular layer, at least to the point where they are verified as being no longer viable. Optional atomic layer by atomic layer disassembly might be utilized to disable the deleterious effects of individual toxic organic/inorganic molecules. (Note: Multiple redundancies in programming and established failsafe protocols would negate the possibility that any "self" healthy cell or biological entity would even be approached by sentinels. Any deviation from established programming would result in immediate nanodevice shutdown and its subsequent retrieval for egress.)

Further in the future as sentinel technologies continue to evolve, most likely with the assistance of augmented human intelligence and advanced artificial intelligence (AI), they may conceivably serve as a robust replacement for the human immune system altogether. In these cases, the innate immune system might be induced to indefinite dormancy, albeit, it could be reactivated if required/desired. (Note: As with all forms of significant nanomedical augmentation, these advanced systems might be offered as available options for a given patient, and thereby would be subject to the legal requirements of patient consent, as well as physician, surgeon, medical board, and ethics committee review and approval.)

17.2.2 Nanomedical Cognitive Enhancement

Bostrom and Sandberg present an aptly put query, "The human brain—the focus of many of the most alluring proposed enhancements—is arguably the most complex thing in the known universe. Given how rudimentary is our understanding of the human organism, particularly the brain, how could we have any realistic hope of enhancing such a system?" [120]. A food for thought question, posed by Bruce asks: "Should nanotechnology make humans better, as in nanomedicine, or should we use it to make 'better' humans, by manipulating our capacities beyond medical conditions?" [121]. It is indeed logical and correct that endeavors toward the prospective augmentation of the "most complex thing" will be fraught with seemingly insurmountable challenges and complexity. The likelihood of failure will be great, at least until an extensive breadth of comprehensive knowledge as to the nuances of brain structure and functionality has been amassed, thoroughly considered, understood, tested, and verified. The acquisition of this requisite exquisitely detailed knowledge of the brain, via the brain itself, is certain to be assisted (in no small measure) by AI, which already has the ability to process vast volumes of data at staggering speeds and run simulations toward the resolution of ultracomplex problems (Chapter 7).

Eliasmith and Anderson offer a glimpse of the complexity of the human brain through the characterization of some of the parameters of neurons, or what they refer to as "fascinating, wildly diverse devices." The human brain is "lit" through a dense neuronal network comprised of $\sim10^{10}$ neurons, which may contain up to thousands of distinct species. The cohesive functionality of this massive population is supported by $\sim10^{13}$ synapses and a cumulative interconnective fiber length of ~45 miles, with communications being enabled by ~100 unique types of neurotransmitters. The lengths of neurons can range from ~100 μm to ~1 m along which communicative action potentials may be transmitted at velocities of from ~2 to 400 km/h, via neural spikes (as with pyramidal cells), or without them (in retinal horizontal cells). Whereas cerebellar cortex-resident purkinje neurons sport $\sim200,000$ input connections, retinal ganglion cells have a mere ~500 [122].

Nanomedicine may well evolve capacities for enabling the first incremental nascent steps toward potential finely controllable and clinically safe cognitive enhancement. However, these capacities will likely be tempered, as they should, by intelligent moral and ethical considerations, hopefully arriving at clarity in regard to what the true motivators should be behind various forms of cognitive augmentation. A broad review culminating in consensus as to what the essence and core values of humanity and humanness should be is warranted, as well as how we are to perceive and conduct ourselves with respect to the prospect of having an ever-increasing influence over the human brain, the human condition, and human evolution itself. A pearl of wisdom on these issues, again from Bostrom and Sandberg: "By understanding both the sense in which there is validity in the idea that nature is wise and the limits beyond which the idea ceases to be valid, we are in a better position to identify promising human enhancements and to evaluate the risk–benefit ratio of extant enhancements" [120].

17.2.2.1 Nanopsychopharmaceuticals

Initial nanomedical modalities for addressing deficits in neurocognitive performance and for the augmentation of what is considered to be normal brain function may likely proceed through nanopsychopharmaceutical enhancement, whereby various species of drug-laden nanocarriers deliver their molecular payloads directly to specific sites within the brain to illicit particular therapeutic and "enhanced-from-nominal" responses. Nanomedical strategies for cognitive augmentation may include the specifically targeted delivery of a wide range of "nootropics" (cognitive enhancers) that interact with neuronal receptors, ion channels, nerve growth factors, enzymes, etc. [123] and strategies that increase the stimulation of neurons, elevate the efficiency and sustainability of synapse firing, and enhance the accessibility and localized delivery of neurotransmitters (e.g., acetylcholine, gamma-aminobutyric acid [GABA], glutamate, dopamine [DOPA], norepinephrine, serotonin). These therapies might assist significantly in the alleviation of depression and anxiety as well as with the modulation of executive function, memory, mood, libido, appetite, and sleep [124].

In the area of memory enhancement, several drug candidates are being investigated that can manipulate explicit neural pathways, such as those that induce long-term potentiation and later phase memory consolidation [124]. The cholinesterase inhibitor, donepezil, which is used in the treatment of Alzheimer's disease, was also seen to enhance the retention performance of healthy middle-aged pilots following training in a flight simulator [125]. Ampakines are benzamide compounds that augment alertness, sustain attention span, and assist in learning and memory, which function by depolarizing AMPA (α-amino-3-hydroxy-5-methyl-4-isoxazole propionic acid) receptors to enhance rapid "excitatory transmission" [126,127]. The drug molecule MEM 1414, activates an increase in the production of the cAMP response element-binding protein (CREB) by inhibiting the PDE-4 enzyme, which typically breaks it down. cAMP response element-binding protein subsequently triggers genes to generate other proteins that fortify the synapses [124,128].

As relates to potential applications and what may be perceived as the misuse of future nanomedical memory enhancers, a case in point may be illustrated by a current (2013) controversy from the halls of academia, where an increasing number of college students are resorting to the illegal acquisition and nonmedical use of prescription drugs to enhance their cognitive abilities in sustaining focus and concentration and boosting study/exam performance. The cognitive enhancing drugs of choice include attention-deficit hyperactivity disorder (ADHD) medications such as Ritalin, Concerta, Metadate, or Methylin (methyphenidate) [129] and amphetamines such as Adderall, Dexedrine, Benzedrine, Methedrine, Preludin, and Dexamyl [129–131].

A positive spin as to general cognitive enhancement is offered by Greely et al. who suggest:

> Like all new technologies, cognitive enhancement can be used well or poorly. We should welcome new methods of improving our brain function. In a world in which human work-spans and lifespans are increasing, cognitive enhancement tools – including the pharmacological – will be increasingly useful for improved quality of life and extended work productivity, as well as to stave off normal and pathological age related cognitive declines. Safe and effective cognitive enhancers will benefit both the individual and society [132].

A proviso added is that proper care should be taken to identify any problems that could be initiated or aggravated through drug-induced cognitive enhancement, presumably by developing a prudent strategy to "...maximize its benefits and minimize its harms" [133]. In what might be considered a polar twist on the cognitive enhancement theme, there are also drugs that have the capacity to block or erase memories. In the therapeutic realm, these agents would target traumatic memories (e.g., posttraumatic stress disorder [PTSD]) which may indeed be considered a welcome cognitive enhancement through the negation of the prospect of lifelong suffering due to disturbing unwanted memories. The targeted delivery of these types of "amnestic agents" via nanocarriers may someday selectively locate and "delete" undesired memories in any individual, as a reversed form of cognitive augmentation. In this vein, as relates to a potential antirelapse therapy against continued drug addiction via the eradication of "drug memories," Milton and Everitt explain "memory reconsolidation" as "... the process by which memories, destabilised at retrieval, require restabilisation to persist in the brain. It has been demonstrated that even old, well-established memories require reconsolidation following retrieval; therefore, memory reconsolidation could potentially be exploited to disrupt, or even erase, aberrant memories that underlie psychiatric disorders, thereby providing a novel therapeutic target." [134]. The NMDA subtype of glutamate receptor (NMDAR) and the b-adrenergic receptor (βAR) are two primary neurotransmitter receptors that are critical in both memory consolidation and reconsolidation processes (Refs. [135–138] from [134]). Hence, drug antagonists such as scopolamine and propranolol, which bind with these receptors, may induce amnestic effects.

17.2.2.2 Nanomedical Neural Implants: Brain/AI Interfaces

It is imaginable that the advanced nanomedical augmentation of human cognitive abilities might convey profound effects relating to enhanced cognitive velocity, learning capacity, attentiveness, associative recall and memory, creativity, visualization, conceptualization, abstract thought, pattern recognition, judgment, interferential reasoning, sensory acumen, motors skills, and pain management, but to name a few. Prospectively, minimally invasive implants or self-assembled nanomedical interfaces could support the formation of communications conduits between the brain and AI, which may circumvent diseased or damage nerve/muscle pathways to, for example, allow for the reestablishment of controlled movement and sensation within the limbs of paralyzed individuals. This might be enabled, on the software side, through the translation of cortically derived intent (e.g., brain signals as functional output) via suitable algorithms into control commands to drive the purposeful tactile articulation of formerly paralyzed, prosthetic, or nanomedically regenerated limbs [139,140]. Stimulus input signals might be detected and delivered by limb or device-resident interfaces as an appropriate code to the brain to "elicit a precept" (touch or vision). As Donoghue puts it, "The use of these inputs and outputs is determined by the individual through the interplay between precept and desired action" [140].

Direct response brain/AI interfaces may be realized via "intracortical recording devices" that are engineered to imprint the output signals of multiple neurons that are associated with movement, or intent of movement. This capacity necessitates much more robust and sophisticated neural interfaces combined with advanced signal processing and algorithms to properly translate spontaneous neural action potentials into command signals [140].

The implantation of nanomedical cognitive "boosters," the establishment of neural interfaces with AI, and uploading the contents of the human brain/mind into AI-driven avatars, or ultradynamic post- and transhuman entities, are surely considered the stuff of science fiction today. However, these far-flung possibilities have been under intense scrutiny by researchers and ethicists around the world for a number of years [141–148]. Their realization would rely heavily on acquired and implemented (AI-facilitated) expertise involving sophisticated nanomaterials, nanotechnological processes, and nanomedicine toward the development of robust and highly efficient nanomedical neural implants.

(NOTE: An intriguing perspective that might be construed as a plausible rationalization for what underlies, and may continue to drive the demand for cognitive enhancement, is provided by Bostrom and Sandberg when they state that "…modern society requires much more study and intellectual concentration than was typical for the human species in its environment of evolutionary adaptation…"; hence individuals today are engaged in the "…struggle to meet the demands of the school or the workplace…." This leads to the premise: "Technological self-modification and the use of cognitive enhancement methods can be seen as an extension of the human species' ability to adapt to its environment" [146].)

Hart et al. endeavored to quantify the velocity of higher mental activity (in this case, verbal object processing and comprehension) through direct cortical electrical interference via an array of electrodes that had been placed subdurally in a patient for clinical purposes. The cortical activation velocity was measured by electrocorticography (brain activity recording via the direct application of electrodes on cortical surface), utilizing dual electrodes at a particular site (left lateral occipitotemporal gyrus) when the subject was naming, subsequent to visual stimulus, and was quantified to be 250–300 ms. It was also found that 450–750 ms was required (following current onset) to complete the processing of a verbal object meaning [147]. Synaptic modulation through nanomedically induced increases in neuron activity or the release of neuromodulators/transmitters might facilitate the enhancement of learning kinetics. Localized increases in the availability of glucose molecules (the brain's primary energy source) may also play a role toward this end [148]. Glucose was shown to moderate the release of acetylcholine in the hippocampus, which had been inhibited by opiates, and had impacts on learning and memory at other sites in the brain, including the amygdala (processes memory and emotional reactivity) and the medial septum (linked to the hippocampus and involved with spatial information processing) [149,150]. D-amphetamine was observed to augment learning, in one case the learning of an artificial language [151]. It is surmised that a rise in neuronal excitability may increase cortical plasticity with the effect of inducing synaptic sprouting and remodeling [152].

17.2.2.2.1 Implantable Aerogel Scaffold

Unique nanomaterials may facilitate the design and fabrication of viable nanomedical implants for neural regeneration and brain repair, which by extension might serve as platforms for the selective enhancement of brain function in humans. Sabri et al. investigated mesoporous (Ø approx. <300 nm pore size) high surface area polyurea cross-linked silica aerogels as potential substrates for the growth and propagation of dorsal root ganglion (DRG) neurons. In terms of their use as implantable brain scaffolds, silica aerogels have a range of attractive features. They are lightweight, yet mechanically robust, and can be utilized as membranes to enable fluid and nutrient exchange to promote cell attachment, while preventing the entrapment of cells within its pores via size exclusion [153–156]. The aerogels were sterilized under exposure (1 h) to UV and IPA (isopropyl alcohol), where the UV light (flux of ~2 W/m^2) enhanced the hydrophilicity of the surface by ~50% (drop contact angle reduced from 61° to 31.20°), which encouraged DRG adhesion. The aerogel was subsequently coated with a thin layer (5 µL drop with ~3.14 mm^2 surface area) of laminin 1 (basal lamina protein that stimulates neurite protrusion/elongation and migration of neuronal growth cones). In comparison to other candidate cell growth enhancers (e.g., poly-L-lysine and basement membrane extract), laminin 1 proved to best facilitate the adhesion and propagation of DRG neurons with long axons and a small number of dendrites [153,157].

17.2.2.2.2 Ultrathin Film Neural Electrodes

Kim et al. explored the use of several types of prefabricated ultrathin flexible neural electrodes that were transfer-printed onto a bioresorbable silk fibroin (derived from *Bombyx mori* silk moth cocoons) substrate, comprising a biointerfaced system, which was shown to conform well to the convoluted surfaces of the cerebral cortex. The applied electrode appeared to follow the indented contours of the sulci (crevasses on the brain surface) to a certain extent. In this study, a feline animal model was employed for visual cortex neural monitoring using this system. The electronic arrays (500 µm × 500 µm) were comprised of 30 (6 × 5) gold contact electrodes that were supported by a polyimide (PI) film, which was adhered to the silk substrate.

An anisotropic conductive film ribbon was bonded to one end of the electrode array and utilized to convey data to a digital acquisition system.The interconnect leads were coated with ~1.2 µm thick PI overcoat to negate exposure to surrounding fluids or contact with tissues. When applied to biological tissue, the silk substrate dissolved (dissolution rates can be tuned) and resorbed, leaving the electrode array, which then, as the researchers state, "initiates a spontaneous, conformal wrapping process driven by capillary forces at the biotic/abiotic interface" [158].

As a possible adjunct to this technology that might improve the capacity for recording neural signals, Bink et al. demonstrated that flexible photolithographically fabricated organic thin film transistors, inclusive of source, drain, and amplification capabilities could be directly interfaced with neural electrode arrays [159]. These ultrathin film neural electrode technologies might serve as a precursor to implantable or eventually self-assembling nanoscale-resolution brain–machine interfaces.

17.2.2.2.3 Carbon Nanotube Enhanced Neural Electrodes

Toward increasing the functional resolution, and thus the localized selectivity and prospective influence of implanted neural electrodes, Keefer et al. electrochemically populated conventional stainless steel and tungsten electrodes with carbon nanotubes. It was found that the carbon nanotube coating served to amplify both the recording of neural signals and the electronic stimulation of neurons in vitro, as well as in rat and monkey models. The clinical electrical excitation of neuronal circuitry can be of significant benefit for human patients with epilepsy, Parkinson disease, and may improve persistent pain, hearing deficits, and depression. The advancement of brain–machine communications will be contingent on increasing the quality of electrode–neuronal interfaces by lowering the impedance and elevating the charge transfer of electrodes [160].

Carbon nanotubes possess a number of advantageous attributes, encompassing nanoscale dimensions (Ø ~2 nm × ~1 µm long), high surface areas (700–1000 m^2/g), extreme conductivity, biocompatibility, and chemical inertness. The deposition of a MWNT suspension with potassium-gold cyanide (KAuCN) onto the wire electrodes (∅ ~5 μm) of a multiple indium-tin oxide electrode array resulted in a decrease in impedance (at 1 kHz), from 940 kΩ (untreated electrode) to 38 kΩ and a ~40-fold increase in charge transfer compared to the untreated electrode. In addition, the carbon nanotube coated electrodes facilitated neuronal growth, exhibited operational stability in physiological milieu for a minimum of 3 months, and well accommodated neural signal recording. When acyl chloride modified nanotubes were deposited onto an amine-coated gold electrode, the charge transfer was shown to increase by 140-fold. Further, when a laser-etched stainless steel electrode was coated with a composite comprised of carbon nanotubes and a conductive polymer (polypyrrole), the charge transfer was boosted by >1600-fold [160].

Eleni et al. formulated unique conductive nanocomposite biomaterials comprised of MWNTs (∅ ~100 nm) that were highly dispersed within polymers (polyhedral oligomeric silsesquioxane-integrated poly(carbonate-urea) urethane (POSS-PCU) and polyhedral oligosilsesquioxane polycaprolactone (POSS-PCL), which are typically highly insulating. The composite MWNT/POSS-PCU was proposed to promote neural cell propagation and the regeneration of axons through the provision of guidance channels/conduits, whereas the MWNT/POSS-PCL may enhance electrode/neural tissue interfaces when applied as a microelectrode coating for neural prosthetics and brain implants [161].

"Buckypapers" are 3D matrices of laterally oriented spaghetti-like mats of nanotubes that have the macroscopic appearance of black paper. Patterned high-density pristine buckypaper islands with high specific capacitance were microfabricated by Ben-Jacob and Hanein via thermal chemical vapor deposition onto a passivated titanium nitride and silicon dioxide microelectrode substrate. The cell bodies of neurons exhibited a preferential and robust anchoring affinity for the carbon nanotube islands and subsequently demonstrated interactive self-organizing connectivity via the extension of single axons or bundles of axons and dendrites to form a functional neural network (Figure 17.7). As relates to neural implant applications, this system has the advantage of supporting neural propagation and the enhancement of tissue–electrode interfaces while negating the requirement of an additional adhesion promoter coating [162].

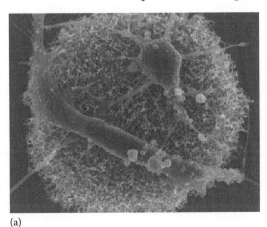
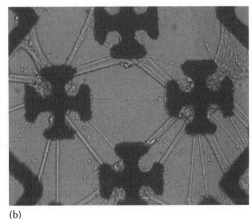

(a)   (b)

FIGURE 17.7
(a) Preferential adhesion of neurons to highly dense pristine buckypaper "island." (b) Neuronal cell bodies adhered to dense carbon nanotube crosses showing extended network of thick bundles of axons and dendrites. (From Ben-Jacob, E. and Hanein, Y., *J. Mater. Chem.*, 18, 5181–5186, 2008. Reproduced by permission of The Royal Society of Chemistry.)

17.2.2.2.4 Nanoparticle-Augmented Neuroprostheses

A strategy for augmenting the surfaces of neuroprostheses such that they would not elicit negative brain tissue responses involved the use of controlled release of drug-eluting nanoparticles (Ø ~80 to 100 nm) that were comprised of a hydrophobic, poly(propylene sulfide) core, surrounded by a hyrdophilic poly(ethylene glycol) exterior, which were dispersed within a poly(ethylene oxide) milieu. The nanoparticles contained the hydrophobic anti-inflammatory drug, dexamethasone, which can impart a positive effect on cells that are disturbed as a consequence of localized implantation damage. The encapsulation efficiency was shown to be 15% *w/w*. Microfabricated platinum/polymide cortical neuroprostheses were coated with the polymeric/nanoparticle composite and implanted within the cortexes of six rats. Subsequent to implantation, the poly(ethylene oxide) matrix dissolved, exposing the surfaces of the electrodes. The nanoparticles were observed to increase in size (to Ø ~800 nm) post-implantation (possibly nanoparticle aggregation or adhered residual polymer chains from matrix) and remained in close proximity to the electrode penetration site. Following an initial "burst" release (40% of total payload) over the first day, the drug was released at a stable rate. In comparison to controls, the nanoparticle-coated microelectrodes exhibited a ~25% decrease in the "impedance magnitude of the tissue reaction" (4.17 MΩ controls/3.15 MΩ coated), respectively, over 46 days [163].

17.2.2.2.5 Nanoengineered Titanium Wire/Titania Nanotube Implant

A nanoengineered brain implantable platform that might allow for the localized release of drugs directly to the brain interstitium has been investigated by Gulati et al., who employed titanium (Ti) wires (Ø ~0.75 mm × 10–20 mm long) upon which arrays of titania nanotubes (TNTs) were grown via a two-step electrochemical anodization technique. The resulting TNTs were present as highly uniform, dense, and vertically aligned arrays with diameters of 170 ± 10 nm × 70 ± 2 μm long. Two model drug compounds, including DOPA (a neurotransmitter) and doxorubicin (DOXO) (an anticancer drug) were loaded into the TNTs to analyze this system in vitro. Each Ti wire implant was found to accommodate loading volumes of 170 μg DOPA and 1200 μg DOXO, with release profiles spanning from one to several weeks. In vitro kinetics studies revealed a dual phase release sequence encompassing an initial burst discharge that consumed 60% (100 μg) DOPA (17 μg/h) and 25% (300 μg) DOXO (50 μg/h) over the first 6 h (the differences were due to solubility variances of the drugs in a buffer solution). This was followed by the protracted diffusion of DOPA and DOXO over the next 8 days (DOPA—9 μg/day and DOXO—112 μg/day) until the TNTs were completely spent [164].

A number of advantages over conventional brain implants may be offered by these diminutive biocompatible nanotube-populated wires, encompassing amenable geometry, ease of insertion via microsurgery, straightforward loading, and sustained/stimulated release of water-soluble and insoluble drugs, tuneable drug release kinetics, and adaptability to a wide range of localized brain therapies and brain enhancements [164]. They may also facilitate the development of stable, reliable, and robust brain/AI interfacial arrays when one envisions the potential addition of neuron growth/propagation factors and the integration of appropriate nanocircuitry.

17.2.2.2.6 Nanoporous Silicon on Ceramic Microelectrode

Conventional microelectrodes intended as brain/computer/machine interface platforms suffer from inconsistent neural recording and brief operational lifetimes that may be due, not to deficiencies in the electrodes themselves, but rather from the formation of nonconductive glial scarring in surrounding neural tissues. This scarring may arise from a lack of biocompatibility with neural tissues of smooth-surfaced microelectrodes. Moxon et al. investigated the potential for improved neurocompatibility of multichannel thin film ceramic microelectrode arrays via the application of a nanoporous silicon coating (~1 µm thick with Ø ~100 nm pores). A reduction in the adhesion of astrocytes (which play a role in the formation of glial scar tissue) and an increase in the extension of neurites were observed on nanoporous silicon in contrast to nonporous silicon. Importantly, the silicon coating imparted minimal interference with the electronic functionality of the microelectrode; hence, this surface modification strategy may allow for long-term microelectrode implantation [165].

17.2.3 Nanomedical Sensory Enhancement

Nanomedical sensory (e.g., visual, auditory, olfactory) enhancements may be possible due to the potentially extreme compactness that is made possible in nanodevices, and amenability for high-resolution connectivity/interfacability with biological sensory elements and associated neural pathways.

17.2.3.1 Visual Enhancement

Nanomedical retinal implants may have the capacity to initiate or restore sight in clinically blind individuals, someday giving them 20/20 full color vision. Appropriately selected and configured nanomaterials may facilitate the establishment of a higher number of electrical contacts within the retina and serve as replacements for damaged photoreceptors, thereby increasing image resolution. Companies such as Second Sight and Bionic Vision (Australia) are endeavoring to attain this goal via the incorporation of nanoscale electrodes within their retinal devices. Israel-based company Nano Retina and U.S.-based Second Sight Medical Products, Inc., are working to develop artificial retinas, which operate via the interactions between an implant and a dedicated pair of glasses that are fitted with a bridge-mounted camera. The implants are powered, in the case of Nano Retina's design, by a small infrared laser that is mounted to glasses, and in Second Sight's design, by a microprocessor and battery pack that is worn on a belt. In operation, the camera captures an image, which is delivered to a microprocessor and converted to electronic signals that are subsequently sent to a glass-mounted transmitter. The implant receives these signals and transfers them to electrodes that are interfaced with the retina, emitting electrical pulses that traverse through to the optic nerve and into the brain, which distinguishes light and dark patterns that correlate to the originally captured image [166].

One of the primary challenges that has prevented efficient ocular drug delivery involves the traversal of restrictive ocular barriers (e.g., blood aqueous barrier (BAB) and the blood retinal barrier (BRB)), which strictly mediate the transfer of solutes and fluids within the eye.

Ophthalmic pharmacotherapies may be utilized to augment various aspects of vision via ocularly implantable microelectromechanical (MEMs) or nanoelectromechanical (NEMs) drug dispensing systems [167,168], which contain highly controllable nanometric electronic and mechanical features. These devices may permit advancements in the sustained delivery, via the vitreous humor or aqueous humor, of nanopharmaceuticals directly to ocular sites (e.g., retina, choroid, ciliary body) that have been compromised via injury or disease. Nanocarriers such as liposomes (Chapter 13), niosomes, and discomes may also be employed to improve the delivery and bioavailability of ophthalmic therapeutics. Interestingly, the negatively charged corneal surface exhibits a selective affinity for nanostructures that carry a positive charge and thus delays the removal of drugs via lacrimal flow [169–172]. The efficacy of nanomedical ocular drug delivery may be improved through the use of site-specific mucoadhesives (e.g., chitosan, HA, adhesive dendrimers, alginates, glyceryl mono-oleate, glyceryl monolinoleate), which can optimize localized drug release through extended residency of drug-eluting nanocarriers or drug-infused thin film implants in the cornea and conjunctiva. Ocularly compatible penetration enhancers such as cyclodextrins may also increase ocular bioavailability. Long-term residency of ocularly adhered drug-eluting nanocarriers will be enabled by virtue of innate biocompatibility, nontoxicity, and the reduction of metabolizing enzymatic action [169,172,173].

17.2.3.1.1 *Nanomedical Expansion of Visual Perception*

Hypothetically, it might be feasible that the appropriate nanomedical ocular enhancements of the retina, lens, and other elements of the natural eye may allow for the expansion of human visual abilities to include completely reversible "mode switching" on demand, to include the perception of additional color hues and photonic wavelengths, such as X-ray (0.01–10 nm), ultraviolet (10–400 nm), and infrared (0.74–300 μm). These capabilities may be expanded even further through the nanoscopically mediated "accommodation" (capacity for sustained visual clarity over a range of distances) of the lens [174], via integrated adaptive lens morphing to negate the requirement of conventional visual aids (glasses, contact lenses). The retina may be enhanced through the potential self-assembly of robust nanophotonic elements that serve as a temporary retinal "overlay" and optic nerve interface, to possibly enable more radically augmented visual modes of perception encompassing night vision, visualization of various forms of radiation, compound eye-like wide field of view, microscopic and/or telescopic vision. In what may seem a quite radical or indeed improbable option today, individuals may select to be fitted with powerfully enhanced nanobionic eyes via total eye replacements [142].

The human eye can typically perceive approximately one million distinct colors via three types of retinal cone cell photoreceptors (trichromats), each of which are activated by specific wavelengths of light with the ability to differentiate roughly 100 hues. A genetic anomaly has been shown to increase color perception via a compliment of four neuronal cone cells in a certain population group (tetrachromats), and is estimated to be present in ~12% of females. This variance endows individuals with the capacity to perceive ~100 million colors [175–177].

Speculatively, the development of implantable and interfaceable biomimetic analogs of neural cone cells might be possible through advances in nanotechnology, nanopharmacology, and nanomedicine. Hence, it is conceivable that the human retina might be modified thus as an optional "augmentory accessory." This particular form of visual amplification might, for example, spur the interest of artists, art gallery curators, interior designers, photographers, and filmmakers. In demonstrating the ability to restore full functionality in damaged photoreceptors, Polosukhina et al. injected a synthetic small-molecule K+ channel photoswitch compound (acrylamide-azobenzene-quaternary ammonium [AAQ]) into the vitreous cavity of the eyes of blind mice to restore retinal light sensitivity and visual response. Potent light reactions were also induced by AAQ in the retinal ganglion cells of mutant mice that were devoid of rods and cones. This drug-like compound conveyed rapid (45 ms light response) and reversible activity to degraded photoreceptors and may have the "potential for the restoration of visual function in humans with end-stage photoreceptor degenerative disease" [179].

The nanomedical manipulation of (elastic and transparent) lens fiber cells (comprised of α-, β-, and γ-crystallin proteins) [180] and thus their enhanced cumulative capacity accommodation in the adaptive focusing on objects, might be augmented through the integration of transparent nanocomputer-controlled artificial muscles [181]. They may assist the activities of the ciliary body that circumscribes the lens, which is made up of ciliary processes and tri-oriented ciliary muscles that are attached to the lens via the zonule of Zinn connective tissue [178] (Figure 17.8). To focus on distant objects, the biconvex lens is radially drawn and flattened, whereas its curvature and thickness increase for close-range focusing [174].

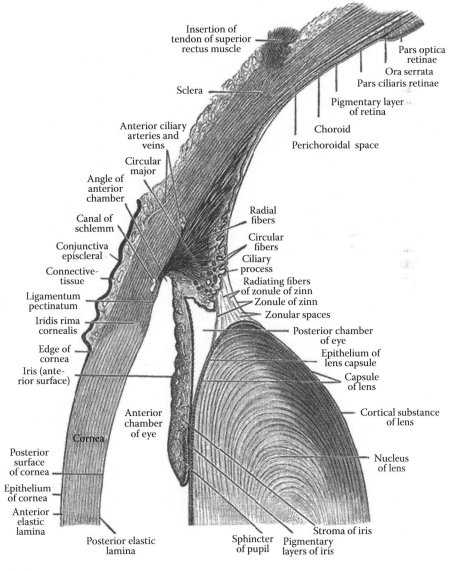

FIGURE 17.8

Detailed depiction of the structural elements that enable the visual accommodation of the lens. (From Gray, H., *Anatomy of the Human Body*, Lea & Febiger, Philadelphia, PA, 1918, Bartleby.com, 2000. www.bartleby.com/107/, accessed December 17, 2012.)

Nanomedically enhanced lenses, corneas, and photoreceptors might be controllably induced to segment into a multifaceted compound eye-like configuration (driven by sophisticated nanodevices) when initiated to do so by "users" to dramatically enhance their visual field of view and to detect rapid movement [182]. Alternately, ultraprecise micro- or nano-lensed compound eye-like goggles, glasses, contact lenses, or ocular implants [183–185] may work in conjunction with the adapted retinas of users. In arthropods, inclusive of insects, arachnids, and crustaceans, up to thousands of ommatidium (distinct optical units consisting of a light-diffracting facet lens, a crystalline cone, and photoreceptor cells with a rhabdom waveguide) [186] comprise the compound eye to cumulatively provide a wide field of view image, albeit at reduced spatial resolution. This arrangement effectively enables rapid motion analysis to provide precise navigation in quickly changing 3D environments. Huang et al. replicated the compound eye of a common housefly using a 100 nm thick alumina thin film that was cast on the fly's compound eye via a low-temperature atomic layer deposition method, which demonstrated comparable optical reflection attributes as the original. Further of a compound eye strategy include high sensitivity, anti-reflection, and increased photon capture [186]. This type of ocular augmentation might offer operational advantages to pilots, astronauts, military personnel, police, security, first responders, and disaster-relief personnel.

Avian species [187]; insects [188]; reindeer, rodents, bats, and marsupials [189]; reptiles [190]; and crustaceans [191] are endowed with visual perception in the ultraviolet (UV) portion of the spectrum through an additional complement of UV-sensitive pigments or UV receptors [190]. Biomimetic analogs of these features might be nanomedically translated to enhance the human eye in the perception of UV wavelengths. Molecular UV-protective elements could be integrated within these constructs, such as aldehyde dehydrogenases (ALDH3A1 and ALDH1A1), which are enzymatic corneal crystallin proteins that can shield internal visual tissues from UV radiation and reactive oxygen-induced degradation [192]. Ascorbic acid has also been shown to serve as a protectant against UV photophthalmic damage to ocular tissue [193].

Human eyes are devoid of the biologic reflector (tapetum lucidum) that is a common feature in many vertebrates, which imparts the capacity for enabling night vision. The tapetum lucidum, in some forms, is positioned directly behind the retina and reflects light back through the photoreceptor layer, in effect augmenting the sensitivity of the retina to enhance vision in dimly lit (mesopic) environments [194,195]. The transducin $\beta\gamma$-complex mediates the amplification of signals involved in the rod phototransduction cascade, and thus is an essential element in imparting nocturnal vision [196]. Rhodopsin visual pigments have an absorption spectrum that can span from the UV to the infrared [197]; hence, biomimetic analogs of rhodopsin [198] may be employed to nanomedically enhance human visual acumen to include a far wider range of photonic wavelengths.

In addition to possessing the capacity to perceive a far wider range of colors, Sutherland explains that tetrachromats "might possess a red photopigment shifted slightly further into infrared wavelengths, enabling them to see beyond the natural limit of human perception, allowing for cat-like night-vision, and perhaps even directly perceiving hints of body heat" [199]. Myriad forms of thermoreceptors are utilized by insects and animals for the detection and acquisition of food and survival. Certain snakes, such as the Crotalinee (pit viper), Boidae (boas), and Pythonidae (pythons) are endowed with infrared (8–10 μm range) imaging receptors called pit organs, which in conjunction with their visual systems, allow them to detect subtle changes in temperature, as proximity sensors, to locate and capture prey. The optic tectum in these snakes integrates pit organ IR with visual sensory stimuli [200,201]. At the subcellular level, the protein, transient receptor potential ankyrin 1 (TRPA1) facilitates the detection of infrared radiation. The molecular processes that enable infrared vision, at least in these snakes, involve simultaneous modifications in three amino acids (L330M, Q391H, and S434T), which function to alter structures within the core regions of ankyrin repeats [202]. Remarkably, forest fire seeking beetles, which can only reproduce by depositing their eggs in the bark of newly destroyed conifers, can detect forest fires at distances of from 60 to 100 miles away, utilizing pit organs that detect IR at wavelengths of from 2 to 4 μm [200].

Sarusi et al. are in the process of developing a thin film (1 μm thick) nanocoating toward the realization of night vision glasses with improved resolution that will convey to the user, the effect of seeing under a full moon. The nanocoating is comprised of a multilayered lamination of nanocolloidal material that absorbs photons in the short-wave infrared segment of the spectrum via nanophotonics and converts them (at approx. >10% efficiency) to visible light photons utilizing high-efficiency organic light-emitting diodes. This is in contrast to conventional night vision technologies that function via the amplification of available light, which varies resolution quality [203]. This technology might be extrapolated for integration into contact lenses or implantable nanomedical epiretinal prosthesis to allow for high-resolution thermal and night vision on demand.

Wong et al. have made an intriguing discovery in that the transmission of specific photonic wavelengths can be caused to "leak" when they traverse longitudinally helically twisted hollow-latticed photonic crystal fibers (Figure 17.9). When forced to transit along the curvatures of the spiralled hollow conduits (somewhat analogously to the trajectory of

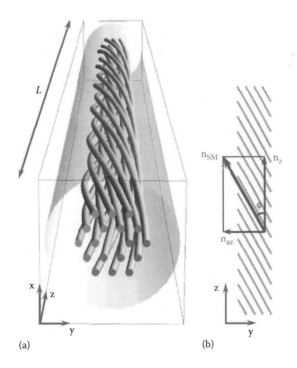

(a)   (b)

FIGURE 17.9
(a) Perspective view of (anticlockwise) helical lattice photonic crystal fiber. Blue tubular structures are hollow channels that run through the glass fiber (twist is exaggerated for clarity). (b) Depiction of axial (n_z) and azimuthal (n_{az}) elements of the refractive index (n_{SM}). The fiber axis/channel angle (φ) increases with the radius ρ giving the proximate correlation $\varphi \approx \alpha\rho$. (Reproduced from Wong, G.K. et al., *Science*, 337(6093), 446, 2012. With permission.)

sound in "whispering gallery mode") configured as a hexagonal array (Ø 900 nm channels at 2.9 µm spacing), a certain portion of the transmitted light spectrum is diverted via transmission loss, causing "power to drain away laterally from the core." Hence, the helical lattice functions as a band-rejection filter. Wavelength transmission can be mediated through the intensity of the helical twist, where a tighter twist will result in a "transmission shift towards longer wavelengths" [204]. It might be possible that ultrathin film arrays of such helical waveguides could serve as components of retinal augmentory devices that allow for the manipulation of light wavelengths to potentially expand the domain of human visual perception.

17.2.3.2 Auditory Enhancement

As with nanomedical visual enhancements, nanotechnological/nanomedical interventions may facilitate the augmentation of human auditory functionality. Preliminary advances may be manifest as miniaturized, highly sensitive, and dynamic nanomaterials enhanced auditory prosthesis that may not only significantly improve nominal hearing (~20 Hz to ~20 kHz) for the patient, but also offer optional on-demand access to an extended range of audio frequencies (infrasound at approx. <20 Hz to ultrasound approx. >200 kHz).

Infrasound (~10 to 20 Hz/17–23 m wavelengths) is employed by elephants (*Loxodonta africana* and *Elephas maximus*) to communicate via ~31 distinct calls, information that is associated with resource utilization, predator avoidance, and social interactions [205]. In humans, infrasound (~2 to 20 Hz) may be perceived as pressure or oscillation of the tympanic membrane or vibrations at certain sites of the body. This sensation is noticeable, for example, from thunder, the emanations of large machinery, or the rumble of distant trains. The lowest sounding pipe organ pipes are tuned to ~17 Hz [206]. Although infrasound frequencies are not audible in the tonal sense, its enhanced perception might hypothetically be possible through implanted or self-assembled nanostructured vibratory/pressure-activated membranes (e.g., possibly incorporating graphene) [207,208] that overlay, interface with, and augment the functionality of the eardrum, or piezo nanowires or nanofibers [209] that enhance the frequency receptivity of cochlear hair cells to resonate at infrasound frequencies or harmonics thereof. The nanomedically augmented capacity in humans for the perception of infrasound may convey critical utility to potentially provide early warnings of significant macro events such as earthquakes, tsunami, tornadoes, hurricanes, bolides, avalanches, or clear air turbulence.

At the other extreme, the human ability to perceive ultrasonic frequencies may be useful for secure communications between similarly enhanced individuals, or mission-associated echolocation in the military, intelligence, or first responder communities. Nanostructured piezoelectric or capacitive ultrasonic transducer arrays may facilitate the realization of these capacities [210]. Nishimura et al. have reported a phenomenon whereby ultrasound may be perceived via bone conduction. When a "...frequency of lower than 120 kHz is delivered via bone conduction, it can create an auditory sensation" [211]. It is surmised that ultrasonic bone conduction may potentially occur, as ultrasound is not transmitted through the middle ear to the cochlea due to "poor impedance" [212], or alternatively, that it might be generated via a nonlinear process [213].

Conventional (peripheral) cochlear implants (bionic ears) (Figure 17.10) are of benefit to patients with severe deafness in that they circumvent inner ear damage through the direct electrical stimulation of auditory nerve fibers via an electrode array that is implanted within the first turn of the spiral/snail-shaped cochlea (Chapter 2). The primary components of cochlear implants include a microphone, an external speech processor, and an implanted

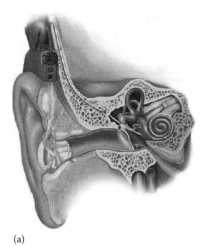
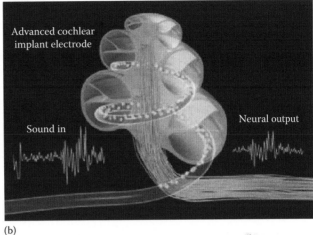

(a)   (b)

FIGURE 17.10
Graphic representations of (a) conventional cochlear implant and (b) advanced conductive polymer cochlear implant electrode. ((a) From Wikimedia Commons. (b) Reproduced from Mats Bjorklund, Magipics. With permission.)

hermetic device that contains an electrode array (~16 to 22 channels). Within the cochlea, multiple spatial domains in the sound-sensitive basilar membrane of the organ of Corti respond tonotopically to specific sound frequencies through spectral analysis. This involves the activation of specific membrane-resident sites that selectively vibrate at particular range of frequencies, which conveys auditory input action potentials along spiral ganglion neurons to the brain. The external speech processor of the cochlear implant converts sound signals into frequency bands, which are translated to pulsed action potentials at the electrode array. Individual electrodes are designed to spatially align with the inherent frequency band configuration of the cochlear basilar membrane "position–frequency map" [214,215].

It may be plausible that the sensitivity and spectral range of cochlear implants can be enhanced through the incorporation of biocompatible nanomaterial-comprised or coated electrode arrays. Hansen et al. explored the use of different materials (silicon and platinum) to assess their biocompatibility with explanted spiral ganglion neurons from newborn rats. It was found that the platinum electrodes exhibited the highest degree of biocompatibility and supported neurite sprouting and outgrowth. In addition, it was learned that not only the materials themselves, but their spatial arrangement can also significantly impact the extension of neurites [216]. Further considerations toward the design of implantable cochlear electrodes beyond their physical composition and mechanical aspects encompass properties such as conductivity, modulus, topologic geometries, surface nanostructure, surface area, and porosity. In the realm of nanomaterials, it might be feasible to utilize platinum nanowires or nanotubes to serve as biologically inert high surface area electrodes toward the establishment of the critical interface between advanced implant electrodes and cochlear neural structures.

Organic conductive polymers (e.g., polypyrroles [217,218], polythiophene [219], poly(3,4-ethylene dioxythiophene) (PEDOT) [220], PEDOT-para-toluene sulfonate [221]) used in cochlear implants facilitate their potential capacity for interfacing with, delivering neurotrophic factors to, and supporting the growth of auditory spiral ganglion neurons [222] (Figure 17.10). The requirement of cochlear implants for low electrical impedance can be hindered (e.g., 2.5–3.5 to >10 kΩ on platinum) by the initial localized formation of scar tissue (fibrous tissue capsule formed via protein adsorption, the incursion of monocytes, and adherence of macrophages) on electrode surfaces at the implantation site [223,224]. It was found that an applied current may temporarily reduce the impedance at cell-covered electrodes, which reverts to an impedance increase, presumably via the further adherence of cells to electrode surfaces when the implant is left dormant [222]. Nanostructured polymeric electrodes have the capacity to lower electrical impedance, improve interactions with bio-entities such as enzymes and antibodies, and be electrically induced to eject bioactive agents such as nerve growth factors, thus having the potential for enhancing implant performance considerably. Carbon nanotubes and graphene might also be utilized as elements of polymeric composite electrode coatings for cochlear implants to improve physiological acceptance and functional efficiency. It was demonstrated by Jan et al. that a laminate of MWNT-polyelectrolyte (MWNT-PE) electrode coating layers significantly surpassed the performance of two state-of-the-art neural interface coatings (iridium oxide (IrOx) and PEDOT) [225].

In cases where the auditory nerve itself is incapacitated, alternate types of implants may be considered such as

1. *Auditory brain stem implant*—employs a grid of surface electrodes to activate the cochlear nucleus [226]
2. *Penetrating auditory brain stem implant*—designed to access cochlear nucleus tonotopic structures [227]
3. *Auditory midbrain implant*—stimulates the cochlear nucleus and inferior colliculus [228]

The functionality of these implant types will also likely benefit from the application of appropriate nanomaterials-based electrode coatings.

Another class of nanomedical auditory enhancements may take the form of nanoscale constructs within the inner ear that serve as highly efficient computer implant-controlled sonic filters, or frequency manipulators to "focus" on user-specified frequencies (e.g., human voices) from a heterogeneous sonic mix in the environment. Metamaterials (engineered materials typically not found in nature) employed to this end could conceivably contain elements that are comprised of DNA-based nanostructures. Lee et al. have developed an intriguing "bird's nest" DNA hydrogel (Figure 17.11) that assumed a solid form when immersed in water, which turned into a liquid gel on exposure to air. Intriguingly, the DNA hydrogel rapidly (~15 s) reverted back to its original (preliquid gel) shape when re-immersed in water, regardless of how many space-filling geometries (in differently shaped containers) it formed while in the liquid gel state. The DNA hydrogel nests were comprised of elongated DNA chains, which were noncovalently "woven" using a Φ29 bacteria phage polymerase. Interestingly, this meta-hydrogel contains a hierarchical internal composition that can act as an electrical circuit that can be activated and deactivated using water [229].

By default, these nanometric selective frequency filters might also instantaneously block high-decibel sound toward the prevention of hearing damage conditions such as tinnitus (which itself might be alleviated via the implantation of nanowires to replace damaged cochlear components). Speculatively, the design of a frequency-discriminating prosthesis might be possible via the biomimetic emulation of the tympanal ridge in the cicada. This unique structure is physically tethered by what is called the tympanal apodeme, to multitudes of neural mechanoreceptors. In conjunction with the tympanal membrane, the tympanal ridge acts to dissipate and decrease maximum deflection amplitudes as they traverse from the apex of the ridge to its base [230,231].

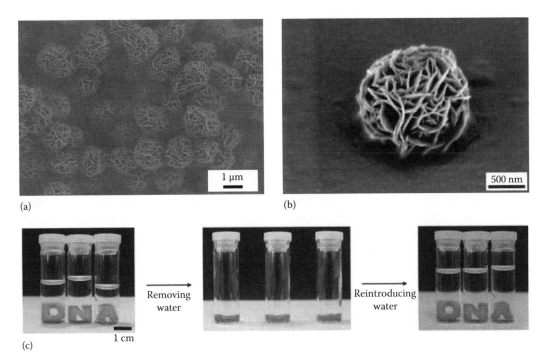

FIGURE 17.11
(a) Aggregate of "bird's nest" DNA hydrogel. (b) Isolated DNA bird's nest. (c) Rapid reconfiguration of original solid gel letters "DNA" from the wet (solid gel) to dry (liquid gel) DNA hydrogel state with return to wet state. (Reproduced from Lee, J.B. et al., *Nat. Nanotechnol.*, 7(12), 816, 2012. With permission.)

17.2.3.3 Olfactory Enhancement

Nanomedically enhanced olfactory capacities might further expand the human capacity for distinguishing the range of ~10,000 species of volatile chemical scent molecules, via ~1000 species of olfactory receptor (OR) neurons that have evolved to date. The human olfactory system is comprised of bilateral pairs of three primary processing elements, namely the olfactory epithelium (within which a cumulative ~24 million ORs are embedded), olfactory bulb, and olfactory cortex [232]. The chief functions of the perception of smell in humans pertain to safety and survival (e.g., fire, pungent chemicals, the "smell" of fear in other humans, evaluation of food, flavor perception, etc., to facilitate mate selection, mood, behavior modification, and other forms of identification). Olfactory inputs are typically paid relatively indirect attention in comparison to visual and auditory inputs, which are the dominantly applied windows of perception of the world. Nevertheless, humans have a remarkably high olfactory resolution for specific chemicals. For instance, ethyl mercaptan, which is combined with propane as an odorant safety feature, can be detected by humans at levels of from 0.009 [233] to 0.2 ppb [234] (parts per billion), whereas isoamyl mercaptan can be discerned at 0.77 ppt (parts per trillion) [235].

Philpott et al. reported on the superosmic phenomenon, where ~12% of 235 subjects involved in the study exhibited a 100,000 times lower olfactory concentration resolution (utilizing phenylethyl alcohol and eucalyptol) than what was considered as average. This apparently random capacity was found in some cases to rapidly be lost. It was hypothesized that this augmented olfactory acumen might be attributed to the activation of an accessory olfactory pathway (e.g., vomeronasal organ), or some "modulation of the existing olfactory apparatus" [236]. Once the underlying mechanisms of naturally occurring superosmic abilities have been definitively ascertained, it seems plausible that the kinetics involved might be nanomedically mimicked to provide similar olfactory enhancements.

Lee et al. have developed a highly sensitive and selective biomimetic nanobioelectronic nose (nbe-nose) that was enabled through the use of carboxylated polypyrrole nanotube transducers, which were functionalized with (dry state) human OR proteins (hOR3A1) as the recognition components. This "nbe-nose," which was manifest as an array of interdigitated microelectrodes that were bridged by the functionalized conductive polymeric nanotubes, demonstrated the ability to detect gas molecules (e.g., 3,4-methylenedioxy dihydrocinnamic acid, piperonal, safrole, and phenyl propanol) on the order of 0.02 ppt. For comparison, the detection threshold of human olfaction has been determined to be 0.01 ppt [237]. It is thought that OR proteins are endowed with exceptional sensitivity and selectivity, as each protein has affinities for a variety of molecules; hence, individual molecular odorants can bind with multiple ORs [238,239]. The efficacy of perception of the nbe-nose was preliminarily posited to be related to the "ionization status of cysteine residues in the OR." It is also theorized that ORs may also have the unique ability to detect a diverse range of molecular vibration energies by means of quantum coherence [240,241].

Nanomedical interventions into olfactory mechanisms may also augment the human capacity for olfactory masking, where the perception of undesired odors can be selectively suppressed or negated. Takeuchi et al. illustrate that there is an association between odor masking and odorant suppression of the transduction current that traverses cyclic nucleotide-gated (CNG) and Ca^{2+}-activated Cl^- ($Cl_{(Ca)}$) channels. They suggest that the inhibition of odorants proceeds subsequent to the evaporation and air/water separation of odorants at the olfactory mucus. Odorant molecules control the CNG channels to initiate masking, whereas the $Cl_{(Ca)}$ channels that richly populate the olfactory cilia amplify and reduce the resulting signals, spanning its entirety. Thus, it may be possible to design manipulative nanostructures to serve as masking "plugs" that target olfactory ciliary membranes [242].

17.2.3.4 Taste Enhancement

The human tongue is populated by four species of papillae (fungiform, filiform, foliate, and circumvallate) that contain onion-shaped taste buds, each of which contain 50–100 taste cells of four different types, which house four kinds of taste receptors that can discern the five taste qualities (sweet, sour, salty, bitter, and umami) [243]. Nanomedically enabled taste enhancement strategies might facilitate the restoration of normal taste for patients who have been afflicted with ageusia (loss of taste) as a result of injury or disease [244]. Beyond clinical regenerative capabilities, they might also have advantages insofar as the further refinement of discernment, appreciation, pleasure, and creativity in the culinary and oenophile domains. Novel, richly complex, or "time-cascading" flavors (those that transition across a nuanced spectrum of flavors over time) that may be formulated in the future [245], which are beyond the perception range of human taste might be experienced through augmented or amplified taste receptors, integrated into the human tongue. These dynamic "ultraflavors" may also be designed to activate multiple sensory experiences, where individuals have opted for synesthetic augmentation (described in the following paragraphs).

Toward these possibilities, a nanobioelectronic tongue, analogous in performance to its human counterpart was developed by Song et al. that incorporated a "human taste receptor-functionalized field effect transistor." Using a similar strategy to that reviewed earlier for the nbe-nose, this hybrid nbe-tongue was comprised of a carboxylated polypyrrole nanotube field effect transistor, which was functionalized with the human taste receptor protein (hTAS2R38). Concentrations as low as 1 fM (femtomolar) of bitterness tastant compounds such as phenylthiocarbamide (PTC) and propylthiouracil (PROP) were shown to be detected with high sensitivity [246]. Associated work included the development of a "bioelectronic super-taster (BST)," which incorporated single-walled carbon nanotube (SWNT) transistors on a SiO_2 substrate for the monitoring of human bitter taste receptor proteins (hTAS2R38) in a lipid membrane. The BST had the ability to perceive bitter tastants (PTC, PROP) at concentrations of 100 fM and could differentiate between bitter and nonbitter tastants that had similar chemical structures, as can be discerned by the human tongue [247].

A synthetic sweetness receptor was developed by Chen et al. that consisted of polyhydroxylated C_{60} fullerenes (fullerenols) toward the study of the thermodynamic properties that direct the binding events in association with the sensation of sweetness. Each of these receptors possessed spherical hydrophobic cores, which were functionalized with ~>18 polyhydroxy groups that served as latent hydrogen bond donors. The molecular kinetics/energies of the system were investigated utilizing an isothermal titration calorimetry (ITC) method. It was found that when synthetic sweeter compounds (sodium cyclamate, acesulfame-K, saccharin, and sucralose) were bound to the fullerenol receptors, a higher exothermic heat release occurred in contrast to natural carbohydrates (D-galactose, maltose, D-trehalose, D-glucose, sucrose, and D-fructose) with lower sweetness. This indicated that in most instances, hydrogen-binding events were initially required to connect the sweetness molecules to the fullerenols, along with hydrophobic core-mediated structural alterations that led to positive entropy transformations. Insights such as these will likely facilitate and have positive utility toward the development of nanomedical taste sensation enablement and/or enhancement strategies [248].

The cross-pollination of sensory perceptions (synesthesia) might serve as an additional nanomedically induced ocular sensory augmentory option as rich fodder for scientific investigation and to nourish insatiable human curiosities. It is estimated that several percentage of the human population are naturally wired this way to a certain extent, via "failure to prune" neural processes that overextend their bounds into adjoining sensory regions, and endowed with the capacity to, for instance, visualize certain shapes or colors in association with specific sounds, or perceive certain tastes in response to spoken words [249]. Suslick observes that almost all sense pairings are possible, and describes efforts in the development of intentional synesthesia systems (e.g., sight-tasting, where optical data is captured by a glass-mounted video camera and translated to an electrode array which rests on the tongue; and a smell-seeing optoelectronic nose, which "converts olfactory-like information into a visual output: smell-seeing through the use of colorimetric sensor arrays") [250].

17.2.4 Physiological Augmentation

Although a comprehensive exploration of all potential nanomedical physiological enhancements is beyond the scope of this chapter, a number of selected primary areas will be explored in the following sections. As is alluded to earlier sections, these augmentations might be regarded as possible optional enhancements that may extend far beyond the realm of nominal human health and well-being. Hence, while the nanomedical technologies might be available to enable particular augmentations, they will also likely be subject to established ethical and moral parameters that serve to ensure personal and public safety and preserve the sensibilities of future societies.

17.2.4.1 Musculoskeletal Augmentation

The significantly increased strength, smoothness, wear resilience, and physiological/biological compatibility of implanted hip [251–253], knee [254], and other joint replacements [255,256] are currently (2013) being realized via the integration of unique nanomaterials (e.g., nanocomposites [251], nanoparticles [252], nanotubes [253], nanofibers [255], nanostructured ceramics [256], and diamondoid [257]). These nearer term applications of nanomedical skeletal enhancement will likely experience wide implementation in the years to come, as nanomaterials synthesis, formulations, and nanomaterial/biological tissue integration techniques evolve and improve.

The improved robustness of frail bones might be possible through the selective delivery of nanopharmaceutical formulations in the treatment of elderly patients with osteoporosis, or patients who are afflicted with other bone-degrading conditions (e.g., osteitis fibrosa cystica, which results in bone dissolution and thinning via an excess of parathyroid hormone from overactive parathyroid glands, which triggers the increased activity of bone-dissolving/resorbing osteoclasts) [258]. These may include hybrid nanocarrier (e.g., liposomes, dendrimers, nanotubes, nanoporous silica, ceramic nanoparticles)/bone marrow stromal cell chaperoned delivery strategies [259], whereby the stem cells might be employed as bone-targeting vectors that are conjugated with nanocarriers. These constructs may serve dual benefits via the combination of stromal cell osteogenic activities [260] and nanocarrier-delivered bone growth factors, such as bone morphogenetic proteins 2 and 7 (BMP-2 [261]; BMP-7 [262]), synthetic BMP-related peptides [263], platelet-derived growth factor (PDGF-BB) [261], and strontium ranelate [264]. A mutation in the low-density lipoprotein receptor-related protein 5 (LRP5) gene was found in a group of rare individuals to impart high bone density via the malfunction of Wnt signaling (a protein network cell signal pathway). Both fibronectin and osteocalcin, which are involved with bone growth, were shown to be elevated. LRP5 might be also delivered to bone tissues via nanotherapeutic carriers to enhance skeletal structures [265].

As nanomedicine matures, it can be envisaged that the mechanical integrity of any of the 206 bones [178] that comprise the structural framework of the human body might be significantly fortified through the incorporation of nanostructures and/or by nanomaterials-based surface modifications. Bone-augmenting nanomaterials could be delivered directly to bone surfaces via the appropriate nanovectors that are endowed with targeting agents, which have a robust affinity for hydroxyapatite (calcium phosphate—$Ca_{10}(PO_4)_6(OH)_2$) (e.g., bisphosphonates [266], helical rosette nanotubes with lysine side chains (HRN-K1) [267], synthetic nanohydroxyapatite [268]), or constituent calcium ions themselves (e.g., proteins parvalbumin [269], calbindin D28k [270], silk fibroin [271]). The nanomaterials of choice for this application may be derived from the diamondoid group, as they are among the strongest and most durable materials known. Diamondoids, which will likely constitute many classes of nanomedical devices, can be manifest as stiff yet flexible and tough covalent composite nanomaterials that contain high-density 3D bond architectures encompassing pure diamond, fullerenes, covalent ceramics (silicon carbide, silicon nitride, and boron nitride), sapphire, and nitrogen-based diamondoids [272], and might be comprised of a range of elements from the periodic table:

> Group I—hydrogen (H)
> Group III—boron (B), aluminum (Al)
> Group IV—carbon (C), silicon (Si), germanium (Ge)
> Group V—nitrogen (N), phosphorus (P)
> Group VI—oxygen (O), sulfur (S)
> Group VII—fluorine (F), chlorine (Cl) [273]

The potential for rapid bone fracture healing via multitudes of dedicated nanomedical devices working under the premise and exploitation of massive parallelism might be possible in the era of mature nanomedicine, making the fracturing and breakage of nanomedically enhanced human bone a rare event indeed. The self-implantation of diamondoid nanodevices within bone matrices, or the self-assembled generation of "nanosteoshield" bone-coating systems, could provide dynamic and robust reinforcement for all components of the human skeleton. Alternately, linked groups of conceptual nanomedical "osteolaminal" nanodevices may function to fill the voids in bone tissues that have been ravaged via osteoporosis, or be tasked with the top dressing of the entire surfaces of selected, or all bones (Chapter 16). As an optional nontherapeutic augmentation, osteolaminals might be employed to impart further robustness to normal bone in healthy individuals.

Insofar as current (2013) advances in nanomedical bone remodeling, nanocrystalline diamond (NCD) that possesses a large nanotopological surface area is receptive to "additional complex chemical refinement" via "functionalization with bioactive molecules." It has been demonstrated by Kloss et al. that oxygen-terminated NCD binds stably and strongly with BMP-2 via physisorption to facilitate bone formation [274,275]. One might conceive of a nanomedical bone enhancement strategy where many multiple interleaved thin film layers comprised of nanocrystalline diamond, natural bone, and other robust nanoscale materials to cumulatively significantly increase the strength and resilience of human bone. Zhou and Lee describe the beneficial attributes of synthetic hydroxyapatite (HAp) nanoparticles in terms of their excellent biocompatibility, robust bone adhesion, and integration. A diverse range of HAp micro and nanopowders have been synthesized to date, including microsphere, microflower, microsheets, nanorod and nanowire morphologies, utilizing sol–gel and mechanochemical techniques, hydrothermal reactions, microemulsions, and coprecipitation. Nanoparticulate HAp may be synthesized via wet chemistry, combustion, mechanochemical methods; precipitation employing chemicals such as ethylenediaminetetraacetic acid (EDTA), amino acids, and citric acid can be used to control HAp nucleation and crystal growth. Important factors encompass nanoparticle dimensions, crystalline morphology, and the capacity for forming composites with additional types of inorganic nanomaterials [276].

Jamilpour et al. explored the effects of replacing collagen fibers in osseous tissues with carbon nanotubes toward the potential augmentation of the mechanical characteristics of human bone. Although the mechanical properties of bone are improved via the presence of carbon nanotubes, they may pose the detrimental destabilization in natural continuous bone remodeling (osteoclast resorption and osteoblast formation) processes. Carbon nanotubes possess mechanical qualities and strain energy densities (SED) (the impetus for bone remodeling) that differ from those of collagen fibers. A resulting study between carbon nanotube/HAp artificial bone and collagen fiber/HAp natural bone indicated that a reduction of 85% in the quantity of SED was present in artificial bone ($\sim$289.6 J/nm^2) in contrast to natural bone ($\sim$1919.6 J/nm^2). Clearly, a range of additional investigations are warranted to resolve the challenge of how the SED of potential nanofibers or nanotubes might be improved to match those of collagen, while not impeding with bone remodeling [277,278].

Though immensely complex and challenging, the prospective nanomedical integration of micro and nanoporous diamondoid, nanoceramic, nanonacre [279], or carbon nanofiber-based materials into human bones may impart significantly enhanced core exoskeletal attributes, while supporting normal bone-related physiologic/metabolic processes. Thus, the development of appropriate intimate interfaces between these potential augmentative nanomaterials and natural bone tissues will be of critical importance. These augmentations might also work synergistically with nanomedical epidermal enhancements that endow the human skin with instantaneous reactivity (e.g., rapid responsive alteration of mechanical properties) to protect individuals against virtually any physical impact or insult (Section 17.2.4.3).

Ligaments, tendons, cartilage, the menisci of the knee, and annulus fibrosus (outer covering) of intervertebral disks, might be nanomedically augmented via the nanocarrier-mediated delivery of advanced nanocomposite materials that imbue fortifying attributes to the existing constituents of these biomaterials. Alternately, pregrown/synthesized or 3D-printed replacements might (initially) be surgically implanted. Advanced nanomedical imaging techniques could allow for the fabrication of dimensionally and morphologically identical replacements for diseased or damaged musculoskeletal elements and facilitate their proper "fitting" via the acquisition of highly accurate spatial coordinate data. Prospectively, in the future, these vital structural biomaterials might be partially or completely replaced in situ (element by element/layer by layer) with enhanced counterparts utilizing a reconstructive strategy similar to sequential quadraplanar whole-organ regeneration (Section 17.1.2.4).

Nerurkar et al. investigated the use of nanofibrous electrospun scaffolds under a dynamic culturing technique to facilitate and support mesenchymal stem cell (MSC) alignment, the increased generation and integration of collagen, and sulfated glycosaminoglycan (GAG) (a vital constituent of extracellular matrix) in vitro, in an effort to biomimetically emulate the microarchitectures of musculoskeletal tissues. An aligned electrospun mesh comprised of poly(ε-caprolactone) nanofibers ($\varnothing$ ~300 nm to 1 µm) was seeded with MSCs, which permeated the entire thickness (0.75 mm) of the nanofiber scaffold within 6 weeks, as did collagen and subsequently GAG. Though the tensile moduli of the construct produced in this study was ~35 MPa, which remains considerably lower than that of natural fibrocartilages found in the annulus fibrosus (80–120 MPa) [280] and menisci of the knee (100–300 MPa) [281], further modifications in nanofiber electrospinning and culturing process are likely to reap continually improved tensile strength [282] (Refs. [280,281] from [282]).

Mujeeb et al. utilized a particular self-assembling short ionic octapeptide (FEFEFKFK (F, phenylalanine; E, glutamic acid; K, lysine), possessing amino acid residues that were variably polar and nonpolar, in the formation of a self-supporting hydrogel, which was found to be comprised of densely entangled b-sheet-rich nanofibers. This mechanically stable nanomaterial construct was shown to support chondrocyte growth and the incorporation of collagen type II. Hence, it was deemed to have utility as a template for the generation of cartilage, which has an inherently weak capacity for self-repair [283]. Zhao et al. describe the use of electrospun PCL nanofiber meshes and PLGA nanofiber scaffolds that can serve as templates for cartilage as well [284].

One may envisage that this type of unique biocompatible/degradable nanobiomaterial could be combined, in addition to chondrocytes and collagen/ECM, with function-boosting chemical compounds and/or the appropriate nanomaterials, and utilized for the "moulding" of customized shapes to therapeutically replace and enhance any cartilage within the human body. In cosmetic or aesthetic applications, these constructs could serve to modify and augment specific sites as might be requested by the patient.

17.2.4.2 Muscle Augmentation

There are three classes of muscle tissue within the human body encompassing skeletal, cardiac, and smooth muscle, each with its own composition and mode of action. The synchronized motion (at ~10 nm increments) of thousands of myosin heads cause bulky myosin filaments to glide along slender actin filaments, which cumulatively initiates sarcomere contraction on the order of 1 μm. Thus, highly parallel nanoscale contractions translate to macroscpic movements [285,286]. The nanomedical replacement and augmentation of different species of human muscle fiber might assist in addressing muscle-related diseases (e.g., muscular dystrophies) or the resolution of serious injuries (paralysis). The normal functionality of healthy muscle elements might also be enhanced so as to significantly improve their loading capacity (strength), resilience, and longevity. Actuatable artificial muscles may be comprised of and enabled through the use of smart materials such as piezoelectrics/ceramics [287,288], shape memory alloys [289,290], giant magnetostrictive materials [291,292], and dielectric elastomers [293,294], which have varied power requirements, actuation velocities, elongation, and repeatability capacities. The evolution of myriad polymeric/nanomaterial composites will likely facilitate the development of highly robust yet elegantly actuatable nanobiosynthetic muscle.

The ability of advanced nanobiomaterials to morph (intelligent and efficient adaptability) or undergo phase transitions (solid/liquid/plasma/gas) at the nano/micro/macro scales under specific stimuli or within particular environments may enable a wide range of possibilities for the augmentation of muscles and myriad other human physiological systems. Nguyen et al. describe a proof of concept for morphing magnet filler–polymer matrix composites that have potential applications in self-healing and as artificial muscle. These morphing composites typically consist of magnetic nanoparticles (e.g., Fe, Fe_3O_4) that are embedded within the matrices of polymers (e.g., polypyrrole, polyurethane), rubbers (e.g., silicone elastomers), or hydrogels (e.g., polyvinyl acetate). When exposed to a magnetic field, the magnetic particles react with the abutting polymeric chains, thereby altering their positions. Cumulatively, this activity alters the morphology of the composite. The benefits of this material include rapid response, self-sensing, and dynamic remote contactless actuation. Modes of actuation include elongation, contraction, deflection, and coiling. When the nanoparticle filler concentration was above 60%, the actuation strain surpassed that of biological skeletal muscle by 100%. Additional response properties may be explored when conductive carbon nanotubes are added as well [295].

Shahinpoor described the use of biomimetic conducting ionic polymeric conductor nanocomposites and ionic polymer metal nanocomposites (IPMNCs) as potentially robust candidates for utility as artificial muscles. Intriguingly, these materials have the capacity for retaining their functionality at the nanoscale, which in addition to their potential use in the fine motor control in artificial muscles, might bode well for the potential development of nanoscale actuators and grippers for nanomedical devices that can be activated under several microvolts. Polymeric species that may be integrated within electrically and chemically active ionic polymer gel muscles include polyacrylonitrile (PAN), poly(2-acrylamido-2-methyl-1-propane sulfonic) acid, and polyacrylic-acid-bis-acrylamide. Using specific fabrication techniques, PAN has been demonstrated to produce artificial muscles in the form of "springloaded fiber bundles, biceps, triceps, ribbon type muscles and segmented fiber bundles" [292,296,297].

Polymer metal composites can be realized using perfluorinated sulfonic or carboxylic ionic membranes, which is a dual-phase system that is comprised of a network of Ø 3–5 nm polar fluid ion nanoclusters encased by hydrophobic polytetrafluoroethylene (PTFE), whose backbones impart mechanical stability to the system. It was found through high-resolution NMR that the perfluoroionomer structure contains unique arrangements of nonpolar backbones that are akin to Teflon, which possess ionic and polar side-branches. Also, in PTFE, the polymer backbones are bound with anions, whereas H+, Na+, and Li+ cations are solvated within the nanocluster ionic or polar fluids. When sheets of IPMNC are mechanically compressed, they can produce a significant voltage. Using a 2 × 2 cm sheet, compressive loads of 200 N (73 psi) generated 80 mV, and 350 N (127 psi) produced 108 mV, giving an average output of ~2 mV per linear centimeter [297].

Synthetic molecular machines have been investigated in the development of molecular muscles. Sauvage et al. reported the first instance of chemically mediated stretching and contraction via unimolecular (doubly-threaded) linear rotaxane dimer arrays (Figure 17.12). The rotaxane dimers contained acrylic filament components that could glide along one another under the initiation of chemical signals, involving the exchange of a dicopper(I) transition metal complex (to obtain an extended state) with a dizinc complex (to obtain a retracted state) [298,299]. Another potential nanometric muscle analog involved an electrochemically triggered redox-active polypyrrole conductive polymer film that underwent significant volumetric alterations and thus movement in aqueous media, when its matrix was oxidized or reduced. The oxidation of polypyrrole initiates the removal of electrons from its polymer chains, the reconfiguration of double bonds, and storage of positive charges (e.g., polarans) along the chains. The polymer chains undergo changes (from coiled to rod-like) in conformation in order to preserve electroneutrality, thereby driving the incorporation of water molecules and counterions (swelling) from solution. In the reduction process, the reverse of this sequence ensues, which causes the polymer film to shrink [300].

Completely reversible electromechanical actuation at the single molecule level may also be realized utilizing thiophene-fused [8] annulenes (tetra(2,3-thienylene), which can undergo conformational modifications (tube to planar) via redox activation. Sufficiently

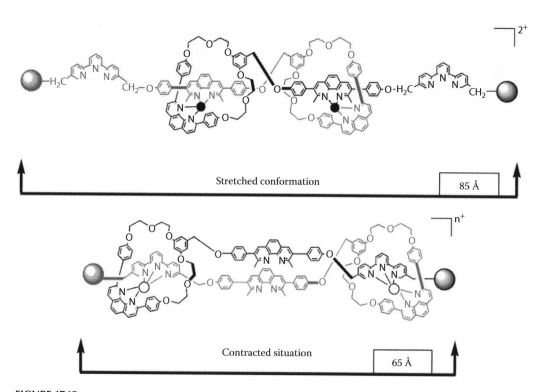

FIGURE 17.12
Extended and retracted states of a rotaxane dimer molecular artificial muscle element. (Reproduced from Jimenez-Molero, M.C. et al., *Chem. Commun. (Camb)*, (14), 1613, 2003. With permission.)

concentrated and configured aggregates of these cyclooctatetraene polymer repeat sub-units might allow for the construction of functional nanomedical synthetic muscles [301,302].

Carbon nanotube yarns might have great potential as augmentative synthetic muscles, contingent on their ability for physiological compatibility. Lima et al. have developed twist-spun carbon nanotube yarns that demonstrated rapid, "high-force, large-stroke torsional and tensile actuation." The actuation of the yarn could be induced photonically, chemically, or electrically. Rather than utilizing electrochemical electrolyte activation, the thermal actuation of MWNT (Ø ~9 nm/6 wall) yarns was enabled through significant volumetric variations (~20% volume increase at between 30° and 90°, and an additional 10% volume increase at between 90° and 210°C) of an actuating paraffin wax guest material that filled the nanometric voids between the nanotubes. Experimental results demonstrated approx. >1.4 million torsional and tensile actuation cycles, where a rotor was spun at ~11,500 revolutions per minute and a 3% tensile stroke at 1200 cycles/min. This coiled Fermat MWNT yarn (Ø ~20 mm) could lift 17,700 times its own weight when a 20 Hz, 18.3 V/cm square-wave voltage was applied. Further, the yarn was shown to lift 175,000 times its own mass in 30 ms under the application of 32 V/cm for 15 ms. The contractile work (0.836 kJ/kg) supplied a power output of 27.9 kW/kg (85 times the optimal output of mammalian skeletal muscle [0.323 kW/kg]) [303]. These values are also 30 times higher than the maximum power density quantified to date for carbon nanotube based synthetic muscles. The nanotube yarns could maintain their integrity and lift heavy loads to a temperature of ~2560°C, which is higher than any other "high-work-capacity" actuator.

A drawback of this system was that at high applied voltages, the life cycles of the nanotube yarns were reduced due to the evaporation of the paraffin wax and extreme heating [304]. The longevity of this class of synthetic muscle for nanomedical applications might be extended significantly when they operate at far lower ambient physiological temperatures, utilizing inert/biocompatible and nonleaching nanotube yarn fillers and encapsulants. Schultz suggests that a further improvement in nanuotube yarns might include opening of the nanotube end caps to enable their being filled with the guest material. Advances in horizontal growth techniques have resulted in carbon nanotubes with lengths of 10 cm [305], and improvements in annealing hold promise for even longer defect-free nanotubes [306]. This may greatly facilitate the fabrication of viable synthetic analogs toward nanomedical muscle augmentation.

A prominent researcher and thought leader in this field (Dr. Mohsen Shahinpoor—Director, Biomedical Engineering Laboratory, University of Maine) offers his perspective on how artificial muscles might advance over the next decade:

> My vision of the future of ionic polymer metal composite (IPMC) artificial muscles may be summarized below in terms of both medical and industrial applications. Note that IPMCs are also excellent sensors that generate huge outputs in terms of millivolts, which can be employed for the sensing, transduction and harvesting of energy from wind or ocean waves. These unique materials work perfectly well in a wet environment and thus they are excellent candidates for medical applications. These might range from endovascular stirrers to enable navigation within the human vasculature; use as deep brain stimulators or micropumps for precision drug delivery, glaucoma and hydrocephalus; artificial muscles for the surgical correction of ptosis (drooping eyelid syndrome); ophthalmological and vision improvement applications; artificial muscles to assist a failing heart; correction of facial paralysis, FacioScapuloHumeral (FSH) and other applications in muscular dystrophy; to mediate the control of drainage or flow

within the human body and myriad additional purposes. On the industrial side, due to the fact that the IPMCs are excellent sensors and low-voltage actuators, they can be used for both sensing and simultaneous actuation for many engineering applications. In the sensing mode they appear to have a very good bandwidth to sense low, as well as high frequencies, in contrast to piezoelectric materials such as PZT or Lithium Niobate, which are only suitable for high frequency sensing. Two emerging visions of the future is to see IPMCs heavily utilized as novel and dynamic probes in scanning probe microscopy and robotic surgery to facilitate the conveyance of specific haptic, force and impedance feedback to surgeons.

17.2.4.3 Cardiovascular and Pulmonary Augmentation

Nanomedicine is likely to enable augmentations of the cardiovascular and pulmonary systems, leading to unprecedented improvements in human health and longevity. Applications might range from the integral fortification (increased flexibility and renewal) and self-cleaning (to negate the accumulation of vascular plaque materials) of arterial and venous walls, to the re-establishment of vascular elements and their permeation at diseased or injured sites via induced angiogenesis (the generation of new capillaries from established blood vessels), to the complete replacement of the vascular system with a highly sophisticated nanomedical "organ" comprised of trillions of interlocking/interacting nanorobots.

The functionality, mechanical integrity, and proper signal transduction within vascular walls are facilitated to a considerable extent by the extracellular matrix complex, whose constituents include collagens, elastin, proteoglycans, and glycoproteins. Hajiali et al. have studied the use of biocompatible and biodegradable composite electrospun scaffolds (Ø ~134 to 864 nm nanofibers) comprised of polyglycolic acid (PGA) blended with gelatin as promising candidates for vascular tissue engineering. These scaffolds were found to possess biomechanical attributes that were appropriate for supporting the attachment, penetration, and propagation of endothelial cells (from human umbilical vein) and smooth muscle cells (from human umbilical artery). An optimized double-layered tubular scaffold construct for the establishment or regeneration of vascular elements is suggested, which utilizes an internal PGA/10 wt% gelatin layer (optimal in this study for endothelial cell support) and external PGA/30 wt% gelatin layer (optimal in this study for smooth muscle cell support) [307].

A potential nanomedical strategy for the induction of angiogenesis/vascular sprouting has been explored by Barui et al. using zinc oxide (ZnO) nanoflowers in vitro and in vivo, with chick embryos. Increased angiogenesis (matured vascular sprouting by proliferating endothelial cells) was observed to be dose-dependent on the concentration (1–20 µg) of nanoflowers, which was shown to be amenable to cellular uptake. It was surmised that the proangiogenic characteristics of the ZnO nanoflowers might be due to the generation of the ROS, hydrogen peroxide (H_2O_2, a known redox signaling molecule) [308]. Inorganic europium (III) hydroxide ($Eu^{III}(OH)_3$) nanorods (Ø 35–50 nm × 200–300 nm long) have been shown by Patra et al. to initiate angiogenesis in a similar manner to other pro-angiogenic cytokines, such as vascular endothelial growth factor (VEGF), at certain concentrations (20–50 µg/mL). These nanomaterials also produce H_2O_2 and superoxide anion ($O2^{\bullet-}$), which are critical in angiogenesis for cell stimulation and migration. Future nanomedical vascular-enhancing therapeutics might encompass severe ischemic heart disease, peripheral and limb ischemic diseases, where blood flow is improved in ischemic tissues through the generation of "collateral" blood vessels [309–311].

In what may be considered a radical nanomedical intervention for the dramatic augmentation of the circulatory system, Freitas and Phoenix hypothesize a "vasculoid personal nanomedical appliance," which would completely supercede the functionality of the innate human vasculature and blood with trillions of highly advanced interactive modular nanorobots, which cumulatively form a sealed/watertight lining that spans the luminal surfaces of the entire vascular tree. As described by the authors

> The vasculoid is a single, complex, multisegmented nanotechnological medical robotic system capable of duplicating all essential thermal and biochemical transport functions of the blood, including circulation of respiratory gases, glucose, hormones, cytokines, waste products, and cellular components. This nanorobotic system, a very aggressive and physiologically intrusive macroscale nanomedical device comprised of ~500 trillion stored or active individual nanorobots, weighs ~2 kg and consumes from 30–200 watts of power in the basic human model, depending on activity level.

This nanomedical system would be powered by glucose and oxygen, as will likely be the case for many medical nanodevices. Luminal endothelial cells, down to capillary level, would be covered with a tightly tessellated array of ~150 trillion "sapphiroid" (sapphire-containing) "basic plate" autonomous ciliated nanorobots (~2 µm^2 × ~1 µm thick). Sapphire is selected over diamond as the nanorobot material due to its superior thermal conductivity. Approximately 16% of this surface area would be functionalized with molecular conveying "docking bays" to enable docking with molecule-distributing "tankers." Biological cells would be transferred by "boxcars" that load and unload their cargoes at "cellulocks" as constituents of 32.6 billion "cellulock plates," each of which take up 60 µm^2 in luminal surface real estate, for utilization as docking bays for cell distribution. A further ~125 trillion basic plates would be reserved for special equipment and for specific physician- or user-defined applications. The internal nanometric components of each basic plate would be modular to facilitate easy restorative repairs and/or replacement if necessary, by mobile vasculocyte repair nanorobots [312].

In terms of nanomedical pulmonary augmentation, the enhancement of pulmonary capacity might be possible through the controllable generation and expansion of new terminal acini, inclusive of bronchiole, distal airways, and air spaces (alveolar sacs). This capability would be based on an intimate knowledge of acini genesis, formation, and functional dynamics. One early study revealed that an acinus contained a single terminal bronchiole, "approximately 14 respiratory bronchioles, 1,200–1,500 ducts, 2,500–4,500 sacs, and 14,000–20,000 alveoli" [313,314]. Pulmonary epithelial injury models have been investigated with the aim of elucidating the molecular events and dedicated stem cell activities that support the regeneration and remodeling of lung tissues. It was discovered that epithelial subsets, including proximal airway-resident basal, secretory, and Clara cells, as well as distal lung parenchyma type 2 alveolar cells have proliferative regenerative abilities in response to injury [315–317]. Investigations with small animal models have revealed rapid reparative activity of the lung epithelium following induced injuries. An essential initial event appeared to be the dedifferentiation and flattening of cells that surrounded the lesion. These flattened cells would then migrate toward the barren area to "restore the barrier function of the epithelium" [318]. Aerosolized nanocarriers that contain payloads of lung epithelial regenerative factors might be inhaled by future patients to not only alleviate a wide range of pulmonary ailments, but also to enhance their pulmonary capacity, efficiency, and resilience.

Perhaps the ultimate in nanomedical pulmonary augmentation, albeit not one that would be integrated into the lungs, but rather, widely distributed throughout the body, might be manifest as nanodevices similar to Freitas' "respirocytes" (Figure 17.13), which would

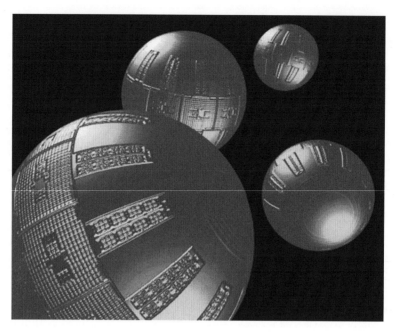

FIGURE 17.13
Artistic representation of respirocyte class artificial red blood cells. (Reproduced from Forrest Bishop and Robert Freitas Jr. With permission.)

serve as highly efficient, nanocomputer-controlled (in combination with external acoustic signal control) artificial red blood cells powered by ambient glucose in vivo. These diamondoid nanodevices would have dimensions of Ø ~1 μm with accommodation for 1.51×10^9 O_2 molecules for release into the bloodstream, and the acquisition of 1.33×10^9 CO_2 molecules for discharge into the lungs, under 1000 atm of pressure. The average respirocyte would have the capacity for delivering 236-fold more O_2 to tissues and CO_2 from tissues than average red blood cells.

Payloads of O_2 and CO_2 would be conveyed via 5184 diamondoid molecular sortation rotors to enable sufficient transfer volume for each molecular species (Chapter 16). Additional sortation rotors would be required for glucose (648) and H_2O (18,144) for a total complement of 29,160 rotors. Freitas estimates that 5.36×10^{12} devices would be required to fully replicate the active oxygenation capacity of human blood, at 8.1×10^{21} O_2 molecules. A therapeutic dose of respirocytes as an aqueous colloidal suspension would amount to ~5.61 cm^3. The recharging of spent respirocytes would occur simultaneously with the release of harvested CO_2 at the pulmonary capillaries within 5–10 s for ~42% of the full respirocyte complement during a single transit cycle, with only 17% of respirocytes that would be present within the lungs at any moment. This is based on the maximum O_2 molecule transmission volume (3.2×10^{21}/s) across the human lung alveoli [319].

17.2.4.4 Epidermal Augmentation

The nanomedical enhancement of the epidermis might include increased suppleness (e.g., wrinkle/scar negation, integrated cosmetics), resilience (e.g., instantaneous wound repair or negation), and the capacity for rapid and unique skin tone (e.g., iridescence [320]) and surface transformations (ridging [321], superhydrophic [322], superhydrophilic [323]) and adaptations in response to different environments and situations. The capacity for initiating a flexible, on demand, "dermal armor" capability might also be envisioned through the integration of biomimetic [324] nanodevice-mediated alterations and hierarchical reinforcement of the epidermis and underlying dermal layers via cross-linked nanostructured domains.

In a conceptual nanoepidermal protective scenario, the skin would retain its natural appearance and suppleness until impacted in some way. It would then become extremely tough and highly resistant against cut, tear, pinch, pressure, wounds, burns, puncturing, etc. This might be seen as analogous to thrusting an object (e.g., finger) into a container that is filled with corn starch and water. If the finger can proceed into the container when penetrated slowly, however, the corn starch will practically turn into a solid when thrusting the finger into the container rapidly. Dedicated nanodevices comprised of ultratough composite materials (diamondoid, sapphire, carbon nanotubes, graphene, hydroxyapatite nanocrystals, collagen nanofibers, etc.) embedded at an appropriate depth and density throughout the various epidermal layers (stratum—corneum, lucidum, granulosum, spinosum, basale) might instantaneously cross-link in response to any mechanical force above a predetermined threshold in the provision of an extremely tough and resilient, yet flexible protective dermal armor.

The virtually instantaneous (within seconds) nanomedical cessation of blood vessel or cutaneous bleeding might be enabled by autonomous (onboard nanocomputer-controlled) nanodevices such as "clottocytes." These nanodevices would rapidly deploy a "coccoon" of nanoscale mesh or netting around themselves, which would entangle with the netting of adjoining clottocytes to swiftly close a wound. They may serve as highly efficient artificial platelets (they would be physically much smaller than their natural platelet counterparts), where upon the detection of a vessel breach or injury would trigger a "progressive controlled mesh-release cascade" [325]. Though human fetal skin (during gestation period only) has the ability to completely regenerate without scarring [326], this is clearly not the case thereafter. Natural wound repair mechanisms (e.g., inflammatory responses, granulation proliferation, and scar formation) may span several months and generate dense unaesthetic scar tissue that remains in a weakened state (by ~15% to 20%) [325,326].

Nanomedicine would aim to accelerate the wound healing process by approx. >1000-fold via dedicated "tissue knitting" nanodevices that might facilitate the complete reconstruction of cutaneous tissues at the molecular and cellular resolution (layer-by-layer), proceeding from the peripheral extents of wound beds and moving inward to complete full regeneration. Though far more rapid, this strategy would be analogous to natural basement-membrane proteins, which "reappear in a very ordered sequence from the margin of the wound inward, in a zipperlike fashion" [327]. This regeneration would be driven by onboard nanodevice data, which would articulate the intimate composition and structure of each cutaneous layer. Required cytokines growth factors and angiogenic factors and biocompatible scaffold nanomaterials (e.g., biodegradable polymeric nanofibers) might be delivered by the appropriate nanocarriers. Ellis-Behnke et al. described the use of self-assembling peptide nanofiber barriers that form an extracellular matrix for the initiation of immediate (within 15 s) hemostasis following the direct application to wounds [328], as well as peptide nanofiber scaffolds for the "neuro knitting" repair of brain tissue, which might also be applied to rapid cutaneous regeneration immediately following trauma [329].

Freitas proposed that a dermal zipper ("zippocyte") with cuboid dimensions of 40 × 40 × 30 µm enabled with ~7000 nanomechanical cilia-like nanorobotic manipulators on five of its six faces might facilitate rapid tissue repair. These manipulators would carry out auxiliary functions inclusive of sensing and mapping, binding to terminating walls of wounds, individual locomotion, stationkeeping via connecting with surrounding nanodevices, and wound debridement. The sixth face might be endowed with larger and more dexterous manipulators for conducting actual reparative tasks. The specific tasking sequence would encompass "(1) activation, (2) entry, (3) immobilization and anti-inflammation, (4) scan surface, (5) debridement, (6) muscle repair, (7) areolar (loose connective) tissue repair, (8) fatty tissue repair, (9) dermis repair, (10) germinative layer restoration, (11) corneum repair, and (12) exit and shutdown" [325].

A number of nanomaterials that may currently facilitate enhanced/accelerated cutaneous wound repair and regeneration include nitric oxide containing nanoparticles, which were shown to lower inflammation, increase collagen deposition and blood vessel formation in immunodeficient mice [330]. Gold nanoparticle (Ø ~1 to 30 nm) carriers, working in conjunction with epigallocatechin gallate (antioxidant polyphenol flavonoid) and α-lipoic acid (antioxidant organosulfur compound), were shown to significantly accelerate wound healing in mice [331]. The topographic configuration of radially aligned poly(ε-caprolactone) nanofiber scaffolds demonstrated increased and faster dural fibroblast cell migration from the periphery of the scaffold to its center, in comparison to random nanofiber nonwoven mats. This type of development might lead to advanced bionanomedical grafts to enhance the speed and efficacy of wound closure or tissue regeneration [332].

17.3 Nanomedicine in Human Longevity

One of the most intriguing and perhaps controversial facets of prospective nanomedical capabilities is its application to the human *disease* of aging. Since humanity first emerged and evolved on Earth, its members have been forced to accept (and adapt their lives accordingly) that the perfectly healthy human body and mind, in its youthful state, will inevitably be subject to physiological and cognitive degradation through cascading biochemical alterations and physical/mental wear and tear, leading to eventual death. With the advent of advanced nanomedical technologies, however, capacities may be developed toward significantly delaying, halting, and perhaps even reversing human aging processes. As biogerontologist and visionary, Aubrey de Grey articulates:

> Aging is a process of decay—the accumulation of various types of molecular and cellular damage that our genetically-programmed metabolism causes but cannot repair. The past century's progress in biology and biotechnology has opened up the possibility that, within decades, we will be able to augment our in-built repair and maintenance processes with a range of "rejuvenation biotechnologies," so that people first given these treatments in middle age can remain youthful perhaps 30 years longer than they naturally would. If these technologies are then refined at a rate typically seen with past technologies, this will confer *indefinite* youth, because residual aspects of aging will be progressively overcome more rapidly than they catch up with us. The consequences for individuals and society would penetrate all aspects of life, but foremost among these consequences will be the alleviation of aging-related suffering and the saving of lives on an unprecedented scale [333].

Worldwide, ~150,000 individuals die every day (approx. two deaths per second), with an estimated ~100,000 of those deaths due to age-related causes. In the developed world, ~90% of all deaths may be attributable to aging [334]. Although forecasts are extremely disparate between current biogerontologists, some are of the opinion that "within as little as 30 years aging will be under a similar degree of control to that which modern medicine exerts over most infectious diseases today" [333]. Three scenarios predominate, as deduced by de Grey, in regard to how this feat might ultimately be achieved:

1. Conversion of the human body to an intrinsically perpetual nonaging condition (maintenance-free), whereby the passage of time becomes inconsequential. This scenario may only be feasible if current biological elements are replaced with essentially solid-state, highly durable materials, and presumably modular components, for simple replacement [333].

2. Development of comprehensive intervallic therapies that have the capacity for negating all cumulative damage in the body, thus enabling a youthful condition over indefinite time lines. This scenario will likely require, as a prerequisite, advanced and highly dynamic AI, in that human research efforts will likely not attain the depth of complex knowledge necessary. This advanced AI, however, may give rise to unforeseen dangers in terms of the potential acquisition and control of major systems (e.g., cities), electronic infrastructures, and economies, coupled with AI capacities for exponential recursive reprogramming and upgrades that will be rapidly unfathomable from the perspective of human comprehension [333,335].

3. Incremental resolution of lowest hanging fruit insofar as anti-aging therapies, utilizing traditional biotechnologies that advance at a characteristic rate. This strategy would likely set in motion a cascading and cumulative effect, whereby imminent therapies will maintain health of the human body for several additional decades, allowing for further advances to be developed and subsequently applied within this time frame to provide even longer spans of healthy life. Eventually, these advances might outpace the human body's degradative capacities [333].

4. The author interjects with a fourth scenario that is somewhat similar to, and indeed may be complementary with (3). This would involve the development and initial implementation of dedicated age-related disease-targeting nanocarriers for advanced drug delivery and specifically engineered nanoparticles for precision hyperthermic therapeutics, which would work in conjunction with pure "first phase" biotechnological anti-aging advances to potentially, further extend their attendant "bought time" [336–339]. As nanomedicine matures with the advent of molecular manufacturing, enabling highly sophisticated autonomous nanodevices, nanomedicine would continue to synergistically work in conjunction with still further advanced biotechnologies, until such time that the distinctions between them begin to blur and they merge [340–342] to become one in the same. The advantage at this juncture, from the nanomedical perspective, is that of the capacity for ultraprecise quantum computer-mediated imaging and mapping, with subsequently programmed manipulations of biomolecular or even atomic events that are increasingly likely to slowdown, stop, or even reverse the aging clock.

17.3.1 Causes of Aging: Brief Summary

Among the most obvious medical manifestations in aging are increased blood pressure, hardening arteries, cerebrovascular disease, renal failure, osteoporosis, osteoarthritis, dementia, type II diabetes, cancer, blindness via retinopathy or cataracts, and immunological decline. There are myriad alterations that occur at the molecular, cellular, tissue, and organ domains, which contribute to human senescence. It appears to some that human aging will forever be an inevitable fate, which cannot be significantly altered by any means, and indeed that it is extremely arrogant for humans to even contemplate tinkering with the result of millions of years of evolution, which has apparently cumulatively anatomically designed in, and thus, hard-programmed the human species for unavoidable decrepitude within a well-defined "expiry date" window [343].

Paradoxically, the vast and seemingly insurmountable challenges that will confront nanomedical conceptualists, designers, and engineers in this domain may actually "spur on" myriad new and bold human endeavors that permeate the visions and vast potentials of nanotechnology and nanomedicine. It is certain that in the era of prehuman flight, many concluded that the concept of human flight was blatantly arrogant and categorically impossible, firmly rooted in the obvious evidence that for millions of years, "humans could not fly," and were clearly anatomically designed and hard-programmed not to do so. "To the people of ancient civilizations, flying was the province of the gods; humankind's place was on earth. For a human to don wings was an expression of the desire to become closer to the divine, but it was also seen as arrogant, a mere mortal's attempt to usurp a prerogative of the gods" [344]. Mere mortals may yet again, in terms of dramatically prolonging human life, rise up to accomplish the impossible. Concomitantly, we must be sure to not be so naive, arrogant, or unrealistic as to think that all of the subtle complexities of the aging process will be "resolved" over a brief decadal time line. It is likely that innumerable incremental nanomedical advances toward the significant extension of human longevity will eventually culminate in remarkable progress.

Historically, human life expectancy has been prolonged through various means by ~50 years over the last two centuries, and as of 2013 the maximum age attained for any human on record is 122 years (Jeanne Calment, France). de Grey predicted that the first person to live for 1000 years might be 60 years old today [345]. To date, there appears to be "no evidence of an upper limit to life expectancy," and while human aging is considered as very complex, it is also thought of as a plastic process. "Although there is no convincing evidence that lifespan is 'programmed' genetically, about one-third of variation in life expectancy can be explained by genetic factors." The remaining two-thirds may be due to "stochastic and environmental factors, including diet." Random cumulative molecular damage that humans sustain throughout their lifetimes is thought to be initiated by chronic stresses brought about by inflammation, oxidative stress/redox alterations, and factors associated with metabolism [346]. A proposed number of primary causes of human aging encompass

1. Noncompensatory cell depletion in the brain, heart, and thymus
2. Proliferation and accumulation of functionally impaired cells
3. Chromosomal/DNA mutations
4. Mitochondrial mutations
5. Accumulation of molecular metabolic derivatives within a wide range of cells (e.g., advanced glycation end-products [AGEs] and lipofuscin)
6. Extracellular accumulation of proteinaceous aggregates
7. Random cross-linking in tissues due to sugar molecule-related chemical reactions [333]

A comprehensive exploration of the various potential nanomedical strategies that might attenuate all of the earlier-mentioned causes of human aging is beyond the scope of this chapter. Hence, a survey of selected lipofuscin eradication approaches will be presented as an exemplar, since this recalcitrant substance may deleteriously impact a broad range of cells, tissues, and organ systems toward the acceleration of aging.

17.3.2 Advanced Glycation End-Products and Lipofuscin

Cumulative degradation processes, as listed earlier, which play a role in the aging of the human body, are initiated in part by metabolic mechanisms, in particular, the formation of compounds such as AGEs and lipofuscin. AGEs are the mutably toxic products of lipids or proteins that nonenymatically form covalent bonds with sugar molecules via glycation (e.g., reducing sugar carbonyl condenses with a protein-reactive amino group) [347], which accumulate within many species of cells and blood vessel walls to negatively impact both intracellular and extracellular biostructures, and hence, their functionality. They have a ubiquitous presence in the vasculature of diabetics and are a factor in the progression of atherosclerosis. Further, they form cross-links between basement membrane molecules within the extracellular matrix, leading to an assortment of micro and macrovascular impediments. AGEs also obstruct nitric oxide function in the endothelium and incite the generation of detrimental ROS [348]. Altogether, AGEs appear to have significant impacts in the advancement of the human aging.

Intriguingly, carbonyl scavenging agents such as aminoguanidine [349–351] and pyridoxamine [352–354] have demonstrated the ability to inhibit the formation and activity of AGEs [347]. They have also, however, exhibited adverse activity in in vivo assays [355,356], hence further fine-tuning of their capacities is warranted. The covalent protein cross-links that are generated by AGEs may also be cleaved via cross-link breakers such as N-phenacylthiazolium bromide [357,358] and ALT-711 (a N-phenacyl-derived thiazolium carbene) [347,359,360].

A further insight is provided by Yin as per AGEs and lipofuscin in that although they are "…produced from different types of biological materials due to different side reactions of essential biology the crosslinking of carbonyl-amino compounds is recognized as a common process during their formation" [361]. Hence, the precision affinity-based targeting of AGEs and lipofuscin, and their associated cross-links by nanocarriers that are laden with these types of beneficial agents might likely go a long way in negating myriad age-related degradation.

Ceroid lipofuscin is an autofluorescent age pigment that constitutes the final breakdown product of, among other bioentities, organelles such as the mitochondria and can also contain AGEs [362]. This yellowish brown granular (Ø ~1 to 5 μm) substance is a heterogeneous mixture, and thus a comprehensive elucidation of its composition is still lacking [363]. Lipofuscin accumulates in cellular lysosomes, within which potent enzymes break down all manner of macromolecular metabolic waste, which is sequestered via autophagy, endocytosis, or phagocytosis. Lipofuscin is what remains at the conclusion of this process and presumably cannot be degraded further.

In aging, lipofuscin accumulates within numerous cell species, resident in the heart (cardiac myocytes), brain (neurons), liver (hepatic cells), kidney (renal tubular cells), skin, and in the retinal pigment epithelium (RPE), where it is a factor in age-associated macular degeneration. It has been learned from the study of purified lipofuscin in RPE, as revealed by Ng et al., that it contains low (~2% *w/w*) protein (e.g., amyloid β-precursor) content, bisretinoids A2E, isoA2E, and all-*trans*-retinal dimer-phosphatidylethanolamine, as well as reactive nitrogen oxide generated nitrotyrosine and reactive lipid segment generated carboxyethylpyrrole and iso[4]levuglandin E(2) adducts. Interestingly, lipofuscin is also a robust generator of ROS [364]. The lipid fraction of lipofuscin is comprised of triglycerides, cholesterol, phospholipids, and peroxidized free fatty acids (4-hydroxy-2-nonenal), with a heterogeneous carbohydrate fraction. Also incorporated are iron, copper, aluminum, zinc, calcium, and magnesium, which also account for 2% of its overall components [365]. The longevity of postmitotic cells is associated with and contingent on the cumulative formation of lipofuscin, which is determined by protein oxidation damage, the efficacy and functionality of mitochondrial repair mechanisms, the proteasomal system, and lysosomes. Interestingly, the cell nuclear compartment, in contrast to the cytosol, is relatively devoid of lipofuscin [366,367].

17.3.2.1 Potential Nanomedical Strategies for Lipofuscin Eradication

The variable compositions of lipofuscin and lipofuscin-related detritic materials that reside within aging humans may likely require the application of a multifaceted nanomedical strategy whose parameters are defined by the particular lipofuscin or lipofuscin-like aggregate species within specific substrates and cell types. For example, in the arteries, "lipofuscin" is comprised primarily of modified (oxidized) cholesterol (oxysterol species 7-ketocholesterol) (7 KC) [368], whereas in the retina it is termed lipofuscin due primarily to its fluorescence. Cardiac lipofuscin aggregates are considered to be the genuine articles (by definition), whereas in the brain, their composition is varied yet again as the majority of intracellular debris that resides here is thought to be other than lysosomal in nature [369]. A number of agents have been shown to have an impact against various lipofuscin aggregates (Table 17.4), which may be delivered to affected areas via precisely targeted nanocarriers or future autonomous nanodevices. In the following section are described a number of potential nanomedically mediated strategies for the eradication of lipofuscin, which may contribute to the quest for enhanced human longevity.

17.3.2.1.1 Enzymatic Eradication of Lipofuscin

It is plausible that lipofuscin aggregates throughout the human body, regardless of their composition, might be targeted via appropriate nanocarriers or nanoreactors [385,386] and eradicated via enzymatic degradation. Dedicated enzyme cargoes may be loaded within nanocarriers, which would encapsulate and protect them until they are queued for release when the nanocarriers are physically tethered to lipofuscin granules. For example, vascular cholesterol and 7 KC can be catalyzed and degraded through the delivery of bacterial enzymes such as cholesterol oxidase from the soil bacteria *Chromobacterium sp.* DS1, which has been shown to function within the low pH environment of lysosomes and boost their activity in the clearance of 7 KC in lysosomes [368].

Nanoreactors are nanometric (Ø ~200 nm) hollow spheres or containers with alternate geometries that are comprised of self-assembling amphiphilic block copolymers (e.g., PMOXA-PDMS-PMOXA or poly(2-methyloxazoline)-poly(dimethylsiloxane)-poly(2-methyloxazoline) triblock copolymer), which encapsulate enzymes within internal aqueous milieu. The walls (~10 nm thick) of the nanoreactors (similar to biological membranes) are made permeable via the integration of channel-forming proteins to enable particulates and substrates to ingress and egress the nanoreactor via diffusion. Thus, catalytic reactions may proceed within the cores of the nanoreactors [386]. If lipofuscin granules can be initially cleaved by dedicated nanodevices into smaller constituents, it may be possible to utilize these types of nanoreactors (with sufficiently accommodating pores) for enzymatic lipofuscin eradication. More sophisticated classes of nanoreactors might contain enzymes that can degrade multiple biodebris substrates to serve as adjunctive artificial lysosomes.

TABLE 17.4

Selection of Antilipofuscin Drugs That Might Be Encapsulated and Delivered by Targeted Nanocarriers or Autonomous Nanodevices

Agent/Compound	Description	Condition	Impact on Lipofuscin	Ref.
ACU-4429	Small nonretinoid molecule, modulates RPE65 enzyme that is required to convert trans-retinol to cis-retinol within the RPE.	Dry age-related macular degeneration.	Prevented the accumulation of A2E in the mouse retina.	[370]
α-Lipoic acid L-Carnitine	Important dithiol antioxidant cofactor in multienzyme mitochondrial complexes. Essential nutrient synthesized from amino acids.	General diseases of aging.	Supplementation of carnitine and lipoic acid reduces lipofuscin accumulation, prevents membrane damage during aging, can prevent age-associated disorders.	[371]
Bacopa monnieri (L.)	Traditional Indian medicinal plant.	Cognitive impairment in aging and senile dementia of Alzheimer type.	Significantly prevented and reduced the aggregation of lipofuscin in the middle-aged and aged rat brain cortex.	[372]
Centrophenoxine	Lipofuscin scavenger.	Lipofuscin accumulation in RPE cells.	Significantly decreased the $Ca^2(+)$ overload, which is associated with lipofuscin formation in human RPE cells.	[373]
Creatine	Natural ergogenic compound with anti-apoptotic, anti-excitotoxic, antioxidative properties.	Parkinson's disease, Huntington's disease, amyotrophic lateral sclerosis.	Significantly lowered lipofuscin accumulation in mouse models.	[374]
Curcumin	Bioactive polyphenolic extract of turmeric.	General diseases of aging.	Decreased lipofuscin levels and increased the life spans of nematode roundworm, *Drosophila* (fruit fly), and mouse.	[375]
Epigallocatechin gallate	Primary active ingredient of green tea.	General diseases of aging.	Decreased the formation of lipofuscin in *Caenorhabditis elegans*.	[376]
Fenretinide	Synthetic derivative of vitamin A.	Dry age-related macular degeneration.	Inhibits accumulation of A2E and lipofuscin in RPE cells.	[370]

(continued)

TABLE 17.4 (continued)

Selection of Antilipofuscin Drugs That Might Be Encapsulated and Delivered by Targeted Nanocarriers or Autonomous Nanodevices

Agent/Compound	Description	Condition	Impact on Lipofuscin	Ref.
Flunarizine	$Ca^2(+)$ channel antagonist.	Lipofuscin accumulation in RPE cells.	Significantly decreased the $Ca^2(+)$ overload, which is associated with lipofuscin formation in human RPE cells.	[373]
Kaempferol			Attenuated the accumulation of lipofuscin in *Caenorhabditis elegans* nematode.	[377]
Piracetam	GABA-derived nootropic (cognitive enhancing) agent.	Alcoholism.	Significant reduction in the formation of neuronal lipofuscin in rats.	[378]
Rapamycin	Macrocyclic triene antibiotic molecule from the soil bacterium *Streptomyces hygroscopicus*.	General diseases of aging.	Inhibition of mammalian target of rapamycin complex 1 (mTORC1) with rapamycin-activated autophagy, which reduced the number of lipofuscin-like particles in human adipocytes.	[379]
			Replicates longevity effects of caloric restriction.	[380]
Resveratrol	Naturally occurring polyphenol found in berries, nuts, and red wine.	General diseases of aging.	Reduction of lipofuscin in the short-lived fish *Nothobranchius furzeri* and decreased protein aggregates in aged fish brains.	[381] [382]
Terminalia chebula (Chebulic myrobalan)	Traditional Indian medicinal plant.	Oxidative stress Liver and kidney aging.	Decreased liver and kidney mitochondrial lipofuscin in aged rats.	[383]
Ubiquinone (CoQ10)	Antioxidant that is a component of the mitochondrial electron transport chain.	Cardiac hypertrophy.	Cardiac content of lipofuscin was decreased in rabbits.	[384]

Enzyme replacement therapies that target enzyme-deficient lysosomes have shown success in the treatment of a number of lysosomal storage diseases [387,388]. Hence, it may be feasible to deliver lipofuscin-degrading enzymes directly into lysosomes utilizing nanocarriers to enable their clearance. The ocular delivery of nanocarriers may be facilitated by the simultaneous delivery of spreading enzymes such as hyaluronidase and collagenase to "rapidly hydrolyze the collagenous and extracellular matrix structure of the sclera" to allow easier access to resident lipofuscin granules [389]. Wu et al. reported that bisretinoid lipofuscin (A2E) that accumulates in RPE cells can be enzymatically cleaved and degraded through the use of horseradish peroxidase [390]. The highly heterogeneous lipofuscin within the heart may require a cascade of multiple species of nanocarrier-delivered potent enzymes for its incremental degradation. Neuronal lipofuscin might be degraded by enzymes that are transported via the cerebrospinal fluid or by nanocarriers that have the capacity for traversing the blood-brain barrier [369].

Another approach toward the eradication of lipofuscin, in addition to the nanomedical delivery of antilipofuscin drugs and enzymes to the lysosomes and cytoplasmic compartments, might be to bolster and increase the functional robustness of the lysosomes themselves. Lysosomes typically take up and process cross-linked proteins and enlarged mitochondria with other bound materials that comprise lipofuscin. Over time, this can lead to lysosomal swelling, destabilization, and rupture, whereupon lipofuscin is released by the lysosomes into the cytosol and causes damage. The lipofuscin is subsequently taken up once again to repeat the cycle [365], which can eventually result in cell death (apoptosis/necrosis). Hence, it may likely be useful to deliver augmentative agents to lysosomes to increase their longevity, and in effect, the longevity of the human host as well.

Baltazar et al. speculated that an increase in lysosomal pH inhibits the capacity of certain lysosome-resident hydrolase enzymes (in mammalian lysosomes there are 50 species) [391] to degrade the influx of various biomaterials that they receive via endocytosis, phagocytosis, or autophagy, and thus has a cumulative negative impact on cell health. They demonstrated that the rapid and sustained restoration of nominal low pH (4.5) in malfunctioning lysosomes through the targeted delivery of acidic polymeric (poly(lactic-co-glycolic acid and poly(DL-lactide)) nanoparticles (Ø ~400 nm) rectified lysosomal enzymatic activity and decreased lipofuscin loads [392]. Koshkaryev et al. showed that lysosomotropic octadecyl-rhodamine B modified liposomes (Chapter 12) facilitated a significant increase in the targeting of lysosomes [393].

An important factor to be mindful of when designing and introducing nanoparticles and other nanomaterials into the human body with the intent of imparting positive outcomes for potentially extending longevity, via the targeting of lysosomes, is that certain species of nanomaterials are indeed toxic [394,395] and can be taken up by and impair their functionality [396,397], thereby completely negating the premise of beneficial nanomedicine. Hence, the stringent testing of nanomaterials that are intended for human nanomedical use should be undertaken as a matter of course to validate their safety, as well as efficacy. The accepted indicators to date of nanomaterial toxicity are inflammation and oxidative stress, albeit the fundamental mechanisms behind these reactions remain inadequately investigated [398].

In this regard, advanced autonomous nanodevices will be comprised of biologically inert/biocompatible materials and/or be endowed with replenishable biocompatible coatings to ensure that there will be zero negative impacts for the patient. An additional advantageous factor is that most nanomedical device residencies within the human body will be on the order of minutes, to several hours, to a day or two for the most complex procedures. Hence, this "surgical strike" style approach for nanomedical practice (rapid deployment/accomplish mission/rapid evacuation) will serve to negate the possibility of toxicity or pathogenic response. Beyond inherent nanodevice biocompatibility, these brief in vivo exposures should not elicit any negative responses from the patient.

17.3.2.1.2 Conceptual Nanomedical Eradication of Lipofuscin

In terms of simplicity, and to facilitate the earliest implementation of feasible therapies, the design of near-term nanomedical lipofuscin removal might undertake a "path of least resistance" approach. This strategy may be warranted in order to initiate nanomedical antilipofuscin treatment regimes as soon as is possible toward the negation of the effects of human aging and the attendant loss of faculties and self-integrity, coupled with untold suffering due to myriad associated diseases. From an economic standpoint, as relates to indefinitely deferred medical expenses brought on by advanced and thorough nanomedical lipofuscin eradication alone (which by extension will significantly delay or negate myriad age-related disease states), may save otherwise enormous per-annum medical expenditures worldwide. For example, Olshansky et al. reported that the annual expenditure on Alzheimer's disease in 2006 was $80–$100 billion, and it is predicted that more than $1 trillion will be spent on Alzheimer's disease and associated dementias by 2050 [399].

Nascent nanomedical therapies involving targeted nanocarriers, nanoreactors, or nanoparticles might employ a number of strategies for the eradication of lipofuscin. One of these might involve hypothermia, whereby metallic (Au) nanoshells [400,401] or magnetic nanoparticles (MNPs) [402,403] would be specifically targeted to cell/lysosome-resident lysosomes. One of these targeting agents may be N-retinylidene-N-retinylethanolamine (A2E), which, paradoxically, is a primary constituent/fluorophore of lipofuscin. A2E on its own, or when coupled with low-density lipoprotein, has been shown to have an affinity for acidic organelles, such as lysosomes. However, when A2E is resident within lysosomes, it can increase their pH, thereby impairing enzymatic activity [404,405]. This alteration in lysosomal pH might be offset or equalized through the concomitant introduction of acidic molecules that either comprise a portion of the decorative elements on the external surfaces of the metallic nanoshells or MNPs, or which are encapsulated within them. Further, the A2E that was utilized for initial lysosome targeting may subsequently be degraded by enzymes such as horseradish peroxidase [406].

Once within the cytosol, a secondary targeting sequence would commence to bind the nanoshells or MNPs to the lipofuscin itself. The monoclonal antibody (AmT-1) was found by Takahashi et al. to bind with lipofuscin pigments in the adrenal gland cells of zona reticulata, liver hepatocytes, and eccrine sweat glands in the skin [407]. Bancher et al. demonstrated that monoclonal antibodies against cerebrovascular amyloid β-protein could bind with neuronal lipofuscin [408]. Heavy metal ions (e.g., copper and iron) were also found to associate with lipofuscin [409]. Subsequently, the nanoshells or MNPs might be thermally activated via external sources (e.g., ultrasound, pulsed NIR laser, or magnetic fields). The initiated thermal energy may serve (theoretically) to effectively "melt" the lipofuscin or its main constituent A2E, thereby degrading it to more elemental constituents, which may be either enzymatically metabolized via attending nanoreactors or otherwise egressed from the body by natural processes.

Although entirely conceptual and seemingly impracticable currently (2013), advanced AI involvement in the design/optimization of sophisticated nanomedical devices working in conjunction with mature nanomanufacturing may indeed bring about much more complex, albeit far more rapid and efficient lipofuscin detection and removal. Advanced autonomous nanodevices might precisely locate lipofuscin granules by exploiting their strong fluorescence signatures (emission spectrum ranges from 450 to 700 nm) [410] to match with onboard reference spectral profiles. The prospective armamentarium at the disposal of these autonomous diamondoid "defuscin" class nanodevices (Figures 17.14 through 17.16) might allow for the complete eradication of lipofuscin aggregates utilizing a feedthrough digestive strategy. These entities may be propelled by arrays of oscillating piezoelectric "fins" or via integrated magnetic nanoparticles, which might be activated and controlled externally. The conical inlet port of the nanodevice would be lined with molecules that possess high affinities for A2E and other lipofuscin elements. Once a lipofuscin

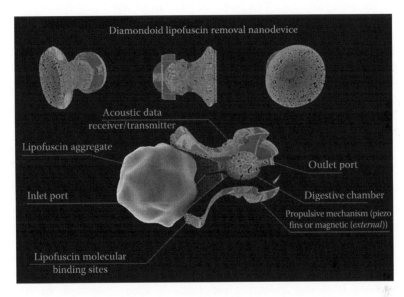

FIGURE 17.14
Artistic representation of one class of "defuscin" diamondoid nanodevice for the removal of lipofuscin. (Reproduced from Svidinenko, Y., DNA-repair nanorobot, Nanobotmodels Company, http://www.nanobotmodels.com/node/48?size=preview, accessed November 22, 2012. With permission.)

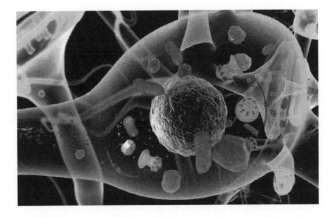

FIGURE 17.15
Artistic representation of "defuscin" diamondoid nanodevices in the process of removing neuronal lipofuscin. (Reproduced from Svidinenko, Y., DNA-repair nanorobot, Nanobotmodels Company, http://www.nanobotmodels.com/node/48?size=preview, accessed November 22, 2012. With permission.)

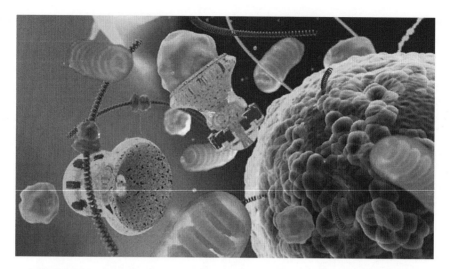

FIGURE 17.16
Artistic (close-up) representation of "defuscin" diamondoid nanodevices in the process of removing lipofuscin from cytoplasm in close proximity to nucleus. (Reproduced from Svidinenko, Y., DNA-repair nanorobot, Nanobotmodels Company, http://www.nanobotmodels.com/node/48?size=preview, accessed November 22, 2012. With permission.)

granule has been captured, it would proceed to be drawn into the core, where it would be digested by potent encapsulated enzymes or nanomechanically minced into a liquid state and subsequently purged from the outlet port. This functionality would be similar to Freitas's microbivore artificial mechanical phagocytes, which operate under a "digest and discharge" protocol [411]. The desired result of this defuscin-mediated digestion would be the fragmentation and ideally dissolution of the chemical cross-links that provide lipofuscin its refractive properties.

Other defuscin-class nanodevice designs may include proboscises that serve dual purposes: as potential electrodes for highly localized hyperthermic interventions, following insertion into the lipofuscin mass, or hollow nanosyringes [412,413] for the injection of powerful cleaving enzymes. The nanomechanical segmentation or disassembly of individual lipofuscin granules at atomic/molecular resolution may be possible employing arrays of diamondoid "debriders" to reduce lipofuscin to its most elemental and harmless fractions. Larger fragments could subsequently be encapsulated for egress through the urinary or gastrointestinal tracts.

The overarching premise here is that treated cells might be thus induced to a more robust state of health (perhaps functioning at more youthful levels) when this cellular burden is extricated.

17.4 Nanomedicine in Radical Human Longevity

The prospect of radical human longevity will likely be enabled via the synergistic melding of mature nanotechnology, molecular manufacturing, nanomedicine, and AI. What might be considered as *radical* in this regard from today's (2013) perspective may be the deliberate quest/challenge for humans to accomplish the 1000 year mark [345] by various means, encompassing

1. Continually incremental and overlapping "escape velocity" advances in biological rejuvenative therapies, such as that proposed by de Grey [414], increasingly assisted by nanomedicines.

2. Integration of/interfacing human physiologies with sophisticated nanomachinery, comprised of diamondoid or other unique and robust nanomaterials, smart materials, and quantum computers driven by AI. Participants would be transforming in essence, to cyborgians. A vivid example of this is the Phoenix and Freitas "vasculoid" nanomedical appliance for the replacement of human blood [312].

3. Uploading the human brain into a nanomanufactured in silico replica within a highly durable, dynamic, robust, and elegant nanosynthetic avatar body/robotic proxy, or in virtual reality, as envisioned by the transhumanist/posthumanist movement [415].

4. Cryonic suspension for the potential reanimation of frozen individuals when sufficiently advanced technologies exist for their transfer/transformation to a posthuman entity [416].

Each of these radical longevity options may theoretically be enabled through the merging of smart nanomaterials and autonomous nanomedical devices, working in conjunction (at this level) with nanotechnologies and AI to facilitate the formation or fabrication of the required atomic and molecular interfaces within complex orchestrations of structure, function, and intimate nanoelectronic interconnectivity. Quantum computation will be indispensible for the flawless operation and maintenance of this multifaceted complex of nanomachinery, particularly when it is interfaced with biological cells and tissues. The development of molecular manufacturing will be an absolute prerequisite and fundamental driver toward the realization of any of these visions. To date (2013), the concept of molecular manufacturing remains as such. Estimates on the time line to the achievement of this keystone technology range from ~2020 to ~2030 [417]. In terms of sophisticated nanodevices, Freitas ventures that the first glimmer of practicable nanorobotics may emerge by 2020 [418].

What we might now consider as extreme human longevity, over an appropriate span of time and experience, may evolve to be as accepted as is our current state of longevity in comparison to the brevity of the human life span as it was some 200 years ago (~50 years) [346]. An individual in the year 1813, one can imagine, would find it totally incomprehensible, and indeed would think it utterly impossible, if told that humans would someday live half a century longer than the nominal life expectancy at that time. The human species possesses an amazing resilience and adaptability to change (again, accrued over time), an unquenchable thirst for knowledge, advancement, and the improvement of our own, and our loved ones lives. For the most part, there is an inherent and sincere desire to endeavor to support the betterment of our kind across the globe, and most importantly, with the unencumbered freedom to do so.

Hence, radical human longevity may indeed come into eventuality, as it is at the core of human nature to unceasingly test and press against the boundaries of the world and life as it is, and yearn for what our hearts and dreams tell us it might be. The prospect of radical longevity, because it is advancing ever closer to actually being possible, will undoubtedly be flared with impassioned arguments from both sides of the issue [419,420], far deeper and much more intense than those discussed earlier as relates to the ethical and moral implications of human cognitive enhancement.

In the larger frame, we live day-to-day on our miraculous and beautiful blue world (at times oblivious to the overwhelming odds for us *not* existing at all) in the midst of the deep and inconceivably vast expanse of darkness speckled with trillions of stars. *Where do our boundaries lie?* It may be suggested that any constraint imposed upon the human imagination and the extent to which we may explore and advance within ourselves and into the without, are entirely self-imposed.

It is likely that the remarkable and truly inestimable possibilities of nanomedicine in serving to benefit human health will progress incrementally forward, until such time that mature nanomanufacturing and AI fuse with reality. Thereafter, the capacity for the attainment of robust human health and unprecedented human longevity will be transformative to an incredible degree, which we will have yet to fathom, as we continue to progress in life's amazing adventure, perhaps one day, to the periphery of the universe.

References

1. Drexler, K.E., Molecular technology and cell repair machines. Paper presented at the *1985 Lake Tahoe Life Extension Festival*, 25 May 1985; reprinted and published in *Claustrophobia Mag* (August–October 1985) and in *Cryonics Mag* (December 1985–January 1986).
2. Wowk, B., Cell repair technology. *Cryonics Mag.* Alcor Foundation, 7–10 July 1988.
3. Gospodinov, A. and Herceg, Z., Shaping chromatin for repair. *Mutat. Res.* pii: S1383–5742(12), 00063–00064, 2012.
4. Swenberg, J.A., Lu, K., Moeller, B.C., Gao, L., Upton, P.B., Nakamura, J., and Starr, T.B., Endogenous versus exogenous DNA adducts: Their role in carcinogenesis, epidemiology, and risk assessment. *Toxicol. Sci.* 120(Suppl. 1) S130–S145, 2011.
5. Jackson, S.P. and Bartek, J., The DNA-damage response in human biology and disease. *Nature* 461, 1071–1078, 2009.
6. Plummer, R., Perspective on the pipeline of drugs being developed with modulation of DNA damage as a target. *Clin. Cancer Res.* 16(18), 4527–4531, 2010.
7. Hoeijmakers, J.H., Genome maintenance mechanisms for preventing cancer. *Nature* 411, 366–374, 2001.
8. Bernstein, C., Bernstein, H., Payne, C.M., and Garewal, H., DNA repair/pro-apoptotic dual-role proteins in five major DNA repair pathways: Fail-safe protection against carcinogenesis. *Mutat. Res.* 511, 145–178, 2002.
9. Dynan, W.S., Takeda, Y., and Li, S., Modifying the function of DNA repair nanomachines for therapeutic benefit. *Nanomedicine* 2(2), 74–81, 2006.
10. Sirzen, F., Nilsson, A., Zhivotovsky, B., and Lewensohn, R., DNA-dependent protein kinase content and activity in lung carcinoma cell lines: Correlation with intrinsic radiosensitivity. *Eur. J. Cancer* 35, 111–116, 1999.
11. Li, S., Takeda, Y., Wragg, S., Barrett, J., Phillips, A.C., and Dynan, W.S., Modification of the ionizing radiation response in living cells by an scFv against the DNA-dependent protein kinase. *Nucl. Acids Res.* 31, 5848–5857, 2003.
12. Nitin, N., LaConte, L.E., Zurkiya, O., Hu, X., and Bao, G., Functionalization and peptide-based delivery of magnetic nanoparticles as an intracellular MRI contrast agent. *J. Biol. Inorg. Chem.* 9, 706–712, 2004.
13. Svidinenko, Y., DNA-repair nanorobot, Nanobotmodels Company. http://www.nanobotmodels.com/node/48?size=preview (accessed November 22, 2012).

14. Hansen, W.K. and Kelly, M., Review of mammalian DNA repair and translational implications. *J .Pharmacol. Exp. Ther.* 295, 1–9, 2000.
15. Hombauer, H., Campbell, C.S., Smith, C.E., Desai, A., and Kolodner, R.D., Visualization of eukaryotic DNA mismatch repair reveals distinct recognition and repair intermediates. *Cell* 147(5), 1040–1053, 2011.
16. Natarajan, A.T. and Palitti, F., DNA repair and chromosomal alterations. *Mutat. Res.* 657(1), 3–7, 2008.
17. Lindahl, T. and Wood, R.D., Quality control by DNA repair. *Science* 1286(5446), 1897–1905, 1999.
18. Cloud, K.G., Shen, B., Strniste, G.F., and Park, M.S., XPG protein has a structure-specific endonuclease activity. *Mutat. Res.* 347(2), 55–60, 1995.
19. Martin, M.J., Juarez, R., and Blanco, L., DNA-binding determinants promoting NHEJ by human Polμ. *Nucl. Acids Res.* 40(22), 11389–403, 2012.
20. Suwaki, N., Klare, K., and Tarsounas, M., RAD51 paralogs: Roles in DNA damage signalling, recombinational repair and tumorigenesis. *Semin. Cell Dev. Biol.* 22(8), 898–905, 2011.
21. Schanz, S., Schuler, N., Lorat, Y., Fan, L., Kaestner, L., Wennemuth, G., Rübe, C., and Rübe, C.E., Accumulation of DNA damage in complex normal tissues after protracted low-dose radiation. *DNA Repair (Amst)* 11(10), 823–832, 2012.
22. Ames, B.N., Micronutrient deficiencies. A major cause of DNA damage. *Ann. N Y Acad. Sci.* 889, 87–106, 1999.
23. Huang, H.B., Chen, G.W., Wang, C.J., Lin, Y.Y., Liou, S.H., Lai, C.H., and Wang, S.L., Exposure to heavy metals and polycyclic aromatic hydrocarbons and DNA damage in Taiwanese traffic conductors. *Cancer Epidemiol. Biomarkers Prev.* 2012.
24. Fallot, G., Neuveut, C., and Buendia, M.A., Diverse roles of hepatitis B virus in liver cancer. *Curr. Opin. Virol.* 2(4), 467–473, 2012.
25. Freitas Jr., R.A., The ideal gene delivery vector: Chromallocytes, cell repair nanorobots for chromosome replacement therapy. *J. Evol. Technol.* 16, 1–97, 2007.
26. Schrlau, M.G., Falls, E.M., Ziober, B.L., and Bau, H.H., Carbon nanopipettes for cell probes and intracellular injection. *Nanotechnology* 19(1), 015101, 2008.
27. Schrlaum, M.G., Dun, N.J., and Bau, H.H., Cell electrophysiology with carbon nanopipettes. *ACS Nano* 3(3), 563–568, 2009.
28. Graham, J. and Gerald, R.W., Membrane potentials and excitation of impaled single muscle fibers. *J. Cell. Comp. Physiol.* 28, 99–117, 1946.
29. Ling, G. and Gerald, R.W., The normal membrane potential of frog sartorious fibers. *J. Cell. Comp. Physiol.* 34, 383–396, 1949.
30. Singhal, R., Orynbayeva, Z., Kalyana Sundaram, R.V., Niu, J.J., Bhattacharyya, S., Vitol, E.A., Schrlau, M.G., Papazoglou, E.S., Friedman, G., and Gogotsi, Y., Multifunctional carbon-nanotube cellular endoscopes. *Nat. Nanotechnol.* 6(1), 57–64, 2011.
31. Orynbayeva, Z., Singhal, R., Vitol, E.A., Schrlau, M.G., Papazoglou, E., Friedman, G., and Gogotsi, Y., Physiological validation of cell health upon probing with carbon nanotube endoscope and its benefit for single-cell interrogation. *Nanomedicine* 8(5), 590–598, 2012.
32. Gupta, A., Avci, P., Sadasivam, M., Chandran, R., Parizotto, N., Vecchio, D., de Melo, W.C., Dai, T., Chiang, L.Y., and Hamblin, M.R., Shining light on nanotechnology to help repair and regeneration. *Biotechnol. Adv.* 31(5), 607–31, 2013.
33. Goldberg, M., Langer, R., and Jia, X., Nanostructured materials for applications in drug delivery and tissue engineering. *J. Biomater. Sci. Polym. Ed.* 18, 241–268, 2007.
34. Verma, S., Domb, A.J., and Kumar, N., Nanomaterials for regenerative medicine. *Nanomedicine (Lond)* 6, 157–181, 2011.
35. Ellis-Behnke, R. and Jonas, J.B., Redefining tissue engineering for nanomedicine in ophthalmology. *Acta Ophthalmol.* 89(2), e108–e114, 2011.
36. Ellis-Behnke, R.G., Liang,Y.X., You, S.W., Tay, D.K., Zhang, S., So, K.F., and Schneider, G.E., Nano neuro knitting: Peptide nanofiber scaffold for brain repair and axon regeneration with functional return of vision. *Proc. Natl. Acad. Sci. USA* 103(13), 5054–5059, 2006.

37. Park, Y.J., Kim, K.H., Lee, J.Y., Ku, Y., Lee, S.J., Min, B.M., and Chung, C.P., Immobilization of bone morphogenetic protein-2 on a nanofibrous chitosan membrane for enhanced guided bone regeneration. *Biotechnol. Appl. Biochem.* 43(Pt 1), 17–24, 2006.

38. Webster, T.J., Ergun, C., Doremus, R.H., Siegel, R.W., and Bizios, R., Specific proteins mediate enhanced osteoblast adhesion on nanophase ceramics. *J. Biomed. Mater. Res.* 51(3), 475–483, 2000.

39. Li, P., Biomimetic nano-apatite coating capable of promoting bone ingrowth. *J. Biomed. Mater. Res. A* 66(1), 79–85, 2003.

40. Spoerke, E.D. and Stupp, S.I., Colonization of organoapatite-titanium mesh by preosteoblastic cells. *J. Biomed. Mater. Res. A* 67(3), 960–969, 2003.

41. Supronowicz, P.R., Ajayan, P.M., Ullmann, K.R., Arulanandam, B.P., Metzger, D.W., and Bizios, R., Novel current-conducting composite substrates for exposing osteoblasts to alternating current stimulation. *J. Biomed. Mater. Res.* 59(3), 499–506, 2002.

42. Li, C., Vepari, C., Jin, H.J., Kim, H.J., and Kaplan, D.L., Electrospun silk-BMP-2 scaffolds for bone tissue engineering. *Biomaterials* 27(16), 3115–3124, 2006.

43. Zong, X., Bien, H., Chung, C.Y., Yin, L., Fang, D., Hsiao, B.S., Chu, B., and Entcheva, E., Electrospun fine-textured scaffolds for heart tissue constructs. *Biomaterials* 26(26), 5330–5338, 2005.

44. Park, J.S., Park, K., Woo, D.G., Yang, H.N., Chung, H.M., and Park, K.H., PLGA microsphere construct coated with TGF-beta 3 loaded nanoparticles for neocartilage formation. *Biomacromolecules* 9(8), 2162–2169, 2008.

45. Li, W.J., Tuli, R., Okafor, C., Derfoul, A., Danielson, K.G., Hall, D.J., and Tuan, R.S., A three-dimensional nanofibrous scaffold for cartilage tissue engineering using human mesenchymal stem cells. *Biomaterials* 26(6), 599–609, 2005.

46. Liu, J. and Zhao, X., Design of self-assembling peptides and their biomedical applications. *Nanomedicine (Lond)* 6(9), 1621–1643, 2011.

47. Zhang, L., Song, H., and Zhao, X., Self-assembling short-peptide hydrogel for three-dimensional culture of rabbit articular chondrocytes *in vitro*. *J. Clin. Rehab. Tiss. Eng. Res.* 12(49), 9779–9782, 2008.

48. Duan, X., McLaughlin, C., Griffith, M., and Sheardown, H., Biofunctionalization of collagen for improved biological response: Scaffolds for corneal tissue engineering. *Biomaterials* 28(1), 780–788, 2007.

49. Zhao, X. and Zhang, S., Designer self-assembling peptide materials. *Macromol. Biosci.* 7(1), 13–22, 2007.

50. Guex, A.G., Kocher, F.M., Fortunato, G., Körner, E., Hegemann, D., Carrel, T.P., Tevaearai, H.T., and Giraud, M.N., Fine-tuning of substrate architecture and surface chemistry promotes muscle tissue development. *Acta Biomater.* 8(4), 1481–1489, 2012.

51. Jin, G.Z., Kim, M., Shin, U.S., and Kim, H.W., Neurite outgrowth of dorsal root ganglia neurons is enhanced on aligned nanofibrous biopolymer scaffold with carbon nanotube coating. *Neurosci. Lett.* 501(1), 10–14, 2011.

52. Nho, Y., Kim, J.Y., Khang, D., Webster, T.J., and Lee, J.E., Adsorption of mesenchymal stem cells and cortical neural stem cells on carbon nanotube/polycarbonate urethane. *Nanomedicine (Lond)* 5(3), 409–417, 2010.

53. Silva, G.A., Czeisler, C., Niece, K.L., Beniash, E., Harrington, D.A., Kessler, J.A., and Stupp, S.I., Selective differentiation of neural progenitor cells by high-epitope density nanofibers. *Science* 303(5662), 1352–1355, 2004.

54. Mattson, M.P., Haddon, R.C., and Rao, A.M., Molecular functionalization of carbon nanotubes and use as substrates for neuronal growth. *J. Mol. Neurosci.* 14(3), 175–182, 2000.

55. Sundaramurthi, D., Vasanthan, K.S., Kuppan, P., Krishnan, U.M., and Sethuraman, S., Electrospun nanostructured chitosan-poly(vinyl alcohol) scaffolds: A biomimetic extracellular matrix as dermal substitute. *Biomed. Mater.* 7(4), 045005, 2012.

56. Meng, H., Chen, L., Ye, Z., Wang, S., and Zhao, X., The effect of a self-assembling peptide nanofiber scaffold (peptide) when used as a wound dressing for the treatment of deep second degree burns in rats. *J. Biomed. Mater. Res.* 89B(2), 379–391, 2009.

57. Brahatheeswaran, D., Mathew, A., Aswathy, R.G., Nagaoka, Y., Venugopal, K., Yoshida, Y., Maekawa, T., and Sakthikumar, D., Hybrid fluorescent curcumin loaded zein electrospun nanofibrous scaffold for biomedical applications. *Biomed. Mater.* 7(4), 045001, 2012.

58. Guo, J., Su, H., Zeng, Y., Liang, Y.X., Wong, W.M., Ellis-Behnke, R.G., So, K.F., and Wu, W., Reknitting the injured spinal cord by self-assembling peptide nanofiber scaffold. *Nanomedicine* 3(4), 311–321, 2007.

59. Harrington, D.A., Sharma, A.K., Erickson, B.A., and Cheng, E.Y., Bladder tissue engineering through nanotechnology. *World J. Urol.* 26, 315–22, 2008.

60. Ma, Z., He, W., Yong, T., and Ramakrishna, S., Grafting of gelatin on electrospun poly(caprolactone) nanofibers to improve endothelial cell spreading and proliferation and to control cell orientation. *Tissue Eng.* 11(7–8), 1149–1158, 2005.

61. Miller, D.C., Thapa, A., Haberstroh, K.M., and Webster, T.J., Enhanced functions of vascular and bladder cells on poly-lactic-co-glycolic acid polymers with nanostructured surfaces. *IEEE Trans Nanobiosci.* 1, 61–66, 2002.

62. Power, C. and Rasko, J.E., Will cell reprogramming resolve the embryonic stem cell controversy? A narrative review. *Ann. Intern. Med.* 155(2), 114–121, 2011.

63. Bongso, A., Fong, C.Y., and Gauthaman, K., Taking stem cells to the clinic: Major challenges. *J. Cell Biochem.* 105(6), 1352–1360, 2008.

64. Janowski, M., Bulte, J.W., and Walczak, P., Personalized nanomedicine advancements for stem cell tracking. *Adv. Drug Deliv. Rev.* 64(13), 1488–1507, 2012.

65. Robinton, D.A. and Daley, G.Q., The promise of induced pluripotent stem cells in research and therapy. *Nature* 481(7381), 295–305, 2012.

66. Ebben, J.D., Zorniak, M., Clark, P.A., and Kuo, J.S., Introduction to induced pluripotent stem cells: Advancing the potential for personalized medicine. *World Neurosurg.* 76(3–4), 270–275, 2011.

67. Robertson, M.J., Gip, P., and Schaffer, D.V., Neural stem cell engineering: Directed differentiation of adult and embryonic stem cells into neurons. *Front Biosci.* 13, 21–50, 2008.

68. Kaji, K., Norrby, K., Paca, A., Mileikovsky, M., Mohseni, P., and Woltjen, K., Virus-free induction of pluripotency and subsequent excision of reprogramming factors. *Nature* 458(7239), 771–775, 2000.

69. Nizzardo, M., Simone, C., Falcone, M., Riboldi, G., Comi, G.P., Bresolin, N., and Corti, S., Direct reprogramming of adult somatic cells into other lineages: Past evidence and future perspectives. *Cell Transplant.* 2012.

70. Kim, J.B., Sebastiano, V., Wum, G., Araúzo-Bravo, M.J., Sasse, P., Gentile, L., Ko, K., Ruau, D., Ehrich, M., van den Boom, D., Meyer, J., Hübner, K., Bernemann, C., Ortmeier, C., Zenke, M., Fleischmann, B.K., Zaehres, H., and Schöler, H.R., Oct4-induced pluripotency in adult neural stem cells. *Cell* 136, 411–419, 2009.

71. Kim, J.B., Greber, B., Araúzo-Bravo, M.J., Meyer, J., Park, K.I., Zaehres, H., and Schöler, H.R., Direct reprogramming of human neural stem cells by OCT4. *Nature* 461, 649–653, 2009.

72. Murtuza, B., Nichol, J.W., and Khademhosseini, A., Micro- and nanoscale control of the cardiac stem cell niche for tissue fabrication. *Tissue Eng. Part B Rev.* 15(4), 443–454, 2009.

73. Santos, T., Maia, J., Agasse, F., Xapelli, S., Ferreira, L., and Bernardino, L., Nanomedicine boosts neurogenesis: New strategies for brain repair. *Integr. Biol. (Camb).* 4(9), 973–981, 2012.

74. Bernardino, L., Eiriz, M.F., Santos, T., Xapelli, S., Grade, S., Rosa, A.I., Cortes, L., Ferreira, R., Bragança, J., Agasse, F., Ferreira, L., and Malva, J.O., Histamine stimulates neurogenesis in the rodent subventricular zone. *Stem Cells* 30(4), 773–784, 2012.

75. Cattaneo, E. and McKay, R., Proliferation and differentiation of neuronal stem cells regulated by nerve growth factor. *Nature* 347(6295), 762–765, 1990.

76. Duester, G., Retinoic acid synthesis and signaling during early organogenesis. *Cell* 134(6), 921–931, 2008.

77. Shah, D.A., Kwon, S.J., Bale, S.S., Banerjee, A., Dordick, J.S., and Kane, R.S., Regulation of stem cell signaling by nanoparticle-mediated intracellular protein delivery. *Biomaterials* 32(12), 3210–3219, 2011.

78. Mironov, V., Boland, T., Trusk, T., Forgacs, G., and Markwald, R.R., Organ printing: Computer-aided jet-based 3D tissue engineering. *Trends Biotechnol.* 21(4), 157–161, 2003.

79. Liu, J.C., A novel strategy for engineering vascularized grafts in vitro. *World J. Stem Cells* 2(4), 93–96, 2010.

80. Jakab, K., Norotte, C., Damon, B., Marga, F., Neagu, A., Besch-Williford, C.L., Kachurin, A., Church, K.H., Park, H., Mironov, V., Markwald, R., Vunjak-Novakovic, G., and Forgacs, G., Tissue engineering by self-assembly of cells printed into topologically defined structures. *Tissue Eng. Part A* 14(3), 413–421, 2008.

81. Lalan, S., Pomerantseva, I., and Vacanti, J.P., Tissue engineering and its potential impact on surgery. *World J. Surg.* 25(11), 1458–1466, 2001.

82. Puhlev, I., Guo, N., Brown, D.R., and Levine, F., Desiccation tolerance in human cells. *Cryobiology* 42(3), 207–217, 2001.

83. Nakahara, Y., Imanishi, S., Mitsumasu, K., Kanamori, Y., Iwata, K., Watanabe, M., Kikawada, T., and Okuda T., Cells from an anhydrobiotic chironomid survive almost complete desiccation. *Cryobiology* 60(2), 138–146, 2010.

84. Xu, T., Binder, K.W., Albanna, M.Z., Dice, D., Zhao, W., Yoo, J.J., and Atala, A., Hybrid printing of mechanically and biologically improved constructs for cartilage tissue engineering applications. *Biofabrication.* 5(1), 015001, 2012.

85. Xu, T., Zhao, W., Zhu, J.M., Albanna, M.Z., Yoo, J.J., and Atala, A., Complex heterogeneous tissue constructs containing multiple cell types prepared by inkjet printing technology. *Biomaterials* 34(1), 130–139, 2013.

86. Murphy, S.V. and Atala, A., Organ engineering—combining stem cells, biomaterials, and bioreactors to produce bioengineered organs for transplantation. *Bioessays* 2012.

87. Murphy, S.V., Skardal, A., and Atala, A., Evaluation of hydrogels for bio-printing applications. *J. Biomed. Mater. Res. A* 101(1), 272–284, 2013.

88. Maffulli, N., Ajis, A., Longo, U.G., and Denaro, V., Chronic rupture of tendo Achillis. *Foot Ankle Clin.* 12(4), 583–596, vi, 2007.

89. Cen, L., Liu, W., Cui, L., Zhang, W., and Cao, Y., Collagen tissue engineering: Development of novel biomaterials and applications. *Pediatr. Res.* 63(5), 492–496, 2008.

90. Lee, B.P., Messersmith, P.B., Israelachvili, J.N., and Waite, J.H., Mussel-inspired adhesives and coatings. *Ann. Rev. Mater. Res.* 41, 99–132, 2011.

91. Uysal, C.A., Tobita, M., Hyakusoku, H., and Mizuno, H., Adipose-derived stem cells enhance primary tendon repair: Biomechanical and immunohistochemical evaluation. *J. Plast. Reconstr. Aesthet. Surg.* pii: S1748–6815(12), 00338-5, 2012.

92. Buschmann, J., Calcagni, M., Bürgisser, G.M., Bonavoglia, E., Neuenschwander, P., Milleret, V., and Giovanoli, P., Synthesis, characterization and histomorphometric analysis of cellular response to a new elastic DegraPol® polymer for rabbit Achilles tendon rupture repair. *J. Tissue Eng. Regen. Med.* 2012.

93. Shah, V., Bendele, A., Dines, J.S., Kestler, H.K., Hollinger, J.O., Chahine, N.O., and Hee, C.K., Dose-response effect of an intra-tendon application of recombinant human platelet-derived growth factor-BB (rhPDGF-BB) in a rat Achilles tendinopathy model. *J. Orthop. Res.* 2012.

94. Strausberg, R.L., Anderson, D.M., Filpula, D., Finkelman, M., Link, R., McCandliss, R., Steve, R., Orndorff, A., Strausberg, S.L., and Wei, T., *Development of a Microbial System for Production of Mussel Adhesive Protein.* ACS Symposium Series., Vol. 385, Ch. 32, 1989, pp. 453–464.

95. Freitas, R.A. Jr., Nanodentistry. *J. Am. Dent. Assoc.* 131(11), 1559–1565, 2000.

96. Lodish, H., Berk, A., Zipursky, S.L., Matsudaira, P., Baltimore, D., and Darnell, J., *Molecular Cell Biology.* 4th edn. W.H. Freeman, New York, 2000.

97. Graham, J.S., Vomund, A.N., Phillips, C.L., and Grandbois, M., Structural changes in human type I collagen fibrils investigated by force spectroscopy. *Exp. Cell Res.* 299(2), 335–342, 2004.

98. Hwang, D.S., Zeng, H., Lu, Q., Israelachvili, J., and Waite, J.H., Adhesion mechanism in a DOPA-deficient foot protein from green mussels. *Soft Matter* 8(20), 5640–5648, 2012.

99. Kadler, K.E., Holmes, D.F., Graham, H., and Starborg, T., Tip-mediated fusion involving unipolar collagen fibrils accounts for rapid fibril elongation, the occurrence of fibrillar branched networks in skin and the paucity of collagen fibril ends in vertebrates. *Matrix Biol.* 19(4), 359–365, 2000.

100. Lauto, A., Mawad, D., Barton, M., Gupta, A., Piller, S.C., and Hook, J., Photochemical tissue bonding with chitosan adhesive films. *Biomed. Eng. Online.* 9, 47, 2010.

101. Brown, R.A., Karamichos, D., Mudera, V., Nazhat, S.N., Cheema, U., and Foroughi, F., Fabricating collagen tissues: Farming versus biomimetic engineering strategies. *Proc. Tissue Eng. Regen. Med. Int. Soc.* 45–45, 2006.

102. Skvorak, K., Gramignoli, R., Hansel, M., Uraz, S., Tahan, V., Dorko, K., Marongiu, F., and Strom S.C., Cell transplantation: A possible alternative to orthotopic liver transplant (OLT). In *Liver Transplantation—Technical Issues and Complications*, Prof. Hesham Abdeldayem (ed.), ISBN: 978-953-51-0015-7, InTech. 2012. http://cdn.intechopen.com/pdfs/28284/InTech-Cell_transplantation_a_possible_alternative_to_orthotopic_liver_transplant_olt_.pdf (accessed July 14, 2013).

103. Kmieć, Z., Cooperation of liver cells in health and disease. *Adv. Anat Embryol. Cell Biol.* 161(III–XIII), 1–151, 2001.

104. de Paepe, B., Mitochondrial markers for cancer: Relevance to diagnosis, therapy, and prognosis and general understanding of malignant disease mechanisms. *Int. Scholar. Res. Network ISRN Pathol.* 2012 (217162), 1–15, 2012.

105. Junqueira, L.C., Carneiro, J., and Robert, O.K., *Basic Histology*. 9th edn. McGraw-Hill, New York, NY, 1998.

106. Kenmochi, N., Kawaguchi, T., Rozen, S., Davis, E., Goodman, N., Hudson, T.J., Tanaka, T., and Page, D.C., A map of 75 human ribosomal protein genes. *Genome Res.* 8(5), 509–523, 1998.

107. Resnik, D.B. and Tinkle, S.S., Ethics in nanomedicine. *Nanomedicine (Lond)* 2(3), 345–350, 2007.

108. Resnik, D.B., Developing drugs for the developing world: An economic, legal, moral, and political dilemma. *Dev. World Bioeth.* 1(1), 11–32, 2001.

109. World Cloning Policies, http://cnx.org/content/m14836/latest/ (accessed December 01, 2012)

110. Rothman, S. and Rothman, D., *The Pursuit of Perfection*. Pantheon Books, New York, 2003.

111. Metcalfe, S.M. and Fahmy, T.M., Targeted nanotherapy for induction of therapeutic immune responses. *Trends Mol. Med.* 18(2), 72–80, 2012.

112. Park, J., Gao, W., Whiston, R., Strom, T.B., Metcalfe, S., and Fahmy, T.M., Modulation of CD4+ T lymphocyte lineage outcomes with targeted, nanoparticle-mediated cytokine delivery. *Mol. Pharm.* 8(1), 143–152, 2011.

113. Demento, S.L., Siefert, A.L., Bandyopadhyay, A., Sharp, F.A., and Fahmy, T.M., Pathogen-associated molecular patterns on biomaterials: A paradigm for engineering new vaccines. *Trends Biotechnol.* 29(6), 294–306, 2011.

114. Perche, F., Benvegnu, T., Berchel, M., Lebegue, L., Pichon, C., Jaffrès, P.A., and Midoux, P., Enhancement of dendritic cells transfection in vivo and of vaccination against B16F10 melanoma with mannosylated histidylated lipopolyplexes loaded with tumor antigen messenger RNA. *Nanomedicine* 7(4), 445–453, 2011.

115. Broos, S., Sandin, L.C., Apel, J., Tötterman, T.H., Akagi, T., Akashi, M., Borrebaeck, C.A., Ellmark, P., and Lindstedt, M., Synergistic augmentation of CD40-mediated activation of antigen-presenting cells by amphiphilic poly(γ-glutamic acid) nanoparticles. *Biomaterials* 33(26), 6230–6239, 2012.

116. Hecht, D. and Fogel, G.B., Modeling the evolution of drug resistance in malaria. *J. Comput. Aided Mol. Des.* 2012.

117. Jordan, M.R., Bennett, D.E., Wainberg, M.A., Havlir, D., Hammer, S., Yang, C., Morris, L., Peeters, M., Wensing, A.M., Parkin, N., Nachega, J.B., Phillips, A., De Luca, A., Geng, E., Calmy, A., Raizes, E., Sandstrom, P., Archibald, C.P., Perriëns, J., McClure, C.M., Hong, S.Y., McMahon, J.H., Dedes, N., Sutherland, D., and Bertagnolio, S., Update on World Health Organization HIV drug resistance prevention and assessment strategy: 2004–2011. *Clin. Infect. Dis.* 54(Suppl 4), S245–S249, 2012.

118. Vergara-Jaque, A., Poblete, H., Lee, E.H., Schulten, K., González-Nilo, F., and Chipot, C., Molecular basis of drug resistance in A/H1N1 virus. *J. Chem. Inf. Model.* 52(10), 2650–2656, 2012.

119. Hao, H., Dai, M., Wang, Y., Huang, L., and Yuan, Z., Key genetic elements and regulation systems in methicillin-resistant Staphylococcus aureus. *Future Microbiol.* 7(11), 1315–1329, 2012.

120. Sandberg, A. and Bostrom, N., The wisdom of nature: An evolutionary heuristic for human enhancement. In *Enhancement of Human Beings*, Bostrom, N., Savulescu, J. (eds.), Oxford University Press, Oxford, U.K., 2007.

121. Bruce, D., White paper: Ethical issues in nano-medicine and enhancement: An overview society, religion and technology project, Church of Scotland. http://www.edinethics.co.uk/nano/nanoeth9a-med.doc (accessed December 04, 2012).

122. Eliasmith, C. and Anderson, C. H., *Neural Engineering: Computation, Representation and Dynamics in Neurobiological Systems.* MIT Press, Cambridge, MA, 2003.

123. Froestl, W., Muhs, A., and Pfeifer, A., Cognitive enhancers (Nootropics). Part 1: Drugs interacting with receptors. Part 2: Drugs interacting with enzymes. Part 3: Drugs interacting with targets other than receptors or enzymes. Disease-modifying drugs. *J. Alzheimers Dis.* 32(4), 793–887, 2012.

124. Farah, M.J., Illes, J., Cook-Deegan, R., Gardner, H., Kandel, E., King, P., Parens, E., Sahakian, B., and Wolpe, P.R., Neurocognitive enhancement: What can we do and what should we do? *Nat. Rev. Neurosci.* 5(5), 421–425, 2004.

125. Yesavage, J.A., Mumenthaler, M.S., Taylor, J.L., Friedman, L., O'Hara, R., Sheikh, J., Tinklenberg, J., and Whitehouse, P.J., Donepezil and flight simulator performance: Effects on retention of complex skills. *Neurology* 59(1), 123–125, 2002.

126. Chang, P.K., Verbich, D., and McKinney, R.A., AMPA receptors as drug targets in neurological disease—Advantages, caveats, and future outlook. *Eur. J. Neurosci.* 35(12), 1908–1916, 2012.

127. Arai, A.C. and Kessler, M., Pharmacology of ampakine modulators: From AMPA receptors to synapses and behavior. *Curr. Drug Targets* 8(5), 583–602, 2007.

128. Solomon, L.D., *The Quest for Human Longevity: Science, Business, and Public Policy.* Transaction Publishers, New Brunswick, NJ, 2006, 197pp.

129. Weyandt, L.L., Janusis, G., Wilson, K.G., Verdi, G., Paquin, G., Lopes, J., Varejao, M., and Dussault, C., Nonmedical prescription stimulant use among a sample of college students: Relationship with psychological variables. *J. Atten. Disord.* 13(3), 284–296, 2009.

130. Varga, M.D., Adderall abuse on college campuses: A comprehensive literature review. *J. Evid. Based Soc. Work* 9(3), 293–313, 2012.

131. Teter, C.J., McCabe, S.E., LaGrange, K., Cranford, J.A., and Boyd, C.J., Illicit use of specific prescription stimulants among college students: Prevalence, motives, and routes of administration. *Pharmacotherapy* 26(10), 1501–1510, 2006.

132. Beddington, J., Cooper, C.L., Field, J., Goswami, U., Huppert, F.A., Jenkins, R., Jones, H.S., Kirkwood, T.B., Sahakian, B.J., and Thomas, S.M., The mental wealth of nations. *Nature* 455(7216), 1057–1060, 2008.

133. Greely, H., Sahakian, B., Harris, J., Kessler, R.C., Gazzaniga, M., Campbell, P., and Farah, M.J., Towards responsible use of cognitive-enhancing drugs by the healthy. *Nature* 456(7223), 702–705, 2008.

134. Milton, A.L. and Everitt, B.J., The psychological and neurochemical mechanisms of drug memory reconsolidation: Implications for the treatment of addiction. *Eur. J. Neurosci.* 31(12), 2308–2319, 2010.

135. Debiec, J. and LeDoux, J.E., Disruption of reconsolidation but not consolidation of auditory fear conditioning by noradrenergic blockade in the amygdala. *Neuroscience* 129, 267–272, 2004.

136. Lee, J.L.C., Milton, A.L., and Everitt, B.J., Reconsolidation and extinction of conditioned fear: Inhibition and potentiation. *J. Neurosci.* 26, 10051–10056, 2006.

137. Ferry, B., Roozendaal, B., and McGaugh, J.L., Role of norepinephrine in mediating stress hormone regulation of long-term memory storage: A critical involvement of the amygdala. *Biol. Psychiatry* 46, 1140–1152, 1999.

138. Sara, S.J., Roullet, P., and Przybyslawski, J., Consolidation of memory for odor-reward association: á-adrenergic receptor involvement in the late phase. *Learn. Mem.* 6, 88–96, 1999.

139. Dornhege, G., Blankertz, B., Krauledat, M., Losch, F., Curio, G., and Müller, K.R., Combined optimization of spatial and temporal filters for improving brain-computer interfacing. *IEEE Trans. Biomed. Eng.* 53(11), 2274–2281, 2006.

140. Donoghue, J.P., Connecting cortex to machines: Recent advances in brain interfaces. *Nat. Neurosci.* 5 (Suppl), 1085–1088, 2002.

141. Verdoux, P., Risk mysterianism and cognitive boosters. *J. Futures Studies* 15(1), 1–20, 2010.

142. Roco, M.C. and Bainbridge, W.S., *Converging Technologies for Improving Human Performance: Nanotechnology, Biotechnology Information Technology and Cognitive Science*. Springer, New York, 2006.

143. Bainbridge, W.S. and Roco, M.C., *Managing Nano-Bio-Info-Cogno Innovations: Converging Technologies in Society*. Springer-Verlag, Inc., New York, 2005.

144. Sententia, W., Neuroethical considerations cognitive liverty and converging technologies for improving human cognition. *Ann. NY. Acd. Sci.* 1013, 221–228, 2004.

145. Clark, A., *Supersizing the Mind: Embodiment, Action, and Cognitive Extension*. Oxford University Press, New York, 2008.

146. Bostrom, N. and Sandberg, A., Cognitive enhancement: Methods, ethics, regulatory challenges. *Sci. Eng. Ethics* 15(3), 311–341, 2009.

147. Hart, J. Jr., Crone, N.E., Lesser, R.P., Sieracki, J., Miglioretti, D.L., Hall, C., Sherman, D., and Gordon, B., Temporal dynamics of verbal object comprehension. *Proc. Natl Acad. Sci. USA* 95(11), 6498–6503, 1998.

148. Sandberg, A. and Bostrom, N., Converging cognitive enhancements. *Ann. N Y. Acad. Sci.* 1093, 201–227, 2006.

149. Gold, P.E., Role of glucose in regulating the brain and cognition. *Am. J. Clin. Nutr.* 61(4 Suppl), 987S–995S, 1995.

150. Mizumori, S.J., Perez, G.M., Alvarado, M.C., Barnes, C.A., and McNaughton, B.L., Reversible inactivation of the medial septum differentially affects two forms of learning in rats. *Brain Res.* 528(1), 12–20, 1990.

151. Breitenstein, C., Wailke, S., Bushuven, S., Kamping, S., Zwitserlood, P., Ringelstein, E.B., and Knecht, S., D-amphetamine boosts language learning independent of its cardiovascular and motor arousing effects. *Neuropsychopharmacology* 29(9), 1704–1714, 2004.

152. Stroemer, R.P., Kent, T.A., and Hulsebosch, C.E., Enhanced neocortical neural sprouting, synaptogenesis, and behavioral recovery with D-amphetamine therapy after neocortical infarction in rats. *Stroke* 29(11), 2381–2393, 1998.

153. Sabri, F., Cole, J.A., Scarbrough, M.C., and Leventis, N., Investigation of polyurea-crosslinked silica aerogels as a neuronal scaffold: A pilot study. *PLoS One* 7(3), e33242, 2012.

154. Mikos, A.G. and Temenoff, J.S., Formation of highly porous biodegradable scaffolds for tissue engineering. *Electron. J. Biotechnol.* 3(2), 1–6, 2000.

155. Christenson, E.M., Soofi, W., Holm, J.L., Cameron, N.R., and Mikos, A.G., Biodegradable fumarate-based polyHIPEs as tissue engineering scaffolds. *Biomacromolecules* 8(12), 3806–3814, 2007.

156. Yoon, J.J., Song, S.H., Lee, D.S., and Park, T.G., Immobilization of cell adhesive RGD peptide onto the surface of highly porous biodegradable polymer scaffolds fabricated by a gas foaming/salt leaching method. *Biomaterials* 25(25), 5613–5620, 2004.

157. Lein, P.J. and Higgins, D., Laminin and a basement membrane extract have different effects on axonal and dendritic outgrowth from embryonic rat sympathetic neurons in vitro. *Dev. Biol.* 136(2), 330–345, 1989.

158. Kim, D.H., Viventi, J., Amsden, J.J., Xiao, J., Vigeland, L., Kim, Y.S., Blanco, J.A., Panilaitis, B., Frechette, E.S., Contreras, D., Kaplan, D.L., Omenetto, F.G., Huang, Y., Hwang, K.C., Zakin, M.R., Litt, B., and Rogers, J.A., Dissolvable films of silk fibroin for ultrathin conformal bio-integrated electronics. *Nat. Mater.* 9(6), 511–517, 2010.

159. Bink, H., Lai, Y., Saudari, S.R., Helfer, B., Viventi, J., Van der Spiegel, J., Litt, B., and Kagan, C., Flexible organic electronics for use in neural sensing. *Conf. Proc. IEEE Eng. Med. Biol. Soc.* 2011, 5400–5403, 2011.

160. Keefer, E.W., Botterman, B.R., Romero, M.I., Rossi, A.F., and Gross, G.W., Carbon nanotube coating improves neuronal recordings. *Nat. Nanotechnol.* 3(7), 434–439, 2008.

161. Eleni, V., Antoniadou, E.V., Ahmad, R.K., Jackman, R.B., and Seifalian, A.M., Next generation brain implant coatings and nerve regeneration via novel conductive nanocomposite development. *Conf. Proc. IEEE Eng. Med. Biol. Soc.* 2011, 3253–3257, 2011.

162. Ben-Jacob, E. and Hanein, Y., Carbon nanotube micro-electrodes for neuronal interfacing. *J. Mater. Chem.* 18, 5181–5186, 2008.

163. Mercanzini, A., Reddy, S.T., Velluto, D., Colin, P., Maillard, A., Bensadoun, J.C., Hubbell, J.A., and Renaud, P., Controlled release nanoparticle-embedded coatings reduce the tissue reaction to neuroprostheses. *J. Control Release* 145(3), 196–202, 2010.

164. Gulati, K., Aw, M.S., and Losic, D., Nanoengineered drug-releasing Ti wires as an alternative for local delivery of chemotherapeutics in the brain. *Int. J. Nanomed.* 7, 2069–2076, 2012.

165. Moxon, K.A., Kalkhoran, N.M., Markert, M., Sambito, M.A., McKenzie, J.L., and Webster, J.T., Nanostructured surface modification of ceramic-based microelectrodes to enhance biocompatibility for a direct brain-machine interface. *IEEE Trans. Biomed. Eng.* 51(6), 881–889, 2004.

166. Daniel, R., Two high-tech approaches to restoring sight. MarketWatch, *The Wall Street Journal*. March 12, 2010. http://www.marketwatch.com/story/two-innovative-views-on-restoring-sight-2010-03-12?pagenumber=1 (accessed December 16, 2012).

167. Staples, M., Daniel, K., Cima, M.J., and Langer, R., Application of micro- and nano-electromechanical devices to drug delivery. *Pharm. Res.* 23(5), 847–863, 2006.

168. Meng, E. and Hoang, T., MEMS-enabled implantable drug infusion pumps for laboratory animal research, preclinical, and clinical applications. *Adv. Drug Deliv. Rev.* 64(14), 1628–1638, 2012.

169. Barar, J., Javadzadeh, A.R., and Omidi, Y., Ocular novel drug delivery: Impacts of membranes and barriers. *Expert Opin. Drug Deliv.* 5(5), 67–81, 2008.

170. Sultana, Y., Maurya, D.P., Iqbal, Z., and Aqil, M., Nanotechnology in ocular delivery: Current and future directions. *Drugs Today (Barc)* 47(6), 441–455, 2011.

171. Bucolo, C., Drago, F., and Salomone, S., Ocular drug delivery: A clue from nanotechnology. *Front Pharmacol.* 3, 188, 2012.

172. du Toit, L.C., Pillay, V., Choonara, Y.E., Govender, T., and Carmichael, T., Ocular drug delivery—A look towards nanobioadhesives. *Expert Opin. Drug Deliv.* 8(1), 71–94, 2011.

173. Nielsen, L.S., Schubert, L., and Hansen, J., Bioadhesive drug delivery systems. I. Characterisation of mucoadhesive properties of systems based on glyceryl mono-oleate and glyceryl monolinoleate. *Eur. J. Pharm. Sci.* 6(3), 231–239, 1998.

174. Atchison, D.A. and Charman, W.N., Thomas Young's contribution to visual optics: The Bakerian lecture "on the mechanism of the eye". *J. Vis.* 10(12), 16, 2010.

175. Greenwood, V., The humans with super human vision, *Discover Mag.* July–August, 2012. http://discovermagazine.com/2012/jul-aug/06-humans-with-super-human-vision (accessed December 16, 2012).

176. de Vries, H., The fundamental response curves of normal and abnormal dichromatic and trichromatic eyes. *Physica* 14(6), 367–380, 1948.

177. Jordan, G., Deebm S.S., Bosten, J.M., and Mollon, J.D., The dimensionality of color vision in carriers of anomalous trichromacy. *J. Vis.* 10(8), 12, 2010.

178. Gray, H., *Anatomy of the Human Body*. Lea & Febiger, Philadelphia, PA, 1918, Bartleby.com, 2000. www.bartleby.com/107/ (accessed December 17, 2012).

179. Polosukhina, A., Litt, J., Tochitsky, I., Nemargut, J., Sychev, Y., De Kouchkovsky, I., Huang, T., Borges, K., Trauner, D., Van Gelder, R.N., and Kramer, R.H., Photochemical restoration of visual responses in blind mice. *Neuron* 75(2), 271–282, 2012.

180. Bloemendal, H., de Jong, W., Jaenicke, R., Lubsen, N.H., Slingsby, C., and Tardieu, A., Ageing and vision: Structure, stability and function of lens crystallins. *Prog. Biophys. Mol. Biol.* 86(3), 407–485, 2004.

181. Aliev, A.E., Oh, J., Kozlov, M.E., Kuznetsov, A.A., Fang, S., Fonseca, A.F., Ovalle, R., Lima, M.D., Haque, M.H., Gartstein, Y.N., Zhang, M., Zakhidov, A.A., and Baughman, R.H., Giant-stroke, superelastic carbon nanotube aerogel muscles. *Science* 323(5921), 1575–1578, 2009.

182. Jeong, K.H., Kim, J., and Lee, L.P., Biologically inspired artificial compound eyes. *Science* 312(5773), 557–561, 2006.

183. Pericet-Camara, R., Dobrzynski, M., L'Eplattenier, G., Zufferey, J.C., Expert, F., Juston, R., Ruffier, F., Franceschini, N., Viollet, S., Menouni, M., Godiot, S., Brückner, A., Buss, W., Leitel, R., Recktenwald, F., Yuan, C., Mallot, H., and Floreano, D., CURVACE—CURVed artificial compound eyes. *Procedia Comp. Sci.* 7, 308–309, 2011.

184. Li, L. and Yi, A.Y., Development of a 3D artificial compound eye. *Opt. Express.* 18(17), 18125–18137, 2010.

185. Duparré, J.W. and Wippermann, F.C., Micro-optical artificial compound eyes. *Bioinspir. Biomim.* 1(1), R1–16, 2006.
186. Huang, J., Wang, X., and Wang, Z.L., Bio-inspired fabrication of antireflection nanostructures by replicating fly eyes. *Nanotechnology* 19(2), 025602, 2008.
187. Carvalho, L.S., Knott, B., Berg, M.L., Bennett, A.T., and Hunt, D.M., Ultraviolet-sensitive vision in long-lived birds. *Proc. Biol. Sci.* 278(1702), 107–114, 2011.
188. Mazza, C.A., Izaguirre, M.M., Curiale, J., and Ballaré, C.L., A look into the invisible: Ultraviolet-B sensitivity in an insect (*Caliothrips phaseoli*) revealed through a behavioural action spectrum. *Proc. Biol. Sci.* 277(1680), 367–373, 2010.
189. Hogg, C., Neveu, M., Stokkan, K.A., Folkow, L., Cottrill, P., Douglas, R., Hunt, D.M., and Jeffery, G., Arctic reindeer extend their visual range into the ultraviolet. *J. Exp. Biol.* 214(Pt 12), 2014–2019, 2011.
190. Shi, Y. and Yokoyama, S., Molecular analysis of the evolutionary significance of ultraviolet vision in vertebrates. *Proc. Natl. Acad. Sci. USA* 100(14), 8308–8313, 2003.
191. Frank, T.M., Johnsen, S., and Cronin, T.W., Light and vision in the deep-sea benthos: II. Vision in deep-sea crustaceans. *J. Exp. Biol.* 215(Pt 19), 3344–3353, 2012.
192. Chen, Y., Thompson, D.C., Koppaka, V., Jester, J.V., and Vasiliou, V., Ocular aldehyde dehydrogenases: Protection against ultraviolet damage and maintenance of transparency for vision. *Prog. Retin. Eye Res.* pii: S1350–9462(12), 00071–00077, 2012.
193. Ringvold, A., Cornea and ultraviolet radiation. *Acta Ophthalmol. (Copenh)*. 58(1), 63–68, 1980.
194. Ollivier, F.J., Samuelson, D.A., Brooks, D.E., Lewis, P.A., Kallberg, M.E., and Komáromy, A.M., Comparative morphology of the tapetum lucidum (among selected species). *Vet. Ophthalmol.* 7(1), 11–22, 2004.
195. Bergmanson, J.P. and Townsend, W.D., The morphology of the cat tapetum lucidum. *Am. J. Optom. Physiol. Opt.* 57(3), 138–144, 1980.
196. Kolesnikov, A.V., Rikimaru, L., Hennig, A.K., Lukasiewicz, P.D., Fliesler, S.J., Govardovskii, V.I., Kefalov, V.J., and Kisselev, O.G., G-protein betagamma-complex is crucial for efficient signal amplification in vision. *J. Neurosci.* 31(22), 8067–8077, 2011.
197. Warrant, E. and Nilsson, D.E., *Invertebrate Vision*. Cambridge University Press, Cambridge, 2006.
198. Dunkelberger, A.D., Kieda, R.D., Shin, J.Y., Rossi Paccani, R., Fusi, S., Olivucci, M., and Crim, F.F., Photoisomerization and relaxation dynamics of a structurally modified biomimetic photoswitch. *J. Phys. Chem. A* 116(14), 3527–3533, 2012.
199. Sutherland, R., Aliens among us: Preliminary evidence of superhuman tetrachromats. April 2001. http://clouds.eos.ubc.ca/~phil/courses/geog373/figures/tetrachromats.pdf (accessed December 18, 2012).
200. Campbell, A.L., Naik, R.R., Sowards, L., and Stone, M.O., Biological infrared imaging and sensing. *Micron* 33(2), 211–225, 2002.
201. Newman, E.A. and Hartline, P.H., The infrared "vision" of snakes. *Sci. Am.* 20, 116–127, 1982.
202. Yokoyama, S., Altun, A., and DeNardo, D.F., Molecular convergence of infrared vision in snakes. *Mol. Biol. Evol.* 28(1), 45–48, 2011.
203. Gonn, A., Nano night vision, *The Jerusalem Post*, December 11, 2012 http://mobiletest.jpost.com/Headlines/Article.aspx?id=98295489&cat=2 (accessed December 27, 2012).
204. Wong, G.K., Kang, M.S., Lee, H.W., Biancalana, F., Conti, C., Weiss, T., and Russell, P.S., Excitation of orbital angular momentum resonances in helically twisted photonic crystal fiber. *Science* 337(6093), 446–449, 2012.
205. Garstang, M., Long-distance, low-frequency elephant communication. *J. Comp. Physiol. A Neuroethol. Sens. Neural Behav. Physiol.* 190(10), 791–805, 2004.
206. Møller, H. and Pedersen, C.S., Hearing at low and infrasonic frequencies. *Noise Health* 6(23), 37–57, 2004.
207. He, X.Q., Kitipornchai, S., and Liew, K.M., Resonance analysis of multi-layered graphene sheets used as nanoscale resonators. *Nanotechnoogy* 16(10), 2086–2091, 2005.
208. Dai, M.D., Kim, C.W., and Eom, K., Nonlinear vibration behavior of graphene resonators and their applications in sensitive mass detection. *Nanoscale Res. Lett.* 7(1), 499, 2012.

209. Fan, Z. and Lu, J.G., Zinc oxide nanostructures: Synthesis and properties. *Nanosci. Nanotechnol.* 5(10), 1561–1573, 2005.

210. Park, K.K. and Khuri-Yakub, B.T., Dynamic response of an array of flexural plates in acoustic medium. *J. Acoust. Soc. Am.* 132(4), 2292–2303, 2012.

211. Nishimura, T., Okayasu, T., Uratani, Y., Fukuda, F., Saito, O., and Hosoi, H., Peripheral perception mechanism of ultrasonic hearing. *Hear. Res.* 277(1–2), 176–183, 2011.

212. Corso, J.F., Bone-conduction thresholds for sonic and ultrasonic frequencies. *J. Acoust. Soc. Am.* 35(11), 1738–1743, 1963.

213. Fujimoto, K., Nakagawa, S., and Tonoike, M., Nonlinear explanation for bone conducted ultrasonic hearing. *Hear. Res.* 204(1–2), 210–215, 2005.

214. Lim, Y.S., Park, S.I., Kim, Y.H., Oh, S.H., and Kim, S.J., Three-dimensional analysis of electrode behavior in a human cochlear model. *Med. Eng. Phys.* 27(8), 695–703, 2005.

215. Versteegh, C.P. and van der Heijden, M., Basilar membrane responses to tones and tone complexes: Nonlinear effects of stimulus intensity. *J. Assoc. Res. Otolaryngol.* 13(6), 785–798, 2012.

216. Hansen, S., Mlynski, R., Volkenstein, S., Stark, T., Schwaab, M., Dazert, S., and Brors, D., Growth behavior of spiral ganglion explants on cochlear implant electrodes and their materials.. Article in German. *HNO* 57(4), 358–363, 2009.

217. Wang, X., Gu, X., Yuan, C., Chen, S., Zhang, P., Zhang, T., Yao, J., Chen, F., and Chen, G., Evaluation of biocompatibility of polypyrrole in vitro and in vivo. *J. Biomed. Mater. Res. A* 68(3), 411–422, 2004.

218. Ateh, D.D., Navsaria, H.A., and Vadgama, P., Polypyrrole-based conducting polymers and interactions with biological tissues. *J. R. Soc. Interf.* 3(11), 741–752, 2006.

219. Widge, A.S., Jeffries-El, M., Cui, X., Lagenaur, C.F., and Matsuoka, Y., Self-assembled monolayers of polythiophene conductive polymers improve biocompatibility and electrical impedance of neural electrodes. *Biosens. Bioelectron.* 22(8), 1723–1732, 2007.

220. Hendricks, J.L., Chikar, J.A., Crumling, M.A., Raphael, Y., and Martin, D.C., Localized cell and drug delivery for auditory prostheses. *Hear. Res.* 242(1–2), 117–131, 2008.

221. Harris, A.R., Morgan, S.J., Chen, J., Kapsa, R.M., Wallace, G.G., and Paolini, A.G., Conducting polymer coated neural recording electrodes. *J. Neural Eng.* 10(1), 016004, 2012.

222. Wallace, G.G., Moulton, S.E., and Clark, G.M., Electrode-cellular interface. *Science* 324(5924), 185–186, 2009.

223. Ni, D., Shepherd, R.K., Seldon, H.L., Xu. S.A., Clark, G.M., and Millard, R.E., Cochlear pathology following chronic electrical stimulation of the auditory nerve: I. Normal hearing kittens. *Hear. Res.* 62 63–81, 1992.

224. Newbold, C., Richardson, R., Huang, C.Q., Milojevic, D., Cowan, R., and Shepherd, R., An in vitro model for investigating impedance changes with cell growth and electrical stimulation: Implications for cochlear implants. *J. Neural Eng.* 1(4), 218–227, 2004.

225. Jan, E., Hendricks, J.L., Husaini, V., Richardson-Burns, S.M., Sereno, A., Martin, D.C., and Kotov, N.A., Layered carbon nanotube-polyelectrolyte electrodes outperform traditional neural interface materials. *Nano Lett.* 9(12), 4012–4018, 2009.

226. Vincent, C., Auditory brainstem implants: How do they work? *Anat. Rec. (Hoboken)* 295(11), 1981–1986, 2012.

227. Otto, S.R., Shannon, R.V., Wilkinson, E.P., Hitselberger, W.E., McCreery, D.B., Moore, J.K., and Brackmann, D.E., Audiologic outcomes with the penetrating electrode auditory brainstem implant. *Otol. Neurotol.* 29(8), 1147–1154, 2008.

228. Lim, H.H., Lenarz, M., and Lenarz, T., Auditory midbrain implant: A review. *Trends Amplif.* 13(3), 149–180, 2009.

229. Lee, J.B., Peng, S., Yang, D., Roh, Y.H., Funabashi, H., Park, N., Rice, E.J., Chen, L., Long, R., Wu, M., and Luo, D., A mechanical metamaterial made from a DNA hydrogel. *Nat. Nanotechnol.* 7(12), 816–820, 2012.

230. Sueur, J., Windmill, J.F., and Robert, D., Tuning the drum: The mechanical basis for frequency discrimination in a Mediterranean cicada. *J. Exp. Biol.* 209(Pt 20), 4115–4128, 2006.

231. Windmill, J.F., Sueur, J., and Robert, D., The next step in cicada audition: Measuring pico-mechanics in the cicada's ear. *J. Exp. Biol.* 212(Pt 24), 4079–4083, 2009.
232. Sela, L. and Sobel, N., Human olfaction: A constant state of change-blindness. *Exp. Brain Res.* 205(1), 13–29, 2010.
233. Nagata, Y., Measurement of odor threshold by triangle odor bag method. *Odor Meas. Rev., Jpn. Minis. Environ.* 118–127, 2003.
234. Whisman, M., Goetzinger, J., Cotton, F., and Brinkman, D., Odorant evaluation: A study of ethanethiol and tetrahdrothiophene as warning agents in propane. *Environ. Sci. Technol.* 12(12), 1285–1288, 1978.
235. Nagata, Y. and Takeuchi, N., Measurement of odor threshold by triangle odor bag method. *Bull. Jpn. Environ. Sanit. Center* 17, 77–89, 1990.
236. Philpott, C.M., Goonetilleke, P., Goodenough, P.C., Clark, A., and Murty, G.E., The superosmic phenomenon. *J. Laryngol. Otol.* 122(8), 805–809, 2008.
237. Keller, A. and Vosshall, L.B., Human olfactory psychophysics. *Curr. Biol.* 14(20), R875–R878, 2004.
238. Lee, S.H., Kwon, O.S., Song, H.S., Park, S.J., Sung, J.H., Jang, J., and Park, T.H., Mimicking the human smell sensing mechanism with an artificial nose platform. *Biomaterials* 33(6), 722–729, 2012.
239. Buck, L.B., Olfactory receptors and odor coding in mammals. *Nutr. Rev.* 62(11 Pt 2), S184–S188, discussion S224–41.
240. Bittner, E.R., Madalan, A., Czader, A., and Roman, G., Quantum origins of molecular recognition and olfaction in drosophila. *J. Chem. Phys.* 137(22), 22A551, 2012.
241. Brookes, J.C., Hartoutsiou, F., Horsfield, A.P., and Stoneham, A.M., Could humans recognize odor by phonon assisted tunneling? *Phys. Rev. Lett.* 98(3), 038101, 2007.
242. Takeuchi, H., Ishida, H., Hikichi, S., and Kurahashi, T., Mechanism of olfactory masking in the sensory cilia. *J. Gen. Physiol.* 133(6), 583–601, 2009.
243. Trivedi, B.P., Gustatory system: The finer points of taste. *Nature* 486(7403), S2–S3, 2012.
244. Fark, T., Hummel, C., Hähner, A., Nin, T., and Hummel, T., Characteristics of taste disorders. *Eur. Arch. Otorhinolaryngol.* 2012.
245. Nanofood 2040- Nanotechnology in Food, Food Processing, Agriculture, Packaging and Consumption State of Science, Technologies, Markets, Applications and Developments to 2015 and 2040 Helmut Kaiser Consultancy http://www.hkc22.com/nanofood2040.html (accessed January 03, 2013).
246. Song, H.S., Kwon, O.S., Lee, S.H., Park, S.J., Kim, U.K., Jang, J., and Park, T.H., Human taste receptor-functionalized field effect transistor as a human-like nanobioelectronic tongue. *Nano Lett.* 2012.
247. Kim, T.H., Song, H.S., Jin, H.J., Lee, S.H., Namgung, S., Kim, U.K., Park, T.H., and Hong, S., "Bioelectronic super-taster" device based on taste receptor-carbon nanotube hybrid structures. *Lab Chip.* 11(13), 2262–2267, 2011.
248. Chen, Z.X., Guo, G.M., and Deng, S.P., Isothermal titration calorimetry study of the interaction of sweeteners with fullerenols as an artificial sweet taste receptor model. *J. Agric. Food Chem.* 57(7), 2945–2954, 2009.
249. Simner, J., Mulvenna, C., Sagiv, N., Tsakanikos, E., Witherby, S.A., Fraser, C., Scott, K., and Ward, J., Synaesthesia: The prevalence of atypical cross-modal experiences. *Perception* 35(8), 1024–1033, 2006.
250. Suslick, K.S., Synesthesia in science and technology: More than making the unseen visible. *Curr. Opin. Chem. Biol.* 16(5–6), 557–563, 2012.
251. Fouad, H. and Elleithy, R., High density polyethylene/graphite nano-composites for total hip joint replacements: Processing and in vitro characterization. *J. Mech. Behav. Biomed. Mater.* 4(7), 1376–1383, 2011.
252. Tsaousi, A., Jones, E., and Case, C.P., The in vitro genotoxicity of orthopaedic ceramic (Al_2O_3) and metal (CoCr alloy) particles. *Mutat. Res.* 697(1–2), 1–9, 2010.
253. Minagar, S., Berndt, C.C., Wang, J., Ivanova, E., and Wen, C., A review of the application of anodization for the fabrication of nanotubes on metal implant surfaces. *Acta Biomater.* 8(8), 2875–2888, 2012.

254. Pal, N., Quah, B., Smith, P.N., Gladkis, L.L., Timmers, H., and Li, R.W., Nano-osteoimmunology as an important consideration in the design of future implants. *Acta Biomater.* 7(7), 2926–2934, 2011.

255. Song, W., Markel, D.C., Wang, S., Shi, T., Mao, G., and Ren, W., Electrospun polyvinyl alcohol-collagen-hydroxyapatite nanofibers: A biomimetic extracellular matrix for osteoblastic cells. *Nanotechnology* 23(11), 115101, 2012.

256. Catledge, S.A., Fries, M.D., Vohra, Y.K., Lacefield, W.R., Lemons, J.E., Woodard, S., and Venugopalan, R., Nanostructured ceramics for biomedical implants. *J. Nanosci. Nanotechnol.* 2(3–4), 293–312, 2002.

257. Catledge, S.A., Borham, J., Vohra, Y.K., Lacefield, W.R., and Lemons, J.E., Nanoindentation hardness, and adhesion investigations of vapor deposited nanostructured diamond films. *J. Appl. Phys.* 91, 5347, 2002.

258. Maina, A.M. and Kraus, H., Successful treatment of osteitis fibrosa cystica from primary hyperparathyroidism. *Case Rep. Orthop.* 2012, 145760, 2012.

259. Li, L., Guan, Y., Liu, H., Hao, N., Liu, T., Meng, X., Fu, C., Li, Y., Qu, Q., Zhang, Y., Ji, S., Chen, L., Chen, D., and Tang, F., Silica nanorattle-doxorubicin-anchored mesenchymal stem cells for tumor-tropic therapy. *ACS Nano* 5(9), 7462–7470, 2011.

260. Deshpande, S.S., Gallagher, K.K., Donneys, A., Tchanque-Fossuo, C.N., Sarhaddi, D., Sun, H., Krebsbach, P.H., and Buchman, S.R., Stem cell therapy remediates reconstruction of the craniofacial skeleton after radiation therapy. *Stem Cells Dev.* 22(11), 1625–32, 2013.

261. Kim, S.E., Yun, Y.P., Lee, J.Y., Shim, J.S., Park, K., and Huh, J.B., Co-delivery of platelet-derived growth factor (PDGF-BB) and bone morphogenic protein (BMP-2) coated onto heparinized titanium for improving osteoblast function and osteointegration. *J. Tissue Eng. Regen. Med.* 2013.

262. Jung, M.R., Shim, I.K., Chung, H.J., Lee, H.R., Park, Y.J., Lee, M.C., Yang, Y.I., Do, S.H., and Lee, S.J., Local BMP-7 release from a PLGA scaffolding-matrix for the repair of osteochondral defects in rabbits. *J. Control Rel.* 162(3), 485–491, 2012.

263. Li, J., Hong, J., Zheng, Q., Guo, X., Lan, S., Cui, F., Pan, H., Zou, Z., and Chen, C., Repair of rat cranial bone defects with nHAC/PLLA and BMP-2-related peptide or rhBMP-2. *J. Orthop. Res.* 29(11), 1745–1752, 2011.

264. Boyd, S.K., Szabo, E., and Ammann, P., Increased bone strength is associated with improved bone microarchitecture in intact female rats treated with strontium ranelate: A finite element analysis study. *Bone* 48(5), 1109–1116, 2011.

265. Boyden, L.M., Mao, J., Belsky, J., Mitzner, L., Farhi, A., Mitnick, M.A., Wu, D., Insogna, K., and Lifton, R.P., High bone density due to a mutation in LDL-receptor-related protein 5. *N. Engl. J. Med.* 346(20), 1513–1521, 2002.

266. Hirabayashi, H. and Fujisaki, J., Bone-specific drug delivery systems: Approaches via chemical modification of bone-seeking agents. *Clin. Pharmacokinet.* 42(15), 1319–1330, 2003.

267. Zhang, L., Chen, Y., Rodriguez, J., Fenniri, H., and Webster, T.J., Biomimetic helical rosette nanotubes and nanocrystalline hydroxyapatite coatings on titanium for improving orthopedic implants. *Int. J. Nanomed.* 3(3), 323–333, 2008.

268. Gopi, D., Nithiya, S., Shinyjoy, E., and Kavitha, L., Spectroscopic investigation on formation and growth of mineralized nanohydroxyapatite for bone tissue engineering applications. *Spectrochim. Acta A Mol. Biomol. Spectrosc.* 92, 194–200, 2012.

269. Vongvatcharanon, S. and Vongvatcharanon, U., Boonyoung, P., Immunohistochemical localization of parvalbumin calcium-binding protein in the heart tissues of various species. *Acta Histochem.* 110(1), 26–33, 2008.

270. Parkash, J., Chaudhry, M.A., and Rhoten, W.B., Calbindin-D28k and calcium sensing receptor cooperate in MCF-7 human breast cancer cells. *Int. J. Oncol.* 24(5), 1111–1119, 2004.

271. Choi, Y., Cho, S.Y., Park, D.J., Park, H.H., Heo, S., and Jin, H.J., Silk fibroin particles as templates for mineralization of calcium-deficient hydroxyapatite. *J. Biomed. Mater. Res. B Appl. Biomater.* 100(8), 2029–2034, 2012.

272. Wang, X., Wang, Y., Miao, M., Zhong, X., Lv, J., Cui, T., Li, J., Chen, L., Pickard, C.J., and Ma, Y., Cagelike diamondoid nitrogen at high pressures. *Phys. Rev. Lett.* 109(17), 175502, 2012.

273. Freitas Jr., R.A. and Merkle, R.C., Nanofactory Collaboration Website http://www.molecularassembler.com/Nanofactory/index.htm (accessed January 06, 2013).

274. Steinmüller-Nethl, D., Kloss, F.R., Najam-Ul-Haq, M., Rainer, M., Larsson, K., Linsmeier, C., Köhler, G., Fehrer, C., Lepperdinger, G., Liu, X., Memmel, N., Bertel, E., Huck, C.W., Gassner, R., and Bonn, G., Strong binding of bioactive BMP-2 to nanocrystalline diamond by physisorption. *Biomaterials* 27(26), 4547–4556, 2006.

275. Kloss, F.R., Gassner, R., Preiner, J., Ebner, A., Larsson, K., and Hächl, O., The role of oxygen termination of nanocrystalline diamond on immobilisation of BMP-2 and subsequent bone formation. *Biomaterials* 29(16), 2433–2442, 2008.

276. Zhou, H. and Lee, J., Nanoscale hydroxyapatite particles for bone tissue engineering. *Acta Biomater.* 7(7), 2769–2781, 2011.

277. Jamilpour, N., Fereidoon, A., and Rouhi, G., The effects of replacing collagen fibers with carbon nanotubes on the rate of bone remodeling process. *J. Biomed. Nanotechnol.* 7(4), 542–548, 2011.

278. Usui, Y., Aoki, K., Narita, N., Murakami, N., Nakamura, I., Nakamura, K., Ishigaki, N., Yamazaki, H., Horiuchi, H., Kato, H., Taruta, S., Kim, Y.A., Endo, M., and Saito, N., Carbon nanotubes with high bone-tissue compatibility and bone-formation acceleration effects. *Small* 4(2), 240–246, 2008.

279. Chen, J.T., Tang, Y.Z., Zhang, J.G., Wang, J.J., and Xiao, Y., Preparation of nano-nacre artificial bone. Article in Chinese. *Nan Fang Yi Ke Da Xue Xue Bao* 28(12), 2171–2173, 2008.

280. Holzapfel, G.A., Schulze-Bauer, C.A., Feigl, G., and Regitnig, P., Single lamellar mechanics of the human lumbar anulus fibrosus. *Biomech. Model. Mechanobiol.* 3(3), 125–140, 2005.

281. Fithian, D.C., Kelly, M.A., and Mow, V.C., Material properties and structure-function relationships in the menisci. *Clin. Orthop. Relat. Res.* (252), 19–31, 1990.

282. Nerurkar, N.L., Sen, S., Baker, B.M., Elliott, D.M., and Mauck, R.L., Dynamic culture enhances stem cell infiltration and modulates extracellular matrix production on aligned electrospun nanofibrous scaffolds. *Acta Biomater.* 7(2), 485–491, 2011.

283. Mujeeb, A., Miller, A.F., Saiani, A., and Gough, J.E., Self-assembled octapeptide scaffolds for in vitro chondrocyte culture. *Acta Biomater.* 9(1), 4609–4617, 2013.

284. Krans, J.L., The sliding filament theory of muscle contraction. *Nature Edu.* 3(9), 66, 2010.

285. Du, G., Moulin, E., Jouault, N., Buhler, E., and Giuseppone, N., Muscle-like supramolecular polymers: Integrated motion from thousands of molecular machines. *Angew Chem. Int. Ed. Engl.* 51(50), 12504–12508, 2012.

286. Zhao, C., Tan, A., Pastorin, G., and Ho, H.K., Nanomaterial scaffolds for stem cell proliferation and differentiation in tissue engineering. *Biotechnol. Adv.* 2012.

287. Ueda, J., Secord, T., and Asada, H.H., Static lumped parameter model for nested PZT cellular actuators with exponential strain amplification mechanisms. In *IEEE International Conference on Robotics and Automation, 2008. ICRA 2008*, 3582–3587, 2008.

288. Ashley, S., Artificial muscles. *Sci. Am.* 289(4), 52–59, 2003.

289. El-Sheikh, M.A., Taher, M.F., and Metwalli, S.M., New optimum humanoid hand design for prosthetic applications. *Int. J. Artif. Organs* 35(4), 251–262, 2012.

290. Hassoulas, I.A., Ladopoulos, V.S., and Kalogerakos, P.D., Study of shape memory alloy fibers for the development of artificial myocardium. *Hellenic J. Cardiol.* 51(4), 301–309, 2010.

291. Chmielus, M., Zhang, X.X., Witherspoon, C., Dunand, D.C., and Müllner, P., Giant magnetic-field-induced strains in polycrystalline Ni-Mn-Ga foams. *Nat. Mater.* 8(11), 863–866, 2009.

292. Shahinpoor, M., Kim, K.J., and Mojarrad, M., *Artificial Muscles: Applications of Advanced Polymeric Nanocomposites.* Taylor & Francis Group, Boca Raton, FL, 2007.

293. Brochu, P. and Pei, Q., Advances in dielectric elastomers for actuators and artificial muscles. *Macromol. Rapid Commun.* 31(1), 10–36, 2010.

294. Stoyanov, H., Kollosche, M., Risse, S., Waché, R., and Kofod, G., Soft conductive elastomer materials for stretchable electronics and voltage controlled artificial muscles. *Adv. Mater.* 2012.

295. Nguyen, V.Q., Ahmed, A.S., and Ramanujan, R.V., Morphing soft magnetic composites. *Adv. Mater.* 24(30), 4041–4054, 2012.

296. Kim, K.J. and Shahinpoor, M., Special issue: Biomimetics, artificial muscles, and nano-bio. *J. Intell. Mater. Syst. Struct.* 18, 101, 2004.

297. Shahinpoor, M., Ionic polymeric conductor nanocomposites (IPCNCs) as distributed nanosensors and nanoactuators. *Bioinspir. Biomim.* 3(3), 035003, 2008.

298. Jimenez-Molero, M.C., Dietrich-Buchecker, C., and Sauvage, J.P., Chemically induced contraction and stretching of a linear rotaxane dimer. *Chemistry* 8(6), 1456–1466, 2002.

299. Jimenez-Molero, M.C., Dietrich-Buchecker, C., and Sauvage, J.P., Towards artificial muscles at the nanometric level. *Chem. Commun. (Camb)* (14), 1613–1616, 2003.

300. Otero, T.F. and Sansieña, J.M., Soft and wet conducting polymers for artificial muscles. *Adv. Mater.* 10(6), 491–494, 1998.

301. Marsella, M.J., Reid, R.J., Estassi, S., and Wang, L.S., Tetra2,3-thienylene: A building block for single-molecule electromechanical actuators. *J. Am. Chem. Soc.* 124(42), 12507–12510, 2002.

302. Bar-Cohen, Y., *Electroactive Polymer (Eap) Actuators as Artificial Muscles: Reality, Potential, and Challenges.* SPIE Press, 2004.

303. Josephson, R.K., Contraction dynamics and power output of skeletal muscle. *Ann. Rev. Physiol.* 55, 527–546, 1993.

304. Lima, M.D., Li, N., Jung de Andrade, M., Fang, S., Oh, J., Spinks, G.M., Kozlov, M.E., Haines, C.S., Suh, D., Foroughi, J., Kim, S.J., Chen, Y., Ware, T., Shin, M.K., Machado, L.D., Fonseca, A.F., Madden, J.D., Voit, W.E., Galvão, D.S., and Baughman, R.H., Electrically, chemically, and photonically powered torsional and tensile actuation of hybrid carbon nanotube yarn muscles. *Science* 338(6109), 928–932, 2012.

305. Schulz, M., Materials science. Speeding up artificial muscles. *Science* 338(6109), 893–894, 2012.

306. Yuan, Q., Xu, Z., Yakobson, B.I., and Ding, F., Efficient defect healing in catalytic carbon nanotube growth. *Phys. Rev. Lett.* 108(24), 245505, 2012.

307. Hajiali, H., Shahgasempour, S., Naimi-Jamal, M.R., and Peirovi, H., Electrospun PGA/gelatin nanofibrous scaffolds and their potential application in vascular tissue engineering. *Int. J. Nanomed.* 6, 2133–2141, 2011.

308. Barui, A.K., Veeriah, V., Mukherjee, S., Manna, J., Patel, A.K., Patra, S., Pal, K., Murali, S., Rana, R.K., Chatterjee, S., and Patra, C.R., Zinc oxide nanoflowers make new blood vessels. *Nanoscale* 4(24), 7861–7869, 2012.

309. Patra, C.R., Abdel Moneim, S.S., Wang, E., Dutta, S., Patra, S., Eshed, M., Mukherjee, P., Gedanken, A., Shah, V.H., and Mukhopadhyay, D., In vivo toxicity studies of europium hydroxide nanorods in mice. *Toxicol. Appl. Pharmacol.* 240(1), 88–98, 2009.

310. Patra, C.R., Bhattacharya, R., Patra, S., Vlahakis, N.E., Gabashvili, A., Koltypin, Y., Gedanken, A., Mukherjee, P., and Mukhopadhyay, D., Pro-angiogenic properties of Europium (III) hydroxide nanorods. *Adv. Mater.* 20(4), 753–756, 2008.

311. Patra, C.R., Kim, J.H., Pramanik, K., d'Uscio, L.V., Patra, S., Pal, K., Ramchandran, R., Strano, M.S., and Mukhopadhyay, D., Reactive oxygen species driven angiogenesis by inorganic nanorods. *Nano Lett.* 11(11), 4932–4938, 2011.

312. Freitas Jr., R.A., and Phoenix, C.J., Vasculoid: A personal nanomedical appliance to replace human blood. *J. Evol. Technol.* 11, 1–139, 2002.

313. Hansen, J.E. and Ampaya, E.P., Human air space shapes, sizes, areas, and volumes. *J. Appl. Physiol.* 38(6), 990–995, 1975.

314. Hansen, J.E., Ampaya, E.P., Bryant, G.H., and Navin, J.J., Branching pattern of airways and air spaces of a single human terminal bronchiole. *J. Appl. Physiol.* 38(6), 983–989, 1975.

315. Kotton, D.N., Next-generation regeneration: The hope and hype of lung stem cell research. *Am. J. Respir. Crit. Care Med.* 185(12), 1255–1260, 2012.

316. Gorissen, S.H., Hristova, M., Habibovic, A., Sipsey, L.M., Spiess, P.C., Janssen-Heininger Y.M., and van der Vliet, A., DUOX1 is required for airway epithelial cell migration and bronchiolar re-epithelialization following injury. *Am. J. Respir. Cell Mol. Biol.* 2012.

317. Vaughan, A.E. and Chapman, H.A., Regenerative activity of the lung after epithelial injury. *Biochim. Biophys. Acta* S0925-4439(12), 00281–00285, 2012.

318. Yahaya, B., Understanding cellular mechanisms underlying airway epithelial repair: Selecting the most appropriate animal models. *Sci. World J.* 2012, 961684, 2012.

319. Freitas. Jr., R.A., Exploratory design in medical nanotechnology: A mechanical artifcial red cell. *Artif. Cells Blood Substit. Immobil. Biotechnol.* 26, 411–430, 1998.

320. Izumi, M., Sweeney, A.M., Demartini, D., Weaver, J.C., Powers, M.L., Tao, A., Silvas, T.V., Kramer, R.M., Crookes-Goodson, W.J., Mäthger, L.M., Naik, R.R., Hanlon, R.T., and Morse, D.E., Changes in reflectin protein phosphorylation are associated with dynamic iridescence in squid. *J. R. Soc. Interf.* 7(44), 549–560, 2010.

321. Salehi, S., Cabibihan, and J.J., Ge, S.S., Artificial skin ridges enhance local tactile shape discrimination. *Sensors (Basel)* 11(9), 8626–8642, 2011.

322. Liu, Y., and Li, G., A new method for producing "Lotus Effect" on a biomimetic shark skin. *J. Colloid Interf. Sci.* 388(1), 235–242, 2012.

323. Comanns, P., Effertz, C., Hischen, F., Staudt, K., Böhme, W., and Baumgartner, W., Moisture harvesting and water transport through specialized micro-structures on the integument of lizards. *Beilstein J. Nanotechnol.* 2, 204–214, 2011.

324. Yang, W., Chen, I.H., Gludovatz, B., Zimmermann, E.A., Ritchie, R.O., and Meyers, M.A., Natural flexible dermal armor. *Adv. Mater.* 2012.

325. Fahy, G.M., West. M.D., Coles, S., and Harris, S.B., *The Future of Aging: Pathways to Human Life Extension*, Springer, New York, 2010.

326. Kishi, K., Okabe, K., Shimizu, R., and Kubota, Y., Fetal skin possesses the ability to regenerate completely: Complete regeneration of skin. *Keio J. Med.* 61(4), 101–108, 2012.

327. Clark, R.A.F., Lanigan, J.M., DellaPelle, P., Manseau, E., Dvorak, H.F., and Colvin, R.B., Fibronectin and fibrin provide a provisional matrix for epidermal cell migration during wound reepithelialization. *J. Invest. Dermatol.* 79, 264–269, 1982.

328. Ellis-Behnke, R.G., Liang, Y.X., Tay, D.K., Kau, P.W., Schneider, G.E., Zhang, S., Wu, W., and So, K.F., Nano hemostat solution: Immediate hemostasis at the nanoscale. *Nanomedicine* 2(4), 207–215, 2006.

329. Ellis-Behnke, R.G., Liang, Y.X., You, S.W., Tay, D.K., Zhang, S., So, K.F., and Schneider, G.E., Nano neuro knitting: Peptide nanofiber scaffold for brain repair and axon regeneration with functional return of vision. *Proc. Natl. Acad. Sci. USA* 103(13), 5054–5059, 2006.

330. Blecher, K., Martinez, L.R., Tuckman-Vernon, C., Nacharaju, P., Schairer, D., Chouake, J., Friedman, J.M., Alfieri, A., Guha, C., Nosanchuk, J.D., and Friedman, A.J., Nitric oxide-releasing nanoparticles accelerate wound healing in NOD-SCID mice *Nanomedicine* 8(8), 1364–1371, 2012.

331. Leu, J.G., Chen, S.A., Chen, H.M., Wu, W.M., Hung, C.F., Yao, Y.D., Tu, C.S., and Liang, Y.J., The effects of gold nanoparticles in wound healing with antioxidant epigallocatechin gallate and α-lipoic acid. *Nanomedicine* 8(5), 767–775, 2012.

332. Xie, J., Macewan, M.R., Ray, W.Z., Liu, W., Siewe, D.Y., and Xia, Y., Radially aligned, electrospun nanofibers as dural substitutes for wound closure and tissue regeneration applications. *ACS Nano* 4(9), 5027–5036, 2010.

333. de Grey, A.D.N.J., Elimination of aging, entry for inclusion. In *Berkshire Encyclopedia of the 21st Century.* http://www.sens.org/files/pdf/Berkshire-PP.pdf (accessed January 20, 2013).

334. CIA World Fact Book, https://www.cia.gov/library/publications/the-world-factbook/fields/2066.html (accessed January 20, 2013).

335. Understanding Artificial Intelligence, Risks and Danger, https://sites.google.com/site/understandai/danger (accessed January 20, 2013).

336. Kanwar, J.R., Sriramoju, B., and Kanwar, R.K., Neurological disorders and therapeutics targeted to surmount the blood-brain barrier. *Int. J. Nanomed.* 7, 3259–3278, 2012.

337. Psarros, C., Lee, R., Margaritis, M., and Antoniades, C., Nanomedicine for the prevention, treatment and imaging of atherosclerosis. *Nanomedicine* 8 (Suppl 1), S59–S68, 2012.

338. Krol, S., Ellis-Behnke, R., and Marchetti, P., Nanomedicine for treatment of diabetes in an aging population: State-of-the-art and future developments. *Nanomedicine* 8 (Suppl 1), S69–S76, 2012.

339. Tamaki, Y., Prospects for nanomedicine in treating age-related macular degeneration. *Nanomedicine (Lond)* 4(3), 341–352, 2009.

340. Ferrer-Miralles, N., Corchero, J.L., Kumar, P., Cedano, J.A., Gupta, K.C., Villaverde, A., and Vazquez, E., Biological activities of histidine-rich peptides; merging biotechnology and nanomedicine. *Microb. Cell Fact.* 10, 101, 2011.

341. Muldoon, L.L., Tratnyek, P.G., Jacobs, P.M., Doolittle, N.D., Christoforidis, G.A., Frank, J.A., Lindau, M., Lockman, P.R., Manninger, S.P., Qiang, Y., Spence, A.M., Stupp, S.I., Zhang, M., and Neuwelt, E.A., Imaging and nanomedicine for diagnosis and therapy in the central nervous system: Report of the eleventh annual Blood-Brain Barrier Disruption Consortium meeting. *Am. J. Neuroradiol.* 27(3), 715–721, 2006.

342. Neves-Petersen, M.T., Duroux, M., Duroux, L., Skovsen, E., and Petersen S.B., Novel photonic technique creates micrometer resolution multi-sensor arrays and provides a new approach to coupling of genes, nucleic acids, peptide hormones and drugs to nanoparticle carriers. *NSTI Nanotech. 2006* 2, 201–204, 2006.

343. Holliday, R., The extreme arrogance of anti-aging medicine. *Biogerontology* 10(2), 223–228, 2009.

344. Century of Flight, Ancient Flying Myths and Legends, http://www.century-of-flight.net/new%20site/frames/myths_frame1.htm (accessed January 20, 2013).

345. de Grey, A.D.N.J., We will be able to live to 1,000, *BBC News*, December 03, 2004. http://news.bbc.co.uk/2/hi/uk/4003063.stm (accessed January 23, 2013).

346. Mathers, J.C., Nutrition and ageing: Knowledge, gaps and research priorities. *Proc. Nutr. Soc.* 1–5, 2013.

347. Raj, D.S., Choudhury, D., Welbourne, T.C., and Levi, M., Advanced glycation end products: A nephrologist's perspective. *Am. J. Kidney Dis.* 35(3), 365–380, 2000.

348. Goldin, A., Beckman, J.A., Schmidt, A.M., and Creager, M.A., Advanced glycation end products: Sparking the development of diabetic vascular injury. *Circulation* 114(6), 597–605, 2006.

349. Brownlee, M., Vlassara, H., Kooney, A., Ulrich, P., and Cerami, A., Aminoguanidine prevents diabetes-induced arterial wall protein cross-linking. *Science* 232(4758), 1629–1632, 1986.

350. Giardino, I., Fard, A.K., Hatchell, D.L., and Brownlee, M., Aminoguanidine inhibits reactive oxygen species formation, lipid peroxidation, and oxidant-induced apoptosis. *Diabetes* 47(7), 1114–1120, 1998.

351. Takino, J., Kobayashi, Y., and Takeuchi, M., The formation of intracellular glyceraldehyde-derived advanced glycation end-products and cytotoxicity. *J. Gastroenterol.* 45(6), 646–655, 2010.

352. Mesías, M., Navarro, M., Gökmen, V., and Morales, F.J., Antiglycative effect of fruit and vegetable seed extracts: Inhibition of AGE formation and carbonyl-trapping abilities. *J. Sci. Food Agric.* 2012.

353. Wu, E.T., Liang, J.T., Wu, M.S., and Chang, K.C., Pyridoxamine prevents age-related aortic stiffening and vascular resistance in association with reduced collagen glycation. *Exp Gerontol.* 46(6), 482–8, 2011.

354. Muellenbach, E.A., Diehl, C.J., Teachey, M.K., Lindborg, K.A., Archuleta, T.L., Harrell, N.B., Andersen, G., Somoza, V., Hasselwander, O., Matuschek, M., and Henriksen, E.J., Interactions of the advanced glycation end product inhibitor pyridoxamine and the antioxidant alpha-lipoic acid on insulin resistance in the obese Zucker rat. *Metabolism* 57(10), 1465–1472, 2008.

355. Thornalley, P.J., Use of aminoguanidine (Pimagedine) to prevent the formation of advanced glycation end products. *Arch. Biochem. Biophys.* 419(1), 31–40, 2003.

356. Williams, M., Clinical studies of advanced glycation end product inhibitors and diabetic kidney disease. *Curr. Diabetes Rep.* 4(6), 441–446, 2004.

357. Vasan, S., Zhang, X., Zhang, X., Kapurniotu, A., Bernhagen, J., and Teichberg, S., An agent cleaving glucose-derived protein crosslinks in vitro and in vivo. *Nature* 382(6588), 275–278, 1996.

358. Cooper, M.E., Thallas, V., Forbes, J., Scalbert, E., Sastra, S., Darby, I., and Soulis, T., The cross-link breaker, N-phenacylthiazolium bromide prevents vascular advanced glycation end-product accumulation. *Diabetologia* 43(5), 660–664, 2000.

359. Kim, T. and Spiegel, D.A., The unique reactivity of N-phenacyl-derived thiazolium salts toward alpha-dicarbonyl compounds. *Rejuv. Res.* 16(1), 43–50, 2013.

360. Kuzan, A., Chwiłkowska, A., Kobielarz, M., Pezowicz, C., and Gamian, A., Glycation of extracellular matrix proteins and its role in atherosclerosis. *Postepy. Hig Med. Dosw (Online)* 66, 804–809, 2012.

361. Yin, D., Biochemical basis of lipofuscin, ceroid, and age pigment-like fluorophores. *Free Radic. Biol. Med.* 21(6), 871–888, 1996.
362. Schutt, F., Bergmann, M., Holz, F.G., and Kopitz, J., Proteins modified by malondialdehyde, 4-hydroxynonenal, or advanced glycation end products in lipofuscin of human retinal pigment epithelium. *Invest. Ophthalmol. Vis. Sci.* 44(8), 3663–3668, 2003.
363. Biesemeier, A., Schraermeyer, U., and Eibl, O., Chemical composition of melanosomes, lipofuscin and melanolipofuscin granules of human RPE tissues. *Exp. Eye Res.* 93(1), 29–39, 2011.
364. Ng, K.P., Gugiu, B., Renganathan, K., Davies, M.W., Gu, X., Crabb, J.S., Kim, S.R., Rózanowska, M.B., Bonilha, V.L., Rayborn, M.E., Salomon, R.G., Sparrow, J.R., Boulton, M.E., Hollyfield, J.G., and Crabb, J.W., Retinal pigment epithelium lipofuscin proteomics. *Mol. Cell Proteomics* 7(7), 1397–1405, 2008.
365. Lois, N. and Forrester, J.V., *Fundus Autofluorescence.* Springer, New York, 2009.
366. Jung, T., Bader, N., and Grune, T., Lipofuscin: Formation, distribution, and metabolic consequences. *Ann. N. Y. Acad. Sci.* 1119, 97–111, 2007.
367. Brunk, U.T. and Terman, A., The mitochondrial-lysosomal axis theory of aging: Accumulation of damaged mitochondria as a result of imperfect autophagocytosis. *Eur. J. Biochem.* 269(8), 1996–2002, 2002.
368. Mathieu, J.M., Wang, F., Segatori, L., and Alvarez, P.J., Increased resistance to oxysterol cytotoxicity in fibroblasts transfected with a lysosomally targeted Chromobacterium oxidase. *Biotechnol. Bioeng.* 109(9), 2409–2415, 2012.
369. de Grey, A.D.N.J., Cambridge University, private communication. 2012
370. Damico, F.M., Gasparin, F., Scolari, M.R., Pedral, L.S., and Takahashi, B.S., New approaches and potential treatments for dry age-related macular degeneration. *Arq. Bras. Oftalmol.* 75(1), 71–76, 2012.
371. Savitha, S., Naveen, B., and Panneerselvam, C., Carnitine and lipoate ameliorates lipofuscin accumulation and monoamine oxidase activity in aged rat heart. *Eur. J. Pharmacol.* 574(1), 61–65, 2007.
372. Porter, R.J., Lunn, B.S., and O'Brien, J.T., Effects of acute tryptophan depletion on cognitive function in Alzheimer's disease and in the healthy elderly. *Psychol. Med.* 33(1), 41–49, 2003.
373. Zhang, L., Hui, Y.N., Wang, Y.S., Ma, J.X., Wang, J.B., and Ma, L.N., Calcium overload is associated with lipofuscin formation in human retinal pigment epithelial cells fed with photoreceptor outer segments. *Eye (Lond)* 25(4), 519–527, 2011.
374. Klopstock, T., Elstner, M., and Bender, A., Creatine in mouse models of neurodegeneration and aging. *Amino Acids* 40(5), 1297–1303, 2011.
375. Shen, L.R., Parnell, L.D., Ordovas, J.M., and Lai, C.Q., Curcumin and aging. *Biofactors* 2013.
376. Abbas. S. and Wink, M., Epigallocatechin gallate inhibits beta amyloid oligomerization in *Caenorhabditis elegans* and affects the daf-2/insulin-like signaling pathway. *Phytomedicine* 17(11), 902–909, 2010.
377. Kampkötter, A., Gombitang Nkwonkam, C., Zurawski, R.F., Timpel, C., Chovolou, Y., Wätjen, W., and Kahl, R., Effects of the flavonoids kaempferol and fisetin on thermotolerance, oxidative stress and FoxO transcription factor DAF-16 in the model organism *Caenorhabditis elegans. Arch. Toxicol.* 81(12), 849–858, 2007.
378. Paula-Barbosa, M.M., Brandão, F., Pinho, M.C., Andrade, J.P., Madeira, M.D., and Cadete-Leite, A., The effects of piracetam on lipofuscin of the rat cerebellar and hippocampal neurons after long-term alcohol treatment and withdrawal: A quantitative study. *Alcohol Clin. Exp. Res.* 15(5), 834–838, 1991.
379. Ost, A., Svensson, K., Ruishalme, I., Brännmark, C., Franck, N., Krook, H., Sandström, P., Kjolhede, P., and Strålfors, P., Attenuated mTOR signaling and enhanced autophagy in adipocytes from obese patients with type 2 diabetes. *Mol. Med.* 16(7–8), 235–246, 2010.
380. Chung, W., Kim, D.H., Park, M.H., Choi, Y.J., Kim, N.D., Lee, J., Yu, B.P., and Chung, H.Y., Recent advances in calorie restriction research on aging. *Exp. Gerontol.* pii: S0531–5565(12), 00304-X, 2012.
381. Luna, C., Li, G., Liton, P.B., Qiu, J., Epstein, D.L., Challa, P., and Gonzalez, P., Resveratrol prevents the expression of glaucoma markers induced by chronic oxidative stress in trabecular meshwork cells. *Food Chem. Toxicol.* 47(1), 198–204, 2009.

382. Valenzano, D.R., Terzibasi, E., Genade, T., Cattaneo, A., Domenici, L., and Cellerino, A., Resveratrol prolongs lifespan and retards the onset of age-related markers in a short-lived vertebrate. *Curr Bio.* l16, 296–300, 2006.

383. Mahesh, R., Bhuvana, S., and Begum, V.M., Effect of *Terminalia chebula* aqueous extract on oxidative stress and antioxidant status in the liver and kidney of young and aged rats. *Cell. Biochem. Funct.* 27(6), 358–363, 2009.

384. Guarnieri, C., Muscari, C., Manfroni, S., Caldarera, I., Stefanelli, C., and Pretolani, E., The effect of treatment with coenzyme Q10 on the mitochondrial function and superoxide radical formation in cardiac muscle hypertrophied by mild aortic stenosis. *J. Mol. Cell. Cardiol.* 19(1), 63–71, 1987.

385. Onaca-Fischer, O., Liu, J., Inglin, M., and Palivan, C.G., Polymeric nanocarriers and nanoreactors: A survey of possible therapeutic applications. *Curr. Pharm. Des.* 18(18), 2622–2643, 2012.

386. De Vocht, C., Polymeric nanoreactors for use in enzyme replacement therapy, PhD Thesis, Uitgeverij VUBPRESS Brussels University Press, Brussels, Belgium, 2010.

387. Ohashi, T., Enzyme replacement therapy for lysosomal storage diseases. *Pediatr. Endocrinol. Rev.* 10 (Suppl 1), 26–34, 2012.

388. Puiu, M., Chirita-Emandi, A., Dumitriu, S., and Arghirescu, S., Hunter syndrome follow-up after 1 year of enzyme-replacement therapy. *BMJ Case Rep.* 2013.

389. Gaudana, R., Ananthula, H.K., Parenky, A., and Mitra, A.K., Ocular drug delivery. *AAPS J.* 12(3), 348–360, 2010.

390. Wu, Y., Zhou, J., Fishkin, N., Rittmann, B.E., and Sparrow, J.R., Enzymatic degradation of A2E, a retinal pigment epithelial lipofuscin bisretinoid. *J. Am. Chem. Soc.* 133(4), 849–857, 2011.

391. Weiss, N., Cross-talk between TRPML1 channel, lipids and lysosomal storage diseases. *Commun. Integr. Biol.* 5(2), 111–113, 2012.

392. Baltazar, G.C., Guha, S., Lu, W., Lim, J., Boesze-Battaglia, K., Laties, A.M., Tyagi, P., Kompella, U.B., and Mitchell, C.H., Acidic nanoparticles are trafficked to lysosomes and restore an acidic lysosomal pH and degradative function to compromised ARPE-19 cells. *PLoS One* 7(12), e49635, 2012.

393. Koshkaryev, A., Thekkedath, R., Pagano, C., Meerovich, I., and Torchilin, V.P., Targeting of lysosomes by liposomes modified with octadecyl-rhodamine B. *J. Drug Target.* 19(8), 606–614, 2011.

394. Maurer-Jones, M.A., and Haynes, C.L., Toward correlation in in vivo and in vitro nanotoxicology studies. *J. Law Med. Ethics* 40(4), 795–801, 2012.

395. Podila, R. and Brown, J.M., Toxicity of engineered nanomaterials: A physicochemical perspective. *J. Biochem. Mol. Toxicol.* 27(1), 50–55, 2013.

396. de Duve, C., de Barsy, T., Poole, B., Trouet, A., Tulkens, P., and Van Hoof, F., Commentary. Lysosomotropic agents. *Biochem. Pharmacol.* 23(18), 2495–2531, 1974.

397. Stern, S.T., Adiseshaiah, P.P., and Crist, R.M., Autophagy and lysosomal dysfunction as emerging mechanisms of nanomaterial toxicity. *Part Fibre Toxicol.* 9, 20, 2012.

398. Li, N., Xia, T., and Nel, A.E., The role of oxidative stress in ambient particulate matter-induced lung diseases and its implications in the toxicity of engineered nanoparticles. *Free Radic. Biol. Med.* 44, 1689–1699, 2008.

399. Olshansky, S.J., Perry, D., Miller, R.A., and Butler, R.N., Pursuing the longevity dividend: Scientific goals for an aging world. *Ann. N.Y. Acad. Sci.* 1114, 11–13, 2007.

400. Lowery, A.R., Gobin, A.M., Day, E.S., Halas, N.J., and West, J.L., Immunonanoshells for targeted photothermal ablation of tumor cells. *Int. J. Nanomed.* 1(2), 149–154, 2006.

401. Bardhan, R., Grady, N.K., Ali, T., and Halas, N.J., Metallic nanoshells with semiconductor cores: Optical characteristics modified by core medium properties. *ACS Nano* 4(10), 6169–6179, 2010.

402. Elsherbini, A.A., Saber, M., Aggag, M., El-Shahawy, A., and Shokier, H.A., Laser and radiofrequency-induced hyperthermia treatment via gold-coated magnetic nanocomposites. *Int. J. Nanomed.* 6, 2155–2165, 2011.

403. Boehm, F.J. and Chen, A., Medical applications of hyperthermia based on magnetic nanoparticles. *Recent Patents Biomed. Eng.* 2(2), 110–120, 2009.

404. Sparrow, J.R., Parish, C.A., Hashimoto, M., and Nakanishi, K., A2E, a lipofuscin fluorophore, in human retinal pigmented epithelial cells in culture. *Invest. Ophthalmol. Vis. Sci.* 40(12), 2988–2995, 1999.

405. Holz, F.G., Schütt, F., Kopitz, J., Eldred, G.E., Kruse, F.E., Völcker, H.E., and Cantz, M., Inhibition of lysosomal degradative functions in RPE cells by a retinoid component of lipofuscin. *Invest. Ophthalmol. Vis. Sci.* 40(3), 737–743, 1999.

406. Wu, Y., Zhou, J., Fishkin, N., Rittmann, B.E., and Sparrow, J.R., Enzymatic degradation of A2E, a retinal pigment epithelial lipofuscin bisretinoid. *J. Am. Chem. Soc.* 133(4), 849–857, 2011.

407. Takahashi, H., Utsuyama, M., Kurashima, C., Mori, H., and Hirokawa, K., Monoclonal antibody to beta peptide, recognizing amyloid deposits, neuronal cells and lipofuscin pigments in systemic organs. *Acta Neuropathol.* 85(2), 159–166, 1993.

408. Bancher, C., Grundke-Iqbal, I., Iqbal, K., Kim, K.S., and Wisniewski, H.M., Immunoreactivity of neuronal lipofuscin with monoclonal antibodies to the amyloid beta-protein. *Neurobiol. Aging* 10(2), 125–132, 1989.

409. Aloj Totáro, E., Cuomo, V., and Pisanti, F.A., Influence of environmental stress on lipofuscin production. *Arch. Gerontol. Geriatr.* 5(4), 343–349, 1986.

410. Eichhoff, G. and Garaschuk, O., Two-photon imaging of neural networks in a mouse model of Alzheimer's disease. *Cold Spring Harb. Protoc.* 2011(10), 1206–1216, 2011.

411. Freitas Jr., R.A., Microbivores: Artificial mechanical phagocytes using digest and discharge protocol, *J. Evol. Technol.* 14, 1–52, 2005.

412. Park, S., Kim, Y.S., Kim, W.B., and Jon, S., Carbon nanosyringe array as a platform for intracellular delivery. *Nano Lett.* 9(4), 1325–1329, 2009.

413. Lopez, C.F., Nielsen, S.O., Moore, P.B., and Klein, M.L., Understanding nature's design for a nanosyringe. *Proc. Natl. Acad. Sci. USA.* 101(13), 4431–4434, 2004.

414. de Grey, A.D.N.J., Escape velocity: Why the prospect of extreme human life extension matters now. *PLoS Biol.* 2(6), 0723–0726, 2004.

415. Bostrom, N., Transhumanist values, ethical issues for the twenty first century. In *Philosophy Documentation Center.* Oxford University, Oxford, U.K., 2005, pp. 3–14. http://www.nickbostrom.com/ethics/values.pdf (accessed January 27, 2013).

416. Shaw, D., Cryoethics: Seeking life after death. *Bioethics* 23(9), 515–521, 2009.

417. Green, R., Molecular manufacturing and grey goo scenario. *Future Tek Science & Technology News*, January 20, 2012. http://www.futuretek.info/molecular-manufacturing-and-grey-goo-scenario/(accessed January 27, 2012).

418. Freitas Jr., R.A., Nanotechnology and radically extended life span, *Life Extension Mag.* 15, 80–85, 2009.

419. Pijnenburg, M.A. and Leget, C., Who wants to live forever? Three arguments against extending the human lifespan. *J. Med. Ethics* 33(10), 585–587, 2007.

420. Partridge, B. and Hall, W., The search for Methuselah. Should we endeavour to increase the maximum human lifespan? *EMBO Rep.* 8(10), 888–891, 2007.

Index

A